Handbook
of
Sensory Physiology

Volume II

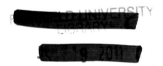
Editorial Board

H. Autrum · R. Jung · W. R. Loewenstein
D. M. MacKay · H. L. Teuber

Somatosensory System

By

D. Albe-Fessard · K.H. Andres · J.A.V. Bates · J.M. Besson · A.G. Brown
P.R. Burgess · I. Darian-Smith · M. v. Düring · G. Gordon · H. Hensel
E. Jones · B. Libet · O. Oscarsson · E.R. Perl · O. Pompeiano · T.P.S. Powell
M. Réthelyi · R.F. Schmidt · J. Semmes · S. Skoglund · J. Szentágothai
A.L. Towe · P.D. Wall · G. Werner · B.L. Whitsel · Y. Zotterman

Edited by

Ainsley Iggo

With 240 Figures

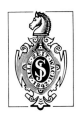

Springer-Verlag Berlin · Heidelberg · New York 1973

ISBN 3-540-05941-5 Springer-Verlag Berlin · Heidelberg · New York
ISBN 0-387-05941-5 Springer-Verlag New York · Heidelberg · Berlin

Typesetting, printing: Joh. Roth sel. Ww., München. Binding: Grimm & Bleicher, München

Preface

The waterproof sensory sheet covering the mammalian body has a rich afferent innervation which provides an abundance of complex information for use by the central nervous system often in conjunction with information from receptors in the joints. This book is an attempt to provide a systematic account of the way in which this somatosensory system works. The properties of the peripheral receptors have been debated in scientific terms for about a century and the resolution of the conflict in favour of the existence of 'specific' receptors for mechanical, thermal and noxious stimuli is reported and discussed in the opening chapters of the book. An awareness of this specificity has forced a re-consideration of the ways in which the central nervous system de-codes the information which is showered upon it.

Advances in knowledge of the fine structure of the central nervous system have raised functional questions about the operation and organisation of the sensory systems in the spinal cord and brain. Fresh insight into the morphological complexity of the dorsal horn and higher levels of the nervous system gives the physiologist a clearer idea of the units with which he works. Progress has been made in understanding the function of sensory relay nuclei in general and individual tracts in particular and is fully decomented. The onflow of sensory or afferent information of skin or joint origin on and through the dorsal horn, spinal cord to the reticular formation and at thalamic, cerebellar and cortical levels is considered critically and thoroughly.

One of the significant recent advances in our understanding of the somatosensory system is the control exerted by the nervous system on the entry of information into and through the dorsal horn and relay nuclei and through reflex pathways. The experimental studies sparked-off by the discovery of primary afferent depolarisation and related mechanisms of descending control have had an impact that is evident in many places in the book.

A recurrent theme, entirely appropriate to its subject, is the question of perception which, however, has only been considered incidentally since a systematic treatment will be given in the final volume of the Handbook. Techniques for electrophysiological stimulation and recording from the nervous system of conscious man are now coming into use and are extensively reported in this volume, alongside new ideas based on neurosurgical experiments on the cerebral cortex.

In an active research field it is both necessary and usual to find conflicts of ideas and no attempt has been made to impose an editorial 'establishment' view on the contributors. As a result the post-graduate student and research worker should find much to stimulate them in the accounts by twenty-five active and productive specialists of the present position in interrelated neuro-anatomical and neurophysiological fields.

Edinburgh, April 1973   A. IGGO

Contents

List of Contributors

ALBE-FESSARD, Denise
Laboratoire de Neurophysiologie Generale,
4 Avenue Gordon-Bennet, Paris-16e, France

ANDRES, Karl H.
Institut für Anatomie II, Ruhr-Universität Bochum, Buscheystraße/MA-6/161,
463 Bochum, West Germany.

BATES, J.A.V.
Medical Research Council, The National Hospital for Nervous Diseases,
Queen Square, London, W.C.1., Great Britain

BESSON, J.M.
Université de Paris, Faculté des Sciences,
4 Avenue Gordon-Bennett, Paris-16e, France

BROWN, A.G.
Department of Veterinary Physiology, University of Edinburgh,
Summerhall, Edinburgh EH9 1QH, Great Britain

BURGESS, P.R.
Department of Physiology, College of Medicine, University of Utah,
Salt Lake City, Utah 84112, USA

DARIAN-SMITH, Ian
Department of Physiology, the John Hopkins University, School of Medicine,
725 N. Wolfe Street, Baltimore, Maryland 21205, USA

DÜRING, Monika von
Institut für Anatomie II, Ruhr-Universität Bochum, Buscheystraße/MA-6/161,
463 Bochum, West Germany

GORDON, George
University Laboratory of Physiology, University Museum,
Oxford, Great Britain

HENSEL, Herbert
Direktor, Physiologisches Institut der Universität,
355 Marburg an der Lahn, Deutschhausstrasse 2, West Germany

JONES, E.G.
   Department of Anatomy, University of Otago, Dunedin, New Zealand

LIBET, Benjamin
   Mt. Zion Neurological Institute, Mt. Zion Hospital, San Francisco,
   California 94115, USA and Department of Physiology,
   University of California School of Medicine, San Francisco,
   California 94122, USA

OSCARSSON, Olov
   Institute of Physiology, University of Lund,
   Sölvegatan 19, 22362 Lund, Sweden

PERL, Edward R.
   Department of Physiology, School of Medicine, University of North Carolina,
   Chapel Hill, North Carolina 27514, USA

POMPEIANO, Ottavio
   Istituto di Fisiologia Umana, Cattedra II, Università di Pisa,
   Via S. Zeno 31, 56100 Pisa, Italy

POWELL, T.P.S.
   Department of Human Anatomy, University of Oxford,
   South Parks Road, Oxford OXI 3QX, Great Britain

RÉTHELYI, M.
   1st Department of Anatomy, Semmelweis University Medical School,
   Tuzolto utca 58, Budapest IX, Hungary

SCHMIDT, Robert F.
   Physiologisches Institut der Universität Kiel,
   23 Kiel, Olshausenstrasse 40/60, West Germany

SEMMES, Josephine
   Section on Perception, Laboratory of Psychology,
   National Institute of Mental Health, Bethesda, Maryland 20014, USA

SKOGLUND, Sten †
   Stockholm, Sweden

SZENTÁGOTHAI, J.
   1st Department of Anatomy, Semmelweis University Medical School,
   Tuzolto utca 58, Budapest IX, Hungary

TOWE, Arnold L.
   Department of Physiology & Biophysics, School of Medicine,
   University of Washington, Seattle, Washington 98105, USA

WALL, Patrick D.
    Department of Anatomy, University College London,
    Gower Street, London, W.C.I., Great Britain

WERNER, Gerhard
    Department of Pharmacology, School of Medicine,
    University of Pittsburgh, Pennsylvania 15213, USA

WHITSEL, Barry L.
    Department of Pharmacology, School of Medicine,
    University of Pittsburgh, Pittsburgh, Pennsylvania 15213, USA

ZOTTERMAN, Yngve
    Kungl Veterinärhögskolan, Stockholm 50, Sweden

Introduction

By

YNGVE ZOTTERMAN, Stockholm (Sweden)

In the 1820-ies in Germany a much notified court proceeding became of great importance for the development of sensory physiology. A prominent citizen had been attacked and beaten one night by a political enemy and subsequently sued him for damages. In the court the judge asked the plaintiff: "In the report you say that the night was so dark that you could not see your hand in front of your face. How could you tell that it was the accused who attacked you?" "Your Honour", said the plaintiff, "it was very easy; in the lightning which occurred when he hit me in the eye I easily recognized the evil face of the accused". This created a fierce debate in the newspapers whether cat's eyes could radiate light and JOHANNES MÜLLER who originally was a comparative anatomist was brought into the discussion. He performed experiments on the eye and the ear which led him to formulate his doctrine of the 'specific nerve energies' in 1826. Ever since then the problems of specificity of the sensory cells and the sensory nerve fibres has been one of the main questions of sensory physiology. When in 1867 LOVÉN in Sweden and SCHWALBE in Germany discovered the taste buds of the tongue and BLIX in 1882 the warm and cold spots in the skin the idea developed that MÜLLER's doctrine should be extended even to the qualities of sensation. In fact HELM-HOLTZ's general idea of colour vision was founded on this basic principle.

When, after the first world war, electronic engineering made it possible to record the information transmitted in single sensory nerve fibres the new data obtained confronted the old ideas developed during the earlier days of psycho-physical research. Gradually the gap has been bridged between the external events working on the receptors and the physical events taking place within the nervous system. It started on a gloomy November morning in 1925 in Cambridge when ADRIAN and I recorded the electrical response of a single sensory nerve fibre to various grades of stimulation of the muscle spindle. That very day we conceived that the nerve fibre transmits information according to the principle of impulse frequency modulation. Consequently the simple code transmitted by the nerve fibre can only inform us about the strength and duration of the stimulus, and the process of adaptation in the receptor.

In this volume prominent research workers from all over the world will give you their views on the function of the Somatosensory System. They review what is known of the processes of excitation occurring in the sensory receptors serving different modalities and qualities, the signalling of afferent fibres, the function of the relays in the central nervous system, the reception of information in the cere-bral cortex as well as descending cortical projections moderating the afferent inflow.

The long list of authors contains names of scientists whose work is familiar to me for their excellent contributions to our knowledge in these particular fields of sensory physiology, granting us a vivid and exciting reading.

Chapter 1

Morphology of Cutaneous Receptors

By

Karl H. Andres and Monika von Düring, Bochum (Germany)

With 20 Figures

Contents

A. Introduction

This and the following three chapters will deal with the morphological and physiological characteristics of cutaneous, joint and tendon receptors that have been identified in vertebrates. A recent historical review of the morphology of cutaneous receptors was given by Munger (1971) in Chapter 17, Volume I of this Handbook and the present morphological account is largely restricted to those receptors which have been studied in detail both electrophysiologically and electron microscopically. This recent work has brought together single unit electrophysiological analysis of cutaneous receptors, which in several instances have been marked and identified during the physiological experiments, and detailed electron microscopical of these same receptors (in some instances those actually identified in the physiological experiments). This very detailed morphological investigation has allowed such accurate detail to be established, that some functions can be postulated on the basis of morphological structure. It is still not possible, however, to account for the transducer function of the receptors in molecular terms, and further technological developments, for example in histochemical technique, may be necessary before it is possible to account for diverse physiological responses from morphologically indistinguishable structures.

B. Axons of Sensory Fibres

The axoplasm of sensory fibres is the same as in motorneurons. The main components are the axoplasmatic reticulum, mitochondria, microtubules and neurofilaments. The relative number of neurofilaments in the axons of group A fibres is higher than in B and C fibres, and in B and C fibres the number of microtubules is greater than in A fibres (Fig. 1). Specific features of the membrane of the axoplasm in electron micrographs are the lack of pinocytotic vesicles and its higher contrast in comparison with the Schwann cell membrane. Coated pits, which are to be found in Ranvier nodes (Fig. 1a) may indicate a special resorption mechanism of the membrane at the nodes.

1. The Node of Ranvier

New results on the ultrastructural organisation of the node of Ranvier provide further support for the hypothesis of saltatory conduction in myelinated nerve fibres. Circular connection of the myelin lamellae with the axoplasm membrane provide a barrier to electrotonic conduction along the axon membrane of the internode (Fig. 1A). The myelin lamellae of the distal part of the internode nearest to the receptor segment have the same cytologic specialisation (Fig. 1B) as at the node. Unmyelinated nerve fibres on the other hand lack such junctional configurations (Fig. 1C).

2. Receptorplasm

Sections of the terminal portion of the sensory fibre, the "receptor axon", show specific morphological differentiation. The specifically differentiated parts are distinguished by a very fine tubular reticulum which arborizes mainly just below the receptor membrane. Small granulated vesicles of 300 Å diameter, and multivesicular bodies are embedded in the matrix. A ring of mitochondria separates the receptor matrix from the central axoplasm (Fig. 2). In the terminal swellings of larger receptor axons a substantial number of lamellated bodies is found (Fig. 2D). Other parts of the receptor axon are not specifically differentiated, and show the structures common to normal axoplasm. One can assume that the specifically differentiated portions are the receptive or transducer part of the receptor axon. Single branches of long straight receptor axons and of branched receptor axons have several receptive portions which are separated by the axonal portions of the receptor axon. In different receptor types the receptor plasm is structurally quite similar, although bundles of very fine filaments can be found in some mechanoreceptors (Fig. 2D). Sensory nerve terminals are morphologically, and presumably in part physiologically, differentiated by their specific envelope or capsule and their specific relation to the surrounding connective tissue. These features will therefore be used for a new morphological classification of the cutaneous receptors.

3. Endoneural Connective Tissue

The perineural sheath accompanies the peripheral nerve and its terminals. Mesothelial cells, which form the main structure of the perineural sheath, enclose the endoneural connective tissue. In free nerve terminals the axon loses its perineural sheath and lies either covered by Schwann cell cytoplasm in the connective tissue of the dermis or naked between epithelial cells of the epidermis. In encapsulated nerve terminals the perineural sheath, which can consist of several mesothelial cell layers, forms the capsule. Previously these lamellae of the capsule were misinterpreted as lamellae of the Schwann cells of the inner core (Fig. 3).

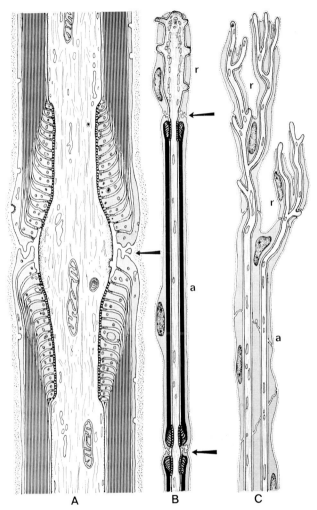

A   B   C

Fig. 1A–C. Schematic representation of sensory nerve fibres. A, High magnification of a node of Ranvier, with clefts between the adjacent Schwann cells marked by arrows. In the paranodal region the pocket-like terminations become closely apposed to the axolemma of Schwann cell lamellae by numerous ringlike barriers. In longitudinal section of the nerve these barriers are seen in cross section. B, Ending of a myelinated sensory nerve fibre, the receptor axon is covered by a Schwann cell. Specifically differentiated axoplasm penetrates the Schwann cell in several locations. The Schwann cell lamellae at the receptor end, that is the distal end of the last internode, are identical in structure with those at the nodes of Ranvier. C, Two unmyelinated sensory fibres embedded in Schwann cells. There are no ringlike adhesions. a = impulse conducting part of axon; r = receptor terminal of axon

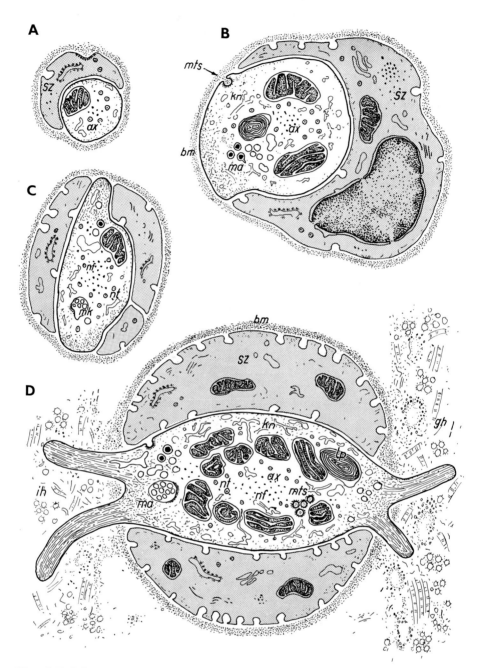

Fig. 2A–D. Schematic representation of receptor terminals in cross section. A and B, Free nerve terminals of the sinus hair in the rat. In A part of the axolemma is in direct contact with the basement membrane of the connective tissue. C, Free nerve terminal in the connective tissue of the duck bill. D, Straight lanceolate terminal of the sinus hair. In D the extensive contact of the sensory axoplasm with the surrounding connective tissue is established by finger-like processes. ax = axoplasm, bm = basement membrane, gh = glassy membrane, ih = hair follicle connective tissue, lp = lamellated particle, ma = receptormatrix, mk = multi-vesicular body, mt = microtubules, mts = coated pits, nf = neurofilaments, sz = Schwann cell, tu = tubular meshwork. (From ANDRES, 1966)

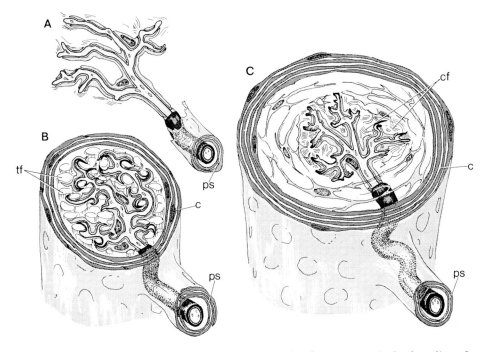

Fig. 3A–C. Schematic representation of free and encapsulated sensory terminals of myelinated fibres. A, Branched lanceolate terminal. The perineural sheath begins at the myelinated part of the axon. B, Golgi tendon organ. The encapsulated nerve endings have a minute capsule space. C, Ruffini corpuscle. The encapsulated ending has a capsule space that separates the terminal from the capsule. cf = collagen fibres of the inner core; ps = perineural sheath which forms the capsule, c; tf = tendon fibres

C. Thermoreceptors

The cold receptor was classically identified as the Krause corpuscle. Electrophysiological investigations (see HENSEL, Chapter 3 of this volume) have now established that cold spots can definitely be identified; specific cold receptors are excited when small areas are cooled and cause a discharge of impulses in a single afferent nerve fibre. Morphological studies of these areas marked during the physiological experiments reveal the presence of specific cold receptors (Figs. 6 and 7 Chapter 3 of this volume). In the glabrous skin of the cat's nose the axons of the cold receptors are myelinated fibres of the A delta type. It seems to be typical of the cold receptor axon that it loses the myelin sheath much earlier than the mechanoreceptor, before it branches in the stratum papillare. Schwann cells accompany the axons until they reach the basement membrane of the epidermis, which is continuous with the basement membrane of the nerve terminals. The receptor terminals penetrate the epithelium for only a few microns. The enlarged terminals contain a specific receptor matrix with small vesicles and an accumulation of mitochondria. The cold receptor is not a Krause corpuscle.

Intraepithelial nerve terminals have also been described in the tongue of several vertebrates. These fibres do not belong to taste buds (Kunze, 1969). Intraepidermal nerve fibres, which penetrate more deeply into the epidermis than the fibres mentioned above, are present in Eimer's organ in the snout of the mole (Fig. 4) (Quilliam, 1966). These intraepithelial terminals may also represent thermoreceptors. Warm receptors in mammals have not so far been identified morphologically. One can be certain, however, that the Ruffini corpuscle (classically regarded as the warm receptor) is not a warm receptor, but rather a mechanoreceptor (Chambers et al., 1972). The warm receptors which lie at the border between cutis and subcutis, probably have unmyelinated axons. The "infra-red" receptor of snakes is represented by free endings in the midst of an amorphous connective tissue matrix (Bleichmar and De Robertis, 1962).

D. Nociceptors

The morphological ultrastructure of pain receptors has so far not been identified unequivocally. Electronmicroscopic results exist mainly for receptors in the dental pulp, in which the myelinated fibres terminate as branched free nerve endings which have contact with the odontocytes (Stockinger and Pritz, 1970; Pritz and Stockinger, 1971). In our electronmicrographs we saw nerve terminals which penetrate into the dental tubules and contain a receptor matrix with the structures described as typical above.

E. Mechanoreceptors

From a morphological point of view one may distinguish two different groups of mechanoreceptors. In the first group the axon terminal represents the receptor or transducer. In the second group the axon terminal forms, together with a specific cell, the Merkel cell-neurite complex, in which the Merkel cell may have a transducer function.

The branched lanceolate terminal. This terminal represents from a morphological point of view a very simple mechanoreceptor. The free receptor axon is encased bilaterally by flattened discs of Schwann cell cytoplasm. Some parts of the arborized nerve terminal show the typical receptor matrix described above (Sect. B2). In these terminals the axoplasm membrane is in direct contact with the basement membrane. The so-called circular lanceolate terminal and the free Ruffini-like endspray endings are structurally similar to the branched lanceolate terminal. Also lanceolate fibres are similar in their internal structure to Ruffini corpuscles and Golgi tendon organs. Typical for these three receptor types is the close contact of their receptive terminals with collagenous fibres (Figs. 2, 3).

1. Ruffini Corpuscle

This receptor is found in the dermis (Ruffini, 1894) of both glabrous and hairy skin as well as in joints (see Skoglund, Chapter 4). A collagenous fibre plexus is present in the Ruffini corpuscle (Goglia and Sklenska, 1969) and the extensively branched endaxons of the Ruffini corpuscle (Fig. 5) are closely associated with the collagenous fibres (Chambers et al., 1972). Collagenous bundles coming

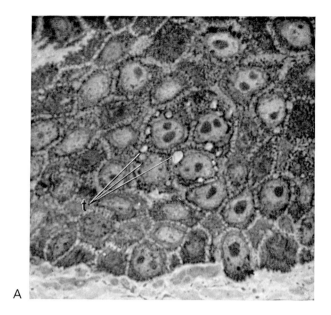

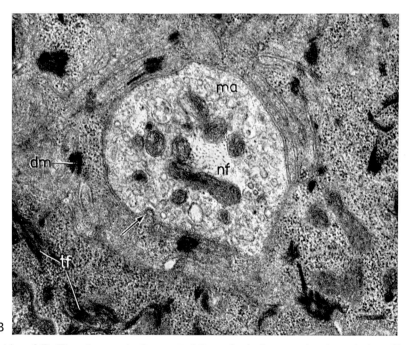

Fig. 4A and B. Eimer's organ in the snout of the mole. A, Cross section through the epidermal papilla of an Eimer's organ. The central cell column is accompanied by several free intra-epidermal terminals (t). Semithin section, magn. 1500 ×. B, Electronmicrograph of a single intraepidermal terminal. ma = receptor matrix containing numerous vesicles of different size, nf = neurofilaments of the axoplasm, tf = tonofibrils, dm = desmosome between epidermal cells, → = coated pit, magnification 30,000 ×

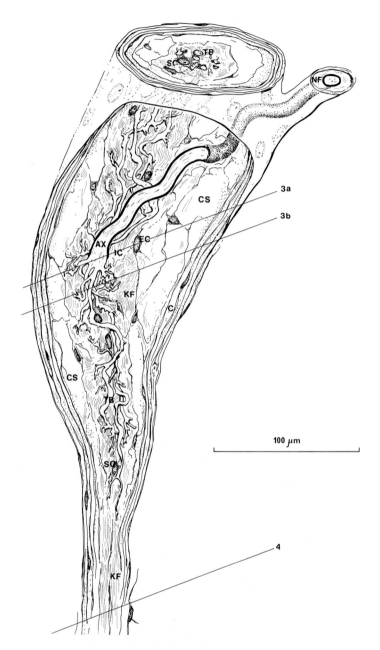

Fig. 5. Reconstruction from serial sections of a Ruffini corpuscle from hairy skin in the cat. The branched terminals lie between the interlaced collagenous fibres of the inner core. AX = axon; C = capsule; CS = capsule space; EC = endoneural cell; IC = inner core; KF = collagenous fibres; NF = myelinated axon with perineural sheath; SC = Schwann cell; TB = branched terminals. (From Chambers et al., 1972)

from the subcutaneous and cutaneous layers enter the spindle-like corpuscle from both poles and therefore unite the receptor complex with the cutis or subcutis to form a functional unit. Stretch of the collagenous fibres also stretches the core of Ruffini corpuscle and these fibres provide the mechanical linkage for the stimulus. Physiological evidence exists that these receptors are slowly adapting (see BURGESS and PERL, Chapter 2). The capsule space of the Ruffini corpuscle is large and extends from the perineural sheath to the receptor complex in the core of the corpuscle. The fluid-filled space may insulate the axon complex from unspecific stimuli (Fig. 5).

2. Golgi Tendon Organ

The Golgi tendon organ, like the Ruffini corpuscle, is spindle-shaped. The fine structure of the receptor complex is similar to the Ruffini endings, with close linkage to collagenous fibres of the tendon bundles (Fig. 6). The direction of its stretch is determined by the tendon bundles which are oriented in parallel with the receptor (Figs. 3B, 6A). The distinct perineural sheath which consists of several mesothelial cell layers and a minute capsule space probably protects the axon terminals from unspecific stimuli from the peritenonium externum or the perimysium (Fig. 6B).

3. Lanceolate Terminals

In the hair shaft of guard hairs and down hairs lanceolate terminals are located in palisades immediately below the sebaceous glands (YAMAMOTO, 1966; ANDRES, 1966; CAUNA, 1969). The terminals are covered by swollen Schwann cells except for narrow slits at their inner and outer sides (Fig. 7A). The combination of receptors forms a cushion-like unit with the receptor terminal sandwiched between Schwann cells and in this respect resembles some lamellated receptors. Therefore, their mechanical behaviour may be similar to that of lamellated receptors and this may account for the rapidly adapting responses of the lanceolate terminals in the down and guard hair follicles (BROWN and IGGO, 1967). In contrast the straight lanceolate endings of sinus hairs are probably slowly adapting receptors (GOTTSCHALDT, IGGO and YOUNG, 1972; Nier pers. comm). In sinus hairs the straight lanceolate endings projects many finger-like processes into the connective tissue of the hair shaft and into the corium of the follicle (Fig. 7B). The sensitivity of these receptors should therefore be multidirectional. In addition, the straight lanceolate endings in the sinus hairs are longer than in other hairs, have a more complex internal structure and each terminal is supplied by a single axon.

4. Lamellated Receptors

Lamellated nerve terminals are distinguished morphologically by a concentric sheath of thin lamellar cells around the axon terminal (Fig. 8). In mammals collagenous fibres of the endoneural connective tissue are present between the lamellae. The lamellated corpuscles show substantial variations in size, and the thickness of the lamellae varies in different corpuscles. They may be swollen and may

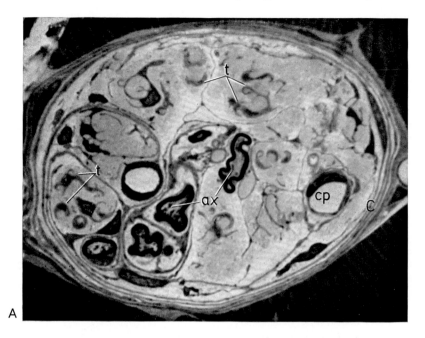

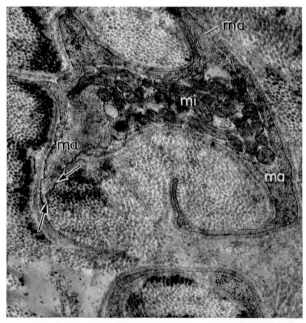

Fig. 6A and B. Golgi Tendon organ. A, Cross section through a Golgi tendon organ of a rat. The terminals (t) and their closely attached Schwann cells clasp the tendon fibres. ax = myelinated axon; c = capsule; cp = capillary. Semithin section, magnification: 1500 ×. B, Electron micrograph of a Golgi tendon terminal. The receptor axon contains numerous mitochondria (mi). Axoplasm-protrusions are filled with the filamentous receptor matrix (ma). The protrusions of the terminal are closely attached to the collagen fibres (arrows). Magn.: 20,000 ×

therefore increase the stiffness and elasticity of the sheath. The rapid adaptation of these receptors probably depends on the elastic sheath of lamellae (Loewenstein and Skalak, 1966). For the special function of the lamellated nerve terminals it might be important whether the perineural sheath completely surrounds the terminal. If it does not, the nerve terminal is in contact with the connective tissue of the surrounding area. This structural organisation is very clear in the

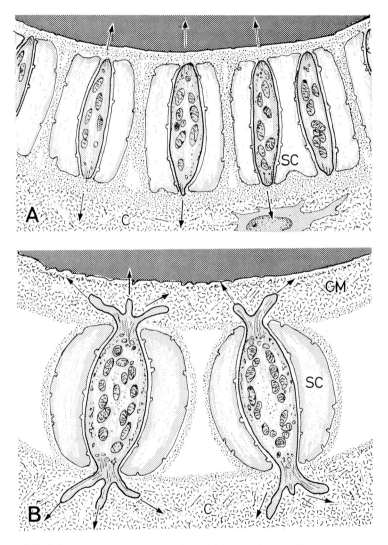

Fig. 7A and B. Schematic representation of straight lanceolate endings, in cross sections of A, Guard and down hairs and B, Sinus hairs. The arrows indicate the probable direction of the effective mechanical stimulus. The straight lanceolate endings form a palisade that is oriented with their long axes parallel with the hair shaft. C = corium of hair follicle; GM = glassy membrane (more conspicuous in sinus lanceolate terminal); SC = Schwann cell

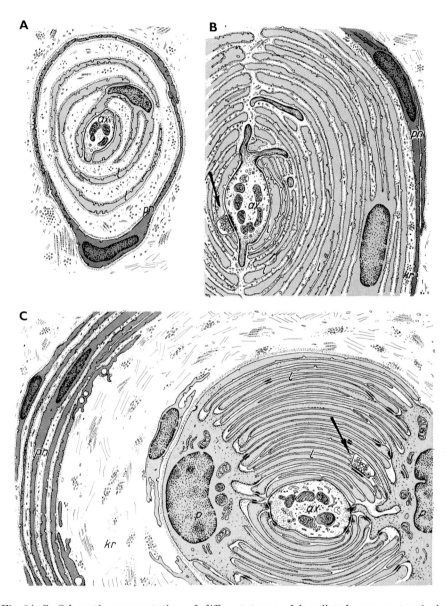

Fig. 8A–C. Schematic representation of different types of lamellated sensory terminals. A, Simple lamellated terminal from the foot-sole skin of *Tupaia*. B, Segment of a Golgi-Mazzoni corpuscle in the hairy skin of the cat. C, Segment of a Herbst corpuscle in the corium of a duck's bill. ax = receptor axon; kr = capsule space; l = Schwann cell lamellae; p = palisade cell; pn = perineural sheath. ↑ = The arrow indicates a terminal of an un-myelinated axon lying on the axon terminal in B, and between the palisade cell lamellae in C. (From Andres, 1969)

Meissner corpuscle which is a rapidly adapting receptor of glabrous skin. The tonofibrils of the epidermis can be followed to the semidesmosomes of the basal cells and then over fine bundles of collagen that enter the Meissner corpuscle (Fig. 9). A small deformation of the epidermis may be sufficient to influence the receptor by being transferred over this tonofibril-collagen-system. Mechanical deformation of deeper skin layers cannot act directly on the receptor complex because of the cup shaped perineural sheath (Fig. 10) at the base of the corpuscle. Lamellated endings with a coiled receptor axon from mechanosensitive muco-

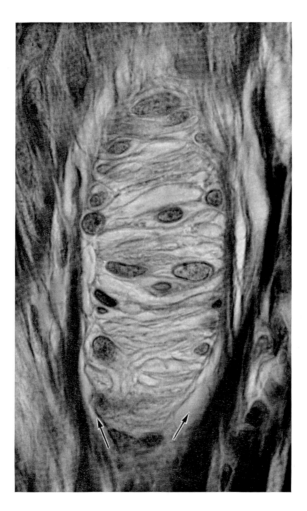

Fig. 9. Meissner corpuscle in glabrous skin from a human finger tip. In this Masson-stained section the tonofibrils of the epidermis are seen to be continuous with collagen fibres entering the upper part of the corpuscle. The lower part of the corpuscle is not connected with the surrounding collagenous lamellae. Arrows indicate a space between the corpuscle and the collagen at the base of the receptor, where there is a cup-shaped perineural sheath (Fig. 10).
Magn.: 1800 ×

cutaneous regions and the genital end bulbs are related to the Meissner corpuscle (Munger, 1965).

Lamellated endings which are completely encapsulated are isolated from the surrounding connective tissue. They are rapidly adapting receptors and respond to high frequency mechanical vibration. Characteristic examples are the lamellated corpuscles (Golgi-Mazzoni corpuscle) in the pig snout (Fig. 19A) and in

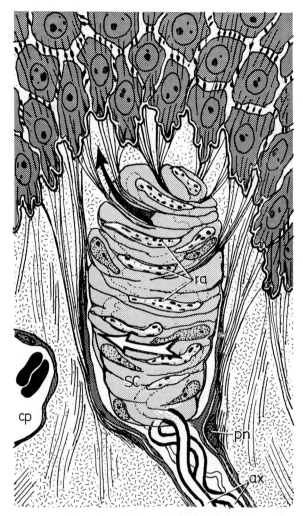

Fig. 10. Schematic representation of a Meissner corpuscle showing the tonofibrilis of the epithelial cells in continuity with collagen fibres of the corium, some of which enter the upper part of the corpuscle. Others are continuous with the endoneural sheath at the basal half of the corpuscle. The tonofibril-collagen system may act directly on the receptor axon (black arrow). The white arrow indicates a possible consecutive movement of the lower part of the corpuscle which could eliminate the mechanical stimulus. Such a mechanism could explain the rapid adaptation of this receptor. Coiled receptor axon (ra); Schwann cells (sc); cup shaped perineural sheath (pn); myelinated axons (ax); capillary (cp)

Eimer's organ of the mole (Figs. 19B, 20). The receptors are similar to but smaller than the Pacinian corpuscle and form two elipsoidal caps which enclose the axon bilaterally. The lamellae are packed very densely and the connective tissue among the lamellae may be absent (Figs. 8B, 11). Lamellated corpuscles of the Pacinian type which are found in birds (Herbst corpuscles) and reptiles lack endoneural connective tissue between the lamellae of the inner core. The two symmetric caps are formed by the so called palisade cells (Figs. 8C, 16). Desmosome-like junctions

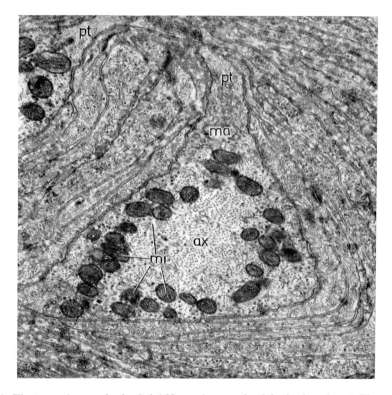

Fig. 11. Electron micrograph of a Golgi-Mazzoni corpuscle of the foreleg of a cat. The receptor axon is covered by lamellae which form several layers. Basement membranes and collagenous fibrils between the lamellae may be absent in close proximity to the axon. The Schwann cell membrane forms numerous pinocytotic vesicles. The receptor axon shows the typical arrangement of the axoplasm (ax), mitochondria (mi) and receptor matrix (ma) with fingerlike protrusions (pt). Magn.: 35,000 ×

and the fingerlike axoplasm-processes are observed between the core lamellae. They probably transmit the mechanical stimulus to the receptor axon membrane. The desmosomes between the core lamellae in the Herbst corpuscle (Fig. 8C) and in the club shaped receptor of reptiles are very distinct, whereas in Pacinian- and Golgi-Mazzoni corpuscles the fingerlike axoplasm processes which project between the lamellae predominate (Fig. 8B). In the Pacinian corpuscle the lamellae of the capsule space are a special differentiation of the perineural sheath (Fig. 12). These lamellae should not be confused with the lamellae of the inner core (Fig. 13). The capsule space of the Herbst corpuscle is not divided into chambers and the connective tissue which is rich in mucoprotein is here very conspicuous (Fig. 16). The capsule space in Golgi-Mazzoni corpuscles and in the club-shaped receptors of reptiles is not very distinct.

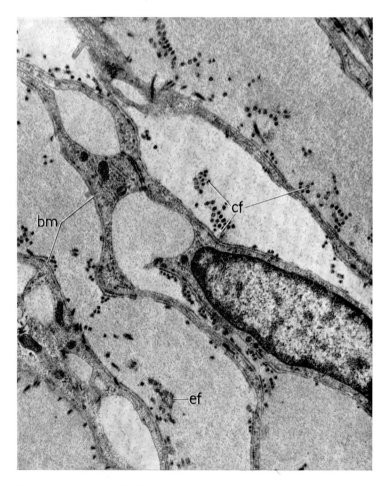

Fig. 12. Electron micrograph of a Pacinian corpuscle to show the fine structure of the capsule space in the neighbourhood of the inner core. Layers of perineural mesothelial cells, which form the lamellae of the capsule space are separated by very loose connective tissue. The collagen fibrils and some elastic fibres are embedded in an amorphous ground substance containing tissue fluid. bm = basement membranes covering the perineural cells; cf = collagen fibrils; ef = elastic fibres. Electronmicrograph Magn.: 3600 ×

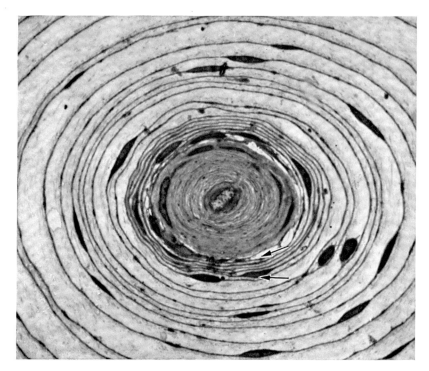

Fig. 13. Photomicrograph of a Pacinian corpuscle, to show the capsule space (outer core) and inner core (Schwann cell lamellae). The inner lamellae (arrow) of the capsule space form a structure that resembles the outer perineural capsule. Semithin section. Magn.: 1500 ×

5. Merkel Cell-Neurite Complex

The second group of mechanoreceptors contains the Merkel cell and the axon terminal (Fig. 14). The Merkel cell is suspected to be the secondary sensory cell of the slowly-adapting type I mechanoreceptor (see BURGESS and PERL, Chapter 2). The Merkel cells of mammals lie in the basal cell layer of the epidermis of both hairy and glabrous skin, whereas Merkel cells of birds lie in the corium of special skin areas. Grandry corpuscles, which are found in ducks, possess features that distinguish them from the mammalian Merkel cell-neurite complex and show substantial variations in size. In the skin of reptiles and amphibians Merkel cell-neurite complexes have only been described on the basis of light microscopy.

A characteristic feature of Merkel- and Grandry cells is the presence of stiff microvilliform cytoplasmic protrusions which contain fine filaments oriented longitudinally. In mammals the microvilli lie in the intercellular space of the epidermis (Fig. 14), whereas in birds they lie in the envelope of Schwann cell cytoplasm. The finger-like processes are oriented horizontally to the surface and may be regarded as a special detector for the sensory cell. Desmosomes, which are

2*

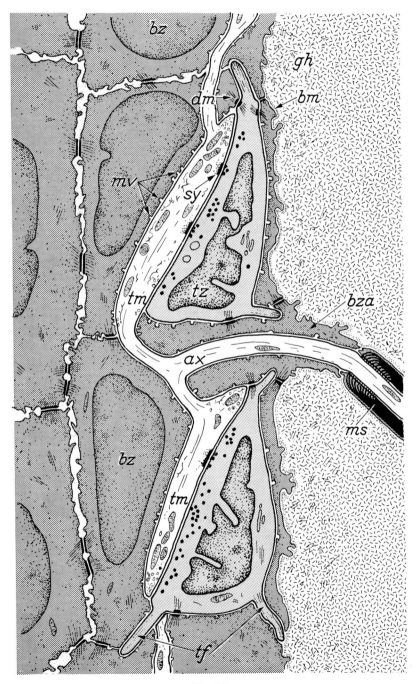

Fig. 14

present between the Merkel cells and the adjacent epidermal cells, do not lie on the finger-like processes. The cytoplasm of the Merkel cells and the Grandry cells contains a meshwork of filaments and granulated vesicles. The content and significance of the latter is still unknown. The myelinated axon branches freely and forms terminals that are enlarged (up to 10 μm diameter). Each forms a roughly

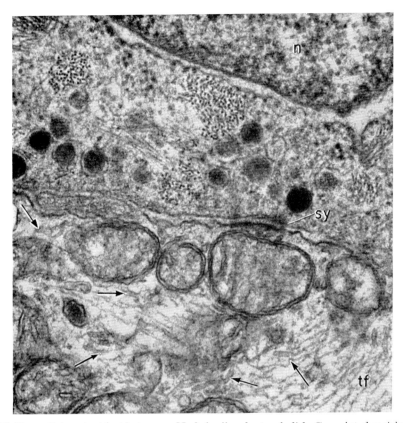

Fig. 15. 'Synaptic' contact (sy) between a Merkel cell and a touch disk. Granulated vesicles are accummulated in the cytoplasm of the Merkel cell above the contact. Thickening of the membrane of the nerve terminal is typical of these contacts. nucleus = n; tonofilaments = tf. In the receptorplasm the tubular meshwork is present (arrows). Electron micrograph. Magn.:
80,000 ×

Fig. 14. Schematic representation of the Merkel cell-neurite complex from the external root sheath of a sinus hair. The myelinated axon loses its myelin and forms contacts, "touch meniscus", or "touch disk", which are in close apposition to the Merkel touch cells. In other situations, e.g. the hairy skin, the Merkel cell is on the opposite side of the Merkel disk, and is therefore closer to the basement membrane of the epidermis. ax = sensory axon; bm = basement membrane; bz = basal cell; dm = desmosome; gh = glassy membrane; tf = fingerlike processes of the touch cell (tz); tm = touch meniscus; sy = contact zone to the Merkel cell, (From ANDRES, 1966)

circular thin plate, the so called "touch meniscus" or "touch disk". The disk-shaped axon terminals of the Grandry corpuscle lie between pairs of sensory cells in the corium, in contrast to the mammalian Merkel disks, each of which is associated with a single Merkel cell and is in the epidermis. Granulated vesicles are concentrated in the cytoplasm subjacent to the nerve terminal and appear to take part in a special contact between sensory cell and axon terminal (Fig. 15). Presynaptic vesicles could not be seen in the nerve-terminal. The axoplasm of the nerve terminal contains microtubules, neurofilaments, accumulations of mitochondria and a tubular meshwork. We know that one axon supplies many Merkel cell-neurite complexes in a circumscribed receptor field, and these complexes in hairy skin have been identified as slowly-adapting type I mechanoreceptors (see Chapter 2). Reconstructions of Grandry corpuscles show that several corpuscles

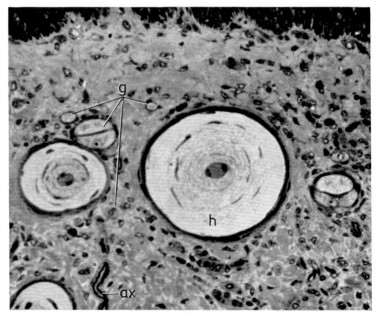

Fig. 16. Herbst corpuscle (h) and Grandry corpuscles (g) in the connective tissue of a duck's bill. Reconstructions from serial sections established that the axon (ax) innervates several Grandry corpuscles of different size. Semithin section. Magn.: 350 ×

of different size can build a functional unit with one axon (Fig. 16). Presumably the Grandry corpuscle acts physiologically as a slowly-adapting mechanoreceptor in the same way as the complex of Merkel.

6. Unmyelinated Axons in Encapsulated Receptors

Unmyelinated nerves associated with the receptor axon are described on electron microscopical evidence for the Pacinian corpuscle (SANTINI, 1968), Herbst corpuscle (NAFSTAD and ANDERSEN, 1970) and the annulospiral ending of the muscle spindle (v. DÜRING and ANDRES unpublished). The terminals of the unmyelinated axons form synaptic contacts with the receptor axon or are distributed among the lamellae of the inner core of the receptor as in the Golgi-Mazzoni and Herbst corpuscles illustrated in Fig. 8B and C. The specific function of these unmyelinated axons is unknown but they may be autonomic post-ganglionic axons and provide centrifugal modulation of the receptor.

F. Complex Sensory Structures

After the classification of the different receptor types their combination to form sensory structures in several specialized and very exposed skin areas will now be considered. *Sinus hairs* (MERKEL, 1880) are present in the perioral facial regions, on the cheeks and around the eyes of many mammals. Familiar examples are the rows of vibrissae on the upper lips of cats, dogs and rats. In the sightless mole, sinus hairs are especially numerous in the hairy skin of the elongated snout of this animal. Not all sinus hairs are as long as the vibrissae and in the cat there are two rows of short sinus hairs on the upper lip, ventral to the vibrissae. Less complex sinus hairs may be present elsewhere, for example, on the inner aspect of the lower foreleg of the cat. The sinus hair follicle is both larger and structurally more complex (Fig. 17) than ordinary hair follicles. There is a prominent venous 'ring sinus' in the upper one-third of the follicle and a spongy vascular sinus in the lower two-thirds. The inner hair follicle receives a very rich sensory nerve-supply which is distributed to receptor terminals in the middle and upper part of the follicle. It is possible on the basis of the detailed results described above to recognise several different kinds of mechanoreceptor. In the rat sinus hairs (Fig. 17) these are A, Merkel receptors adjacent to the glassy membrane in the upper root sheath; B, straight lanceolate terminals adjacent to the glassy membrane in the intermediate zone of the inner hair follicle; C, branched lanceolate terminals, more deeply located in the inner hair follicle; D, branched circular lanceolate terminals in the inner conus of the inner hair follicle just below the sebaceous gland; E, Golgi-Mazzoni lamellated corpuscles adjacent to the branched lanceolate terminals and F, endings of unmyelinated fibres. Special operating characteristics would be predicted for these various receptor terminals because of their specific fine structure and location, and GOTTSCHALDT et al. (1972) have attributed specific physiological functions to them in the cat (see Chapter 2).

A conventional hair (guard hair) has straight lanceolate terminals, without fingerlike projections (Fig. 7A) that form a palisade around the hair shaft. These are presumably receptors for the rapidly-adapting hair follicle afferent units. In addition to this it has branched lanceolate terminals in the connective tissue of the hair shaft. The guard hairs of the eye-lash have, in addition to these two receptors, a touch papillae (Iggo corpuscle) just besides the hair pore (Fig. 18) and in this respect are similar to the tylotrich follicles (STRAILE, 1960).

In glabrous skin of mammals one finds frequently the combination of Merkel cell-neurite complexes, branched lanceolate terminals and lamellated corpuscles as for example in the snout of the pig (Fig. 19A). In the *Eimer's organ* of the mole the above mentioned receptor types are combined with the intraepidermal axon in a regular array (Figs. 19B, 20). The lamellated receptor is presumably a vibration detector and the Merkel cell and lanceolate terminals are presumably slowly-

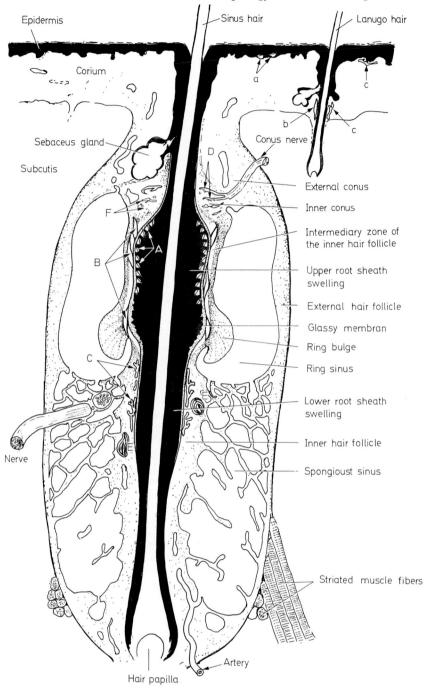

Fig. 17. Schematic representation of a rat's sinus hair with the location of the different sensory receptors. A, Merkel receptor; B, straight lanceolate terminal; C, branched lanceolate ending; D, branched circular lanceolate receptor ending; E, lamellated corpuscle; F, endings of unmyelinated nerve fibres. In the region of a down hair Merkel cells (a) straight (b) and branched (c) lanceolate terminals occur. (From Andres, 1966)

adapting receptors. The intraepidermal axon may be a cold receptor on analogy with structure of the cold receptors in the nose of the cat. One can assume that the mole investigates with this receptor the heat conduction of the objects it touches and thereby perceives something about the object's quality in addition to its form which is perceived with the other receptor types.

In future studies additional histochemical methods will have to be used in addition to the analysis of the fine structure. The topographic distribution of different receptors is just as important as the quantitative analysis of the physiological function of the single receptor type. We have to clarify for example how many single receptors belong to one sensory neuron.

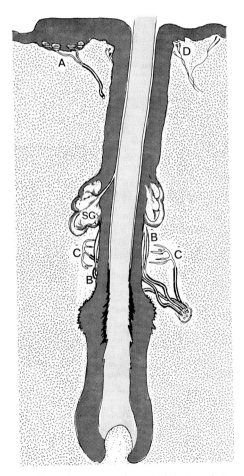

Fig. 18. Schematic representation of a macaque's eyelash hair with its sensory nerve supply. A, Touch papillae (Iggo corpuscle) containing Merkel cells; B, Straight lanceolate terminals; C, Branched circular lanceolate receptor axons; D, Spray-like endings from unmyelinated fibres.
sg = sebaceus gland

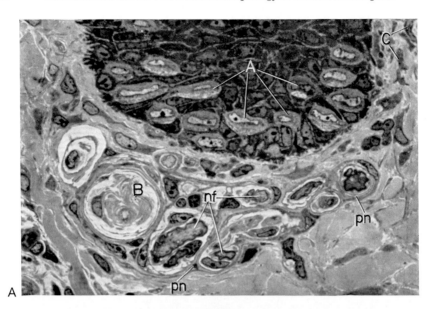

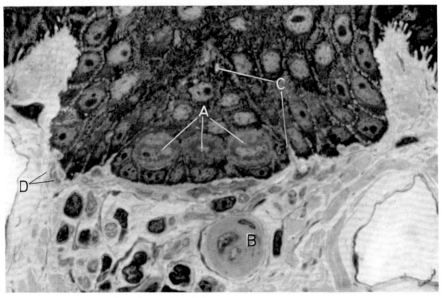

Fig. 19A–B. Two examples of specialized arrays of receptors in glabrous skin. A) Sensory inner-vation pattern in the glabrous snout skin of the pig. The skin is ridged and the basal part of one ridge is shown. A, Merkel cell-neurite complexes in the basal part of the epidermal ridge. B, Lamellated encapsulated corpuscle in the corium immediately below the epidermis and C, Branched lanceolate terminals. nf = nerve fibres; pn = perineural sheath which surrounds the myelinated fibres. Semithin section. Magn.: 900 × B) Basal region of an Eimer's organ from the glabrous skin of the snout of a mole. A, Merkel cell-neurite complexes in the basal region of the epidermis; B, A lamellated encapsulated corpuscle in the corium adjacent to the epidermis; C, Intraepidermal receptoraxons which penetrate to the surface of the epidermis, and D, Spray-like terminals of unmyelinated nerve fibres at the dermo-epidermal border. Semithin section. Magn.: 1500 ×

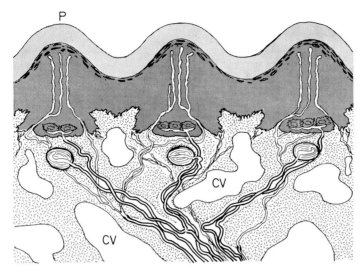

Fig. 20. Diagram of the sensory innervation of the glabrous skin of the mole's nose tip. The Eimer papillae are uniformly supplied, in a regular pattern, by four different kinds of receptor terminals as indicated in Fig. 19 B. A, Merkel cell-neurite complexes; B, lamellated encapsulated corpuscles; C, intraepidermal receptor axons and D, unmyelinated fibres. The different kinds of receptors are supplied by separate axons, but an individual axon may supply several receptors of the same type. cv = cavernous vein system, p = papilla

Acknowledgment

This work has been supported by the Deutsche Forschungsgemeinschaft (Sonderforschungsbereich — Bionach).

References

ANDRES, K.H.: Über die Feinstruktur der Rezeptoren an Sinushaaren. Z. Zellforsch. **75**, 339–365 (1966).

ANDRES, K.H.: Zur Ultrastruktur verschiedener Mechanorezeptoren von höheren Wirbeltieren. Anat. Anz. **124**, 551–565 (1969).

BLEICHMAR, H., DE ROBERTIS, E.: Submicroscopic morphology of the infra-red receptor of pit vipers. Z. Zellforsch. **56**, 748–761 (1962).

BROWN, A.G., IGGO, A.: A quantitative study of cutaneous receptors and afferent fibres in the cat and rabbit. J. Physiol. (Lond.) **193**, 707–733 (1967).

CAUNA, N.: The fine morphology of the sensory receptor organs in the auricle of the rat. J. comp. Neurol. **136**, 81–98 (1969).

CHAMBERS, M.R., ANDRES, K.H., DUERING, M. VON, IGGO, A.: Structure and function of the slowly adapting type II mechanoreceptor in hairy skin. Quart. J. exp. Physiol. **57**, 417–445 (1972).

GOGLIA, G., SKLENSKA, A.: Ricerche ultrastrutturali sopra i corpuscoli di Ruffini delle capsule articoloni nel coniglio. Quad. Anat. prat. **25**, 14–27 (1969).

GOTTSCHALDT, K.-H., IGGO, A., YOUNG, D.W.: Electrophysiology of the afferent innervation of sinus hairs, including vibrissae, of the cat. J. Physiol. (Lond.) **220**, 60–61 P.

KUNZE, K.: Die Papilla filiformis des Menschen als Tastsinnesorgan. Ergebn. Anat. Entwickl.-Gesch. **41** (1969).

LOEWENSTEIN, W.R., SKALAK, R.: Mechanical transmission in a Pacinian corpuscle. J. Physiol. (Lond.) **182**, 346–378 (1966).

Merkel ,F.: Über die Endigungen der sensiblen Nerven in der Haut der Wirbeltiere. Rostock: H. Schmidt 1880.

Munger, B.C.: Patterns of organisation of peripheral sensory receptors. In: Handbook of Sensory Physiology, Vol. I, pp. 524–553. Berlin-Heidelberg-New York: Springer 1971.

Nafstad, P.H., Andersen, A.E.: Ultrastructural investigation on the innervation of the Herbst corpuscle. Z. Zellforsch. **103**, 109–114 (1970).

Pritz, W., Stockinger, L.: Über den Zahnschmerz. Öst. Z. Stomat. **5**, 170–178 (1971).

Quilliam, T.A.: Unit design and array patterns in receptor organs. In: Touch, Heat and Pain, Ciba Foundation Symposium, pp. 86–116. Ed. by A.V.S. de Reuck and J. Knight. London: Churchill 1966.

Ruffini, A.: Sur un nouvel organe nerveux terminal et sur la présence des corpuscules Golgi-Mazzoni dans le conjonctif sous-cutane de la pulpe des doigts de l'homme. Arch. ital. Biol. **21**, 249–265 (1894).

Santini, M.: Noradrenergic fibres in Pacinian corpuscles. Anat. Rec. **160**, 494 (1968).

Stockinger, L., Pritz, W.: Morphologische Aspekte der Schmerzempfindung im Zahn. Dtsch. zahnärztl. Z. **25**, 557–565 (1970).

Straile, W.: Sensory hair follicles in mammalian skin: the tylotrich follicle. Amer. J. Anat. **106**, 133–147 (1960).

Yamamoto, T.: The fine structure of the palisade type sensory endings in relation to hair follicles. J. Electr. Micr. **15**, 158–166 (1966).

Chapter 2

Cutaneous Mechanoreceptors and Nociceptors

By

P. R. Burgess, Salt Lake City (USA) and E. R. Perl, Chapel Hill (USA)

With 8 Figures

Contents

A. Introduction

Although information from sense organs is used by all animals, only man can verbally report his sensory experience. A brief consideration of these experiences may be useful in providing insight into cutaneous sensory mechanisms. Non-noxious deformation of the human skin with a stimulator having a small surface area (2–3 mm²) evokes sensations usually referred to as "touch". If the stimulator remains stationary, the sensation fades. Movement of the stimulator perpendicular to the skin produces changes in the sensory process which allow even rapidly repeated stimuli (e.g. 500 Hz) to be distinguished from stationary ones. When larger stimulators are used, some appreciation of texture can be obtained, and this is enhanced by movement of the stimulating surface across the skin. A smooth stimulator or an insect moving slowly and gently over the skin evokes distinctive sensations usually referred to as "tickle". A sharp object such as a pin lightly pressed against certain points in the skin leads to an unpleasant experience which differs from touch but is equivocally painful; when the pin is pressed against the skin more firmly it usually elicits pain. Thus, sensations induced by mechanical events can be diverse. Moreover, common experience indicates that they may occur with greater or lesser intensity. On the other hand, neurophysiological experiments defining the properties of cutaneous sense organs have most often been done on animals other than man. Behavioral studies generally support the idea that upon stimulation of their integument, other animals distinguish details similar to those appreciated by man. Consideration of the data on this latter point is beyond the scope of this article; however, the properties of cutaneous sense organs in different species, including primates, can be shown to be similar and, on this basis, it may be presumed that general principles derived from their examination apply to man and his sensory mechanisms.

The following material concerns mammalian cutaneous *mechanoreceptors*, sense organs (receptors) that respond vigorously to innocuous mechanical deformation of the skin, and *nociceptors*, a class of cutaneous receptors that distinguishes between innocuous mechanical (or thermal) stimuli and tissue-damaging stimuli. With increasing knowledge, it has become clear that a single criterion is not sufficient to distinguish a cutaneous sense organ. By drawing on data collected from somatic sense organs in various tissues, a framework for discussing cutaneous sensory elements can be formed; within such a context, a set of features serves to separate primary sensory neurons into different groups or classes with remarkably little overlap on grounds meaningful from behavioral considerations. In other words, the functional characteristics of cutaneous sense organs show substantial specialization. This does not mean that one and only one kind of grossly defined stimulus, such as contact with the skin, will excite a given primary afferent neuron. For instance, large thermal stimuli, particularly cooling, will initiate activity from several types of sensory elements which otherwise behave as mechanoreceptors; however, the response to temperature is usually only a fraction of that to one of the varieties of mechanical stimuli. The significance of this dual responsiveness is not known. In terms of input to the central nervous system a response to such different kinds of stimuli may represent uncertainty or noise; alternatively, it may aid in the discrimination of both mechanical and thermal stimuli.

The first of the following sections (B) deals with those cutaneous receptors that are consistently and effectively excited by non-damaging mechanical disturbances of the skin, the *mechanoreceptors*. The second section (C) considers those receptors most responsive to mechanical or other events destructive of tissue, the *nociceptors*.

B. Cutaneous Mechanoreceptors

1. Considerations in the Classification of Cutaneous Mechanoreceptive Neurons

Primary sensory neurons (synonyms: primary afferent neurons or units) extend from the skin and other tissues to the central nervous system. The terminal portions of the neuron lying in the peripheral tissue constitute the receptive or dendritic part of the cell (BODIAN, 1962), receive the stimulus and translate it into nerve impulses which propagate along the afferent fibre or conductive portion of the neuron to synaptic junctions in the spinal cord or brain. Since morphological and physiological features of the conductive and receptive parts are important for distinguishing mechanoreceptive neurons, both will be used for classification.

a) Primary Afferent Fibres

Diameter. The peripheral fibres of a single primary neuron are relatively uniform in diameter for considerable lengths, but vary in diameter from one to another; most of those supplying the skin of the cat (and other mammals) fall into three major categories (GASSER, 1955, 1960): Aα (alpha) myelinated fibres (diameter 6–17 μ including myelin), Aδ (delta) myelinated fibres (diameter 1–5 μ including myelin), and unmyelinated or C fibres (diameter 0.3–1.5 μ). Mechanoreceptors are associated with fibres in all three categories.

The *conduction velocity* of a fibre is related to its diameter. Multiplying an Aα fibre's diameter in μ by a factor of six gives a value approximating its conduction velocity in m/sec (HURSH, 1939). A factor near four seems appropriate for Aδ fibres (see BURGESS, PETIT and WARREN, 1968). Unmyelinated (C) fibres lack saltatory conduction and propagation is relatively slower; a conversion factor of 1.7 has been suggested (GASSER, 1955). Myelinated afferent fibres in muscle nerves have distributions of diameters that fall into three groups (LLOYD and CHANG, 1948) labeled by LLOYD (1943) as I, II, III on the basis of peaks in the compound action potential. Non-myelinated fibres constituted group IV. Cutaneous nerves do not have the same grouping of diameters; however, this muscle nerve

Table 1. *Afferent fibres and cutaneous receptor type*

Fibre Classification	– – – – – Aα – – – – – – – –		Aδ	C
	(Group I)	(Group II)	(Group III)	(Group IV)
Diameter	– – 17–6 μ – – – – – – – – –		5–1 μ	1.5–0.3 μ
	(20–12 μ)	(11–6 μ)		
Conduction Velocity	– – 100–30 m/sec – – – – –		30–4 m/sec	2–0.4 m/sec
	(120–72 m/sec)	(72–30 m/sec)		
Receptor type	G₁ Hair	mechanical nociceptors		C mechano-
	Glabrous Transient	D hair		receptors
	Type I	Mechanical-thermal		Thermoreceptors
	Type II	nociceptors		Polymodal
	Pacinian and	(primate/cat facial)		nociceptors
	paciniform	Thermoreceptors-cool		
	Glabrous	(primate/cat		
	position and	glabrous		
	velocity	and facial)		
	[Type I & II]			
	G₂ Hair			
	Field			

The earliest fibre classification scheme proposed (GASSER and ERLANGER, 1927; ERLANGER and GASSER, 1937) included β and γ fibres in addition to the α, δ and C groups shown in Table 1 and was applied to both motor and sensory fibres. Subsequently, the Type I, II, III and IV classification was devised specifically for the sensory fibres in muscle nerves (LLOYD, 1943). GASSER (1960) later reexamined the classification for cutaneous nerves; the γ elevation in the compound potential of the cat saphenous nerve appeared largely artifactual and the β elevation was not consistent enough to justify special designation. The receptor correlations are only meant to indicate the typical or most common relationship to fibre characteristics

classification has been applied by some to cutaneous afferent fibres. Table 1 compares conduction velocity, fibre diameter, classification nomenclature and receptor type.

b) Receptive Portion of the Neuron

The *disposition of the nerve terminals* in the skin varies with receptor type; it includes the number of branches and their types as well as the relation of the terminal processes to other tissue.

The *receptive field* of a sensory neuron is defined as the peripheral area from which it can be excited by a stimulus that exceeds threshold by a stated amount. In many cases, this area appears to be coextensive with the region wherein the receptive terminals are located while in others remotely applied stimuli may effectively activate the neuron.

Non-neural elements associated with nerve terminals, such as encapsulating cells or hair follicles, are the structures which must be deformed to excite the nerve endings; they may select the nature of the effective stimulus by their mechanical properties and location. The so-called "receptor" cell is a non-neural specialization deserving of special mention. Specialized epithelial cells (Merkel cells) are found in association with certain sensory nerve terminals; the relationship has some features suggestive of a synapse, the epithelial cell being presynaptic (ANDRES, 1966). Cells of this type may be important in the transduction of the stimulus and they have been called receptors. In the following discussion the sensory nerve terminals proper are considered the *receptor* since non-neural elements like the Merkel cell have not been identified in association with most mechanoreceptive endings and a causal relation between cutaneous epithelial cells and excitation of neural structures is still tenuous.

c) Nature of the Exciting Stimulus

The *adequate stimulus* of a receptor can be defined as the stimulus for which it shows the greatest responsiveness (HALL, 1850; SHERRINGTON, 1906). This definition implies that stimuli other than the one to which the receptive apparatus is best adapted to respond are capable of evoking activity. A description of the mechanical status of a structure at any moment in time can be made in terms of (1) the position of the structure, (2) the rate at which the position is changing (velocity), (3) the rate at which the velocity is changing (acceleration), (4) the rate at which the acceleration is changing (jerk), *etcetera*. Each of these terms will be considered a mode of mechanical stimulation and potentially an adequate stimulus for a mechanoreceptor. When mechanoreceptors are examined in terms of the nature of the adequate stimulus, three main classes of behavior can be distinguished: (1) position detection, (2) velocity detection, and (3) detection of rapid transients. A major problem with classifying receptors in this fashion is that many show more than one form of behavior (for example, both position and velocity detection). However, the analysis of receptors with mixed properties is facilitated by the fact that under certain stimulus conditions often they are dominated by a particular type of response.

d) Responsive Characteristics

Other physiological criteria to be used in mechanoreceptor classification can be illustrated by a hypothetical example. Consider a receptor that provides information only about the position of some body part and assume that the innervated structure (a hair follicle, for example) can move back and forth in more than one direction. Position information could be signalled if the receptor's discharge frequency were proportional to displacement. When external forces on the structure are minimal, the structure will assume a certain "rest" position, a position at which its activity (discharge) is generally at its lowest level. This suggests that nerve terminal deformation is least under these conditions, and defines a physiological zero point from which receptor output can be measured as a function of displacement. Various factors influence the precision with which the position of a structure can be specified by receptor activity.

a) Adaptation. For greatest precision the discharge frequency should be time independent for a particular position. Thus, adaptation, a decline in the discharge of a receptor while the stimulus is unchanging (ADRIAN and ZOTTERMAN, 1926), would reduce precision.

b) Fatigue. Similarly, precision will suffer when the response is not identical at given positions on different occasions. Thus, fatigue, a less vigorous response on repeated applications of the same stimulus, can be a source of systematic variability.

c) Linear and Spatial Directionality. For precision, the frequency should be independent of the direction moved to arrive at a particular position; i.e., the receptor should not show "linear directionality". Linear directionality can be evaluated by moving the innervated structure away from the rest position and returning it along the same path and testing the response when a given position is approached from one direction and the opposite. Directional sensitivity of this sort should be distinguished from the responsiveness of a receptor to movements in different directions from the rest position. A receptor that responds when a structure is moved away from the rest position in certain directions, but not others, can be said to show "spatial directionality".

d) Dynamic Range and Input-Output Correlations. The dynamic range of the receptor influences the precision with which position can be specified. Assuming that information is coded in terms of frequency of discharge (Hartline and Ratliff, 1957; Werner and Mountcastle, 1965; Mountcastle, Talbot and Kornhuber, 1966; Jansen, Nicolaysen and Rudjord, 1966; Harrington and Merzenich, 1970), the dynamic range of a position receptor can be defined as the discharge frequency when deformation is greatest minus the frequency when deformation is least. The change in frequency for a given change in position (sensitivity) need not be uniform over the entire range of displacement. The response of the receptor at different positions along the movement continuum can be defined by an input-output function, an expression which relates the frequency of discharge of the receptor to the position of the innervated structure. Various input-output functions have been proposed for cutaneous receptors, of the following general types: linear function, $y = a + bx$ (where y = frequency of discharge, x = suprathreshold stimulus, a and b are constants); power function, $y = ax^b$; log or exponential functions, $y = a + b \log x$ or $\log y = a + bx$ (equivalent to $x = a.e^{by}$ and $y = a.e^{bx}$); log hyperbolic tangent function, $y = \tanh \log x$.

e) Pattern of Discharge. The accuracy with which the position of the structure is specified as a function of time influences precision. When the intervals between successive nerve impulses do not differ much from one another (i.e., are regular), less time is required to establish the frequency than for an irregular pattern.

f) Recovery from Past Activity. The recovery of excitability following an impulse, often referred to as the *recovery cycle*, is a factor influencing the dynamic range and pattern of a receptor's activity. Recovery cycles are readily measured by exciting the receptor with two short duration mechanical pulses separated by varying intervals. At a particular interstimulus interval, the threshold is determined for the second of the two stimuli (the conditioned stimulus) and this threshold is compared with that obtained when the first stimulus of the pair is not given (the unconditioned stimulus). Another interval is chosen and the process repeated until the range of intervals for which the conditioned and unconditioned stimuli differ in threshold has been explored.

The significance of the recovery cycle of a receptor for its pattern of discharge and dynamic range can be appreciated by considering a receptor's generation of nerve impulses. Studies of various mechanoreceptors have indicated the following steps (see Vol. I of this series): (1) The stimulus deforms the sensory nerve terminals, causing their depolarization. This depolarization (the generator potential) increases with increasing stimulus strength. (2) The generator potential spreads electrotonically to a low threshold portion of the sensory neuron where, provided that the depolarization is suprathreshold, nerve impulses are initiated. The rate at which nerve impulses recur will be influenced by the magnitude and duration of the depression of receptor excitability which follows each impulse. If the excitability depression following an impulse lasts only a few msec the effective dynamic range of the receptor will be reduced, should there be no other means for the generation of a low frequency discharge. (Alternatives to depression of the impulse mechanism after its excitation for low frequency generation of impulses include a) oscillation of a near-threshold generator potential and b) destruction of the generator potential by the impulse with its rate of subsequent formation being a function of stimulus strength.)

e) Recapitulation of Theoretical Considerations

From the above, we can predict that the precision with which position can be specified along the movement continuum will be limited by the dynamic range of a receptor whose response is a) time and rate independent, b) without linear directionality and c) completely reproducible. Any deviation from time independence or reproducibility, or any tendency toward directional sensitivity will reduce the number of positions that can be uniquely specified. For a perfectly regular discharge (i.e., all interspike intervals the same size), the time required to determine a particular position would be a simple function of frequency; the analysis period need only be long enough to include at least one interspike interval. For an irregular discharge, the accuracy with which frequency is determinable from a single interspike interval is reduced, and therefore, fewer positions on the movement continuum can be uniquely indicated without increasing the period of analysis and averaging successive intervals.

This preliminary discussion has been used to cast light on some of the factors influencing information transmission from a single position receptor. Pure position receptors are rare in nature and are not found in the skin. However, the principles that govern information transmission are of general significance and apply whether a receptor signals position, velocity or transients. Mathematical expressions can be derived from information theory that allow quantitative descriptions of information transmission by individual sensory fibres (see STEIN, 1967). It is important to bear in mind that while activity initiated by a single receptor may have important behavioral consequences in animals with few neurons, in vertebrates and especially in mammals, populations of receptors are often brought into play by a stimulus and the information transmitted by their collective activity will be increased over that conveyed by the component elements.

f) Determination of Adequate Stimuli for Mechanoreceptors

Real cutaneous receptors signalling position depart from ideal behavior since they are influenced by the rate of skin indentation. Adaptation and specific responsiveness to velocity or higher derivatives of displacement are factors influencing receptor sensitivity to the dynamic aspects of a stimulus. Adaptation after an abrupt displacement is not a simple process; a description of the decline in frequency generally requires three or four exponential terms (Pringle and Wilson, 1952; Houk and Simon, 1967; Chambers, Andres, v. Duering and Iggo, 1972). The time constants defining the process become larger as adaptation progresses and adaptation may ultimately cease leaving a time independent discharge which is a function of the magnitude of the displacement. For present purposes any receptor which discharges when a stimulator is stationary is defined as a *position detector*, even when this discharge ultimately adapts to zero; a

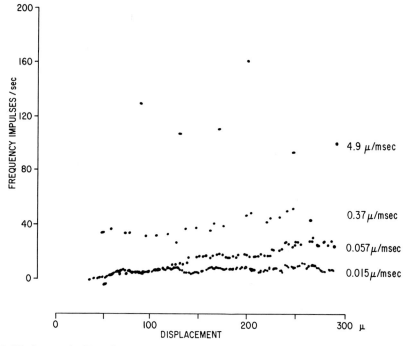

Fig. 1. Discharge of a Type I cutaneous receptor as a function of skin displacement (abscissa). Each plot shows results from a single displacement at the velocity indicated to the right. At 4.9 μ/msec each point represents the reciprocal of the interval between two successive impulses plotted at the displacement of the second impulse. At the lower velocities a sliding average (the averaged value of an odd number of intervals plotted at the displacement corresponding to the central interval) has been plotted to reduce irregularities in the discharge. (Values for 7 intervals at 0.37 μ/msec and 11 intervals at the other velocities were averaged.) See text for additional comment

receptor showing a non-adapting position response shows *static displacement detection*. When a position detector is subjected to a constant velocity (ramp) indentation, the frequency of discharge will increase as a function of displacement without being influenced by velocity, provided that no adaptation takes place. In the presence of adaptation, the response of the receptor will also depend upon velocity. Low velocity ramps will evoke a discharge whose frequency will be a time independent function of displacement because there is time for adaptation to occur. When ramp velocities exceed the decay of adaptation, the response versus displacement curves will steepen increasing the dynamic range (Figs. 1 and

2). *(Throughout the subsequent discussion it is assumed that frequency is plotted on the ordinate and displacement on the abscissa with increasing displacement to the right, as in Figs. 1 and 2.)* Thus, adaptation may impart rate sensitivity to a position receptor. The rate sensitivity of the receptor will be enhanced still further if the receptor also has specific *velocity detector* properties.

A sense organ lacking position detection and producing a non-adapting response proportional to stimulus velocity will generate impulses whose frequency plotted against increasing displacement gives a horizontal line at a constant velocity as illustrated by Fig. 3 (LINDBLOM, 1962; BROWN and IGGO, 1967). Should the

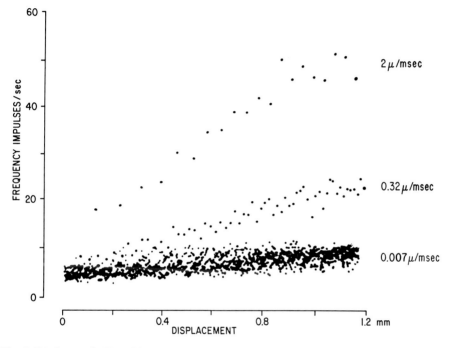

Fig. 2. Discharge of a Type II cutaneous receptor plotted against skin displacement at different velocities as indicated on the right. Results from a single stimulus repetition are plotted at each velocity. A "resting" discharge of approximately 5 impulses/sec was present in the absence of intentional stimulation. See text for additional comment

velocity response adapt, a curve sloping downwards with increasing displacement will be formed. With increasing stimulus velocity, the curves, whatever their shape, are displaced upward as the receptor discharges at progressively higher frequencies. These properties define a velocity detector. A receptor functioning as a pure position detector, with adaptation, does not show this form of velocity response; as velocity increases, the steepening curves of discharge frequency versus displacement are not displaced upward (Fig. 2; Fig. 1 at low velocities; see also Fig. 2 in COOPER, 1961). Such responses are predicted by transfer functions which describe an adapting response to an abrupt stimulus for a cockroach position receptor (PRINGLE and WILSON, 1952) and mammalian Golgi tendon organs (Houk and Simon, 1967). Position receptors, both in the skin and deeper tissues, commonly do have velocity detection characteristics. When a receptor possesses both an adapting position response and velocity detection, plots of frequency versus displacement will steepen for increasing velocities and, once the velocity threshold of the receptor is exceeded, be displaced upward as well, as in Fig. 1 (Cooper, 1961; Lindblom, 1962, 1963; Crowe and Matthews, 1964; Lennerstrand, 1968; Iggo and Muir, 1969; Chambers et al., 1972).

The relative magnitude of these effects will depend upon the rate and extent of the adaptation of the position response and the degree of specific response to

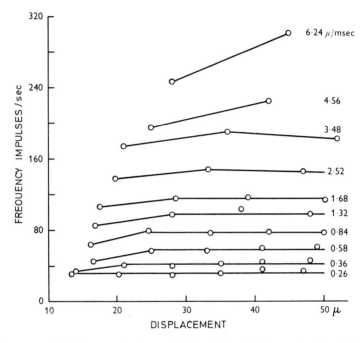

Fig. 3. Responses of a hair receptor to constant velocity displacement of a single hair as a function of displacement. The displacement velocities in μ/msec are given to the right. Frequency was calculated from the reciprocal of impulse interval; each point represents the average of 10 consecutively obtained records. (From Brown and Iggo, 1967)

velocity. In general, only alterations in the inclination of the curves are seen at low velocities since the velocity term is small. As would be expected, the velocity fraction of the response becomes more pronounced in a progression to higher velocities and, at some point, position-velocity receptors may fail to indicate position altogether (B.H.C. Matthews, 1933; Lindblom, 1962; P.B.C. Matthews, 1963). Thus not only do frequency versus displacement curves move upwards at higher velocities, but they also assume a horizontal orientation (Fig. 1). A similar loss of position detection can be seen when the velocity of movement is increased by increasing the frequency of sinusoidal stimuli (Lippold, Redfearn and Vučo, 1958; Lowenstein and Finlayson, 1960; Stuart, Ott,

ISHIKAWA and ELDRED, 1965). Sensory units in which the ratio of velocity to position responsiveness is high are more readily converted to "pure" velocity receptors during stimulator movement than those in which this ratio is lower (LINDBLOM, 1963; P. B. C. MATTHEWS, 1963; STUART et al., 1965).

In the absence of long-term hysteresis, directional differences are absent in responses of receptors with static displacement detection when movements are sufficiently slow. On the other hand, as the velocity is increased, typically linear directionality appears. This has been studied systematically for the primary and secondary endings of mammalian muscle spindles (COOPER, 1961; HARVEY and MATTHEWS, 1961; LENNERSTRAND, 1968) and the properties they exhibit are likely to be of general significance (see WIERSMA and BOETTIGER, 1959). The secondary endings correspond more closely to pure position receptors; both velocity response and linear directionality are less well developed than in primary endings. Thus, the movement used to reach a new position alters the curve relating discharge to position for secondary endings less than for primary endings. This is a further indication that position and velocity detection represent distinct receptor specializations; velocity discharge seems to be best suited to detect deviations *away from* the rest position while position responses show less directional sensitivity.

In addition to receptors that signal position or velocity, certain receptors can be classed as "transient" detectors. Transient detectors respond preferentially to rapid stimuli and do not signal position. They may be thought of as "tuned" to high frequencies. Two general categories are found among receptors of this type. Some behave as velocity detectors with high velocity thresholds while others appear to detect acceleration or its derivative (jerk). Both transient detector types are found in or near the skin of mammals, and although they differ in certain respects they have a number of properties in common.

The bases for describing mechanoreceptors as detectors of position, velocity or transients have been discussed in broad terms. This formulation will now be extended to mammalian cutaneous receptors. Receptor types whose properties suggest a particular responsiveness to similar stimuli will be considered together. Sensory units of hairy skin will be presented first, followed by a discussion of elements of glabrous skin and those associated with specialized structures. Among the mammals, the cat has been the most thoroughly studied, particularly the hairy skin of the hindlimb and will provide a point of departure for consideration of related cutaneous mechanoreceptors of other species.

2. Mechanoreceptors in Hairy Skin

a) Receptors Detecting Position and Velocity

Two cutaneous mechanoreceptor types in the hairy skin of mammals detect both static displacement and velocity. They were first differentiated as Type I and Type II units by IGGO (1966). Type I afferent fibres have diameters in the Aα range and are among the most rapidly conducting (55–75 m/sec) in cutaneous nerves. Type II afferent fibres conduct at somewhat lower Aα velocities (45 to 65 m/sec).

1. Historical Considerations and Morphology. Early electrophysiological investigations of mammalian hairy skin by Adrian (1931, 1932) and Zotterman (1939) described receptors responding to hair movement but did not mention position detectors. In recordings from the rabbit sural nerve, Frankenhaeuser (1949) reported prolonged discharge in response to steady skin deformation, probably of Type I units. (In some studies no distinction was made between Type I and Type II elements; however, differences in discharge pattern of the two types often allows determination of their identity in illustrations.) Witt and Hensel (1959) described responses now recognised as derived from Type II receptors in the cat and directed their attention primarily to activity evoked by temperature changes. Hunt and McIntyre (1960b) did not distinguish between Type I and Type II endings in their study of highly responsive "touch" receptors in the cat sural area, although both Type I and Type II discharges are illustrated. Werner and Mountcastle (1965) also included both types in a detailed quantitative study of position receptors in the cat and monkey; most of their quantitative results were apparently obtained from Type II receptors (see Iggo and Muir, 1969). An important advance occurred when Iggo (1963) and Tapper (1964) independently reported that a single Type I fiber in cat characteristically supplies two or three small dome-like elevations (200–500 μ diameter) excited by the gentlest of mechanical stimuli (5–15 μ of skin displacement). Iggo and Muir (1969; see also Iggo, 1963) showed that the nerve fibre in each dome branches to supply a number of specialized epithelial cells (Merkel cells) located at the base of the thickened epithelium investing the structure. Other studies (Iggo, 1966; Chambers et al., 1972) have demonstrated that Type II fibres are not associated with domes and that the skin spot with the lowest mechanical threshold overlies a Ruffini ending (see Andres, Chapter 1).

Distinct receptor populations with properties like Type I and Type II receptors of the cat have been found in the hairy skin of rabbits (Brown and Iggo, 1967; Brown and Hayden, 1971), primates, including man (Lindblom and Tapper, 1967; Perl, 1968; Harrington and Merzenich, 1970; Knibestöl and Vallbo, 1970) and in the skin of reptiles (Kenton, Kruger and Woo, 1971). In the rabbit and other rodents, Type I fibres also terminate in distinct dome-like elevations morphologically similar to the Type I receptors of carnivores (Straile, 1960; Smith, 1967). The domes are less elevated in primates but otherwise are structurally similar (Smith, 1970). The structure of the endings in reptiles is unknown and thus far Type II receptor properties have been correlated to Ruffini endings only in carnivores.

2. Position and Velocity Detection. Although both Type I and Type II receptors detect position and velocity, Type II receptors are biased more strongly to position and Type I units to velocity detection. The position response of these receptors can be demonstrated by abruptly applying a maintained stimulus as in Fig. 4; the response of both adapts, first rapidly and then more slowly (see Chambers et al., 1972) with a static displacement component evident 2–4 min after stimulus onset. The range of the static Type I response is only about 10 impulses/sec whereas some Type II units have static responses with a dynamic range of 20–25 impulses/sec (Burgess et al., 1968). Thus, Type I receptors cannot provide as much information about skin position under steady-state conditions as individual Type II elements;

even the latter's position responsiveness is not comparable to that of secondary muscle spindle endings (LENNERSTRAND, 1968; MATTHEWS and STEIN, 1969).

For constant velocity displacements, both Type I and Type II receptors show frequency versus displacement responses expected for adapting position receptors with velocity sensitivity (Figs. 1 and 2). As pointed out above, low velocities plot the steady-state response. With increasing stimulus velocities, the frequency versus displacement curves steepen and are displaced upward (IGGO and MUIR, 1969; CHAMBERS et al., 1972). The upward displacement is less marked for Type II, indicating a lower velocity sensitivity (compare Figs. 1 and 2). With still further increases in stimulus velocity, Type I receptors first lose their position response with the frequency versus displacement curves assuming a horizontal orientation (Fig. 1) and then a downward slope may become apparent at very high velocities (TAPPER, 1965, Fig. 3; NILSSON, 1969b). Type II receptors, as would be expected

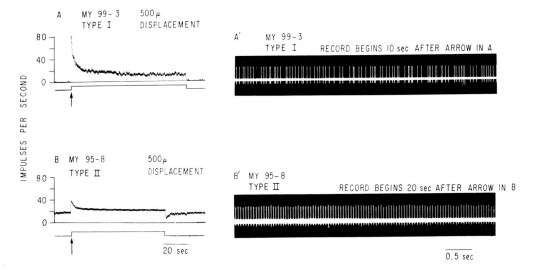

Fig. 4. Examples of activity evoked from Type I and Type II cutaneous receptors. (From BURGESS, PETIT and WARREN, 1968)

from their lesser velocity response, are less readily converted to pure velocity detection.

Type I units may discharge briefly at frequencies as high as 1000/sec to high velocity stimulation and Type II receptors respond to comparable stimuli at frequencies up to 800/sec (see CHAMBERS et al., 1972). As a result of adaptation, the dynamic range of the response is greater the sooner it is sampled after stimulus application.

3. *Linear Directionality.* Type I and Type II cutaneous receptors resemble other receptors with both position and velocity sensitivity in that the velocity response occurs only during movement away from the rest position (BURGESS and HORCH, unpublished). Thus directionality in their velocity response is pronounced. Moreover, since Type II receptors emphasize position detection more than Type I

they would be expected to show less linear directionality in their position response. Detailed studies of direction determined responses of mammalian tactile receptors are not available; however, Kenton, Kruger and Woo (1971) found that Type II reptilian receptors fatigue less readily than Type I. When a receptor fatigues, its threshold increases during a maintained response (B.H.C. Matthews, 1931; Jänig, Schmidt and Zimmermann, 1968) and this should contribute to linear directionality.

4. *Input-Output Functions and Dynamic Range.* In determining input-output functions for receptors signalling both position and velocity, it is important to specify the aspect being measured. There is disagreement in evaluation of position responsiveness of Type I and Type II units by abrupt indentations. In the monkey, Harrington and Merzenich (1970) concluded that the increase in discharge frequency as a function of indentation was best fit by a power function (log frequency linearly related to log indentation) with exponents that fell between 0.35 and 0.75 for both Type I and Type II elements. Similar data had been reported by Werner and Mountcastle (1965) for what apparently were mainly Type II receptors in the cat and monkey, although almost half the examples they illustrate could be equally well described by a logarithmic relationship (frequency linearly related to log indentation). In contrast, Kenton, Kruger and Woo (1971) in the reptile, and Tapper (1964) in the cat, argued that the frequency of Type I discharge increases in a linear fashion with indentation. Moreover, Kenton et al. (1971) determined that the responses of about half of the Type II receptors they tested were best described by a relationship in which the frequency was an exponential function of the stimulus (log frequency linearly related to the indentation); their remaining Type II activity was best matched by power functions with exponents less than one. In input-output relationships described by a power function with an exponent less than one, the sensitivity of a receptor decreases with increasing indentation. Sensitivity remains uniform with indentation in linear correlation between discharge and stimulus while sensitivity increases with indentation in exponential input-output functions. The first and second of these relationships have been suggested for Type I receptors and the first and third for Type II receptors. The reasons for this diversity are not clear although species differences may be partially responsible.

The position response of Type II receptors some time after an abrupt indentation has a limited dynamic range and demonstrates largely uniform sensitivity at different levels of indentation; the input-output functions approach linearity (Werner and Mountcastle, 1965). It is possible that linear input-output functions are a general property of adapted position responses (Eldred, Granit and Merton, 1953; Terzuolo and Washizu, 1962; Lindblom, 1963; Houk and Simon, 1967; Jänig et al., 1968).

The discharge frequency of Type I receptors is a linear function of indentation during low velocity displacement (Iggo and Muir, 1969). The *intervals* between successive impulses from Type II receptors decrease during progressive indentation in a fashion that is equally well described by linear, logarithmic and power functions (Chambers et al., 1972). Chambers et al. (1972) also found the change in the intervals between Type II impulses several seconds after a step indentation equally well described by logarithmic or power functions. On the other hand, for rapidly moving stimuli, the discharge frequency of Type I receptors is closely fit by a power function (exponents 0.3 to 0.5) of stimulus velocity; therefore, the sensitivity to velocity decreases with progressively higher velocities (TAPPER, 1965).

5. *Discharge Pattern and Recovery Cycle.* As shown in Fig. 4, Type II units generate a relatively regular train of impulses under constant stimulus conditions (IGGO, 1966; BURGESS et al., 1968; IGGO and MUIR, 1969; CHAMBERS et al., 1972); the standard deviation of the interval distribution histogram is typically 5–10 % of the mean interval in the range from 15–50 impulses/sec. In contrast, the standard deviation of a Type I interval distribution histogram is typically about 50 % of the mean in the range from 15–50 impulses/sec.

Type I and Type II receptors differ in their recovery from an impulse. Excitability may be depressed in Type II receptors for over 100 msec after an action potential, and at intervals of 10 msec, threshold may be 3 times control values (BURGESS and HORCH, unpublished). This depression of excitability has a similar time course regardless of whether the impulse is initiated orthodromically, by a natural stimulus, or propagates antidromically (see LINDBLOM, 1958). Thus, it is the impulse itself which initiates the excitability change and impulse conduction in the receptor appears to be bidirectional (see PRINGLE, 1938). This explains the observation that an impulse conducting antidromically into the receptor region can reset the discharge pattern during periods of rhythmic activity (B. H. C. MATTHEWS, 1931). As would be predicted from this observation, antidromic impulses entering the receptor at a frequency greater than an ongoing orthodromic discharge silence the orthodromic impulses, an observation which cannot be explained by collision of orthodromic and antidromic impulses; the absolute refractory period occupies too small a fraction of the interspike interval.

Type I receptors have substantially shorter recovery cycles than Type II elements, those of Type II being the longest while those of Type I are intermediate in the range of recovery cycles for cutaneous mechanoreceptors. Depression of excitability cannot be detected after 40–50 msec following a Type I orthodromic impulse; at intervals of 10 msec the threshold is typically $1^1/_2$ to 2 times control values (LINDBLOM and TAPPER, 1967).

The irregularity of Type I discharge compared to Type II activity is apparently due both to a shorter recovery cycle and a more variable generator potential. The latter may be deduced from the facts that, during sustained discharge to a just liminal stimulus, Type II receptors do not exhibit intervals between impulses shorter than 80 msec (BURGESS and HORCH, unpublished), an interval at which the threshold is increased by less than $1^1/_2$ times. Type I units under similar conditions have impulse intervals of 5 msec which yield thresholds that are $2^1/_2$ to 3 times control values. One must conclude that Type I receptors increase their discharge frequency by increasing the frequency and/or amplitude of fluctuations of the generator potential. The origin of such fluctuations is uncertain, but the relationship between Type I nerve terminals and Merkel cells has some features suggestive of a synapse (ANDRES, 1966; IGGO and MUIR, 1969). Although direct evidence is lacking for synaptic excitation of mechanoreceptor endings in the skin, the Merkel cell cytoplasm near the nerve terminal has dense core vesicles which conceivably could contain excitatory transmitter to be liberated for action on the nerve terminal.

Whether the difference in discharge pattern between Type I and Type II receptors is important in the subsequent transmission of sensory information is not known. Less information per unit time is transmitted by irregular interspike intervals than by a regular impulse train (Matthews and Stein, 1969). On the other hand, the irregular Type I discharge favours the occurrence of closely spaced impulses onto second order systems, especially when Type I fibres converge.

6. Spatial Directionality and Sensitivity to Skin Stretch. Type I receptors are not readily excited unless the stimulator makes direct contact with the dome; stretching the dome by remote traction provokes little activity. While Type II receptors are also excited more readily by a stimulator that encounters the centre of their receptive field, they can also be activated when this area of skin is stretched by distant stimulation. Type II receptors show spatial directionality when stimulated by skin stretch. Stretch applied at an angle of 90° to that most effectively exciting it will cause a decrease in activity (Knibestöl and Vallbo, 1970; Chambers et al., 1972). Type II receptors commonly have a resting discharge, sometimes as high as 20 impulses/sec in the absence of deliberate stimulation, possibly caused by some persistent tension on the focal region. Type I receptors rarely have a resting discharge in excess of 1–2 impulses/sec.

7. Overview. Type I and Type II cutaneous mechanoreceptors are similar in several respects (Table 2); 1) both detect position and velocity; 2) their nerve terminals are localized to a small area so that the receptive fields appear focussed or punctate; 3) displacements of the order of 5–15 μ are sufficient to elicit activity when applied to the focus. There also are differences between them: a) Type I endings have less capacity for static displacement detection and have a more vigorous velocity response than Type II endings; b) Type I units usually have receptive fields consisting of 2 or 3 foci while Type II units have only one; c) the morphology of the terminals differs; d) Type II endings are excited by skin stretch and show spatial directionality when stimulated in this fashion while Type I endings have little sensitivity to skin stretch; e) Type II elements have longer recovery cycles and a more regular pattern of discharge than Type I terminals.

Type II endings have properties that are comparable in many respects to static displacement detectors in the deeper tissues of mammals. Such receptors in muscles, tendons, ligaments, etc. have confined terminations, often of the Ruffini type (Boyd, 1954; Skoglund, Chapter 4). Their static responses are typically well developed, consisting of trains of impulses at regular intervals; they have long recovery cycles and are activated when the tissue that contains them is stretched. Type I and other Merkel cell receptors emerge as unique (see below); no other mammalian mechanoreceptors, when subjected to a stationary stimulus, respond with an irregular discharge containing short intervals.

b) Receptors Detecting Velocity

The receptors included in this section have little or no position response and alter their discharge primarily as a function of stimulus velocity. They are derived from fibres that span the entire diameter range present in cutaneous nerves: Aa fibres, Aδ fibres and C fibres.

1. Velocity Detectors with Aα Fibres. Two main classes of velocity detectors are innervated by Aα fibres, "hair" and field receptors. Hair receptors are distinguished by a vigorous response to hair movement. Their response is appreciable if a single isolated hair shaft is displaced either at its tip or base. Afferent fibres giving rise to hair receptors branch to and around several follicles. Field receptor fibres also branch before terminating and each fibre supplies an area (field) of skin. Field receptors differ from hair receptors by not responding to movements of isolated hairs but some field receptors are excited when a number of hairs are moved together, particularly when the stimulator is applied near the base of the hairs. The latter activation is presumably secondary to skin distortion since direct contact with the cutaneous surface produces a markedly more vigorous response.

Hair receptors with Aα fibres were described in the earliest electrophysiological studies of mammalian hairy skin (ADRIAN, 1931) and have been observed since by most investigators who have recorded from cutaneous primary sensory neurons. Several studies in different species have provided evidence that different Aα hair units are not uniform in their response to hair movement (HUNT and McINTYRE, 1960c; BROWN and IGGO, 1967; BURGESS et al., 1968; PERL, 1968; MERZENICH and HARRINGTON, 1969; CREMERS, 1971). Differences have also been noted in the morphology of the hairs innervated by different afferent fibres (BROWN and IGGO, 1967). These morphological differences will be considered after the physiological properties of the receptors have been outlined. Field receptors were not distinguished until recently (BURGESS et al., 1968; PERL, 1968). In the cat, they are most numerous in the hairy skin that surrounds the foot and toe pads.

Physiological characteristics. Velocity detectors with Aα fibres differ from the position-velocity detectors in several ways: 1) They lack static displacement detection; 2) With constant velocity displacements, frequency versus displacement curves assume a horizontal orientation at relatively low discharge frequencies and are then displaced upward as velocity increases (see Fig. 3 and discussion above; LINDBLOM, 1962; BROWN and IGGO, 1967); 3) If a position response can be demonstrated it requires a larger amplitude displacement (by a factor of 10–20) than is needed to produce a comparable response from receptors of the position-velocity type. Velocity detecting receptors differ in the degree to which the position response is developed and a continuum of properties is found from receptors with a distinct but low frequency position response to receptors which respond only to relatively high velocity movements with no position discharge even to abrupt displacement. The velocity at which a receptor first begins to discharge as the rate of displacement is increased will be referred to as its *velocity threshold*. Since even velocity receptors with the best developed position responses lack static displacement detection, no impulses occur to low velocity movements. With progressively increasing stimulus velocity, a response will be obtained first from those velocity receptors with the largest slowly-adapting position responses. With further increases in velocity, the latter are converted to velocity detectors during the movement, although if the displacement is maintained, some discharge will continue after it terminates. The post-movement response becomes larger as velocity increases since with rapid displacements there is less time for adaptation to occur. With a movement lasting only a few msec it becomes difficult to distinguish between the velocity response and a subsequent position response. In general, position responses of cutaneous velocity detectors do not represent an appreciable fraction of their maximal dynamic range.

Hair receptors. Although there apparently is a continuous distribution of certain physiological properties among the Aa hair receptors (Table 2), they can be arbitrarily divided into categories with different features. The subcategories can be distinguished in several ways, including the degree to which the position response is developed, which in turn is related to velocity threshold. Some hair receptors respond to slow (less than 0.5 mm/sec) hair movement (called guard$_2$ or G_2 receptors), others require a more rapid displacement ("intermediate" hair receptors) and still others respond only if high velocity (greater than 20 mm/sec) stimuli are used (G_1 receptors). G_2, intermediate and G_1 hair receptors are derived from Aa fibres that increase progressively in average conduction velocity. G_1 receptors are classified in this article as transient detectors because of their high velocity or velocity derivative thresholds and will be discussed in the next section (C).

The distinction between G_2 and intermediate hair sensory units can be appreciated when both supply the same follicle. Moving the hair slowly away from the rest position and then releasing it excites the G_2 endings during the initial deviation and the intermediate endings during the rapid movement as the hair springs back. With rapid movements away from and back to the rest position the intermediate ending shows little linear directionality, a well-developed feature of G_2 endings. When the hair is moved rapidly and held displaced, G_2 receptors typically show a rapidly declining discharge for 1–2 sec after the hair becomes stationary. Little or no persistent discharge is recorded from intermediate receptors when stimulated in this fashion. Moving hairs of the receptive field in different directions, demonstrates a poorly developed spatial directionality in the G_2 population (Cremers, 1971) while little is seen for intermediate hair elements.

Impulses from the G_2 receptors are evenly spaced during a constant velocity stimulus (Fig. 3), implying a long and significant post-impulse depression of responsiveness. A detectable depression of G_2 responsiveness persists for at least 100 msec after a discharge; ten msec after a preceding impulse, thresholds are increased by 2 to $2^1/_2$ times the control value. Intermediate hair receptors, on the other hand, discharge in a less regular fashion and closely spaced impulses may occur when the rate of a constant velocity displacement exceeds threshold, suggesting a shorter recovery cycle than G_2 units; in fact, a decrease in responsiveness is not apparent after 30–50 msec. Brown and Iggo (1967) have shown that various hair receptors increase frequency of discharge with increasing stimulus velocity in a way that is well described by power functions with exponents of less than one.

Field receptors. Field receptors show a continuum of properties similar to hair receptors (Table 2). All field afferent fibres conduct at Aa velocities; the more rapidly conducting fibres have receptive terminals with little position response or linear directionality (F_1 field) and resemble intermediate hair receptors in velocity threshold and recovery cycle. Field receptors with more slowly conducting fibres (F_2) have some position response and linear directionality. Due to the latter, responses are evoked on deviations from the rest position (skin indentation) but not on return.

The position response of F_2 receptors is somewhat better developed than for G_2 endings and a low frequency discharge may persist for 10–15 sec after a sudden displacement. F_2 receptors have relatively long and large depressions of responsiveness after an impulse which is reflected by a tendency for the receptor to discharge in a regular fashion.

Morphological characteristics of Aa velocity detectors. There is no obvious difference in the receptive field organization of F_1 and F_2 field receptors. On the other hand, different hair follicles are reported to be specially innervated. The general body hair of the cat can be divided into three major but overlapping types (DANFORTH, 1925): (1) down, the most numerous hairs, are thin and flexible throughout their length and form the undercoat; (2) awn hairs, which are nearly as thin at the base as down hairs but thicken near the tip; (3) guard hairs, which are thicker than awn and down hairs at the base and expand still more toward the end of the shaft. Guard hairs differ somewhat in length and thickness but generally extend above the rest of the coat. A class of guard hairs, called tylotrich hairs, has been distinguished from other hairs of the guard type on the basis of their proximity to Type I domes and certain morphological features of the follicle (STRAILE, 1960; MANN and STRAILE, 1965) although they do not form a distinct group on the basis of diameter measurements made at a number of points from base to tip (BURGESS, HORCH and BURGESS, unpublished). Tylotrich follicles and hairs in the rabbit are more distinct than in the cat (STRAILE, 1960) but have not been distinguished in primates. BROWN and IGGO (1967) have described alpha hair receptors in the cat and rabbit associated exclusively with a limited number of tylotrich follicles (T hair receptors) and others that are activated predominantly by movement of a relatively large number of guard hairs other than tylotrichs (G hair receptors). Movement of down hairs is not effective in exciting Aa hair receptors nor is an appreciable response obtained from awn hairs (BROWN and IGGO, 1967; BURGESS et al., 1968; MERZENICH and HARRINGTON, 1969). The relation, if any, between the type of hair innervated and the physiological properties of the receptor is uncertain since receptors classed as G or T on morphological grounds have a range of physiological properties (BROWN and IGGO, 1967). There seems to be a tendency for receptors with higher velocity thresholds to be associated with longer and stiffer hairs (BROWN and IGGO, 1967; BURGESS et al., 1968). Some "matching" between mechanical properties of innervated hairs and the information signalled by the receptors might be expected but additional study is necessary to establish whether such a correlation exists.

Summary of Aa velocity detectors. In comparison to G_2 receptors the intermediate hair receptors show less linear directional characteristics, shorter recovery cycles, higher velocity thresholds, a less well developed position response and fibres that conduct more rapidly. F_1 and F_2 field receptors show a similar separation of properties. A low velocity stimulus excites receptors of the F_2 or G_2 types and higher rates of stimulation not only increase the discharge of such units but also recruit intermediate hair and F_1 endings. These facts suggest a tendency for a continuum between the Type II position detector on the one hand and the transient detector on the other, with the various Aa velocity detectors between.

2. *Velocity Detectors with Aδ Fibres.* Some Aδ units are hair receptors in the sense that they respond readily to movements of individual hairs (Zotterman, 1939; Hunt and McIntyre, 1960c). Recently it has been suggested that the terminals of these afferent fibres are not, in fact, associated with hair follicles (Merzenich, 1968) because there is little tendency for the lowest threshold points to be associated with hair follicles when the skin is mapped with a small stimulator, an association which can be demonstrated in the case of Aα hair receptors. Be that as it may, Aδ hair receptors are readily excited by movements of small groups of down or isolated guard hairs. The response to down hair movement earned them the label *D hair* receptors (Brown and Iggo, 1967) but this belies their ready excitation by guard hair movement; the term, however, is also appropriate as a label for their fibres' conduction velocities.

The properties of D hair units are quite uniform. They are more responsive to slow hair displacement than G_2 endings (Table 2) and the frequency of discharge increases with increasing velocity of hair displacement. Power functions with exponents less than one match the stimulus-discharge relationship closely (Brown and Iggo, 1967). As would be expected from their low velocity threshold, some position responsiveness occurs; it is more marked in primate than cat (Perl, 1968; Merzenich, 1968). In addition to differences in velocity threshold, fibre conduction velocity and excitation by down hair, D hair units differ from G_2 elements in their minimal linear and spatial directionality (Merzenich, 1968) possibly related to down hairs' lack of a fixed "rest" position. Thus the sensory information Aδ hair receptors provide may be less discriminative than other velocity receptors and they seem suited to detect, with great sensitivity, any hair movement.

3. *Velocity Detectors with C Fibres.* In 1939, Zotterman attributed certain responses produced in cat by gentle mechanical stimulation of the skin to receptors with C fibres (hereafter called C mechanoreceptors). Several subsequent studies (Douglas and Ritchie, 1957; Douglas, Ritchie and Straub, 1960; Iggo, 1960; Iggo and Kornhuber, 1968; Bessou, Burgess, Perl and Taylor, 1971) have established a number of their properties. Potentials from their fibres make up the bulk of the first C deflection elicited by electrical stimulation of cutaneous nerve (Douglas and Ritchie, 1957; Bessou et al., 1971).

C mechanoreceptors contrast markedly with myelinated fibre velocity detectors in lacking the ability to signal rapidly changing stimuli (Table 2). A stimulator must remain in contact with the skin for a surprisingly long time (150–200 msec at six times threshold) if a consistent response is to be obtained from them in comparison to minimal contact times of less than 3 msec for mechanoreceptors with myelinated fibres (Bessou et al., 1971). C mechanoreceptors fatigue readily (Iggo, 1960) and if any appreciable activity has occurred in the preceding minute, minimal contact times for a single impulse are increased beyond 500 msec (Bessou et al., 1971). Thus, when C mechanoreceptors are subjected to sinusoidal movements, frequencies in excess of 1–2 Hz evoke little activity. They, therefore, are unable to signal changes in a continuously varying displacement unless the changes are slow relative to the spectrum of mechanical events that animals respond to in natural surroundings.

C mechanoreceptors have a position response; if a displacement is abruptly applied and maintained, the discharge declines rapidly for 3–4 seconds with an occasional impulse occurring thereafter for 15–20 seconds. The C mechanoreceptor position response adapts in about the same time as the position discharge of an F_2 receptor after a comparable stimulus. As the rate of skin indentation is decreased, C mechanoreceptors do not show a decrease in peak discharge frequency until velocities are reached that are low relative to other mechanoreceptors. As might be expected from the long skin contact necessary to excite C mechanoreceptors, a stimulator that moves quickly across the receptive field evokes fewer impulses, at lower frequency, than one which moves more slowly, in contrast to field and other velocity detecting receptors with myelinated fibres. For this reason C mechanoreceptors indicate a range of changing mechanical stimuli that are not precisely signalled by velocity detectors with myelinated fibres.

IGGO and KORNHUBER (1968) and SASSEN and ZIMMERMANN (1971) have examined the input-output functions of C mechanoreceptors, measuring the first 1–2 seconds of activity produced by an abrupt stimulus. Since the velocity response of the receptor would be saturated under these conditions, changes in discharge frequency as a function of changes in stimulus amplitude would presumably represent an alteration in the position response. The frequency of discharge was found to be linearly related to indentation. C mechanoreceptors, however, transmit less quantitative information than mechanoreceptors with myelinated fibres, due in part to a smaller dynamic range. The diameter of an afferent fibre is related to the maximum frequency at which it can conduct impulses; larger Aa fibres can transmit impulses separated by 1 msec or less while Aδ fibres can conduct impulses 2 msec apart. In contrast, C fibres rarely convey impulses separated by less than 6–7 msec. Fluctuation of the response also limits information transmission. Even when fatigue is minimized by stimulating at intervals of 3 min or more, considerable variability and corresponding reduction of precision is the rule (ZIMMERMANN, 1972).

C mechanoreceptors have linear directionality; position and velocity responses occur during skin indentation but are weak or absent during the initial part of stimulator retraction. Sudden withdrawal of a deforming stimulus often gives rise to activity after contact with the skin ceases: i.e., after discharge (ZOTTERMAN 1939, DOUGLAS and RITCHIE, 1957; IGGO, 1960), a behavior not shown by mechanoreceptors with myelinated fibers. After discharge is especially prominent when a stimulator moves across the receptive field.

C mechanoreceptors make up about 50% of the unmyelinated fibre afferent spectrum in proximal nerves of the hindlimb of the cat. They are less common in distal nerves and have not been found with receptive fields in cat glabrous skin in spite of systematic search (BESSOU et al., 1971). The situation for primates is not as well understood. Low threshold C mechanoreceptors with some similar properties do exist in *Macaca mulatta*, but their frequency of occurrence seems less and they are rare in distally distributed nerves; as in cat, none have had receptive fields in glabrous areas (KUMAZAWA and PERL, unpublished). Moreover, while the velocity, absolute mechanical thresholds and afterdischarge are comparable for cat and primate units, certain differences exist (KUMAZAWA and PERL, unpublished). Cat C mechanoreceptors often show a considerable activity after sudden, marked (5–15°C) cooling, but are routinely unresponsive to heating, even to temperatures that sear the skin. Primate C mechanoreceptors are weakly excited by cooling and some give a response to noxious heat (skin surface temperatures of 55 to 70°C).

C mechanoreceptor recovery cycles cannot be measured in the usual way because of the long contact required for activation. Since their impulses tend to occur at evenly spaced intervals, arguments advanced above for other units suggest a considerable excitability depression after an impulse. Their terminals are confined to a small area which is comparatively uniform in sensitivity (Iggo, 1960). C mechanoreceptors do not respond to movements of isolated hairs, although a moderate response can be obtained if a number of hairs are moved simultaneously near their base, an activation probably secondary to skin deformation. Thus, other than size the receptive field organization resembles that of field units with myelinated fibres.

In summary, C mechanoreceptors are effective for detecting lingering mechanical stimuli. Best activation is produced by a slowly moving stimulator, rapidly changing stimuli are not sensed and the precise time of onset and cessation of a brief stimulus is obscured by a long minimal contact time and the presence of after discharge. The unmyelinated fibres that convey impulses from C mechanoreceptors to the central nervous system conduct so slowly that the input is greatly dispersed in time when it reaches central synapses where summation is presumably required for transmission. All these factors contribute to making them a part of a sensing system with slow responses.

c) Receptors Detecting Transients

Two basic receptor types are included in this category, Pacinian corpuscle receptors and G_1 hair receptors. G_1 receptors are found in the skin whereas Pacinian corpuscle (PC) endings are typically located in deeper tissues. Nevertheless, Pacinian units are easily excited from the skin surface (Hunt and McIntyre, 1960a; C.R. Skoglund, 1960; Lindblom and Lund, 1966; Merzenich and Harrington, 1969). Pacinian corpuscles have been found in a number of mammals, as well as in birds (C.R. Skoglund, 1960) and G_1 hair receptors have been described in cats (Hunt and McIntyre, 1960c; Brown and Iggo, 1967; Burgess et al., 1968; Cremers, 1971) and monkeys (Perl, 1968; Merzenich and Harrington, 1969). G_1 and PC receptors have characteristics in common (Table 2) but also differ in certain aspects.

1. *Pacinian Corpuscle Receptors.* Morphologically, Pacinian and the similar paciniform corpuscles are distinctive. The nerve terminal is surrounded by a multilamellated accessory structure of non-neural tissue. The accessory structure has mechanical filtering properties which effectively prevent slow displacements of the outer lamellae from deforming the nerve ending while transmitting abrupt displacements to them (Hubbard, 1958; Loewenstein and Mendelson, 1965; Ozeki and Sato, 1965). Thus, Pacinian or PC receptors display no position response even with rapidly applied stimuli, although at one time it was thought that they did (Adrian and Umrath, 1929).

PC units respond readily to vibrations transmitted from remote stimulus locations (C. R. SKOGLUND, 1960; HUNT and MCINTYRE, 1960a; LINDBLOM and LUND, 1966; MERZENICH and HARRINGTON, 1969; LYNN, 1971) and have been referred to as vibration receptors. In terms of the present classification, vibration is considered a repeated mechanical transient. PC receptors are difficult to excite even with large amplitude sinusoidal displacements at frequencies below 40–60 Hz but will respond to vibrations as small as 1 μ applied to the skin surface at frequencies of 150–400 Hz (HUNT, 1961; SATO, 1961; LINDBLOM and LUND, 1966; TALBOT, DARIAN-SMITH, KORNHUBER and MOUNTCASTLE, 1968; JÄNIG et al., 1968; NILSSON, 1969b; MERZENICH and HARRINGTON, 1969). At frequencies higher than 300–400 Hz, the displacement required to elicit a discharge is again increased. Thus the receptors are "tuned" to frequencies in the range of 150–300 Hz in the sense that at these frequencies, displacements of the smallest amplitude are effective for excitation. If the threshold displacement required for some form of response (e.g., one impulse per stimulus cycle) is determined as a function of stimulus frequency (a "tuning curve") the relationship suggests that above 100 Hz these receptors actually respond to a derivative of velocity, i.e. acceleration or jerk (ZIMMERMANN, personal communication). This concept is supported by the observation that Pacinian corpuscle endings discharge preferentially at the onset or termination of the constant velocity portions of a ramp movement; i.e., at those times when velocity is changing. Acceleration detection implies tuning to high frequencies since acceleration is greatest when position changes rapidly (see AUTRUM, 1941). The properties of the corpuscle and nerve ending are alone sufficient to endow the receptor with acceleration detection since tuning curves have the same general shape whether obtained by stimulating tissues remote from the corpuscle or by stimulating the corpuscle itself (SATO, 1961; MERZENICH, 1968). The mechanical characteristics of the corpuscle are presumably responsible, at least in part, for acceleration detection (see NISHI and SATO, 1968), but as discussed below, the rate of change of the generator potential must also reach a certain critical value.

Pacinian corpuscles lack linear directionality. If a stimulator is positioned to move at right angles to the skin, discharge occurs on indentation and retraction under similar stimulus conditions (ARMETT and HUNSPERGER, 1961; LYNN, 1971). A response of this type is also obtained when isolated corpuscles are stimulated directly (GRAY and MALCOLM, 1950; GRAY and SATO, 1953; ALVAREZ-BUYLLA and RAMIREZ DE ARELLANO, 1953). Fatigue is not prominent; the receptors have approximately the same tuning curve whether they respond for a few or many consecutive stimulus cycles (LINDBLOM and LUND, 1966; TALBOT et al., 1968). Recovery cycles are short; it is often difficult to detect any change in excitability at interstimulus intervals longer than 5–6 msec (GRAY and MALCOLM, 1950; LOEWENSTEIN and ALTAMIRANO-ORREGO, 1958; ARMETT and HUNSPERGER, 1961; OZEKI and SATO, 1964) and short interspike intervals are the rule for suprathreshold transients.

It is difficult to contrive a smoothly increasing stimulus that evokes more than 2 or 3 impulses from PC receptors. Even constant acceleration displacements only initiate an impulse or two, generally at the onset of movement when acceleration is greatest (HORCH, CORNWALL and BURGESS, unpublished). Pacinian corpuscles are known to accommodate rapidly; i.e., even though the generator potential is maintained at a high value, the threshold for impulse initiation increases so rapidly that only a few impulses can be produced (GRAY and MATT-HEWS, 1951; LOEWENSTEIN, 1958; LOEWENSTEIN and MENDELSON, 1965; OZEKI and SATO, 1965). Therefore, as in other receptors with short recovery cycles, the PC generator potential is suprathreshold for short periods only.

Pacinian corpuscles have a particular cluster of properties: high frequency tuning or transient detection, a lack of linear or spatial directionality, short recovery cycles, and little fatigue. Due to a short recovery cycle and absence of fatigue, corpuscles are unhindered in responding repeatedly at short intervals to the higher frequency components (rapid changes) of a stimulus. These characteristics are in striking contrast to Type II units in which prolonged depression of excitability after an impulse regulates the discharge.

Afferent fibres from Pacinian corpuscles fall into the upper half of the $A\alpha$ range. Most of the PC fibres innervating the hindlimb have a central branch which extends the length of the spinal cord to synapse with cells of the nucleus gracilis in the medulla (PERL, WHITLOCK and GENTRY, 1962; PERL, 1964; PETIT and BURGESS, 1968). Although other hindlimb cutaneous mechanoreceptor fibres reach the medulla (see PETIT and BURGESS, 1968; BROWN, 1968), Pacinian fibres are distinctive in that there is no decrease in the conduction velocity after entrance into the central nervous system (WHITEHORN, CORNWALL and BURGESS, unpublished). For this reason, synchronous activity in a population of PC fibres will show little temporal dispersion, favoring a high signal to noise ratio when summation is required for synaptic transmission and information with high temporal resolution is to be transmitted.

2. G_1 *Hair Receptors.* Like PC receptors, G_1 hair receptors are tuned to high frequencies and require rapid hair displacement for activation. Even large amplitude sinusoidal displacements do not produce a discharge at frequencies below 60–80 Hz. Although threshold amplitude declines as stimulus frequency increases from 80–200 Hz, small amplitude sinusoidal oscillations (less than 50 μ) applied to either skin or hair do not evoke responses at any frequency. In this respect they differ from PC receptors in that the shape of their tuning curves are consistent with response to high velocity and do not imply acceleration or jerk detection. In addition, G_1 receptors fatigue, showing increasing threshold amplitude on frequently repeated activation. As a consequence of these several properties, G_1 receptors do not respond to transients propagating from distant regions and are effectively activated only by the larger amplitude movements of stiff hair shafts (see above).

G_1 hair receptors resemble Pacinian receptors in showing little linear or spatial directionality (Table 2). Recovery cycles are also short; there is little decrease in G_1 excitability after 10 msec. It can be argued, as in the case of PC receptors, that short recovery cycles are appropriate for transient detectors to respond with multiple discharges to a single event because the rapidity of the required displacement makes the stimulus duration short. Even so, G_1 receptors rarely produce more than 2–3 impulses to high velocity, large hair movements.

G_1 endings are well adapted to signal rapid displacements with high temporal resolution and resemble PC receptors in high frequency tuning, little directional

Table 2. *Properties of cutaneous mechanoreceptors*

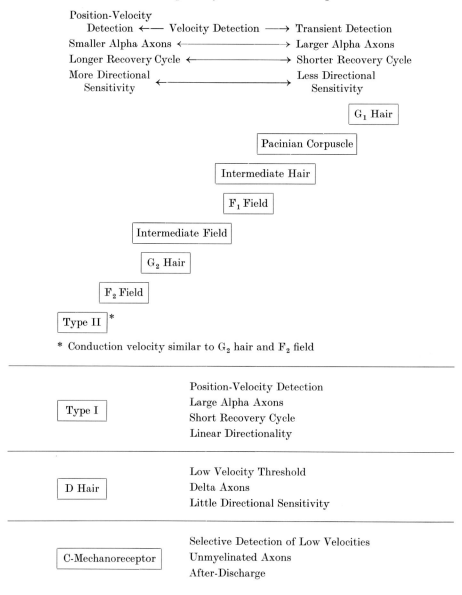

Position-Velocity
Detection ←— Velocity Detection —→ Transient Detection
Smaller Alpha Axons ←————————————→ Larger Alpha Axons
Longer Recovery Cycle ←————————————→ Shorter Recovery Cycle
More Directional ←————————————→ Less Directional
Sensitivity   Sensitivity

G₁ Hair

Pacinian Corpuscle

Intermediate Hair

F₁ Field

Intermediate Field

G₂ Hair

F₂ Field

Type II *

* Conduction velocity similar to G_2 hair and F_2 field

Type I
Position-Velocity Detection
Large Alpha Axons
Short Recovery Cycle
Linear Directionality

D Hair
Low Velocity Threshold
Delta Axons
Little Directional Sensitivity

C-Mechanoreceptor
Selective Detection of Low Velocities
Unmyelinated Axons
After-Discharge

sensitivity, a short recovery cycle, and rapidly conducting axons. They differ from PC receptors by responding to velocity rather than acceleration, and by not detecting low amplitude displacements of the innervated area.

3. Mechanoreceptors in Glabrous Skin

Receptor types present in glabrous skin are most conveniently considered according to species because of substantial differences in glabrous skin and the absence of comparative information on similar elements in different animals.

a) Cat

Receptors with F_1 and F_2 properties are common in the glabrous skin of the cat's foot and toe pads (JÄNIG et al., 1968; LYNN, 1969; JÄNIG, 1971; PETIT, CORNWALL, HORCH and BURGESS, unpublished). There are, of course, no hair receptors. Low threshold receptors derived from delta fibres are present but are relatively less common than D hair receptors in the adjacent hairy skin. C mechanoreceptors appear to be entirely absent from the glabrous skin of the cat's foot (BESSOU et al., 1971). Type II receptors are rarely found and pad position is signalled almost exclusively by receptors which discharge with an irregular pattern similar to that of Type I units of hairy skin. Domes are not visible on the pad but collections of Merkel cells are present at the junction of the epithelium and dermis; JÄNIG (1971) has provided evidence that an irregular position detecting discharge originates from endings associated with these cells. In addition to discharge pattern, position units in pad skin resemble Type I receptors in their recovery cycle, adaptation rate, dynamic range of the position response, linear directionality of position and velocity responses, and the conduction velocity of their afferent fibres. The central projection pattern from the hindlimb is identical to that of Type I units from hairy skin; an ascending collateral extends in the dorsal columns to upper lumbar or lower thoracic levels but not to upper cervical levels (WHITEHORN, CORNWALL and BURGESS, 1971). Thus it appears appropriate to refer to these receptors as Type I pad receptors.

b) Raccoon

Two populations of receptors have been described in the glabrous skin of the raccoon snout and palm (BARKER and WELKER, 1969; BARKER, HAZELTON and WELKER, 1970; PUBOLS, PUBOLS and MUNGER, 1971; MUNGER, PUBOLS and PUBOLS, 1971). One responds to an abrupt displacement with a weak position response that adapts within a few seconds and is similar to F_2 receptors of hairy skin. If ramp displacements of constant velocity are applied, the impulses tend to be either uniformly spaced along the ramp or to occur with higher frequency as displacement increases. PUBOLS et al. (1971) report that such units have discharge frequency versus displacement functions which are horizontal over a considerable range of stimulus velocities. The second type of receptor has little or no position response and a tendency to give the highest frequency discharge just after the onset of a constant velocity displacement. The latter type detects velocity since the response occurs during a constant velocity displacement, but the velocity response apparently adapts and therefore will be influenced by the derivative of rate (acceleration); in addition specific acceleration detection properties may be present. Relatively pure acceleration or jerk receptors such as the Pacinian corpuscles, on the other hand, have little capacity to signal velocity since they tend to respond at the onset and termination of a ramp displacement rather than during the constant velocity portion. The raccoon receptors also differ from the

Pacinian type in that the former produce fairly uniformly spaced impulses during displacements of constant velocity or acceleration whereas smoothly increasing stimuli do not generate a stream of impulses from PC receptors. Moreover, the raccoon receptors do not respond readily to vibrations transmitted from remote stimulus locations. Both raccoon sensory units noted by PUBOLS et al. (1971) yielded an increase of impulse frequency approximated by a power function of stimulus velocity with an exponent of less than one.

MUNGER et al. (1971) suggested that the receptors with a weak position response were associated with Merkel cells in the raccoon palm. The properties of these receptors differ in two major respects from those JÄNIG (1971) related to Merkel cells in the pad skin of the cat: 1) The raccoon receptor shows no static displacement detection and the position response adapts rapidly relative to cat units. 2) The discharge of the raccoon receptor is comparatively regular. Thus, the raccoon receptor has F_2 field receptor properties rather than the sustained irregular position response characteristic of Merkel type endings in the hairy skin of the cat, rabbit and primate and the glabrous skin of the cat. If the morphological correlation of MUNGER et al. (1971) is correct, Merkel cell receptors do not have uniform physiological properties.

c) Primates

The receptors in the glabrous skin of the primate hand and foot are similar to those in the foot and toe pads of cats. Merkel cells are common in primate glabrous skin and by analogy to the cat might be expected to contribute to a static displacement response with irregular discharge i.e., Type I. Such activity has been recorded from the monkey palm (IGGO, personal communication) and from the human hand (KNIBESTÖL and VALLBO, 1970). Receptors with Type II properties have also been observed (IGGO, 1963; PERL, 1968; TALBOT et al., 1968), although they are apparently less common than those with Type I properties (KNIBESTÖL and VALLBO, 1970; IGGO, personal communication). It might be predicted that an ending of the Ruffini type would be responsible for Type II activity since that presumptive correlation has been made for hairy skin. Receptors with F_1 and F_2 field properties are present in monkeys (LINDBLOM, 1965; TALBOT et al., 1968) and in man (HAGBARTH, HONGELL, HALLIN and TOREBJÖRK, 1970; KNIBESTÖL and VALLBO, 1970). Meissner corpuscles are plentiful in primate glabrous skin and could give rise to F_1 and F_2 type discharge. Encapsulated endings similar to Meissner corpuscles are found in comparable locations in cat glabrous skin (MALINOVSKÝ, 1966); JÄNIG (1971) has associated these with F_1 and F_2 types of activity.

4. Mechanoreceptors Associated with Sinus Hairs

Many mammals have specialized tactile hairs such as vibrissae. They are generally the longest and thickest hairs on the body and originate from follicles that have a number of distinctive morphological features, including a blood sinus that envelops the external root sheath and gives them the name sinus hairs. In the cat, they are found not only around the nose and mouth but also just above the wrist on the volar aspect of the forelimb (carpal hairs). Vibrissae and carpal hairs are structurally similar and have generally similar receptor complements. Individual position-velocity and velocity neurons are each activated from only one sinus hair regardless of location.

a) Receptors Detecting both Position and Velocity

Sinus hairs are associated with receptors having static displacement detection (Fitzgerald, 1940; Kerr and Lysak, 1964; Nilsson and Skoglund, 1965; Iggo, 1968; Nilsson, 1969a; Zucker and Welker, 1969) in contrast to sensory units of the general body hair which show little position response. Sinus hair shafts are thick over much of their length and displacement of the shaft will be more precisely transmitted to the follicle and nerve endings than for the more flexible hairs of the general body surface. In addition to the vibrissae and carpal hairs proper, there are other instances in which static displacement detectors are associated with relatively stiff hairs. Some of the short, sturdy hairs around the lip and snout in the cat and dog have receptors of this type (Kerr and Lysak, 1964; Iggo, 1968) as do some of the thick hairs on the back of the fingers in monkeys (Merzenich and Harrington, 1969).

If the rate of sinus hair displacement is progressively increased, plots of frequency versus displacement move upwards in a fashion typical of receptors detecting both position and velocity (Nilsson, 1969a). The velocity input-output relationship for these sinus hair units can be approximated by power functions with exponents between 0.3 and 1.1 (Nilsson, 1969a). As is often the case, the position response is more nearly linear; the receptor discharge as a function of displacement can be described by power functions with exponents between 0.6 and 1.5 (Nilsson, 1969a). The dynamic range of the velocity response is greater than that of the position response and in the ratio of position to velocity activity, the tested receptors resemble Type II units of hairy skin.

Spatial directionality is characteristic of sinus hair receptors with static displacement detection (Fitzgerald, 1940; Kerr and Lysak, 1964; Nilsson, 1969a; Zucker and Welker, 1969). Different receptors vary in the size of the angle of displacement necessary for activation, but a common pattern is for a response to appear when the hair is displaced from the rest position in one quadrant of a circle but not in others. Nilsson (1969a) illustrates both regular and irregular activity from cat sinus position receptors. Gottschaldt, Iggo and Young (1972) noted a similar difference in discharge pattern among sinus receptors and suggested that the irregular discharge is associated with the Merkel cell units known to be present in the external root sheath of sinus hairs; they found that the receptors with an irregular firing pattern had little resting discharge and pronounced spatial directionality. Those receptors with regular activity had less spatial directionality, a better developed position response and resting discharge that could be as high as 20/sec.

The velocity response of sinus hair position receptors is obtained only during movements away from the rest position. Linear directionality of the position response is dependent upon the rate of the return movement. Typical of cutaneous receptors responsive to position and velocity, activity during return to the rest position is inversely related to the rate of return (NILSSON, 1969a; ZUCKER and WELKER, 1969).

b) Receptors Detecting Velocity

Sinus hair receptors detecting velocity have properties that resemble those of velocity detectors in other tissues. A series of impulses are produced as the hair is displaced from the rest position, as long as the rate of movement exceeds a threshold value. These receptors show little spatial directionality and while some velocity response may be obtained if the hair returns to the rest position rapidly enough, linear directionality can be demonstrated (ZUCKER and WELKER, 1969; NILSSON, 1969a).

c) Receptors Detecting Rapid Mechanical Transients

Clusters of Pacinian corpuscles are found near carpal hairs, and in the cat, they respond without linear or spatial directionality (NILSSON, 1969b). Movement of any carpal hair in the group will excite a particular Pacinian corpuscle because of the great sensitivity of these receptors to transmitted vibrations. PC receptors are not found in association with vibrissae, although endings surrounded by a few lamellae are present in the follicle (ANDRES, 1966). A vibrissae receptor with the brief discharge and high frequency tuning characteristic of a transient detector has been described in the rat by ZUCKER and WELKER (1969) and in cats by GOTTSCHALDT et al. (1972). Linear and spatial directionality are apparently absent. A single vibrissae transient detector is excited by movement of one hair only, which is consistent with the idea that they are not typical PC endings.

5. Comments

a) Position Detection

The receptors found in association with sinus hairs possess the same specializations as do static displacement detectors in other locations. It seems to be a principle that relatively sturdy body projections such as sinus hairs, claws and teeth are associated with static position receptors. In the most general sense, the appendages of an animal may be considered projections from the axial frame and each articulation of the appendage may be considered the base of another projecting part. Claws are rigidly attached to the terminal phalangeal joint in the cat and, thus, receptors that sense claw position are in fact articular receptors. Certain common features are evident in the design of those receptive units that signal the static position of projecting structures. There is minimal sustained activity when the innervated structure is in the rest position. In the case of teeth and most sinus hairs, the rest position of the structure is at or near the mid-position. Most articulations also occupy an intermediate position at rest. Thus, when a joint or tooth is displaced in one direction, particular receptors begin to discharge, or increase their discharge if already active, and this discharge is graded with displacement. Return of the structure to the mid-position and displacement in the opposite direction, evokes progressively increasing activity in a different population of receptors. This organization might be termed an opponent system in contrast to one with receptors exhibiting maximal activity at one extreme, intermediate activity at intermediate positions and minimal activity at the opposite extreme. Greater numbers of receptors are required to establish opponent populations than would apparently be needed if individual receptors responded over the whole range of movement, but activity at intermediate positions is minimal in the first case and would be appreciable with full range receptors. Many factors may have dictated the evolution of opponent rather than full range receptors, some are possibly dependent on the way in which the stimulus can be transmitted to the sensory nerve endings while others may reflect the value of a minimal level of ongoing activity in the neutral (rest) state for subsequent central processing.

In contrast to a special sense organ like the cochlea, spatial tuning does not emerge in the receptors of appendages. It is possible that a particular slowly-adapting receptor could show maximal activity at some intermediate or partially offset position with a decline in discharge occurring as the projecting structure is moved to either side of this position, a situation analogous to some cochlear nerve units which apparently give a maximal response to sound activating a particular part of the basilar membrane with lesser responses to activation of adjacent regions. A population of receptors tuned to different positions could specify the position of the structure. Receptors of this type have not been reported from sinus hairs, teeth or claws. A few have been described in association with the knee joint, but they must be comparatively rare (S. Skoglund, 1956; Burgess and Clark, 1969). Rather, the somatic position receptors display an end position "bias": they progressively increase discharge as the structure they innervate is moved from an intermediate to its end or maximally displaced position.

b) General

The classification proposed assumes that mechanoreceptors are specialized to detect different modes of mechanical stimulation and may be considered an outgrowth of the concept of receptor specificity. Support for the classification comes from the fact that some receptor characteristics are distributed in a way that is systematically correlated with the mode or modes of mechanical stimulation occurring in nature. However, Type I and D hair receptors have properties which do not contribute in an obvious way to an indication of features of the effective mode of stimulation (Table 2). Ultimately, the usefulness of the scheme proposed here will be determined by the generality with which it can be applied.

One consequence of treating mechanoreceptors as specifically designed to respond to certain modes of mechanical stimulation is that the term *adaptation* takes on a new meaning. As originally used (Adrian and Zotterman, 1926), slowly adapting receptors were those with static displacement detection and rapidly adapting receptors were those with little or no position response. In the context of the present classification, adaptation is considered to occur if the discharge of a receptor declines while the mode of mechanical stimulation it detects is held constant. Thus, a receptor that detects velocity would show no adaptation by this criterion if the discharge did not decline during constant velocity stimulation, whereas it might be considered rapidly adapting according to original usage. As more investigators have begun to treat receptors in terms of sensitivity to particular aspects of mechanical stimulation, adaptation as a descriptive term has been less used. The terms "dynamic" and "static" have been applied to muscle spindles (see P. B. C. MATTHEWS, 1964). LINDBLOM's important studies (1962, 1963) on frog skin mechanoreceptors clearly embody the concept of velocity and position sensitivity as distinct aspects of a receptor's response to mechanical stimulation. BROWN and IGGO (1967), IGGO and MUIR (1969), BARKER, HAZELTON and WELKER (1970), and CHAMBERS et al. (1972) have also taken this approach. ZIMMERMANN (personal communication) has explicity proposed that the mechanoreceptors of the cat's glabrous pad skin be treated in terms of position, velocity and acceleration detection.

Further insight on this proposed classification of mechanoreceptive neurons will await knowledge of how their central fibres are organized after entrance into the central nervous system. Support for it would be provided should the information specifically encoded by peripheral terminals be utilized by central systems in a fashion making appropriate use of the information.

C. Cutaneous Nociceptors

1. Criteria for Nociceptors

Noxious and its Latin parent *noxius* mean hurtful, harmful or damaging. An early use of this term for stimuli appeared in SHERRINGTON's attempt (1906) to formulate a common ground between the sensory experience that man calls pain and animal experimentation on related phenomena. Turning to everyday observation, he commented that cutaneous pain could readily be elicited by stimuli of quite different characteristics, mechanical, thermal and electrical. In spite of this, he noted that "excitants of skin pain, have all a certain character in common, namely this, that they become *adequate* as excitants of pain when they are of such intensity as threatens damage to the skin."

Classification of a given primary afferent unit as a nociceptor by some authors has presumed that they should respond only when the skin is damaged. While such receptors do exist, it is clear that a broader view must be taken. For animals to adapt and survive in the face of a hostile environment, cutaneous receptors, to serve well the function of nociception, must warn of events that *threaten* cutaneous integrity without overt damage. Only in this circumstance can an organism react to avoid injury. Psychophysical experiments long ago demonstrated that non-damaging mechanical stimulation to certain spots on the skin could elicit a pricking, unpleasant sensation while at other spots the same stimulation would evoke simply a tactile sensation (VON FREY, 1894). These considerations suggest that rather than relying upon excitation exclusively by skin damage as the criterion for a nociceptor, another feature need be weighed, namely, the ability of the sensory unit effectively and reliably to distinguish between noxious and innocuous events in the signals it provides to the central nervous system.

Before it can be securely argued that nociceptors are a separate and distinctive class of primary afferent units, different from the mechanoreceptors discussed above and the thermoreceptors treated in Chapter 3, it is necessary to consider the response of various cutaneous receptors to stimuli graded from the innocuous to the noxious level. In addition, many of the standards used in the classification of mechanoreceptors need be applied to determine whether nociception represents an extension of the functional attributes of mechanoreceptors and thermoreceptors.

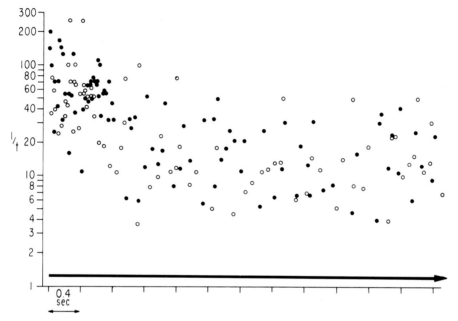

Fig. 5. Discharge pattern evoked by innocuous but firm pressure (filled circles) and noxious pressure (open circles) from a receptor in primate glabrous skin. (From Perl, 1968)

a) Response of Mechanoreceptors and Thermoreceptors to Noxious Stimuli

The bulk of the sensory units in a mammalian cutaneous nerve are mechanoreceptors (Brown and Iggo, 1967; Burgess, Petit and Warren, 1968; Perl, 1968; Bessou, Burgess, Perl and Taylor, 1971). A relatively small percentage, all with slowly-conducting afferent fibres, respond vigorously to small temperature changes. These thermoreceptors (see Chapter 3) respond weakly to all but noxious mechanical stimuli which in turn tend to inactivate them for subsequent thermal or mechanical stimuli. Mechanoreceptors and thermoreceptors may be considered low-threshold sensory units, since they are excited by quite small stimuli of the appropriate type, stimuli that are at or below the threshold for man's perception or behavioral evidence of an animal's recognition.

Experiments testing the effects of stimuli graded from near threshold for any cutaneous sensory unit through the overtly damaging level have demonstrated that individual low threshold receptors do not provide signals reliably differentiating noxious from innocuous stimuli (PERL, 1968; BESSOU and PERL, 1969; BESSOU et al., 1971). Given two mechanical stimulators, such as a small probe with a rounded edge several mm² in area and one formed to a sharp point, clear differences exist in the responses they evoke with submaximal stimuli. For a variety of mechanoreceptors, including hair, field, and Type I and Type II contact receptors, a particular displacement of the skin surface with fixed dynamic features caused by the pointed probe usually evokes a greater response (i.e., higher frequency and/or more impulses) than the same displacement with the blunt probe. Stated in general terms low threshold mechanoreceptors ordinarily respond more vigorously, at submaximal intensities, to a sharply pointed than to a blunt stimulator. On the other hand, any response *pattern* elicited from a particular receptor by a noxious stimulus with a sharp probe, including those producing skin damage, can be readily mimicked by an innocuous stimulus with particular velocity and position properties from a blunt probe.

An example of a comparison between responses to innocuous and to noxious stimuli is shown in Fig. 5 for a receptor of the Type I class from monkey glabrous skin. The filled circles show the pattern of activity produced by moderate pressure across the fold of skin containing the unit's receptive field; this was an innocuous stimulus as judged by the absence of residual effects and by the lack of discomfort when similarly applied to human skin. Subsequently, a device of similar shape, but exerting much greater pressure, was applied to the same skin area. The latter left evidence of enduring disturbance of the skin's structure and was quite painful when applied to the skin of a man's hand; no systematic difference in the discharge pattern for these two stimuli is apparent in Fig. 5. Tests using a variety of stimuli bridging the noxious range repeatedly gave similar results for all known forms of low threshold mechanoreceptors in evaluations that considered maximal frequency, the duration of activity to stimuli of varying time course and the existence of special patterns of discharge.

Inasmuch as sensory units with slowly conducting afferent fibres (0.3 to 30 m/sec) have long been known to have some special part in the production of pain (HEINBECKER, BISHOP and O'LEARY, 1933; ZOTTERMAN, 1933; CLARK, HUGHES and GASSER, 1935; LEWIS, 1942; COLLINS, NULSEN and RANDT, 1960), comparison of responses to innocuous relative to noxious stimulation were particularly important for sensory units with unmyelinated fibres. Fig. 6 A and B show the discharge of a C fibre mechanoreceptor when a disc of some 2 mm diameter was pressed against the receptive field by an electromagnetic device. The same velocity and deflection of a sharp probe making contact with the centre of the field evoked the responses illustrated by Fig. 6 A′ and B′. The average response to the moderate innocuous stimuli and the damaging stimuli are indistinguishable. These examples serve to emphasize the inability of individual mechanoreceptors to provide appropriate information for distinguishing noxious from innocuous mechanical stimuli.

The situation for the low-threshold thermoreceptors is somewhat less clear. Thermoreceptors generally have very high thresholds for mechanical stimuli, although an intense mechanical stimulus may evoke an appreciable transient response which is then followed by inactivation of the receptor. On the other hand, many cold receptors show reproducible activity to noxious heat stimuli; a response labeled "paradoxical" (Dodt and Zotterman, 1952). Warm thermoreceptors also may show marked activity to noxious heat; in some instances, the discharge frequency may be as high to mildly noxious heat 45–47° C as for innocuous levels of warming (Hensel and Huopaniemi, 1969; Kumazawa and Perl, unpublished). The importance of thermoreceptor responses to high temperatures

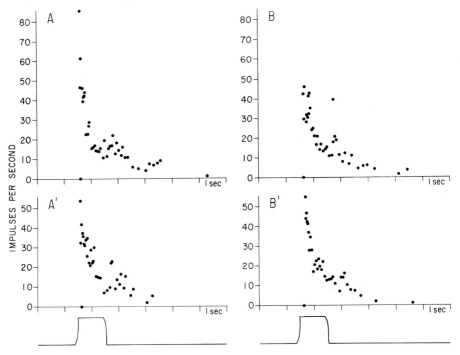

Fig. 6. Responses evoked from a C mechanoreceptor by innocuous (*A* and *B*) and noxious (*A'* and *B'*) mechanical stimuli. The stimulus time and form are shown in the lowermost traces; velocity and displacement were identical for all tests. *A* (*A'*) and *B* (*B'*) were first and third of a series at 100 sec intervals. A blunt probe was used for *A* and *B* and a needle tip contacting the center of the same area for *A'* and *B'*. (From Bessou et al., 1971)

is not clear, although it does seem that they do not uniquely indicate noxious stimuli since the same unit's response to innocuous temperature stimuli mimic those to noxious ones.

b) High Threshold Receptors and Noxious Stimuli

In contrast to the poor differentiation between innocuous and noxious stimuli provided by the signals from low threshold mechanoreceptors and thermoreceptors, several types of receptive units provide unequivocal information about the presence of noxious stimuli. An example is shown in Fig. 7 from a sensory unit of primate glabrous skin; this element did not respond to pressures exceeding 100 gm with a blunt probe (Fig. 7A), but was excited by pressure with a sharp probe

(Fig. 7 B), and gave a still more vigorous response to forcible pinching of the receptive field with a sharp-toothed tissue forceps (Fig. 7 C).

Cutaneous sensory elements with elevated thresholds in comparison to other receptors, or with special responses to noxious stimuli were first reported early in the history of electrophysiology on the basis of multiunit recordings from fine peripheral nerves (ADRIAN, 1931; ZOTTERMAN, 1933, 1936). The activity of one fibre as opposed to another was difficult to discern in such recordings so that

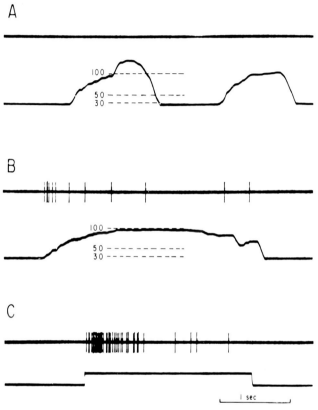

Fig. 7. Responses (upper trace) of a mechanical nociceptor with a myelinated afferent fibre to graded mechanical stimuli. Lower trace in *A* and *B* shows output of calibrated probe in grams; *A* – blunt tip of 2 mm, *B* – needle tip, *C* – pinch to receptive field with a serrated forceps. (From PERL, 1968)

characteristics of individual units could not be determined. This point became particularly important when it was learned that some fibres of similar small diameter stemmed from receptors responding to innocuous mechanical stimuli (ZOTTERMAN, 1939). Study of cutaneous sensory elements one by one led to better evidence for elements with elevated thresholds for all stimuli (MARUHASHI, MIZUGUCHI and TASAKI, 1952; DODT, 1954). With emergence of techniques for recording from single fibres of the slowest conduction (C or non-myelinated), several reports suggested that receptors with generally elevated thresholds could have different features (Iggo, 1959, 1960; Iriuchijima and Zotterman, 1960; Witt, 1962). Surveys of the functional characteristics of relatively large numbers of sensory units in both cat and monkey have confirmed the existence of several types of cutaneous sensory units which meet requirements for specific nociceptive function (Burgess and Perl, 1967; Perl, 1968; Bessou and Perl, 1969; Kumazawa and Perl, unpublished).

2. Classification of Nociceptors

The present evidence is consistent with two major types of cutaneous nociceptors.

a) Mechanical Nociceptors

Certain cutaneous receptors respond only to strong mechanical stimuli and are excited weakly, if at all, by any form of thermal stimuli including those destroying the skin. They are also unresponsive to irritant chemicals. A prominent group have myelinated afferent fibres conducting between 5 and 50 m/sec with mean values of 15 to 25 m/sec ($A\delta$). They have been found in both carnivore and primate and their receptive fields include hairy and glabrous skin (Hunt and McIntyre, 1960c; Burgess and Perl, 1967; Perl, 1968). Their fibres make up approximately 20 % of the $A\delta$ group. The threshold of these elements is greatly elevated (5 to 1000 X) for any mechanical stimulus in comparison to the mechanoreceptors described in the previous section. Some units of this type give weak (threshold) or moderate responses to non-damaging stimuli while others are not excited unless stimuli are well above the level necessary for overt damage. All, however, progressively increase their discharge as mechanical stimuli are graded from near damaging to overtly damaging. Their receptive fields consist of 3 to 20 spots (<1 mm^2) scattered over 1 to 8 cm^2 from which responses can be evoked, separated by skin areas where equivalent stimuli are ineffective. Each responsive spot associated with a given afferent fibre has a similar but not identical threshold. Repeated stimulation of a given spot causes fatigue and inactivation while the excitability of other spots remains unchanged. In spite of the range of threshold and afferent fibre conduction velocities for these units, their unique receptive field structure suggests that they represent variations of one basic receptor type. As a group such elements respond with somewhat irregularly spaced discharges and are best classified as velocity and position detectors with some systematic grading of characteristics according to threshold. The highest threshold units of this type are activated only by moving stimuli and show no after-discharge; consequently they are rapidly adapting to position even when the stimulus consists of a sharp object penetrating the skin. At the other end of the distribution, the most responsive mechanical nociceptors, while retaining velocity sensitivity, continue to respond after a stimulator stops moving, presenting both velocity and position detecting properties. There is a rough tendency for conduction velocity to be inversely related to threshold; the highest threshold units have fibres with the lowest conduction velocity. The central terminations of mechanical nociceptors with myelinated fibres also seem to be distributed differently according to conduction velocity; those with the lowest conduction velocity terminate within a segment or two after entering the spinal cord whereas the more rapidly conducting fibres with lower threshold terminals run rostrally in the dorsal columns for several segments (BURGESS and WHITEHORN, unpublished).

Mechanical nociceptors with unmyelinated (C) fibres have been reported in cutaneous nerves (IGGO, 1960; BESSOU and PERL, 1969). The least uncertainty is attached to a type with terminals in the subcutaneous fatty tissue (BESSOU and PERL, 1969); these respond to strong mechanical stimuli that produce distorting pressure to the subcutaneous tissue with a slowly adapting, regular discharge of relatively low frequency (1–15/sec). Because of their protected subcutaneous position, dynamic characteristics are difficult to judge; however, they have position detection properties in view of their persisting discharge. As long as the skin remains unbroken, this type is unaffected by skin temperature (from 0 to 60°C) and by irritant chemicals. If the skin is broken, allowing penetration of chemicals placed on the surface, a variety of substances such as strong acids, hypertonic salt solutions, acetylcholine and bradykinin may initiate long-lasting discharges (BESSOU and PERL, 1969; BURGESS and PERL, unpublished). It is possible though far from proven that this category of nociceptors represents a type that is widely distributed in subcutaneous tissue.

One group of C fibre receptors are reported to be excited by very intense mechanical stimuli to give small responses consisting of a few impulses (1–5) from receptive fields of 2–5 mm². Adequate thermal stimuli for nociceptor evaluation (skin freezing and surface temperatures over 70°C) were not routinely used as tests in initial observations of these units (IGGO, 1960; BESSOU and PERL, 1969) raising the possibility that responses to grossly insulting thermal events were missed. More recent work has uncovered essentially similar units that also respond to very low cutaneous temperatures (BESSOU and PERL, 1969; BURGESS and PERL, unpublished); all of this group may represent inadequately defined mechanical-cold units.

b) Mechanical and Thermal Nociceptors

Three categories of sensory units respond as nociceptors to both thermal and mechanical stimuli. One group, the polymodal nociceptors, will be treated separately below because of several special features.

In the primate, receptors with fine myelinated fibres conducting between 4 and 10 m/sec are excited to persistent activity by noxious heat (over 45°C) and damaging mechanical stimuli (IGGO and OGAWA, 1971; PERL, unpublished). Noxious heat evokes a discharge that adapts slowly to a given temperature and consistently evokes more impulses than any mechanical stimulus. Cold, including freezing, is weakly effective. Receptive fields are small (2–3 mm²).

In both cats and monkeys C fibre receptors have been found that respond to noxious cold and to strong mechanical stimuli (IGGO, 1959; IRIUCHIJIMA and ZOTTERMAN, 1960; BURGESS and PERL, unpublished; KUMAZAWA and PERL, unpublished). The terminals seem to be more deeply located than the mechanical nociceptors with myelinated fibres or the polymodal nociceptors (see below). Mechanical thresholds are very high, a response usually requiring penetration of the skin with a sharp object. Repeated mechanical stimuli usually inactivate the unit for some time. Stimuli cooling the skin to below 15°C evoke a low frequency (1–5/sec) discharge. In some units the response adapts to maintained cold while in others a persisting discharge is generated. Receptive fields consist of oval areas of 2–8 mm² longitudinally distributed along the axis of a limb and frequently along the course of a subcutaneous vein.

   1. Polymodal Nociceptors. A large fraction of cutaneous unmyelinated fibre afferent units have elevated but not extreme thresholds for mechanical stimuli, promptly respond to noxious heat and usually are excited by irritant chemicals applied to the skin. They differ from mechanical and heat responsive nociceptors with myelinated fibres in being activated as effectively by strong mechanical as they are by thermal stimuli. They have been found in both cat and monkey and represent from 40 to over 90 % of randomly sampled C fibre afferent units (Bessou and Perl, 1969; Bessou, Burgess, Perl and Taylor, 1971; Kumazawa and Perl, unpublished). Nerves supplying distal portions of the limb seem to contain relatively high proportions of such units, probably because of the paucity of low threshold C mechanoreceptors. Conduction velocities of polymodal units are among the slowest of all sensory units. Receptors of this category probably made up the heat sensitive C fibre receptors described by Iggo (1959), Iriuchijima and Zotterman (1960) and Witt (1962).

   Polymodal nociceptors usually have a receptive field consisting of one area of 1–2 mm² although units in both cat and monkey have been found with two such fields separated by over 10 mm of tissue from which responses cannot be evoked. Like mechanical nociceptors with myelinated fibres, polymodal nociceptors display a range of mechanical thresholds. Gentle mechanical stimuli such as stroking the receptive field with a brush or light (<5 gm) pressure with a blunt object generally will not evoke a response. The most sensitive elements require stronger, though still not overtly noxious, stimuli and increase their discharge as the stimulus increases to damaging intensities. The least sensitive are not excited until the skin is visibly injured. There is a rough positive correlation between a polymodal receptor's threshold to mechanical stimuli and the threshold to heat. Mechanically induced responses show a dynamic component reminiscent of that exhibited by the C fibre mechanoreceptors. The discharge elicited by maintained pressure with a needle dies off in 0.3 to several sec with the briefer responses produced by the higher threshold units. Repeated mechanical insults to the receptive field often are followed by a low frequency background discharge.

   The polymodal elements usually do not respond to sudden or slow cooling of even 20°C to temperatures of 10–15°C. Freezing of the skin may evoke a few impulses in some units of the group. Heating, however, is consistently effective. Threshold thermode temperature for heat responses varies from 42°C to about 60°C. Radiant heat thresholds measured by a radiometer technique fall into the same range. The response to heat is prompt (i.e., within 1–2 sec of a change in thermode temperature) and graded for 5 to 15°C above the liminal value. The response to heat is persistent though often cyclical; bursts of impulses are followed by periods of quiescence. At the upper range of responsiveness to heat, impulses often appear in groups of 2 to 3 with intervals of less than 15 msec between the discharges of a burst; when present the bursts appear at rates of 1 to 10/sec. Irritant chemicals, such as strong acids, applied to unbroken skin also provoke a low frequency, long-lasting discharge.

A striking feature of the majority of polymodal nociceptors is a change in responsiveness and appearance of background activity, particularly after noxious

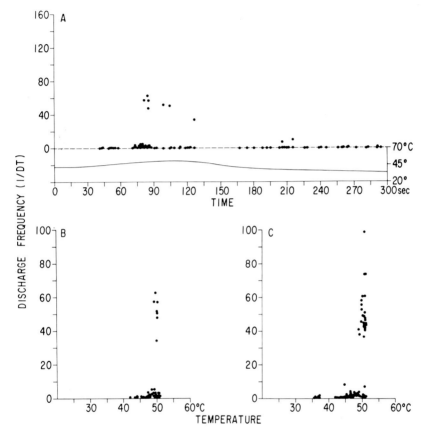

Fig. 8. Discharge of a polymodal nociceptor to contact heating of the skin. Heat applied with a thermode of approximately 2 mm² contact surface. *A* – Dots show discharge as 'instantaneous frequency' as function of time; continuous trace below indicates thermode temperature. *B* – plot of discharge as a function of thermode temperature for first 150 sec of *A*. *C* – Plot of discharge as function of thermode temperature for 150 sec of a second heating of same receptive field area with a similar time course and terminal temperature as in *A*. (From PERL, 1972)

heat (BESSOU and PERL, 1969; KUMAZAWA and PERL, unpublished; see also WITT, 1962). Heat of liminal intensity is often followed by a drop in threshold for subsequent heating of 2 to 8°C and/or a higher frequency or larger number of impulses at a given temperature. Repeated cycles of heating to just threshold levels make this effect more prominent. An example is shown in Fig. 8; in the upper graph the instantaneous frequency is plotted as a function of time in parallel with

5*

a record of skin surface temperature. In the two graphs in the lower part of Fig. 8 the discharge frequency is plotted as a function of temperature for the first 150 sec of the upper graph (lower left) and the first 150 sec of a second trial with similar time course of heating started 5 min after the first. The graphs of Fig. 8 emphasize the appearance of background discharge and the enhanced response to a particular temperature on a second trial. Background discharge and sensitization can be demonstrated in the majority of polymodal units provided that the initial stimulation is not strongly supraliminal (5°C or less suprathreshold). High skin temperatures (over 55°C), particularly if maintained, lead to receptor inactivation lasting from minutes to hours. Decreases in mechanical threshold often accompany the changes in heat threshold. With sensitization, responses to sudden cooling of 10–20°C regularly appear. These sensitizing effects can be demonstrated within 60 sec after a stimulus and can last for hours.

3. Chemical Intermediaries

Long-lasting changes of responsiveness bring forth the question of some enduring agent or mediator between noxious stimulus and nociceptor activation. Although persistent changes in sensitivity have been demonstrated so far under conditions that have meaning for natural circumstances only in the case of polymodal elements, such effects may occur with other nociceptors as well. If the receptive field of a relatively responsive mechanical nociceptor is heated slowly to temperatures of 50–55°C and maintained, a response may be evoked after a relatively long latency (20–30 sec); thereafter, slow heating may initiate a response with a shorter delay (Burgess and Whitehorn, unpublished).

Direct evidence for a chemical transmitter exciting nociceptors is lacking and those indications that do exist are circumstantial. It has long been postulated that a chemical intermediary exists for human pain. Among the candidates are histamine (Rosenthal and Minard, 1939; Rosenthal, 1968), Lewis' substance P (Lewis, 1942), potassium release from injured cells (Benjamin, 1968), bradykinin and other polypeptides (Keele and Armstrong, 1964; Lim, 1970), acidity (Lindahl, 1961) and acetylcholine (see Keele and Armstrong, 1964). Histamine is capable of producing pain when applied to abraided skin and is released by damage to skin (Rosenthal and Minard, 1939; Rosenthal, 1968); however, in concentrations expected for the skin it ordinarily provokes itch rather than pain (Lewis, 1942). Polymodal nociceptors are weakly excited by bradykinin injected into or placed on abraided skin of the receptive field. Histamine similarly applied is even less effective, while acetylcholine (10^{-5} gm/liter) evokes a vigorous discharge as does K^+ in concentrations 2 to 4 X higher than extracellular fluid (Bessou and Perl, 1969; Burgess and Perl, unpublished). Under comparable conditions mechanical nociceptors are not activated by such agents.

An interesting common ground exists between the neurophysiological data on nociceptors and observations on certain kinds of inflammation. Jancsó (1960), in studies on the neurogenic component in inflammation, found that repeated parenteral applications of capsaicin and related pungent acetylamides to rodents, depressed the inflammatory reaction to local application of these compounds. Animals so desensitized no longer exhibited inflammatory responses or signs of discomfort after chemical agents. Moreover, a lowering of heat threshold for cutaneous nociceptive reactions secondary to local application of chemicals also disappeared. At the same time, the reactions initiated by strong mechanical stimuli were unaltered. These observations are another indication of a possible difference between mechanically and chemical-heat evoked nociceptive mechanisms.

4. Comments on Nociceptors

In summary, the present indications are that a group of mammalian cutaneous receptors are specialized for nociception. In both carnivore and primates two major groups emerge: a class responding principally, if not exclusively, to strong mechanically induced distortion of the skin and a class responsive to both strong mechanical and intense thermal stimulation. The most common of the latter in both carnivore and primate responds to chemical insults of the unbroken skin as well. In primates each class is represented by a type with myelinated afferent fibres of slow conduction (under 40 m/sec) and a type with C afferent fibres. In the absence of previous insults to the skin or subcutaneous tissue, sensory units fitting the criteria for nociceptors do not have background activity.

There is no direct evidence on the factors underlying the elevated thresholds that nociceptors have for various stimuli. "Pain" receptors have long been considered bare nerve endings, but support for this view is entirely circumstantial. Furthermore, what appears "bare" under the light microscope of earlier histologists may look quite different when examined with the electronmicroscope. The latter point is especially pertinent since neural elements of the skin are difficult to stain histologically. In any case, at the present we are no closer to an understanding of the morphological basis of nociceptor specificity than we were after BISHOP's (1943) histological analysis of "pain" spots in his own skin or WOOLARD, WEDDELL and HARPMAN's (1940) studies incriminating the subepithelial plexus of unmyelinated fibres in pain responses.

D. Receptors and Sensation

Putting together the evidence for systematic differences among cutaneous mechanoreceptors and nociceptors provides a mass of information which leaves little room for challenge to the concept of their specialization. A relationship between receptor morphology and physiological characteristics is less extensively documented, however convincing in some instances. Therefore, a part of the argument for cutaneous sense organ specificity advanced at the turn of the century by VON FREY is supportable, although the direct correlation he proposed between a particular kind of cutaneous receptor and a particular human sensation needs additional consideration.

Before tackling the problem of sensation, some other implications of receptor specificity should be discussed. An overview of mechanoreceptor characteristics indicates that while one type differs from another to a greater or lesser degree, their functional features span the variety of mechanical events which may disturb an animal's skin in its natural environment remarkably well. Distant disturbances of the terrain can be detected (Pacinian corpuscles), the rate and direction of objects brushing the hairy coat or the skin can be sensed (Aα hair, field, D hair, C mechanoreceptor units), and the intensity and change of pressure against the skin signalled (Type II, Type I units). Not only is this array of cutaneous transducers suitable for signalling a wide range of mechanical events, but also each element is attuned or best adapted to a limited fraction of this spectrum so that the presence of a response in one or another serves to indicate features of the mechanical disturbance. Viewed in another way, a major step in information processing occurs in the selective activation of the population that follows from receptor specificity. This does not mean that a given stimulus excites one and only one type of receptor; on the contrary, a stimulus from nature may excite several kinds of receptors in an area of skin. The view best fitting the known facts suggests that as stimuli differ in intensity and dynamic features (velocity, acceleration, duration), different proportions of various receptor types will be excited and within the excited population differing degrees of activity will result. Only when particular stimuli act within constrained frames of location and time will the afferent input be dominated by one kind of receptor.

Although these considerations make it appear unlikely that any cutaneous sensation is uniquely related to a particular sense organ, nevertheless, such a relationship does seem to exist for certain cutaneous sensory experiences. The cases in point involve those receptors whose characteristics set them apart from all others: Pacinian corpuscles, Type II, C mechanoreceptors and the nociceptors.

Vibration has come to be considered a special subcategory of somatic sensation as a consequence of findings in the neurological clinic where it occasionally is noted to be dissociated from other senses. Since the ability to detect the presence of vibration extends over a sinusoidal frequency range paralleling that for which Pacinian corpuscles have a particular sensitivity, Hunt and McIntyre (1960a) and Hunt (1961) proposed that vibration sense was related to their activity. In an elegant quantitative analysis, Talbot et al. (1968) compared human threshold for different frequencies of vibration and the behavior of different receptors from a comparable skin area of monkey; a close fit was demonstrated between the threshold for human flutter-vibration sensation and the average threshold of two receptor types for a response of one impulse to one stimulus cycle. One of the two receptors had features matching those of Pacinian corpuscles and the other fits that of the F_1 type (see p. 50). While conclusions from such work involve broad assumptions, Talbot et al's correlations are impressive and convincing.

The position detecting features of Type I and Type II receptors are an invitation for a comparison between their features and the sense of skin pressure. Merzenich and Harrington (1968) could not evoke a distinct sensation from stimulation of a single haarscheibe (dome) of man but found a good fit between the discharges evoked by graded skin indentation from Type II units of the monkey and judgements on the intensity of pressure on human hairy skin produced by similar stimuli. Their results imply a sensory function for Type II units, but leave mysterious the functional significance of the more numerous Type I units and the ascending sensory systems they project upon.

In the first description of low threshold C fibre mechanoreceptors, Zotterman (1939) suggested a role for them in the peculiar sensation that man calls tickle. This idea is supported by the unique responsiveness of C mechanoreceptors to slowly-moving stimuli, the type particularly effective in evoking tickle. Moreover, the afterdischarge from C mechanoreceptors is reminiscent of the aftersensation, often accompanying tickle, produced by a light brushing of the skin by a slowly moving blunt object.

Quantitative comparison of pain sensation in man and the activity evoked in receptors by closely similar stimuli is not available; nevertheless, there are features of the two that can be compared on the basis of separately acquired data. The fact that nociceptor afferent fibre conduction velocities match the dependence of pain on slowly conducting afferent fibres has already been referred to. Another point is that short latency pain produced by a sharp object pressed against the skin can only be evoked from certain small areas (spots) whose dimensions are consistent with those of the receptive fields of the myelinated mechanical nociceptors. In this regard, pinprick pain is usually described as a "sharp" sensation that rapidly fades during a maintained stimulus; this behavior is akin to the discharge pattern of the myelinated mechanical nociceptors to needle pressure. The pain reported by human subjects to Aδ fibre activation is said to be sharp or bright while that due to C fibre activity is more dull and aching (LANDAU and BISHOP, 1958). The dual representation of nociceptors in the myelinated and C fibre portions of the afferent spectrum supports LEWIS and POCHIN's (1937) argument that a double pain response to a single sudden stimulus is due to differences in conduction time (see also LANDAU and BISHOP, 1958). The usual thresholds given for heat pain in human beings, 45–46°C (HARDY and STOLWIJK, 1966), and its changes with repeated stimuli (HARDY, 1966) compare closely with the threshold and behavior of polymodal nociceptors. Finally, the sensitization of polymodal nociceptors has intriguing implications for the pain associated with inflammation. For example, ordinary experience shows that human skin after mild injury such as sunburn has a lower threshold for pain to both heat and mechanical stimuli. Acute inflammation of the skin or other tissues commonly is associated with lowered pain threshold for mechanical stimuli. Thus, JANCSÓ's (1960) evidence for a mechanism common to inflammation and certain nociceptive reactions represents another link between pain and nociception, one best fit by the excitatory process for polymodal nociceptors and the attendant property of sensitization.

Any attempted correlation between human sensation and the first step in the process, the activity of a sense organ, contains assumptions of massive proportions, including a principal one on the properties of neural mechanisms underlying perception and consciousness. Therefore, as suggested earlier, this kind of hypothesized relationship becomes less precarious if the information contained in the activity of a given type of sense organ is transmitted by ascending sensory pathways which are separate from those concerned with activity of another type. To this point, the observation that certain dorsal column nuclear cells respond to higher frequencies of vibration as if principally or exclusively excited by Pacinian corpuscles (PERL et al., 1962; PERL, 1964) is consistent with attribution of a special significance to their input. A closer tie to perception appears in the report of a parallel between entrainment of cortical somatosensory region neurons to sinusoidal stimuli and the evocation of a learned response to that stimulus (CARLI et al., 1971). Returning to the relationship between pain and nociceptor activation, recent evidence has demonstrated that high threshold mechanoreceptors provide the sole or major excitatory input to certain spinal dorsal horn neurons of lamina I (posteriomarginal cells) while other spinal cells of the same nucleus receive projections from polymodal nociceptors (Christensen and Perl, 1970). The finding that some lamina I cells form part of a spinal projection system classically considered a tract important for pain in man gives these results a probable relevance to the sensation (Kumazawa et al., 1971).

Thus, the evidence does suggest the origin of certain cutaneous sensory experiences from the activation of a specific kind of sense organ. This point should not be surprising for, after all, there is little doubt that vision begins from the eye and hearing from the ear. On the other hand, the importance of a number of identified skin receptors for sensation is not clear. For example, how do the various hair receptors fit into the picture of cutaneous sensation? We do appreciate the presence of stimuli moving across the skin, but is this a separate sense? Still another unanswered point is the influence of activity of sense organs other than the type specifically evoking a sensation on conscious experience; recent interest in pain mechanisms brings this forcibly to mind. Among the problems blocking an understanding of somatic sensation these are but two; they and numerous others await solutions that depend upon information from experiments on various levels of neural activity which have been designed with proper attention to the properties of sensory receptors.

References

Adrian, E.D.: The messages in sensory nerve fibres and their interpretation. Proc. roy. Soc. B. **109**, 1–18 (1931).

Adrian, E.D.: The Mechanism of Nervous Action; Electrical Studies of the Neurone. Philadelphia: Univ. of Pennsylvania Press 1932.

Adrian, E.D., Umrath, K.: The impulse discharge from the Pacinian corpuscle. J. Physiol. (Lond.) **68**, 139–154 (1929).

Adrian, E.D., Zotterman, Y.: The impulses produced by sensory nerve endings. Part III. Impulses set up by touch and pressure. J. Physiol. (Lond.) **61**, 465–483 (1926).

Alvarez-Buylla, R., Ramirez de Arellano, J.: Local responses in Pacinian corpuscles. Amer. J. Physiol. **172**, 237–244 (1953).

Andres, K.H.: Über die Feinstruktur der Rezeptoren an Sinushaaren. Z. Zellforsch. **75**, 339–365 (1966).

Armett, C.J., Hunsperger, R.W.: Excitation of receptors in the pad of the cat by single and double mechanical pulses. J. Physiol. (Lond.) **158**, 15–38 (1961).

Autrum, H.: Über Gehör und Erschütterungssinn bei Locustiden. Z. vergl. Physiol. **28**, 580–637 (1941).

Barker, D.J., Hazelton, D.W., Welker, W.I.: Neural coding of skin displacement and velocity in raccoon Rhinarium. Fed. Proc. **29**, 522 (1970).

Barker, D.J., Welker, W.I.: Receptive fields of first-order somatic sensory neurons innervating Rhinarium in coati and raccoon. Brain Res. **14**, 367–386 (1969).

Benjamin, F.G.: Release of intracellular potassium as a factor in pain production. In: The Skin Senses, pp. 466–479. Ed. by D.R. Kenshalo. Springfield: C.C. Thomas 1968.

Bessou, P., Burgess, P.R., Perl, E.R., Taylor, C.B.: Dynamic properties of mechanoreceptors with unmyelinated (C) fibers. J. Neurophysiol. **34**, 116–131 (1971).

Bessou, P., Perl, E.R.: Response of cutaneous sensory units with unmyelinated fibers to noxious stimuli. J. Neurophysiol. **32**, 1025–1043 (1969).

Bishop, G.H.: Response to electrical stimulation of single sensory units of skin. J. Neurophysiol. **6**, 361–382 (1943).

BODIAN, D.: The generalized vertebrate neuron. Science **137**, 323–326 (1962).

BOYD, I.A.: The histological structure of the receptors in the knee-joint of the cat correlated with their physiological response. J. Physiol. (Lond.) **124**, 476–488 (1954).

BROWN, A.G.: Cutaneous afferent fibre collaterals in the dorsal columns of the cat. Exp. Brain Res. **5**, 293–305 (1968).

BROWN, A.G., HAYDEN, R.E.: The distribution of cutaneous receptors in the rabbit's hind limb and differential electrical stimulation of their axons. J. Physiol. (Lond.) **213**, 495–506 (1971).

BROWN, A.G., IGGO, A.: A quantitative study of cutaneous receptors and afferent fibres in the cat and rabbit. J. Physiol. (Lond.) **193**, 707–733 (1967).

BURGESS, P.R., CLARK, F.J.: Characteristics of knee joint receptors in the cat. J. Physiol. (Lond.) **203**, 317–335 (1969).

BURGESS, P.R., PERL, E.R.: Myelinated afferent fibres responding specifically to noxious stimulation of the skin. J. Physiol. (Lond.) **190**, 541–562 (1967).

BURGESS, P.R., PETIT, D., WARREN, R.M.: Receptor types in cat hairy skin supplied by myelinated fibers. J. Neurophysiol. **31**, 833–848 (1968).

CARLI, G., LAMOTTE, R.H., MOUNTCASTLE, V.B.: A simultaneous study of somatic sensory behavior and the activity of somatic sensory cortical neurons. Fed. Proc. **30**, 664 (1971).

CHAMBERS, M.R., ANDRES, K.H., DUERING, M. VON, IGGO, A.: The structure and function of the slowly adapting Type II receptor in hairy skin. Quart. J. exp. Physiol. **57**, 417—445 (1972).

CHRISTENSEN, B.N., PERL, E.R.: Spinal neurons specifically excited by noxious or thermal stimuli. Marginal zone of the dorsal horn. J. Neurophysiol. **33**, 293–307 (1970).

CLARK, D., HUGHES, J., GASSER, H.S.: Afferent function in the group of nerve fibers of slowest conduction velocity. Amer. J. Physiol. **114**, 69–76 (1935).

COLLINS, W.F., JR., NULSEN, F.E., RANDT, C.T.: Relation of peripheral nerve size and sensation in man. Arch. Neurol. (Chic.) **3**, 381–385 (1960).

COOPER, S.: The responses of the primary and secondary endings of muscle spindles with intact motor innervation during applied stretch. Quart. J. exp. Physiol. **46**, 389–398 (1961).

CREMERS, P.F.L.J.M.: Responses of single units in the nervus suralis and the nucleus gracilis to stimulation of a hair receptor of cat and rat. Ph. D. Thesis, The Catholic University, Nijmegen, The Netherlands 1971.

CROWE, A., MATTHEWS, P.B.C.: The effects of stimulation of static and dynamic fusimotor fibres on the response to stretching of the primary endings of muscle spindles. J. Physiol. (Lond.) **174**, 109–131 (1964).

DANFORTH, C.H.: Studies in hair. Arch. Derm. Syph. (Chic.) **11**, 637–653 (1925).

DODT, E.: Schmerzimpulse bei Temperaturreizen. Acta physiol. scand. **31**, 83–96 (1954).

DODT, E., ZOTTERMAN, Y.: The discharge of specific cold fibres at high temperatures. (The paradoxical cold). Acta physiol. scand. **26**, 358–365 (1952).

DOUGLAS, W.W., RITCHIE, J.M.: Non-medullated fibres in the saphenous nerve which signal touch. J. Physiol. (Lond.) **139**, 385–399 (1957).

DOUGLAS, W.W., RITCHIE, J.M., STRAUB, R.W.: The role of non-myelinated fibres in signalling cooling of the skin. J. Physiol. (Lond.) **150**, 266–283 (1960).

ELDRED, E., GRANIT, R., MERTON, P.A.: Supraspinal control of the muscle spindles and its significance. J. Physiol. (Lond.) **122**, 498–523 (1953).

ERLANGER, J., GASSER, H.S.: Electrical signs of nervous activity. Philadelphia: University Pennsylvania Press 1937.

FITZGERALD, O.: Discharges from the sensory organs of the cat's vibrissae and the modification in their activity by ions. J. Physiol. (Lond.) **98**, 163–178 (1940).

FRANKENHAEUSER, B.: Impulses from a cutaneous receptor with slow adaptation and low mechanical threshold. Acta physiol. scand. **18**, 68–74 (1949).

FREY, M. VON: Beiträge zur Physiologie des Schmerzsinns. Ber. kgl. sächs. Ges. Wiss. Leipzig 185–196 (1894).

GASSER, H.S.: Properties of dorsal root unmedullated fibers on the two sides of the ganglion. J. gen. Physiol. **38**, 709–728 (1955).

GASSER, H.S.: Effect of method leading on the recording of the nerve fibre spectrum. J. gen. Physiol. **43**, 927–940 (1960).

Gasser, H.S., Erlanger, J.: The rôle played by the sizes of the constituent fibers of a nerve trunk in determining the form of its action potential wave. Amer. J. Physiol. **80**, 522–547 (1927).

Gottschaldt, K.-M., Iggo, A., Young, D.W.: Electrophysiology of the afferent innervation of sinus hairs, including vibrissae, of the cat. J. Physiol. (Lond.) **222**, 60–61 P (1972).

Gray, J.A.B., Malcolm, J.L.: The initiation of nerve impulses by mesenteric Pacinian corpuscles. Proc. roy. Soc. B. **137**, 96–114 (1950).

Gray, J.A.B., Matthews, P.B.C.: A comparison of the adaptation of the Pacinian corpuscle with accommodation of its own axon. J. Physiol. (Lond.) **114**, 454–464 (1951).

Gray, J.A.B., Sato, M.: Properties of the receptor potential in Pacinian corpuscles. J. Physiol. (Lond.) **122**, 610–636 (1953).

Hagbarth, K.-E., Hongell, A., Hallin, R.G., Torebjörk, H.E.: Afferent impulses in median nerve fascicles evoked by tactile stimuli of the human hand. Brain Res. **24**, 423–442 (1970).

Hall, M.: Synopsis of the Diastaltic System. London 1850.

Hardy, J.D.: In: Touch, Heat and Pain. Ciba Foundation Symposium, p. 78. Ed. by A.V.S. de Reuck and J. Knight. Boston: Little, Brown and Co. 1966.

Hardy, J.D., Stolwijk, J.A.J.: Tissue temperature and thermal pain. In: Touch, Heat and Pain. Ciba Foundation Symposium, p. 27–56. Ed. by A.V.S. de Reuck and J. Knight. Boston: Little, Brown and Co. 1966.

Harrington, T., Merzenich, M.M.: Neural coding in the sense of touch: human sensations of skin indentation compared with the responses of slowly adapting mechanoreceptive afferents innervating the hairy skin of monkeys. Exp. Brain Res. **10**, 251–264 (1970).

Hartline, H.K., Ratliff, F.: Inhibitory interaction of receptor units in the eye of limulus. J. gen. Physiol. **40**, 357–376 (1957).

Harvey, R.J., Matthews, P.B.C.: The response of de-efferented muscle spindle endings in the cat's soleus to slow extension of the muscle. J. Physiol. (Lond.) **157**, 370–392 (1961).

Heinbecker, P., Bishop, G.H., O'Leary, J.: Pain and touch fibers in peripheral nerves. Arch. Neurol. Psychiat. (Chic.) **29**, 771–789 (1933).

Hensel, H., Huopaniemi, T.: Static and dynamic properties of warm fibres in the infra-orbital nerve. Pflügers Arch. **309**, 1–10 (1969).

Houk, J., Simon, W.: Responses of Golgi tendon organs to forces applied to muscle tendon. J. Neurophysiol. **30**, 1466–1481 (1967).

Hubbard, S.J.: A study of rapid mechanical events in a mechanoreceptor. J. Physiol. (Lond.) **141**, 198–218 (1958).

Hunt, C.C.: On the nature of vibration receptors in the hind limb of the cat. J. Physiol. (Lond.) **155**, 175–186 (1961).

Hunt, C.C., McIntyre, A.K.: Characteristics of responses from receptors from the flexor longus digitorum muscle and the adjoining interosseous region of the cat. J. Physiol. (Lond.) **153**, 74–87 (1960a).

Hunt, C.C., McIntyre, A.K.: Properties of cutaneous touch receptors in cat. J. Physiol. (Lond.) **153**, 88–98 (1960b).

Hunt, C.C., McIntyre, A.K.: An analysis of fibre diameter and receptor characteristics of myelinated cutaneous afferent fibres in cat. J. Physiol. (Lond.) **153**, 99–112 (1960c).

Hursh, J.B.: Conduction velocity and diameter of nerve fibers. Amer. J. Physiol. **127**, 131–139 (1939).

Iggo, A.: Cutaneous heat and cold receptors with slowly-conducting (C) afferent fibres. Quart. J. exp. Physiol. **44**, 362–370 (1959).

Iggo, A.: Cutaneous mechanoreceptors with afferent C fibres. J. Physiol. (Lond.) **152**, 337–353 (1960).

Iggo, A.: New specific sensory structures in hairy skin. Acta neuroveg. (Wien) **24**, 175–180 (1963).

Iggo, A.: Cutaneous receptors with a high sensitivity to mechanical displacement. In: Touch, Heat and Pain, pp. 237–256. Ed. by A.V.S. de Reuck and J. Knight. Boston: Little, Brown and Co. 1966.

Iggo, A.: Electrophysiological and histological studies of cutaneous mechanoreceptors. In: Skin Senses, pp. 84–111. Ed. by D.R. Kenshalo. Springfield: C.C. Thomas 1968.

IGGO, A., KORNHUBER, H.H.: A quantitative analysis of non-myelinated cutaneous mechano-receptors. J. Physiol. (Lond.) **198**, 113P (1968).

IGGO, A., MUIR, A.R.: The structure and function of a slowly adapting touch corpuscle in hairy skin. J. Physiol. (Lond.) **200**, 763–796 (1969).

IGGO, A., OGAWA, H.: Primate cutaneous thermal nociceptors. J. Physiol. (Lond.) **216**, 77–78P (1971).

IRIUCHIJIMA, J., ZOTTERMAN, Y.: The specificity of afferent cutaneous C fibres in mammals. Acta physiol. scand. **49**, 267–278 (1960).

JÄNIG, W.: Morphology of rapidly and slowly adapting mechanoreceptors in the hairless skin of the cat's hind foot. Brain Res. **28**, 217–232 (1971).

JÄNIG, W., SCHMIDT, R.F., ZIMMERMANN, M.: Single unit responses and the total afferent outflow from the cat's foot pad upon mechanical stimulation. Exp. Brain Res. **6**, 100–115 (1968).

JANCSÓ, N.: Role of the nerve terminals in the mechanism of inflammatory reactions. Bull. Millard Fillmore Hosp. Buffalo N. Y. **7**, 53–77 (1960).

JANSEN, J.K.S., NICOLAYSEN, K., RUDJORD, T.: Discharge pattern of neurons of the dorsal spinocerebellar tract activated by static extension of primary endings of muscle spindles. J. Neurophysiol. **29**, 1061–1086 (1966).

KEELE, C.A., ARMSTRONG, D.: Substances Producing Pain and Itch. London: Arnold 1964.

KENTON, B., KRUGER, L., WOO, M.: Two classes of slowly adapting mechanoreceptor fibres in reptile cutaneous nerve. J. Physiol. (Lond.) **212**, 21–44 (1971).

KERR, F.W.L., LYSAK, W.R.: Somatotopic organization of trigeminal-ganglion neurones. Arch. Neurol. (Chic.) **11**, 593–602 (1964).

KNIBESTÖL, M., VALLBO, Å.B.: Single unit analysis of mechanoreceptor activity from the human glabrous skin. Acta physiol. scand. **80**, 178–195 (1970).

KUMAZAWA, T., PERL, E.R., BURGESS, P.R., WHITEHORN, D.: Excitation of posteromarginal cells (Lamina I) in monkey and their projection in lateral spinal tracts. Proc. Intl. Union Physiol. Sci. **9**, 972 (1971).

LANDAU, W.M., BISHOP, G.H.: Evidence for a double peripheral pathway for pain. Science **128**, 712–714 (1958).

LENNERSTRAND, G.: Position and velocity sensitivity of muscle spindles in the cat. I. Primary and secondary endings deprived of fusimotor activation. Acta physiol. scand. **73**, 281–299 (1968).

LEWIS, T.: Pain. New York: MacMillan 1942.

LEWIS, T., POCHIN, E.E.: The double pain response of the human skin to a single stimulus. Clin. Sci. **3**, 67–76 (1937).

LIM, R.K.S.: Pain. Ann. Rev. Physiol. **32**, 269–288 (1970).

LINDAHL, O.: Experimental skin pain induced by injection of water-soluble substances in humans. Acta physiol. scand. **51**, 1–90 (1961).

LINDBLOM, U.: Excitability and functional organization within a peripheral tactile unit. Acta physiol. scand. **44**, Suppl. 153, 1–84 (1958).

LINDBLOM, U.: The relation between stimulus and discharge in a rapidly adapting touch receptor. Acta physiol. scand. **56**, 349–361 (1962).

LINDBLOM, U.: Phasic and static excitability of touch receptors in toad skin. Acta physiol. scand. **59**, 410–423 (1963).

LINDBLOM, U.: Properties of touch receptors in distal glabrous skin of the monkey. J. Neurophysiol. **28**, 966–985 (1965).

LINDBLOM, U., LUND, L.: The discharge from vibration-sensitive receptors in the monkey foot. Exp. Neurol. **15**, 401–417 (1966).

LINDBLOM, U., TAPPER, D.N.: Terminal properties of vibro-tactile sensor. Exp. Neurol. **17**, 1–15 (1967).

LIPPOLD, O.C.J., REDFEARN, J.W.T., VUČO, J.: The effect of sinusoidal stretching upon the activity of stretch receptors in voluntary muscle and their reflex responses. J. Physiol. (Lond.) **144**, 373–386 (1958).

LLOYD, D.P.C.: Neuron patterns controlling transmission of ipsilateral hindlimb reflexes in cat. J. Neurophysiol. **6**, 293–326 (1943).

LLOYD, D.P.C., CHANG, H.-T.: Afferent fibers in muscle nerves. J. Neurophysiol. **11**, 199–208 (1948).

LOEWENSTEIN, W.R.: Generator processes of repetitive activity in a Pacinian corpuscle. J. gen. Physiol. **41**, 825–845 (1958).

LOEWENSTEIN, W.R., ALTAMIRANO-ORREGO, R.: The refractory state of the generator and propagated potentials in a Pacinian corpuscle. J. gen. Physiol. **41**, 805–824 (1958).

LOEWENSTEIN, W.R., MENDELSON, M.: Components of receptor adaptation in a Pacinian corpuscle. J. Physiol. (Lond.) **177**, 377–397 (1965).

LOWENSTEIN, O., FINLAYSON, L.H.: The response of the abdominal stretch receptor of an insect to phasic stimulation. Comp. Biochem. Physiol. **1**, 56–61 (1960).

LYNN, B.: The nature and location of certain phasic mechanoreceptors in the cat's foot. J. Physiol. (Lond.) **201**, 765–773 (1969).

LYNN, B.: The form and distribution of the receptive fields of Pacinian corpuscles found in and around the cat's large foot pad. J. Physiol. (Lond.) **217**, 755–771 (1971).

MALINOVSKÝ, L.: Variability of sensory nerve endings in foot pads of a domestic cat *(Felis ocreata L., F. domestica)*. Acta anat. (Basel) **64**, 82–106 (1966).

MANN, S.J., STRAILE, W.E.: Tylotrich (hair) follicle: association with a slowly adapting tactile receptor in the cat. Science **147**, 1043–1045 (1965).

MARUHASHI, J., MIZUGUCHI, K., TASAKI, I.: Action currents in single afferent nerve fibres elicited by stimulation of the skin of the toad and the cat. J. Physiol. (Lond.) **117**, 129–151 (1952).

MATTHEWS, B.H.C.: The response of a single end organ. J. Physiol. (Lond.) **71**, 64–110 (1931).

MATTHEWS, B.H.C.: Nerve endings in mammalian muscle. J. Physiol. (Lond.) **78**, 1–53 (1933).

MATTHEWS, P.B.C.: The response of de-efferented muscle spindle receptors to stretching at different velocities. J. Physiol. (Lond.) **168**, 660–678 (1963).

MATTHEWS, P.B.C.: Muscle spindles and their motor control. Physiol. Rev. **44**, 219–288 (1964).

MATTHEWS, P.B.C., STEIN, R.B.: The regularity of primary and secondary muscle spindle afferent discharges. J. Physiol. (Lond.) **202**, 59–82 (1969).

MERZENICH, M.M.: Some observations on the encoding of somesthetic stimuli by receptor populations in the hairy skin of primates. Ph.D. Thesis, Johns Hopkins Univ., 1968.

MERZENICH, M.M., HARRINGTON, T.: The sense of flutter-vibration evoked by stimulation of the hairy skin of primates: comparison of human sensory capacity with the responses of mechanoreceptive afferents innervating the hairy skin of monkeys. Exp. Brain Res. **9**, 236–260 (1969).

MOUNTCASTLE, V.B., TALBOT, W.H., KORNHUBER, H.H.: The neural transformation of mechanical stimuli delivered to the monkey's hand. In: Touch, Heat and Pain, pp. 325 to 345. Ed. by A.V.S. DE REUCK and J. KNIGHT. Boston: Little, Brown and Co. 1966.

MUNGER, B.L., PUBOLS, L.M., PUBOLS, B.H., Jr.: The Merkel rete papilla — a slowly adapting sensory receptor in mammalian glabrous skin. Brain Res. **29**, 47–61 (1971).

NILSSON, B.Y.: Structure and function of the tactile hair receptors on the cat's foreleg. Acta physiol. scand. **77**, 396–416 (1969a).

NILSSON, B.Y.: Hair discs and Pacinian corpuscles functionally associated with the carpal tactile hairs in the cat. Acta physiol. scand. **77**, 417–428 (1969b).

NILSSON, B.Y., SKOGLUND, C.R.: The tactile hairs on the cat's foreleg. Acta physiol. scand. **65**, 364–369 (1965).

NISHI, K., SATO, M.: Depolarizing and hyperpolarizing receptor potentials in the non-myelinated nerve terminal in Pacinian corpuscles. J. Physiol. (Lond.) **199**, 383–396 (1968).

OZEKI, M., SATO, M.: Initiation of impulses at the non-myelinated nerve terminal in Pacinian corpuscles. J. Physiol. (Lond.) **170**, 167–185 (1964).

OZEKI, M., SATO, M.: Changes in the membrane potential and the membrane conductance associated with a sustained compression of the non-myelinated nerve terminal in Pacinian corpuscles. J. Physiol. (Lond.) **180**, 186–208 (1965).

PERL, E.R.: Études sur la sensibilité tactile et sur la sensibilité vibratoire. Actualités neurophysiol. 91–110 (1964).

PERL, E.R.: Myelinated afferent fibres innervating the primate skin and their response to noxious stimuli. J. Physiol. (Lond.) **197**, 593–615 (1968).

PERL, E. R.: Mode of action of nociceptors. In: Cervical Pain, pp. 157–164. C. Hirsch and Y. Zotterman, Eds. Oxford: Pergamon Press 1972.

PERL, E. R., WHITLOCK, D. G., GENTRY, J. R.: Cutaneous projection to second order neurons of the dorsal column system. J. Neurophysiol. **25**, 337–358 (1962).

PETIT, D., BURGESS, P. R.: Dorsal column projection of receptors in cat hairy skin supplied by myelinated fibers. J. Neurophysiol. **31**, 849–855 (1968).

PRINGLE, J. W. S.: Proprioception in insects. I. A new type of mechanical receptor from the palps of the cockroach. J. exp. Biol. **15**, 101–113 (1938).

PRINGLE, J. W. S., WILSON, V. J.: The response of a sense organ to a harmonic stimulus. J. exp. Biol. **29**, 220–234 (1952).

PUBOLS, L. M., PUBOLS, B. H., JR., MUNGER, B. L.: Functional properties of mechanoreceptors in glabrous skin of the raccoon's forepaw. Exp. Neurol. **31**, 165–182 (1971).

ROSENTHAL, S. R.: Histamine as the chemical mediator for referred pain. In: The Skin Senses, pp. 480–498. Ed. by D. R. KENSHALO. Springfield: C. C. Thomas 1968.

ROSENTHAL, S. R., MINARD, D.: Experiments on histamine as the chemical mediator for cutaneous pain. J. exp. Med. **70**, 415–425 (1939).

SASSEN, M., ZIMMERMANN, M.: Capacity of cutaneous C fibre mechanoreceptors to transmit information on stimulus intensity. Proc. Inter. Union Physiol. Sci. **9**, 493, 1466 (1971).

SATO, M.: Response of Pacinian corpuscles to sinusoidal vibration. J. Physiol. (Lond.) **159**, 391–409 (1961).

SHERRINGTON, C. S.: The Integrative Action of the Nervous System. New Haven: Yale University Press 1906.

SKOGLUND, C. R.: Properties of Pacinian corpuscles of ulnar and tibial location in cat and fowl. Acta physiol. scand. **50**, 385–386 (1960).

SKOGLUND, S.: Anatomical and physiological studies of knee joint innervation in the cat. Acta physiol. scand. **36**, 1–101 (1956).

SMITH, K. R., JR.: The structure and function of Haarscheibe. J. comp. Neurol. **131**, 459–474 (1967).

SMITH, K. R., JR.: The ultrastructure of the human *Haarscheibe* and Merkel cell. J. invest. Derm. **54**, 150–159 (1970).

STEIN, R. B.: The information capacity of nerve cells using a frequency code. Biophys. J. **7**, 797–826 (1967).

STRAILE, W. E.: Sensory hair follicles in mammalian skin: the tylotrich follicle. Amer. J. Anat. **106**, 133–147 (1960).

STUART, D., OTT, K., ISHIKAWA, K., ELDRED, E.: Muscle receptor responses to sinusoidal stretch. Exp. Neurol. **13**, 82–95 (1965).

TALBOT, W. H., DARIAN-SMITH, I., KORNHUBER, H. H., MOUNTCASTLE, V. B.: The sense of flutter-vibration: comparison of the human capacity with response patterns of mechanoreceptive afferents from the monkey hand. J. Neurophysiol. **31**, 301–334 (1968).

TAPPER, D. N.: Cutaneous slowly adapting mechanoreceptors in the cat. Science **143**, 53–54 (1964).

TAPPER, D. N.: Stimulus-response relationships in the cutaneous slowly-adapting mechanoreceptor in hairy skin of the cat. Exp. Neurol. **13**, 364–385 (1965).

TERZUOLO, C. A., WASHIZU, Y.: Relation between stimulus strength, generator potential and impulse frequency in stretch receptor of Crustacea. J. Neurophysiol. **25**, 56–66 (1962).

WERNER, G., MOUNTCASTLE, V. B.: Neural activity in mechanoreceptive cutaneous afferents: stimulus-response relations, Weber functions and information transmission. J. Neurophysiol. **28**, 359–397 (1965).

WHITEHORN, D., CORNWALL, M. C., BURGESS, P. R.: Central course of identified cutaneous afferents from cat hindlimb. Fed. Proc. **30**, 433 (1971).

WIERSMA, C. A. G., BOETTIGER, E. G.: Unidirectional movement fibres from a proprioceptive organ of the crab, *Carcinus maenas*. J. exp. Biol. **36**, 102–112 (1959).

WITT, I.: Aktivität einzelner C-Fasern bei schmerzhaften und nicht schmerzhaften Hautreizen. Acta neuroveg. (Wien) **24**, 208–219 (1962).

WITT, I., HENSEL, H.: Afferente Impulse aus der Extremitätenhaut der Katze bei thermischer und mechanischer Reizung. Pflügers Arch. ges. Physiol. **268**, 582–596 (1959).

Woolard, H.H., Weddell, G., Harpman, J.A.: Observations on the neurohistological basis of cutaneous pain. J. Anat. (Lond.) **74**, 413–440 (1940).

Zimmermann, M.: Cutaneous C-fibres: peripheral properties and central connections. In: The Somatosensory System. Ed. by V. Aschoff and H.H. Kornhuber. Stuttgart: Thieme-Verlag (1972, in press).

Zotterman, Y.: Studies in the peripheral nervous mechanism of pain. Acta med. scand. **80**, 1064 (1933).

Zotterman, Y.: Specific action potentials in the lingual nerve of cat. Skand. arch. **75**, 105–120 (1936).

Zotterman, Y.: Touch, pain and tickling: an electrophysiological investigation on cutaneous sensory nerves. J. Physiol. (Lond.) **95**, 1–28 (1939).

Zucker, E., Welker, W.I.: Coding of somatic sensory input by vibrissae neurons in the rat's trigeminal ganglion. Brain Res. **12**, 138–156 (1969).

Chapter 3

Cutaneous Thermoreceptors

By

Herbert Hensel, Marburg/Lahn (Germany)

With 20 Figures

Contents

A. General Concept of Thermoreceptors

The concept of thermoreceptors is based originally on human sensory physiology, in particular on the fact that thermal sensations can be elicited from localized sensory spots in the skin (Blix, 1882). Detailed investigations have revealed a differentiation of "warm" and "cold" spots, that is, local areas responding only with warm or cold sensations. In some cases these spots also responded with thermal sensations to inadequate electrical stimulation. It seems thus justified to speak of specific thermoreceptors in the classical sense of Müller (1840). This means that temperature sensations (E_T) are correlated with localized neural structures (N)

$$E_T \to N.$$

$\to$ is the symbol of a probability implication (Reenpää, 1962; Hensel, 1966). This type of specificity could be called "*sensory specificity*".

As a result of modern neurophysiological methods it has become possible to define thermoreceptors in biophysical terms, namely, as nerve endings (N) excited only or preferably by temperature stimuli (S_T)

$$S_T \to N.$$

Here we can speak of "*biophysical specificity*". It is obvious that this concept reaches far beyond the realm of conscious temperature sensation. The biophysical definition holds for any thermosensitive structure, irrespective of whether its excitation is correlated with temperature sensations, or whether conscious experiences are difficult to establish, as it is the case in animal experiments.

Although both concepts are closely related, they are not identical, the criterion being a quality of *sensation* (E) in the first case and a quality of *stimulus* (S) in the second case. A clear distinction between both is necessary, especially when the relationship between temperature sensation and neural code or the question of specificity is concerned. For example, a receptor excited by cooling as well as by application of menthol might be classified as a specific cold receptor in terms of sensation (E), but it has at best a relative specificity or selective sensitivity with respect to the thermal stimulus (S).

On the one hand, cutaneous thermoreceptors are the source of conscious temperature information but on the other hand they are perhaps even more important in connection with behavioural and thermoregulatory responses. Thus the physiology of thermoreceptors implies various approaches, namely (1) temperature sensations in human subjects, (2) afferent impulses from units responding to thermal stimulation in animals and, to some extent, in man, (3) behavioural responses to thermal stimulation in animals, and (4) thermoregulatory reflexes in animals and human subjects.

The following chapter will be concerned mainly with sensory and neurophysiological aspects of temperature receptors in the skin of homeotherms, with some implications for behavioural responses and thermoregulation.

B. Thermal Sensations

1. Structure of Temperature Sensation

It is relatively easy to discriminate the phenomenal qualities of *warm* and *cold* from the manifold of cutaneous sensations. Both qualities form a sensory continuum of various intensities: "indifferent" — "lukewarm" — "warm" — "hot" — "heat pain" on the warm side and "indifferent" — "cool" — "cold" — "cold pain" on the cold side.

Whether the sensation of "*heat*" is only a more intense warm sensation or a mixture of various qualities is not quite clear. According to Alrutz (1900) heat is a combination of warmth and "paradoxical" cold. The sensory quality brought about by simultaneous application of warm and cold stimuli was interpreted by several authors as "heat" but statistical investigations in untrained subjects have shown that the number of "heat" judgements decreased when cold stimuli were added to pure warm stimuli (For references see HENSEL, 1952a). Perhaps "heat" might be a quality of its own, its neurophysiological correlate being the activity of particular "heat" fibres excited by high temperatures (IGGO, 1959).

The experience of thermal comfort and discomfort when larger areas of the body are exposed to various temperatures is not only due to the function of cutaneous thermoreceptors but reflects an integrated state of the thermoregulatory system.

2. Cold and Warm Spots

Since the discovery by BLIX (1882) of sensory spots from which adequate or electrical stimuli elicited cold and warm sensations, respectively, numerous authors have described the distribution of *cold* and *warm spots* in the skin of man. In general, cold spots seem to be distributed more densely than warm spots (Table 1). Investigations on the topography of warm spots in the external skin of human subjects have been made by REIN (1925b), of cold spots by STRUGHOLD and PORZ (1931). For further references see v. SKRAMLIK (1937) and HENSEL (1952a).

Table 1. *Number of cold and warm spots per square centimetre in human skin*

	Cold spots[a]	Warm spots[b]
Forehead	5.5– 8	
Nose	8	1
Lips	16 –19	
Other parts of face	8.5– 9	1.7
Chest	9 –10.2	0.3
Abdomen	8 –12.5	
Back	7.8	
Upper arm	5 – 6.5	
Forearm	6 – 7.5	0.3–0.4
Back of hand	7.4	0.5
Palm of hand	1 – 5	0.4
Finger dorsal	7 – 9	1.7
Finger volar	2 – 4	1.6
Thigh	4.5– 5.2	0.4
Calf	4.3– 5.7	
Back of foot	5.6	
Sole of foot	3.4	

[a] From STRUGHOLD and PORZ (1931).
[b] From REIN (1925b).

From experiments in human subjects alone it is difficult to decide whether the temperature spots represent discontinuous cold and warm sensitive fields in an otherwise thermally insensitive area, or whether they are maxima in a thermosensitive continuum. Electrophysiological evidence is in favor of the first alternative (p. 94).

3. Thermal Sensation and Temperature

Because of their intracutaneous site, thermoreceptors have neither the temperature of the skin surface nor that of the blood. Any reliable metrics of thermal stimuli has thus to account for the temperatures in different layers of the skin. By

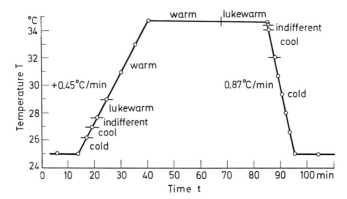

Fig. 1. Temperature sensation on linear warming and cooling of the foot. (From HENSEL. 1952a)

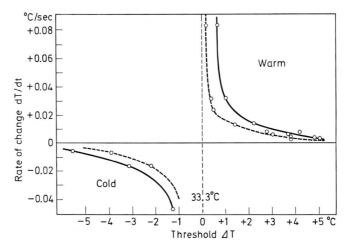

Fig. 2. Average thresholds (ΔT) of warm and cold sensations on the forearm (20 cm²) as a function of rate of temperature change (dT/dt). Initial temperature 33.3°C. Dashed lines: thresholds; solid lines: distinct sensations. (From HENSEL, 1950b)

means of fine thermocouples it has been possible to measure directly the intracutaneous temperature field under stationary and non-stationary conditions (HENSEL, 1950a, b; 1952a).

When a cutaneous area, such as hand or foot, is adapted to a constant temperature of 25°C, linear temperature rises will cause a sequence of sensations from "cool" to "warm" (Fig. 1). After having reached a constant temperature level, the intensity of sensation decreases considerably. On linear cooling with a similar slope, the cold sensation starts at the same temperature at which a warm sensation occurs when the temperature is rising. Starting with indifferent temperatures of 33.5°C, the threshold (Δ T) deviates the more from this point, the slower the temperature is changed. By plotting the rate of change (dT/dt) versus the thermal threshold (Δ T), a hyperbolic function is obtained (Fig. 2). Similar results have been found by KENSHALO, HOLMES and WOOD (1968). At high and low temperatures the threshold rate of change finally reaches zero which means that steady temperature sensations occur at constant skin temperatures. The limits for this steady sensations are 24 and 35°C according to GERTZ (1921). With controlled intracutaneous temperature and 20 cm² stimulus area, the limit for steady cold sensations was 20°C and for steady warm sensations 40°C (HENSEL, 1950b).

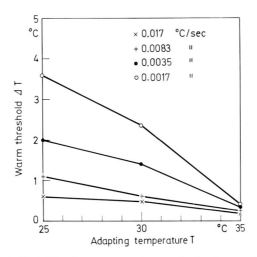

Fig. 3. Average thresholds (ΔT) of warm sensation on the hand as a function of adapting temperature (T) for linear temperature rises from 0.0017 to 0.017°C/sec. (From HENSEL, 1952a)

Starting from adapting temperatures of 34°C, cooling the skin with temperature transients of approximately rectangular shape elicited a cold sensation, the estimated magnitude of which was a linear function of the magnitude of the cold stimulus over a range of 10°C. 4 categories of magnitude could be correctly identified over this range with 95% confidence. Warming the skin from 34°C with rectangular stimuli revealed a similar relationship between sensation and stimulus, the number of categories being 5 over the 10°C range (DARIAN-SMITH and DYKES, 1971).

Starting from various adapting temperatures, the threshold (Δ T) for warm sensations at equal rates of warming increases with decreasing adapting temperature. In the diagram Fig. 3 the warm thresholds (Δ T) are depicted as a function of adapting temperature for various rates of stimulus temperature changes. An analogous behaviour has been found for cold sensations as well. The fact that the warm thresholds increase with decreasing adapting temperatures, whereas the highest cold thresholds are found at high adapting temperatures is in good agreement with numerous investigations (Hahn, 1927, 1949; Ebaugh and Thauer, 1950; Thauer and Ebaugh, 1952; Lele, 1954; Kenshalo, 1969) and also with the observation of daily life that we feel less cold when the body was well warmed up previously to cooling (Thauer, 1958).

4. Stimulus Area

Numerous investigations have revealed a considerable influence of stimulus area on the thresholds and intensities of temperature sensation (Weber, 1846; Hardy and Oppel, 1937, 1938; Hensel, 1950b). Fig. 4 shows the warm thresholds at uniform rates of linear temperature increases as a function of stimulus area from 1 to 1000 cm². Within this range the threshold can vary by several degrees. It

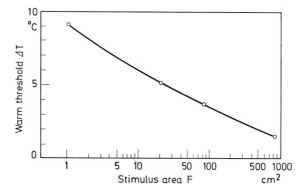

Fig. 4. Average thresholds (ΔT) of warm sensations on the forearm for linear temperature rises of 0.017°C/sec as a function of stimulus area (F). Initial temperature 30°C. (From Hensel, 1950b)

should be mentioned here that the results from stimulus areas less than 1 cm² are difficult to interpret, since the factor of three-dimensional heat flow becomes decisive at small areas. Thus the dependence of thresholds on stimulus area might be rather a physical than a physiological effect (Hensel, 1952a).

In connection with the biological importance of thermoreception in man, the results obtained by stimulation of large cutaneous areas or of the whole body surface are of particular interest. Maréchaux and Schäfer (1949) have measured the warm thresholds when the whole body was warmed up in a climatic chamber with linear temperature rises from 0.001 to 0.01°C/sec. Under these conditions even extremely slow rates of changes of 0.001°C/sec led to warm sensations at skin temperatures of 35°C. This corresponds well with the observation that thermal comfort is restricted to a relatively narrow range of integral skin temperature, approximately from 32 to 34°C.

5. The Adequate Stimulus

As a result of the previously described findings, the threshold and intensity of warm and cold sensations are dependent (1) on the absolute temperature (T) of the skin, (2) on the rate of change (dT/dt) and (3) on the stimulus area (F).

Stimulation of thermoreceptors by intravenous injection of cold and warm solutions leads to the same sensations as when the receptors were stimulated from the skin surface (HENSEL, 1950b). Thermoelectric measurements at various depth of the skin have shown that on intravenous cooling and warming the spatial temperature gradient in the skin is reversed in comparison with the gradient on stimulation from the skin surface. Thus the general condition for warm and cold sensations is warming or cooling *per se*, independent of direction and slope of the intracutaneous spatial temperature gradient (dT/dx). Investigations with microwave and infrared heating of the skin have led to similar results (VENDRIK and VOS, 1958).

6. Inadequate Stimulation

a) "Paradoxical" Sensations. On strong heat stimulation one can feel a peculiar quality of cold that has been called *"paradoxical"* cold sensation by v. FREY (1895). This well established phenomenon (ALRUTZ, 1897; THUNBERG, 1901; HAHN, 1927, 1949) is observed when the skin is heated to temperatures above 45°C.

It is not certain whether a *"paradoxical"* warm sensation exists (REIN, 1925a; GRUNDIG, 1930).

b) Chemical Stimulation. A well known substance with specific action on thermoreceptors is *menthol*. It elicits a cold sensation at otherwise indifferent skin temperatures. GOLDSCHEIDER (1898) has proved that this cold sensation is not due to evaporative cooling but to a chemical action. Menthol also acts on intravenous application (SCHWENKENBECHER, 1908).

Calcium gives rise to a distinct warm sensation when given intracutaneously or intravenously; it lowers the warm threshold and increases the cold threshold at the same time (HIRSCHSOHN and MAENDL, 1922; SCHREINER, 1936). Other substances causing warm sensations are locally applied *carbon dioxide* or carbonic acid (LILJESTRAND and MAGNUS, 1922; GOLLWITZER-MEIER, 1937), and *chloroform*, which seems to lower the warm thresholds but also to act on other cutaneous receptors (REIN, 1925a; SCHMIDT, 1949). Finally, certain substances extracted from *spices*, such as capsaicine, cinnamonylic-acrylic acid piperidide and undecylenic acid vanillylamide elicit strong warm sensations but also pain (STARY, 1925; SANS, 1949).

C. Neurophysiology of Thermoreceptors

1. Biophysical Specificity and Classification

Since any biological process is dependent on temperature, and any neural structure in the skin is exposed to thermal stimuli, qualitative data alone are not sufficient to classify a nerve ending as thermoreceptor. For this decision, quantitative measurements of the response to various kinds of stimuli are required.

Certain receptors in the tongue and external skin of the cat served by myelinated nerve fibres respond to both mechanical and thermal stimulation (Hensel and Zotterman, 1951d; Witt and Hensel, 1959; Iggo, 1968). The same holds for various myelinated fibres in the skin of monkeys (Iggo, 1969) and man (Hensel and Boman, 1960). These "spurious" thermoreceptors are, in fact, slowly adapting mechanoreceptors. In the monkey, their mechanical indentation thresholds tested by von Frey hairs were 5 to 20 μm (Iggo, 1969). Further, the conduction velocities of slowly adapting mechanoreceptors sensitive to cooling were 30 to 80 m/sec and thus considerably higher than those of specific thermoreceptors. Finally, the mechanosensitive fibres did not exhibit a group discharge pattern on cooling which is a typical property of many cold receptors (p. 94).

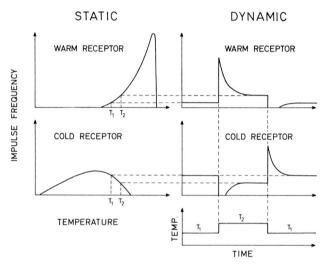

Fig. 5. Generalized response of cutaneous single warm and cold receptors to constant temperatures (static response) and to rapid temperature changes (dynamic response)

There are also unmyelinated C fibres that are stimulated by mechanical deformation and cooling as well (Douglas, Ritchie and Straub, 1960). Iriuchijima and Zotterman (1960) and Witt (1963) have found cutaneous C fibres responding to almost any kind of stimulation, such as pressure, cooling, warming and application of histamine. The function of this group of nerve endings is not yet known.

Other non-myelinated cutaneous fibres in the cat and dog are excited only by intense heating (Iggo, 1959; Hensel, Iggo and Witt, 1960; Iriuchijima and Zotterman, 1960; Bessou and Perl, 1969). The large majority of these "heat" fibres had thresholds above 46°C, sometimes as high as 55°C and responded also to strong mechanical stimuli. This receptor population can rather clearly be distinguished from the group of warm fibres since most of the "heat" receptors, besides being mechanically sensitive, were active at temperatures at which the warm fibres had ceased to discharge.

The first specific thermoreceptors identified by electrophysiological methods were the cold receptors in the tongue of the cat served by small myelinated fibres

Table 2. *Specific thermoreceptors in the external skin*

Species	Nerve	Receptive field	Type of receptor	Author
Man	radial	hairy skin, hand dorsum	cold	HENSEL and BOMAN (1959)
Monkey	median, ulnar saphenous	hairy and glabrous skin, arm and leg	cold	IGGO (1963, 1969), KENSHALO and GALLEGOS (1967), PERL (1968)
	saphenous, radial	hairy skin, hand and foot dorsum	warm	HENSEL (1969), HENSEL and IGGO (1971)
Dog	infra-orbital	hairy and marginal skin, face	cold	HENSEL (1952a), IRIUCHIJIMA and ZOTTERMAN (1960), IGGO (1969)
			warm	IRIUCHIJIMA and ZOTTERMAN (1960)
Cat	infra-orbital	hairy and marginal skin	cold	HENSEL (1952b), BOMAN (1958), IRIUCHIJIMA and ZOTTERMAN (1960
			warm	IRIUCHIJIMA and ZOTTERMAN (1960), HENSEL (1968), HENSEL and KENSHALO (1969)
	saphenous	hairy skin, leg	cold, warm	HENSEL, IGGO and WITT (1960), IRIUCHIJIMA and ZOTTERMAN (1960), STOLWIJK and WEXLER (1971)
Rat	infra-orbital	hairy and marginal skin, face	cold	BOMAN (1958)
	saphenous	hairy skin, leg	cold, warm	IRIUCHIJIMA and ZOTTERMAN (1960)
	scrotal	hairy skin, scrotum	cold, warm	IGGO (1969)

(ZOTTERMAN, 1935, 1936). Their high selective sensitivity was firmly established by numerous investigations (HENSEL and ZOTTERMAN, 1951b; DODT and ZOTTERMAN, 1952b; ZOTTERMAN, 1953; HENSEL, 1966). In the following, lingual thermoreceptors only will be dealt with as far as no corresponding results are available for thermoreceptors in the external skin.

In neurophysiological terms, the *general properties* of cutaneous thermoreceptors can be described as follows: (1) they have a static discharge at constant temperatures (T), (2) they show a dynamic response to temperature changes (dT/dt), with either a positive temperature coefficient (warm receptors) or a negative coefficient (cold receptors), (3) they are not excited by mechanical stimuli within reasonable limits of intensity.

The variety of cutaneous thermoreceptors can be divided, by the criterion of their dynamic response, into well defined classes of *warm* and *cold receptors* (Fig. 5). Irrespective of the initial temperature, a warm receptor will always show an overshoot of its discharge on sudden warming and a transient inhibition on cooling, whereas a cold receptor will respond in the opposite way, namely, with an inhibition on warming and an overshoot on cooling. Besides this dynamic behaviour there are also typical differences in the static frequency curves of both types of cutaneous receptors, in that the temperature of the maximum discharge is much lower for cold receptors than it is for warm receptors.

Table 2 shows the occurrence of specific thermoreceptors in the skin of various homeotherms. Only those receptors have been included whose specificity has been tested according to the above criteria.

In the skin of *human subjects* only very few cold receptors have been identified by electrophysiological methods (HENSEL and BOMAN, 1960). As far as can be judged from the relative spike height, they belonged to the group of myelinated fibres. No warm receptors have been found as yet. It seems quite certain from recent experiments in primates (HENSEL, 1969; HENSEL and IGGO, 1971) that warm receptors in man are served by unmyelinated C fibres.

2. Localization and Structure

a) **Physiological Measurement of Depth.** As long as no morphological evidence was available, one has tried to measure the intracutaneous depth of thermoreceptors by means of physiological methods. These investigations are based on a number of rather vague assumptions and the results thus at best approximative. By use of thermo-electrically controlled intracutaneous temperature movements and measurements of reaction time an average depth of 0.15 to 0.17 mm for cold receptors and 0.3 to 0.6 mm for warm receptors in human subjects was found (BAZETT and McGLONE, 1930; BAZETT, McGLONE and BROCKLEHURST, 1930). The results suggest that the layer of cold receptors is immediately beneath the epidermis, whereas the site of warm receptors is in the upper layers of the corium. A subcutaneous site is out of the question.

Electrophysiological measurements of the depth of thermoreceptors are more accurate, as they exclude any error caused by central information processing. When rapid cold jumps with precise start are applied to the cat's tongue, and the thermal diffusion coefficient of the tissue is known, one can calculate the velocity of the cold wave penetrating the tongue. From the latency of the first cold impulse, amounting to only a few hundredths of a second after the onset of cooling, and the threshold temperature change, a minimum depth of 0.18 ± 0.05 mm for the cold receptors is obtained, whereas the maximum depth is ca. 0.22 mm (HENSEL, STRÖM and ZOTTERMAN, 1951). This means that the receptors must be situated in a rather superficial subepidermal layer.

b) **Morphological Structures.** VON FREY'S (1895) hypothesis that specific corpuscular nerve terminals were the anatomical substrate of thermal receptors has started numerous attempts to identify histologically the underlying neural structures of cold and warm spots in human subjects. The results of these endeavours were negative (For references see HENSEL, 1952a).

Later cold and warm sensitive cutaneous areas in man have been found without any encapsulated or corpuscular nerve endings (HAGEN et al., 1953; WEDDELL, PALMER and PALLIE, 1955; WEDDELL and MILLER, 1962). This rules out v. FREY's original concept but does not disprove, of course, the functional specialization of cold and warm receptors. As SINCLAIR (1955) admits, it remains possible that specialized endings exist, but that the differences are too subtle to be revealed by present histological methods.

Recent electron microscopical studies (CAUNA, 1968, 1969) have given valuable insight into the fine structure of various cutaneous nerve endings but, because of a lack of functional correlation, have not revealed the morphological substrate of thermoreceptors. Further progress in this direction can only be expected by a direct combination of electrophysiological and electron microscopical methods.

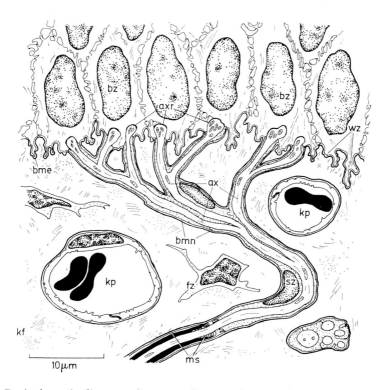

Fig. 6. Semi-schematic diagram of nerve endings at the site of an electrophysiologically identified cold receptor in the hairy skin of the cat's nose. (*ms*) myelin sheath of afferent nerve fibre; (*sz*) non-myelinated Schwann cell accompanying terminal axons (*ax*) to the basal membrane (*bme*) of epidermis; (*bmn*) basement membrane of nerve terminals; (*axr*) receptive endings with mitochondria; (*bz*) basal epidermal cells; (*wz*) root feet of basal cells; (*kp*) capillaries; (*fz*) fibrocyte; (*kf*) collagen fibrils of stratum papillare. (From ANDRES, v. DÜRING and HENSEL, unpublished)

An attempt in this direction was made in the nasal area of cats (KENSHALO et al., 1970). Afferent impulses from single cold and warm fibres dissected from the infra-orbital nerve were led off, and the spot-like receptive fields were localized under the microscope by means of small thermal stimulators with a tip diameter of 0.05 to 0.07 mm. All receptors were carefully tested for specificity. The accuracy of localization was about 0.05 to 0.1 mm. In most cases the cold spots even responded when the stimulator approached without touching the skin, which proves that

A

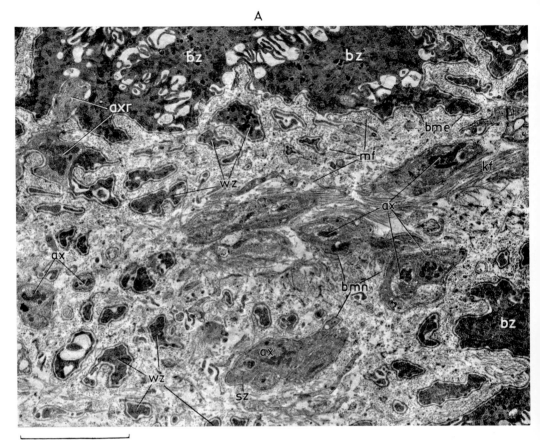

5μm

Fig. 7. *A* electron micrograph of nerve endings at the site of an electrophysiologically identified cold receptor in the hairy skin of the cat's nose. Section through the boundary between stratum papillare and basal epidermis parallel to the skin surface. (*ax*) non-myelinated terminal axons; (*axr*) receptive ending; (*sz*) Schwann cell; (*bmn*) basement membrane of nerve terminals; (*bme*) basement membrane of epidermis; (*bz*) basal epidermal cells; (*wz*) root feet of basal cells; (*kf*) collagen fibrils. ×5000. *B* non-myelinated terminal axon (from Fig. 7*A*, lower edge, middle). (*mi*) mitochondria; (*v*) vesicles in the axoplasm of receptor; (*mv*) membrane vesicles of Schwann cell. For further explanation see Fig. 7*A*. ×32000. Fixation with glutaraldehyde-formalin perfusion and osmium tetroxide, embedding with araldite, staining with uranyl acetate and lead citrate. (From Andres, v. Düring and Hensel, unpublished)

the receptor site must be very superficial. After marking the receptive fields, the skin was excised and prepared for electron microscopy. Further investigations of the ultrastructures of thermoreceptors with an improved technique of intra-vital fixation were carried out by Andres, v. Düring and Hensel (unpublished).

In the hairy skin of the cat's nose the receptive structures at the site of cold spots are served by thin myelinated axons dividing into several non-myelinated terminals within the stratum papillare (Figs. 6 and 7). The terminal axons are

B

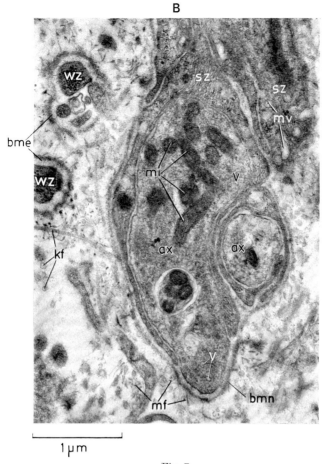

1 μm

Fig. 7

accompanied by unmyelinated Schwann cells as far as the epidermal basement membrane. A continuous connection between the basement membrane of the epidermis and that of the nerve terminals is seen. The receptive endings which penetrate a few microns deep into the basal epidermal cells contain numerous mitochondria as well as an axoplasmatic matrix with fine filaments and micro-vesicles (Fig. 7 B).

With a certain variability such structures were found regularly at the site of electrophysiologically identified cold receptors in the hairy skin of the cat's nose. In the glabrous skin, however, it was difficult to discriminate between the cold-sensitive structures and the axons serving Merkel cells. An analysis of the anatom-ical substrate of warm receptors is in progress but definite results have not been obtained as yet.

c) **Afferent Innervation and Receptive Fields.** Judging from the relative spike height ZOTTERMAN (1936) suggested that the cold fibres of the tongue of the cat

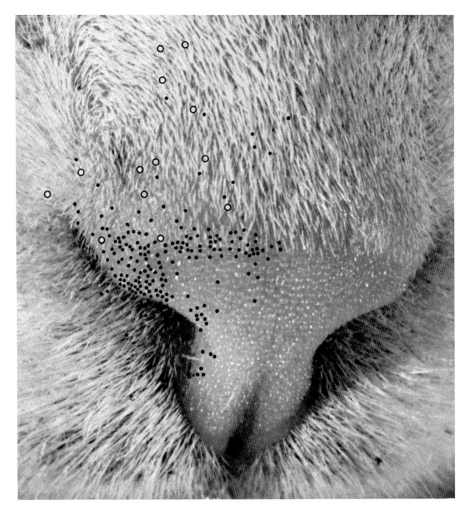

Fig. 8. Spot-like receptive fields of specific single cold fibres (dots) and warm fibres (circles) in the nasal region of the cat. Results from several preparations of the lateral nasal branches of the infra-orbital nerve

were fairly thin myelinated fibres belonging to the A δ group according to Erlanger and Gasser's (1937) nomenclature. The specific cold and warm fibres in the saphenous nerve of the cat belong mainly to the group of non-myelinated C fibres, whereas in the infra-orbital nerve of cat and dog numerous myelinated cold fibres are found. In monkeys the cutaneous cold fibres are myelinated and unmyelinated, the warm fibres only unmyelinated. The distribution of thermal fibres in man is not known; on the basis of available evidence (Hensel and Boman, 1960) it seems probable that part of the cold fibres are myelinated and the warm fibres are non-myelinated. Table 3 summarizes the conduction velocities of single cold and warm fibres in the external skin of several species. We can conclude that cutaneous cold fibres with the highest conduction velocities of 20 m/sec (Iggo, 1959) have diame-

Table 3. *Average conduction velocities of single cold and warm fibres in several species*

Species	Nerve	Receptive field	Cold fibres[a] myelinated m/sec	non-myelinated m/sec	Warm fibres non-myelinated m/sec	Author
Monkey	saphenous	hairy skin, leg and foot dorsum	6.3±2.5 (8)	0.7±0.3 (6)	0.7±0.2 (9)	HENSEL and IGGO (1971)
	radial	hairy skin, hand	8.0±3.0 (16)			PERL (1968)
	musculo-cutaneous	hairy skin, arm	5.2±1.8 (5)	0.6 (1)		IGGO (1969)
	median	glabrous skin, hand	10.7±3.0 (5)			IGGO (1969)
Cat	saphenous	hairy skin, leg		1.0 (3)	0.8 (1)	HENSEL et al. (1960)
	post. fem. cut.	hairy skin, leg		0.8–1.1 (8)	0.8 (2)	BESSOU and PERL (1969)
Dog	saphenous	hairy skin, leg			0.4–0.6 (2)	IRIUCHIJIMA and ZOTTERMAN (1960)
	infra-orbital	hairy and marginal skin, face	14 (3)			IGGO (1969)
Rat	saphenous	hairy skin		0.9±0.1 (6)	1.0±0.2 (7)	IRIUCHIJIMA and ZOTTERMAN (1960)

[a] Number of units indicated in brackets.

ters of 3 to 4 μm (Maruhashi, Mizuguchi and Tasaki, 1952), whereas the diameters of the slowly conducting C fibres are in the range of 1 μm.

In most cases single cold and warm fibres, respectively, innervate one peripheral spot in the skin (Perl, 1968, Iggo, 1969; Hensel and Kenshalo, 1969; Hensel, 1969). Only for primates Kenshalo and Gallegos (1967) have reported single cold fibres to innervate up to 8 multiple spots, the whole field amounting to about 1.7 cm². Fig. 8 shows a map of the tip of the cat's nose with specific cold and warm spots, each of them innervated by a single fibre. In a few cases the cold-sensitive areas were somewhat larger, up to a few tenths of a millimeter, and had a spatially inhomogenous cold sensitivity.

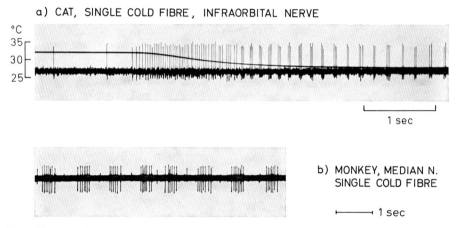

Fig. 9. Burst discharges of single cutaneous cold fibres. *a* Dynamic discharge of a fibre from the cat's infra-orbital nerve and temperature of the thermode when cooling the nose from 32 to 27°C. At constant temperatures of 32 and 27°C the discharge was regular. (From Hensel and Wurster, 1970). *b* Static discharge of a fibre from the median nerve in the monkey at constant temperature of the hairy skin of the forearm. (From Iggo, 1969)

3. Thermoreceptor Excitation and Temperature

a) Static and Dynamic Response of Cold Receptors. At constant skin temperatures in the normal range all cutaneous cold receptors exhibit a static discharge with a constant impulse frequency. The temporal sequence of impulses can be more or less regular, or it can consist of periodic bursts of 2 to 10 impulses separated by silent intervals (Fig. 9). Such bursts have been described for cold fibres in the lingual nerve of cats (Hensel and Zotterman, 1951b; Dodt, 1953), the infra-orbital nerve of cats (Hensel and Kenshalo, 1969; Hensel and Wurster, 1970) and dogs (Iggo, 1969), and the saphenous and trigeminal nerve of monkeys (Iggo, 1963, 1969, 1970; Iggo and Iggo, 1971; Kenshalo and Gallegos, 1967; Poulos, 1971).

The temperature range of static activity varies for different cold fibres, the extremes being about 5°C and 43°C. Low thermal limits of activity were found in cold receptors served by C fibres (Hensel, Iggo and Witt, 1960), whereas for A δ fibres the lowest temperature was about 10°C. The static impulse frequency of individual cold fibres rises with temperature, reaches a maximum and falls again at high temperatures. Sometimes a second maximum is seen at low temperatures in connection with the transition from regular to burst discharges (Fig. 19). Myelinated cutaneous cold fibres have static temperature ranges of more than 20°C and maximum frequencies of 6 to 20 imp/sec (IGGO, 1969; HENSEL and WURSTER, 1970), whereas in non-myelinated cold fibres the static ranges and maximum frequencies may be somewhat smaller (HENSEL, IGGO and WITT, 1960). The temperatures of the maximum discharge are different for each unit and vary in most cases

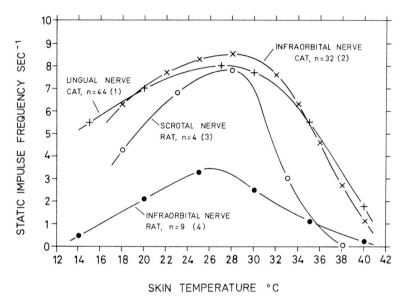

Fig. 10. Comparison of average static frequencies of various cutaneous cold receptor populations as a function of skin temperature. (1) from BENZING et al. (1969), (2) from HENSEL and WURSTER (1970), (3) from IGGO (1969), (4) from BOMAN (1958)

from 18 to 34°C. As Fig. 10 shows, the average temperatures for the maximum activity of various cutaneous cold receptor populations are rather similar, ranging from 26 to 30°C in monkeys, cats and rats. Only in the lip of dogs the average value was near 35°C (IGGO, 1969, 1970; IGGO and IGGO, 1971).

Similar static response characteristics of cold-sensitive units to peripheral thermal stimulation have been obtained by extracellular recording with microelectrodes inserted into different levels of the trigeminal pathway in squirrel and rhesus monkeys. The levels of the system studied were (1) the trigeminal ganglion (POULOS and LENDE, 1970a, b); (2) the descending trigeminal nuclear complex of the medulla (POULOS, 1971); and (3) the ventrobasal complex of the thalamus (POULOS and BENJAMIN, 1968; POULOS, 1971).

Considering the average frequency of cold impulses, there is no possibility of discrimination between static temperatures below and above the maximum, say, 18 and 34°C (Fig. 10). However, the burst discharge might carry additional temperature information independent of the average impulse frequency and thus allow differentiation between lower and higher temperatures. For example, in monkeys the average impulse frequency of cutaneous cold fibres has a positive temperature coefficient in the low temperature range, whereas the number of impulses in a burst as well as the ratio of impulses within a burst to the number of bursts per second has a negative temperature coefficient (Iggo, 1969).

On sudden cooling to a lower temperature level, the cold receptors respond with a transient overshoot in frequency, followed by adaptation to the new static discharge (Figs. 5 and 11). When the skin is warmed up again to the initial level, a transient decrease in frequency or silent period is seen, after which the frequency

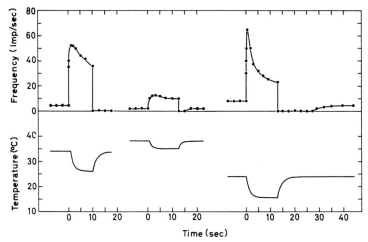

Fig. 11. Impulse frequency of a single cold fibre from the superficial branch of the radial nerve in man and skin temperature as a function of time when applying thermal stimuli to the dorsum of the hand. (From Hensel and Boman, 1960)

rises again and finally reaches the initial static value. The highest dynamic over-shoot observed in a single cutaneous cold fibre was 300 imp/sec (Iggo, 1969), the highest ratio of static to dynamic frequencies 1:30. Cutaneous cold receptors in the trigeminal area of cats often respond with a burst discharge on cooling even when the static discharges are fairly regular (Fig. 9a).

The higher the rate of cooling at a given temperature, the higher is the dynamic overshoot (Hensel, 1953a). On rectangular cooling of single cold units, the magnitude of this overshoot is a linear function of the stimulus magnitude within a range of 5 to 10°C (Hensel, 1953b; Darian-Smith and Dykes, 1971). When equal temperature changes are applied at various adapting temperatures, the dynamic overshoot is a function of temperature and follows approximately the shape of the static activity curve (Hensel and Zotterman, 1951b; Iggo, 1969; Kenshalo et al., 1971), as shown in Fig. 12 for a population of cold units from the Gasserian ganglion in the cat, the receptive fields of which were localized in the nasal region.

From the slope of the static and dynamic frequency curves we can derive the static and dynamic *differential sensitivity* ($\Delta v / \Delta T$), i.e., the change in frequency (Δv) for a small change in temperature (ΔT). Of course, the dynamic differential

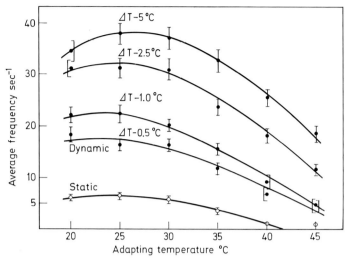

Fig. 12. Average static frequency and average dynamic peak frequencies of 25 specific cold units in the Gasserian ganglion of the cat as a function of adapting temperature when applying cold stimuli of −0.5 to −5.0 °C to the nose at a cooling rate of −0.4 °C/sec. The amount of cooling (ΔT) is indicated on the dynamic curves. (From KENSHALO et al., 1971)

sensitivity increases with the rate of temperature change. Some extreme values of dynamic differential sensitivities obtained with high rates of change are given in Table 4.

b) Static and Dynamic Response of Warm Receptors. The quantitative relationship between temperature stimulus and activity of cutaneous warm receptors has been studied recently in the infra-orbital nerve of cats (HENSEL, 1968; HENSEL and KENSHALO, 1969; HENSEL and HUOPANIEMI, 1969) and, to some extent, in the radial and saphenous nerve of monkeys (HENSEL, 1969). In addition, a few quantitative data are available from non-myelinated warm fibres in the cat saphenous nerve (HENSEL, IGGO and WITT, 1960; STOLWIJK and WEXLER, 1971) and the scrotal nerve of rats (IGGO, 1969).

Warming the nasal region of cats elicits a mass discharge of warm impulses in the lateral nasal branch of the infra-orbital nerve serving the apical hairy skin of the nose (Figs. 8 and 13). Similar multi-fibre discharges on warming have been

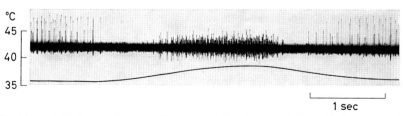

Fig. 13. Afferent discharge of a multi-fibre preparation from the infra-orbital nerve of the cat and skin temperature during thermal stimulation of the nose. The activity of specific cold and warm fibre populations is clearly distinguishable. (From HENSEL and HUOPANIEMI, 1969)

recorded from the scrotal nerve in rats (Iggo, 1969) and from the saphenous nerve in cats (Stolwijk and Wexler, 1971).

In the experiment shown in Fig. 14, the nerve preparation contained a single warm fibre and a single cold fibre. Both units had different receptive fields and could be stimulated separately.

Fig. 15 shows the average static frequencies of warm and cold receptor populations in the infra-orbital nerve of the cat as a function of skin temperature. There is some overlap in the static temperature ranges of both groups, the curves crossing near 37°C. The population of infra-orbital warm receptors is surprisingly homogenous, the maximum discharges being between 45 and 47°C. In the whole temperature range the sequence of impulses is fairly regular, in contrast to the burst discharge of cold receptors. When the temperature exceeds that at which activity is maximal the impulse discharge stops rather abruptly, this inhibition being completely reversible. A summary of quantitative data for populations of cold and warm receptors in the nasal area of cats is given in Table 4.

Table 4. *Properties of single cold and warm fibres from the nasal area of cats*[a]

Property	Cold fibres	Warm fibres
Number of units	26	22
Static temperature limits	5 ... 43°C	30 ... 48°C
Maximum static frequency (average)	9 impulses/sec	36 impulses/sec
Temperature of static maximum (average)	27°C	46°C
Maximum static differential sensitivity (average)	–1 impulses/sec°C	+14 impulses/sec°C
Highest dynamic differential sensitivity	–50 impulses/sec°C	+70 impulses/sec°C
Highest dynamic frequency	240 impulses/sec	200 impulses/sec

[a] From Hensel and Kenshalo (1969).

In primates, specific warm receptors have been discovered only recently in the dorsum of hand and foot (Hensel, 1969). Their spot-like fields are served by non-myelinated fibres (Hensel and Iggo, 1971) which show a rather regular discharge pattern at temperatures below the static maximum. The primate warm receptors differ in some respect from those in the cat's nose (Fig. 16). One group seems to have a similar temperature dependence of static activity as has been found for infra-orbital warm receptors, the maximum being near 45°C, but another group has their maximum discharge at temperatures between 40 and 42°C. At higher temperatures the discharge slows down and changes from a regular to a more irregular or a burst pattern.

The limited amount of quantitative data for other warm receptors does not allow detailed comparisons. A non-myelinated unit in the saphenous nerve of the cat had a static sensitivity range from 38.5 to 43°C and a sharp maximum at 41.2°C (Hensel, Iggo and Witt, 1960) whereas the respective data for another unit in the scrotal nerve were 37 to 45°C and 42°C (Iggo, 1969).

On sudden temperature changes the warm receptors behave in the opposite way than do the cold receptors, in that they respond to warming with an overshoot

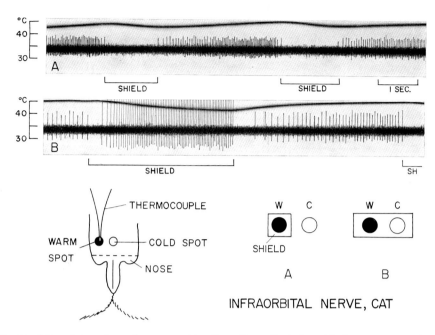

Fig. 14. Afferent impulses of a preparation from the cat's infra-orbital nerve containing a single warm fibre and a single cold fibre. A when the warm (W) spot on the nose is shielded from heat radiation the warm fibre discharge stops. B simultaneous shielding of warm (W) and cold (C) spot causes inhibition of warm fibre and excitation of cold fibre. (From HENSEL and KENSHALO, 1969)

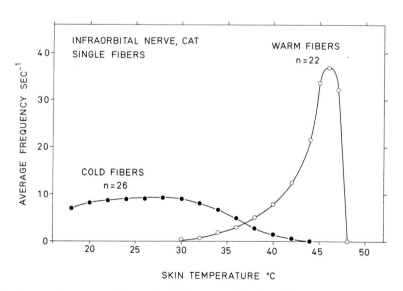

Fig. 15. Average frequency of the static discharge as a function of temperature for populations of single warm and cold fibres from the cat's infra-orbital nerve supplying the nose. (From HENSEL and KENSHALO, 1969)

7*

and to cooling with transient inhibition (Fig. 5). The highest dynamic response of a single warm fibre from the cat's nose was 200 imp/sec, that is 5.5 times higher than the average static maximum of 36 imp/sec.

The diagram in Fig. 17 shows the static frequency as well as the dynamic maximum on sudden warming as a function of temperature for 3 single warm fibres. At temperatures below the static threshold, dynamic responses can still be

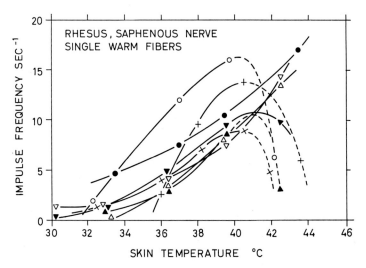

Fig. 16. Static frequency of single warm fibres from the monkey's saphenous nerve as a function of constant temperatures. The receptive fields were in the hairy skin on the dorsum of foot and toes. Solid lines: regular discharge pattern; dashed lines: irregular discharge or periodic bursts

elicited. When the adapting temperature increases between 28 and 44°C, the overshoot caused by equal amounts of warming (Δ T) becomes higher, the slope of the dynamic curves being steeper than that of the static ones. These results are analogous to those found for cold receptors.

4. The Adequate Stimulus

From the neurophysiological data we can conclude that the excitation of cutaneous thermoreceptors is dependent (1) on the absolute temperature (T) and (2) on the rate of temperature change (dT/dt) or the temporal gradient.

The hypothesis of *spatial* temperature gradients (dT/dx) being the adequate stimulus of thermosensitive nerve endings could not be verified by cooling the tongue of the cat with reversed gradients (Hensel and Zotterman, 1951e; Hensel and Witt, 1959). When a cold receptor on the surface of the tongue is cooled from above, its discharge frequency will increase (Fig. 18). On cooling the tongue from the lower surface, however, the resting discharge of the cold receptor will increase as well, in spite of a reversed spatial temperature gradient. Thus we come

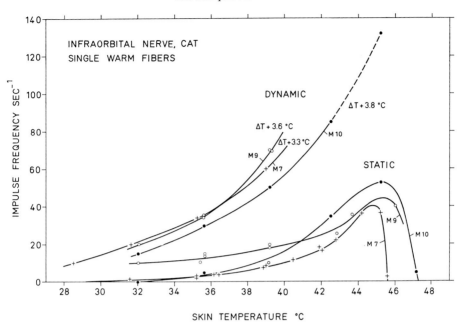

Fig. 17. Static impulse frequency and dynamic peak frequency on sudden warming as a function of skin temperature for 3 single warm fibres from the cat's nose. The amount of warming (ΔT) is indicated on the dynamic curves. The dashed part of the curve is extrapolated from warming by 2.8°C. (From HENSEL and HUOPANIEMI, 1969)

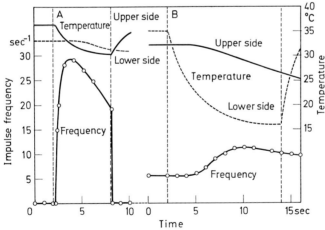

Fig. 18. Impulse frequency of a single cold fibre in the lingual nerve of the cat and temperature on both sides of the tongue when cooling the upper and lower surface, respectively. (From HENSEL and WITT, 1959)

to the conclusion that in accordance with sensory experiments (p. 85) the adequate stimulus of thermoreceptors is temperature and its temporal change *per se* and not the direction or slope of a spatial gradient.

5. Inadequate Stimulation

a) Paradoxical Discharge. The occurrence of "paradoxical" excitations at extreme temperatures has not been studied systematically in cutaneous thermoreceptors but was reported in cold fibres from the lingual nerve of cats (Dodt and Zotterman, 1952b). Whereas at temperatures between 40 and 45°C no static discharge of these fibres is seen, they start again discharging at lingual temperatures above 45°C (Fig. 19). On further warming, the frequency of this "paradoxical" excitation rises and reaches a maximum at about 50°C. Above this value the receptors will be damaged.

No "paradoxical" discharge of cutaneous warm receptors has been observed as yet; however, as Dodt and Zotterman (1952a) and Dodt (1953) have reported, fibres in the chorda tympani sensitive to warming respond with a phasic burst of impulses when the tongue is cooled rapidly by more than 8°C.

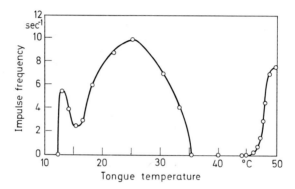

Fig. 19. Impulse frequency of a single cold fibre from the cat's tongue as a function of constant temperatures. Above 45°C a "paradoxical" discharge occurs. (From Zotterman, 1953)

b) Chemical Stimulation. *Menthol* causes a shift of the activity range of lingual cold receptors towards higher temperatures. When the cat tongue is kept at 40°C there is no static activity in most cases. Application of menthol dissolved in water (1:10^4) elicits a strong discharge of cold impulse which can be stopped by further warming of the tongue (Hensel and Zotterman, 1951c). Further investigations have shown that menthol not only enhances the normal activity of cold receptors but also the paradoxical discharge at 45 to 50°C (Dodt, Skouby and Zotterman, 1953).

Dodt, Skouby and Zotterman (1953) have tested the action of cholinergic substances on single cold fibres in the lingual nerve of the cat. *Acetylcholine* in small doses extended the static activity range towards higher temperatures, whereas higher doses inhibited the static discharge.

Increased concentrations of CO_2 reduce the discharge frequency of lingual cold receptors in the cat and stimulate at the same time receptors sensitive to warming (Dodt, 1956; Boman, Hensel and Witt, 1957). This corresponds well with the subjective experiences in a CO_2 bath. When the *blood supply* to the tongue is arrested, the steady discharge of cold receptors in the tongue gradually diminishes and often falls to zero within 2 or 4 min (HENSEL, 1953c). Release of the arterial occlusion is followed by a transient overshoot and complete restoration of the initial discharge within 1 min. This behaviour of cold receptors is in accordance with the subjective experiences known as "Ebbecke's phenomenon" (EBBECKE, 1917): When an extremity is exposed to low temperatures and its arterial blood supply arrested, the cold sensation diminishes gradually. After releasing the occlusion the inflow of blood is accompanied by an intense cold sensation.

6. Theoretical Considerations

It is obvious that thermoreceptors show a continuous discharge even when the temporal and spatial temperature gradient is zero, that is, no thermal energy is transferred between the environment and the receptor. Of course, no static discharge is possible without energy but this energy may be derived from chemical processes within the receptor rather than from the transfer of thermal energy, the temperature being only a controlling factor for metabolic rates.

The fundamental mechanisms of thermoreceptor excitation are still unknown. Several hypothetic models have been proposed but these are so far only formal in nature. In order to describe formally the behaviour of thermoreceptors, such a model should at least account for (1) the difference between warm and cold receptors, (2) the static response at constant temperatures and (3) the dynamic response to temperature changes.

The course of the receptor discharge at constant temperatures and particularly the effect of temperature changes suggest that we have to deal with at least two interacting processes. SAND (1938) has assumed an exciting (E) and an inhibiting (I) process, the condition for the initiation of impulses being $E > I$. This model would principally account for the static behaviour of cold as well as of warm receptors since the static frequency curves of both are of similar shape with static maxima at certain temperatures. The time dependence of the discharge could be introduced by the assumption that E and I change exponentially with different time constants k_E and k_I when the temperature is changed between two levels. The temporal course of the impulse frequency would thus follow from the difference of two exponential functions.

For lingual cold receptors k_E was found to be 0.3 to 2.2 sec (HENSEL, 1963a), whereas k_I was smaller than 0.1 sec. By varying k_E and k_I, the dynamic response of both cold and warm receptors could be described. For further details see HENSEL (1952a) and ZOTTERMAN (1953).

A more recent model (ZERBST and DITTBERNER, 1970; ZERBST, 1972) is based on the assumption that a chemical reaction of transmitter release is coupled with the diffusion transport of the transmitter to the excitable membrane. In the membrane compartment the transmitter is inactivated by some chemical process and also removed by diffusion. Temperature alters the velocity coefficients of the chemical reactions whilst the diffusion coefficients are unaltered by temperature. This model was found to agree well with the stimulus response characteristics of cold receptors.

D. Comparison of Various Approaches to Thermoreceptor Function

In the present state of research it is difficult to arrive at a synopsis of experiments dealing with sensory, neurophysiological, behavioural and thermoregulatory aspects of the function of cutaneous thermoreceptors. Only very few measurements of afferent impulses from cutaneous thermoreceptors in human subjects have been made as yet (Hensel and Boman, 1960). The results prove that specific cold receptors exist but do not allow a quantitative correlation between the properties of thermoreceptor populations with the data of temperature sensation. Any conclusion from animal experiments must remain more or less hypothetical because (1) the structure of animal and human skin and hence the distribution and behaviour of thermoreceptors might differ considerably and (2) animals have no verbal communication and, therefore, will hardly give detailed informations about the quality of their sensations. Provided that thermoreceptors in man are comparable with those in homeothermic animals, there would be a good agreement between thermoreceptor activity and the facts of human temperature sensation.

At skin temperatures near $33°$ C cold and warm receptors are continously active (Figs. 11 and 15) but no conscious temperature sensation is observed. The latter begins only when a relatively high number of thermal impulses per unit of time reaches the central nervous system. Thus the threshold of thermal sensations is correlated with an integrative central process rather than with the activity of single peripheral receptors. This *"central threshold"* may possibly be expressed as the magnitude of a slow cortical potential (P_T), which, in turn, is dependent on the average impulse frequency (v) and the number (n) of simultaneously active receptors. Since the frequency of single temperature fibres is a function of absolute temperature (T) and rate of change (dT/dt), whereas the number of active units depends on the surface area (F), the condition for conscious temperature sensations (E_T) can be expressed as follows

$$E_T \rightarrow P_T \rightarrow f(n, v) \rightarrow \varphi(T, dT/dt, F).$$

In accordance with this concept is the observation that in human subjects the warm thresholds fluctuate statistically and the relative number of positive answers is a probability function of the temperature stimulus (Eijkman and Vendrik, 1963; Vendrik and Eijkman, 1968). This suggests that, according to the "detection theory", the sensory threshold for warmth is dependent on the signal-to-noise ratio of nervous activity. The sub-threshold static discharge of cutaneous thermoreceptors can be considered as "internal noise" of the system.

Järvilehto (unpublished) has tried recently to determine the central threshold of conscious temperature sensation when stimulating a single cold spot in human skin. After having determined the threshold of sensation, identical stimuli were applied to single cold spots in the skin of the cat's nose and the impulses in single afferent fibres recorded. The threshold of conscious cold sensations corresponded to an average impulse frequency of 65 sec^{-1}. This is much higher than the conscious threshold of hair receptors in human subjects which might correspond to only a single impulse in a single fibre (Hensel and Boman, 1960).

The presence of separate cold and warm spots in human skin and the electrophysiological findings of specific cutaneous cold and warm receptors support the theory that the sensory qualities of "cold" and "warmth" can be ascribed to a *dual* set of receptors. However, it remains possible that, for example, inhibition of the static cold receptor discharge might be associated with certain warm sensations, but the assumption of only one cold-sensitive receptor system accounting for all facts of human temperature sensation would be incompatible with several experimental findings, e.g. with the fact that blocking of A fibres by pressure on the radial nerve in human subjects abolishes the cold sensation, whereas the warm sensation persists (Torebjörk and Hallin, 1972).

   Behavioural measurements of the thresholds for thermal stimulation of the face of cats have revealed a temperature sensitivity comparable with that of the

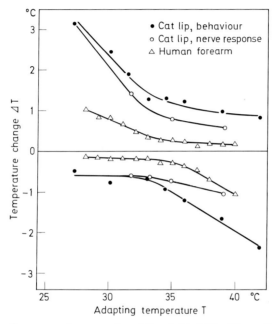

Fig. 20. Behaviourally measured warm and cool thresholds (ΔT) of the cat's upper lip (1.7 cm²) and electrophysiologically measured "thresholds" (equal magnitudes of integrated nerve potential) as a function of adapting temperature (T). Thermal thresholds on human forearm (14.4 cm²) are also shown for comparison. (From Kenshalo and Brearley, 1970; human threshold data from Kenshalo, 1969)

human forearm (Kenshalo, Duncan and Weymark, 1967; Brearley and Kenshalo, 1970). When the thresholds (ΔT) were plotted as a function of adapting temperature (T), and the larger surface area in human experiments was accounted for, the curves for cat and man were surprisingly similar (Fig. 20). In contrast to the face, other cutaneous regions, such as back and thigh, were less sensitive to cooling and highly insensitive to warming, the cats responding only to noxious heat (Kenshalo, 1964; Kenshalo, Duncan and Weymark, 1967).

   When the activity of multi-fibre preparations supplying the cat's upper lip is recorded, the integrated steady discharge shows a phasic increase on cooling and a phasic decrease on warming. By using equal magnitudes of the integrated response as a criterion, one can obtain electrophysiological "threshold" curves as a function of adapting temperatures (Kenshalo, 1968; Kenshalo and Brearley, 1970). A comparison of electrophysiological and behavioural thresholds is shown in Fig. 20. The question remains open whether a decrease in the integrated discharge means a quality of "warmth" or of "less cool" for the cat. In addition, the possibility cannot be excluded that the integrated potential also contained small impulses from warm fibres being masked by the larger spikes from cold fibres.

Afferents from cutaneous thermoreceptors are not only a source of conscious information but also a very important input for the system of *temperature regulation* (Thauer, 1958; Hardy, 1961; Hensel, 1966; Hammel, 1968). They can signal thermal disturbances from the skin before the central temperature of the body has been influenced. This function of cutaneous receptors is favoured by the fact that they have a high dynamic sensitivity and thus respond in particular to rapid thermal disturbances.

It should be emphasized that thermoregulatory reflexes from cutaneous cold and warm receptors may be elicited even when no conscious sensations or behavioural responses are present, e. g., during sleep. Experiments in unanesthetized cats have shown that warming the leg in water of 40°C causes a marked reflex vasodilatation in the ear. The peripheral origin of this reflex is proved by the fact that the central body temperature, as measured in the hypothalamus, drops at the same time (Kundt, Brück and Hensel, 1957). However, as shown by Kenshalo (1964), warming the cat's leg to 40°C does not lead to any behavioural response. Thus the behavioural threshold for thermal stimuli seems to be considerably higher than the threshold for thermoregulatory reflexes.

References

Alrutz, S.: Studien auf dem Gebiet der Temperatursinne. I. Skand. Arch. Physiol. **7**, 321–340 (1897).

Alrutz, S.: Studien auf dem Gebiet der Temperatursinne. II. Skand. Arch. Physiol. **10**, 340–352 (1900).

Bazett, H.C., McGlone, B.: Experiments on the mechanism of stimulation of end-organs for cold. Amer. J. Physiol. **93**, 632 (1930).

Bazett, H.C., McGlone, B., Brocklehurst, R.J.: The temperatures in the tissues which accompany temperature sensations. J. Physiol. (Lond.) **69**, 88–112 (1930).

Benzing, H., Hensel, H., Wurster, R.D.: Integrated static activity of lingual cold receptors. Pflügers Arch. **311**, 50–54 (1969).

Bessou, P., Perl, E.R.: Response of cutaneous sensory units with unmyelinated fibres to noxious stimuli. J. Neurophysiol. **32**, 1025–1043 (1969).

Blix, M.: Experimentala bidrag till lösning af frågan om hudnervernas specifika energi. I. Upsala Läk.-Fören. Förh. **18**, 87–102 (1882–1883).

Boman, K.K.A.: Elektrophysiologische Untersuchungen über die Thermoreceptoren der Gesichtshaut. Acta physiol. scand. **44**, Suppl. 149 (1958).

Boman, K.K.A., Hensel, H., Witt, I.: Die Entladung der Kaltreceptoren bei äußerer Einwirkung von Kohlensäure. Pflügers Arch. ges. Physiol. **264**, 107–112 (1957).

Brearley, E.A., Kenshalo, D.R.: Behavioural measurements of the sensitivity of cat's upper lip to warm and cool stimuli. J. comp. physiol. Psychol. **70**, 1–4 (1970).

Cauna, N.: Light and electron microscopical structure of sensory end-organs in human skin. In: The skin senses (ed. D.R. Kenshalo), pp. 15–37. Springfield, Ill.: Charles C. Thomas 1968.

Cauna, N.: The fine morphology of the sensory receptor organs in the auricle of the rat. J. comp. Neurol. **136**, 81–98 (1969).

DARIAN-SMITH, I., DYKES, R.W.: Peripheral neural mechanisms of thermal sensation. In: Oral-facial sensory and motor mechanisms (ed. R. DUBNER and Y. KAWAMURA), p. 7–22. New York: Appleton-Century-Crofts, Meredith. Corp. 1971.

DODT, E.: The behaviour of thermoreceptors at low and high temperatures with special reference to Ebbecke's temperature phenomena. Acta physiol. scand. 27, 295–314 (1953).

DODT, E.: Die Aktivität der Thermoreceptoren bei nichtthermischen Reizen bekannter thermoregulatorischer Wirkung. Pflügers Arch. ges. Physiol. 263, 188–200 (1956).

DODT, E., SKOUBY, A.P., ZOTTERMAN, Y.: The effect of cholinergic substances on the discharges from thermal receptors. Acta physiol. scand. 28, 101–114 (1953).

DODT, E., ZOTTERMAN, Y.: Mode of action of warm receptors. Acta physiol. scand. 26, 345–357 (1952a).

DODT, E., ZOTTERMAN, Y.: The discharge of specific cold fibres at high temperatures. (The paradoxical cold.) Acta physiol. scand. 26, 358–365 (1952b).

DOUGLAS, W.W., RITCHIE, J.M., STRAUB, R.W.: The role of non-myelinated fibres in signalling cooling of the skin. J. Physiol. (Lond.) 150, 266–283 (1960).

EBAUGH, F.G., Jr., THAUER, R.: Influence of various environmental temperatures on the cold and warm threshold. J. appl. Physiol. 3, 173–182 (1950).

EBBECKE, U.: Über die Temperaturempfindungen in ihrer Abhängigkeit von der Hautdurchblutung und von den Reflexzentren. Pflügers Arch. ges. Physiol. 169, 395–462 (1917)

EIJKMAN, E.G., VENDRIK, A.J.H.: Detection theory applied to the absolute sensitivity of sensory systems. Biophys. J. 3, 65–78 (1963).

ERLANGER, J., GASSER, H.S.: Electrical signs of nervous activity. Philadelphia (Pa.): Philadelphia University Press 1937.

FREY, M. von: Beiträge zur Sinnesphysiologie der Haut. III. Ber. sächs. Ges. (Akad.) Wiss. 47, 166–184 (1895).

GERTZ, E.: Psychophysische Untersuchungen über die Adaptation im Gebiet der Temperatursinne und über ihren Einfluß auf die Reiz- und Unterschiedsschwellen. II. Hälfte. Z. Sinnesphysiol. 52, 105–156 (1921).

GOLDSCHEIDER, A.: Gesammelte Abhandlungen. Leipzig: Johann Ambrosius Barth 1898.

GOLLWITZER-MEIER, K.: Beiträge zur Wärmeregulation auf Grund von Bäderwirkungen. Klin. Wschr. 1937 II, 1418–1421.

GRUNDIG, J.: Zur Frage der paradoxen Warmempfindungen. Z. Biol. 89, 547–554 (1930).

HAGEN, E., KNOCHE, H., SINCLAIR, D.C., WEDDELL, G.: The role of specialized nerve terminals in cutaneous sensibility. Proc. roy. Soc. B 141, 279–287 (1953).

HAHN, H.: Die Reize und die Reizbedingungen des Temperatursinnes. I. Der für den Temperatursinn adäquate Reiz. Pflügers Arch. ges. Physiol. 215, 133–169 (1927).

HAHN, H.: Beiträge zur Reizphysiologie. Heidelberg: Scherer 1949.

HAMMEL, H.T.: Regulation of internal body temperature. Ann. Rev. Physiol. 30, 641–710 (1968).

HARDY, J.D.: Physiology of temperature regulation. Physiol. Rev. 41, 521–606 (1961).

HARDY, J.D., OPPEL, TH.W.: Studies in temperature sensation. III. J. clin. Invest. 16, 535–540 (1937).

HARDY, J.D., OPPEL, TH.W.: Studies in temperature sensation. IV. J. clin. Invest. 17, 771–778 (1938).

HENSEL, H.: Die intracutane Temperaturbewegung bei Einwirkung äußerer Temperaturreize. Pflügers Arch. ges. Physiol. 252, 146–164 (1950a).

HENSEL, H.: Temperaturempfindung und intracutane Wärmebewegung. Pflügers Arch. ges. Physiol. 252, 165–215 (1950b).

HENSEL, H.: Physiologie der Thermoreception. Ergebn. Physiol. 47, 166–368 (1952a).

HENSEL, H.: Afferente Impulse aus den Kältereceptoren der äußeren Haut. Pflügers Arch. ges. Physiol. 256, 195–211 (1952b).

HENSEL, H.: The time factor in thermoreceptor excitation. Acta physiol. scand. 29, 109–116 (1953a).

HENSEL, H.: Das Verhalten der Thermoreceptoren bei Temperatursprüngen. Pflügers Arch. ges. Physiol. 256, 470–487 (1953b).

HENSEL, H.: Das Verhalten der Thermoreceptoren bei Ischämie. Pflügers Arch. ges. Physiol. 257, 371–383 (1953c).

HENSEL, H.: Allgemeine Sinnesphysiologie, Hautsinne, Geschmack, Geruch. Berlin-Heidel-berg-New York: Springer 1966.

HENSEL, H.: Spezifische Wärmeimpulse aus der Nasenregion der Katze. Pflügers Arch. **302**, 374–376 (1968).

HENSEL, H.: Cutane Wärmereceptoren bei Primaten. Pflügers Arch. **313**, 150–152 (1969).

HENSEL, H., BOMAN, K. K.A.: Afferent impulses in cutaneous sensory nerves in human subjects. J. Neurophysiol. **23**, 564–578 (1960).

HENSEL, H., HUOPANIEMI, T.: Static and dynamic properties of warm fibres in the infra-orbital nerve. Pflügers Arch. **309**, 1–10 (1969).

HENSEL, H., IGGO, A.: Analysis of cutaneous warm and cold fibres in primates. Pflügers Arch. **329**, 1–8 (1971).

HENSEL, H., IGGO, A., WITT, I.: A quantitative study of sensitive cutaneous thermoreceptors with C afferent fibres. J. Physiol. (Lond.) **153**, 113–126 (1960).

HENSEL, H., KENSHALO, D. R.: Warm receptors in the nasal region of cats. J. Physiol. (Lond.) **204**, 99–112 (1969).

HENSEL, H., STRÖM, L., ZOTTERMAN, Y.: Electrophysiological measurements of depth of thermoreceptors. J. Neurophysiol. **14**, 423–429 (1951).

HENSEL, H., WITT, I.: Spatial temperature gradient and thermoreceptor stimulation. J. Physiol. (Lond.) **148**, 180–189 (1959).

HENSEL, H., WURSTER, R.D.: Static properties of cold receptors in nasal area of cats. J. Neurophysiol. **33**, 271–275 (1970).

HENSEL, H., ZOTTERMAN, Y.: The response of the cold receptors to constant cooling. Acta physiol. scand. **22**, 96–113 (1951a).

HENSEL, H., ZOTTERMAN, Y.: Quantitative Beziehungen zwischen der Entladung einzelner Kältefasern und der Temperatur. Acta physiol. scand. **23**, 291–319 (1951b).

HENSEL, H., ZOTTERMAN, Y.: The effect of menthol on the thermoreceptors. Acta physiol. scand. **24**, 27–34 (1951c).

HENSEL, H., ZOTTERMAN, Y.: The response of mechanoreceptors to thermal stimulation. J. Physiol. (Lond.) **115**, 16–24 (1951d).

HENSEL, H., ZOTTERMAN, Y.: Action potentials of cold fibres and intracutaneous temperature gradient. J. Neurophysiol. **14**, 377–385 (1951e).

HIRSCHSOHN, J., MAENDL, H.: Studien zur Dynamik der endovenösen Injektion bei Anwendung von Calcium. Wien. Arch. inn. Med. **4**, 379–414 (1922).

IGGO, A.: Cutaneous heat and cold receptors with slowly-conducting (C) afferent fibres. Quart. J. exp. Physiol. **44**, 362–370 (1959).

IGGO, A.: An electrophysiological analysis of afferent fibres in primate skin. Acta neuroveg. (Wien) **24**, 225–240 (1963).

IGGO, A.: Electrophysiological and histological studies of cutaneous mechanoreceptors. In: The skin senses (ed. D.R. KENSHALO), pp. 84–111. Springfield, Ill.: Charles C. Thomas 1968.

IGGO, A.: Cutaneous thermoreceptors in primates and sub-primates. J. Physiol. (Lond.) **200**, 403–430 (1969).

IGGO, A.: The mechanisms of biological temperature reception. In: Physiological and beha-vioural temperature regulation (ed. J.D. HARDY, A.P. GAGGE and J.A.J. STOLWIJK), pp. 391–407. Springfield, Ill.: Charles C. Thomas 1970.

IGGO, A., IGGO, B.J.: Impulse coding in primate cutaneous thermoreceptors in dynamic thermal conditions. J. Physiol. (Paris) **63**, 287–290 (1971).

IRIUCHIJIMA, J., ZOTTERMAN, Y.: The specificity of afferent cutaneous C fibres in mammals. Acta physiol. scand. **49**, 267–278 (1960).

KENSHALO, D.R.: The temperature sensitivity of furred skin of cats. J. Physiol. (Lond.) **172**, 439–448 (1964).

KENSHALO, D.R.: Behavioural and electrophysiological responses of cats to thermal stimuli. In: The skin senses (ed. D.R. KENSHALO), pp. 400–422. Springfield, Ill.: Charles C. Thomas 1968.

KENSHALO, D.R.: Psychophysical studies of temperature sensitivity. In: Contributions to sensory physiology (ed. W.D. NEFF). New York: Academic Press 1969.

KENSHALO, D.R., BREARLEY, E.A.: Electrophysiological measurements of the sensitivity of cat's upper lip to warm and cool stimuli. J. comp. physiol. Psychol. **70**, 5–14 (1970).

KENSHALO, D.R., DUNCAN, D.G., WEYMARK, C.: Thresholds for thermal stimulation of the inner thigh, footpad, and face of cats. J. comp. physiol. Psychol. **63**, 133–138 (1967).

KENSHALO, D.R., GALLEGOS, E.S.: Multiple temperature-sensitive spots innervated by single nerve fibres. Science **158**, 1064–1065 (1967).

KENSHALO, D.R., HENSEL, H., GRAZIADEI, P., FRUHSTORFER, H.: On the anatomy, physiology and psychophysics of the cat's temperature sensing system. In: Oral-facial sensory and motor mechanisms (ed. R. DUBNER and Y. KAWAMURA), p. 23–45. New York: Appleton-Century-Crofts, Meredith. Corp. 1971.

KENSHALO, D.R., HOLMES, CH.E., WOOD, P.B.: Warm and cool thresholds as a function of rate of stimulus temperature change. Perception and Psychophysics **3**, 81–84 (1968).

KUNDT, H.W., BRÜCK, K., HENSEL, H.: Hypothalamustemperatur und Hautdurchblutung der nichtnarkotisierten Katze. Pflügers Arch. ges. Physiol. **264**, 97–106 (1957).

LELE, P.P.: Relationship between cutaneous thermal thresholds, skin temperature and cross-sectional area of the stimulus. J. Physiol. (Lond.) **126**, 191–205 (1954).

LILJESTRAND, G., MAGNUS, R.: Die Wirkungen des Kohlensäurebades beim Gesunden nebst Bemerkungen über den Einfluß des Hochgebirges. Pflügers Arch. ges. Physiol. **193**, 527–554 (1922).

MARÉCHAUX, E.W., SCHÄFER, K.E.: Über Temperaturempfindungen bei Einwirkung von Temperaturreizen verschiedener Steilheit auf den ganzen Körper. Pflügers Arch. ges. Physiol. **251**, 765–784 (1949).

MARUHASHI, I., MIZUGUCHI, K., TASAKI, I.: Action currents in single afferent nerve fibres elicited by stimulation of the skin of the toad and the cat. J. Physiol. (Lond.) **117**, 129–151 (1952).

MÜLLER, J.: Handbuch der Physiologie des Menschen, Bd. 1. Koblenz: J. Hölscher 1840.

PERL, E.R.: Myelinated afferent fibres innervating the primate skin and their response to noxious stimuli. J. Physiol. (Lond.) **197**, 593–615 (1968).

POULOS, D.A.: Trigeminal temperature mechanisms. In: Oral-facial sensory and motor mechanisms (ed. R. DUBNER and Y. KAWAMURA), p. 47–72. New York: Appleton-Century-Crofts, Meredith. Corp. 1971.

POULOS, D.A., BENJAMIN, R.M.: Response of thalamic neurons to thermal stimulation of the tongue. J. Neurophysiol. **31**, 28–43 (1968).

POULOS, D.A., LENDE, R.A.: Response of trigeminal ganglion neurons to thermal stimulation of oral-facial regions. I. Steady-state response. J. Neurophysiol. **33**, 508–517 (1970a).

POULOS, D.A., LENDE, R.A.: Response of trigeminal ganglion neurons to thermal stimulation of oral-facial regions. II. Temperature change response. J. Neurophysiol. **33**, 518–526 (1970b).

REENPÄÄ, Y.: Allgemeine Sinnesphysiologie. Frankfurt a.M.: V. Klostermann 1962.

REIN, H.: Beiträge zu der Lehre von der Temperaturempfindung der menschlichen Haut. Z. Biol. **82**, 189–212 (1925a).

REIN, H.: Über die Topographie der Warmempfindung. Beziehungen zwischen Innervation und receptorischen Endorganen. Z. Biol. **82**, 513–535 (1925b).

SAND, A.: The function of the ampullae of Lorenzini, with some observations on the effect of temperature on sensory rhythms. Proc. roy. Soc. B **125**, 524–553 (1938).

SANS, K.: Die Heißempfindung bei chemischer Reizung der äußeren Haut. Inaug.-Diss. Heidelberg 1949.

SCHMIDT, R.: Die Empfindung der äußeren Haut bei Reizung durch Säuren, Laugen und Chloroform. Inaug.-Diss. Heidelberg 1949.

SCHREINER, H.J.: Das Wärmegefühl nach Calciuminjektionen. Inaug.-Diss. Göttingen 1936.

SCHWENKENBECHER, A.: Über Mentholvergiftung des Menschen. Münch. med. Wschr. **1908**, 1495–1496.

SINCLAIR, D.C.: Cutaneous sensation and the doctrine of specific energy. Brain **78**, 584–614 (1955).

SKRAMLIK, E. von: Psychophysiologie der Tastsinne. In: Arch. Psychol., Erg.-Bd. 4, Teil 1 u. 2. Leipzig: Akademische Verlagsgesellschaft 1937.

Stary, Z.: Über Erregung der Wärmenerven durch Pharmaka. Naunyn-Schmiedeberg's Arch. exp. Path. Pharmak. **105**, 76–87 (1925).

Stolwijk, J.A.J., Wexler, I.: Peripheral nerve activity in response to heating the cat's skin. J. Physiol. (Lond.) **214**, 377–392 (1971).

Strughold, H., Porz, R.: Die Dichte der Kaltpunkte auf der Haut des menschlichen Körpers. Z. Biol. **91**, 563–571 (1931).

Thauer, R.: Probleme der Thermoregulation. Klin. Wschr. **36**, 989–998 (1958).

Thauer, R., Ebaugh, F.G., Jr.: Die Unterschiedsschwelle der Kalt- und Warmempfindung in Abhängigkeit von der absoluten Luft- bzw. Hauttemperatur. Pflügers Arch. ges. Physiol. **225**, 27–45 (1952).

Thunberg, T.: Untersuchungen über die relative Tiefenlage der kälte-, wärme- und schmerz-perzipierenden Nervenenden in der Haut und über das Verhältnis der Kältenervenenden gegenüber Wärmereizen. Skand. Arch. Physiol. **11**, 382–435 (1901).

Torebjörk, H.E., Hallin, R.G.: Activity in C fibres correlated to perception in man. In: Cervical pain (ed. C. Hirsch and Y. Zotterman), p. 171–178. Oxford: Pergamon Press 1972.

Vendrik, A.J.H., Eijkman, E.G.: Psychophysical properties determined with internal noise In: The skin senses (ed. D.R. Kenshalo), pp. 178–194. Springfield, Ill.: Charles C. Thomas 1968.

Vendrik, A.J.H., Vos, J.J.: Comparison of the stimulation of the warmth sense organ by microwave and infrared. J. appl. Physiol. **13**, 435–444 (1958).

Weber, E.H.: Der Tastsinn und das Gemeingefühl. In: Wagners Handwörterbuch der Physiologie, Bd. III/2, S. 481–588. Braunschweig: F. Vieweg & Sohn 1846.

Weddell, G., Miller, S.: Cutaneous sensibility. Ann. Rev. Physiol. **24**, 199–222 (1962).

Weddell, G., Palmer, E., Pallie, W.: Nerve endings in mammalian skin. Biol. Rev. **30**, 159–195 (1955).

Witt, I.: Aktivität einzelner C-Fasern bei schmerzhaften und nicht schmerzhaften Hautreizen. Acta neuroveg. (Wien) **25**, 208–219 (1963).

Witt, I., Hensel, H.: Afferente Impulse aus der Extremitätenhaut der Katze bei thermischer und mechanischer Reizung. Pflügers Arch. ges. Physiol. **268**, 582–596 (1959).

Zerbst, D.: Analyse der Nachrichtenverarbeitung durch biologische Rezeptoren. Leipzig: VEB Georg Thieme 1972.

Zerbst, D., Dittberner, K.H.: Analytical approach to the excitation mechanisms of thermal cold receptors. Pflügers Arch. **319**, R 126 (1970).

Zotterman, Y.: Action potentials in the glossopharyngeal nerve and in the chorda tympani. Skand. Arch. Physiol. **72**, 73–77 (1935).

Zotterman, Y.: Specific action potentials in the lingual nerve of cat. Skand. Arch. Physiol. **75**, 105–119 (1936).

Zotterman, Y.: Special senses: thermal receptors. Ann. Rev. Physiol. **15**, 357–372 (1953).

Zotterman, Y.: Thermal sensations. In: Handbook of physiology, vol. I, sect. 1, Neuro-physiology, pp. 431–458. Washington, D.C.: American Physiological Society 1959.

Chapter 4

Joint Receptors and Kinaesthesis

By

Sten Skoglund, Stockholm (Sweden)

With 12 Figures

Contents

A. Introduction

In his classical study Goldscheider 1889 attributed most of the sensations involved in kinaesthesis to the joints. He stated that minute changes of joint position of less than one angular degree is perceived as a movement and not as a set of successive positions. He further stated that for passive movements the minimal perceptible excursion in the knee joint is 0.5–0.7 degrees if the speed reaches 1–2.5 degrees/sec. The limit for perception of willed movements is slightly lower.

Sherrington in a textbook article in 1900 pointed out that kinaesthesis means recognition of position of active and passive movement and of resistance to movement. These sensations must according to him arise in muscles, joints and bones. The contribution of muscle receptors to the perception of these sensations has been questioned in modern neurophysiology whereas the role of the joint receptors has never been in any doubt. The recognition of the role of joint receptors in kinaesthesis is thus very old and information on the morphology of joint innervation dates even further back whereas a knowledge of the exact physiology of joint receptors is a fairly recent achievement. It is not the intention of the present author to give any complete survey of the morphology of joint innervation, thus papers which do not contribute anything new will be omitted, especially if they use a terminology which is different from that of all other authors in the field. The reader will instead be referred to several review articles. However, a brief account of the innervation of joints, especially the knee joint of the cat will be given to serve as a background for the presentation of physiological data.

B. Articular Nerve Distribution and Calibre Spectra

The first systematic study of the innervation of joints was performed by Rüdinger in 1857. He dissected most of the nerves to the diarthrodial joints in man. Subsequent studies have to a great extent been confirmations of this basic work. The first to study the distribution of joint nerves in an experimental animal was Gardner (1944) who described the knee joint nerves in cat fetuses. His observations were to a great extent confirmed and extended by Skoglund (1956). A very extensive survey on joint innervation has been published by Poláček (1966).

With regard to the distribution of joint nerves it can generally be stated that articular branches arise from the main nerve trunks, especially from cutaneous nerves but also from muscular branches. Some direct articular nerves have been described for most joints investigated, like the posterior and medial articular nerves to the knee joint in the cat and these direct nerves either emanate from main mixed nerve trunks or from cutaneous nerves. In addition there are articular nerve branches arising from muscle nerves which might even travel with the muscular branches piercing the muscles in reaching a joint.

Some data have been presented with regard to the fibre spectra of joint nerves. Gardner (1944) and Skoglund (1956) made calibre spectra of both the medial and the posterior knee joint nerves in the cat. Burgess and Clark (1969a) presented data on the posterior nerve in the cat. The biggest fibres in both nerves were found to be 17–18 microns with a peak around 6 microns. Since as pointed out by Skoglund (1956) there are great differences from animal to animal, no further descriptions seem valid other than stating that the articular nerves resemble cutaneous nerves in their composition, containing in addition to the myelinated fibres a large number of unmyelinated ones, both of sympathetic origin and C-fibres of dorsal root origin.

C. Articular Nerve Terminals

Some of the old anatomists like Rauber, Krause, Nicoladoni and Hagen-Torn (for ref. see Gardner, 1950a; Skoglund, 1956) saw modified Pacinian corpuscles in the connective tissue of joints, that is Pacinian corpuscles with fewer layers than usual in their capsule. Some of these authors also described other types of endings. Sfameni (1902) was the first to describe Ruffini-like endings and small terminal plaques in the fibrous parts of the joint capsules. He also claimed that such plaques were present in the synovial layer but did not describe any Pacinian-like corpuscles. Gardner (1942) studied the endorgans in the knee joint of the mouse and found free nerve endings and specialized encapsulated endings in the connective tissue. Pacinian corpuscles were not found within or associated with the articular capsule but occurred commonly in the fibrous periosteum near articular or ligamentous attachments. Gardner (1944) also investigated the knee joint innervation of the adult cat using a methylene blue staining technique as well as fetal material stained with Bodian's activated protargol method.

Gardner found that branches of the femoral nerve formed extensive plexuses in the medial and lateral part of the knee joint capsule whereas branches of the

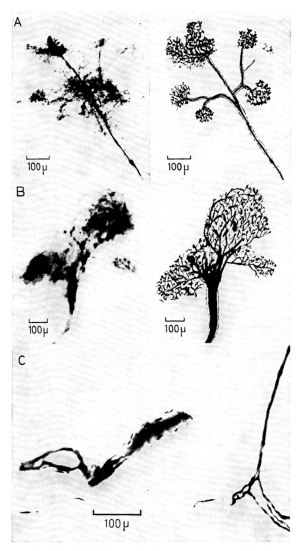

Fig. 1. A. A sensory unit of the Ruffini-type in the posterior part of the joint capsule. Five endings arising from the same axon. Photomicrograph, gold stain. To the right a camera lucida
drawing of the endings seen in A to the left. B. Golgi-ending in the anterior cruciate ligament.
Photomicrograph, gold stain. To the right a camera lucida drawing of the ending at the same
magnification. C. Modified Vater-Pacini corpuscle in the capsule. Gold stain. (From SKOGLUND,
1956)

common peroneal nerve supplied the lateral part of the capsule. These nerves
according to GARDNER contribute nonmyelinated axons which end in relation to
the smooth muscles of articular blood vessels. Free nerve endings are found in the
adventitia of the vessels and in the joint capsule. GARDNER also described myelinated axons which he thought were sensory in function supplying the blood vessels.
Later on EKHOLM and SKOGLUND (1963) demonstrated myelinated postganglionic

sympathetic fibres in the knee joint nerves of the cat. Finally Gardner described Ruffini-endings located mainly in the posterior capsule.

Samuel (1952) found encapsulated bodies in the fibrous capsule of the knee joint in the cat. He also described terminal expansions, nerve sprays or loops or simple endings. Andrew (1954a) studied the sensory innervation of the medial ligament in the knee joint of the cat using methylene blue. He found one type of ending resembling the Golgi-tendon organ associated with the ligament and another resembling the Ruffini-like ending in the joint capsule. No Pacinian corpuscles were described.

In 1954 Boyd studied the receptors in the knee joint of the cat in correlation with their physiological response. Boyd used the gold chloride method and found two types of sensory units which he called a "spray" type and a "lamellated" type. The spray type is obviously identical with the Ruffini-like receptor and the lamellated type with the modified Pacinian corpuscle. Occasionally he found Golgi-tendon organs in the cruciate ligaments.

Skoglund (1956) demonstrated three types of sensory endings in various parts of the feline knee joint in gold stained material. In the medial collateral ligament, the medial patellar ligament and the cruciate ligaments but never outside these structures Golgi-tendon organs were found. In the fibrous part of the joint capsule Ruffini-endings were found which were smaller than the Golgi-tendon organs in the ligaments but more numerous. In addition a few modified Vater-Pacinian corpuscles were found in the capsule.

In 1966 Poláček published an extensive review on the receptors of joints, their structure, variability and classification. His evaluations are based on a long series of personal investigations (for ref. see Poláček, 1966). Poláček states that there are great variations not only in the distribution of nerves to the joints but also in the appearance of the joint receptors. The latter may vary with age and species but Poláček states that mainly three types of endings are present in joints. Firstly the free endings, secondly the spray type and thirdly the encapsulated Pacinian-like receptor. Furthermore, he suggests that these receptors should be classified according to their structure, phylogenetical development and data on their function. It is obvious that Poláček considers both the Ruffini-like and the Golgi-tendon organ to belong to the spray type. Although one might not agree with all of Poláček's opinions, it is obvious that his work and that of his group have clarified several of the discrepancies regarding the differences in the innervation of different joints found by different authors. Consequently, it appears unnecessary to review the literature on all the different joints that have been investigated, the more so since most of the work that concerns us here, namely the physiology of joint receptors, has been performed on the first order afferents from the knee joint of the cat.

In summary, it can be concluded that three types of joint receptors are present in most joints. Firstly the spray type which when situated in the capsule has been called a Ruffini-like receptor (Fig. 1A). (Sfameni, 1902; Gardner, 1944; Skoglund, 1956) and when situated in the ligaments has been called a Golgi-tendon organ (Andrew, 1954; Skoglund, 1956) (Fig. 1B), secondly the encapsulated Pacinian-like corpuscle (Fig. 1C) and thirdly the free nerve ending.

D. Response Characteristics of Joint Receptors

In view of all the morphological work done in the field of joint receptors the physiological studies on first order afferents from these receptors are relatively few and nearly all of them have been performed on the knee joint of the cat. There is good reason, though, to believe that the results obtained in this particular joint are valid for all joints since central neurons responding to joint rotation behave similarly, regardless of which joint is activated (see below).

GARDNER (1947) recorded from the posterior articular nerve in the knee joint of the cat and showed that the frequency increases when pressure is applied to the

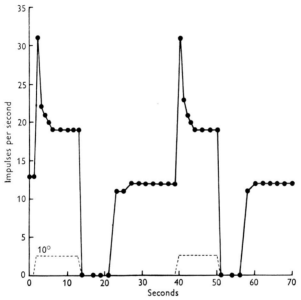

Fig. 2. Graph of the impulse frequency of a single afferent neurone innervating the capsule of the knee joint of the cat. Graph plots frequency of impulses against time as the joint is moved through 10 degrees of flexion and back again, as indicated by the dashed line. Note onset transient during movement, adaptation to a more or less steady frequency of discharge during steady joint displacement, rapid drop in frequency when joint moves away from excitatory position, postexcitatory silent period, recovery to resting frequency of discharge and almost exact repetition of the pattern of discharge when the movement is repeated. (From BOYD and ROBERTS, 1954)

joint capsule. ANDREW and DODT (1953), recording from the medial articular nerve to the knee joint of the cat, described slowly adapting endings having an arc of maximum sensitivity covering a few degrees of angular movement, the ranges being different for individual endings. They also reported that the patellar and medial collateral ligaments were equipped with endings which signalled tension. The responses of these endings to steady tension were also measured. ANDREW and DODT demonstrated that these joint receptors can be activated by increasing the intra-articular pressure.

8*

Andrew (1954) recorded action potentials from the medial articular nerve in cats, rabbits and rats when applying tension to the medial collateral ligament both *in situ* and in isolated preparations. He found slowly adapting endings connected to large myelinated fibres which responded to tensions applied to the ligament. Andrew's histological studies led him to believe that these endings resemble Golgi-tendon organs whereas he found Ruffini-type endings in the connective tissue of the capsule. Andrew concluded that the slowly adapting responses from the Golgi-tendon organs of the ligaments were responsible for recording tension changes in the ligaments. These tensions changes in the ligaments are not influenced by changes in the tension of the muscles at the joint.

Andrew (1954) also studied the thyroepiglottis joint in the cat. He used an isolated larynx preparation to study the responses to position changes and passive movement. The responses to movement produced by muscular action were recorded in anaesthetized animals. The proprioceptors were found to be slowly adapting stretch receptors responding either to extension only or to a deviation either towards extension or flexion from a midposition. Andrew concluded that the receptors could give information for a central mechanism to gauge accurately the position and movement of the epiglottis and furthermore that these receptors were in many respects similar to the previously described proprioceptors in the knee joint of the cat.

Boyd and Roberts (1953) described the proprioceptive discharges from stretch receptors in the knee joint of the cat. They recorded from the posterior articular nerve in decerebrate cats with the joint in different positions and during various movements. These authors described two types of responses: rapidly and slowly adapting. The slowly adapting response was more frequently encountered. Boyd and Roberts stated that these discharges show characteristic frequencies during movements (Fig. 2). They furthermore found that the degree of exaggeration depends on the rate of movement and the exaggerated response is followed by adaptation to the appropriate new steady impulse frequency. These authors also demonstrated that the endorgans giving the slowly adapting discharges were located in the posterior part of the joint capsule and had a distribution similar to that of the typical Ruffini-endings described by Gardner (1944). They concluded that the slowly adapting sense organs in the joint capsule are capable of providing accurate information about the relative position of the bones forming the joint (Fig. 3) and in doing so they may play an important part in the control of fine movements.

Boyd (1954) correlated the two types of discharges in the posterior articular nerve to the histological structure of the receptors in the knee joint and concluded that the slowly adapting response emanates from what he called the spray type, the typical Ruffini-ending of Gardner. The rapidly adapting response, on the other hand, arises from the lamellated type of sensory unit, the Pacinian-like corpuscle.

Cohen (1955) recorded the activity of knee joint proprioceptors from the undivided posterior articular nerve in decerebrate cats in response to the full physiological range of flexion-extension type movements of the joint. Cohen found proprioceptive firing at all angles of the knee joint but stated that proprioceptive activity was usually most intense at the extremes of the flexion-extension

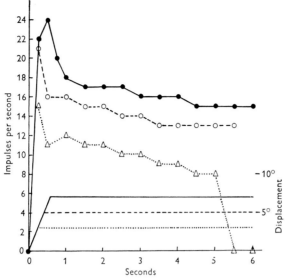

Fig. 3. Graphs of the impulse frequency in a single afferent fibre innervating the capsule of the knee joint of the cat, showing frequency of discharge against time during flexion at a rate of 10 degrees per sec carried through three different angles: open triangles, 10 degrees; open circles, 12 degrees; closed circles, 14 degrees. The upper curves show the frequencies of the impulses, the lower ones the angular displacements from a position of 132 degrees of extension, where this receptor did not discharge. Note that steady state frequency is higher for greater joint displacements. (From Boyd and Roberts, 1953)

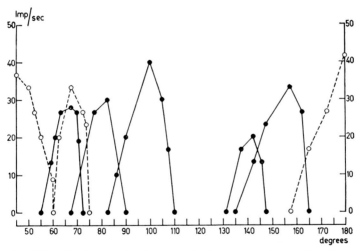

Fig. 4. Graphs of impulse frequencies for eight single neurones innervating slowly adapting receptors in the capsule of the knee joint of the cat. The adapted impulse frequency is plotted against position of the joint in degrees. Solid lines show values for five units in one experiment; dotted lines show those of three units in another. *The figure is not representative for the distribution of endings* which are successively activated during full movement, since in general activation of endings occurs more often immediately before or at full flexion or full extension than in the intermediate positions of the joint. The sensitive ranges (15 to 30 degrees) are representative of the behaviour of most endings. (From Skoglund, 1956)

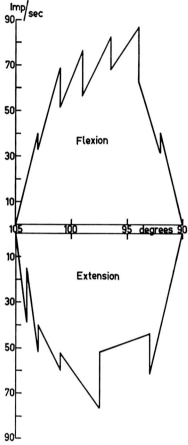

Fig. 5. Graphs of the impulse frequency in a single afferent neurone innervating the capsule of the knee joint of the cat, as the joint is moved in steps through the "excitatory angle" for the receptor, in opposite directions. After each small step of the movement the frequency is allowed to reach an adapted rate. The two curves are almost mirror images. (From Skoglund, 1956)

range, as measured by both the number and the rate of firing of the active proprioceptors. Any individual proprioceptor had only a limited range of knee joint angle during which it fired and its threshold angle for firing was quite precise. Once a proprioceptor was activated its rate of firing normally increased until the joint reached a point of maximum sensitivity for that receptor after which the frequency usually decreased until firing ceased entirely. Static position of the joint at an angle which was within the sensitivity range of a receptor usually revealed very slow adaptation of the receptor. Cohen suggested that there is only one type of proprioceptor in the knee joint of the cat.

In 1956 Skoglund showed that there is a maximum of impulses from the medial articular nerve when the tibia is at full flexion or full extension and in the posterior nerve as the tibia reaches full extension. In the posterior nerve the situation at full flexion could not be analysed with the recording technique used.

SKOGLUND also showed that the slowly adapting sensory endings covered fairly small angular deviations of the joint, usually 15–30 degrees (Fig. 4) (cf. ANDREW and DODT, 1953; BOYD and ROBERTS, 1953). SKOGLUND also recorded responses from both slowly and rapidly adapting receptors in the two above mentioned nerves. He divided the responses into three categories which could be related to the different types of endings present in the joint. In accordance with the findings of ANDREW (1954) SKOGLUND showed that the ligaments are equipped only with

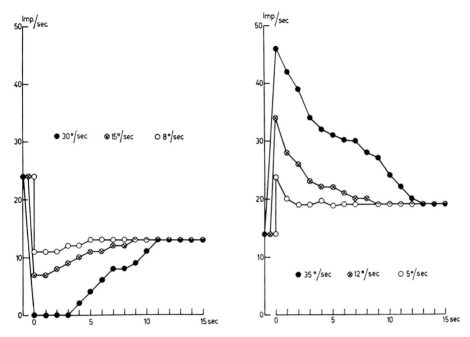

Fig. 6. Graph of the response of a slowly adapting sense organ to a movement of 5 degrees with different speeds. Impulse frequency is plotted against time in seconds. Each plot shows the decline in impulse frequency from the peak value attained at the completion of the movement (right). Graph of the response of the same slowly adapting sense organ to a movement of 5 degrees in the opposite direction with different speeds (left). (From SKOGLUND, 1956)

the so-called Golgi-tendon organs. These endings are responsible for one type of slowly adapting response. The other slowly adapting response arises from the Ruffini-endings in the joint capsule. The rapidly adapting response emanates from the modified Pacinian corpuscles. SKOGLUND concluded, as did ANDREW, that the activity of the Golgi-endings is not influenced by the muscles inserting at the joint and are thus able to record the exact position of the joint. They could also record the direction of movement but their low sensitivity to movement makes them less adequate to signal the speed of the movement. The slowly adapting Ruffini-endings which lie in the capsule signal the direction of movement (Fig. 5) and owing to their considerable sensitivity to movement they can also signal speed of movement (Fig. 6). The activity of the Ruffini-endings in the capsule, however, is in-

fluenced by the action of the muscles which alter the tension of the joint capsule
(Fig. 7), hence they cannot be regarded as true position receptors although they
will signal minor variations of position as movement. Additionally, the change of
frequency induced by the muscles inserting at the joint might be a tool in discriminating between active and passive movements. The Pacinian corpuscles eventually give rise to the rapidly adapting response. Skoglund considered this
receptor as an acceleration receptor since it is sensitive to quick movements independent of their direction.

Eklund and Skoglund (1960) studied the response pattern of Ruffini-like
receptors in isolated knee joint capsules, which were exposed to a linear increase

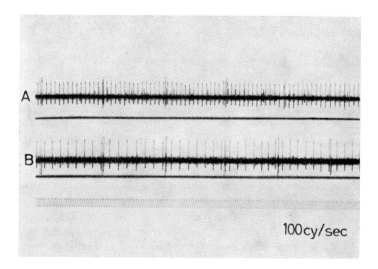

Fig. 7. Decerebrate cat. A. The response of three sensory endings connected to the medial
nerve at a position of a few degrees flexion. The nerve supply to the muscles is intact. B. The
response of the three sensory endings at the same position of the tibia after cutting the quadriceps nerve. (Amplification is increased somewhat in B to secure the response after dener-
vation.) Time: 100 cy/sec. Note that the biggest spike retains the same frequency whereas the
smallest spikes disappear and the medium sized spikes have a different frequency after nerve
section. (From Skoglund, 1956)

of tension. The response pattern was also studied while applying an additional
tension increase at angles to the linear one and by applying pressure to the preparation. The frequency response obtained with linearly increasing tensions
showed that the investigated sense organs behave like other slowly adapting
mechanoreceptors in general (Fig. 3). By applying additional tensions at right
angles to the linearly increasing one when the latter produced a high or maximum
frequency in a single organ, temporary alterations of frequencies could be produced but the impulse discharge could never be silenced. The authors concluded
that the sensitivity bands displayed by the investigated sense organs *in vivo* are
only a reflection of the tension variations in the capsule during movements, i.e.
variations of stimulus strength.

BURGESS and CLARK (1969 b) recorded from posterior articular nerve fibres in dorsal root filaments of the cat and determined the conduction velocities and the characteristics of the joint receptors. These authors found that the conduction velocities were distributed similarly to posterior articular nerve fibre diameters as determined histologically (BURGESS and CLARK, 1969 a). They recorded from a total of 278 units out of which 209 were slowly adapting. Of these 140 responded at both marked flexion and marked extension, 47 responded only during extension. Four slowly adapting fibres were activated specifically at intermediate joint positions. Outward twist of the tibia (abducting the foot) enhanced the discharge of most slowly adapting joint fibres. BURGESS and CLARK also found two types of rapidly adapting receptors. One which they called Pacinian corpuscle-like receptor (fourteen fibres) responded transiently to joint movement in any direction regardless of initial position. The other type was called phasic joint receptor (thirty fibres) and was rapidly adapting at most joint positions but could give a low rate sustained discharge when strongly stimulated. Furthermore, BURGESS and CLARK obtained slowly adapting posterior articular nerve fibres that responded to succinylcholine and which they considered to originate from muscle spindles. Eleven of their slowly conducting myelinated fibres responded only to extreme joint movement which was considered noxious.

On the basis of the data presented it seems safe to state that there are at least three types of responses from the joint receptors; two types of slowly adapting receptor responses and one rapidly adapting type. The slowly adapting responses are activated by limited ranges of joint positions and movements. Most of them exhibit a maximum of discharge at either full flexion or full extension and can be designated as single-ended. There are, however, also receptors having their maximum discharge in between the extremes of flexion and extension, such receptors can be designated double-ended. The Golgi-tendon receptors of the ligaments being mostly single-ended and giving slowly adapting responses and not influenced by tension changes in the muscles inserting at the joint would signal the exact position of the joint and the direction of movement. Owing to their low sensitivity they are less able to signal speed of movement. The slowly adapting Ruffini-endings in the capsule having small angles of activity, being either single- or double-ended, and having high sensitivity would signal small movements, speed and direction of movement. Since their responses are under the influence of the tension of the muscles inserting at the joint they would also signal resistance to movement and possibly be able to discriminate between active and passive movement. The Pacinian-like corpuscles having rapidly adapting responses and being activated by all movements of the joint regardless of initial position, their frequency of response being a function of the speed of movement, would serve as movement detectors and may be some sort of acceleration receptor.

The statement of BURGESS and CLARK that 140 of their 209 isolated slowly responses were activated at both "marked flexion" and "marked extension" raises the question of the angular specificity of the joint receptors. Since it was shown by EKLUND and SKOGLUND (1959) that the restricted angular activity of Ruffini-endings is not due to any specificity in the receptors, but to the change in tension of the capsule during movement of the joint and that the joint receptors, as shown already by GARDNER (1944), can be activated by exerting pressure on the joint capsule, it might be asked whether the movements induced by Burgess and Clark caused tension variations both at flexion and extension in those parts of the capsule where the 140 receptors were stimulated. Such tension variations in the capsule could also be induced by pressure. Since the authors state that these responses appeared at "marked" flexion and extension, it is the opinion of the present author that under the experimental conditions prevailing great caution has to be taken not to overextend a joint and not to force it into such a flexed position in which surrounding tissues might exert unphysiological pressure on the joint capsule. One is therefore apt to inquire, whether the response at both flexion and extension from the same endorgans would occur under physiological conditions. Burgess and Clark furthermore do not state whether the receptors activated by both flexion and extension were situated only in the joint capsule. It is thus possible that unnatural movements would exert tension on the ligaments causing the sensory endings in them to fire at both flexion and extension. If, however, the observation is correct that many joint receptors are activated at both flexion and extension, one must question the function of these receptors in serving kinaesthesis unless central mechanisms of discrimination, which will be further discussed later on, are presumed. Burgess and Clark (1969b) raised this question from a somewhat different angle in questioning the rationale for the accumulation of responses at the extreme of flexion and extension which was observed by both Cohen (1955) and Skoglund (1956). They suggested that the receptors being activated at those positions would hardly take part in the discrimination of position but instead serve some reflex function. However, their finding that many receptors are activated at both flexion and extension also appear to be incompatible with the idea that such receptors fulfil a meaningful function in reflex regulation.

E. Reflex Effects from Joint Receptors

Gardner (1950b) studied the reflex muscular responses to stimulation of articular nerves in decerebrate and decapitate cats. He directly observed the reflex muscular responses to single and repetitive electrical stimulation of articular nerves. Gardner compared his results with the effects of stimulating muscle nerves. He also recorded the responses to articular nerve stimulation from ventral roots. Simultaneous stimulation of all the fibres in an articular nerve usually resulted in withdrawal and in decerebrate animals in crossed extension as well. Gardner considered these responses as due to nociceptive stimuli since they were best developed when nonmyelinated and small myelinated fibres were activated. Stimulation of the large fibres only gave multineuron arc discharges over several ventral roots to the flexors of the thigh and leg. The responses obtained in decerebrate animals were, however, very variable. They were often absent and when present they were usually flexor in nature although in two instances, there was primarily extension of the hindlimb. Decerebrate animals, if subsequently decapitated, showed constant flexor reflexes at lower stimulation intensities irrespective of the responses present during decerebration. Gardner postulated that the larger articular fibres and their central connections may subserve phasic mechanisms such as locomotion. He also thought that the reflexes from the articular nerves would in such case be more easily demonstrated in spinal animals and more likely inhibited in decerebrate animals.

BESWICK et al. (1955) found like GARDNER that stimulation of articular nerves by single shocks evokes a polysynaptic reflex discharge in lumbar and sacral ventral roots. They reported that a conditioning volley in an articular nerve may cause inhibition of the motoneurones of some extensor muscles for about 30 msec following the stimulus. A similar conditioning volley may facilitate the motoneurones of some limb flexors for a similar length of time.

SKOGLUND (1956) studied both the effects of electrical and adequate stimulation of knee joint afferents on the monosynaptic reflex of both flexors and extensors of the hindlimb in both decerebrate and decerebrate and low spinal cats. He, like GARDNER, found the effects of electrical stimulation of the large articular nerve fibres to be very variable in different animals giving sometimes inhibition and sometimes facilitation of flexors and the reciprocal effect on extensors. The effects were small and sometimes absent, but when present they were always reciprocal on the flexors and extensors of the joint. Adequate stimulation of the endings connected to the medial nerve also gave variable effects which were also always reciprocal. SKOGLUND explained the great variability of joint reflexes on muscles as being due to a combination of the mass test used (the monosynaptic potential from a whole ventral root) and the great variability in the nerve supply to the same joint. The great variation of the reflex effects in response to electrical stimulation of the articular nerves was explained as being due to the fact that the endings stimulated at extension are not the same as those stimulated at flexion and consequently they may have different effects. A simultaneous stimulation of all the fibres will then, if they are evenly distributed to endings active at flexion and at extension, give no or undetectable effects on the monosynaptic mass test. Sometimes one of the components is better represented than the other and a small effect will result.

ANDERSSON and STENER (1954) showed that a strong increase of the tension of the medial collateral ligament in the knee joint of the decerebrate rat gave no reflex motor effects in the muscles of the thigh. That the absence of reflex motor effects was not due to absence of afferent discharge from the ligament was shown by recording action potentials from the medial and posterior articular nerves while increasing the tension in the ligament. On the other hand, these authors always obtained "control reflexes" by gentle pressure against certain points within the ventromedial region of the knee joint. These "control reflexes" disappeared after severing the medial articular nerve.

EKHOLM et al. (1960) studied the response of knee flexors and extensors to stimulation of knee joint receptors in decerebrate and spinalized decerebrate cats. When stimulating the joint receptors by increasing the intra-articular pressure or by probing the anterior part of the knee, the extensors were always inhibited while the flexors were facilitated. When the receptors of the medial collateral ligament were stimulated by increasing its tension a facilitation of the flexors was always obtained in the spinal animal and sometimes in the decerebrate animal. The difference in the results of ANDERSSON and STENER (1959) and EKHOLM et al. (1960) must be due to differences in the central excitability state of the animals used, especially since EKHOLM et al. always obtained reflex effects from the medial collateral ligament in the spinal animal.

In summary it can then be stated that the joint receptors are capable of eliciting reflex effects as evidenced by the polysynaptic discharges obtained in the ventral roots on stimulation of articular nerves (Gardner, 1947; Beswick et al., 1955). Most authors seem to have obtained facilitation of flexors and inhibition of extensors (Gardner, 1947; Beswick et al., 1955; Skoglund, 1956) although the opposite effect was also sometimes observed. This again raises the question whether different endings are active at flexion and extension or not. The observation of Burgess and Clark (1969 b) that very many receptors are active at both flexion and extension would be compatible with the idea that articular nerves give facilitation of flexors and inhibition of extensors, i.e. they would be giving the same reflex effects at both flexion and extension of the knee joint. On the other hand, there are observations (Gardner, 1950 b; Skoglund, 1956) that stimulation of articular nerves sometimes give the opposite effect. One might question the role of the joint receptors in locomotion if they only gave facilitation of flexors and inhibition of extensors, in particular one must ask what would be the reason to inhibit extensors at the flexed position of the knee in a movement. Apart from the explanation given by Skoglund (1956) for the variability of the reflex effects elicited from the articular nerves of the knee, especially that one or the other of two components of the articular nerve might be dominant, usually the one giving flexion reflexes, there is also the possibility that electrical stimulation of the articular nerves in order to cause measurable reflex effects with the testing methods used often has to be so strong that some pain fibres causing flexion are included, adding to those afferents giving flexor reflexes. However, it must be stated that the conditions under which the reflex effects of the joint afferents are analysed are far from the ones prevailing under physiological conditions while still other possibilities are at hand. Assuming quite naturally that the joint receptors have a given set of fixed central connections it is quite possible that alterations of the central excitability state in different parts of these connections caused both by peripheral and central influences might allow the joint receptors to work in purposeful reflex functions, regardless of whether they are activated at several positions of the joint. Thus, inhibition or facilitation of different central connections from the same receptor would compensate for their being active at several joint positions. The final effects from the joint receptors would be determined by the much more powerful innervation of the muscles. Mechanisms like those suggested above might also be at work with regard to the central integration of the afferent discharges serving kinaesthesis but before discussing these problems the spinal pathways and central representation of joint afferents will be surveyed.

F. Spinal Pathways and Supraspinal Connections of Joint Afferents

Gardner et al. (1949) stimulated the dorsal funiculi at various levels and recorded antidromically conducted impulses from articular nerves. Gardner et al. concluded that their experimental results indicated that most, if not all, of the articular fibres synapse with internuncial neurones shortly after entering the spinal cord. They concluded, however, that the larger myelinated fibres, those probably arising from Ruffini-type endings, also continue rostrally in the ipsilateral dorsal funiculi to the medulla oblongata. Maximum conduction rates at levels of entry were 90–100 m/sec but only 20–30 m/sec at cervical levels. The decrease was, by these authors, held to be due to a decrease in diameter of the parent fibres as collaterals are given off. No evidence of conduction over spino-cerebellar tracts was obtained. However, this latter conclusion was based on the observation that no activity could be recorded from these tracts when stimulating the articular nerves, but this was also the case when recording from the dorsal funiculi rostral to the level of the entrance of the articular nerves. The conclusion that the articular nerve fibres ascend in the dorsal funiculi was thus mainly based on the experiments using antidromic stimulation.

GARDNER and NOER (1952) studied the projection of afferent fibres from muscles and joints to the cerebral cortex. In cats anaesthetized with sodium pentobarbital, surface positive potential changes were evoked in the contralateral somatic area I and ipsilateral and contralateral somatic area II following stimulation of various muscle, joint and cutaneous nerves. The results of selective sectioning of the cord indicated that with regard to area I all these nerves have several ascending paths in the spinal cord. These findings were confirmed by GARDNER and HADDAD (1953).

HADDAD (1953) reported that stimulation of articular nerves gave evoked potentials in the anterior lobe of the cerebellum. Selective cord incisions showed that there are crossed and uncrossed paths in each ventral and lateral region of the cord. Impulses can reach either cerebellar hemisphere by any of these paths. Impulses may cross at brainstem and cerebellar levels and there is evidence that spino-olivary and spinoreticular as well as spinocerebellar fibres are concerned.

SKOGLUND (1956) confirmed that both the medial and posterior knee joint nerves in the cat are represented in the contralateral sensory areas I and II and in the ipsilateral sensory area II. The latencies for these responses were with optimal recording conditions 10–15 msec. SKOGLUND controlled the stimulation of the articular nerves and restricted it to the largest fibres connected to the mechanoreceptors. With such stimulation no cortical responses were obtained after cutting the dorsal funiculi.

BURGESS and CLARK (1969a) reported that stimulation of the cervical dorsal columns excited an average of nine knee joint fibres in the cat posterior articular nerve, eleven fibres in the cat medial nerve and thirteen fibres in the monkey posterior articular nerve. The numerous slowly adapting fibres could not be antidromically excited from the cervical dorsal columns. Recordings from single fibres in the dorsal columns failed to yield any number of slowly adapting joint fibres except from the terminal phalangeal (claw) joints. Several control experiments should, according to these authors, suggest that the antidromic stimulation method accurately defined the dorsal column projection of joint fibres. However, in connection with their control experiments BURGESS and CLARK describe that "when the dorsal columns are stimulated caudal to the cervical cord, additional posterior articular nerve fibres with longer latencies are activated, the first of these usually appearing at midthoracic levels".

MOUNTCASTLE (1957) described cells in the cat's somatic sensory cortex related to deep structures, which were activated from deep fascia and connective tissue

and the regions of the joints and joint capsules but never from muscle. These cells
driven by joint movement signal the steady position and phasic changes in position
of joints and are suitably arranged to subserve position sense. Mountcastle observed pairs of closely adjacent cells which responded reciprocally to alternating joint
movements (Fig. 8).

MOUNTCASTLE and POWELL (1959) described the functional properties of a
class of neurones of the postcentral gyrus in monkeys. These cells are sensitive
to movements and steady angles of the joints. Such neurones discharge rapid onset

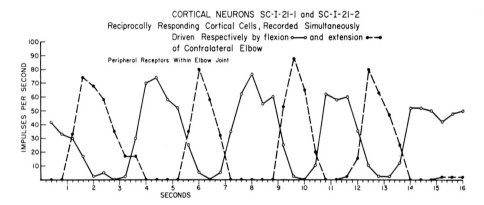

Fig. 8. Impulse frequency graphs of two neurones of postcentral homologue of the cerebral
cortex of the cat. Discharges of the two units observed simultaneously at a single microelectrode position. Units responded reciprocally to alternating flexions and extensions of the
contralateral elbow. Graphs plot continuously the average frequencies for each consecutive
400 msec period. Impulse frequency reaches zero for each unit when the joint reaches the
position maximally excitatory for the other unit. During fourteenth and fifteenth seconds the
joint was held in steady extension, and the extension unit fires steadily, while the flexion unit
is almost completely silent. (From MOUNTCASTLE, 1957)

transients when the joint to which they are related is moved in the excitatory
direction for the cell. The large majority of cells thereafter discharge at steady
rates with steady joint positions within the excitatory range of the joint angle.
The level of that steady rate is determined by the joint angle and is independent
of the speed or direction of movement bringing the joint to that angle. Movement
of a joint away from the excitatory direction causes a decrease in the discharge rate
of such a cortical cell. Closely adjacent cells responding in reciprocal manner, one
being excited and the other inhibited to a given movement were also observed.
MOUNTCASTLE and POWELL (1959) stated that this class of neurones together with
their relevant peripheral receptors, afferent nerves and relay neurones constitute
the essential neural substratum serving the somatic sensory component of the
sense of position and kinaesthesis.

POGGIO and MOUNTCASTLE (1960, 1963) and PERL and WHITLOCK (1961)
reported on thalamic neurones in the ventrobasal complex that were activated by
joint rotation. MOUNTCASTLE et al. (1963) using deafferented-head macaque

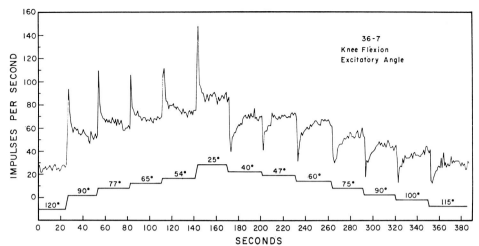

Fig. 9. Graph plotting, continuously, impulses per second versus time for the excitatory angle study of a ventrobasal thalamic cell sensitive to flexion of the contralateral knee. For a statistical analysis of homogeneity the counting period used was 200 msec. Analyses of variance between successive 5-sec periods of the last 15 sec of each plateau showed that the populations were homogeneous. (From MOUNTCASTLE et al., 1963)

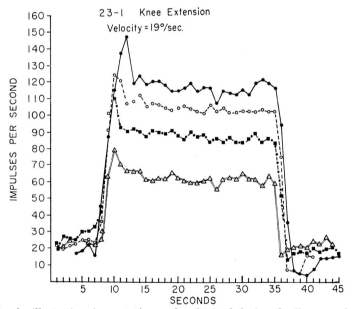

Fig. 10. Graphs illustrating, in part, the results obtained during the "one speed to several angles" experiment for a ventrobasal thalamic cell driven by extension of the contralateral knee. For each angle five trials were made, and the data listed in terms of impulses per 200 msec counting period. The five lists were then oriented correctly in time, averaged and summed for each second, and finally plotted, as shown, as impulses per second. The knee was rotated from a position well outside the excitatory angle to true joint angles of, from above downward, 180°, 125°, 100° and 80°, respectively. Movements towards extension were begun at the 7th sec, and those towards flexion at the 35th sec. (From MOUNTCASTLE et al., 1963)

monkeys and recording from cells in the ventrobasal nuclear complex of the thalamus, found in every case that the joint neurones are maximally activated at the
extremities of the range of movement of a joint. For example, neurones driven by
rotation of the contralateral knee reach their highest rates at either full flexion
or full extension and never at any intermediate position. Less extreme positions
evoked successively lower frequencies of discharge until threshold position was
reached when the neurone discharges at its "spontaneous" rate. Further displacements produce no further change in that rate of discharge (Fig. 9). The thalamic

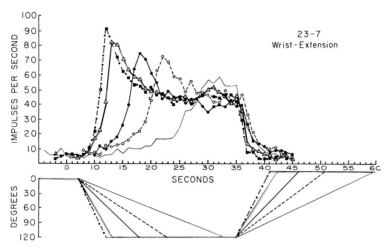

Fig. 11. Graphs illustrating the results of the "several speeds to one angle" experiment for a
ventrobasal thalamic cell driven by extension of the contralateral wrist. Scale for angle shown
below, is arbitrary: 120° on this scale equals 85° extension of the wrist from its midposition.
The edge of the excitatory angle was 55° on this arbitrary scale, or 20° extension of the wrist
from its midposition. Five trials were made at each speed, the results oriented in time and
averaged, and the averages are plotted as the curves show. Angular velocities were 23, 19,
11, 7.5 and 4 degrees per second, respectively, for the curves with peaks successively from left
to right, as indicated by identical lines above and below. (From Mountcastle et al., 1963)

cells thus mirror the behaviour of the peripheral sense organs, but they have
active angles about four times those of the latter. Within their active angle the
thalamic cells also signal position by their adapted frequencies (Fig. 10). The
excitatory angle as depicted by this relation of frequency to angle is a continuous
monotonic, and thus single-ended, function. The transient increase of frequency
varies with the speed of movement just as in the peripheral receptors (Fig. 11).
These and other results will be further taken up in the final discussion of joint
receptors and kinaesthesis.

From the experiments reviewed it appears safe to conclude that articular nerve
fibres reach the anterior lobe of the cerebellum and both the contralateral sensory
areas I and II and the ipsilateral area II, by way of the ventrobasal complex, where
the responding cells, though having 4 times as large active angles, obviously exhibit
the same characteristics of discharge as single-ended peripheral receptors. That the

rapidly adapting mechanoreceptor responses ascend through the dorsal funiculi is also obvious from the experiments of BURGESS and CLARK (1969a). However, the exact spinal pathway for the slowly adapting afferents, except those reaching the anterior lobe of the cerebellum through the spinocerebellar tracts (HADDAD, 1953), appears obscure.

Although GARDNER and NOER (1952) and GARDNER and HADDAD (1953) obtained cortical responses with articular stimulation after cutting the dorsal funiculi, the possibility remains that the ascending activity was mediating pain since no control of the afferent stimulation was made. With regard to the experiments of BURGESS and CLARK (1969) one must inquire into the possibility of studying other than the directly ascending fibres with the antidromic technique. All impulses being mediated in the dorsal columns after one synapse are of course excluded, providing such fibres exist. Several authors have reported cells responsive to joint movements in the rostral part of the dorsal column nuclei (GORDON and PAINE, 1960; KRUGER et al., 1961; PERL et al., 1962; WINTER, 1965). Actually KRUGER et al. (1961) describe both rapidly and slowly adapting neurones in the dorsal column nuclei. They furthermore state that these neurones "displayed a steadily increasing rate as the joint angle was increased over the entire range of angular displacement and were classified as slow-adapting". According to OSWAL-DO-CRUZ and KIDD (1964) the third pathway from the periphery via the lateral cervical nucleus does not convey any impulses from the receptors subserving kinaesthesis. Consequently, it has still to be inferred that the spinal route for kinaesthetic impulses is via the dorsal column although this path might not be a monosynaptic one other than for the rapidly adapting joint receptors. Before finally discussing the central representation of joint receptors we will first reconsider some of the new evidence for a contribution of muscle receptors to kinaesthesis.

G. Muscle Receptors and Kinaesthesis

For a long time it was the generally held idea that the receptors of the muscles made an important contribution to the afferent inflow in kinaesthesis. After the demonstration of MOUNTCASTLE et al. (1952) that there is no cortical representation of muscle afferents of group I, the earlier opinion had to be changed, as emphasized by ROSE and MOUNTCASTLE (1959). However, since then new evidence has been put forward for a cortical representation of muscle receptors.

Actually some workers like GARDNER and NOER (1952), GARDNER and MORIN (1953) and McINTYRE (1953) found cortical responses from group II muscle afferents and possibly group I afferents. The explanation for this finding, however, was generally held to be the presence of joint and other deep structure fibres in muscle nerves, as described in an earlier paragraph.

GARDNER and MORIN (1953), however, stated that they were only stimulating group I and II afferents and, furthermore, that responses were also obtained from the precentral gyrus in monkeys. ALBE-FESSARD et al. (1965) confirmed that evoked potentials were obtained in both motor and sensory cortices in monkeys after group I afferent stimulation.

AMASSIAN and BERLIN (1958) were the first to report that group I afferents originating from slowly adapting stretch receptors in the forelimb do project to the sensorimotor cortex. This observation was confirmed by Oscarsson and Rosén (1963) who in addition demonstrated that the forelimb group I path is activated by primary muscle spindle afferents and projects through the dorsal funiculus medial lemniscal system to a small area located rostral to the postcruciate dimple in the posterior sigmoid gyrus. Hindlimb group I afferents have also been shown to project to the cat cerebral cortex in a projection pattern that is very similar to that of forelimb afferents. Thus, Landgren and Silfvenius (1969a) showed a projection field rostromedial to the postcruciate dimple overlapping the corresponding forelimb area. They also showed a second projection field on the medial side of the hemisphere, extending from area 3a into the sensory cortex (area 1 of Hassler and Muhs-Clement). Landgren et al. (1967) also reported group I hindlimb responses in the region of the anterior suprasylvian sulcus.

The group I paths from the forelimb and the hindlimb differ in their spinal course. As mentioned above the forelimb path travels in the dorsal columns as shown by Oscarsson and Rosén (1963) and by Landgren et al. (1967). The hindlimb path, on the other hand, has a spinal course that closely agrees with the location of the dorsal spinocerebellar tract, which according to Landgren and Silfvenius leaves two alternative possibilities: 1) the spinal component of this path is the dorsal spinocerebellar tract neurones or 2) this path utilizes other neurones with ascending axons travelling together with the dorsal spinocerebellar tracts. The brainstem relay is according to Landgren and Silfvenius (1969b) localized in the nucleus Z of Brodal and Pompeiano (1957).

Regardless of the similarities and the differences between the fore- and hindlimb projections of group I muscle spindle afferents the above mentioned authors seem to agree that the weight of all evidence is against an assumption of a role of this afferent inflow in kinaesthesis. Supporting this opinion is the finding of Giaquinto et al. (1963) who showed that stimulation of group I forelimb or hindlimb afferents in waking or sleeping cats did not cause any change of the behavior or the electroencephalogram. Furthermore, group I afferent volleys can not be used for triggering of instrumental conditioned reflexes as found by Swett and Bourassa (1967). In addition Gelfan and Carter (1967) showed that stretching of exposed muscle tendons in man at tensions that apparently activated primary as well as secondary muscle spindle afferents failed to evoke sensations of change in muscle tension or joint position. Blocking of impulses from joint and skin receptors without affecting the transmission from muscle receptors eliminated the kinaesthesis according to Provins (1958) and Merton (1964).

On the basis of the above quoted evidence it still seems valid to conclude that muscle receptors do not contribute to kinaesthesis. Paillard and Brouchon (1968), however, who confirmed Goldscheider's original finding from 1889 that the accuracy of limb localization after active movements is significantly higher than after passive ones, use this observation to argue for a contribution of muscle afferents over the gamma loop or the motor outflow. They conclude that the significant information derived from self-induced movement is related to the dynamic phase of the movement and seem to base their conclusion on the assumption that information of articular origin is the same under both active and passive conditions. They simply state that although a change in muscle tension alters the sensitivity of some joint receptors, this may be considered of little importance and, furthermore, that it is doubtful whether such an effect can explain the better calibration of position in the case of active displacements. Actually, it would be just during the dynamic phase of a movement that the joint receptors would be influenced by the muscles inserting at the joint.

It is certainly difficult to follow the arguments of PAILLARD and BROUCHON in view of the experimental data at hand with regard to the change of proprioceptive information demonstrated under various muscle tensions (SKOGLUND, (1956). Since PAILLARD and BROUCHON in 1968 brought up the old hypothesis of "sensation of innervation" in connection with the difference between active and passive movement, it is certainly worth while to recollect that the objection to this hypothesis forwarded by SHERRINGTON in 1900 was that "it sunders sharply the sensations of passive from those of active movement whereas there is strong ground for believing the two intimately allied". This statement of SHERRINGTON seems still to be valid. The functional role of the cortical representation of muscle spindle afferents might not be settled but the opinion expressed by PROVINS (1958) that "the present evidence provides no justification for assuming that the threshold appreciation of active limb movement or joint position with the muscles tensed is based on information derived from a source different from that used in the operation of passive movement" has the advantage of resting on an experimental basis. With regard to the interaction between joint and muscle afferents necessary for motor performance in the way discussed by PAILLARD and BROUCHON (1967) the cerebellum ought to be the place.

H. Joint Receptors and Kinaesthesis

From the analyses of the joint receptors it is obvious that the Golgi-tendon organs in the ligaments being uninfluenced by the muscles inserting at the joint are able to signal the exact position of the joint and probably also the direction of movement. The Ruffini-endings being very sensitive would be able to signal speed of movements and their direction, but since they are influenced by the tension of the muscles inserting at the joints they would also be able to signal resistance to movement and possibly discriminate between active and passive movements. The Pacinian corpuscles would most likely be able to detect very small movements and may signal acceleration of movement.

These functions of the joint receptors appear very simple and quite intelligible if one considers the activity of single peripheral endorgans under the prerequisite that they have a certain localization within the joint tissue which in turn suggests that they are activated at a certain position of the joint or by movements within a restricted angle. Considering, however, that the active angle of several joint receptors are overlapping and the possibility, that some receptors are active at both flexion and extension, the problem of the perception of kinaesthetic stimuli is certainly a more complicated one. So far little data with regard to the function of cortical cells is available whereas the study of MOUNTCASTLE et al. (1963) on thalamic neurones gives some interesting information about the central transformation of the sensory inflow from joint receptors.

9*

As pointed out by Mountcastle et al. (1963) a change in position must be signalled by variations in the spatial pattern of activity in large groups of neurones. These authors state that of the thalamic nerve cells related to a given joint, some will be driven by movement in one direction, some by the other. Furthermore, all those activated by a given movement will discharge along monotonically increasing functions reaching their maximal firing rates at the limit of movement which is either full flexion or full extension, regardless of the increasing rates of discharge in the relevant group of cells. Mountcastle et al. (1963) pointed out that this state of affairs is of a certain interest since the study of the first order afferents suggests that the situation there is quite different, whereby they most likely must mean the double-ended receptors. Hence they conclude there must take place a remarkable transformation between first and third-order elements in the system mediating kinaesthesis.

In Fig. 12, from Mountcastle et al. (1963) it is obvious that the thalamic neurones have receptive angles greater than one half of the total range of angular movement, overlapping in the middle region. Since the first order afferents have active angles over less than a fourth of the thalamic ones, it must mean that those activated on the other side of the neutral position cannot belong to those having their maximum activity in the opposite direction. Hence it can be concluded that double-ended receptors contribute to the discharge of the thalamic neurones and when some drop out others are recruited and in an increasing amount while the joint is approaching an extreme position. With regard to the receptors which are lying at the extreme of flexion or extension there would be no problems and since they are the most numerous, as shown by Cohen (1955), Skoglund (1956) and Burgess and Clark (1969b), their behavior would fit in well with the description of the thalamic neurones given by Mountcastle et al. (1963). The double-ended receptors, on the other hand, cannot signal position by frequency with the exception of that position which produces the maximum discharge (Fig. 4) since within the sensitive range of any of these receptors there are always two different positions which evoke the same signal. Mountcastle et al. suggest that such receptors, if signalling position, could only be detected by determining which fibres of the total population were active. In the first place this must apply to all receptors of course, since several peripheral receptors converge on to the same thalamic neurones as evidenced by their wider receptive angle of joint movement. This means that each thalamic neurone can only signal position by frequency of response, a frequency which for each neurone must be a function of the position of the joint and thus the number of first order afferents activated as well as their firing rate. The number of active peripheral receptors increases towards the extremes of joint positions, consequently the thalamic neurones should quite logically have their maximum discharge at the extreme of flexion or extension.

Some problems in the central transformation of the afferent input from joints might concern us in this connection, namely the number of thalamic neurones involved and their mode of behaviour in between each other with regard to the discrimination of kinaesthetic stimuli. Just as there is a set of peripheral receptors overlapping, there is obviously a set of both thalamic and cortical neurones overlapping and not having either the same receptive angle or the same frequency of response at a fixed position. The question then inevitably arises how discrimination between these neurones is achieved in the end. This question can be extended to inquire into which receptor is connected to which central neurone or whether they are connected to many of them in an orderly way, thus conveying at the same time something of the peripheral place where they are situated. In that way a collection of central neurones will not only vary intensively in the domain of frequency which for a single neurone reflects a spatial pattern in the periphery, but this very same spatial pattern is also transferred to a number of central neurones being activated during a particular movement or at a particular position. The action of the overlapping active receptors in the periphery has thus been transformed into

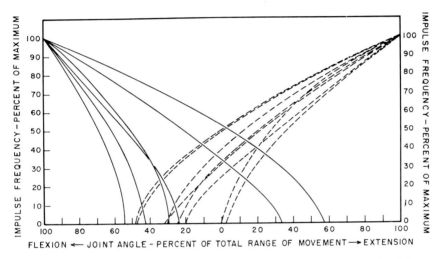

Fig. 12. Plots of the best fitting power function for each of 14 hinge joint ventrobasal thalamic neurones. Abscissa scale normalized for different joints by correcting values for each to percent of the maximal possible movement in either direction from a middle, or neutral position of the joint. (From MOUNTCASTLE et al., 1963)

a series of frequency codes in several central neurones signalling position and movement.

Under the prerequisite that all joint receptors have a certain fixed set of connections the fact that endings might fire at both flexion and extension as described by BURGESS and CLARK (1969b) would not hamper their recognition, providing that they alone are not able to drive a neurone at one of these positions. If the summation of many receptors is necessary to drive for instance a flexor neurone, it would not be driven only by those that are active at extension but these could well contribute to the spontaneous activity outside the active angle. Such an explanation, though highly speculative, should mean that they only fulfil a reinforcing, conditioning function to keep the central pathway open.

MOUNTCASTLE et al. (1963) furthermore emphasized the importance of the observations that the transformations of the peripheral receptor activity occurs as early as in the thalamic stage. These authors expected the subsequent neural transformation after the thalamic relay to the cortical cells to occur along linear coordinates as far as the value intensity was concerned. From the data presented by Mountcastle and Powell (1959) about cortical neurones, although incomplete with respect to several of the parameters studied in thalamic neurones, it appears that such an expectation might be true. However, one might ask whether the transformation seen in thalamic neurones does not take place as early as at the second order neurones (cf. Kruger et al., 1961) and thus being but a reflection of the transfer of the first order afferents at the first synapse, integrating the activity of overlapping active joint receptors and from there on it is just a linear transfer.

Mountcastle et al. (1963) described the neural transform from the periphery to the thalamic neurones as a lawful relation obeying a power function with regard to the steady joint position (Fig. 12). The central neurones, however, like the joint receptors, show transient increases during movement (Fig. 11). These transients varying with speed and range of movement have so far not been analysed in detail. However, this behaviour of central neurones would well explain the better perception of position following a movement. The adaptation of the central neurones to the steady discharge might well explain the well-known temporal degradation of position sense, and why no contribution of either muscle afferents or motor outflow is necessary. Still, though, we must inquire into the mechanism by which the frequency codes of central neurones are transformed into awareness or kinaesthetic sensations.

References

Albe-Fessard, D., Liebeskind, J., Lamarre, Y.: Projection au niveau du cortex somatomoteur du singe d'afférences provenant des récepteurs musculaires. C.R. Acad. Sci. (Paris) **261**, 3891–3894 (1965).

Amassian, V.E., Berlin, L.: Early cortical projection of group I afferents in the forelimb muscle nerves of the cat. J. Physiol. (Lond.) **143**, 61P (1958).

Andersson, S., Stener, B.: Experimental evaluation of the hypothesis of ligamento-muscular protective reflexes. II. A study in cat using the medial collateral ligament of the knee joint. Acta physiol. scand. **48**, Suppl. 166, 27–49 (1959).

Andrew, B.L.: The sensory innervation of the medial ligament of the knee joint. J. Physiol. (Lond.) **123**, 241–250 (1954a).

Andrew, B.L.: Proprioception at the joint of the epiglottis of the rat. J. Physiol. (Lond.) **126**, 507–523 (1954b).

Andrew, B.L., Dodt, E.: The development of sensory nerve endings at the knee joint of the cat. Acta physiol. scand. **28**, 287–296 (1953).

Beswick, F.B., Glockey, N.J., Evanson, J.M.: Some effects of the stimulation of articular nerves. J. Physiol. (Lond.) **128**, 83–84 (1955).

Boyd, I.A.: The histological structure of the receptors on the knee joint of the cat correlated with their physiological response. J. Physiol. (Lond.) **124**, 476–488 (1954).

Boyd, I.A., Roberts, T.D.M.: Proprioceptive discharges from stretch-receptors in the knee joint of the cat. J. Physiol. (Lond.) **122**, 38–58 (1953).

Brodal, A., Pompeiano, O.: The vestibular nuclei of the cat. J. Anat. (Lond.) **91**, 438–454 (1957).

Burgess, P.R., Clark, F.J.: Characteristics of knee joint receptors in the cat. J. Physiol. (Lond.) **203**, 301–317 (1969a).

Burgess, P.R., Clark, F.J.: Dorsal column projection of fibres from the cat knee joint. J. Physiol. (Lond.) **203**, 281–299 (1969b).

Cohen, L.A.: Activity of knee joint proprioceptors recorded from the posterior articular nerve. Yale J. Biol. Med. **28**, 225–232 (1955/1956).

EKHOLM, J., EKLUND, G., SKOGLUND, S.: On the reflex effects from the knee joint of the cat. Acta physiol. scand. **50**, 167–174 (1960).

EKHOLM, J., SKOGLUND, S.: Autonomic contributions to myelinated fibres in peripheral nerves. Acta morph. neerl.-scand. **6**, 55–63 (1963).

EKLUND, G., SKOGLUND, S.: On the specificity of the Ruffini like joint receptors. Acta physiol. scand. **49**, 184–191 (1960).

GARDNER, E.: Nerve terminals associated with the knee joint of the mouse. Anat. Rec. **83**, 401–420 (1942).

GARDNER, E.: The distribution and termination of nerves in the knee joint of the cat. J. comp. Neurol. **80**, 11–32 (1944).

GARDNER, E.: Conduction rates and dorsal root inflow of sensory fibres from the knee joint of the cat. Amer. J. Physiol. **152**, 436–445 (1948).

GARDNER, E.: Physiology of movable joints. Physiol. Rev. **30**, 127–176 (1950a).

GARDNER, E.: Reflex muscular responses to stimulation of articular nerves in the cat. Amer. J. Physiol. **161**, 133–141 (1950b).

GARDNER, E., HADDAD, B.: Pathways to the cerebral cortex for afferent fibres from the hindleg of the cat. Amer. J. Physiol. **172**, 476–482 (1953).

GARDNER, E., LATIMER, F., STILWELL, D.: Central connections for afferent fibres from the knee joint of the cat. Amer. J. Physiol. **159**, 195–198 (1949).

GARDNER, E., MORIN, F.: Spinal pathways for projections of cutaneous and muscular afferents to the sensory motor cortex of the monkey (Macaca mulatta). Amer. J. Physiol. **174**, 149–153 (1953).

GARDNER, E., NOER, R.: Projection of afferent fibres from muscles and joints to the cerebral cortex of the cat. Amer. J. Physiol. **168**, 437–441 (1952).

GELFAN, S., CARTER, S.: Muscle sense in man. Exp. Neurol. **18**, 469–473 (1967).

GIAQUINTO, S., POMPEIANO, O., SWETT, J.E.: EEG and behavioural effects of fore- and hindlimb muscular afferent volleys in unrestrained cats. Arch. ital. Biol. **101**, 133–148 (1963).

GOLDSCHEIDER, A.: Untersuchungen über den Muskelsinn. Arch. Anat. u. Physiol. **13**, 369–502 (1889).

GORDON, G., PAINE, C.H.: Functional organization in the nucleus gracilis of the cat. J. Physiol. (Lond.) **153**, 331–349 (1960).

HADDAD, B.: Projection of afferent fibres from the knee joint to the cerebellum of the cat. Amer. J. Physiol. **172**, 511–514 (1952).

KRUGER, L., SIMINOFF, R., WITKOVSKY, P.: Single neuron analysis of dorsal column nuclei and spinal nucleus of trigeminal in cat. J. Neurophysiol. **24**, 333–349 (1961).

KUHN, R.A.: Topographical pattern of cutaneous sensibility in the dorsal column nuclei of the cat. Trans. Amer. neurol. Ass. **74**, 227–230 (1949).

LANDGREN, S., SILFVENIUS, H.: Projection to cerebral cortex of group I muscle afferents from the cat's hindlimb. J. Physiol. (Lond.) **200**, 353–372 (1969a).

LANDGREN, S., SILFVENIUS, H.: The medullary relay in the path from hindlimb muscle spindles to the cerebral cortex. Acta physiol. scand. Suppl. 330 (1969b).

LANDGREN, S., SILFVENIUS, H., WOLSK, O.: Somato-sensory paths to the second cortical projection area of the group I muscle afferents. J. Physiol. (Lond.) **191**, 543—559 (1967).

MERTON, P.A.: Human position sense and sense of effort. Symp. Soc. exp. Biol. 387–400 (1964).

MOUNTCASTLE, V.B.: Modality and topographic properties of single neurons of cat's somatic sensory cortex. J. Neurophysiol. **20**, 408–434 (1957).

MOUNTCASTLE, V.B., COVIAN, M.R., HARRISON, C.R.: The central representation of some forms of deep sensibility. Proc. Ass. Res. Nerv. Ment. Dis. **30**, 339–370 (1952).

MOUNTCASTLE, V.B., POGGIO, G.F., WERNER, G.: The relation of thalamic cell response to peripheral stimuli varied over an intensive continuum. J. Neurophysiol. **26**, 807–834 (1963).

MOUNTCASTLE, V.B., POWELL, T.P.S.: Central nervous mechanisms subserving position sense and kinesthesis. Bull. Johns Hopk. Hosp. **105**, 173–200 (1959).

OSCARSSON, O., ROSÉN, I.: Projection to cerebral cortex of large muscle spindle afferents in forelimb nerves of the cat. J. Physiol. (Lond.) **169**, 924–945 (1963).

PAILLARD, J., BROUCHON, M.: Active and passive movements in the calibration of position sense. In: The neuropsychology of spatially oriented behavior, ed. S.J. FREEDMAN. Homewood, Ill.: Doresy Press 1968.

Perl, E. R., Whitlock, D. G.: Somatic stimuli exciting spinothalamic projections to thalamic neurons in cat and monkey. Exp. Neurol. **3**, 256–296 (1961).

Perl, E. R., Whitlock, D. G., Gentry, J. R.: Cutaneous projection to second order neurons of the dorsal column system. J. Neurophysiol. **25**, 337–358 (1962).

Poggio, G. F., Mountcastle, V. B.: The functional properties of ventro-basal thalamic neurons studied in unanaesthetized monkeys. J. Neurophysiol. **26**, 775–806 (1963).

Poláček, P.: Receptors of the joints. Their structure, variability and classification. Acta Facul. Med. Univ. Bruneneis (1966).

Provins, K. A.: The effect of peripheral nerve block on the appreciation and execution of finger movements. J. Physiol. (Lond.) **143**, 55–67 (1958).

Rose, J. E., Mountcastle, V. B.: Touch and kinesthesis. In: Handbook of Physiol. Section I Neurophysiol. 387–429 (1959).

Rüdinger, N.: Die Gelenknerven des menschlichen Körpers. Erlangen: Verlag Ferdinand Enke 1857.

Samuel, E. P.: The autonomic and somatic innervation of the articular capsule. Anat. Rec. **113**, 53–70 (1952).

Sfameni, A.: Researches anatomiques sur l'existence des nerfs et sur leur mode de se terminer dans le tissu adipeux, dans le périoste, dans le périchondre et dans les tissus qui renforcent les articulations. Arch. ital. Biol. **38**, 49–101 (1902).

Sherrington, C. S.: The muscular sense. Schäfer: Textbook of Physiol. **2**, 1002–1025 (1900).

Skoglund, S.: Anatomical and physiological studies of knee joint innervation in the cat. Acta physiol. scand. **36**, Suppl. 124 (1956).

Swett, J. E., Bourassa, C. M.: Comparison of sensory discrimination thresholds with muscle and cutaneous nerve volleys in the cat. J. Neurophysiol. **30**, 530–545 (1967).

Winter, D. L.: N. gracilis of cat. Functional organization and corticofugal effects. J. Neurophysiol. **28**, 48–70 (1965).

Chapter 5

The Concept of Relay Nuclei

By

GEORGE GORDON, Oxford (Great Britain)

With 1 Figure

Contents

A. Introduction

All sensory pathways directed to the cerebral cortex contain at least two synaptic interruptions which provide sites for access and interaction. When these occur in compact nuclear regions like the dorsal column nuclei, sensory trigeminal nucleus, lateral cervical nucleus, or the ventroposterior nucleus of the thalamus one calls such regions *relay nuclei* and the cells projecting out of them *relay cells*. When the cells of origin of an ascending tract are distributed segmentally, like those giving rise to the spinocervical or spinothalamic tracts, one may call such cells *tract cells*.

The definition of the various somaesthetic relay nuclei is primarily anatomical. Electrophysiological study, involving an examination of the receptive properties of single relay cells, and of their projection as determined by antidromic excitation, has shown that single nuclei usually contain several semi-independent functional elements. For example, the output of the main cell-masses of the dorsal column nuclei travels in the medial lemniscus to the thalamus, whereas some fibres from the rostral poles of these nuclei diverge from the lemniscus in the upper midbrain and probably end on a variety of cell-groups in this region (GORDON and JUKES, 1964a; KUYPERS and TUERK, 1964; HAND and LIU, 1966). A very small part of the rostral pole of the gracile nucleus projects to the cerebellum (GORDON and HORRO-BIN, 1967). The lemniscal projection of the cuneate nucleus contains both a cutaneous and a muscle afferent system which connect with different regions of the ventroposterior nucleus and are there relayed to different regions of the sensory cortex (Oscarsson and Rosén, 1963; Andersson et al., 1966). These apparently disparate components of a single sensory nucleus both receive a projection, in the cuneate nucleus, from the same regions of the sensorimotor

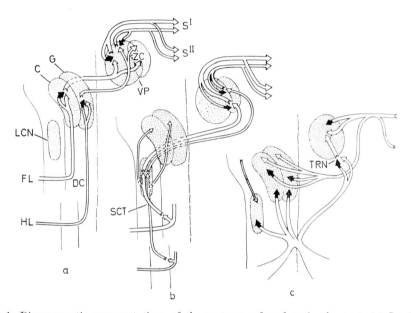

Fig. 1. Diagrammatic representations of the systems referred to in the text. (a) Intrinsic connections of the dorsal column-lemniscothalamic system. (b) Intrinsic connections of the spinocervico-lemniscothalamic system. This figure also shows extrinsic afferent inputs to the dorsal column nuclei, carried in the dorsolateral fascicle and possibly arising from the spino-cervical tract. (c) Extrinsic ascending and descending influences on relay nuclei. No attempt is made to define the ascending paths precisely, but it is thought that these are predominantly in the ventral spinal quadrants. Conventions: — arrow-heads and arrow-tails are used to indicate inputs and outputs, respectively, of relay nuclei or cortex. Open arrow-heads represent excitation, black arrow-heads inhibition: a shaded arrow indicates a path of unknown nature. Interneurones are not represented, and pre- and post-synaptic inhibition are not distinguished. The vertical dotted line in each figure indicates the midline. Abbreviations: — C, cuneate nucleus; DC, dorsal column; FL, forelimb; G, gracile nucleus; HL, hind limb; LCN, lateral cervical nucleus; S I and S II, areas of somaesthetic cortex; SCT, spinocervical tract; TRN, thalamic reticular nuclei; VP, ventroposterior nucleus; ZC, thalamic zone of con-vergence

cortex, and there is a striking resemblance in the patterns of action of the descend-ing paths (cf. Rosén, 1969; Gordon and Jukes, 1964b and Levitt et al., 1964). In this instance the similarity between cutaneous and muscle afferent paths, as appearing in their corticofugal control, may be related to the well-known associa-tion between tactile acuity and exploratory movement. The function of any nucleus should therefore be considered in terms of the control systems acting on it as well as in terms of its simpler transmitting functions.

In the cat, the animal so far most intensively studied, the sensory input from skin receptors, apart from those in the trigeminal area, is projected to the cerebral cortex through at least two major systems in parallel — the dorsal column-lemniscothalamic and the spinocervicothalamic systems. Much of this article will deal with the often contrasting functional characteristics of relay nuclei in these two systems. The schematic diagrams in Fig. 1 identify the nuclei and some of the inter-relationships to be described. The special features of the trigeminal system are described elsewhere in this volume (DARIAN-SMITH, Chapter 9). My purpose is to review concepts of the functioning of relay nuclei which have emerged from recent anatomical and electrophysiological evidence, without prejudice as to their precise sensory functions, which have for long been the subject of controversy (SHERRINGTON, 1900; NORRSELL, 1966; WALL, 1970). The posterior group of thalamic nuclei (see POGGIO and MOUNTCASTLE, 1960), one part of which receives a somatic input, will not be considered here in the context of a relay nucleus. This interesting region, only a quarter or so of whose output has so far been defined, is known to receive its input through converging branches of the other known afferent paths (CALMA, 1965; ROWE and SESSLE, 1968; CURRY, 1971).

B. Receptive Fields

The study of receptive fields of individual relay cells gives important information about the functioning of a nucleus providing that the receptive characteristics of its incoming fibres are already well known. Clearly the evidence will be easiest to interpret in studies of first-order nuclei like the dorsal column nuclei and progressively more difficult at succeeding relays in a serially connected system.

1. Dorsal Column-Lemniscothalamic System

The relay cells of the dorsal column nuclei which give rise to the main lemniscal projection lie mostly in the central portions of these nuclei in the region of the cell-nests (GORDON and JUKES, 1964a; KUYPERS and TUERK, 1964; HAND and LIU, 1966). They are arranged in an accurate somatotopic fashion, which is reproduced in the part of the thalamic ventroposterior nucleus to which they project, but is not seen in other somaesthetic nuclei except in analogous regions of the trigeminal system. The somatotopic arrangement has been demonstrated in great detail in the raccoon (JOHNSON et al., 1968). Excitatory receptive fields increase in size with distance from the apices of the limbs, cells with proximal fields having considerable excitatory spatial convergence (GORDON and JUKES, 1964a; WINTER, 1965). Receptive fields are in general larger than those of corresponding incoming fibres (WINTER, 1965). Size of field also depends on the type or types of receptor by which the cell is activated: cells driven by claw receptors in the cat have minute spot-like excitatory fields, but the fields of cells driven from hairs or pads in the extremities are always larger (GORDON and JUKES, 1964a).

The dorsal column nuclei are remarkable in that their output contains a high proportion of "pure lines" in which the response properties of individual types of superficial receptor are preserved. Four groups of cells have been recognized on this basis in the cat's gracile nucleus, all represented in the lemniscal output — those excited by rapidly adapting hair receptors, or pad receptors, by slowly adapting mechanoceptors in skin, or by slowly adapting claw receptors (PERL et al., 1962; GORDON and JUKES, 1964a). Corresponding classes of relay cell have been recognized in the thalamic ventroposterior nucleus (ROSE and MOUNTCASTLE, 1959; NAKAHAMA et al., 1966; MANSON, 1969); and representatives of all these classes have been shown to project from this nucleus to the somaesthetic cortex (MANSON, 1969). There is at present no evidence of relay cells in the dorsal column nuclei requiring noxious stimuli to excite them.

The commonest type of cell seen in the gracile output with obvious excitatory convergence from more than one kind of skin receptor was that excited by hair and adjacent pad receptors in a single coherent receptive field (GORDON and JUKES, 1964a), an arrangement ensuring continuity in the representation of the body surface in the nucleus. More precise studies of the degree of specificity in the receptive characteristics of gracile and cuneate cells were made by recording from single lemniscal axons of cells receiving an excitatory input from the dorsal columns (BROWN et al., 1970): recording is then possible for the longer period needed for adequate study of the receptive field. It was found that some cells are more specialized in this sense than was previously thought. Some were excited exclusively from tylotrich hairs in receptive fields of only a few mm^2; and these had stimulus-velocity/impulse-frequency relations like those of primary tylotrich fibres (see BROWN and IGGO, 1967). Another group responded exclusively to stimulating small groups of touch corpuscles and showed their characteristic response properties; and another had punctate pressure-sensitive fields and responded to stretching skin, like Type II corpuscles (see CHAMBERS and IGGO, 1967). This specificity must depend on precise excitatory connections in the nuclei rather than on any gating action applied by a descending control system, because such systems are probably inactive under the deep anaesthesia used in these experiments; though it is possible that minor contributions from other receptors could be suppressed by afferent inhibition. It should be noted that this order of receptor specificity has been seen in the postcentral cortex of the unanaesthetized monkey with respect to Pacinian corpuscles and to rapidly adapting skin touch receptors (MOUNTCASTLE et al., 1969); and it seems likely that these are served by the dorsal column-lemniscothalamic system.

Records from single lemniscal fibres have also shown that nearly all the relay cells had a resting discharge, even under deep anaesthesia, which is not present in most primary afferent fibres (SCHWARTZ et al., 1964). This discharge must have been generated by intranuclear mechanisms, if only because in a majority of cells it could be totally inhibited by appropriate peripheral stimuli (BROWN et al., 1970). This has removed the suspicion that such activity seen in records from the nuclei might be largely the result of the presence of the electrode there. Such resting discharge may be significant as a background against which to signal inhibitory actions.

The great majority of relay cells in the central regions of the dorsal column nuclei have inhibitory components in their receptive fields (GORDON and PAINE, 1960; GORDON and JUKES, 1964a). This inhibition is elicited by light mechanical stimulation of hairs or pads in an area which partly or completely surrounds the excitatory field and always exceeds it in size. The effectiveness of inhibition diminishes with distance from the excitatory centre. This "surround inhibition" has also been seen in the fields of cells in the part of the thalamic ventroposterior nucleus to which this system projects, but not in as high a proportion of them as might have been expected. The reasons for this obscuring of the inhibitory fields are not fully known, though the fact that they were observed in 47 % of cells investigated under chloralose compared with only 10 % of all cells investigated under barbiturate (GORDON and MANSON, 1967) suggests that additional factors including some mechanism differentially sensitive to anaesthetics is operative in the thalamus, and there is independent evidence for this (KING et al., 1957; ANGEL, 1964, 1967). Inhibitory components were found in the fields of only 5 % of cells in this region of the thalamus of the unanaesthetized monkey (POGGIO and MOUNTCASTLE, 1963).

One interesting reason for the obscuring of simple inhibitory field components in the ventroposterior nucleus could be that more complex receptive fields are being developed, as they are at different levels of the visual system, and that techniques of observation have not been adequate to reveal them. It is well known that human tactile discrimination is greatly increased when relative movement can occur between the skin and the stimulating object; and the simple receptive fields of the dorsal column nuclei, in which both excitatory and inhibitory components are predominantly velocity-sensitive, seem appropriate units from which to build fields containing, for instance, directional preference. In spite of general awareness of this possibility, there is as yet no experimental support for any systematic organization on these lines: only isolated examples of cells with some form of directional sensitivity have been reported, in the ventroposterior nucleus of the anaesthetized cat (GORDON and MANSON, 1967) and in the postcentral cortex of the unanaesthetized monkey (MOUNTCASTLE et al., 1969). Appropriate conditions for a proper study of this question may require that the animal is conscious, unrestrained and therefore free to explore its surroundings.

2. Spinocervico-Lemniscothalamic System

The spinocervical tract relays in the lateral cervical nucleus (Fig. 1), which projects through a distinct part of the contralateral medial lemniscus (BUSCH, 1961) to the contralateral ventroposterior nucleus where the projection terminates in a dorsolateral zone of convergence with that of the dorsal column-lemniscal system (LANDGREN et al., 1965), and this in turn projects to the cortical areas S I and S II (ANDERSEN et al., 1966). The lateral cervical nucleus is specially well developed in carnivores: it is also present in primates, and it has been suggested that the cells distributed through the length of the spinal dorsolateral white matter in rodents and insectivores represent a dispersed homologue of this nucleus (see WALDRON, 1969).

The nuclei of this system differ in several respects from those of the dorsal column-lemniscothalamic system, first in size — considered in terms of numbers of fibres and relay cells the spinocervicothalamic system is smaller by an order of magnitude than the latter. Secondly these nuclei seem to lack the somatotopic precision of the dorsal column system. In the cat's lateral cervical nucleus the forelimb was found to predominate and to lie lateral to that of the hind limb, but no more detailed somatotopic relation was recognized in the very thin transverse profile or in the rostrocaudal axis (Horrobin, 1966), nor could Boivie (1970) find any anatomical evidence of somatotopic order in the rostrocaudal axis. Similarly the main thalamic relay of this system is diffusely organized in somatotopic terms, at least for the hind limb which alone has been investigated at this level (Land-gren et al., 1965).

The receptive fields of fibres of the spinocervical tract are described in another article in this volume (Brown, p. 315). The features which particularly distinguish them from those in, for example, the main output of the dorsal column nuclei are the absence of units with an input from only one type of receptor, and the absence of inhibitory components in a surround pattern. The receptive fields of cells in the lateral cervical nucleus of the cat are certainly larger than those of spinocervical tract fibres, and their average size is considerably larger than that for relay cells in the dorsal column nuclei: as in the dorsal column nuclei, size of receptive field increases with distance from the apex of a limb (Horrobin, 1966). This nucleus therefore represents a region of considerable spatial convergence. The nature of the receptor convergence on to these cells has not yet been so precisely determined as in the spinocervical fibres; but it is generally agreed that some 80 % of cells have an input from hair receptors (Horrobin, 1966; Morin et al., 1963; Oswaldo-Cruz and Kidd, 1964). There are often other components in addition, such as those derived from fibres of high electrical threshold in muscle nerves (Fedina et al., 1968). Surround inhibition has not been seen.

C. Mechanisms for Surround Inhibition

It is believed that the mechanisms responsible for surround inhibition in the dorsal column nuclei are activated by the *intrinsic* afferent input to these nuclei — that is, by the dorsal column which is the main afferent tract of this relay system. Strong presynaptic and postsynaptic inhibition occurs in the nuclei when the cervical dorsal column is stimulated. Very much weaker effects occur when other afferent tracts are stimulated after section of the dorsal column at cervical level; and the inhibition now produced by peripheral stimuli does not have either the low mechanical threshold or the peripheral distribution characteristic of surround inhibition (Davidson and Smith, 1970; Dart and Gordon, 1970).

Eccles and his colleagues made an extensive study of the inhibitory actions, particularly presynaptic inhibitory actions, produced in the cuneate nucleus by electrical stimulation of cutaneous and mixed nerves in the forelimb, their evidence suggesting that the interneurones required for inhibition of relay cells lay within or adjacent to the nucleus (see Andersen et al., 1964a). More recently, similar techniques were used to show that both pre- and postsynaptic inhibition of relay cells in the dorsal column nuclei is produced by light mechanical stimulation of the appropriate area of skin, even by deflection of a few hairs (Andersen et al., 1968, 1970). The magnitude of presynaptic inhibitory action has been found to be greatest in the regions of both the trigeminal nucleus (Darian-Smith, 1965) and of the dorsal column nuclei (ANDERSEN et al., 1968, 1970) where cells with surrounding inhibitory fields occur most densely. It was pointed out by ANDERSEN et al. (1964b) and by GORDON and JUKES (1964a) that it is improbable that the inhibitory action in the receptive field of a single cell was initiated only from an area surrounding the excitatory component of the field, but rather that the excitatory field is superimposed on a larger area, the whole of which generates inhibition. This has been shown to be true for presynaptic inhibition in single primary fibres entering the trigeminal nucleus (DARIAN-SMITH, 1965) and for postsynaptic inhibition in single relay cells of the cuneate nucleus (ANDERSEN et al., 1970). It is clear that both types of inhibitory action must participate in surround inhibition. As both actions are apparently initiated through the same primary afferent fibres, and act in sequence along a common relay path, only a highly specific method for blocking one or other action would allow an estimate of their relative importance.

The inhibitory actions in the dorsal column nuclei are exerted against an excitatory transmitting action of great intensity, in which two or three of the large unitary EPSPs may be sufficient to fire a relay cell (ANDERSEN et al., 1964b). It has generally been assumed that such inhibitory actions contribute to spatial sharpening in the system.

It seems unlikely that recurrent inhibition from collaterals of the lemniscal axons of relay cells plays an essential part in the generation of surround inhibition in the dorsal column nuclei. Little inhibitory effect could be produced by stimulating the rostral end of the medial lemniscus, which caused antidromic excitation of the main mass of cuneate relay cells, compared with the massive primary afferent depolarization and IPSPs produced in the same nucleus by dorsal column stimulation (ANDERSEN, ETHOLM and GORDON, unpublished observations). In these experiments, spread of stimulus to the cerebral peduncle was avoided by using a single critically placed focal electrode. Inhibition of relay cells in the dorsal column nuclei is nevertheless produced by stimulating in an area of the upper brainstem which corresponds quite closely with the transverse lemniscal profile (GORDON and JUKES, 1964b): these effects were not confined to cells with inhibitory field components and were therefore not thought likely to be concerned in surround inhibition. Furthermore a similar inhibition, produced in this way, is seen in the lateral cervical nucleus, which does not show surround inhibition (HORROBIN, 1966). It is possible that such effects might have been in part the result of activating cells or descending axons whose distribution at this level is superimposed on the lemniscal profile: activation of a recurrent inhibitory system remains a possibility.

In very marked contrast to the situation in the dorsal column nuclei, the cells in the thalamic ventroposterior nucleus are strongly affected by recurrent inhibition, which is seen as a large prolonged IPSP resulting from stimulating thalamocortical fibres (ANDERSEN et al., 1964c). That this is genuinely a recurrent effect is shown by its surviving chronic cortical ablation and consequent degeneration of corticothalamic fibres. This recurrent inhibition was considered in the context of a mechanism capable of sustaining slow rhythmic action of thalamocortical neurons, but its sensory significance is unknown. Nor is anything known of the function of the remarkable synaptic glomeruli, found in this nucleus and in the medial and lateral geniculate nuclei (Jones and Powell, 1969). It has already been said that little is understood of any modifications in somatic receptive fields which occur at a thalamic level.

The fact that relay nuclei possess intrinsic inhibitory systems, with the interneuronal organization that this implies, and also receive extrinsic ascending and descending fibres which terminate in them (see below), must explain, for example, the observation that only some 20 % of boutons in the cuneate nucleus were seen with electron microscopy to degenerate after section of the dorsal column (Walberg, 1966).

D. Extrinsic Afferent Effects on Transmission through Relay Nuclei

It has recently become clear that somaesthetic relay nuclei are subject to facilitatory and inhibitory influences through pathways other than their main afferent tracts: these will be called *extrinsic* afferent influences.

Reasons were given for believing that the surround inhibition seen in the dorsal column nuclei is intrinsic, requiring intact dorsal column fibres. After section of the dorsal columns, inhibition of relay cells in these nuclei was still produced, but only by noxious peripheral stimuli (Davidson and Smith, 1970; Dart and Gordon, 1970). Such extrinsic afferent inhibition, partly at least presynaptic, can be produced by stimulating the ipsilateral dorsolateral fascicle (which contains among others the spinocervical tract) after dorsal column section (Dart and Gordon, 1970), but the afferent paths may well be more extensive than this because the peripheral inhibitory field is very large and bilateral. It is possible that the inhibitory effects seen by Jabbur and Banna (1968) and by Andersen et al. (1970) on electrical stimulation of contralateral limbs, involved the same pathways and mechanisms.

It has also been found that relay cells of the lateral cervical nucleus can be inhibited from fields which include wide areas of both sides of the body (Fedina et al., 1968). This inhibition was exerted both pre- and postsynaptically on the nucleus itself, independently of actions earlier in this pathway. Skin receptors with a wide range of mechanical thresholds, including noxious thresholds, were involved, and also muscle afferents of high electrical threshold. The principal afferent path for this inhibition ran in the ventral spinal quadrants. Bilateral inhibition from "flexor reflex afferents" also occurs on spinocervical tract cells whose axons terminate in the lateral cervical nucleus (Hongo et al., 1968). It is interesting, in view of the widespread extrinsic effects on the lateral cervical nucleus, that only some 15 % of its boutons degenerate after section of its afferent input through the spinocervical tract (Westman, 1969).

Extrinsic *facilitatory* interaction has been described at the thalamic level by Angel and Dawson (1963), who showed that transmission through the thalamic relay nucleus in the anaesthetized rat can be greatly increased by the previous application of strong peripheral stimuli, like pinching or rubbing, anywhere on the body. Angel (1964) considered that these facilitatory effects were mediated by cells of the adjacent thalamic reticular nuclei, which were affected by strong and widespread peripheral stimuli with an appropriate time-course. At first sight it seems paradoxical that strong cutaneous stimuli, applied anywhere on the body, should increase transmission through the ventroposterior thalamus to the cortex, but should at the same time reduce transmission through spinal and medullary nuclei. It must however be emphasized that such an increase or decrease in transmission could only be understood if one knew not only the pattern of response being transmitted in each case and its significance, but also what patterns of peripheral stimulation would operate these extrinsic mechanisms in the conscious unrestrained animal. The apparently nociceptive threshold for most of these effects is only known so far to apply in the anaesthetized animal.

E. Interaction between Tactile Sensory Systems

It has been assumed so far that the two major chains of somaesthetic relay nuclei were functionally independent; but it is now known that this is not strictly true, even at the level of the dorsal column nuclei. An excitatory tactile input to both dorsal column nuclei has been seen after total section of the cervical dorsal columns, the afferent fibres concerned ascending in the ipsilateral dorsolateral fascicle, some possibly as collaterals of the spinocervical tract (TOMASULO and EMMERS, 1970; DART and GORDON, 1970). This input terminates at least in part on relay cells in these nuclei and is driven by tactile rather than noxious stimuli (DART and GORDON, 1970, 1972): it must therefore be regarded as having a different character from the extrinsic inhibitory input described above. It has also been shown that some cells in the dorsal column nuclei give rise to axons *descending* in the dorsolateral fascicle: the destination of these fibres is not known but it may be supposed that they terminate in the dorsal horn and possibly on neurons of an ascending system such as the spinocervical tract (DART, 1971; DART and GORDON, 1972). These new findings suggest the existence of a close reciprocal inter-relationship between the spinal components of the somaesthetic system in the dorsal part of the cord, so that one is no longer justified in thinking of a functionally isolated "dorsal column system" even at this level. It should be noted that the discovery of such cross-connections creates a new practical difficulty in designing appropriate electrophysiological or behavioural experiments to investigate the functions of different components of the somaesthetic system, since it can no longer be assumed, for instance, that section of the dorsal column isolates the dorsal column nuclei from a peripheral sensory input.

Excitatory convergence also occurs between the dorsal column-lemniscothalamic system and the spinocervicothalamic system in the border zone identified in the ventroposterior nucleus by LANDGREN et al. (1965), on cells shown to relay to the cortical areas S I and S II (ANDERSEN et al., 1966).

F. Descending Control

Many studies of somaesthetic relay nuclei have been carried out under conditions where the relay cells were fairly free of any influences except those exerted by their own main afferent tracts. It was pointed out above that all these nuclei are under the influence of extrinsic afferent inputs: they are also all under some form of descending control, whose full range is still not known in detail. This is known partly from anatomical evidence, which is particularly clear-cut in the case of corticofugal connections, and partly from electrophysiological evidence, usually in acute experiments in which such systems were either excited electrically, or, in the case of a tonically active system, reversibly or irreversibly blocked. Such experiments unfortunately throw no light on the contexts in which these systems normally operate.

Descending control systems are discussed in detail elsewhere in this volume (TOWE, Chapter 17). The main point to emphasize here is the contrast between the powerful somatotopically arranged corticofugal systems operating on the dorsal column and thalamic ventroposterior nuclei on the one hand; and on the other, the lateral cervical nucleus, receiving no descending fibres from above the midbrain (GRANT and WESTMAN, 1969), but receiving some from below this level (GRANT, personal communication), and on which relatively little corticofugal action has been detected in electrophysiological experiments (GORDON and JUKES, 1963). Cells of the spinocervical tract have been shown to be under a tonic inhibitory control, in the decerebrate cat, which can selectively reduce the number of types of receptor activating them and can thus exert a profound effect on the character of their receptive fields (see BROWN, Chapter 19). It is possible that the fibres descending on to the lateral cervical nucleus operate in the same way, but no information exists about this. The corticofugal systems operating on the dorsal column and ventroposterior nuclei are most unlikely to operate in this way because, as said earlier, a large majority of elements in these nuclei are so "pure" receptively as to leave little scope for this type of modification of their receptive fields: inhibition of certain of these elements at the expense of others could certainly be used to select which types of receptor had access to the sensory cortex, though it is not known if the descending systems operate in this way. The topographical organization of these particular corticofugal systems suggests that they have a *spatially* organized mode of operation in the population of relay cells and within the receptive fields of individual cells. It has been suggested, for instance, that the predominantly inhibitory corticofugal action on the cat's dorsal column nuclei, which was found to act on virtually all relay cells in the gracile nucleus with inhibitory components in their receptive fields (GORDON and JUKES, 1964b), might modify the degree of spatial sharpening by interacting with afferent inhibition (GORDON and JUKES, 1964b; LEVITT et al., 1964).

It is not clear that the corticofugal actions on the dorsal column nuclei and ventroposterior nucleus constitute a feedback in the true sense, with the control properties which this concept implies, although they are often referred to in this way. Some corticofugal cells projecting to one or other dorsal column nucleus have cutaneous receptive fields and these lie in a corresponding part of the body (McCOMAS and WILSON, 1968; GORDON and MILLER, 1969). It has been shown that the dorsal column system contributes at least some of the excitation to corticofugal cells affecting these nuclei (TOWE and ZIMMERMAN, 1962; GORDON and MILLER, 1969); but it is not known if the descending system acts on the same cells as were responsible for its upstream excitation, nor whether other afferent systems such as the spinocervicothalamic can also contribute to excitation, or inhibition, of corticofugal cells acting on the dorsal column nuclei.

The last ten years have seen considerable advances in detailed knowledge of the relay nuclei of the somaesthetic system. These nuclei, while having in common a relay function, differ widely in a single species in such features as somatotopic organization, receptive specificity, inhibitory components of receptive fields, and extrinsic ascending and descending control. Even the apparently equivalent cuneate and gracile nuclei differ, in the cat, in that the former contains a representation of muscle afferents from the appropriate limb and the latter does not. It can be inferred that these sometimes radical differences in physiological organization are reflected in differences in sensory function; but the parts played by individual nuclei in sensory function remains to be defined, and in view of the cross-connections now believed to exist between the different nuclear systems, such definition may prove to be elusive. It seems likely that progress in this direction could only be made by investigating their activity in conscious unrestrained animals of a variety of species, and where possible in Man.

References

ANDERSEN, P., ANDERSSON, S. A., LANDGREN, S.: Some properties of the thalamic relay cells in the spino-cervico-lemniscal path. Acta physiol. scand. **68**, 72–83 (1966).

ANDERSEN, P., ECCLES, J.C., OSHIMA, T., SCHMIDT, R.F.: Mechanisms of synaptic transmission in the cuneate nucleus. J. Neurophysiol. **27**, 1096–1116 (1964b).

ANDERSEN, P., ECCLES, J.C., SCHMIDT, R.F., YOKOTA, T.: Identification of relay cells and interneurons in the cuneate nucleus. J. Neurophysiol. **27**, 1080–1095 (1964a).

ANDERSEN, P., ECCLES, J.C., SEARS, T.A.: The ventro-basal complex of the thalamus: types of cells, their responses and their functional organization. J. Physiol. (Lond.) **174**, 370–399 (1964c).

ANDERSEN, P., ETHOLM, B., GORDON, G.: Presynaptic depolarization of dorsal column fibres by adequate stimulation. J. Physiol. (Lond.) **194**, 83–84P (1968).

ANDERSEN, P., ETHOLM, B., GORDON, G.: Presynaptic and postsynaptic inhibition elicited in the cat's dorsal column nuclei by mechanical stimulation of skin. J. Physiol. (Lond.) **210**, 433–455 (1970).

ANDERSSON, S.A., LANDGREN, S., WOLSK, D.: The thalamic relay and cortical projection of Group I muscle afferents from the forelimb of the cat. J. Physiol. (Lond.) **183**, 576–591 (1966).

ANGEL, A.: Evidence for cortical inhibition of transmission at the thalamic sensory relay nucleus in the rat. J. Physiol. (Lond.) **169**, 108–109P (1963).

ANGEL, A.: The effect of peripheral stimulation on units located in the thalamic reticular nuclei. J. Physiol. (Lond.) **171**, 42–60 (1964).

ANGEL, A.: The effect of "attention" and anaesthesia on evoked somatosensory cortical responses. J. Physiol. (Lond.) **192**, 6–7P (1967).

ANGEL, A., DAWSON, G.D.: The facilitation of thalamic and cortical responses in the dorsal column sensory pathway by strong peripheral stimulation. J. Physiol. (Lond.) **166**, 587–604 (1963).

BOIVIE, J.: The termination of the cervicothalamic tract in the cat. An experimental study with silver impregnation methods. Brain Res. **19**, 333–360 (1970).

Brown, A.G., Gordon, G., Kay, R.H.: Cutaneous receptive properties of single fibres in the cat's medial lemniscus. J. Physiol. (Lond.) **211**, 37–39P (1970).

Brown, A.G., Iggo, A.: A quantitative study of cutaneous receptors and afferent fibres in the cat and rabbit. J. Physiol. (Lond.) **193**, 707–732 (1967).

Calma, I.: The activity of the posterior group of thalamic nuclei in the cat. J. Physiol. (Lond.) **180**, 350–370 (1965).

Chambers, M.R., Iggo, A.: Slowly-adapting cutaneous mechanoreceptors. J. Physiol. (Lond.) **192**, 26P (1967).

Curry, M.J.: An electrophysiological study of the somatic posterior group. J. Physiol. (Lond.) **216**, 56–57P (1971).

Darian-Smith, I.: Presynaptic component in the afferent inhibition observed within trigeminal brain-stem nuclei of the cat. J. Neurophysiol. **28**, 695–709 (1965).

Dart, A.M.: Cells of the dorsal column nuclei projecting down into the spinal cord. J. Physiol. (Lond.) **219**, 29 P (1971).

Dart, A.M., Gordon, G.: Excitatory and inhibitory afferent inputs to the dorsal column nuclei not involving the dorsal columns. J. Physiol. (Lond.) **211**, 36–37P (1970).

Dart, A.M., Gordon, G.: Some properties of spinal connections of the dorsal column nuclei which do not involve the dorsal columns. In: The Somatosensory System: ed. H. Kornhuber. Stuttgart: Thieme, in preparation.

Davidson, N., Smith, C.A.: Second-order neurone inhibition in the rat cuneate nucleus evoked from the contralateral periphery. J. Physiol. (Lond.) **210**, 60P (1970).

Fedina, L., Gordon, G., Lundberg, A.: The source and mechanisms of inhibition in the lateral cervical nucleus of the cat. Brain Res. **11**, 694–696 (1968).

Gordon, G., Horrobin, D.F.: Antidromic and synaptic responses in the cat's gracile nucleus to cerebellar stimulation. Brain Res. **5**, 419–421 (1967).

Gordon, G., Jukes, M.G.M.: An investigation of cells in the lateral cervical nucleus of the cat which respond to stimulation of the skin. J. Physiol. (Lond.) **169**, 28–29P (1963).

Gordon, G., Jukes, M.G.M.: Dual organization of the exteroceptive components of the cat's gracile nucleus. J. Physiol. (Lond.) **173**, 263–290 (1964a).

Gordon, G., Jukes, M.G.M.: Descending influences on the exteroceptive organizations of the cat's gracile nucleus. J. Physiol. (Lond.) **173**, 291–319 (1964b).

Gordon, G., Manson, J.R.: Cutaneous receptive fields of single nerve cells in the thalamus of the cat. Nature (Lond.) **215**, 597–599 (1967).

Gordon, G., Miller, R.: Identification of cortical cells projecting to the dorsal column nuclei of the cat. Quart. J. exp. Physiol. **54**, 85–98 (1969).

Gordon, G., Paine, C.H.: Functional organization in nucleus gracilis of the cat. J. Physiol. (Lond.) **153**, 331–349 (1960).

Grant, G., Westman, J.: The lateral cervical nucleus in the cat. IV. A light and electron microscopical study after midbrain lesions with demonstration of indirect Wallerian degeneration at the ultrastructural level. Exp. Brain Res. **7**, 51–67 (1969).

Hand, P., Liu, C.N.: Efferent projections of the nucleus gracilis. Anat. Rec. **154**, 353 (1966).

Hongo, T., Jankowska, E., Lundberg, A.: Postsynaptic excitation and inhibition evoked from primary afferents in neurones of the spinocervical tract. J. Physiol. (Lond.) **198**, 569–592 (1968).

Horrobin, D.F.: The lateral cervical nucleus of the cat; an electrophysiological study. Quart. J. exp. Physiol. **51**, 351–371 (1966).

Jabbur, S.J., Banna, N.R.: Presynaptic inhibition of cuneate transmission by widespread cutaneous inputs. Brain Res. **10**, 273–276 (1968).

Johnson, J.R., Welker, W.I., Pubols, B.H.: Somatotopic organization of raccoon dorsal column nuclei. J. comp. Neurol. **132**, 1–44 (1968).

King, E.E., Naquet, R., Magoun, H.W.: Alterations of somatic afferent transmission through the thalamus by central mechanisms and barbiturates. J. Pharmacol. exp. Ther. **119**, 48–63 (1957).

KUYPERS, H.G.J.M., TUERK, J.D.: The distribution of the cortical fibres within the nuclei cuneatus and gracilis in the cat. J. Anat. (Lond.) **98**, 143–162 (1964).

LANDGREN, S., NORDWALL, A., WENGSTRÖM, C.: The location of the thalamic relay in the spino-cervico-lemniscal path. Acta physiol. scand. **65**, 164–175 (1965).

LEVITT, M., CARRERAS, M., LIU, C.N., CHAMBERS, W.W.: Pyramidal and extrapyramidal modulation of somatosensory activity in gracile and cuneate nuclei. Arch. ital. Biol. **102**, 197–229 (1964).

MANSON, J.R.: The somatosensory cortical projection of single nerve cells in the thalamus of the cat. Brain Res. **12**, 489–492 (1969).

McCOMAS, A.J., WILSON, P.: An investigation of pyramidal tract cells in the somatosensory cortex of the rat. J. Physiol. (Lond.) **194**, 271–288 (1968).

MORIN, F., KITAI, J.T., PORTNOY, H., DEMIRJIAN, C.: Afferent projections to the lateral cervical nucleus: a micro-electrode study. Amer. J. Physiol. **204**, 667–672 (1963).

MOUNTCASTLE, V.B., TALBOT, W.H., SAKATA, H., HYVÄRINEN, J.: Cortical neuronal mechanisms in flutter-vibration studied in unanaesthetized monkeys. Neuronal periodicity and frequency discrimination (1969).

NAKAHAMA, H., NISHIOKA, S., OTSUKA, T.: Excitation and inhibition in ventrobasal thalamic neurons before and after cutaneous input deprivation. Progr. Brain Res. **21A**, 180; Amsterdam: Elsevier Publ. Co.1966.

NORRSELL, U.: The spinal afferent pathways of conditioned reflexes to cutaneous stimuli in the dog. Exp. Brain Res. **2**, 269–282 (1966).

OSCARSSON, O., ROSÉN, I.: Projection to cerebral cortex of large muscle spindle afferents in forelimb nerves of the cat. J. Physiol. (Lond.) **169**, 924–945 (1963).

OSWALDO-CRUZ, E., KIDD, C.: Functional properties of neurones in the lateral cervical nucleus of the cat. J. Neurophysiol. **27**, 1–14 (1964).

PERL, E.R., WHITLOCK, D.G., GENTRY, J.R.: Cutaneous projection to second-order neurons of the dorsal column system. J. Neurophysiol. **25**, 337–358 (1962).

POGGIO, G.F., MOUNTCASTLE, V.B.: A study of the functional contributions of the lemniscal and spinothalamic systems to somatic sensibility. Central nervous mechanisms in Pain. Bull. Johns Hopk. Hosp. **106**, 266–316 (1960).

POGGIO, G.F., MOUNTCASTLE, V.B.: The functional properties of ventrobasal thalamic neurons studied in unanaesthetized monkeys. J. Neurophysiol. **26**, 775–806 (1963).

ROSE, J.E., MOUNTCASTLE, V.B.: Touch and Kinesthesis. In: Handbook of Physiology, Sect. 1, 1. Neurophysiology, pp. 387–429. Washington: American Physiological Society 1959.

ROSÉN, I.: Afferent connexions to Group I activated cells in the main cuneate nucleus of the cat. J. Physiol. (Lond.) **205**, 209–236 (1969).

ROWE, M.J., SESSLE, B.J.: Somatic afferent input to posterior thalamic neurones and their axon projection to cerebral cortex in the cat. J. Physiol. (Lond.) **196**, 19–35 (1968).

SCHWARTZ, S., GIBLIN, D., AMASSIAN, V.E.: Resting activity of cuneate neurons. Fed. Proc. **23**, 466 (1964).

SHERRINGTON, C.S.: In: Textbook of Physiology, ed. E.A. SCHÄFER. pp. 862–863 and 977–978. Edinburgh and London: Pentland 1900.

TOMASULO, K., EMMERS, R.: A spinocervical input to the gracile nucleus. Anat. Rec. **166**, 390 (1970).

TOWE, A.L.: Somatosensory cortex: Descending influences on ascending systems (This volume).

TOWE, A.L., ZIMMERMAN, I.D.: Peripherally evoked cortical reflex in the cuneate nucleus. Nature (Lond.) **194**, 1250–1251 (1962).

WALBERG, F.: The fine structure of the cuneate nucleus in normal cats and following interruption of afferent fibres. An electron microscopical study with particular reference to findings made in Glees and Nauta sections. Exp. Brain Res. **2**, 107–128 (1966),

WALDRON, H. A.: The morphology of the lateral cervical nucleus in the hedgehog. Brain Res. **16**, 301–306 (1969).

WALL, P. D.: The sensory and motor role of impulses travelling in the dorsal columns towards cerebral cortex. Brain **93**, 505–524 (1970).

WESTMAN, J.: The lateral cervical nucleus in the cat. III. An electron microscopical study after transection of spinal afferents. Exp. Brain Res. **7**, 32–50 (1969).

WINTER, D. L.: Nucleus gracilis of cat. Functional organization and corticofugal effects. J. Neurophysiol. **28**, 48–70 (1965).

Chapter 6

Control of the Access of Afferent Activity to Somatosensory Pathways

By

ROBERT F. SCHMIDT, Kiel (Germany)

With 20 Figures

Contents

I. Introduction

The central nervous system of a mammal, or any other vertebrate for that matter, is continuously exposed to a barrage of afferent impulses coming from the receptors of its various sense organs. For instance, the dorsal roots of the cat's spinal cord contain on each side roughly 500,000 fibres (DUNCAN and KEYSER, 1938; HOLMES and DAVENPORT, 1940), and many of these will be active even in the absence of a sensory stimulus. Although practically no data are available on either the temporal and spatial profile of afferent impulses reaching the spinal cord after a sensory stimulus, or on its overall information processing capabilities, I should like to assume that in most circumstances the afferent input is greater than the maximal number of impulses the spinal cord input system can deal with, and that the central action of the "surplus" inflow is reduced or abolished by inhibition. For example, many stimulus continua range through several orders of magnitude. Thus, the central apparatus connected to the peripheral receptors has to react as appropriately to one or a few impulses from a single receptor as to the maximal discharge rates which the receptor population involved will eventually produce. Since several properties of the neuronal elements put rather narrow limits on the range of responses of a neuronal network, the central nervous system is forced to adapt its input sensitivity to the range of the peripheral stimuli by inhibiting the inflow: the greater the afferent inflow, the greater the inhibition.

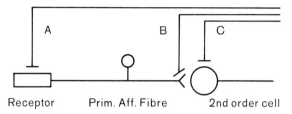

Fig. 1. Earliest possible sites to modify afferent input. See text

Suppression of afferent inflow is not only necessary for the adaptation on the stimulus intensity level but may also serve many other purposes such as to concentrate on vital afferent inputs by suppressing those which are trivial to the organism at that moment ("focussing the attention"). It is not surprising, therefore, that inhibition of afferent activity can be induced from a great number of places in the central nervous system ranging from the afferent fibres themselves up to the most complex cortical structures.

Inhibition of afferent activity can be exerted at any place in the centripetal pathways but it appears most economical to do it at the earliest possible sites, even before the unwanted afferent activity has produced any appreciable disturbance in the central nervous system. Fig. 1 illustrates that there are three prime locations in the afferent pathway which can be used for this task: (a) the receptor, (b) the primary afferent terminal, and (c) the second order cell. Whereas in invertebrates direct inhibition of peripheral receptors is a rather common feature it has been practically completely abandoned in the somaesthetic and kinaesthetic receptor systems of vertebrates in favour of presynaptic inhibition. This offers the same advantages as receptor inhibition plus the added advantage that the presynaptic inhibitory axons do not have to travel out to the periphery. Thus the presynaptic inhibitory synapses of afferent terminals and the postsynaptic inhibitory synapses of second order cells are the prime targets for all nervous activity aimed at inhibiting afferent input in vertebrates.

In addition to the inhibition of afferent activity, many examples have been described of central facilitation of afferent input. Such facilitation can be induced by the removal of a tonic presynaptic inhibition of afferent fibres, by the removal of postsynaptic inhibition, or by postsynaptic excitation of second order (or later) cells. (In the vertebrate CNS there is as yet no evidence for an active facilitation of afferent fibre efficacy via an axo-axonal mechanism.) Often, facilitation of a given afferent input is accompanied by attenuation of other inputs. With or without this concomitant attenuation, afferent facilitation increases the central effectiveness of an input relative to its competitors. Thus, functionally speaking, central facilitation of afferent inflow subserves the same selective function as central inhibition of afferent input.

In this review the emphasis will be on the segmental and descending control of the access to afferent pathways via presynaptic inhibition of afferent fibre terminals of the somatosensory system. It is only within the last decade that the ubiquity and potency of presynaptic inhibition of primary afferents has come to light, thanks to a considerable body of work done in many laboratories throughout the world, particularly in regard to its synaptic mechanism, its pharmacology and the organization and mode of operation of its various reflex pathways both at the segmental and suprasegmental level. Less detailed reference will be made to postsynaptic inhibition of second order or later neurones in somato-sensory pathways, although it is appreciated that postsynaptic inhibition is also of eminent importance in the control of afferent input. Fortunately, this latter aspect of input control is taken up in several other contributions to this volume, particularly in those of BROWN, DARIAN-SMITH, GORDON, OSCARSSON, TOWE, WALL, to which the reader is referred to. It has to be recognized that the separation of the input controlling mechanisms into those exerting their influence on afferent fibres and those doing so at second order or later neurones is solely done on practical and methodological grounds, and is probably meaningless from the functional point of view. At several locations, such as in the dorsal column nuclei, it has already been shown that both systems are operative simultaneously during peripherally evoked as well as during corticofugal activity. But, here as elsewhere, the relative significance of presynaptic versus postsynaptic inhibition is still difficult to evaluate and at present largely a matter of speculation.

II. Anatomical and Physiological Basis of the Control of Afferent Input

A. Postsynaptic Inhibitory Synapses of Second Order Cells and Their Pathways

For several reasons it will be sufficient merely to quote some relevant literature on this topic rather than to write a comprehensive review on it. First of all, as is well summarized in several reviews, monographs and symposium proceedings (cf. ECCLES, 1964; ECCLES and SCHADÉ, 1964; EULER et al., 1968; BRAZIER, 1969; HUBBARD et al., 1969; McLENNAN, 1970) none of the basic properties of the synaptic mechanism and mode of operation of inhibitory synapses of second order cells seems to differ from those of other central neurones. Actually, the inhibitory synapses of motoneurones offer a very good example for this statement since this neurone is a second order cell for Ia afferent fibres from muscle spindles, and it is also the target of many inhibitory paths, including those coming from agonist Ib and antagonist Ia afferent fibres. Secondly, our present knowledge on the post-synaptic inhibitory pathways in the spinal cord and at higher levels of the central nervous system, has been well documented in the literature quoted above (cf. LUNDBERG, 1969) and, particularly, in the recent Sherrington Lectures of ECCLES (1969). Finally, the pharmacology and neurochemistry of mammalian central postsynaptic inhibition has been reviewed recently (CURTIS, 1968, 1969, 1970; cf. also ECCLES, 1964; HUBBARD et al., 1969; McLENNAN, 1970) and there is no need for further repetition.

B. Presynaptic Inhibitory Synapses, Anatomical Aspects

Originally axo-axonic synapses were postulated on the basis of physiological evidence only (ECCLES, 1961; ECCLES et al., 1962a). Since that time this type of structure has been found in the spinal cord and in several other regions of the nervous system. It is thus justified to assume that axo-axonic synapses are the morphological substrate of primary afferent depolarization and presynaptic inhibition, although the histological results are equivocal: the presynaptic synapses cannot always be found in those regions where the physiological results would locate them, and the functional polarity of the synapse as judged by presently accepted electronmicroscopical criteria is sometimes the wrong way round, the primary afferent fibre appearing as presynaptic to the presumed interneuronal axon.

The first histological description of axo-axonic contacts in the mammalian spinal cord was given by GRAY, 1962 (see also GRAY, 1963). Meanwhile axo-axonic contacts have been seen in ventral (KHATTAB, 1968) and in dorsal regions of the spinal grey matter (RALSTON, 1965, 1968a, b; KERR, 1966), and the investigations of SCHEIBEL and SCHEIBEL (1968), CONRADI (1969), RÉTHELYI and SZENTÁGOTHAI (1969) and RÉTHELYI (1970) have made it likely that such contacts exist between primary afferent collaterals and axons originating from interneurones of the spinal cord. For instance, in the substantia gelatinosa RÉTHELYI and SZENTÁGOTHAI (1969) found axo-axonic synapses between the presynaptic endings of the axons of intraspinal neurones and the terminals of myelinated afferent fibres. At the motoneuronal level it was shown by CONRADI (1969) that on the convex side of dorsal root boutons there were regularly apposed small boutons containing synaptic vesicles of irregular shape. These latter boutons established a synaptic complex with the big boutons of dorsal root (Group Ia) fibres. A similar arrangement can be found on the Ia fibres terminating on Clarke's column neurones (Fig. 2). There, the very large (so called "giant") axon terminals with spheric vesicles of primary muscle afferents (Ia fibres) establish multiple (climbing-type) contacts with dorsal spinocerebellar tract neurones. Smaller nerve terminals originating from local neurones, and characterized by flattened vesicles, establish axo-axonic synapses with the giant terminals of the Ia fibres.

In the cuneate nucleus, WALBERG (1965) found axo-axonic synapses in configurations corresponding exactly to those predicted on the basis of physiological

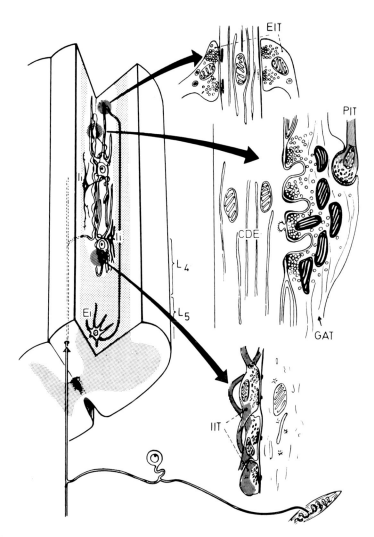

Fig. 2. Diagram illustrating the configuration of axo-axonal synapses on Ia terminals in Clarke's column at light microscopic (left) and at electron microscopic level (right). The large clear neurones are dorsal-spino-cerebellar-tract neurones (DSCT-neurones), which are accompanied by smaller, probably inhibitory, interneurones (black, Ii). The Ia afferent fibre entering from a lower lumbar segment terminates by giant axon terminals (GAT). The ultrastructure of a synapse between GAT and a dendrite of a DSCT neurone (CDE) can be recognized at centre right. An axo-axonic synapse is established between GAT and a small axon terminal (presynaptic inhibitory terminal, PIT) containing flattened synaptic vesicles. It is assumed to derive from the inhibitory interneurones, Ii, of the Clarke's column. The excitatory spinal interneurone, Ei, establishes axodendritic synaptic terminals, EIT, with remote parts of dendrites of DSCT neurones (top right). IIT are presumed inhibitory interneuronal terminals on DSCT cells stemming from the Ii interneurones (bottom right). (From RÉTHELYI, 1970)

observations (Andersen et al., 1964a–c). The presynaptic bouton participating in the axo-axonic contact was usually small, the other one large. Degeneration experiments established that the large boutons were axon terminals of cuneate tract fibres. Furthermore, evidence was presented that the small presynaptic boutons did not originate from neurones located outside the cuneate nucleus, a finding well in agreement with the physiological results (cf. chapter III C, Fig. 19). There is as yet no physiological correlate for the frequent finding of Walberg and other histologists that the presynaptic axon of the axo-axonic contacts often also forms axo-dendritic contacts on the same dendrites as the postsynaptic axon. These arrangements suggest that a combined presynaptic and postsynaptic inhibition can be exerted by these axons. (At the crayfish neuromuscular junction, activation of the inhibitory nerve fibres always produces pre- and postsynaptic inhibition, Dudel and Kuffler, 1961).

The presence of axo-axonic contacts in the *trigeminal brain stem nuclei* has been described by Kerr (1966) and by Gobel and Dubner (1968, 1969). It was clearly established (Kerr, 1970) that in the majority of cases the primary afferent fibres are postsynaptic to presynaptic knobs of unknown origin containing flattened vesicles. The existence of axo-axonic contacts at the relay nuclei of primary afferents of other nerves has not been reported so far. But it has been known for some time that axo-axonic contacts exist in the *lateral geniculate body* (Szentá-gothai, 1962; Colonnier and Guillery, 1964). The synaptic endings of the optic afferents are of complex glomerular structure (Szentágothai, 1963; Peters and Palay, 1966), and numerous axo-axonic contacts are found on the optic nerve terminals in the glomeruli. Presynaptic depolarization of optic nerve terminals has frequently been reported (cf. Angel et al., 1965, 1966; Kahn et al., 1967; Marchiafava and Pompeiano, 1966a, b), and it might be assumed that this depolarization was due to an activation of the axo-axonic contacts of the glomerular complexes. At various other sites in the *thalamus*, axo-axonic contacts having specific structural differentiations have been found (Majorosso et al., 1965; Pappas et al., 1965; Tömböl, 1967). They are particularly frequent in the complex synaptic groupings first described in the pulvinar and designated synaptic glomeruli by Majorosso et al. (1965). So far no physiological results are available in regard to the functional role of these axo-axonic contacts except for the findings of Andersen, Eccles and Sears (1964b), who presented evidence that in the ventro-basal complex of the thalamus, presynaptic inhibition is exerted onto the terminals of lemniscal fibres, presumably by a pathway leading from lemniscal collaterals to a local interneurone, which in turn makes presynaptic axo-axonic contact on lemniscal terminals (see section IV).

C. Presynaptic Inhibitory Synapses, Physiological Mechanism

Eccles and his co-workers observed that the presynaptic inhibition of Ia induced motoneuronal EPSPs (Frank and Fuortes, 1957) precisely correlated with a depolarization of presynaptic fibres (primary afferent depolarization (PAD), Eccles, Eccles and Magni, 1961; Eccles, Magni and Willis, 1962). This finding led to the postulate that presynaptic depolarization was responsible for the EPSP depression because it reduced the size of the presynaptic impulse and hence decreased the liberation of the excitatory transmitter. It was further postulated that the depolarization was due to the activation of an axo-axonic synapse located near the terminal of the recipient afferent fibre (as later confirmed by electron-microscopy, see section II B), and that this synapse was activated through poly-synaptic reflex pathways involving at least two interneurones. Furthermore, the observations made on Ia afferent fibres were extended to other types of spinal primary afferents and it was postulated that the depolarization of Ib afferent fibres and of Group II and III cutaneous afferent terminals also indicate a presy-naptic inhibition of the excitatory action of these fibres (Eccles et al., 1962a, b; Eccles et al., 1963a).

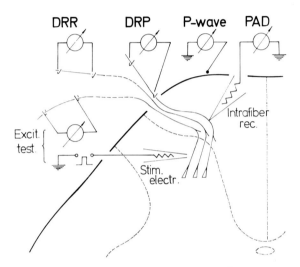

Fig. 3. Methods for detecting primary afferent depolarization, PAD. From right to left these methods are: The intrafibre recording of the PAD from primary afferents with glass capillary microelectrodes; the recording of the positive potential wave, P-wave, from the dorsum of the spinal cord near the dorsal root entry zone; the recording of dorsal root potentials, DRP, with bipolar Pt or Ag/AgCl wire electrodes from dorsal rootlets cut off a few mm distal to their dorsal root entry; the recording of dorsal root reflexes, DRR, either in dorsal root filaments, or preferentially in peripheral nerves; and the testing of the excitability of the terminal sections of primary afferent fibres. Not included in the figure is the recording of slow potentials inside the spinal cord with an extracellular microelectrode. (From Schmidt, 1971)

Fig. 3 shows schematically the principal methods used in the investigation of primary afferent depolarization. Each of the methods shown has its particular potentialities and limitations. All of them are able to detect the occurrence of PAD, but they differ greatly in their capability to signal what types of fibres are depolarized. Two of them, the recording of dorsal root potentials (DRP) and the recording of slow positive potentials from the cord dorsum (P-waves) give no hint at all as to the fibre types receiving the depolarization, while two others, the recording of dorsal root reflexes (DRR) and the testing of intraspinal excitability changes of fibre populations, allow the classification of the depolarized fibres in regard to their conduction velocity and their origin from muscle or cutaneous nerves. But only the most sophisticated ones, intracellular recording and testing of the excitability of single afferent fibres, can be used for the exact determination of the modality to which the fibre under observation belongs. (For a detailed discussion of the various methods of recording PAD see Schmidt, 1971.)

So far the mode of operation of the presumed axo-axonic synapse is not well understood. For instance, by analogy with other chemically operated depolarizing synapses, it would be expected that the depolarizing mechanism would have an equilibrium potential. However, as summarized by Schmidt (1971, pp. 42–45) several experimental attempts have failed to produce conclusive evidence for the existence of such an equilibrium potential. Somewhat more decisive results have been obtained in regard to the duration of the presumed transmitter action by testing the effect of an action potential propagating down an afferent fibre to its central terminals on the PAD of that fibre. Such an action potential is expected to erase all electrotonic potentials in the fibre. Yet, if an action potential was super-imposed at various times during the PAD of a Group Ia nerve fibre, the reduction in amplitude of the PAD was very small indeed, particularly when the impulse was interpolated early with respect to the PAD (Eccles et al., 1963c; Schmidt et al., 1967a). Somewhat comparable observations have been reported for the action of an interpolated afferent volley in partly destroying the dorsal root potentials recorded from a frog dorsal root (Eccles and Malcolm, 1946). Eccles et al. (1963c) suggested that the simplest hypothesis to explain these findings is that the interpolated action potential destroys all the PAD that is preformed in that fibre, but that subsequently the lingering transmitter rebuilds much of the depolarization. Thus it would be envisaged that the transmitter continues to act throughout the whole duration of the PAD. This mechanism ensures that repetitive afferent impulses appearing at the fibre terminals during PAD are all effectively inhibited.

Although all experimental results reviewed in the preceding paragraph are in accordance with the hypothesis that PAD can be attributed to the prolonged action of a chemical transmitter substance which operates in a manner comparable with other excitatory transmitters, namely by effecting a high permeability to ions, it has to be appreciated that the mechanism generating the PAD is far from understood. Generally speaking, little further experimental evidence in regard to the synaptic mechanism of PAD has been brought forward since the experiments of Eccles and his co-workers in the early 1960s (cf. Schmidt, 1971). There is one additional observation of Decima and Goldberg (1970; cf. also Grinnell, 1970) that antidromic activation of motoneurones increases the excitability of the presynaptic terminals, but the mechanism and physiological significance of this motoneurone-presynaptic interaction is also not clear at present.

During PAD a reduced amount of transmitter is liberated when an impulse propagates down to a depolarized nerve terminal. In the extreme situation the impulse is blocked before reaching some or all of the terminals, but in most in-stances the terminals are invaded by a spike potential of decreased size, which releases a reduced amount of transmitter. As shown by Kuno (1964) in motoneu-rones, the unit size of the EPSP remains unchanged during PAD but the probabi-lity of generation of the unit EPSP components is reduced. Other experimental evidence in support of this relation between spike size and transmitter release, both at central and peripheral synapses, has been reviewed by SCHMIDT (1971). Fig. 4 shows the results of an attempt to mimick the PAD of Ia fibre terminals on motoneurones by an electrical polarization of the spinal cord. It is seen that polarization of the presynaptic terminals induces reductions of the EPSP amplitudes

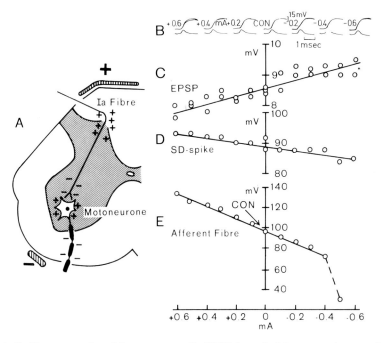

Fig. 4 A–E. Changes produced in monosynaptic EPSP by polarizing current across the cord. As shown in A, the polarizing current was applied through two electrodes, one situated medial to the dorsal root entrance, the other just lateral from the ventral roots. B–D, intracellular recording from a motoneurone, the membrane potential being –70 mV. B shows specimen records of EPSPs under the influence of increasing currents, as indicated in mA for each record, CON being the control value. Each record consists of many superimposed faint traces. The upper traces are the intracellular records which are differentiated in the lower traces. In C the amplitudes of the EPSPs (in mV) for the series partly shown in A are plotted against the direction and strength of the polarizing currents. D shows the amplitudes of the antidromically evoked SD-spike measured under the influence of the same currents. Similarly E gives the changes in spike potential amplitude which the polarizing currents produced in a primary afferent fibre from the nerve to flexor digitorum longus muscle. The fibre was impaled by a micro-electrode at about 0.5 mm below the dorsal cord surface. In B–E the signs (+) and (–) indicate the polarity of the dorsal surface electrode (see A). (From ECCLES, KOSTYUK and SCHMIDT, 1962 c)

in a manner comparable with that seen during PAD, although the reduction of the EPSP amplitude with depolarizing currents was always much smaller than during strong presynaptic inhibition. There are several possible explanations for this difference. In the first place, in presynaptic inhibition the depolarization of the presynaptic terminals may be larger. Secondly, since with presynaptic inhibition the depolarization of the afferent fibres is actively produced by a transmitter substance, the presynaptic spike would be decreased not only by the diminution of the membrane potential (as occurs with the depolarizing current), but also as a consequence of the increased ionic conductance, just as occurs with the muscle impulse at an activated motor end-plate (FATT and KATZ, 1951; DEL CASTILLO and KATZ, 1954) and also with synaptic actions on nerve cells (FADIGA and BROOK-HART, 1960; NISHI and KOKETSU, 1960). The conductance increase may be even more important than the membrane potential change in decreasing the presynaptic action potential (as for instance at the presynaptic inhibitory synapse of the cray-fish, DUDEL, 1963, 1965). Furthermore, during strong PAD, collision with an antidromic dorsal root reflex or block of conduction may prevent altogether the invasion of some or all of the synaptic terminals of primary afferent fibres, a possibility firmly advocated by WALL and his colleagues (HOWLAND et al., 1955; WALL et al., 1955; WALL, 1964). Finally, it should be pointed out that the libera-tion of transmitter may have a very steep relationship to the size of the spike potential in the synaptic terminals, even a fourth power relationship (LILEY, 1956); spike augmentations of 10–25% have been shown to enlarge the transmitter output at the neuromuscular junction by 200–300% (HUBBARD and SCHMIDT, 1962, 1963). KATZ (1962) has suggested that, as a consequence, the relatively small depolarization produced in presynaptic inhibition may nevertheless have a large depressant action on transmitter liberation and so on the EPSP.

D. General Properties of Presynaptic Inhibitory Pathways

The neuronal pathways for presynaptic inhibition have properties correspond-ing to those of other polysynaptic somatosensory and motor reflex pathways of the spinal cord. First of all, there is a central latency of several milliseconds. The shortest central latencies were found in the cuneate nucleus, where 2.0–2.2 msec elapsed between the arrival time of the fastest component of the afferent volley at the cuneate nucleus, and the onset of PAD recorded intracellularly from a cuneate tract fibre (ANDERSEN et al., 1964b). At the lumbar segmental level the central latency of the PAD ranged from 2.0 to 3.0 msec for cutaneous primary afferent fibres (KOKETSU, 1956; ECCLES and KRNJEVIĆ, 1959), and from 4.0 to 5.0 msec for muscle primary afferents (ECCLES, MAGNI and WILLIS, 1962). Further-more, there are other features of polysynaptic pathways such as temporal and spatial facilitation, post-tetanic potentiation, and depression during repetitive stimulation (ECCLES, ECCLES and MAGNI, 1961; ECCLES, MAGNI and WILLIS, 1962; ECCLES et al., 1963b; DECANDIA, GASTEIGER and MANN, 1968, 1971; DECANDIA, ELDRED and GROVER, 1971). Temporal and spatial facilitation can be more easily demonstrated in those pathways leading from Group I muscle afferents to Group Ia afferents, than in those from cutaneous to cutaneous afferent fibres, mainly because the latter reflex pathways require only very few impulses for maximal activation (SCHMIDT et al., 1967b; JÄNIG et al., 1968).

The interneuronal pathway of presynaptic inhibition thus has properties which correspond to polysynaptic reflex pathways having at least two synapses in serial order, and such pathways have been postulated for the simplest pathways for PAD production in the spinal cord and the cuneate nucleus (ECCLES et al., 1962a; ANDERSEN et al., 1964b). In the unanaesthetized spinal animal these pathways exhibit considerable spontaneous activity which causes excitability fluctuations of the fibre terminals (RUDOMIN and DUTTON, 1968, 1969a, b; RUDOMIN et al., 1969; RUDOMIN, 1972; ROWE, 1970). The spontaneous changes of the presynaptic membrane potentials reflected by the excitability fluctuations seem to be mainly responsible for the variability of the excitatory actions (such as monosynaptic reflex responses) of primary afferent fibres observed under these conditions.

The last interneurones of the reflex pathways of presynaptic inhibition, i.e. those whose axons make synaptic contacts with afferent terminals, have not yet been clearly identified. Their properties, particularly their excitatory synaptic inputs have to be in agreement with the functional organisation of presynaptic inhibition which will be dealt with later in this review and which is summarized

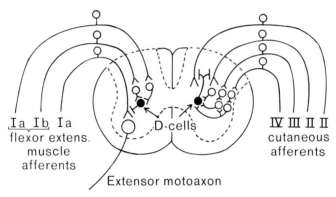

Fig. 5. Schematic diagram illustrating interneuronal pathways of PAD. The left-hand side illustrates the convergence of flexor Ia and IB fibres onto a D type interneurone which in turn makes axo-axonic contacts on the terminals of an afferent Ia fibre from extensor muscle. On the right-hand side pathways for presynaptic inhibitory actions on cutaneous primary afferents are shown. Further discussion in the text

in Figs. 9, 10 and 12–14. ECCLES et al. (1962a) carried out a search for such interneurones. Those cells that could be classified as belonging to one or the other reflex chain of presynaptic inhibition were labelled D-cells. The majority of these cells were located at the base of the dorsal horn at a depth of 1.65–2.5 mm from the dorsal surface. Some of the simplest possible pathways of PAD and presynaptic inhibition are shown diagramatically in Fig. 5. It has to be appreciated that there exist much more complex paths of activation of the interneurones making axo-axonic contacts on myelinated afferents than the simplest possible pathways in the diagram (cf. the section on the functional organisation of presynaptic inhibition, III). In addition, there are many descending pathways interacting with those at the segmental level, cf. section III A.

WALL (1962, 1964) has proposed that the activity of the small cells of the substantia gelatinosa (lamina II, SG-cells) controls the membrane potentials of the cutaneous afferent terminals and that these cells are in turn excited monosynaptically by large afferents. Since it has not been possible, so far, to record from the small SG-cells, only indirect evidence has been presented to support this hypothesis. The findings described above and summarized in Fig. 5 do not exclude the possibility that SG-cells act as D-cells, i.e. as the final and possibly the only interneurone in the PAD pathway, but the more attractive suggestion appears to be that the axons of the SG-cells make excitatory synaptic contacts with the dendrites of those lamina IV cells which send their axons to the synaptic complexes in lamina II to establish axo-axonic contacts with primary afferents (RÉTHELYI and SZENTÁGOTHAI, 1969). The D-cells, i.e. the pyramidal cells postulated by these authors, would thus act as the final common path for segmental as well as suprasegmental influences resulting in presynaptic inhibition of myelinated cutaneous afferents.

E. Pharmacological Aspects of Presynaptic Control of Access to Afferent Pathways

The pharmacology of presynaptic inhibition is quite distinct from that of postsynaptic inhibition, both at the segmental and at higher levels of the central nervous system. During the last decade, there have been numerous investigations dealing with the influence of a great variety of drugs on primary afferent depolarization and presynaptic inhibition. In this section only a brief outline of the major results of these investigations will be given. For a more detailed discussion and a more complete review of the literature the reader is referred to SCHMIDT (1971).

Barbiturates such as pentobarbitone (Nembutal) greatly prolong the time course of PAD and of presynaptic inhibition and increase the effectiveness of the presynaptic inhibitory action (ECCLES et al., 1963f; BANNA and JABBUR, 1969). Chloralose has similar effects, whereas the great number of other anaesthetics so far tested (cf. SCHMIDT, 1963; MIYAHARA et al., 1966; RICHENS, 1969) showed no definite effect on presynaptic inhibition. Regularly with smaller doses of these anaesthetics (for instance chloral-hydrate, paraldehyde, ether, urethane, chloroform, halothane, ethylchloride, nitrous oxide) the time course of presynaptic inhibition was shortened and its effectiveness was increased. The most likely explanation for these phenomena is that the anaesthetics curtail the after-discharges of the interneurones in the pathways responsible for the PAD and that they remove some of the background activity in the presynaptic inhibitory pathways thus giving rise to a hyperpolarization of primary afferent fibres. Such a hyperpolarization (i.e. a removal of tonic presynaptic inhibitory action) will increase the efficiency of an afferent volley activating the presynaptic inhibitory pathways. In the intact cat, ethanol induces preterminal depolarization of trigeminal primary afferents and increases the amount of cortically induced PAD (SAUERLAND et al., 1970).

Depressant drugs had diverse effects on presynaptic inhibition. Mephenesin always blocked presynaptic inhibition, even in concentrations that had little effect on unconditioned responses (LLINÁS, 1964; RUDOMIN, 1966; MIYAHARA et al., 1966). The last authors reported that the anticonvulsant drug trimethiadone showed actions similar to those exhibited by anaesthetics, whereas procaine enhanced presynaptic inhibition in low doses and blocked it in high doses (cf. also GRINNELL, 1966). Amidopyrine diminished the amplitude of the DRP in spinal and decerebrate cats (JURNA, 1966). The tranquillizing muscle relaxant agent, diazepam, had particularly pronounced actions on PAD (SCHMIDT, 1965; PIXNER, 1966; SCHMIDT, VOGEL and ZIMMERMANN, 1967; STRATTEN and BARNES, 1968). It was shown that this substance both increased and prolonged considerably presynaptic inhibition and primary afferent depolarization (Fig. 6). The amount and time course of postsynaptic inhibition of motoneurones was not altered by diaze-

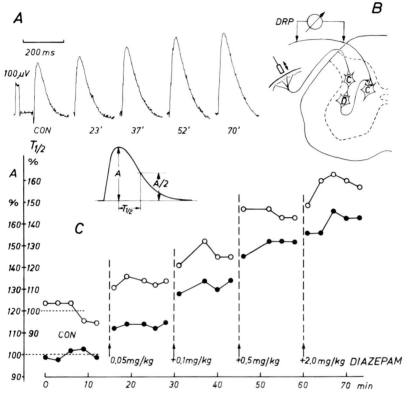

Fig. 6 A–C. Action of diazepam on DRPs. B. The DRPs were recorded from a L_7 dorsal rootlet following mechanical stimulation of the central foot pad (700 μm indentation for 5 msec). The specimens in A are x-y-plots of averaged DRPs (20 trials each) recorded before (CON) and after 4 consecutive diazepam administrations. The indicated time in minutes corresponds to that shown in the abscissa of C. As indicated in the inset the filled circles and the left-hand ordinate plot the amplitude of the DRPs, the open circles and the right-hand ordinate give the time to half decay. (From SCHMIDT, VOGEL and ZIMMERMANN, 1967)

pam, nor were the polysynaptic spinal reflex pathways strongly depressed (NGAI et al., 1966; SCHMIDT, VOGEL and ZIMMERMANN, 1967) except when very high doses were used (HUDSON and WOLPERT, 1970b). It appears that the muscle relaxant effect of diazepam is at least partly due to the increase and prolongation of presynaptic inhibition (SCHMIDT, VOGEL and ZIMMERMANN, 1967; HUDSON and WOLPERT, 1970a), i.e. a reduction of the excitatory effects of the sensory input into the motor systems.

11*

The convulsive action of picrotoxin and similarly acting drugs (bemegride, pentylentetrazol) seems at least partly be due to the depression of PAD and presynaptic inhibition produced by these substances. Thus, in the isolated toad spinal cord, picrotoxin depressed dorsal root potentials in concentrations which enhanced the ventral root reflex discharges (Schmidt, 1963; Grinnell, 1966; Tebēcis and Phillis, 1969a). Furthermore, Eccles et al. (1963f) found in the spinal cord of the cat that picrotoxin reduced the dorsal root potentials and diminished presynaptic inhibition (Fig. 7). With higher concentrations the depressed presynaptic inhibition was accompanied by convulsant activity of the preparation.

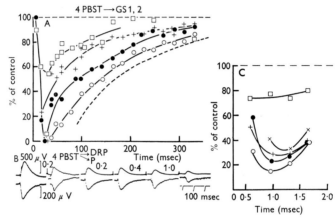

Fig. 7 A–C. Action of picrotoxin on the presynaptic and postsynaptic inhibition of monosynaptic reflexes and on DRPs and P-waves. In A, the presynaptic inhibitory action of 4 hamstring nerve (PBST) Group I volleys (300/s) was tested by monosynaptic reflexes evoked by 2 gastrocnemius-soleus (GS) volleys at 1.5 msec interval and recorded monophasically in the S_1 ventral root. The symbols show the relation of the successive i.v. injection of picrotoxin to the inhibitory curves. ---- control; ○ after picrotoxin 0.2 mg/kg; ● after further 0.6 mg/kg; + after further 1 mg/kg; □ 10 min later. The DRPs and P-waves in B were obtained concurrently with the inhibitory curves in A. C shows the action of successive i.v. injection of picrotoxin on the postsynaptic inhibition, one quadriceps (Q) Group I afferent volley inhibiting the monosynaptic reflex produced by a PBST volley. ○ control; ● after picrotoxin 0.08 mg/kg; + after further 0.16 mg/kg; × after further 0.5 mg/kg; □ after strychnine 0.08 mg/kg. (From Eccles, Schmidt and Willis, 1963f)

In the decerebrate cat the depression of segmental dorsal root potentials and the removal of presynaptic inhibition of monosynaptic reflexes by picrotoxin appeared even more pronounced than in the spinal animals (Llinás, 1964). At the cuneate nucleus, picrotoxin as well as bemegride and pentylentetrazol depressed the P-wave and the increased excitability of cuneate presynaptic terminals produced by conditioning cortical or cutaneous volleys (Banna and Jabbur, 1969, 1970; Banna and Hazbun, 1969). Further, it reduced the inhibition of the lemniscal discharge by conditioning cutaneous sources (Boyd et al., 1966; Banna and Jabbur, 1968, 1969).

The mode of action of picrotoxin on presynaptic inhibition is not yet fully elucidated. Possibly it is a competitive occupation of the receptor sites for the presynaptic inhibitory transmitter substance. Such a mechanism has already been proposed to account for the blocking action of picrotoxin at the inhibitory synapse of the crayfish neuromuscular junction, where GABA is the transmitter. Further, a GABA-picrotoxin interaction has recently been demonstrated by GALINDO (1969) in the mammalian central nervous system and by TEBĒCIS and PHILLIS (1969 a, b) in the toad spinal cord. And bicuculline, which has been shown to be a relative selective GABA antagonist, and to suppress certain strychnine-insensitive inhibitions in the feline central nervous system (CURTIS et al., 1971 b; ENGBERG and THALLER, 1970; see however GODFRAIND et al., 1970), appears to have a powerful blocking action on presynaptic inhibition (CURTIS et al., 1971 a; LEVY et al., 1971). Nevertheless, there are reports which do not support these ideas. For instance, TEBĒCIS and PHILLIS (1969 a) pointed out that, in some of their experiments, picrotoxin even at high concentrations had no effects on dorsal root potentials and they concluded that the action of picrotoxin is more complex than has been suggested above. BESSON et al. (1971, 1972) found that at the lumbar level picrotoxin depresses segmental DRPs but facilitates DRPs evoked by descending influences (forelimb nerve volleys, acoustic, visual and cortical stimuli). Similarly, pentylentetrazol seems to depress DRPs of local origin and to enhance those of central origin (BESSON and ABDELMOUNÈNE, 1970). Furthermore, GRANIT and his co-workers have failed to find appreciable amounts of presynaptic inhibition (cf. GRANIT, 1968), but instead have described a strychnine-resistant, picrotoxin-sensitive postsynaptic inhibition (KELLERTH, 1965, 1968; KELLERTH and SZUMSKI, 1966 a, b). Their conclusions depend heavily upon the significance of the "synaptic activation noise" recorded during muscle stretch and on the assumption that changes in firing rate of artificially depolarized neurones reflect only postsynaptic actions, and, therefore, these results are in need of further confirmation. Nevertheless it may be postulated from their findings that the strychnine-resistant, picrotoxin-sensitive postsynaptic inhibition occurs in parallel to presynaptic inhibition. This possibility is suggested by the histological findings (cf. WALBERG, 1965) that the presynaptic parts of axo-axonic synapses often also have specific synaptic contacts with those neurones on which the afferent terminals end. It is thus envisaged (CURTIS et al., 1971 a) that at least two types of spinal inhibitory interneurones have synapses on motoneurones: those blocked by strychnine (transmitter glycine) and those blocked by picrotoxin and bicucilline (transmitter GABA ?). At the neuromuscular junction of the crayfish pre- and postsynaptic inhibition are always exerted by the same inhibitory axon (DUDEL and KUFFLER, 1961; ATWOOD and MORIN, 1970).

Strychnine seems to have only indirect actions on PAD and presynaptic inhibition due to the removal of postsynaptic inhibition on the cells of the pathways of PAD. In the early stages of strychnine poisoning the removal of postsynaptic inhibition results in an enhanced and prolonged interneuronal discharge and a consequently enhanced and prolonged PAD, whereas in the later stages the PAD is reduced because of the occlusion produced in the PAD pathways by the considerable spontaneous and convulsive interneuronal activity. The extensive literature on the effects of strychnine on PAD and presynaptic inhibition has recently been summarized and reviewed (SCHMIDT, 1971).

Several amino acids have been proposed as possible transmitter substances in the central nervous system (for reviews see CURTIS, 1968, 1969). For instance, in crustaceae the neutral amino acid, γ-amino-butyric acid (GABA), has an action which is identical with that of the inhibitory transmitter substance at several pre- and postsynaptic inhibitory synapses. Picrotoxin and bicuculline act as blocking agents at these synapses, depressing both the inhibitory synaptic action and the action of GABA. Since presynaptic inhibition in the cat is reversibly antagonized by picrotoxin, the effect of topically administered GABA on PAD has been tested by Eccles et al. (1963f). It was found that GABA reduced and shortened the dorsal root potentials and increased the dorsal root reflexes. GABA also depressed the dorsal root potential in the isolated toad spinal cord (Phillis, 1960; Schmidt, 1963; Tebēcis and Phillis, 1969a). Simultaneously it increased the excitability of the primary afferent fibres. However, Curtis and Ryall (1966) tested the action of electrophoretically administered GABA upon the excitability of the preterminal region of spinal afferent fibres and found under these conditions that GABA did not increase, but actually decreased, the electrical excitability of the terminals, and this has been confirmed on cuneate primary afferent fibre terminals (Galindo, 1969). These results underline the original assumptions of Eccles et al. (1963f) and Schmidt (1963) that topically administered GABA reduced the dorsal root potentials not only by depolarizing the presynaptic fibre terminals but also by actions at other sites of the PAD pathway. Certainly, further clarification of the situation is needed, particularly in view of the reports that the pre- and postsynaptic depressant actions of GABA could be fully blocked by picrotoxin (Galindo, 1969), that the GABA antagonist bicuculline effectively depressed presynaptic inhibition (Curtis et al., 1971a; Levy et al., 1971) and that in cats depletion of GABA by semicarbazide results in reduced presynaptic inhibition of monosynaptic reflexes (Bell and Anderson, 1970).

Acidic amino acids such as glutamic acid excite postsynaptic elements. Curtis et al. (1961) found that glutamic acid increased the ventral root reflex discharge of isolated toad spinal cords and that it depolarized motoneurones. Phillis (1960) reported that, in the same preparation, glutamic acid reduced the dorsal root potential evoked by dorsal root stimulation and this finding has been confirmed (Schmidt, 1963; Phillis and Tebēcis, 1967; Tebēcis and Phillis, 1967, 1969a, b). A comparison of the depression of the dorsal root potential and the excitability increase of primary afferent fibres showed that, unlike GABA, glutamic acid probably directly depolarized the primary afferent fibres. Curtis and Ryall (1966) in their microelectrophoretic study also found excitability increases of presynaptic fibres upon glutamic acid (or DL-homocysteic acid) injection. Nevertheless the significance of the results obtained with acidic amino acids remains just as obscure as that of the changes measured upon GABA administration.

Catecholamines have profound actions on presynaptic inhibitory actions in the spinal cord, presumably because some of the descending pathways which exert a presynaptic inhibitory control on primary afferents are noradrenergic. Lundberg and his co-workers found that the PAD induced in ipsi- and contralateral flexor reflex afferents (FRA) by volleys in other FRA were markedly reduced after intravenous injection of DOPA (L-3, 4 dihydroxyphenylalanine), whereas the dorsal root potentials induced in Group I muscle afferents were not affected. (The transmission from the FRA to motoneurones and ascending pathways was also depressed.) Under these conditions volleys in FRA evoked a long latency PAD in ipsi- and contralateral Group Ia fibres from flexors and extensors (together with a powerful long latency flexor reflex). A detailed physiological and pharmacological analysis of these phenomena revealed that, most probably, descending inhibitory noradrenergic tracts end on interneurones of the FRA interneuronal pathways, and that DOPA mimicks activity in these descending tracks by inducing synthesis and overflow of noradrenaline from their synaptic terminals (ANDÉN et al., 1963, 1964, 1966a, b; ANDÉN, JUKES and LUNDBERG, 1964, 1966; JANKOWSKA et al., 1966; LUNDBERG, 1966; ENGBERG et al., 1968).

The diagrams in Fig. 8 show schematically the proposed pathways of FRA fibres to the presynaptic terminals of FRA and muscle Group Ia afferent fibres.

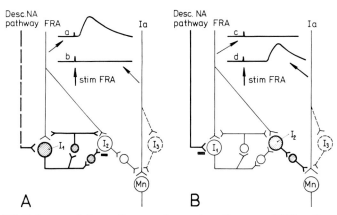

Fig. 8 A and B. Influence of descending noradrenergic pathway on PAD pathways. The diagrams were constructed to illustrate the findings and conclusions of LUNDBERG and collaborators quoted in the text. A gives the situation in the acute spinal cat, B that in a cat with an intact descending noradrenergic pathway. For further discussion of the diagrams see text. (From SCHMIDT, 1971)

The situation in the acute spinal cat is given in A. A volley in the FRA fibres evokes activity in the interneuronal chains starting at the interneuron I_1 and this activity results in PAD of FRA fibres (DRP specimen a in A), and in inhibition of the pathway starting at interneurone I_2 and leading to the Ia preterminals. No PAD is induced in these terminals (specimen b in A). Activation of the descending inhibitory pathway (NA) or injection of DOPA results in the situation shown in B; the interneuronal chain I_1 is inhibited. Thus no PAD can be recorded from FRA fibres (specimen c) but the Ia fibres are depolarized via I_2 (specimen d). The pathway I_3 leading from Group Ia afferents to Group Ia afferents remains unaffected.

The existence of descending noradrenergic pathways and the absence of segmental noradrenergic neurones have been suggested by the use of histochemical and biochemical methods (CARLSSON et al., 1964; DAHLSTRÖM and FUXE, 1965). The proposal that DOPA acts not directly on PAD interneurones but by liberating transmitter (mostly noradrenaline) from such descending pathways is largely based on pharmacological evidence. First of all DOPA has little or no effect after inhibition of DOPA decarboxylase (by meta-hydroxy-benzylhydrazine), and its effect is potentiated by monoamino-oxidase inhibition (by nialamide). These findings suggest that DOPA acts only after decarboxylation (to dopamine which is converted to noradrenaline) and not directly. Furthermore, reserpine pretreatment prevents the effects of DOPA. Finally the effects of DOPA can be antagonized by the blockers of adrenergic α-receptors (phenoxybenzamine and chlorpromazine), but not by the β-blocker, pronethalol (Nethalide). Injection of 5-HTP (5-hydroxytryptophane, precursor of 5-HT, 5-hydroxytryptamine) has actions similar to those seen after DOPA injection (Andén, Jukes and Lundberg, 1964). As summarized by Lundberg (1966) there is pharmacological evidence that, as with DOPA, the effects of 5-HTP are due to liberation of 5-HT from terminals of a descending pathway, and that these terminals have receptor sites different from those activated by DOPA (or its derivatives).

The effect of tetrodotoxin (TTX) on dorsal root potentials (DRPs) generated by dorsal root stimulation or by direct stimulation of the dorsal horn was studied by Rudomin and Muñoz-Martinez (1969). It was shown that the DRP produced by dorsal root stimulation completely disappeared upon intra-arterial TTX administration (40–80 μg/kg), whereas the DRP generated by dorsal horn stimulation was depressed but not abolished. Several explanations of this phenomenon were offered by the authors. To them the most likely explanation appeared to be that, by analogy with the effects of depolarizing currents at TTX poisoned synapses and neuromuscular junctions (Bloedel et al., 1966, 1967; Katz and Miledi, 1967a–c), the stimulating current released transmitter from the presynaptic terminals of axo-axonic synapses and that this transmitter evoked the observed TTX-resistant DRPs.

Carlsson (1964) tested the effects of Na^+-reduction on the DRP. Frog spinal cords were perfused with Ringer's solution (normal colloid osmotic pressure achieved by addition of dextran) and the Na^+-concentration of the perfusion fluid was varied. The DRP was shown to vary linearly with the $\log_{10}$ of the Na^+-concentration (Na^+ replaced by sucrose). These results were interpreted as evidence for the role of an internuncial system in the generation of the DRP.

Different types of prostaglandins depolarize amphibian dorsal root fibres and reduce the size of DRPs (Phillis and Tebēcis, 1968). This effect has an extremely slow rate of recovery (0.5–1 h). The site of action is unknown. Increases in the H^+-concentration caused a depolarization of dorsal root terminals and a simultaneous decrease in amplitude and increase in duration of the DRP.

III. Local and Descending Influences on Transmission from Primary Afferents to Second-Order Cells

A. Inhibitory Influences Exerted onto Primary Afferents of the Spinal Cord

Three general comments should be made before starting a detailed consideration of the functional organization of presynaptic inhibition. *First*, it should be pointed out that in most of the studies concerned with these questions the various manifestations of primary afferent depolarization (PAD) have usually been used as indicators for presynaptic inhibitory processes. The inhibition itself was rarely measured. It was generally assumed that the amount and time course of PAD was directly related to the amount and time course of the presynaptic inhibition exerted onto the depolarized fibres. *Secondly*, it should be mentioned that nearly all results reported here have been obtained from the central nervous system of the cat. It has to remain open, therefore, to what extent the organisation of the PAD reflex pathways in other mammals resembles that described here. *Thirdly*, it should be made clear that on the one hand it is usually possible to discover the relative amounts of presynaptic depolarization exerted from various inputs onto a given fibre population, whereas on the other hand, when a given input acts on different fibre populations it is difficult to judge the relative amounts of the respective depolarizations. Comparisons of the latter type can only be made when the depolarization is measured directly by intrafibre recording, and this has only been done systematically when testing the relative potency of spinal afferents in depolarizing other spinal afferents (ECCLES, MAGNI and WILLIS, 1962; ECCLES et al., 1963a, e).

1. Presynaptic Inhibitory Pathways Ending on Muscle Primary Afferent Terminals

Presynaptic Inhibition of Ia Afferents from Muscle Spindles. A considerable amount of effort in various laboratories throughout the world has been devoted to the investigation of the segmental pathways leading to Group Ia afferent fibre terminals from muscle. The general conclusion is that Ia fibres from primary endings of muscle spindles of flexor and extensor muscles are presynaptically inhibited, i.e. depolarized, by volleys mainly in Group Ia and Group Ib afferent fibres of ipsilateral flexor muscles, and little if at all by Group II (from secondary muscle spindle endings) and Group III afferent impulses (ECCLES, ECCLES and MAGNI, 1961; ECCLES, KOZAK and MAGNI, 1961; ECCLES, MAGNI and WILLIS, 1962; ECCLES et al., 1963a, b; ECCLES and WILLIS, 1962; SCHMIDT and WILLIS, 1963a, b; VOORHOEVE and VERHEY, 1963; COOK et al., 1965; VERHEY et al., 1966; DECANDIA, GASTEIGER and MANN, 1968, 1971; BARNES and POMPEIANO, 1970a, c). The PAD was exerted both onto those Ia terminals making monosynaptic excitatory contacts on motoneurones and onto those conveying excitation to neurones of ascending tracts (ECCLES et al., 1963d; JANKOWSKA et al., 1965). Volleys in Ib fibres often proved to be slightly more effective than volleys in Ia fibres in depolarizing Ia fibres. The greater effectiveness of flexor Ib fibres compared to flexor Ia fibres in depolarizing Ia fibres was also seen when the presynaptic inhibitory effects upon stretch and contraction of ipsilateral muscles were studied (DEVANANDAN et al., 1964, 1965a, b, 1966; cf. also DECANDIA, ELDRED and GROVER, 1971). Under conditions of particularly strong activation of tendon organs from flexor muscles (maximum stretch and contraction), the PAD of Ia fibres exceeded considerably that seen after activation of primary muscle spindle endings only (slight stretch).

Volleys in extensor Group I fibres generated very little or no PAD in Ia fibres of flexor muscles. However, contraction of extensor muscles did induce PAD in agonist extensor muscles (DEVANANDAN, ECCLES and STENHOUSE, 1966). Experiments with electrical stimulation of extensor nerves (Decandia et al., 1966) or activation of primary muscle spindle endings by vibratory stimuli (Gillies et al., 1969; Barnes and Pompeiano, 1970b, d) confirmed that stimulation of Group I agonist fibres depolarized Ia extensor terminals, and evidence was presented that this depolarization was parallelled by a presynaptic inhibition of the agonist monosynaptic reflex (Decandia, Provini and Táboříková, 1967; Gillies et al., 1969; Barnes and Pompeiano, 1970b, d; cf. Eccles, Schmidt and Willis, 1962). Usually, repetitive activation had to be used to obtain appreciable effects, single afferent volleys were mostly ineffective (Wall, 1958). The results indicate that the PAD produced by extensor Group I fibres has a more circumscribed feedback character than that evoked by activity in flexor Group I fibres, although there seem to be some exceptions to this rule (cf. Eccles et al., 1963d).

Several types of muscle and cutaneous afferent volleys have proved to be ineffective in the spinal animal in evoking presynaptic inhibition in Group Ia afferent fibres. First of all, all types of contralateral afferent volleys from muscle and skin nerves had no depolarizing effect on Ia afferents and did not depress the size of Ia EPSPs (Devanandan, Holmqvist and Yokota, 1965). Secondly, volleys in ipsilateral flexor reflex afferents, FRA, i.e. certain myelinated cutaneous afferents and high threshold muscle afferents (Group II and III fibres), did not induce PAD in Ia fibres (Eccles, Kozak and Magni, 1961; Eccles, Magni and Willis, 1962; Lund et al., 1965). They did, however, inhibit the PAD evoked in Ia afferents by volleys in Ia afferents (Lund et al., 1965). This is one of several examples indicating that afferent activity not only produces PAD, but is also able to inhibit it. This inhibition presumably takes place on the interneurones of the PAD pathway, possibly presynaptically through depolarization of interneuronal terminals. In the intact animal, cutaneous nerve volleys activate spino-bulbo-spinal reflex mechanism which operate on monosynaptic reflexes via presynaptic inhibition of Ia terminals (Shimamura et al., 1967; Shimamura and Aoki, 1969).

Several descending pathways induce PAD in Ia afferent terminals. Stimulation of the ipsi- or contralateral sensorimotor cortex or of the pyramidal tract remained ineffective (Andersen, Eccles and Sears, 1962, 1964a; Carpenter, Lundberg and Norsell, 1962, 1963), but in a systematic investigation of the PAD evoked by repetitive stimulation of the brain stem and of the cerebellum it was seen that upon stimulation of a dorsal midline region of the medulla a depolarization was induced in lumbar Ia terminals of flexor and extensor muscles (Carpenter, Engberg and Lundberg, 1962, 1966). This PAD disappeared after transection of the ventral quadrants of the spinal cord and it was concluded that it was due to the activation of the ipsilateral medial longitudinal fasciculus. Similar effects were obtained by Cook et al. (1969b) and Barnes and Pompeiano (1970e) when stimulating the ipsilateral VIIIth cranial nerve. They attributed these effects to the vestibular nuclei and their descending afferent projection pathway, because the same results were obtained when stimulating the vestibular complex, especially the medial and descending vestibular nuclei and the medial longitudinal fasciculus at mesencephalic levels. Further, complete lesions of the vestibular nuclei (Cook et al., 1969a) or of the lateral vestibular nucleus (Barnes and Pompeiano, 1970e) abolished the dorsal root potentials evoked by stimulation of the IIIth nerve. Stimulation of the contralateral caudal part of the closely related fastigial nucleus also elicited PAD in Ia fibres of flexor and extensor muscles (CANGIANO et al., 1969a).

The diagram shown in Fig. 9 gives schematically the various segmental and suprasegmental inputs producing inhibition of flexor and extensor Ia afferent fibre terminals. On the left hand side the thicknesses of the arrows give an estimate of the potencies of the segmental pathways in producing PAD and presynaptic inhibition. These estimates are based on an appreciation of the results reviewed in the preceding paragraphs and indicate merely that, according to the evidence at present available, not all types of Group I muscle afferents are equally potent

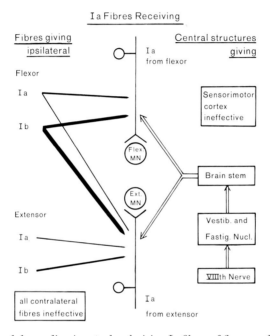

Fig. 9. Segmental and descending inputs depolarizing Ia fibres of flexor and extensor muscles. The approximate relative amount of depolarization contributed by each segmental input has been estimated from the results quoted in the text and is indicated by the width of the arrows. No estimates are available for the relative amounts of depolarization induced by centrifugal activity. MN, motoneurone

in producing PAD of either flexor or extensor Ia fibres. The potency of the descending presynaptic inhibitory influences (right hand side in Fig. 9) and their significance for the regulation of movement and posture is even more difficult to evaluate (cf. LUNDBERG, 1966, 1967). Generally it appears that (unlike Ib and cutaneous afferents, see below) Ia fibres cannot be activated by stimulation of cortical areas, whereas some subcortical descending pathways seem to be quite effective. Most probably further investigations will reveal additional and even more complex pathways involved in the control of the excitatory input from Ia afferents. For instance, in the unrestrained, unanaesthetized cat, a PAD of Ia terminals has been observed during the phasic events of the desynchronized phase of sleep (Morrison and Pompeiano, 1965a, b; Baldissera, Cesa-Bianchi and Mancia, 1966; Baldissera and Broggi, 1967). Possibly this PAD is responsible for the transient depression of the homonymous monosynaptic reflexes that occurs during these periods of desynchronized sleep.

Presynaptic Inhibition of Ib Afferents from Golgi Tendon Organs. The main *ipsilateral* segmental sources from which flexor and extensor Ib endings are depolarized are the Ib fibres of both flexor and extensor muscles (Eccles et al., 1963a). It is noteworthy that the extensor Group I volleys were just as effective in depolarizing Ib fibres as the flexor Group I volleys. By various stimulating and recording procedures it was established that volleys in Ia fibres of all types of muscle nerves did not produce any PAD of Ib fibres. There were, however, definite contributions to the PAD of Ib fibres when high threshold muscle afferents (Group II and III fibres) were included in the volley or when cutaneous nerves were stimulated. The predominance of Ib fibres in inhibiting Ib fibre afferents was confirmed in experiments evoking activity in Ia and Ib fibres by muscle stretch (Devanandan et al., 1965a). *Contralateral* volleys in certain types of afferent fibres also depolarize Ib terminals. Devanandan, Holmqvist and Yokota (1965) showed that the crossed PAD of Ib fibres originated from high threshold (II and III) muscle afferents and from cutaneous fibres. Their results also indicated that Ib fibres have a weak inhibiting action onto the contralateral Ib nerve terminals.

Several *suprasegmental* structures seem to exert a powerful inhibitory influence on Ib afferent terminals. First of all, it was recognized that stimulation of the sensorimotor cortex produced PAD of Ib afferent fibres, the effective cortical areas being the somatosensory areas I and II (Andersen, Eccles and Sears, 1962, 1964a; Carpenter, Lundberg and Norrsell, 1962, 1963; Abdelmoumène et al., 1970; Calma and Quayle, 1971). The effect was predominantly contralateral from SI, whereas the SII effect was bilateral. The SI arm and leg areas acted specifically on the arm and leg afferent fibres respectively. Single cortical stimuli were relatively ineffective, whereas repetitive stimulation caused a large recruitment of responses. This summation took place in the spinal cord, not at the cortical level. The effects were shown to be mediated by pyramidal and by extrapyramidal pathways (Hongo and Jankowska, 1967; Hongo and Okada, 1967). Spatial facilitation between the paths from primary afferents and cortex was observed. In addition, interneurones of the D-type (cf. Fig. 5) were found in the dorsal horn and in the intermediate nucleus of Cajal that were fired by cortical stimulation and otherwise had properties making them possible candidates for the mediation of the cortically evoked presynaptic inhibition. All these findings indicate that an interneuronal system mediates the transmission from the synaptic terminals of the cortico-spinal fibres to the presynaptic inhibitory axo-axonal synapses.

Repetitive electrical stimulation of wide areas of the brain stem of decerebrate cats also evoked considerable PAD of Ib fibres (Carpenter, Engberg and Lundberg, 1962, 1966). Two main regions were recognized. One is a very distinct area in the midline region about 1 mm ventral to the 4th ventricle in the medulla. Stimulation of this area also produced PAD in Ia (see above) and cutaneous fibres. The second area is a more widespread ventromedial region. Stimulation of this area produced PAD of Ib and cutaneous fibres only. These effects may be due in part to the activation of pathways descending from higher centres, but it is interesting to note that the lowest thresholds for evoking these effects were found in a region corresponding to Magoun's inhibitory center. The complex presynaptic inhibitory effects which can be elicited from the VIIIth cranial nerve and the vestibular and fastigial nuclei are not only exerted onto Ia (see above) but also onto Ib fibres (COOK et al., 1968, 1969a, b; CANGIANO et al., 1969a). In decerebrate cats, stimulation of the lateral parts of the intermediate region on both sides of the anterior cerebellar cortex also induced large PAD of Ib (and cutaneous) afferents (CARPENTER et al., 1966; CANGIANO et al., 1969b).

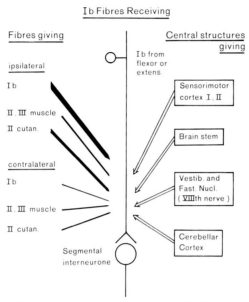

Fig. 10. Segmental and descending inputs depolarizing Ib fibres from Golgi tendon organs. The approximate relative amount of depolarization contributed by each segmental input has been estimated from the results quoted in the text and is indicated by the width of the arrows. No estimates are available for the relative amounts of depolarization induced by descending activity

The left hand side of the diagram in Fig. 10 summarizes the results obtained when testing the presynaptic depolarizing action of segmental afferent input onto Ib primary afferent fibres. As in Fig. 9 the afferent inputs were assembled to give the basic types (ipsi- and contralateral) Groups Ib, II, III and cutaneous. Since it was not possible to discover any topographical relationship, or any difference between flexor and extensor Ib fibres, a single Ib afferent fibre in the middle of the diagram represents the Ib fibre population receiving the inhibition, and the Ib-fibres giving the depolarization are also pooled. Again the thicknesses of the arrows give approximate measures of the potencies of the various pathways. For the ipsilateral input these estimates are based on the results of ECCLES et al. (1963a), whereas the contralateral estimates are given according to the findings of DEVANANDAN et al. (1965). On the right hand side of the diagram the principal supraspinal regions from which Ib fibres can be inhibited are given. Here no evidence is available on the potency of these pathways relative to each other and relative to the segmental input.

Presynaptic Inhibition of Group II and III Afferent Fibres from Muscle. Very little is known of the conditions which may induce PAD and presynaptic inhibition in myelinated high threshold muscle afferents. It is generally assumed that these fibres not only contribute to the FRA system (as defined by ECCLES and LUNDBERG, 1959), thus evoking PAD in Ib and cutaneous afferents (cf. ECCLES et al., 1962a, b; ECCLES et al., 1963a, e) but also receive PAD from flexor reflex afferents. The only direct evidence to support this assumption has been reported by ECCLES et al. (1963a), who recorded intracellularly from a small number of Group II fibres the PAD induced by cutaneous and muscle nerve stimulation. The results suggested that Group II muscle afferents are depolarized by cutaneous volleys as well as by Group I muscle volleys. Descending systems also seem to be able to evoke PAD in Group II afferents: CARPENTER et al. (1963) observed that of 12 muscle Group II fibres, 6 displayed an increased excitability after stimulation of the sensorimotor cortex.

2. Presynaptic Inhibitory Pathways Ending on Cutaneous Primary Afferent Terminals

In the early investigations on PAD, it was recognized that volleys in myelinated cutaneous afferents were particularly powerful in evoking a large PAD of spinal afferents. Indirect methods such as the recording of dorsal root reflexes (TOENNIES, 1938, 1939; MEGIRIAN, 1968, 1970, 1971) and the testing of the excitability of the spinal axon terminals (WALL, 1958), indicated that this PAD was mainly exerted onto the cutaneous fibres themselves, both those that have been primarily activated and those initially passive. These original observations were fully confirmed by the subsequent intrafibre studies of cutaneous PAD (KOKETSU, 1956; ECCLES and KRNJEVIĆ, 1959, Table 2; ECCLES et al., 1963e). A typical example for such measurements is illustrated in Fig. 11.

Apart from the predominant influence of cutaneous afferents onto the cutaneous PAD system, several other *ipsilateral* segmental inputs are able to depolarize cutaneous fibres. *First*, activation of muscle Ib fibres, both of flexor and extensor muscles, usually gave appreciable PAD in cutaneous fibres (see Fig. 11), whereas stimulation of Ia fibres almost always remained completely ineffective (ECCLES et al., 1963e). *Secondly*, Group II and III fibres from muscle, which in many respects work in synergy with cutaneous fibres, also exert a considerable depolarizing influence on cutaneous afferent terminals (ECCLES et al., 1962a, b, 1963e). The effectiveness of these fibres, and of all the other "flexor reflex afferents" of cutaneous and joint nerves, depends on the experimental situation: they are much more powerful in the spinal than in the decerebrate animal (CARPENTER and ENGBERG et al., 1963). *Third*, volleys in cutaneous unmyelinated fibres (Group IV fibres) lead to depolarizations of cutaneous myelinated fibres which are often just as powerful as those induced by cutaneous Group II fibres (JÄNIG and ZIMMERMANN, 1971). Further, in cats anaesthetized with chloralose, heterosegmental presynaptic depolarization of cutaneous afferents has been reported (MALLART, 1965; CALMA and QUAYLE, 1971). Finally, visceral afferents in the caudal sympathetic chain also

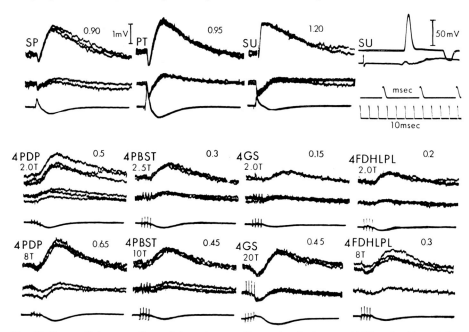

Fig. 11. Intracellular recording of the primary afferent depolarization (PAD) of a fibre of the sural (SU) nerve at 0.7 mm depth. The SU record in the upper right-hand corner shows in the upper trace the intracellular spike, and in the lower the cord dorsum potential. All other records were at a higher amplification and at a much slower sweep speed in order to display the depolarizations produced by afferent volleys in various cutaneous and muscle nerves of the hind limb, as indicated by the symbols. Upper traces are the intracellular records, depolarization being upward. Middle traces show the field potentials similarly recorded, but with the microelectrode just outside the fibre; the lower traces show the cord dorsum potentials, but with upward deflexion negative. All records are formed by the superposition of several traces, usually three. Subtraction of the extracellular fields from the intracellular potentials gives the PAD, which are shown in mV for each record. The cutaneous nerves in the first row have been stimulated with single shocks of four times threshold strength. All other nerves were stimulated with four shocks at 300/s and the stimulus strength is indicated on each record relative to the threshold (T). The 1 mV calibration is for the intracellular and extracellular records. The 10 msec time marker is for all except the spike record, which was recorded at the faster sweep speed. SP is a cutaneous nerve, PDP and PBST are flexor muscle nerves, GS and FDHLPL are extensor muscle nerves, and PT is a mixed nerve. (From ECCLES, SCHMIDT and WILLIS, 1963e)

induce presynaptic depolarization in cutaneous afferents of the lumbar spinal cord (SELZER and SPENCER, 1969). The results for PAD effects from contralateral afferent inputs onto cutaneous afferents resemble those from the ipsilateral side (ECCLES et al., 1964a, b). In general, the effects were always much weaker and, as always with contralateral actions, their latency was longer. Furthermore, when contralateral muscle nerves were stimulated, volleys in Ia and Ib fibres remained ineffective, while Group II and III volleys evoked a presynaptic depolarization.

In regard to descending presynaptic inhibitory influences it has been a general finding that those supraspinal structures exerting presynaptic depolarization on muscle Ib fibres usually also depolarized spinal cutaneous afferents. The reader is referred, therefore, to page 172 where the relevant papers have been reviewed. Presynaptic depolarization initiated from supraspinal structures and restricted to cutaneous afferents has not yet been described. In a short note Calma (1966) reported that stimulation of the ventral thalamo-diencephalic region caused bilateral presynaptic depolarization of cutaneous afferents but he did not specifically state that a simultaneous presynaptic depolarization of muscle Ia or Ib afferents had been excluded.

The inhibitory effects of presynaptic depolarization of cutaneous afferents should manifest themselves as a reduction of the monosynaptic EPSP in the appropriate segmental interneurones, without any other detectable change of the postsynaptic membrane. Because of the small size of these interneurones very few observations of this type have been reported (Eccles et al., 1962b). In all other cases the conclusion that an inhibitory action was due to presynaptic depolarization was based on the close parallelism observed between the depolarization and the inhibition in regard to their various properties such as time course, mode of generation, operational relationships, pharmacology, and so forth. Inhibitory actions of cutaneous afferent volleys that have been attributed in whole or in part to presynaptic inhibition include: the flexor reflex inhibition produced by ipsilateral (Eccles et al., 1962b; Schmidt and Willis, 1963b) as well as by contralateral afferent volleys (Eccles et al., 1964a, b); the inhibition of the monosynaptic and polysynaptic discharges into the ipsilateral dorsolateral funiculus (Eccles et al., 1962b); the inhibition of dorsal root potentials and dorsal root reflexes (Eccles et al., 1962b; Schmidt and Willis, 1963b); the inhibition of discharges of cuneate neurones into the medial lemniscus and the depression of cuneate P-waves (Andersen, Eccles, Oshima and Schmidt, 1964; Carli et al., 1966; Cesa-Bianchi et al., 1968); and the inhibition of discharges in second order trigeminal nuclei (Darian-Smith, 1965; Rowe and Carmody, 1970). Furthermore, it has been generally assumed that the presynaptic depolarization in cutaneous afferents produced by other inputs, for example high threshold muscle afferents or supraspinal structures, is always accompanied by a depression of the excitatory actions of the depolarized terminals.

The parallelism between presynaptic depolarization (primary afferent depolarization, PAD) and presynaptic inhibition has been accepted so universally that many authors use both expressions synonymously. Even if it had been established beyond reasonable doubt that PAD always reflects presynaptic inhibition and that presynaptic inhibition is always accompanied by PAD, this synonymous usage should be avoided to prevent misunderstandings. Since at present the rôle of PAD in presynaptic inhibition relative to other factors, such as impedance changes at the terminal regions, is far from being clarified (cf. section II C) it appears even more important not to confuse the terminal depolarization with the accompanying inhibitory process.

The various inputs producing PAD of segmental cutaneous afferents are summarized in Fig. 12. The upper part of the left hand side shows diagramatically the ipsilateral segmental inputs. Except for arrow "IV cutan" the thicknesses of the arrows are proportional to the average PAD measured by Eccles and Krnjević (1959) and by Eccles et al. (1963e) in a population of about 100 fibres. The thickness of arrow "IV cutan" was taken from intracellular measurements of Jänig

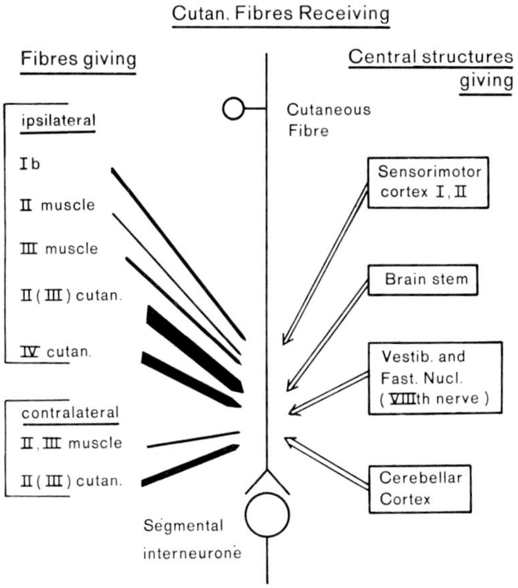

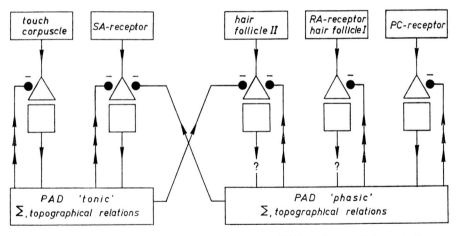

Fig. 12. Segmental and descending inputs depolarizing spinal cord cutaneous afferent fibres. The approximate relative amount of depolarization contributed by each segmental input has been estimated from the results quoted in the text and is indicated by the width of the arrows. No estimates are available for the relative amounts of depolarization induced by descending activity

Fig. 13. The operational relationships of the cutaneous PAD pathways. Schematic diagram illustrating the presynaptic inhibitory connections within the cutaneous mechanoreceptor afferent population. The boxes in the upper row stand for the various receptor types, the slowly adapting receptors being assembled on the left-hand side. The middle row complex indicates the first synapses in the spinal cord onto which the receptors project, the closed circles showing the presynaptic control. The PAD generating systems are shown in the lower row. The number of arrows in the feedback lines denote the feedback gain. SA and RA designate slowly and rapidly adapting receptors respectively. PC are Pacinian corpuscles. (From JÄNIG, SCHMIDT and ZIMMERMANN, 1968b)

and Zimmermann (1971) who compared the PAD produced by sural Group II (and III) volleys with that produced by sural Group IV volleys during block of the myelinated fibres. Thus this part of the diagram gives an approximate measure of the relative potencies of the various ipsilateral segmental inputs giving PAD of cutaneous afferent fibres. It should be added in parenthesis that so far no evidence for PAD of cutaneous or muscle Group IV fibres has been brought forward. The observations on PAD effects from contralateral afferent fibres are given in the lower left hand-side of the diagram. Again, the relative effectiveness of these inputs is given by the thickness of the arrows, the estimates being based on the results of Eccles et al. (1964a, b). Finally, on the right-hand side of the diagram the principal supraspinal regions from which cutaneous afferents can be depolarized are given. These regions correspond to those from which Ib fibres can be depolarized (cf. Fig. 10). As in Figs. 9 and 10 the thickness of the descending arrows does not indicate the potency of the pathways which they symbolize.

Several lines of evidence indicate that the depolarizing action of cutaneous afferents onto cutaneous afferents is not an indiscriminative feedback mechanism but possesses a high degree of modality specificity and a complex functional organisation. Most of the work related to this problem has been done using various types of mechanical stimuli to the skin. Dorsal root potentials evoked by mechanical stimuli were first seen by Barron and Matthews (1938) in the frog and in the cat, and by Fuortes (1951) in the frog. They have also been described in the cat by Mendell and Wall (1964), Vyklický and Tabin (1966); Schmidt et al. (1966) and Jänig et al. (1967), see also Fig. 15. These observations indicated that activity in mechano-sensitive units did produce presynaptic inhibition. In order to study which cutaneous sensory modalities received the inhibition, the PAD of single afferent fibres of known modality had to be measured within the spinal cord. Such a method, together with carefully controlled mechanical stimuli, was used to study the PAD in different types of mechanoreceptor afferents of the cat's hind limb (Jänig et al., 1968). It was found that two separate systems generate PAD in cutaneous afferents, both being of negative feed-back character. As schematically shown in Fig. 13, one system is activated by impulses from rapidly adapting low-threshold receptors, and preferentially depolarizes the terminals of such afferents, and correspondingly, the other system is activated by and operates on the slowly adapting units. In both PAD systems the size of the depolarization is graded, depending on the stimulus strength. Further, the PAD of mechanoreceptor afferents of the hind limb is organized in a "surround" fashion. As seen in Fig. 14, the mechanical stimuli exerted their greatest depolarizing influence onto the afferents of those receptors which were nearest to the point of the stimulus application, and the PAD decreased when the conditioning stimulus was moved away from the receptive field of the fibre under study.

Painful radiant heat applied to the plantar pad of spinal cats produced PAD of cutaneous fibres and also, to a lesser extent, of Ib muscle afferents, whether or not the posterior tibial nerve was cooled to block the activity in cutaneous Group II fibres (Vyklický et al., 1969; Burke et al., 1971). Whitehorn and Burgess (personal communication) also observed that damaging skin stimuli, such as radiant heat and the application of noxious clips, depolarized cutaneous mechanoreceptor afferents. It was suggested by both groups of authors that these

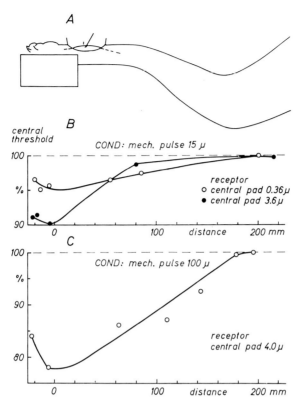

Fig. 14. Topographic organization of PAD of mechanoreceptor afferents. In B the central excitability changes of single mechanoreceptor afferents from the central food pad were measured 50 msec (open circles) and 30 msec (points) after a mechanical stimulus of 15 μ indentation and 4 msec duration applied to various positions along the leg. These distances are given on the abscissa and can be related to the limb in A which is drawn to scale. The afferent fibres came from touch receptors having mechanical thresholds as indicated in microns. C is from another receptor. The conditioning stimulus produced a 100 μ skin indentation. (From SCHMIDT, SENGES and ZIMMERMANN, 1967b)

PAD resulted from the afferent activity mainly in small myelinated (Group III) and unmyelinated (Group IV) cutaneous afferents. (For a more detailed discussion of the presynaptic effects of Group III and IV afferent fibres see section III B).

B. Disinhibition of Primary Afferents of the Spinal Cord during Tonic Presynaptic Depolarization – Positive Dorsal Root Potentials

Several experimental conditions have been reported in the literature, where afferent activity gave rise not only to a phasic dorsal root potential (DRP, see Figs. 3, 6, 17) but to a more prolonged depolarization lasting throughout the stimulation. Examples are the prolonged dorsal root potentials evoked either by repetitive stimulation of cutaneous nerves (Eccles et al., 1963e), or by the squeezing of the cat's foot by hand (Mendell and Wall, 1964) or by applying constant pressure to the cat's foot pads (Jänig, Schmidt and Zimmermann, 1967; Fig. 15). These results suggest that *in vivo* some or all of the presynaptic inhibitory pathways are capable of exerting not only transient (phasic), but also more persistent

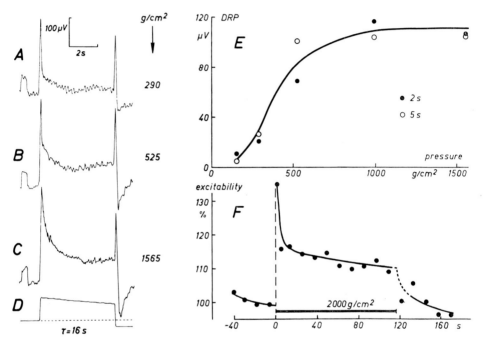

Fig. 15 A–F. A, B, C show DRPs during stimulation of the large pad of the left hind foot by constant pressure pulses of 5.5 sec duration and with the indicated strength. The records were taken from a L₇ dorsal rootlet. The AC-coupled preamplifier had a time constant of 16 sec, resulting in a square pulse deformation as demonstrated in D. For each specimen 10 consecutive measurements were averaged in a computer at a repetition rate of 1/30 sec. In E the DRP size 2 sec (●) and 5 sec (○) after the stimulus onset is plotted versus stimulus strength. In F the intraspinal excitability (ordinate) of the lateral plantar nerve was measured before, during and after a 200 g/cm² pressure stimulus 115 sec in duration (horizontal bar above the abscissa). (From Jänig, Schmidt and Zimmermann, 1967)

(tonic), inhibitory influences on the primary afferent terminals. Temporary removal of such a tonic presynaptic depolarization would lead to a transitory hyperpolarization of primary afferent terminals (primary afferent hyperpolarization, PAH) which, for example, could be recorded as a "positive" dorsal root potential.

Positive dorsal root potentials (PAH) have been observed in a variety of experimental situations. They were first reported by Lundberg and Vyklický (1963) and illustrated by Lundberg (1964, his Fig. 17). Another example is shown in Fig. 16 (Lundberg and Vyklický, 1966). The tonic dorsal root potentials evoked by tetanic stimulation of a certain brain stem area were temporarily depressed by single afferent volleys in high-threshold afferents (Group III) of the gastrocnemious soleus nerve. The same effect was produced by volleys in cutaneous afferents but never by single volleys or a train of volleys in Group I afferents from flexors or extensors (LUNDBERG and VYKLICKÝ, 1963, 1966; cf. also CHAN and BARNES, 1971). These effects were seen in decerebrate, decerebellate cats. In precollicular

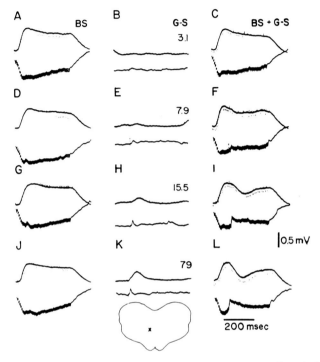

Fig. 16 A–L. Removal of the DRP evoked from the brain stem by volleys in high threshold muscle afferents. The DRPs (upper traces in A–L) in the left column are evoked by stimulation of the brain stem (BS) in the region shown in the drawing at the bottom of the middle column. The middle column shows the effect of stimulation of the gastrocnemius-soleus (G–S) nerve at the strength indicated for each record in multiples of thresholds for the nerve. In the corresponding records of the right column there is combined stimulation of the brain stem and the G–S nerve at strength given in the corresponding records in the middle column. The voltage calibration is for the DRPs. The lower traces in A–L were recorded from the surface of the spinal cord at the L₇ dorsal root entry zone. (From LUNDBERG and VYKLICKÝ, 1966)

decerebrate cats CANGIANO et al. (1969 b) observed that stimulation of the vermal cortex of the anterior lobe of the cerebellum, evoked positive dorsal root potentials in lumbar dorsal roots (their Fig. 2), and that such stimulation was able to inhibit temporarily the tonic negative dorsal root potential evoked by tetanic stimulation of the VIIIth nerve (their Fig. 3). By stimulation and ablation experiments they were able to show that this PAH reflected a tonic inhibitory control of the cerebellar cortex on the vestibular nuclei, which in turn generated a tonic PAD of

Group I as well as cutaneous afferents. (No effort was made to distinguish between effects on Ia and Ib afferent fibres.) Removal of a tonic presynaptic inhibition of Ia fibres restores the monosynaptic EPSP to its control height (Lund et al., 1965).

Positive dorsal root potentials were also seen in spinal unanaesthetized animals. Mendell and Wall (1964) recorded pure positive dorsal root potentials following single stimuli to high threshold cutaneous afferents during preferential block of conduction in the larger fibres (their Fig. 2), and these results were confirmed later on (Dawson et al., 1970, their Fig. 2). Similarly, stimulation of high threshold afferents of flexor and extensor muscle nerves gave rise to positive dorsal root potentials in spinal unanaesthetized cats (Mendell, 1970). In all three papers it was agreed that the short latency (25–50 msec) positive dorsal root potentials were due to activity in small (A delta, Group III) myelinated afferents. In addition, Mendell and Wall (1964) claimed to have shown that, "if a pure C-fibre volley is fired into the cord, an entirely positive DRP is generated". This somewhat premature statement, partly withdrawn in 1970 (Dawson et al.), gave rise to an exciting controversy and still ongoing experimental activity on the effects of Group IV afferent fibres (C-fibres) on presynaptic inhibition, mainly because Melzack and Wall (1965) suggested that the disinhibition reflected in the positive DRPs might play a rôle in the perception of noxious stimuli (gate control theory of pain). Zimmermann (1968b) and Jänig and Zimmermann (1971) in nembutalized and in unanaesthetized spinal cats were unable to repeat the results of Mendell and Wall but instead always recorded negative C-DRPs which were particularly well developed in the absence of A-fibre activity due to block (Fig. 17). Similar results were reported by Franz and Iggo (1968) who used a cold block for the suppression of Group II and III afferent activity instead of the different types of current blocks employed by Mendell and Wall (1964); Zimmermann (1968a) and Dawson et al. (1970). Vyklický et al. (1969) and Burke et al. (1971) used intense (noxious) radiant heat to the central plantar pad instead of electrical stimuli to cutaneous nerves to induce activity in Group III and IV afferents. Again, they were only able to record negative DRP and concomitant excitability increases in cutaneous and Ib fibre terminals even in those preparations in which electrical stimuli to cutaneous or muscle nerves clearly gave positive DRP components (DRP VI Lloyd, 1952; cf. also Lloyd and McIntyre, 1949) or purely positive DRPs (with muscle nerve stimuli, cf. Mendell, 1970, 1971). Cold block of the large myelinated afferents did not influence the results. It was concluded by Burke et al. (1971) that their results provided no support for a presynaptic gating mechanism operating during painful stimuli but that the results have no bearing on the question of gates operating via postsynaptic mechanisms.

Apart from the speculation on the presence or absence of a presynaptic gate control mechanism and in the complete absence of information on the exact modalities transmitted via cutaneous and muscle Group III and IV afferent fibres, our present knowledge on the effects of these afferents on segmental presynaptic inhibition may be summarized as follows: It has been shown that depending on the experimental situation afferent volleys in Group III fibres from skin, joint and muscle nerves produce either negative DRPs (Eccles et al., 1962a, their Figs. 1 and 2; Carpenter and Engberg et al., 1963), or no DRPs (Mendell, 1970), or positive DRPs (MENDELL and WALL, 1964; MENDELL, 1970; DAWSON et al., 1970; BURKE et al., 1971). Group IV afferents from skin seem to induce mainly negative DRPs both following electrical and natural stimulation (ZIMMERMANN, 1968b; JÄNIG and ZIMMERMANN, 1971; BURKE et al., 1971), and there is some indication of positive DRPs from Group IV muscle afferents (MENDELL, 1970). There seems to be general agreement that positive DRPs always reflect a hyperpolarization of primary afferent terminals due to the removal of a tonic presynaptic depolariza-

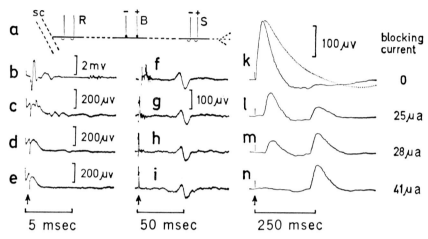

Fig. 17 a–n. Dorsal root potentials evoked by afferent volleys in Group IV cutaneous fibres. (a) Arrangement on the sural nerve of the electrodes for stimulation, (S) blocking of the Group II and III fibres (B), and recording (R); sc, sciatic. (b, f), Nerve records taken at R and displayed at different gains and sweep speeds appropriate to depict the Group II and III and Group IV volleys respectively. The stimulus given at S was 10 V, 0.5 msec. (k), DRP (average of five successive records) evoked by the volleys shown to the left in b and f. The sequences arranged below b, f, k correspond to these records, but a blocking current of increasing strength (as indicated at right) was applied at B before the stimuli were given. Note reduction and disappearances of Group II and III activity in b–e and the appearance of the late DRP in l–n. Stimuli are indicated by arrows below the records. Unanaesthetized cat with spinal cord cut at C_3. The dotted line in k indicates the time course of the DRP after i.v. injection of 30 mg/kg nembutal. (From ZIMMERMANN, 1968b)

tion, and this also applies to those PAH seen after stimulation of brain stem and cerebellar structures (see Fig. 16). It is envisaged that the discrepancies, as far as they still exist between the reports from the various laboratories, can be resolved by applying a triad of experimental measures: (a) standardization and careful control of the experimental situation, (b) activation of the various Group III and IV fibre populations by adaequate stimulation, and (c) use of recording methods which allow the precise determination of the types of afferent fibres receiving the depolarization or its removal. Certainly, the existence of segmental and descending pathways for the induction and for the (transient) removal of prolonged (tonic) presynaptic inhibition offers to the organism a powerful tool for the long term suppression and graded modulation of somatosensory input into the central nervous system. These tonic presynaptic mechanisms may well have a functional significance exceeding that of the more phasic PAD which, for technical reasons, has been analysed much more carefully in the past. In this respect it is worth noting that habituation and sensitization do not seem to be parallelled by longlasting changes of the presynaptic membrane potential (Groves et al., 1970).

Outside the spinal cord PAH has been observed on primary afferents of the trigeminal nucleus (Scibetta and King, 1969; Nakamura and Wu, 1970; Sessle and Dubner, 1970; Dubner and Sessle, 1971). Furthermore, evidence has been presented for presynaptic hyperpolarization of non-primary axon terminals in the thalamus (Sessle and Dubner, 1970, 1971) and of corticofugal axons ending in the trigeminal nuclei (Dubner and Sessle, 1971). On the other hand, afferent volleys in the Group III fibres of the tooth pulp always elicited PAD in other tooth pulp afferents (Davies et al., 1971, see also section III D).

C. Inhibitory Influences Exerted onto Primary Afferents Ending in the Dorsal Column Nuclei

Since the cuneate and gracile nuclei are first synaptic relays receiving ipsilateral tactile and kinaesthetic inputs from forelimb and hindlimb body regions respectively, they are particularly well suited to study afferent inhibition in the somatosensory pathways. Basically, only four types of neuronal elements are present in the nuclei: (a) the primary afferents of the dorsal columns which end on (b) relay cells which projects to the contralateral ventrobasal nuclei of the thalamus; in addition the afferent terminals make excitatory synaptic contacts with (c) interneurones which project inside the dorsal column nuclei; finally (d) projections from various ascending and descending pathways make excitatory and/or inhibitory synaptic contacts both on relay cells and on interneurones. It is not surprising, therefore, that many efforts have been devoted to an analysis of the inhibitory phenomena taking place in these nuclei either by afferent activity or by descending influences.

A centripetal volley in the dorsal columns is followed by a deep and prolonged depression of transmission in the dorsal column nuclei. Marshall (1941) first demonstrated this depression in cats by stimulating the superficial radial nerve and recording mass responses from the medial lemniscus. Later on, this inhibition of about 100–200 msec duration was also observed in the discharges that a testing volley evoked from individual cells of the gracile and cuneate nuclei. In the gracile nucleus Gordon and Paine (1960) frequently found spatial inhibition of individual relay cells, particularly with cells having small receptive fields (in addition, they also found examples of spatial facilitation). The afferent inhibition was most often produced by electrical or mechanical stimuli applied near the receptive area but outside it. This afferent inhibition is mainly exerted onto those relay cells receiving their input from hair receptors (Perl et al., 1962; Gordon and Jukes, 1964a). Inhibition of the surround type was also seen in the dorsal column nuclei of the rat (Dawson et al., 1963; McComas, 1963). More recently, it has also been shown in the cat that afferent inhibition in the dorsal column nuclei can be produced by stimulation of widespread cutaneous areas that do not project directly to the nucleus under observation (JABBUR and BANNA, 1968, 1970), a finding partly anticipated by GORDON and PAINE (1960). However, inhibition from these widespread cutaneous sources was consistently less than that exerted by cutaneous areas surrounding the receptive field. Widespread afferent inhibition is also present in the rhesus monkey (BIEDENBACH, JABBUR and TOWE, 1971). Auditory and visual inputs also seem to depress transmission in the dorsal column nuclei (JABBUR, 1972).

An influence of descending fibres on slow wave activity (N-wave) in the dorsal column nuclei was first observed by SCHERRER and HERNÁNDEZ-PEÓN (1955, 1958; cf. also HERNÁNDEZ-PEÓN et al., 1956). Repetitive stimulation of the pontine or mesencephalic reticular formation caused a depression of the negative N-wave for periods up to 80 sec. Single shocks to the cerebral cortex will also attenuate the postsynaptic response in the dorsal column nuclei (DAWSON, 1958a, b). This effect is most marked when the stimulus to the contralateral sensorimotor cortex precedes the onset of the postsynaptic activity by 5 msec. Subsequent investigators observed both facilitation and depression of the N-wave as a consequence of cortical or reticular stimulation (GUZMAN-FLORES et al., 1960, 1962; CHAMBERS et al., 1963; FELIX and WIESENDANGER, 1970). Similarly, single unit studies have shown both excitatory and inhibitory cortifugal effects (CARRERAS et al., 1960; LEVITT et al., 1960, 1964; JABBUR and TOWE, 1960, 1961a, b; TOWE and JABBUR, 1961; GORDON and JUKES, 1962, HARRIS et al., 1965; WINTER, 1965). Stimulation of reticular structures also influences unitary activity of dorsal column nuclei (CESA-BIANCHI and SOTGIU, 1969) as does stimulation of cerebellar structures and of non-specific thalamic nuclei (SOTGIU and CESA-BIANCHI, 1970). For a variety of reasons, the results of these detailed studies are not always in complete agreement. *First*, as pointed out by NORTON (1970), the terms excitation, excitatory effect, inhibition and inhibitory effect are used by different investigators to describe slightly different effects brought about by slightly different techniques. *Secondly*, there are also differences in excitatory and inhibitory effects between species (rat, cat, monkey). For instance, in the cat, inhibitory corticofugal influences are seen only in cells also subject to afferent inhibition and in all cells in which afferent inhibition is observed (mainly hair sensitive cells; GORDON and JUKES, 1964b). The cells receiving corticofugal excitatory influences, on the other hand, are principally touch-pressure cells, none of which is subject to afferent inhibition. In the monkey, the pattern of corticofugal influences is far more variable (HARRIS et al., 1965; BIEDENBACH, JABBUR and TOWE, 1971).

Is the afferent inhibition in the dorsal column nuclei exerted via pre- or postsynaptic inhibition? THERMAN (1941) first reported that cutaneous volleys passing up the dorsal columns produced, on the surface of the cuneate and gracile nuclei, N- and P-waves resembling those produced at the segmental level. In the subsequent investigations on the origin of the P-waves evoked by cutaneous volleys it was clearly shown that, as at the segmental level, the P-waves reflected a depolarization of the primary afferent terminals. *First*, WALL (1958) reported that, synchronously with the P-wave on the surface of the nucleus gracilis, there was an increased excitability of the gracilis tract fibres in that nucleus: *second* it was shown that, during the P-wave, the distribution of the potential fields within the cuneate nucleus was as expected on the assumption that during PAD the afferent terminal regions act as sinks for the current sources on the shafts of the cuneate tract fibres (Andersen et al., 1964a); *third*, by intracellular recording from the presynaptic fibres of the cuneate nucleus, the depolarization was directly demonstrated and shown to conform with the other more indirect observations (Fig. 18). When the recording microelectrode was within or close to the large synaptic knobs of the cuneate tract fibres, the PAD had a very rapid onset with a latency of 2 msec and a summit as early as 5 msec later. Often these steep depolarizations gave rise to impulses which were generated near to the synaptic terminals in the cuneate nucleus (dorsal column reflexes, Fig. 18E, F, G).

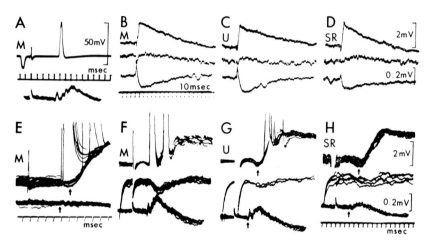

Fig. 18 A–H. Intracellular recording of dorsal root reflexes. A. Identification of the fibre of the median nerve (M) in the cuneate nucleus. B–D. Primary afferent depolarizations (PAD) in response to single volleys in the median (M), ulnar (U), and superficial radial nerve (SR) respectively. E. Spike and onset of PAD with dorsal root reflexes (DRR) taken at fast sweep speed. Since these DRR were generated in the cuneate nucleus they were termed dorsal column reflexes (DCR). F–H. Spikes, PAD and DCR to single M, U and SR volleys. Latency of PAD onset indicated as the time between the first spike in surface record and the second arrow.
(From Andersen, Eccles, Schmidt and Yokota, 1964b)

The rapid onset of PAD is suggestive of a very short reflex pathway having one to two local interneurones. Interneurones with the requisite properties have been described (Andersen et al., 1964c) and pharmacological evidence has been adduced that this reflex pathway has a distinctive pharmacology: Boyd et al. (1966) after testing the effects of convulsants on the recovery cycles of the cuneate nucleus, came to the conclusion that the presynaptic inhibitory pathway is blocked by picrotoxin and pentylentetrazol. Banna and Jabbur (1969) arrived at similar conclusions when testing the effects of picrotoxin, strychnine and pentobarbitone on the increase in excitability of cuneate presynaptic terminals produced by cortical or cutaneous volleys.

Afferent volleys undoubtedly also activate local short reflex pathways ending in inhibitory synapses on the relay cells of the dorsal column nuclei (Andersen, Eccles, Oshima and Schmidt, 1964). In its general features the postsynaptic

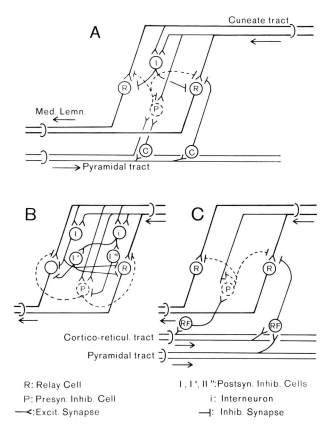

R: Relay Cell   I, I ', II ":Postsyn. Inhib. Cells
P: Presyn. Inhib. Cell   i: Interneuron
—<:Excit. Synapse   —|: Inhib. Synapse

Fig. 19 A–C. Pathways for pre- and postsynaptic inhibition in the dorsal column nuclei. A. Schematic diagram illustrating the suggested connections between the primary afferent collaterals, the fibres of the pyramidal tract, and the relay neurones as suggested by ANDERSEN et al. (1964c). B. Modification proposed by BOYD, MERITT and GARDNER (1966) of the postsynaptic inhibitory pathways based on pharmacological evidence. C. Modification proposed by WIESENDANGER (1969) of the descending presynaptic inhibitory pathways. RF, reticular formation. For detailed discussion see text. (From SCHMIDT, 1971)

inhibition of cuneate neurones seems to be comparable with that with other neurones in the spinal cord and brain. The latency differential of 0.85–1.6 msec with respect to monosynaptic excitation is in accord with the general postulate of one interneurone on the postsynaptic inhibitory pathway. The time course shows the characteristic feature of a relatively brief rise to the summit from which there is a much slower decay, so that the total duration is usually 15–20 msec. However some neurones exhibit much longer IPSPs with a duration even in excess of 100 msec, and the same neurone may give evidence of both the brief and the long IPSP, which presumably are generated by two types of inhibitory synapses. There is pharmacological evidence that there are at least two postsynaptic inhibitory pathways, the shorter one being blocked by strychnine, the other one by strychnine plus mephenesin (BOYD et al., 1966; cf. also BANNA and JABBUR, 1969).

Fig. 19 summarizes in diagrammatic form the presumed interconnections of the local pre- and postsynaptic inhibitory pathways in the dorsal column nuclei. Both the presynaptic and the postsynaptic inhibitory interneurones can be activated not only by the dorsal column afferents but also by activity in descending pathways coming from various parts of the brain stem and higher regions of the brain. Thus these local interneurones form the "final common path" for peripherally and centrally induced inhibition of afferent input.

The corticofugal influences seem to be transmitted to the dorsal column nuclei via the pyramidal tracts. Corticofugal effects can be induced by stimulation of the pyramidal tract in the midbrain (Towe and Zimmermann, 1962; Winter, 1965) and they are also abolished by section of the tract (Levitt et al., 1960, 1964). Brain stem sections which spare only the pyramidal tracts do not block the effects of cortical stimulation (Jabbur and Towe, 1960, 1961a, b; Magni et al., 1959). There is, however, more recent evidence that the cortico-dorsal column nuclei projections are a specific projection rather than collaterals from cortico-spinal fibres (Gordon and Miller, 1969). Anatomically fibre tracts have been demonstrated, by degeneration methods, to pass from the somatosensory cortex in the contralateral hemisphere with the motor fibres to the dorsal column nuclei (Chambers and Liu, 1957; Walberg, 1957; Kuypers, 1958a, b; Levitt et al., 1964; Kawana, 1969). As summarized by Wiesendanger (1969) and by Schmidt (1971), there is circumstantial evidence that the inhibitory interneurones of the dorsal column nuclei not only receive direct excitatory contacts from pyramidal axon collaterals, but that these neurones also can be activated from the pyramidal tract via the reticular formation (Fig. 19C, cf. also Felix and Wiesendanger, 1970). Similarly, the PAD observed in the cuneate nucleus after stimulation of cerebellar and non-specific thalamic nuclei also seems to be mediated by the bulbo-pontine reticular formation (Sotgiu and Cesa-Bianchi, 1970).

D. Inhibitory Influences Exerted onto Trigeminal Afferent Fibres

Darian-Smith (1965) first described PAD of trigeminal afferents and a concurrent depression of second-order neurones following electrical and tactile stimulation of the skin at and around the receptive field under observation. He concluded that at least part of the surround inhibition is of presynaptic origin, and this conclusion has been accepted by subsequent investigators (Baldissera et al., 1967; Stewart et al., 1967; Vyklický et al., 1967; Rowe, 1970; Rowe and Carmody, 1970; Dubner and Sessle, 1971; cf. also Darian-Smith, this volume). The general features of peripherally evoked PAD of trigeminal afferents closely resemble those seen in the spinal cord and, particularly, in the dorsal column nuclei. In addition, evidence has been presented that interactions between the various trigeminal nuclei can be exerted via variations of the level of PAD of trigeminal afferents (Scibetta and King, 1969).

The corticofugal inhibitory effects on synaptic transmission in the trigeminal nuclei (Hernández-Peón and Hagbarth, 1955) parallel in every respect the PAD of trigeminal afferents (Darian-Smith and Yokota, 1966a, b; Hammer et

al., 1966; WIESENDANGER et al., 1967a, b; STEWART et al., 1967; SHENDE and
KING, 1967; HEPP-REYMOND and WIESENDANGER, 1969; SAUERLAND and MIZU-
NO, 1969a), whereas no signs of postsynaptic inhibition have been detected (WIE-
SENDANGER and FELIX, 1969). Stimulation of the brain stem gives similar effects
(BALDISSERA et al., 1967). It has been inferred from these findings that the inhibitory corticofugal control is largely presynaptic in nature and that the pathways
are similar to or even identical with those leading to the afferent terminals in the
dorsal column nuclei (cf. Fig. 19). The PAD of trigeminal afferents during desynchronized sleep (BALDISSERA et al., 1966) also has its analogue in the cuneate nucleus (CARLI et al., 1966) and the spinal cord (BALDISSERA, CESA-BIANCHI and
MANCIA, 1966).

Recent anatomical (GOBEL and DUBNER, 1969) and physiological (DUBNER et
al., 1969; DUBNER and SESSLE, 1971) evidence suggests that the corticofugal
fibres leading to the trigeminal brain stem nuclei, while producing PAD of trigeminal primary afferent fibres, are themselves subjected to presynaptic depolarization after either stimulation of trigeminal nerve branches or following cortical
stimulation (facial somatosensory projection areas I–II and III). The depolarizations were observed on cortico-bulbar endings both in the main sensory nucleus
and in nucleus caudalis. The cortical neurones receiving this presynaptic depolarization at their axonal endings in the brain stem usually had short-latency cutaneous input from the face and mouth. The neurones seem to be involved in a rapidly
conducting feedback loop between the sensorimotor cortex and the trigeminal
nuclei. This feedback loop presumably takes part in the control of trigeminal
afferent input.

Marked primary afferent depolarization of the tooth pulp afferent terminals
ending in the rostral part of the trigeminal nuclear complex has recently been
observed by DAVIES et al. (1971). This PAD was seen following a conditioning
volley in low threshold (Group II) afferent fibres of the infraorbital nerve or in the
afferent fibres of another tooth. Contrary to the former the latter volley did not
induce appreciable PAD in Group II trigeminal afferents. Since the tooth pulp
afferents are of the Group III fibre type (Aδ-fibres, diameter 1–7 μ), and since
pain seems to be the only modality of sensation transmitted by these fibres, these
observations are of importance in several respects: first of all they confirm that
Group III somatic afferents are under a presynaptic control analogous to that of
the Group II afferents; secondly it is remarkable that Group II volleys induce
large excitability changes in the Group III (pain) afferents, whereas Group III
volleys give no appreciable depolarization of Group II terminals; finally, it is
interesting to note that in these experiments under pentobarbitone anaesthesia,
practically pure Group III afferent volleys only gave PAD, never PAH (see
section III B).

The reciprocal control of jaw-opening and jaw-closing reflexes to a marked
extent also seems to be exerted via presynaptic inhibition of the afferent fibres of
these reflex arcs. NAKAMURA and WU (1970; see also SAUERLAND and MIZUNO,
1969b) observed that volleys in Group II and III and possible Ib afferents of the
masseter muscle nerve induced presynaptic depolarization in the mechanoreceptor
fibres of the lingual nerve. With the same time course, there was a depression of
the second order neurones in the nucleus oralis as well as of the linguo-digastric

reflex. All three effects were abolished by picrotoxin. These effects indicate that masseteric nerve stimulation inhibited the linguo-digastric reflex presynaptically at the first synaptic relay of this reflex pathway. (The facilitation of the linguo-digastric reflex preceding the inhibitory phase was not accompanied by any sign of presynaptic hyperpolarization, i.e. it was presumably due to postsynaptic excitation.) Similar results were obtained by Sauerland and Thiele (1970) who in addition studied the effects of proprioceptive input from masticatory muscles on glossopharyngeal afferents and who used not only electrical stimulation but also muscle stretch as a conditioning input.

IV. Inhibitory Influences on Transmission from Second Order Axons to Third Order Cells

The results reviewed in sections II and III permit the assumption that in the vertebrate central nervous system all types of myelinated somaesthetic primary afferent fibres are subject to PAD and thus to a presynaptic inhibitory control of their excitatory synaptic actions. This presynaptic inhibition effectively replaces receptor inhibition (cf. section I and Fig. 1). Very little is known about presynaptic inhibition of axon terminals stemming from other than primary afferent axons. It is generally felt among neurophysiologists that presynaptic inhibition is restricted mainly to primary afferent terminals but this opinion probably only reflects a lack of evidence. There are some indications of presynaptic inhibition of axons of second order cells in somaesthetic pathways (see below) and also of axon terminals of central neurones in the trigeminal nuclei (see III D) and in the lateral geniculate nucleus (cf. Schmidt, 1971).

At the segmental level very few observations have been made in regard to a possible presynaptic inhibition of second order or later axon terminals. Lundberg and Vyklický (1963) and Lund et al. (1965) observed that volleys in flexor reflex afferents (or cortical stimulation) effectively depressed the PAD generated in Ia fibre terminals by volleys in other Ia fibres without generating a PAD of Ia fibre terminals (see section III A, 1). It was postulated, that this inhibition from the flexor reflex afferents occurred on the interneurones transmitting effects from Group Ia fibres to Group Ia fibres. Furthermore, since the time course of the inhibition was practically identical with the PAD evoked from the flexor reflex afferents, and since the inhibition survived large doses of strychnine (see section II E) it was tentatively suggested that the inhibition was presynaptic through depolarization of interneuronal terminals.

More direct evidence for a presynaptic inhibition of second order axon terminals was obtained in the lateral cervical nucleus. This nucleus receives its excitatory input from the fibres of the spinocervical tract, which have their cells of origin in the spinal dorsal horn and ascend in the dorsolateral funiculus (cf. Brown, this volume). Fedina et al. (1968) presented evidence that the excitatory transmission from the spinocervical tract to the cells of the lateral cervical nucleus is both under presynaptic and postsynaptic inhibitory control. Two indications for presynaptic inhibition were found: electrical stimulation of cutaneous nerves of ipsi- and contralateral fore- and hindlimbs and of the skin of the cat's forepaw increased the excitability of spinal cervical tract axons; at the same time the monosynaptically evoked EPSPs in cells of the lateral cervical nucleus were reduced without any change of the membrane potential of the cells. Light tactile stimulation of the forepaw was ineffective in producing a detectable depolarization, but strong pinching produced a definite effect (the spino-cervical tract carries mainly information from receptors innervated by Group III and IV nerve fibres and not from sensitive receptors in the foot pads or slowly adapting mechanoreceptors innervated by large myelinated afferents, cf. BROWN and IGGO, 1967; BROWN and FRANZ, 1969, 1970; BROWN, this volume). Supraspinal mechanisms were not necessary for these effects, which were still seen after section of the cord at the spino-medullary junction. In contrast to the dorsal column nuclei, no evidence for a "surround" pattern of inhibition was found.

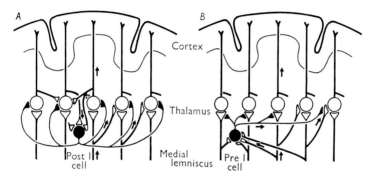

Fig. 20 A and B. Pathways for postsynaptic (A) and presynaptic inhibition (B) in the ventro-basal complex of the thalamus. In A axon collaterals of thalamocortical relay cells (TRC) are seen to excite both TRC and the postsynaptic inhibitory interneurone (Post I cell). In B branches of lemniscal fibres excite the presynaptic inhibitory interneurone (Pre I cell), which is widely distributed to the synaptic knobs of lemniscal fibres. (From ANDERSEN, ECCLES and SEARS, 1964b)

The axons of the second-order cells of the dorsal column nuclei projects to the thalamus through the contralateral medial lemniscus. Excitability testing of the axon terminals of cuneate tract fibres in the ventro-basal complex of the thalamus (VPL) before and after conditioning stimuli to forelimb nerves, revealed a depolarization with a time course characteristic for PAD of spinal afferents. It was concluded that this depolarization reflected presynaptic inhibition of lemniscal terminals, which added to the powerful postsynaptic inhibition of the thalamo-cortical relay cells observed under these conditions (ANDERSEN, BROOKS et al., 1964). There were no clear indications of presynaptic inhibition induced by cortical stimulation. The pathways of postsynaptic and presynaptic inhibition (Fig. 20) have been further analyzed by ANDERSEN, ECCLES and SEARS (1964b). By employing lemniscal and cortical stimulation it was shown that ventro-basal cells could be identified either as thalamo-cortical relay cells or as cells which qualified as being postsynaptic or presynaptic inhibitory interneurones. More recently, SESSLE and DUBNER (1971) observed that the presynaptic terminals of trigeminothalamic neurones in the nucleus ventralis posteriomedialis thalami (VPM) regularly showed a sequence of presynaptic depolarization followed by presynaptic hyperpolarization after conditioning stimuli applied to the infraorbital nerve, the facial skin (mechanical stimuli), or the sensorimotor cortex. The sequence of depolarization and hyperpolarization of these terminals correlated with the time course of afferent and cortically induced inhibition and facilitation of VPM neurones. The authors concluded from their findings that presynaptic mechanisms play a rôle in the modification of thalamic neuronal activity.

These latter results as well as those obtained in the VPL, in the lateral cervical nucleus, and on segmental interneurones await further electrophysiological and, particularly, histological support and confirmation.

V. Summarizing and Concluding Remarks

A. Synaptic Mechanisms of the Control of Afferent Input at First Order Cells

Our present state of knowledge of the mechanisms producing presynaptic depolarization of primary afferent fibres (primary afferent depolarization, PAD), and of the inhibitory effects induced thereby, may be summarized as follows:

1. Primary afferent fibres, and possibly the axons of several other types of neurones, can be subjected to a prolonged depolarization which can be recorded both with intracellular (cf. Figs. 11, 18) and extracellular techniques (Figs. 5–7, 15–17).

2. Physiological evidence indicates that this depolarization is exerted at or near the terminals of the axon (section II C).

3. The presynaptic depolarization blocks or decreases the action potentials propagating towards the axon terminals.

4. As a consequence, a reduced amount of transmitter is released by the presynaptic action potential (section II C). This inhibitory process has been called presynaptic inhibition.

5. All phenomena are in good agreement with the concept that presynaptic depolarization is due to the activation of chemically mediated synapses situated at or near the preterminal endings of the axons subjected to presynaptic depolarization (axo-axonic synapses). Anatomical evidence support this concept originally derived from physiological findings (section II B).

6. The axo-axonal synapses can be activated through reflex pathways consisting of two to several interneurones (section II D).

7. The pharmacology of presynaptic inhibition differs remarkably from that of postsynaptic inhibition (section II E).

There are several aspects of this concept which are in need of further experimental support. *First*, the mode of operation of the axo-axonal synapses both in regard to their transmitter substance and in regard to the subsynaptic actions of this transmitter substance have to be clarified. *Second*, the changes which the presynaptic spike undergoes during presynaptic depolarization are not known in any detail. And *third*, so far only indirect evidence has been brought forward in favour of the postulated steep relationship between presynaptic spike size and transmitter release.

B. Functions of the Inhibitory Control of Somatosensory Primary Afferents

The considerable work done on the reflex connections of axo-axonal synapses on primary afferents and on the excitation and/or inhibition of these pathways by peripherally or centrally evoked activity, has given some insight on the rôle which presynaptic inhibition may play in the control of afferent input:

1. The most remarkable feature of segmental presynaptic inhibition seems to be its negative feedback character. The various muscle and cutaneous afferents preferentially activate those reflex paths leading to the afferent terminals of their own sensory modality or quality (cf. Figs. 9, 10, 12). The advantages of this type of negative feedback include both a central input adjustment to the stimulus intensity level, and the automatic suppression of trivial inputs so that the central mechanism is cleared in readiness for significant input.

2. Within the Group I afferents from the muscles of a given limb those coming from flexor muscles are generally more powerful than those coming from extensors, and the Ib fibres are much more powerful than the Ia fibres (Figs. 9, 10). The significance of these findings for the reflex control of movement and posture (LUNDBERG, 1966; HOUK and HENNEMAN, 1967) is an open question, much as is the functional significance of the postsynaptic Renshaw inhibition.

3. For the cutaneous afferents coming from mechano-receptors it has been demonstrated that the negative feedback is organized in a "surround" fashion, thus creating a system of lateral or afferent inhibition at the earliest possible level of the somatic afferent system (Fig. 14). This arrangement gives, for instance, the possibilities of restoration of spatial contrast in the stimulus pattern, and it facilitates the localization of the stimulus.

4. Several types of peripheral receptors and some supramedullary areas tend to induce tonic presynaptic depolarizations which in turn, depending on the situation, are either increased (enhancement of inhibition) or decreased (disinhibition) by other segmental or descending influences. Particularly, the effects of small myelinated and of unmyelinated afferents seem to depend a great deal on the experimental situation (section III B).

5. Descending presynaptic inhibitory influences from various parts of the brain stem and the cortex are able to increase or decrease selectively the efficacy of somaesthetic and proprioceptive input channels thus providing a mechanism of "focussing the attention" on important messages. The sensitivity of the channels can be decreased through PAD, whereas it can be increased by a removal or suppression of presynaptic inhibition (disinhibition) coming from other sources.

Acknowledgement

The experiments quoted from the authors laboratory in Heidelberg have been supported by the Deutsche Forschungsgemeinschaft. Thanks are due to those authors and publishers who have allowed us to reproduce illustrations previously published elsewhere. The author is also greatly indebted to Fräulein A. Huxhagen for help with the bibliography, Frau E. Tallone for the production of the illustrations and Frau L. Vosgerau for the typing of the manuscript.

References

ABDELMOUMÈNE, M., BESSON, J.-M., ALÉONARD, P.: Cortical areas exerting presynaptic inhibitory action on the spinal cord in cat and monkey. Brain Res. **20**, 327–329 (1970).

ANDÉN, N.E., JUKES, M.G.M., LUNDBERG, A.: Spinal reflexes and monoamine liberation. Nature (Lond.) **202**, 1222–1223 (1964).

ANDÉN, N.E., JUKES, M.G.M., LUNDBERG, A.: The effect of Dopa on the spinal cord. 2. A pharmacological analysis. Acta physiol. scand. **67**, 387–397 (1966).

ANDÉN, N.E., JUKES, M.G.M., LUNDBERG, A., VYKLICKÝ, L.: A new spinal flexor reflex. Nature (Lond.) **202**, 1344–1345 (1964).

ANDÉN, N.E., JUKES, M.G.M., LUNDBERG, A., VYKLICKÝ, L.: The effect of Dopa on the spinal cord. 1. Influence on transmission from primary afferents. Acta physiol. scand. **67**, 373–380 (1966a).

ANDÉN, N.E., JUKES, M.G.M., LUNDBERG, A., VYKLICKÝ, L.: The effect of Dopa on the spinal cord. 3. Depolarization evoked in the central terminals of ipsilateral Ia afferents by volleys in the flexor reflex afferents. Acta physiol. scand. **68**, 322–336 (1966b).

ANDÉN, N.E., LUNDBERG, A., ROSENGREN, E., VYKLICKÝ, L.: The effect of Dopa on spinal reflexes from the FRA (flexor reflex afferents). Experientia (Basel) **19**, 654–655 (1963).

ANDERSEN, P., BROOKS, C. McC., ECCLES, J.C., SEARS, T.A.: The ventro-basal nucleus of the thalamus: potential fields, synaptic transmission and excitability of both presynaptic and post-synaptic components. J. Physiol. (Lond.) **174**, 348–369 (1964).

ANDERSEN, P., ECCLES, J.C., OSHIMA, T., SCHMIDT, R.F.: Mechanisms of synaptic transmission in the cuneate nucleus. J. Neurophysiol. **27**, 1096–1116 (1964).

ANDERSEN, P., ECCLES, J.C., SCHMIDT, R.F., YOKOTA, T.: Slow potential waves produced in the cuneate nucleus by cutaneous volleys and by cortical stimulation. J. Neurophysiol. **27**, 78–91 (1964a).

ANDERSEN, P., ECCLES, J.C., SCHMIDT, R.F., YOKOTA, T.: Depolarization of presynaptic fibers in the cuneate nucleus. J. Neurophysiol. **27**, 92–106 (1964b).

ANDERSEN, P., ECCLES, J.C., SCHMIDT, R.F., YOKOTA, T.: Identification of relay cells and interneurons in the cuneate nucleus. J. Neurophysiol. **27**, 1080–1095 (1964c).

ANDERSEN, P., ECCLES, J.C., SEARS, T.A.: Presynaptic inhibitory action of cerebral cortex on the spinal cord. Nature (Lond.) **194**, 740–743 (1962).

ANDERSEN, P., ECCLES, J.C., SEARS, T.A.: Cortically evoked depolarization of primary afferent fibers in the spinal cord. J. Neurophysiol. **27**, 63–77 (1964a).

ANDERSEN, P., ECCLES, J.C., SEARS, T.A.: The ventro-basal complex of the thalamus: types of cells, their responses and their functional organization. J. Physiol. (Lond.) **174**, 370–399 (1964b).

ANGEL, A., MAGNI, F., STRATA, P.: Evidence from pre-synaptic inhibition in the lateral geniculate body. Nature (Lond.) **208**, 495–496 (1965).

ANGEL, A., MAGNI, F., STRATA, P.: Excitability of intra-geniculate optic tract fibres after reticular stimulation in the midpontine pretrigeminal cat. Arch. ital. Biol. **103**, 668–693 (1966).

ATWOOD, H.L., MORIN, W.A.: Neuromuscular and axo-axonal synapses of the crayfish opener muscle. J. Ultrastruct. Res. **32**, 351–369 (1970).

BALDISSERA, F., BROGGI, G.: An analysis of potential changes in the spinal cord during desynchronized sleep. Brain Res. **6**, 706–715 (1967).

BALDISSERA, F., BROGGI, G., MANCIA, M.: Presynaptic inhibition of trigeminal afferent fibres during the rapid eye movements of desynchronized sleep. Experientia (Basel) **22**, 754–755 (1966).

BALDISSERA, F., BROGGI, G., MANCIA, M.: Depolarization of trigeminal afferents induced by stimulation of brain-stem and peripheral nerves. Exp. Brain Res. **4**, 1–17 (1967).

BALDISSERA, F., CESA-BIANCHI, M.G., MANCIA, M.: Phasic events indicating presynaptic inhibition of primary afferents to the spinal cord during desynchronized sleep. J. Neurophysiol. **29**, 871–887 (1966).

BANNA, N.R., HAZBUN, J.: Analysis of the convulsant action of pentylenetetrazol. Experientia (Basel) **25**, 382–383 (1969).

BANNA, N.R., JABBUR, S.J.: Antagonism of presynaptic inhibition in the cuneate nucleus by picrotoxin. Nature (Lond.) **217**, 83–84 (1968).

BANNA, N.R., JABBUR, S.J.: Pharmacological studies on inhibition in the cuneate nucleus of the cat. Int. J. Neuropharmacol. **8**, 299–308 (1969).

BANNA, N.R., JABBUR, S.J.: The action of bemegride on presynaptic inhibition. Int. J. Neuropharmacol. **9**, 553–560 (1970).

BARNES, C.D., POMPEIANO, O.: Presynaptic inhibition of extensor monosynaptic reflex by Ia afferents from flexors. Brain Res. **18**, 380–383 (1970a).

BARNES, C.D., POMPEIANO, O.: Effects of muscle vibration on the pre- and postsynaptic components of the extensor monosynaptic reflex. Brain Res. **18**, 384–387 (1970b).

BARNES, C.D., POMPEIANO, O.: Inhibition of monosynaptic extensor reflex attributable to presynaptic depolarization of the group Ia afferent fibers produced by vibration of flexor muscle. Arch. ital. Biol. **108**, 233–258 (1970c).

BARNES, C.D., POMPEIANO, O.: Presynaptic and postsynaptic effects in the monosynaptic reflex pathway to extensor motoneurons following vibration of synergic muscles. Arch. ital. Biol. **108**, 259–294 (1970d).

BARNES, C.D., POMPEIANO, O.: Dissociation of presynaptic and postsynaptic effects produced in the lumbar cord by vestibular volleys. Arch. ital. Biol. **108**, 295–324 (1970e).

BARRON, D.H., MATTHEWS, B.H.C.: The interpretation of potential changes in the spinal cord. J. Physiol. (Lond.) **92**, 276–321 (1938).

BELL, J.A., ANDERSON, E.G.: A comparison of the actions of semicarbazide and picrotoxin on spinal synaptic activity. Pharmacologist **12**, 252 (1970).

BESSON, J.M., ABDELMOUMÈNE, M.: Modifications of the dorsal root potentials during cortical seizures. Electroenceph. clin. Neurophysiol. **29**, 166–172 (1970).

BESSON, J.M., ABDELMOUMÈNE, M., RIVOT, J.-P.: Some pharmacological effects on the transmission of afferent impulses on the interneurons in the cat lumbar dorsal horn. In: The Somato-sensory System. Ed. by H.H. KORNHUBER, J. ASCHOFF. Stuttgart: Georg Thieme Verlag 1973 (in press).

BESSON, J.M., RIVOT, J.-P., ALEONARD, P.: Action of picrotoxin on presynaptic inhibition of various origins in the cat's spinal cord. Brain Res. **26**, 212–216 (1971).

BIEDENBACH, A., JABBUR, S.J., TOWE, A.L.: Afferent inhibition in the cuneate nucleus of the rhesus monkey. Brain Res. **27**, 179–182 (1971).

BLOEDEL, J., GAGE, P.W., LLINÁS, R., QUASTEL, D.M.J.: Transmitter release at the squid giant synapse in the presence of tetrodotoxin. Nature (Lond.) **212**, 49–50 (1966).

BLOEDEL, J., GAGE, P.W., LLINÁS, R., QUASTEL, D.M.J.: Transmission across the squid giant synapse in the presence of tetrodotoxin. J. Physiol. (Lond.) **188**, 52–53P (1967).

BOYD, E., S., MERITT, D.A., GARDNER, L.C.: The effect of convulsant drugs on transmission through the cuneate nucleus. J. Pharmacol. exp. Ther. **154**, 398–409 (1966).

BRAZIER, M.A. (Editor): The Interneuron. UCLA Forum in Medical Sciences Nr. 11, pp. 1–552. Berkeley and Los Angeles: University of California Press 1969.

BROWN, A.G., FRANZ, D.N.: Responses of spinocervical tract neurones to natural stimulation of identified cutaneous receptors. Exp. Brain Res. **7**, 231–249 (1969).

BROWN, A.G., FRANZ, D.N.: Patterns of response in spinocervical tract neurones to different stimuli of long duration. Brain Res. **17**, 156–160 (1970).

BROWN, A.G., IGGO, A.: A quantitative study of cutaneous receptors and afferent fibres in the cat and rabbit. J. Physiol. (Lond.) **193**, 707–733 (1967).

Burke, R. E., Rudomin, P., Vyklický, L., Zajac III, F. E.: Primary afferent depolarization and flexion reflexes produced by radiant heat stimulation of the skin. J. Physiol. (Lond.) **213**, 185–214 (1971).

Calma, I.: Presynaptic inhibition of the terminals of cutaneous nerve fibres by stimulation of the ventral thalamo-diencephalic region. J. Physiol. (Lond.) **185**, 58–60 P (1966).

Calma, I., Quayle, A. A.: Supraspinal control of the presynaptic effects for forepaw and hindpaw skin stimulation in the cat under chloralose anaesthesia. Brain Res. **33**, 101–114 (1971).

Cangiano, A., Cook, W. A., Pompeiano, O.: Primary afferent depolarization in the lumbar cord evoked from the fastigial nucleus. Arch. ital. Biol. **107**, 321–340 (1969a).

Cangiano, A., Cook, W. A., Pompeiano, O.: Cerebellar inhibitory control of the vestibular reflex pathways to primary afferents. Arch. ital. Biol. **107**, 341–364 (1969b).

Carli, G., Diete-Spiff, K., Pompeiano, O.: Presynaptic and postsynaptic inhibition on transmission of cutaneous afferent volleys through the cuneate nucleus during sleep. Experientia (Basel) **22**, 239–240 (1966).

Carlson, C. B.: Sodium and the dorsal root potential. J. Physiol. (Lond.) **172**, 295–304 (1964).

Carlsson, A., Falck, B., Fuxe, K., Hillarp, N.: Cellular localization of monoamines in the spinal cord. Acta physiol. scand. **60**, 112–119 (1964).

Carpenter, D., Engberg, I., Funkenstein, H., Lundberg, A.: Decerebrate control of reflexes to primary afferents. Acta physiol. scand. **59**, 424–437 (1963).

Carpenter, D., Engberg, I., Lundberg, A.: Presynaptic inhibition in the lumbar cord evoked from the brain stem. Experientia (Basel) **18**, 450–451 (1962).

Carpenter, D., Engberg, I., Lundberg, A.: Primary afferent depolarization evoked from the brain stem and the cerebellum. Arch. ital. Biol. **104**, 73–85 (1966).

Carpenter, D., Lundberg, A., Norrsell, U.: Effects from the pyramidal tract on primary afferents and on spinal reflex actions to primary afferents. Experientia (Basel) **18**, 337–338 (1962).

Carpenter, D., Lundberg, A., Norrsell, U.: Primary afferent depolarization evoked from the sensorimotor cortex. Acta physiol. scand. **59**, 126–142 (1963).

Carreras, M., Levitt, M., Chambers, W. W., Liu, C. N.: Unit activity in the posterior column nuclei and cortofugal influences upon it. Anat. Rec. **136**, 174–175 (1960).

Castillo, J. Del, Katz, B.: The membrane change produced by the neuromuscular transmitter. J. Physiol. (Lond.) **125**, 546–565 (1954).

Cesa-Bianchi, M. G., Mancia, M., Sotgiu, M. L.: Depolarization of afferent fibers to the Goll and Burdach nuclei induced by stimulation of the brain stem. Exp. Brain Res. **5**, 1–15 (1968).

Cesa-Bianchi, M. G., Sotgiu, M. L.: Control by brain stem reticular formation of sensory transmission in Burdach nucleus. Analysis of single units. Brain Res. **13**, 129–139 (1969).

Chambers, W. W., Liu, C. N.: Cortico-spinal tract of the cat. An attempt to correlate the pattern of degeneration with deficits in reflex activity following neocortical lesions. J. comp. Neurol. **108**, 23–56 (1957).

Chambers, W. W., Liu, C. N., McCouch, G. P.: Inhibition of the dorsal column nuclei. Exp. Neurol. **7**, 13–23 (1963).

Chan, S. H. H., Barnes, C. D.: Presynaptic facilitation: positive dorsal root potentials evoked from brain stem reticular formation in lumbar cord. Brain Res. **28**, 176–179 (1971).

Colonnier, M., Guillery, R. W.: Synaptic organization in the lateral geniculate nucleus of the monkey. Z. Zellforsch. **62**, 333–355 (1964).

Conradi, S.: On motoneuron synaptology in adult cats. Acta physiol. scand. Suppl., **332**, 1–115 (1969).

Cook, W. A., Cangiano, A., Pompeiano, O.: Vestibular influences on primary afferents in the spinal cord. Pflügers Arch. ges. Physiol. **299**, 334–338 (1968).

Cook, W. A., Cangiano, A., Pompeiano, O.: Dorsal root potentials in the lumbar cord evoked from the vestibular system. Arch. ital. Biol. **107**, 275–295 (1969a).

Cook, W. A., Cangiano, A., Pompeiano, O.: Vestibular control of transmission in primary afferents to the lumbar spinal cord. Arch. ital. Biol. **107**, 296–320 (1969b).

COOK, W.A., NEILSON, D.R., BROOKHART, J.M.: Primary afferent depolarization and mono-synaptic reflex depression following succinylcholine administration. J. Neurophysiol. **28**, 290–311 (1965).

CURTIS, D.R.: Pharmacology and neurochemistry of mammalian central inhibitory processes. In: Structure and Function of Inhibitory Neuronal Mechanisms, pp. 429–456. Oxford and New York: Pergamon Press 1968.

CURTIS, D.R.: The pharmacology of spinal postsynaptic inhibition. Progr. Brain Res. **31**, 171–189 (1969).

CURTIS, D.R.: Central synaptic transmitters. Proc. Aust. Assoc. Neurologists **7**, 55–60 (1970).

CURTIS, D.R., DUGGAN, A.W., FELIX, D., JOHNSTON, G.A.R.: Bicuculline, an antagonist of GABA and synaptic inhibition in the spinal cord of the cat. Brain Res. **32**, 69–96 (1971a).

CURTIS, D.R., DUGGAN, A.W., FELIX, D., JOHNSTON, G.A.R., McLENNAN, H.: Antagonism between bicuculline and GABA in the cat brain. Brain Res. **33**, 57–73 (1971b).

CURTIS, D.R., PHILLIS, J.W., WATKINS, J.C.: Actions of amino acids on the isolated hemisect-ed spinal cord of the toad. Brit. J. Pharmacol. **16**, 262–283 (1961).

CURTIS, D.R., RYALL, R.W.: Pharmacological studies upon spinal presynaptic fibres. Exp. Brain Res. **1**, 195–204 (1966).

DAHLSTRÖM, A., FUXE, K.: Evidence for the existence of monoamine neurons in the central nervous system. II. Experimentally induced changes in the intraneuronal amine levels of bulbo-spinal neuron systems. Acta physiol. scand. **64**, Suppl. 247, 1–85 (1965).

DARIAN-SMITH, I.: Presynaptic component in the afferent inhibition observed within trige-minal brain-stem nuclei of the cat. J. Neurophysiol. **28**, 695–709 (1965).

DARIAN-SMITH, I., YOKOTA, T.: Cortically evoked depolarization of trigeminal cutaneous afferent fibres in the cat. J. Neurophysiol. **29**, 170–184 (1966a).

DARIAN-SMITH, I., YOKOTA, T.: Corticofugal effects on different neuron types within the cat's brain stem activated by tactile stimulation on the face. J. Neurophysiol. **29**, 185–206 (1966b).

DAVIES, W.I.R., SCOTT, D., JR., VESTERSTRØM, K., VYKLICKÝ, L.: Depolarization of the tooth pulp afferent terminals in the brain stem of the cat. J. Physiol. (Lond.) **218**, 515–532 (1971).

DAWSON, G.D.: The effect of cortical stimulation on transmission through the cuneate nucleus in the anaesthetized rat. J. Physiol. (Lond.) **142**, 2–3P (1958a).

DAWSON, G.D.: The central control of sensory inflow. Proc. roy. Soc. Med. **51**, 531–535 (1958b).

DAWSON, G.D., MERRILL, E.G., WALL, P.D.: Dorsal root potentials produced by stimulation of fine afferents. Science **167**, 1385–1387 (1970).

DAWSON, G.D., PODACHIN, V.P., SCHATZ, S.W.: Facilitation of cortical responses by com-peting stimuli. J. Physiol. (Lond.) **166**, 363–381 (1963).

DECANDIA, M., ELDRED, E., GROVER, F.S.: Effects of prolonged stretch of flexor muscles upon excitability of an extensor reflex arc. Exp. Brain Res. **12**, 161–170 (1971).

DECANDIA, M., GASTEIGER, E.L., MANN, M.D.: Escape of the extensor monosynaptic reflex from presynaptic inhibition. Brain Res. **7**, 317–319 (1968).

DECANDIA, M., GASTEIGER, E.L., MANN, M.D.: Excitability changes of extensor motoneurons and primary afferent endings during prolonged stimulation of flexor afferents. Exp. Brain Res. **12**, 150–160 (1971).

DECANDIA, M., PROVINI, L., TÁBOŘÍKOVÁ, H.: Excitability changes in the Ia extensor termi-nals induced by stimulation of agonist afferent fibres. Brain Res. **2**, 402–404 (1966).

DECANDIA, M., PROVINI, L., TÁBOŘÍKOVÁ, H.: Presynaptic inhibition of the monosynaptic reflex following the stimulation of nerves to extensor muscles of the ankle. Exp. Brain Res. **4**, 34–42 (1967).

DECIMA, E.E., GOLDBERG, L.J.: Centrifugal dorsal root discharges induced by motoneurone activation. J. Physiol. (Lond.) **207**, 103–118 (1970).

DEVANANDAN, M.S., ECCLES, R.M., STENHOUSE, D.: Presynaptic inhibition evoked by muscle contraction. J. Physiol. (Lond.) **185**, 471–485 (1966).

DEVANANDAN, M.S., ECCLES, R.M., YOKOTA, T.: Presynaptic inhibition induced by muscle stretch. Nature (Lond.) **204**, 996–998 (1964).

DEVANANDAN, M.S., ECCLES, R.M., YOKOTA, T.: Depolarization of afferent terminals evoked by muscle stretch. J. Physiol. (Lond.) **179**, 417–429 (1965a).

Devanandan, M.S., Eccles, R.M., Yokota, T.: Muscle stretch and the presynaptic inhi-
    bition of the group Ia pathway to motoneurones. J. Physiol. (Lond.) 179, 430–441
    (1965b).
Devanandan, M.S., Holmqvist, B., Yokota, T.: Presynaptic depolarization of group I
    muscle afferents by contralateral afferent volleys. Acta physiol. scand. 63, 46–54 (1965).
Dubner, R., Sessle, B.J.: Presynaptic excitability changes of primary afferent and cortico-
    fugal fibers projecting to trigeminal brain stem nuclei. Exp. Neurol. 30, 223–238 (1971).
Dubner, R., Sessle, B.J., Gobel, S.: Presynaptic depolarization of corticofugal fibres parti-
    cipating in a feedback loop between trigeminal brain stem nuclei and sensorimotor cortex.
    Nature (Lond.) 223, 72–73 (1969).
Dudel, J.: Presynaptic inhibition of the excitatory nerve terminal in the neuromuscular
    junction of the crayfish. Pflügers Arch. ges. Physiol. 277, 537–557 (1963).
Dudel, J.: The mechanism of presynaptic inhibition at the crayfish neuromuscular junction.
    Pflügers Arch. ges. Physiol. 284, 66–80 (1965).
Dudel, J., Kuffler, S.W.: Presynaptic inhibition at the crayfish neuromuscular junction. J.
    Physiol. (Lond.) 155, 543–562 (1961).
Duncan, D., Keyser, L.L.: Further determinations of the number of fibers and cells in the
    dorsal roots and ganglia of the cat. J. comp. Neurol. 68, 479–490 (1938).
Eccles, J.C.: The mechanism of synaptic transmission. Ergebn. Physiol. 51, 299–430
    (1961).
Eccles, J.C.: The Physiology of Synapses. pp. 1–316. Berlin-Göttingen-Heidelberg-New York:
    Springer 1964.
Eccles, J.C.: The inhibitory pathways of the central nervous system. The Sherrington Lec-
    tures IX. Springfield, Ill.: Charles C. Thomas 1969.
Eccles, J.C., Eccles, R.M., Magni, F.: Central inhibitory action attributable to presynaptic
    depolarization produced by muscle afferent volleys. J. Physiol. (Lond.) 159, 147–166
    (1961).
Eccles, J.C., Kostyuk, P.G., Schmidt, R.F.: Central pathways responsible for depolariza-
    tion of primary afferent fibres. J. Physiol. (Lond.) 161, 237–257 (1962a).
Eccles, J.C., Kostyuk, P.G., Schmidt, R.F.: Presynaptic inhibition of the central actions
    of flexor reflex afferents. J. Physiol. (Lond.) 161, 258–281 (1962b).
Eccles, J.C., Kostyuk, P.G., Schmidt, R.F.: The effect of electric polarization of the spinal
    cord on central afferent fibres and on their excitatory synaptic action. J. Physiol. (Lond.)
    162, 138–150 (1962c).
Eccles, J.C., Kozak, W., Magni, F.: Dorsal root reflexes of muscle Group I afferent fibres.
    J. Physiol. (Lond.) 159, 128–146 (1961).
Eccles, J.C., Krnjević, K.: Potential changes recorded inside primary afferent fibres within
    the spinal cord. J. Physiol. (Lond.) 149, 250–273 (1959).
Eccles, J.C., Magni, F., Willis, W.D.: Depolarization of central terminals of Group I
    afferent fibres from muscle. J. Physiol. (Lond.) 160, 62–93 (1962).
Eccles, J.C., Malcolm, J.L.: Dorsal root potentials of the spinal cord. J. Neurophysiol. 9,
    139–160 (1946).
Eccles, J.C., Schadé, J.P. (Editors): Physiology of Spinal Neurons. Progress in Brain Res.
    Vol. 12, pp. 1–317. Amsterdam-London-New York: Elsevier Publishing Comp. 1964.
Eccles, J.C., Schmidt, R.F., Willis, W.D.: Presynaptic inhibition of the spinal monosy-
    naptic reflex pathway. J. Physiol. (Lond.) 161, 282–297 (1962).
Eccles, J.C., Schmidt, R.F., Willis, W.D.: Depolarization of central terminals of Group Ib
    afferent fibers from muscle. J. Neurophysiol. 26, 1–27 (1963a).
Eccles, J.C., Schmidt, R.F., Willis, W.D.: The location and the mode of action of the pre-
    synaptic inhibitory pathways on to Group I afferent fibers from muscle. J. Neurophysiol.
    26, 506–522 (1963b).
Eccles, J.C., Schmidt, R.F., Willis, W.D.: The mode of operation of the synaptic mecha-
    nism producing presynaptic inhibition. J. Neurophysiol. 26, 523–538 (1963c).
Eccles, J.C., Schmidt, R.F., Willis, W.D.: Inhibition of discharges into the dorsal and
    ventral spinocerebellar tracts. J. Neurophysiol. 26, 635–645 (1963d).
Eccles, J.C., Schmidt, R.F., Willis, W.D.: Depolarization of the central terminals of cuta-
    neous afferent fibers. J. Neurophysiol. 26, 646–661 (1963e).

ECCLES, J.C., SCHMIDT, R.F., WILLIS, W.D.: Pharmacological studies on presynaptic inhibition. J. Physiol. (Lond.) 168, 500–530 (1963f).

ECCLES, R.M., HOLMQVIST, B., VOORHOEVE, P.E.: Presynaptic inhibition from contralateral cutaneous afferent fibres. Acta physiol. scand. 62, 464–473 (1964a).

ECCLES, R.M., HOLMQVIST, B., VOORHOEVE, P.E.: Presynaptic depolarization of cutaneous afferents by volleys in contralateral muscle afferents. Acta physiol. scand. 62, 474–484 (1964b).

ECCLES, R.M., LUNDBERG, A.: Synaptic actions in motoneurones by afferents which may evoke the flexion reflex. Arch. ital. Biol. 97, 199–221 (1959).

ECCLES, R.M., WILLIS, W.D.: Presynaptic inhibition of the monosynaptic reflex pathway in kittens. J. Physiol. (Lond.) 165, 403–420 (1962).

ENGBERG, I., LUNDBERG, A., RYALL, R.W.: Reticulospinal inhibition of transmission in reflex pathways. J. Physiol. (Lond.) 194, 201–223 (1968).

ENGBERG, I., THALLER, A.: On the interaction of picrotoxin with GABA and glycine in the spinal cord. Brain Res. 19, 151–154 (1970).

EULER, C. VON, SKOGLUND, S., SÖDERBERG, U. (Editors): Structure and function of inhibitory neuronal mechanisms, pp. 1–563. Oxford: Pergamon Press 1968.

FADIGA, E., BROOKHART, J.M.: Monosynaptic activation of different portions of the motor neuron membrane. Amer. J. Physiol. 198, 693–703 (1960).

FATT, P., KATZ, B.: An analysis of the end-plate potential recorded with an intracellular electrode. J. Physiol. (Lond.) 115, 320–370 (1951).

FEDINA, L., GORDON, G., LUNDBERG, A.: The source and mechanisms of inhibition in the lateral cervical nucleus of the cat. Brain Res. 11, 694–696 (1968).

FELIX, D., WIESENDANGER, M.: Cortically induced inhibition in the dorsal column nuclei of monkeys. Pflügers Arch. 320, 285–288 (1970).

FRANK, K., FUORTES, M.G.F.: Presynaptic and postsynaptic inhibition of monosynaptic reflexes. Fed. Proc. 16, 39–40 (1957).

FRANZ, D.N., IGGO, A.: Dorsal root potentials and ventral root reflexes evoked by nonmyelinated fibers. Science 162, 1140–1142 (1968).

FUORTES, M.G.F.: Potential changes of the spinal cord following different types of afferent excitation. J. Physiol. (Lond.) 113, 372–386 (1951).

GALINDO, A.: GABA-picrotoxin interaction in the mammalian central nervous system. Brain Res. 14, 763–767 (1969).

GILLIES, J.D., LANGE, J.W., NEILSON, P.D., TASSINARI, C.A.: Presynaptic inhibition of the monosynaptic reflex by vibration. J. Physiol. (Lond.) 205, 329–339 (1969).

GOBEL, S., DUBNER, R.: Axo-axonic synapses in the main sensory trigeminal nucleus. Experientia (Basel) 24, 1250–1251 (1968).

GOBEL, S., DUBNER, R.: Fine structural studies of the main sensory trigeminal nucleus in the cat and rat. J. comp. Neurol. 137, 459–494 (1969).

GODFRAIND, J.M., KRNJEVIĆ, K., PUMAIN, R.: Doubtful value of bicuculline as a specific antagonist of GABA. Nature (Lond.) 228, 675–676 (1970).

GORDON, G., JUKES, M.G.M.: Correlation of different excitatory and inhibitory influences on cells in the nucleus gracilis of the cat. Nature (Lond.) 196, 1183–1185 (1962).

GORDON, G., JUKES, M.G.M.: Dual organization of the exteroceptive components of the cat's gracile nucleus. J. Physiol. (Lond.) 173, 263–290 (1964a).

GORDON, G., JUKES, M.G.M.: Descending influences on the exteroceptive organizations of the cat's gracile nucleus. J. Physiol. (Lond.) 173, 291–319 (1964).

GORDON, G., MILLER, R.: Identification of cortical cells projecting to the dorsal column nuclei of the cat. Quart. J. exp. Physiol. 54, 85–98 (1969).

GORDON, G., PAINE, C.H.: Functional organization in nucleus gracilis of the cat. J. Physiol. (Lond.) 153, 331–349 (1960).

GRANIT, R.: The case for presynaptic inhibition by synapses on the terminals of motoneurons. In: Structure and function of inhibitory neuronal mechanisms, pp. 183–196. Ed. by C. VON EULER, S. SKOGLUND and U. SÖDERBERG. Oxford and New York: Pergamon Press 1968.

GRAY, E.G.: A morphological basis for pre-synaptic inhibition? Nature (Lond.) 193, 82–83 (1962).

Gray, E.G.: Electron microscopy of presynaptic organelles of the spinal cord. J. Anat. (Lond.) **97**, 101–106 (1963).

Grinnell, A.D.: A study of the interaction between motoneurones in the frog spinal cord. J. Physiol. (Lond.) **182**, 612–648 (1966).

Grinnell, A.D.: Electrical interaction between antidromically stimulated frog motoneurones and dorsal root afferents: enhancement by gallamine and TEA. J. Physiol. (Lond.) **210**, 17–44 (1970).

Groves, P.M., Glanzman, D.L., Patterson, M.M., Thompson, R.F.: Excitability of cutaneous afferent terminals during habituation and sensitization in acute spinal cat. Brain Res. **18**, 388–391 (1970).

Guzman-Flores, C., Buendia, N., Anderson, C., Lindsley, D.B.: Cortical and reticular influences upon evoked responses in dorsal column nuclei. Exp. Neurol. **5**, 37–46 (1962).

Guzman-Flores, C., Buendia, N., Lindsley, D.B.: Cortical and reticular influences upon evoked responses in dorsal column nuclei. Fed. Proc. **20**, 330 (1960).

Hammer, B., Tarnecki, R., Vyklický, L., Wiesendanger, M.: Corticofugal control of presynaptic inhibition in the spinal trigeminal complex of the cat. Brain Res. **2**, 216–218 (1966).

Harris, F., Jabbur, S.J., Morse, R.W., Towe, A.L.: Influence of the cerebral cortex on the cuneate nucleus of the monkey. Nature (Lond.) **208**, 1215–1216 (1965).

Hepp-Reymond, M.-C., Wiesendanger, M.: Pyramidal influence on the spinal trigeminal nucleus of the cat. Arch. ital. Biol. **107**, 54–66 (1969).

Hernández-Peón, R., Hagbarth, K.E.: Interaction between afferent and cortically induced reticular responses. J. Neurophysiol. **18**, 44–55 (1955).

Hernández-Peón, R., Scherrer, H., Velasco, M.: Central influences on afferent conduction in the somatic and visual pathways. Acta neurol. lat.-amer. **2**, 8–22 (1956).

Holmes, F.W., Davenport, H.A.: Cells and fibers in spinal nerves; number of neurites in dorsal and ventral roots of cat. J. comp. Neurol. **73**, 1–5 (1940).

Hongo, T., Jankowska, E.: Effects from the sensorimotor cortex on the spinal cord in cats with transected pyramids. Exp. Brain Res. **3**, 117–134 (1967).

Hongo, T., Okada, Y.: Cortically evoked pre- and postsynaptic inhibition of impulse transmission to the dorsal spinocerebellar tract. Exp. Brain Res. **3**, 163–177 (1967).

Houk, J., Henneman, E.: Feedback control of skeletal muscles. Brain Res. **5**, 433–451 (1967).

Howland, B., Lettvin, J.Y., McCulloch, W.S., Pitts, W.H., Wall, P.D.: Reflex inhibition by dorsal root interaction. J. Neurophysiol. **18**, 1–17 (1955).

Hubbard, J.I., Llinás, R., Quastel, O.M.J.: Electrophysiological analysis of synaptic transmission. London: E. Arnold 1969.

Hubbard, J.I., Schmidt, R.F.: Repetitive activation of motor nerve endings. Nature (Lond.) **196**, 378–379 (1962).

Hubbard, J.I., Schmidt, R.F.: An electrophysiological investigation of mammalian motor nerve terminals. J. Physiol. (Lond.) **166**, 145–165 (1963).

Hudson, R.D., Wolpert, N.K.: Central muscle relaxant effects of diazepam. Neuropharmacology **9**, 481–488 (1970a).

Hudson, R.D., Wolpert, N.K.: Anticonvulsant and motor depressant effects of Diazepam. Arch. int. Pharmacodyn. **186**, 388–401 (1970b).

Jabbur, S.J.: The effect of the visual and the auditory systems on the dorsal-column medial-lemniscal system. In: The Somato-sensory System. Ed. by H.H. Kornhuber, J. Aschoff. Stuttgart: Georg Thieme Verlag 1972 (in press).

Jabbur, S.J., Banna, N.R.: Presynaptic inhibition of cuneate transmission by widespread cutaneous inputs. Brain Res. **10**, 273–276 (1968).

Jabbur, S.J., Banna, N.R.: Widespread cutaneous inhibition in dorsal column nuclei. J. Neurophysiol. **33**, 616–624 (1970).

Jabbur, S.J., Towe, A.L.: Effect of pyramidal tract activity on dorsal column nuclei. Science **132**, 547–548 (1960).

Jabbur, S.J., Towe, A.L.: Cortical excitation of neurons in dorsal column nuclei of cat, including an analysis of pathways. J. Neurophysiol. **24**, 499–509 (1961a).

JABBUR, S.J., TOWE, A.L.: The influence of the cerebral cortex on the dorsal column nuclei. In: Nervous Inhibition Proc. Int. Symp. Ed. by E. FLOREY. New York: Pergamon Press 1961b.

JÄNIG, W., SCHMIDT, R.F., ZIMMERMANN, M.: Presynaptic depolarization during activation of tonic mechanoreceptors. Brain Res. **5**, 514–516 (1967).

JÄNIG, W., SCHMIDT, R.F., ZIMMERMANN, M.: Two specific feedback pathways to the central afferent terminals of phasic and tonic mechanoreceptors. Exp. Brain Res. **6**, 116–129 (1968).

JÄNIG, W., ZIMMERMANN, M.: Presynaptic depolarization of myelinated afferent fibres evoked by stimulation of cutaneous C fibres. J. Physiol. (Lond.) **214**, 29–50 (1971).

JANKOWSKA, E., JUKES, M.G.M., LUND, S.: The pattern of presynaptic inhibition of transmission to the dorsal spinocerebellar tract. J. Physiol. (Lond.) **178**, 17–18P (1965).

JANKOWSKA, E., LUND, S., LUNDBERG, A.: The effect of DOPA on the spinal cord. 4. Depolarization evoked in the central terminals of contralateral Ia afferent terminals by volleys in the flexor reflex afferents. Acta physiol. scand. **68**, 337–341 (1966).

JURNA, I.: Depression of the dorsal root potential of the cat spinal cord by amidopyrine. Int. J. Neuropharmacol. **5**, 361–365 (1966).

KAHN, N., MAGNI, F., PILLAI, R.V.: Depolarization of optic fibre endings in the lateral geniculate body. Arch. ital. Biol. **105**, 573–582 (1967).

KATZ, B.: The transmission of impulses from nerve to muscle, and the subcellular unit of synaptic action. Proc. roy. Soc. B. **155**, 455–477 (1962).

KATZ, B., MILEDI, R.: Tetrodotoxin and neuromuscular transmission. Proc. roy. Soc. B. **167**, 8–22 (1967a).

KATZ, B., MILEDI, R.: The release of acetylcholine from nerve endings by graded electric pulses. Proc. roy. Soc. B. **167**, 23–28 (1967b).

KATZ, B., MILEDI, R.: A study of synaptic transmission in the absence of nerve impulses. J. Physiol. (Lond.) **192**, 407–436 (1967c).

KAWANA, E.: Projections of the anterior ectosylvian gyrus to the thalamus, the dorsal column nuclei, the trigeminal nuclei and the spinal cord in cats. Brain Res. **14**, 117–136 (1969).

KELLERTH, J.-O.: A strychnine-resistant postsynaptic inhibition in the spinal cord. Acta physiol. scand. **63**, 469–471 (1965).

KELLERTH, J.-O.: Aspects on the relative significance of pre- and postsynaptic inhibition in the spinal cord. In: Structure and functions of inhibitory neuronal mechanisms, pp. 197–212. Ed. by C. VON EULER, S. SKOGLUND and U. SÖDERBERG. Oxford and New York: Pergamon Press 1968.

KELLERTH, J.-O., SZUMSKI, A.J.: Two types of stretch-activated post-synaptic inhibitions in spinal motoneurons as differentiated by strychnine. Acta physiol. scand. **66**, 133–145 (1966a).

KELLERTH, J.-O., SZUMSKI, A.J.: Effects of picrotoxin on stretch-activated postsynaptic inhibitions in spinal motoneurons. Acta physiol. scand. **66**, 146–156 (1966b).

KERR, F.W.L.: The ultrastructure of the spinal tract of the trigeminal nerve and the substantia gelatinosa. Exp. Neurol. **16**, 359–376 (1966).

KERR, F.W.L.: The organization of primary afferents in the subnucleus caudalis of the trigeminal: A light and electron microscopic study of degeneration. Brain Res. **23**, 147–165 (1970).

KHATTAB, F.J.: A complex synaptic apparatus in spinal cord of cats. Experientia (Basel) **24**, 690–691 (1968).

KOKETSU, K.: Intracellular potential changes of primary afferent nerve fibers in spinal cords of cats. J. Neurophysiol. **19**, 375–392 (1956).

KUNO, M.: Mechanism of facilitation and depression of the excitatory synaptic potential in spinal motoneurones. J. Physiol. (Lond.) **175**, 100–112 (1964).

KUYPERS, H.G.J.M.: An anatomical analysis of the cortico-bulbar connexions to the pons and lower brain stem in the cat. J. Anat. (Lond.) **92**, 198–218 (1958a).

KUYPERS, H.G.J.M.: Corticobulbar connexions to the pons and lower brain stem in man. An anatomical study. Brain Res. **81**, 364–388 (1958b).

LEVITT, M., CARRERAS, M., CHAMBERS, W.W., LIU, C.N.: Pyramidal influences on unit activity in posterior column nuclei of cat. Physiologist **3**, 103 (1960).

Levitt, M., Carreras, M., Liu, C.N., Chambers, W.W.: Pyramidal and extrapyramidal modulation of somatosensory activity in gracile and cuneate nuclei. Arch. ital. Biol. **102**, 197–229 (1964).

Levy, R.A., Repkin, A.H., Anderson, E.G.: The effect of bicuculline on primary afferent terminal excitability. Brain Res. **32**, 261–265 (1971).

Liley, A.W.: The effects of presynaptic polarization on the spontaneous activity at the mammalian neuromuscular junction. J. Physiol. (Lond.) **134**, 427–443 (1956).

Llinás, R.: Mechanisms of supraspinal actions upon spinal cord activities. Pharmacological studies on reticular inhibition of alpha extensor motoneurons. J. Neurophysiol. **27**, 1127–1137 (1964).

Lloyd, D.P.C.: Electrotonus in dorsal root nerves. Cold Spr. Harb. Symp. quant. Biol. **17**, 203–218 (1952).

Lloyd, D.P.C., McIntyre, A.K.: On the origin of dorsal root potentials. J. gen. Physiol. **32**, 409–443 (1949).

Lund, S., Lundberg, A., Vyklický, L.: Inhibitory action from the flexor reflex afferents on transmission to Ia afferents. Acta physiol. scand. **64**, 345–355 (1965).

Lundberg, A.: Supraspinal control of transmission in reflex paths to motoneurones and primary afferents. In: Progress in Brain Research, Vol. 12, pp. 197–221. Ed. by J.C. Eccles and J.P. Schadé. Physiology of Spinal Neurons (1964).

Lundberg, A.: Integration in the reflex pathway. In: Nobel Sympos. I: Muscular afferents and motor control, pp. 275–305. Ed. by R. Granit. Stockholm: Almquist & Wiksell; New York-London-Sydney: J. Wiley & Sons 1966.

Lundberg, A.: The supraspinal control of transmission in spinal reflex pathways. Electroenceph. clin. Neurophysiol. Suppl. **25**, 35–46 (1967).

Lundberg, A.: Convergence of excitatory and inhibitory action on interneurones in the spinal cord. In: The interneurone. UCLA Forum Med. Sci. No. 11. Ed. by M.A.B. Brazier. Los Angeles: University of California Press 1969.

Lundberg, A., Vyklický, L.: Inhibitory interaction between spinal reflexes to primary afferents. Experientia (Basel) **19**, 247 (1963).

Lundberg, A., Vyklický, L.: Inhibition of transmission to primary afferents by electrical stimulation of the brain stem. Arch. ital. Biol. **104**, 86–97 (1966).

Magni, F., Melzack, R., Moruzzi, G., Smith, C.J.: Direct pyramidal influences on the dorsal-column nuclei. Arch. ital. Biol. **97**, 357–377 (1959).

Majorossy, K., Réthelyi, M., Szentágothai, J.: The large glomerular synapse of the pulvinar. J. Hirnforsch. **7**, 415–432 (1965).

Mallart, A.: Heterosegmental and heterosensory presynaptic inhibition. Nature (Lond.) **206**, 719–720 (1965).

Marchiafava, P.L., Pompeiano, O.: Excitability changes of the intrageniculate optic tract fibres produced by electrical stimulation of the vestibular system. Pflügers Arch. ges. Physiol. **290**, 275–278 (1966a).

Marchiafava, P.L., Pompeiano, O.: Enhanced excitability of intra-geniculate optic tract endings produced by vestibular volleys. Arch. ital. Biol. **104**, 459–479 (1966b).

Marshall, W.H.: Observations on subcortical somatic sensory mechanism of cats under Nembutal anaesthesia. J. Neurophysiol. **4**, 25–43 (1941).

McComas, A.J.: Responses of the rat dorsal column system to mechanical stimulation of the hind paw. J. Physiol. (Lond.) **166**, 435–448 (1963).

McLennan, H.: Synaptic Transmission. Philadelphia: W.B. Saunders 1970.

Megirian, D.: Centrifugal discharges in cutaneous nerve fibers evoked by cutaneous afferent volleys in the acutely spinal phalanger "Trichosurus vulpecula". Arch. ital. Biol. **106**, 343–352 (1968).

Megirian, D.: Centrifugal cutaneous nerve discharges in the decerebrate phalanger "Trichosurus vulpecula". Arch. ital. Biol. **108**, 388–399 (1970).

Megirian, D.: Vestibular and somatosensory evoked centrifugal cutaneous nerve discharges in the decerebrate-decerebellate phalanger "Trichosurus vulpecula". Arch. ital. Biol. **109**, 152–165 (1971).

Melzack, R., Wall, P.D.: Pain mechanisms: A new theory. Science **150**, 971–979 (1965).

MENDELL, L.M.: Positive dorsal root potentials produced by stimulation of small diameter muscle afferents. Brain Res. **18**, 375–379 (1970).

MENDELL, L.M.: Inhibition of the negative DRP during a steady positive DRP. Fed. Proc. **30**, 433 (1971).

MENDELL, L.M., WALL, P.D.: Presynaptic hyperpolarization: a role for fine afferent fibres. J. Physiol. (Lond.) **172**, 274–294 (1964).

MIYAHARA, J.T., ESPLIN, D.W., ZABLOCKA, B.: Differential effects of depressant drugs on presynaptic inhibition. J. Pharmacol. exp. Ther. **154**, 118–127 (1966).

MORRISON, A.R., POMPEIANO, O.: Corticospinal influences on primary afferents during sleep and wakefulness. Experientia (Basel) **21**, 660–661 (1965a).

MORRISON, A.R., POMPEIANO, O.: Central depolarization of group Ia afferent fibers during desynchronized sleep. Arch. ital. Biol. **103**, 517–537 (1965b).

MORRISON, A.R., POMPEIANO, O.: Depolarization of central terminals of group Ia muscle afferent fibres during desynchronized sleep. Nature (Lond.) **210**, 201–202 (1966).

NAKAMURA, Y., WU, C.Y.: Presynaptic inhibition of jaw-opening reflex by high threshold afferents from the masseter muscle of the cat. Brain Res. **23**, 193–211 (1970).

NGAI, S.H., TSENG, D.T.C., WANG, S.C.: Effect of diazepam and other central nervous system depressants on spinal reflexes in cats: A study of site of action. J. Pharmacol. exp. Ther. **153**, 344–351 (1966).

NISHI, S., KOKETSU, K.: Electrical properties and activities of single sympathetic neurons in frogs. J. cell. comp. Physiol. **55**, 15–30 (1960).

NORTON, A.C.: The dorsal column system of the spinal cord: Its anatomy, physiology, phylogeny and sensory function. An updated review. Los Angeles: UCLA Brain Information Service 1970.

PAPPAS, G.D., COHEN, E.B., PURPURA, D.P.: Electron microscope study of synaptic and other neuronal interrelation in the feline thalamus. 8th International Congress of Anatomists, Wiesbaden, 8–13 August 1965. Georg Thieme-Verlag: Stuttgart.

PERL, E.R., WHITLOCK, D.G., GENTRY, J.R.: Cutaneous projection to second-order neurons of the dorsal column system. J. Neurophysiol. **25**, 337–358 (1962).

PETERS, A., PALAY, S.L.: The morphology of laminae A and A_1 of the dorsal nucleus of the lateral geniculate body of the cat. J. Anat. (Lond.) **100**, 451–486 (1966).

PHILLIS, J.W.: Assay methods for transmitter substances of the central nervous system. Ph. D. Thesis, Australian National University, Canberra (1960).

PHILLIS, J.W., TEBĒCIS, A.K.: The effects of topically applied cholinomimetic drugs on the isolated spinal cord of the toad. Comp. Biochem. Physiol. **23**, 541–552 (1967).

PHILLIS, J.W., TEBĒCIS, A.K.: Prostaglandins and toad spinal cord responses. Nature (Lond.) **217**, 1076–1077 (1968).

PIXNER, D.B.: The effect of some drugs upon synaptic transmission in the isolated spinal cord of the frog. J. Physiol. (Lond.) **189**, 15P (1966).

RALSTON III, H.J.: The organization of the substantia gelatinosa Rolandi in the cat lumbosacral cord. Z. Zellforsch. **57**, 1–23 (1965).

RALSTON III, H.J.: The fine structure of neurons in the dorsal horn of the cat spinal cord. J. comp. Neurol. **132**, 275–302 1968a).

RALSTON III, H.J.: Dorsal root projections to dorsal horn neurons in the cat spinal cord. J. comp. Neurol. **132**, 303–330 (1968b).

RÉTHELYI, M.: Ultrastructural synaptology of Clarke's column. Exp. Brain Res. **11**, 159–174 (1970).

RÉTHELYI, M., SZENTÁGOTHAI, J.: The large synaptic complexes of the substantia gelatinosa. Exp. Brain Res. **7**, 258–274 (1969).

RICHENS, A.: The action of general anaesthetic agents on root responses of the frog isolated spinal cord. Brit. J. Pharmacol. **36**, 294–311 (1969).

ROWE, M.J.: Reduction of response variability in the somatic sensory system by conditioning inputs. Brain Res. **22**, 417–420 (1970).

ROWE, M.J., CARMODY, J.J.: Afferent inhibition over the response range of secondary trigeminal neurones. Brain Res. **18**, 371–374 (1970).

RUDOMIN, P.: Pharmacological evidence for the existence of interneurons mediating primary afferent depolarization in the solitary tract nucleus of the cat. Brain Res. **2**, 181–183 (1966).

Rudomin, P.: Some presynaptic mechanisms controlling impulse transmission in mono-synaptic pathways. In: The Somato-sensory System. Ed. by H.H. Kornhuber and J. Aschoff. Stuttgart: Georg Thieme Verlag 1972 (in press).

Rudomin, P., Dutton, H.: The effects of primary afferent depolarization on excitability fluctuations of Ia terminals within the motor nucleus. Experientia (Basel) 24, 48–50 (1968).

Rudomin, P., Dutton, H.: Effects of conditioning afferent volleys on variability of mono-synaptic responses of extensor motoneurons. J. Neurophysiol. 32, 140–157 (1969a).

Rudomin, P., Dutton, H.: Effects of muscle and cutaneous afferent nerve volleys on excita-bility fluctuations of Ia terminals. J. Neurophysiol. 32, 158–169 (1969b).

Rudomin, P., Dutton, H., Muñoz-Martinez, J.: Changes in correlation between monosy-naptic reflexes produced by conditioning afferent volleys. J. Neurophysiol. 32, 759–772 (1969).

Rudomin, P., Muñoz-Martinez, J.: A tetrodotoxin-resistant primary afferent depolarization. Exp. Neurol. 25, 106–115 (1969).

Sauerland, E.K., Mizuno, N.: Cortically induced presynaptic inhibition of trigeminal pro-prioceptive afferents. Brain Res. 13, 556–568 (1969a).

Sauerland, E.K., Mizuno, N.: Effect of trigeminal proprioceptive input on the lingual-hypoglossal reflex. Anat. Rec. 163, 322–323 (1969b).

Sauerland, E.K., Mizuno, N., Harper, R.M.: Presynaptic depolarization of trigeminal cutaneous afferent fibers induced by ethanol. Exp. Neurol. 27, 476–489 (1970).

Sauerland, E.K., Thiele, H.: Presynaptic depolarization of lingual and glossopharyngeal nerve afferents induced by stimulation of trigeminal proprioceptive fibers. Exp. Neurol. 28, 344–355 (1970).

Scheibel, M.E., Scheibel, A.B.: Terminal axonal patterns in cat spinal cord. II. The dorsal horn. Brain Res. 9, 32–58 (1968).

Scherrer, H., Hernández-Peón, R.: Inhibitory influence of reticular formation upon synaptic transmission in gracilis nucleus. Fed. Proc. 14, 132 (1955).

Scherrer, H., Hernández-Peón, R.: Hemmung postsynaptischer Potentiale im Nucleus gracilis. Pflügers Arch. ges. Physiol. 267, 434–445 (1958).

Schmidt, R.F.: Pharmacological studies on the primary afferent depolarization of the toad spinal cord. Pflügers Arch. ges. Physiol. 277, 325–346 (1963).

Schmidt, R.F.: Die Wirkung von Diazepam (Valium "Roche") auf synaptische Funktionen des Rückenmarks. Communicationes, VI. Internat. Congr. Electroenceph. Clin. Neuro-physiol., Wien 1965, pp. 627–630 (1965).

Schmidt, R.F.: Presynaptic inhibition in the vertebrate central nervous system. Ergebn. Physiol. 63, 20–101 (1971).

Schmidt, R.F., Senges, J., Zimmermann, M.: Excitability measurements at the central terminals of single mechano-receptor afferents during slow potential changes. Exp. Brain Res. 3, 220–233 (1967a).

Schmidt, R.F., Senges, J., Zimmermann, M.: Presynaptic depolarization of cutaneous me-chanoreceptor afferents after mechanical skin stimulation. Exp. Brain Res. 3, 234–247 (1967b).

Schmidt, R.F., Trautwein, W., Zimmermann, M.: Dorsal root potentials evoked by natural stimulation of cutaneous afferents. Nature (Lond.) 212, 522–523 (1966).

Schmidt, R.F., Vogel, M.E., Zimmermann, M.: Die Wirkung von Diazepam auf die präsy-naptische Hemmung und andere Rückenmarksreflexe. Naunyn-Schmiedebergs Arch. Pharmak. exp. Path. 258, 69–82 (1967).

Schmidt, R.F., Willis, W.D.: Intracellular recording from motoneurones of the cervical spinal cord of the cat. J. Neurophysiol. 26, 28–43 (1963a).

Schmidt, R.F., Willis, W.D.: Depolarization of central terminals of afferent fibers in the cervical spinal cord of the cat. J. Neurophysiol. 26, 44–60 (1963b).

Scibetta, C.J., King, R.B.: Hyperpolarizing influence of trigeminal nucleus caudalis on pri-mary afferent preterminals in trigeminal nucleus oralis. J. Neurophysiol. 32, 229–238 (1969).

Selzer, M., Spencer, W.A.: Interactions between visceral and cutaneous afferents in the spinal cord: Reciprocal primary afferent fiber depolarization. Brain Res. 14, 349–366 (1969).

SESSLE, B.J., DUBNER, R.: Presynaptic hyperpolarization of fibers projecting to trigeminal brain stem and thalamic nuclei. Brain Res. **22**, 121–125 (1970).

SESSLE, B.J., DUBNER, R.: Presynaptic excitability changes of trigeminothalamic and corticothalamic afferents. Exp. Neurol. **30**, 239–250 (1971).

SHENDE, M.C., KING, R.B.: Excitability changes of trigeminal primary afferent preterminals in brain-stem nuclear complex of squirrel monkey (Saimiri sciureus). J. Neurophysiol. **30**, 949–963 (1967).

SHIMAMURA, M., AOKI, M.: Effects of spino-bulbo-spinal reflex volleys on flexor motoneurons of hindlimb in the cat. Brain Res. **16**, 333–349 (1969).

SHIMAMURA, M., MORI, S., YAMAUCHI, T.: Effects of spino-bulbo-spinal reflex volleys on extensor motoneurons of hindlimb in cats. J. Neurophysiol. **30**, 319–332 (1967).

SOTGIU, M.L., CESA-BIANCHI, M.G.: Primary afferent depolarization in the cuneate nucleus induced by stimulation of cerebellar and thalamic non-specific nuclei. Electroenceph. clin. Neurophysiol. **29**, 156–165 (1970).

STEWART, D.H., SCIBETTA, C.J., KING, R.B.: Presynaptic inhibition in the trigeminal relay nuclei. J. Neurophysiol. **30**, 135–153 (1967).

STRATTEN, W.P., BARNES, C.D.: Spinal effect of diazepam. Fed. Proc. **27**, 571 (1968).

SZENTÁGOTHAI, J.: Anatomical aspects of junctional transformation. In: Information Processing in the Nervous System. Ed. by R.W. GERAD and J.W. DUYFF. Proc. Internat. Union Physiol. Sciences, Vol. 3, pp. 119–136. Amsterdam: Excerpta Medica Foundation 1962.

SZENTÁGOTHAI, J.: The structure of the synapse in the lateral geniculate body. Acta anat. (Basel) **55**, 166–185 (1963).

TEBĒCIS, A.K., PHILLIS, J.W.: The effects of topically applied biogenic monoamines on the isolated spinal cord of the toad. Aust. J. exp. Biol. med. Sci. **45**, 23–24P (1967).

TEBĒCIS, A.K., PHILLIS, J.W.: Reflex response changes of the toad spinal cord to variations in temperature and pH. Comp. Biochem. Physiol. **25**, 1035–1047 (1968).

TEBĒCIS, A.K., PHILLIS, J.W.: The use of convulsants in studying possible functions of amino acids in the toad spinal cord. Comp. Biochem. Physiol. **28**, 1303–1315 (1969a).

TEBĒCIS, A.K., PHILLIS, J.W.: The pharmacology of the isolated toad spinal cord. Experiments in Physiology and Biochemistry **2**, 361–395 (1969b).

THERMAN, P.O.: Transmission of impulses through the Burdach nucleus. J. Neurophysiol. **4**, 153–166 (1941).

TÖMBÖL, T.: Short neurons and their synaptic relations in the specific thalamic nuclei. Brain Res. **3**, 307–326 (1967).

TOENNIES, J.F.: Reflex discharge from the spinal cord over the dorsal roots. J. Neurophysiol. **1**, 378–390 (1938).

TOENNIES, J.F.: Conditioning of afferent impulses by reflex discharge over the dorsal roots. J. Neurophysiol. **2**, 515–525 (1939).

TOWE, A.L., JABBUR, S.J.: Cortical inhibition of neurons in dorsal column nuclei of cat. J. Neurophysiol. **24**, 488–498 (1961).

TOWE, A.L., ZIMMERMANN, I.D.: Peripherally evoked cortical reflex in the cuneate nucleus. Nature (Lond.) **194**, 1250–1251 (1962).

VERHEY, B.A., VAN KEULEN, L.C.M., VOORHOEVE, P.E.: An extreme form of presynaptic inhibition by Ia afferents. Acta physiol. pharmacol. neerl. **14**, 1 (1966).

VOORHOEVE, P.E., VERHEY, B.A.: Pre- and postsynaptic effects on fusimotor- and alpha motoneurones of the cat upon activation of muscle spindle afferents by succinylcholine. Acta physiol. pharmacol. neerl. **12**, 12–22 (1963).

VYKLICKÝ, L., MAKSIMOVÁ, E.V., JIROUSEK, J.: Neurones in the reflex pathway between trigeminal sensory fibres in the cat. Physiol. bohemoslov. **16**, 285–296 (1967).

VYKLICKÝ, L., RUDOMIN, P., ZAJAC III, F.E., BURKE, R.E.: Primary afferent depolarization evoked by a painful stimulus. Science **165**, 184-186 (1969).

VYKLICKÝ, L., TABIN, V.: Primary afferent depolarization evoked by adequate stimulation of skin receptors. Physiol. bohemoslov. **15**, 89–97 (1966).

WALBERG, F.: Corticofugal fibres to the nuclei of the dorsal columns. An experimental study in the cat. Brain **80**, 273–287 (1957).

Walberg, F.: Axoaconic contacts in the cuneate nucleus, probable basis for presynaptic depolarization. Exp. Neurol. **13**, 218–231 (1965).

Wall, P.D.: Excitability changes in afferent fibre terminations and their relation to slow potentials. J. Physiol. (Lond.) **142**, 1–21 (1958).

Wall, P.D.: The origin of a spinal cord slow potential. J. Physiol. (Lond.) **164**, 508–526 (1962).

Wall, P.D.: Presynaptic control of impulses at the first central synapse in the cutaneous pathway. In: Progress in Brain Research, Vol. 12, pp. 92–118. Physiology of Spinal Neurons. Ed. by J.C. Eccles and J.P. Schadé. Amsterdam: Elsevier Publ. Comp. 1964.

Wall, P.D., McCulloch, W.S., Lettvin, J.Y., Pitts, W.H.: Factors limiting the maximum impulse transmitting ability of an afferent system of nerve fibres. 3rd. London Symp. on Information Theory, pp. 329–344. London: Butterworth 1955.

Wiesendanger, M.: The pyramidal tract. Recent investigations on its morphology and function. Ergebn. Physiol. **61**, 72–136 (1969).

Wiesendanger, M., Felix, D.: Pyramidal excitation of lemniscal neurons and facilitation of sensory transmission in the spinal trigeminal nucleus of the cat. Exp. Neurol. **25**, 1–17 (1969).

Wiesendanger, M., Hammer, B., Tarnecki, R.: Cortifugal control of presynaptic inhibition in the spinal trigeminal nucleus of the cat. The effect of pyramidotomy and barbiturates. Schweiz. Arch. Neurol. Neurochir. Psychiat. **100**, 255–276 (1967a).

Wiesendanger, M., Hammer, B., Tarnecki, R.: Corticale Beeinflussung der synaptischen Übertragung im Trigeminuskern der Katze. Helv. Physiol. Acta **25**, CR 237–239 (1967b).

Winter, D.L.: N. gracilis of cat. Functional organization and cortifugal effects. J. Neurophysiol. **28**, 48–70 (1965).

Zimmermann, M.: Selective activation of C-fibers. Pflügers Arch. ges. Physiol. **301**, 329–333 (1968a).

Zimmermann, M.: Dorsal root potentials after C-fiber stimulation. Science **160**, 896–898 (1968b).

Chapter 7

Distribution and Connections of Afferent Fibres in the Spinal Cord

By

M. Réthelyi and J. Szentágothai, Budapest (Hungary)

With 22 Figures

Contents

1. Course of Primary Afferents in the White Matter

1.1 Entrance into the Spinal Cord of the Dorsal Roots

Upon entering the spinal cord through the dorsolateral sulcus the dorsal root fibers penetrate into various depths along the dorsomedial border of the dorsal grey column. The narrow strip occupied in the dorsal funiculus (dorsal white column) by the primary sensory fibers at or near the level of their entrance (the so-called root entrance zone) closely follows the medial borderline of the dorsal horn, its length and orientation thus varies in different regions of the cord. The concepts of a lateral division of the rootlets entering Lissauer's tract and containing mainly small calibered fibers (Ranson, 1913) has been questioned recently (Earle, 1952; Wall, 1962) but with certain modifications appears to be still acceptable (Szentágothai, 1964a) (see paragraph 1.4).

1.2 Bifurcation of the Primary Afferents

The bifurcation in Y-shape fashion (Nansen, 1886; Ramón y Cajal, 1890) occurs at the approximate depth in the dorsal funiculus at which one of the branches begins its ascent and the other its descent. No convincing evidence for non bifurcating fibers, or for those entering the grey matter directly, has ever been reported.

1.3 Distribution and Course of Ascending and Descending Branches of Primary Afferents in the Dorsal Funiculus

Pertinent information is based chiefly on the classical myelinization (Flechsig, 1876, 1890; Trepinski, 1898), demyelinization (rev.: Bok, 1928) and on Marchi degeneration studies (rev.: Foerster, 1936). Rather incomplete data on propriospinal dorsal tract fibers (Marie, 1892; Tower, 1937) complicate the picture considerably; most of this material being beyond the scope of this review and the reader is referred to the reviews quoted above.

1.3.1 The Ascending Branches of the Dorsal Root Fibers

The general principle of arrangement in the dorsal funiculus of the ascending primary afferent branches according to segmental origin, is simple and generally referred to as the rule of Kahler (1882). According to this the ascending branches of the primary afferent fibers belonging to the same segment occupy thin bands on the cross section of the dorsal funiculus, oriented approximately in parallel with the dorsomedial border of the posterior horn. These bands are gradually shifted during their ascent in dorso-medial direction due to new parallel bands of ascending branches of the dorsal roots entering from the successive cranial segments. They are wedged progressively between the dorsomedial border of the dorsal horn and the band of ascending branches having entered the cord one segment below. In fact, however, the situation is not that simple: myelinization studies have shown (Flechsig, 1876, 1890; Trepinski, 1898) that each band of fibers of common segmental origin consists of an earlier developing deeper and later developing more superficial fiber system. It is assumed (rev.: Bok, 1928) that while the superficial part of the segmental band reaches the dorsal column nuclei of the medulla oblongata, the deep fiber system may be, at least partially, exhausted before reaching the medulla by issuing collaterals to the spinal grey matter.

1.3.2 The Descending Branches of the Dorsal Root Fibers

The descending branches of primary afferents accumulate in an inverse comma-shaped bundle (Schultze, 1883), situated between Goll's and Burdach's tracts, in the lower cervical and the thoracic segments. During their descent the fibers are shifting position — similar to the ascending branches — in medial direction. In the lumbar segments the descending fibers accumulate at both sides of the median septum of the posterior funiculus in a symmetric fusiform field: in the sacral segments this field is reduced to a triangular area on the surface of the posterior funiculus at both sides of the median septum. Recent degeneration studies (Imai and Kusama, 1969) establish that the descending branches of the primary afferents of the upper cervical segments descend until the level C_6, those from the lower cervical segments to that of T_6. The descending branches of the thoracic roots bridge only 2–3 segments, while according to a single observation on segment L_1 the descending fibers may reach the lower end of the lumbar enlargement.

1.4 The Primary Afferent Component of Lissauer's Tract

Lissauer's tract, a fine calibered bundle situated immediately laterad to the entering dorsal rootlets and with an ill-defined border towards the lateral funiculus, has been thought for some time to consist largely of dorsal root fibers for pain conduction (Ranson, 1913, 1914; Ranson and Billingsley, 1916; Ranson and Hess, 1915). It appears now to be established that the majority of the Lissauer tract fibers are propriospinal (Earle, 1952), probably only the most medial fibers are primary afferents (Szentágothai, 1964a). The primary afferents ascend and descend one or two segments, at the highest, before terminating in the substantia gelatinosa (Schimert, 1939). The propriospinal fibers of this tract are somewhat longer and may bridge five-six segments (Szentágothai, 1964a).

2. Collaterals of the Primary Afferents

2.1 Modes of Origin, Initial Course, Bundling, and Segmental Distribution

Primary afferents entering the spinal grey matter are almost exclusively collaterals, excepting the terminal parts of the descending dorsal root branches, and those of the assumed short primary afferent branches of the deep ascending (1.3.1) posterior funiculus system. The collaterals of the primary afferents enter the grey substance of the dorsal horn along its entire border with the dorsal funiculus. Corresponding to the rule of Kahler (1.3.1) collaterals arising from more medial (and ventral) parts of the posterior funiculus belong to fibers that have entered a few segments below (or above), while those entering from the most lateral area originate from dorsal root fibers of the same segment. Collaterals arising from the ventromedial area of the dorsal funiculus are thought to be of propriospinal nature (Pierre Marie's bundle [1892]), except for the collaterals of the nucleus of Clarke (2.4.4, Fig. 6), which are undoubtedly of primary afferent nature. Most of the primary afferent collaterals penetrate through the three dorsal laminae of the grey matter (Rexed, 1952), and begin their various courses in the centre (lamina IV) or at the base (lamina V) of the dorsal horn. A special group of generally more delicate primary afferent collaterals arising from the medial part of Lissauer's tract (Ramón y Cajal, 1909 [Fig. 120]) and others arising from a superficial area immediately medially from the dorsal root entrance (Szentágothai, 1964a) enter the substantia gelatinosa from its entire dorsal circumference after having participated in a flat marginal plexus at the border of the grey matter. They arborize in the superficial layers (laminae I–III) of the dorsal horn. While pene-trating into the spinal grey matter, collaterals of different origin and destination gather into bundles (of 3–20 axons). Scheibel and Scheibel (1969) have called attention to the possible functional significance of fasciculation through pre-synaptic interaction within these bundles.

Segmental distribution: On the basis of Golgi pictures it has been assumed that primary afferents issue most collaterals in the segment of their entrance (Ramón y Cajal, 1909), while the number of collaterals already shows a sharp drop in the neighbouring segments. This has been substantiated essentially by the early degeneration studies (Schimert, 1939) and on the lumbosacral cord with more advanced degeneration (Nauta-Gygax) methods (Szentágothai, 1961a; Sprague and Ha, 1964). The only systematic study now available on the cervical roots (Imai and Kusama, 1969) shows that the total range of collaterals issued by a single root spreads over six segments in the upper and over up to fourteen segments (six ascending and seven descending) in the lower cervical region.

2.2 Somatotopic Termination of Primary Afferent Collaterals

There are two seemingly conflicting types of somatotopic arrangement in the termination of primary afferents in the spinal grey matter: (a) A successive shift in medial direction of the termination fields in the dorsal horn of collaterals issued by the ascending, and a successive lateral shift of the terminal fields of the col-laterals given by the descending dorsal root branches. (b) Projection of the ventral part of the dermatome (distal parts of limbs) medially, and of its dorsal part laterally in the substantia gelatinosa.

(a) Indications for a medial shift of the termination fields of the collaterals corresponding to ascending distance from the root entrance were already found in the early degeneration studies (Schimert, 1939), and this became particularly clear in Clarke's column (Szentágothai, 1961b). However, the general principle of the medial shift of the termination field of primary afferents in the dorsal horn in ascending, and lateral shift in descending direction only became apparent in recent observations in the cervical cord (Imai and Kusama, 1969).

(b) The existence of a true somatotopic projection of the dermatome in the spinal grey matter has been assumed on the basis of glove-type distributions of thermanaesthesia in syringomyelia. Using the favourable extraspinal location of the second spinal cervical ganglion in the cat Szentágothai and Kiss (1949) have differentiated two separate regions of this ganglion, the cells of which contribute fibers mainly either to the dorsal or to the ventral branch of the second cervical nerve. The results appeared to show quite consistently that the ventral branch of the 2nd cervical nerve projects preferentially to the medial, and the greater occipital nerve to the lateral half of the substantia gelatinosa. The termination of fibers from the greater occipital nerve (Kruger et al., 1961; see also Imai and Kusama, 1969) in the ventralmost part of the spinal trigeminal nucleus agrees well with this projection principle. Developmental studies in the chick and the lizard (Szentágothai and Székely, 1956) show the same crossed projection of the dorsal spinal nerve branches upon the lateral, and of the ventral nerve branches upon medial cellular masses of the dorsal horn.

It might seem at first sight that these two projection principles (a) and (b) are conflicting and mutually exclusive. Fig. 1 shows a hypothetical model of the dorsal horn cellular mass, made — as an attempt to reconcile the two principles — under the assumption that it is built of three medially sloping sagittal discs, each belonging to a cervical segment. In reality there is an extensive overlap between the discs belonging to neighbouring segments (IMAI and KUSAMA, 1969) but this has been neglected in the diagram. It is assumed additionally that the ventral part of each dermatome projects upon the dorsal, and the dorsal part upon the

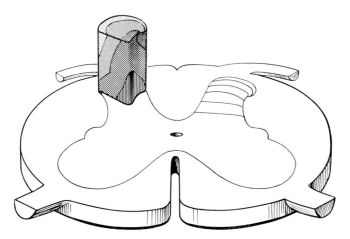

Fig. 1. Attempt at illustrating stereodiagramatically the dual projection principle (discussed in the text) of the periphery upon the dorsal horn cellular mass. The lightly stippled region corresponds to the termination field of collaterals of primary afferents that have entered the cord one segment above the illustrated disc. The densely stippled region would correspond to the terminal field occupied by collaterals of fibers entered through the illustrated segment, the obliquely hatched to the termination field of the collaterals belonging to the segment below, and the vertically hatched to those having entered two segments below

ventral half of each disc. If now this group of discs were bent in the way the laminated cellular mass of the dorsal horn might be supposed to be bent by the development of the dorsal funiculi (SZENTÁGOTHAI and KISS, 1949), to become an inverse trough, with the convexity in the dorsal and the concavity in the ventral direction[1], one may get the very rough idea of how the two projection principles might be combined in the dorsal horn. Our understanding of these general principles is probably still extremely crude and marginal, however, such reasoning shows at least as much that the general principles of somatotopic arrangement prevailing in most parts of the CNS exists, in distorted form, also in the spinal cord.

Since the most motoneurons are arranged somatotopically[2] in an order reverse to that of rule (b) on the projection of the dermatomes upon the dorsal laminae of

1 This bending applies fully only to the dorsalmost part of the dorsal horn cellular mass.

2 Motoneurons supplying the axial dorsal musculature are situated medially and the motoneurons of distal limb muscles laterally in the ventral horn.

the dorsal horn, it stands to reason that primary afferents directed towards the ventral horn ought to cross somewhere in the intermediate region. Such a crossing of the primary afferent collaterals had been illustrated very clearly by v. Lenhossék (1895) and by Ramón y Cajal (1909 [Fig. 115]) at a time when the possible

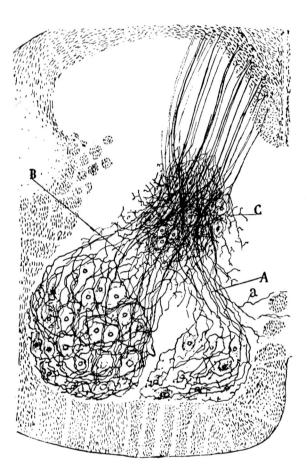

Fig. 2. Reproduction of a drawing of Ramón y Cajal (1909, Fig. 115) illustrating the crossing in the intermediate region (C) of a more medial group of collaterals destined for the lateral motor nucleus (B) and of a group arising from more lateral part of the posterior funiculus directed towards the medial motor cell group (A). (See also Fig. 5 B)

implications of this were completely unknown. The illustration of Ramón y Cajal is reproduced here in Fig. 2. The tendency for the overcrossing of primary afferent collaterals with destinations in the ventral horn can also be seen in a photomicrograph published some time ago by one of the present authors (J. Szentágothai, 1967a [Fig. 3]). A photograph of the same material is added here in Fig. 5 B.

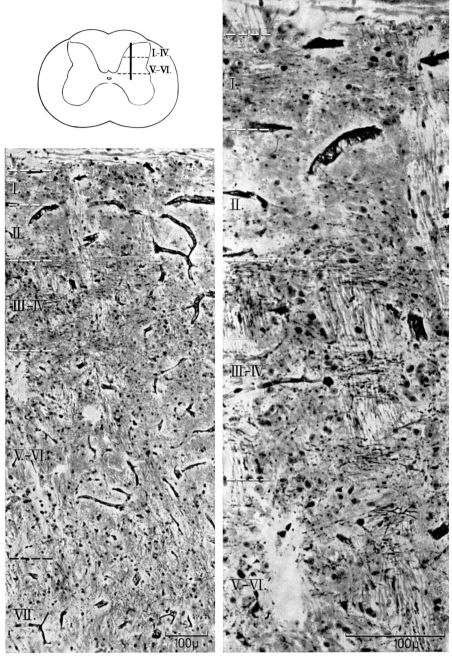

Fig. 3. Paramedian sagittal section of the segment L_5 two days after transection of the L_5 dorsal root, Fink-Heimer stain. Situation of the section is shown in small diagram in upper left corner. Photomicrograph at left is with smaller magnification for general survey, right photograph at somewhat higher magnification shows intensive degeneration of longitudinally oriented axons in lamina I, while only very fine degeneration fragments are found in lamina II. Lamina III and IV contain coarse, predominantly longitudinally oriented rows of fragments, from lamina V on degeneration rows become transversally (perpendicularly) oriented

2.3 The General Distribution of Primary Afferent Collaterals in the Grey Matter[3]

The over-all arborization of primary afferents in the grey matter can be studied most favourably with modern axonal degeneration methods after the transection of dorsal roots. For reference to the distribution of these collaterals in transverse sections the excellent semi-diagrammatic illustrations of Sprague and Ha (1964) should be consulted. Sterling and Kuypers (1967a) have drawn attention to the importance of longitudinal (particularly of sagittal) sections in which important details of the general arborization can be studied. As the overall distribution in the sagittal plane of degeneration after dorsal radicotomy is less known, an example of this is presented in Fig. 3 in two different magnifications. It becomes apparent at higher magnification that there is a dense, predominantly longitudinally oriented, plexus of delicate degenerated fibers in lamina I. The degeneration appears to be less dense in lamina II, although a substantial number of very delicate degeneration fragments are still present (Heimer and Wall, 1968; Réthelyi and Szentágothai, 1969). Lamina III and IV are characterized by a dense longitudinally oriented plexus of coarser degenerated fibers. In lamina V the longitudinally oriented fibers undergoing degeneration disappear and the rows of fragments become gradually oriented in dorsoventral direction. The orientation of the neuropil in various parts of the grey matter will be discussed in more detail in subsequent paragraphs.

2.4 The Different Types of Primary Afferent Collaterals

Attempts at separating different types of primary afferent collaterals had already been made in the early classical investigations of the cord. Ramón y Cajal (1909) divided them into six distinct groups: (1) so called "reflex collaterals" to the ventral horn, (2) collaterals to the head (center) of the dorsal horn, (3) collaterals to the intermediary nuclei, (4) collaterals to the column of Clarke, (5) commissural collaterals, and (6) collaterals to the substantia gelatinosa. In the following paragraphs the different types of collaterals will be discussed in the same order.

2.4.1 Direct Primary Afferent Collaterals to Motoneurons. There is a vast body of evidence available for the assumption that only the primary Ia afferents of the muscle spindle issue direct collaterals to motoneurons. Most of this evidence is of physiological nature and will, therefore, not be discussed in this chapter. Direct anatomical evidence for this assumption is available only in the proprioceptive reflex arc of the masticatory muscles (Szentágothai, 1948) but there is no reason anatomically why it should be otherwise in any other part of the CNS.

Two recent Golgi studies on direct (i.e. Ia) primary afferent collaterals to motoneurons (Szentágothai, 1967a; Scheibel and Scheibel, 1969) are in fair agreement with respect to the observations but are at variance in interpretation. While Scheibel and Scheibel (1969) argue that about 30% of the Ia afferent collaterals may reach directly — i.e. without intercalated interneurons — motor

---

3 In the description of any structural detail or elements of the grey matter the lamination concept and subdivisions of Rexed (1952, 1954) are employed.

cells that supply antagonistic pairs of muscles, no evidence from this emerges from the sample analysed by SZENTÁGOTHAI (1967a). This may be caused by different interpretation of "motor" and "non-motor" branches of the main collaterals (compare Fig. 4A with the figures of SCHEIBEL and SCHEIBEL, 1969).

Fig. 4A shows two representative Ia collaterals and interpretation of branches reaching motoneurons by slightly overstressing their thickness, and of the "non-

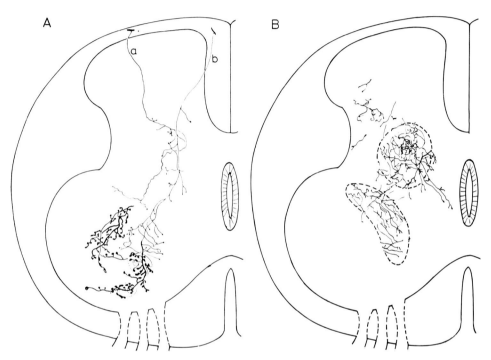

Fig. 4. A. Two collaterals of Ia primary afferents from a newborn kitten: Golgi stain. Terminal branches ending in the motor nucleus are in fact somewhat coarser than those directed to non-motor nuclei of the grey matter, but this difference has been exaggerated in the drawing. B. Superimposed drawing of the "non motor" terminal branches of ten Ia collaterals. The two regions containing massive termination of such branches are encompassed by dashed lines.
From SZENTÁGOTHAI (1967a)

motor" branches by leaving them as thin as seen in the preparation. Fig. 4B shows the "non-motor" side branches of ten Ia collaterals selected from the same lumbar segment of a kitten. The arborization fields (indicated by dashed lines) are more informative for the interneurons that are reached potentially by the side branches (to be discussed under the headings 3.2.4 and 3.3).

STERLING and KUYPERS (1967b) assumed on the basis of degeneration results that the terminal branches synapsing with motoneurons would turn into longi-tudinal direction and then might establish climbing type synapses with the motoneuron dendrites. This is denied by SCHEIBEL and SCHEIBEL (1969), who, on the contrary, emphasize that the final arborization of the Ia collaterals is restricted to neuropil sheets of transversal orientation. Collaterals to the motor nucleus are issued by Ia afferents not only in the segment of entrance but also in the two neighbouring segments, their number appears to fall off very quickly in the second neighbouring segment both in ascending and descending direction (Szent-ágothai, 1961 a).

2.4.2 Collaterals to the Centre of the Dorsal Horn. This is a special group of collaterals of smallish caliber, arising from the depth of the root entrance zone of the dorsal funiculus. They have an almost horizontal course before breaking up into the dense neuropil predominantly in the medial part of the neck and the head of the dorsal horn (laminae IV and V). These collaterals are illustrated in much the same way both in early classical studies (see Fig. 113 by Ramón y Cajal, 1909) and in recent investigations (Scheibel and Scheibel, 1969 [Fig. 1]).

As cutaneous afferents according to physiological studies (Wall, 1967) reach both laminae IV and V, it is reasonable to assume that many of these collaterals are the branches of small and medium size calibered cutaneous afferents. However, visceral afferents were recently found to send collaterals specifically to lamina V (Selzer and Spencer, 1969) and since they are delta fibers, some of the collaterals belonging to this set may be visceral afferents.

2.4.3 Collaterals to the Intermediary Region. This group is the most diverse and hence the least known. Among a number of unknown types only one can be identi-fied with certainty: (a) the side branches of Ia collaterals. Another with reasonable confidence (b): the collaterals of Ib (tendon organ) afferents. And finally (c) a more ambiguous medial marginal group of primary afferent collaterals can be separated.

(a) *The side branches of Ia (muscle spindle) collaterals* to the intermediary region have been mentioned already in paragraph 2.4.1 and appear to belong to two distinct populations (Fig. 4 B). The more dorsal side branches have a focus of arborization in the middle third of lamina VI (Szentágothai, 1967 a; Scheibel and Scheibel, 1969). The ventral group of side branches has a focus of termination in a half-moon shaped area of lamina VII, immediately adjacent to the medial border of the motoneuron pool. The possible significance of this latter group in conveying reciprocal inhibition in the stretch reflex has been shown recently by Hultborn et al. (1968).

(b) *Ib (tendon organ) afferent collaterals can be* identified tentatively (Fig. 5 A) as relatively large calibered collaterals that do not reach motoneurons and arborize in a more extended field of laminae VI and VII. There is a good agreement between the dorsal arborization field of the Ia collateral side branches and an area of above 20 % maximum focal potential found by Eccles et al. (1954 c, 1960) for Ia afferents on one hand, and between the larger termination territory of the assumed Ib (Fig. 5 A) collaterals and the area of above 20 % maximum potentials generated by Ib afferents (see also Sprague and Ha, 1964). Additional evidence for the Ib nature of this group of collaterals will be presented in connexion with the primary afferent collaterals of Clarke's column (Fig. 6 B); see paragraph 2.4.4.

(c) *The medial marginal group* of primary afferent collaterals is well recogniz-able in dorsal radicotomy degeneration material (Sprague and Ha, 1964 [Figs. 6

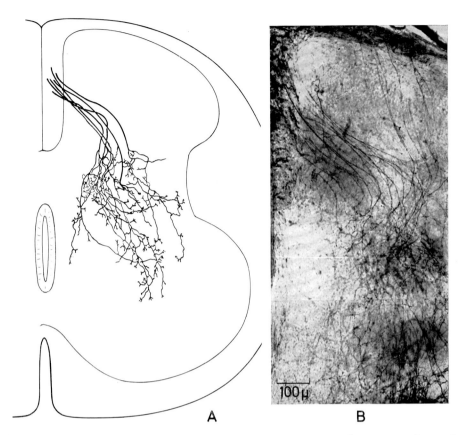

Fig. 5. A. Camera lucida drawings of coarse collaterals not entering the motor nucleus and hence considered as originating from Ib primary afferents. The termination field extends over a wide central area of laminae VI and VII. Kitten lumbar enlargment, rapid Golgi stain. B. Photomicrograph of a Golgi preparation of the lumbar enlargement of a kitten (series from which Figs. 4 and 5 A have been extracted), showing the tendency of the coarse dorsal funiculus collaterals to cross in the intermediate region (see RAMÓN Y CAJAL's drawing in Fig. 2).
Both Ia and Ib collaterals are stained in this material. Medial is to the left

and 8]). Some authors interpret them as reflex collaterals contacting medioventral motoneurons (SPRAGUE and HA, 1964; SCHEIBEL and SCHEIBEL, 1969), other results (SCHIMERT, 1939; SZENTÁGOTHAI, 1966a; IMAI and KUSAMA, 1969) would rather indicate that they are a separate group. This is born out by recent Golgi studies (RÉTHELYI, 1968) according to which this — at least in the upper lumbar and lower thoracic cord — is a well identified specific group of collaterals terminating in the medial part of lamina VII and in lamina VIII (Fig. 6D).

Unfortunately there is no identified anatomical counterpart of flexor reflex afferents that according to physiological evidence (HONGO et al., 1966) ought to have a wider field of arborization than found by any collateral arborization known in the Golgi picture. This field ought to be even wider than permitted by the degeneration results after dorsal radicotomy. The only anatomical explanation of

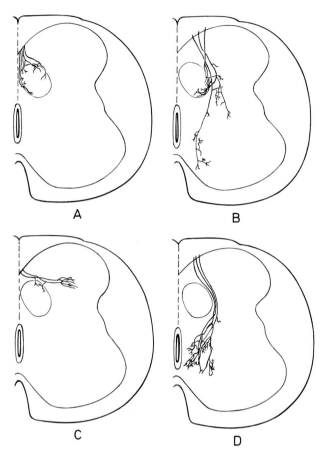

Fig. 6. Four sets of primary afferent collaterals from the level of Clarke's column (upper lumbar segments). A = main group considered as Ia collaterals, B = group of the supposed Ib collaterals (see text). C = collaterals directed to the centre of the dorsal horn and giving side branches to Clarke's column. D = medial bundles of primary afferent collaterals, directed to lamina VII and VIII. Branches of this set do not seem to make contact with the medial motoneurons. Réthelyi (1968)

this discrepancy would be to assume that flexor reflex afferents contact in many cases distal parts of dendrites.

2.4.4 Primary Afferent Collaterals to Clarke's Column. The primary afferent collaterals to Clarke's column arise from the depth of Burdach's tract somewhat mediad to the root entrance zone (v. Lenhossék, 1895; Ramón y Cajal, 1909). This corresponds to the fact that before giving collaterals to the column, primary afferents of lumbar and sacral origin have to ascend for at least two segments after having entered the cord (Schimert, 1939; Szentágothai, 1961b); this is not so upward from Th_9 (Szentágothai, 1966a) where collaterals are already issued to neurons situated in the region comparable to Clarke's column in the segment of entrance. Primary afferents entering the column turn immediately into longitudinal direction and give rise to a longitudinally oriented terminal plexus (RAMÓN Y CAJAL, 1909 [Fig. 118]). Synaptic relations will be discussed in paragraph 3.4.2. The primary afferent fibers give several collaterals to Clarke's column during their ascent (LLOYD and McINTYRE, 1950; SZENTÁGOTHAI and ALBERT, 1955; SZENTÁGOTHAI, 1961 b; RÉTHELYI, 1968); these collaterals are shifted more mediad the longer the distance of their ascent. Primary afferents belonging to any given lumbosacral segment thus occupy an almost sagittal disc in Clarke's column sloping upwards slightly in medial direction (SZENTÁGOTHAI, 1961 b). For the segment L_4, for example, this disc starts in L_1 at the lateral side of the column and reaches the level of Th_{10} on its medial side. There is, of course, considerable overlap between neighbouring and even some between second neighbouring segments.

Three different types of primary afferent collaterals (Fig. 6) have been separated recently, which can be identified with fair probability with three specific types of afferents (RÉTHELYI, 1968): (i) A main group (Fig. 6A) occupying the dorsomedial three quarters of the nucleus, and hence (LUNDBERG and OSCARSSON, 1956) are undoubtedly collaterals of Ia (muscle spindle) afferents; (ii) another group — originating more laterally in the dorsal funiculus and directed rather indiscriminately to a wide area of the intermediate region — give side branches to a ventrolateral sector of the column (Fig. 6 B). Identification of this group with Ib (tendon organ) afferents is based on the following evidence: (a) they are relatively coarse, (b) their main termination is similar to the group shown in Fig. 5 (paragraph 2.4.3), (c) they have contacts with a smaller fraction of Clarke neurons (LUNDBERG and OSCARSSON, 1956), (d) lack convergence upon the same neurons with Ia afferents (LUNDBERG and OSCARSSON, 1956; JANSEN et al., 1966), and finally (e) the first collaterals given to the column by any segment during the ascent of its fibers belong to this group (OSCARSSON, 1957; RÉTHELYI, 1968 [Fig. 6]). (iii) A third group are collaterals, giving side branches to the column, directed to the center (lamina IV) of the dorsal horn (Fig. 6C). Their primary afferent nature has not been verified by degeneration but it is likely that they correspond to cutaneous afferents (LUNDBERG and OSCARSSON, 1960).

2.4.5 Commissural Collaterals. Commissural axons of primary afferent nature have been assumed to occur in the dorsalmost arciform bundle of the posterior commissure (RAMÓN Y CAJAL, 1909). This has been verified by degeneration (SCHIMERT, 1939), however, the abundance of commissural afferent collaterals in the caudal segments (S_2 and S_3) has been detected only much later (SPRAGUE, 1958; SZENTÁGOTHAI, 1961 a). Some of these in S_2 have been thought by these authors to reach motoneurons directly, but this is not, so far, supported by Golgi studies (SCHEIBEL and SCHEIBEL, 1969).

2.4.6 Collaterals to the Substantia Gelatinosa. Two types of primary afferent collaterals to the substantia gelatinosa[4] can be distinguished: (a) coarse collaterals entering laminae II and III from the ventral side — they are certainly primary afferents, and (b) fine collaterals entering the dorsal horn from the dorsal side (from Lissauer's tract and the lateral superficial part of the Burdach tract); such collaterals are only partially of primary afferent origin.

---

4 See footnote 6 (on page 229) concerning cytoarchitectonic equivalents of the substantia gelatinosa.

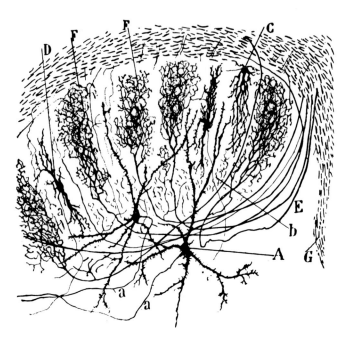

Fig. 7. Ramón y Cajal's (1909, Fig. 121) drawing of the arborization in the substantia gelatinosa of the coarse collaterals (E). Large antenna type neuron (A) of lamina IV and somewhat smaller one of Lamina III, both of whose axons (a) join the dorsal part of the lateral funiculus. C and D̊ are cells of the substantia gelatinosa proper

(a) *The coarse collaterals* have been described and illustrated first by Ramón y Cajal (1909 [Fig. 121]) reproduced here in Fig. 7. They originate from lateral parts of Burdach's tract and either penetrate through the medial part of the substantia gelatinosa or curve around its medio-ventral margin. Upon reaching lamina IV they turn back and enter laminae III and II from the ventral side. In lamina III they break up into ascending flame shaped arborizations that in transversal sections appear to separate the neuropil into lobuli (Szentágothai, 1964a) cutting vertically (or more correctly radially) through laminae II and III. It has not been recognized until the recent Golgi study of Scheibel and Scheibel (1968) that the flame-shape arborizations of Ramón y Cajal in fact are narrow sagittally (radially) oriented sheets (or discs) of neuropil, about 200 μm long and 20–30 μm wide. The relevant histological information is assembled in a plate in Fig. 8, and some transverse sections from different regions of the cord are shown in Fig. 9. Secondary degeneration after radicotomy shows that these collaterals are undoubtedly primary afferents (Szentágothai, 1964a[5]). From a large body

5 This has been questioned on the basis of alleged lack in secondary degeneration (although the degeneration shown by Szentágothai [1964a, Fig. 15] was clear enough) by Ralston (1965) and Sterling and Kuypers (1967a). With the improved degeneration techniques for fine unmyelinated axons (Fink and Heimer, 1967) the termination of primary afferents in lamina II could be shown beyond doubt (Heimer and Wall, 1968; Réthelyi and Szentágothai, 1969).

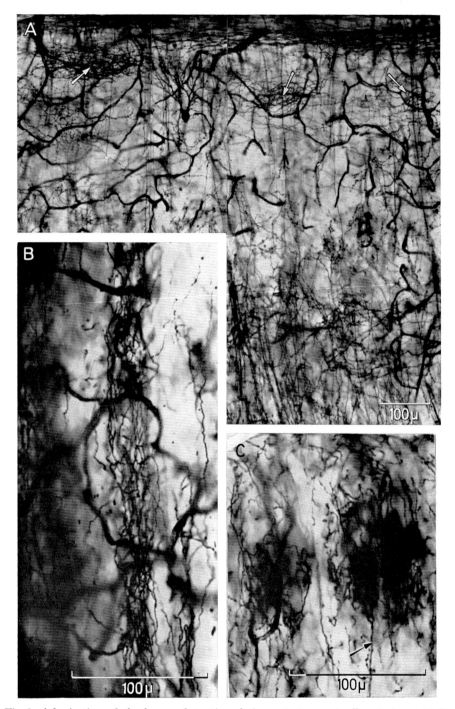

Fig. 8. Arborization of the large substantia gelatinosa (cutaneous) afferents in sagittally (radially) oriented brick-shape spaces (lobuli) of the neuropil. A = sagittal section in small magnification, showing three arborization "lobules" (arrows) and a small antenna type neuron of lamina III. B = horizontal (longitudinal perpendicular to the sagittal) plane; C = transverse section with several neighbouring lobuli, the preterminal axon branch of one is visible (arrow) entering from the ventral side. 5–7 days old kitten, lumbar cord

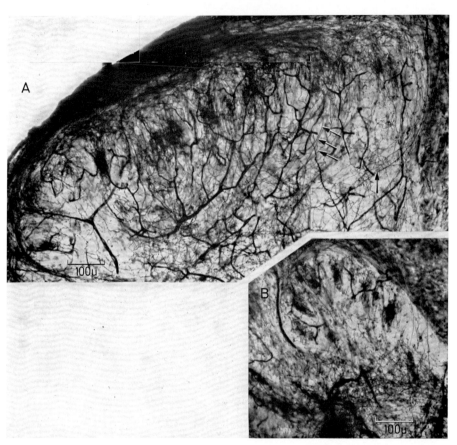

Fig. 9. Lobular arrangement of the neuropil in the substantia gelatinosa. A = transverse section from the lumbar enlargement, B = from thoracic region. 5–7 days old kitten. During later development the neuropil lobuli become elongated in dorsoventral direction. Rapid Golgi stain. Arrows point to dorsal funiculus collaterals recurving into dorsal direction

of physiological evidence it is also obvious that these collaterals correspond to low threshold cutaneous afferents.

(b) *The small calibered primary afferents* entering the substantia gelatinosa from the dorsal side are more controversial. Their primary afferent origin has been emphasized by S. W. Ranson and co-workers (Ranson, 1913, 1914; Ranson and Hess, 1915; Ranson and Billingsley, 1916) and has led to a general concept on the spinal pain pathway. Doubts against this theory (Wall, 1962) arose from the propriospinal origin of these fibers (v. Lenhossék, 1895; Ramón y Cajal, 1909; Earle, 1952). However, the primary afferent nature of part of the Lissauer tract plexus (see paragraph 1.4) has been shown by degeneration (Schimert, 1939; Szentágothai and Kiss, 1949; Szentágothai, 1964a). Due to the mixed origin of the fine calibered Lissauer's tract fibers, it is difficult to decide from Golgi pictures, whether the smaller axonal arborizations occupying the outer part of the substantia gelatinosa ("capping plexus" of SCHEIBEL and SCHEIBEL, 1968) are propriospinal or primary afferents. In the diagram given in Fig. 13 (see paragraph 3.2.1) it is assumed that they are both (SZENTÁGOTHAI, 1964a [Figs. 2 and 3]).

2.4.7 Primary Afferent Terminals in Lamina I. Little attention has been paid until very recently to the thin tangentially oriented axonal plexus (having some preference for the longitudinal direction) and nerve cells with tangentially oriented dendrites (v. LENHOSSÉK, 1895; RAMÓN Y CAJAL, 1909 [Figs. 147, 148, 149]). Degeneration after dorsal radicotomy shows clearly (Fig. 3 B) that the fine axons are mainly of primary afferent nature. Axo-somatic synapses established between the axonal plexus and the marginals cells of lamina I have been interpreted (SZENTÁGOTHAI, 1964a [Fig. 12]) as being of primary afferent origin. This lamina appears most recently to gain crucial importance through the observation by CHRISTENSEN and PERL (1970) on cells localized in lamina I of the caudal and the lumbosacral cord responding specifically to noxious mechanical and thermal stimuli.

3. Spinal Nuclei Involved in Ascending Relay, and Their Synaptic Connectivity

3.1 Cells of Origin of Second Order Sensory (and Other Ascending) Spinal Pathways

Due to technical difficulties, anatomical information about the cells of origin of various ascending tracts was scanty and rather uncertain until very recently when intracellular techniques in neurophysiology contributed greatly to the clarification of the situation. As the ascending tracts themselves are outside the scope of this review the problem of their origin will be discussed in the following paragraphs mainly from the viewpoint of possible connexions with primary afferents.

3.1.1 Cells of the Spinocervical Tract. It has been realized only recently that part of the tactile (and perhaps also pain) information is relayed through an ascending tract in the dorsal part of the lateral funiculus (MORIN, 1955) that has been identified as the spinocervical tract (NORSELL and VOORHOEVE, 1962; ANDERSSON, 1962). The tract terminates in the upper cervical segments (ECCLES et al., 1960; LUNDBERG and OSCARSSON, 1961; LUNDBERG, 1964; TAUB and BISHOP, 1965).

A comparison of (i) the origin of axons entering the area of this tract from spinal neurons in the Golgi picture (v. LENHOSSÉK, 1895; RAMÓN Y CAJAL, 1890; MATSUSHITA, 1969; and also from our own unpublished material), (ii) the cyto-architectonic lamination (REXED, 1954), and (iii) the localization of thirty-six spinocervical tract neurons established by intracellular recording (HONGO et al., 1968) leads to the conclusion that the cells of origin of the spinocervical tract are localized in laminae III, IV and V.

There is one specific group of neurons at the dorsal border of lamina IV: the *large antenna type neurons* (Figs. 7 and 10) that can be identified quite easily with the cells of origin of the spinocervical tract. They are arranged in a neat row

(Fig. 10) and send their dendrites vertically (or more correctly radially) through the entire depth of the substantia gelatinosa (Fig. 7). The dendrites would thus have ample opportunity to get into multiple contacts with the sagittally oriented neuropil sheets ("lobuli") brought about by the terminal arborization of the large cutaneous afferents (2.4.6). According to the localization of spinocervical tract neurons established with intra- and extracellular recording (HONGO et al., 1968) the antenna type neurons could contribute only to a small fraction of the total neuron population giving rise to this tract. Many of the cells identified as giving rise to spinocervical tract fibers appear to be localized in the deeper strata of lamina IV and in lamina V, some even in lamina III.

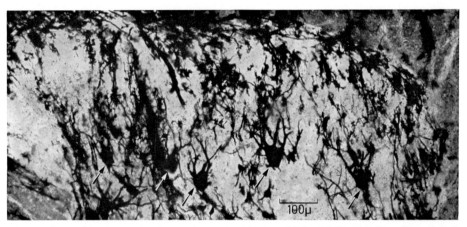

Fig. 10. Large antenna type neurons (arrows) of lamina IV (and III) with dorsally oriented dendrites. Adult cat, L₇ perfusion Golgi-Kopsch stain

A substantial number of medium size and even larger cells in the "head of the dorsal horn" (corresponding to laminae III [ventral part] — lamina IV — dorsal part of lamina V) have very long, longitudinally oriented, dendrites (Fig. 11) and axons joining the dorsal part of the lateral funiculus. They are embedded into the longitudinally oriented axonal plexus of the dorsal horn, which is largely primary afferent in origin (STERLING and KUYPERS, 1967a). As seen in Fig. 3, this plexus extends from lamina III well into lamina V, however, it is difficult to judge how much of the plexus is preterminal (note relative coarseness of degenerated fragments) and how much is really terminal. Taking into account the criteria for identification of spinocervical tract neurons by HONGO et al. (1968), it is reasonable to assume that large cutaneous afferents also have other collaterals than the large flame-shape arborizations of the substantia gelatinosa. The longitudinal plexus in the dorsal horn centre is undoubtedly fed partially by cutaneous afferents.

3.1.2 Cells of Origin of the Crossed Anterolateral (Spinothalamic) Tract. The exact site of origin of the crossed anterolateral ascending tract fibers (the classical spinothalamic tract of EDINGER) is still controversial. Lack of degeneration changes in the anterior commissure following lesions placed into the dorsal horn, and appearance of degenerated commissural fibers whenever the lesion included the

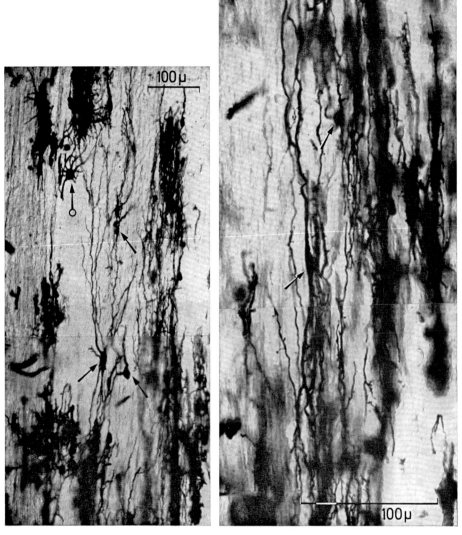

Fig. 11. Cells with longitudinally oriented dendrites in the head (center) of the dorsal horn (arrows). Cell indicated by ringed arrow in left part of left photomicrograph belongs to the lateral surface of the dorsal horn. Adult cat, Th_{13}, perfusion Golgi-Kopsch procedure

intermediate region was interpreted by assuming that the dorsal horn proper does not contribute significantly to the antero-lateral ascending tract (SZENTÁGOTHAI, 1951, 1964b). This appears not quite correct in the light of new observations on the localization of some cells giving rise to some crossed fibers of the ventral spinocerebellar tract in the lateral part of lamine V (HUBBARD and OSCARSSON, 1962). From a recent systematic study of the crossed and uncrossed initial portions of spinal interneuron axons (MATSUSHITA, 1970) it appears that the vast majority of cells contributing axons to the crossed ascending tracts are localized in the intermediate region and the ventral horn (Fig. 12).

As two ascending tracts at least originate from the commissural cells shown in Fig. 12: the spinothalamic and the ventral spinocerebellar tract, the corresponding two cell populations ought somehow to be separated. There are reliable data only for the cells giving rise to the ventral spinocerebellar tract (to be discussed in

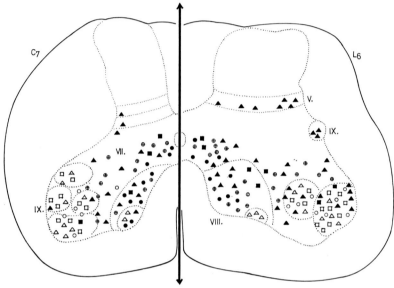

Fig. 12. Locations of interneurons in the 7th cervical (left) and the 6th lumbar (right) segments, giving rise to crossed ascending fibers (solid symbols) and to ventral root fibers (open symbols). Symbols containing crosses indicate cells with unidentified destination of their axons. Large neurons are indicated by quadrats, medium sized neurons by triangles, and small ones by circles. From Matsushita (1970)

paragraph 3.1.4) which appear to arise mainly from the lateral part of laminae V and VI as well as from the lateral part of the ventral horn. This leaves for the origin of the classical spinothalamic tract mainly the larger commissural cells in the medial part of lamina VII and in lamina VIII. It will be recalled that this region receives a quite massive inflow of primary afferent collaterals (Fig. 6D), termed the medial marginal group (2.3.4c).

3.1.3 Clarke's Column and the Dorsal Spinocerebellar Tract. The origin of the dorsal spinocerebellar tract from the large neurons of Clarke's column is well known (see early bibliography in Ramón y Cajal, 1909). A unique feature (in the spinal tract) of this nucleus is its "close" character, i.e. that practically all dendrites of its neurons arborize within the territory of the nucleus, and few dendrites of other cells enter this territory. This makes it easy to trace the course of various types of afferents to their specific regions of termination (2.4.4). Interneurons and synaptic relation of Clarke's column will be discussed in paragraph 3.2.3.

Very unfortunately the relatively well known character and connectivity of Clarke's column (Szentágothai and Albert, 1955; Szentágothai, 1961b;

RÉTHELYI, 1968, 1970) applies only to its lower part (T$_9$–L$_3$). Virtually nothing is known about apparently similar large neurons having exactly the same positions in the middle and upper thoracic segments, and receiving a very substantial inflow from collaterals of primary afferents that have entered both through the same and in the neighbouring dorsal roots (SZENTÁGOTHAI, 1966a). Two mainly longitudinal terminal plexuses of primary afferent origin have been distinguished in the intermediomedial region (IMAI and KUSAMA, 1969): a ventro-medial and a dorso-lateral. The dorso-lateral is fed only by dorsal roots arising from the roots of the intumescentiae, while the ventromedial plexus is ubiquitous. Clarke's column can be partially, but not completely, identified with the dorsolateral plexus, but it is unknown what type of secondary cells correspond to the dorso-lateral plexus fed by the roots of the brachial plexus. The ventro-medial primary afferent plexus of IMAI and KUSAMA (1969) may contact partly the anterior ascending tract neurons (3.1.2), however, there are numerous relatively large neurons in this region (see for example Fig. 145 of RAMÓN Y CAJAL, 1909) sending their axons into the ipsilateral lateral funiculus.

3.1.4 Cells of Origin of the Ventral Spinocerebellar Tract. As this is a crossed tract of mainly large calibered fibers (HÄGGQVIST, 1936; SZENTÁGOTHAI-SCHIMERT, 1941a) any large (and perhaps also some medium size) cell(s) in the lumbar enlargement (and below) can be considered as a potential ventral spinocerebellar cell(s). Comparing the positions of large and medium size commissural cells (Fig. 12) as found by MATSUSHITA (1970) and the localization of physiologically-identified intermediate region ventral spinocerebellar neurons (HUBBARD and OSCARSSON, 1962) a fairly good agreement is found for large commissural neurons in the lateral part of laminae V, VI and VII. If additionally the field of terminal arborization of Ib primary afferents deduced from Fig. 5 is considered there is a substantial common territory even for the cell bodies, without taking into account the dendrites. This is in good agreement with the fact that Ib afferents are the chief monosynaptic primary afferent source of a physiologically well defined group of spinocerebellar tract fibers (ECCLES et al., 1961a; HUBBARD and OSCARSSON, 1962). The assumption that the border cells of Cooper and SHERRINGTON (1940) of the ventral horn might be cells of origin of the ventral spinocerebellar tract is in acceptable agreement with the location of some medium size commissural cells at the lateral border of the ventral horn (Fig. 12). Recently, direct anatomo-physiological evidence for the origin of ventral spinocerebellar tract fibers from the border cells has become available (JANKOWSKA and LINDSTRÖM, 1970). Physiological studies (BURKE et al., 1971) seem to indicate that the spinal border cells are the main source of the ventral spinocerebellar tract. The fact that this group of cells receives considerable monosynaptic input from Ia muscle afferents is also in fair agreement with the arborization of their collaterals (Fig. 4). However, their synaptic input appears to be much more complex than assumed hitherto (LUNDBERG and WEIGHT, 1971): some more dorsally located cells of this group receive monosynaptic convergence from Ia and Ib afferents, some even have no monosynaptic input from primary afferents. The location of the cells receiving monosynaptic Ib input (BURKE et al., 1971) can be reconciled with the arborization of the supposed Ib afferents as shown in Fig. 5 if it is assumed that the synapses are in contact with the dendrites. A remarkable new hypothesis has been for-

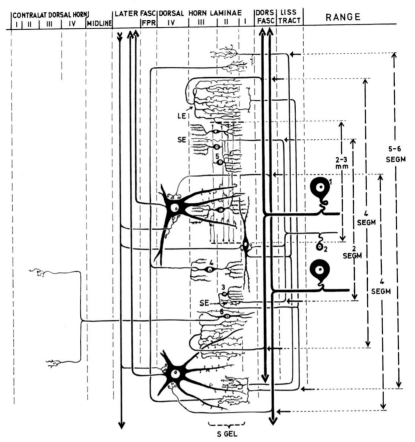

Fig. 13. Diagram illustrating neuronal connections of the substantia gelatinosa in an imaginary longitudinal section plane that runs through all relevant structures, to illustrate maximal distances bridged (at right). The several tracts of the white, and the laminae of the grey matter are indicated above. 1 = spinal ganglion cell of large cutaneous afferent, 2 = cell of small "C" afferent, 3 = substantia gelatinosa neuron giving rise to Lissauer tract, and 4 = issuing lateral tract propriospinal fibers, 5 = substantia gelatinosa neurons giving rise to the longitudinal fine axonal plexus of the substantia gelatinosa itself, 6 = commissural substantia gelatinosa neuron. LE are large (lobular) end arborizations of the large calibered cutaneous afferents, SE are small end arborizations of C or delta fibers. The connections of the large antenna type neurons in lamina IV are shown tentatively, particularly in the upper cell. Slightly modified from Szentágothai (1964a)

warded by Lundberg (1971) most recently on the basis of the synaptic inputs for the spinal border cells about the possible role of ventral spinocerebellar neurons as comparing and feeding back information about the excitatory and inhibitory influences conveyed onto motoneurons. This hypothesis is well in accord with all known anatomical facts.

3.2 Interneurons and Synaptic Arrangements Involved in Ascending Relay

Interneurons are involved in two different ways in the relay of sensory impulses towards higher levels: (a) either truly intercalated into the pathway as an essential neuronal link for the transmission of impulses from the primary afferents to the ascending tract neurons, or, conversely, (b) arranged in parallel with (or superimposed upon) the main chain of transmission, subserving various mechanisms of parallel (collateral), recurrent, and/or reciprocal inhibition (or perhaps reinforcement). Arrangement (a) is present, obviously, wherever transmission from primary afferents to ascending tract neurons is di- or multisynaptic; type (b) occurs where the transmission is predominantly monosynaptic, as for example in Clarke's column. As the relay to the ascending tracts is, in most cases, monosynaptic as well as di- and multisynaptic, this distinction is largely of theoretical value and the two types of arrangements occur generally in combination. The specific interneuron groups of the monosynaptic reflex pathway will be discussed briefly in a separate subdivision (3.3).

3.2.1 The Substantia Gelatinosa. Due to various types of neurons, showing highly specific arborization patterns of dendrites, as well as due to similarly specific arrangement of the neuropil, neuronal architectonics and connectivity of the substantia gelatinosa was relatively well explored by the early neurohistologists (v. LENHOSSÉK, 1895; RAMÓN Y CAJAL, 1909); a recent combined Golgi and degeneration study (SZENTÁGOTHAI, 1964a) yielded the neuron connectivity as shown diagrammatically in Fig. 13. The important new observation by SCHEIBEL and SCHEIBEL (1968) on the sagittal (radiate) laminar organization of both dendritic and terminal axonal arborizations (mentioned already in paragraph 2.4.6) has been taken into account in this diagram, which is thus a somewhat modified version of our original drawing (SZENTÁGOTHAI, 1964a [Fig. 3]). The diagram in Fig. 13 is largely self explanatory and has to be understood as an imaginary longitudinal (sagittal or radial) section passing through all relevant structures[6]. There are three predominant features in this neuron system: (a) The self contained (or circular) neuron arrangement, i.e. most neurons feed back to the same system either by axons ascending and descending in Lissauer's tract or in the most dorso-medial part of the lateral funiculus (SZENTÁGOTHAI, 1964a). (b) The "crossing-over" type synaptic arrangement between many of the terminal axon branches[7] and dendrites. On analogy with the molecular layer of the cerebellar cortex it can be assumed that the longitudinally oriented dense axonal neuropil — mainly propriospinal (local) in origin (SZENTÁGOTHAI, 1964a) — could drive (or influence) synaptically the neurons in lamina III (Fig. 11) and the large antenna type neurons (Fig. 10) over their spiny dendrites ascending through the substantia gelatinosa (Fig. 14). (c) The neuron network is fed by two types of primary afferents, of which the coarse at least are probably mainly cutaneous (2.4.6).

---

6 It has been a matter of argument, whether only lamina II ought to be considered as substantia gelatinosa as originally described by REXED (1954) or, conversely, lamina III be included (SZENTÁGOTHAI, 1964a; RALSTON, 1965; STERLING and KUYPERS, 1967a; SCHEIBEL and SCHEIBEL, 1968). This is more a matter of viewpoint: in certain respects lamina II is indeed different from lamina III (RALSTON, 1965; RÉTHELYI and SZENTÁGOTHAI, 1969) while in others, for example in cell types, lamina III is a gradual transition towards lamina IV.

7 This expression is taken over from the characteristic synaptic relation between parallel fibers and spines of Purkinje cell dendrites in the cerebellar cortex (HÁMORI and SZENTÁGOTHAI, 1964) which this arrangement strongly resembles.

Since there is no ascending axonal system originating directly from the substantia gelatinosa, forward conduction through the spinocervical tract may depend on, or at least be influenced by, the synaptic stimulation of lamina III and IV neuron dendrites by the "crossing-over" synaptic system of the substantia gelatinosa. The same might apply in inverse manner to the large tangential neurons in lamina I, the dendrites of which may enter the substantia gelatinosa too (v. Lenhossék, 1895; Ramón y Cajal, 1909).

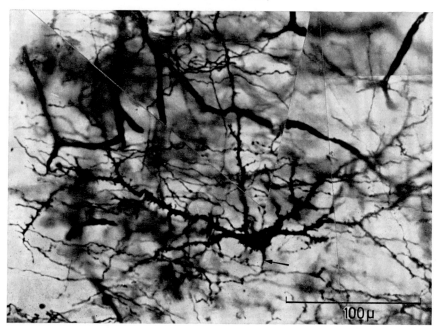

Fig. 14. Medium size antenna type neuron of lamina III, with characteristic "spiny" dendrites ascending through the fine longitudinal axonal plexus of the substantia gelatinosa. Sagittal sections from the lumbar cord of a kitten, rapid Golgi procedure. The origin of the longitudinally oriented axon is indicated by an arrow

Specific synaptic arrangements have been found in electron microscope studies (Ralston, 1965; Réthelyi and Szentágothai, 1965; Kerr, 1966) in lamina II. These are synaptic complexes organized in characteristic manner around large sinuous axon terminals of intraspinal origin, and with the participation of primary afferent axon terminals as well as of dendrite endings and dendritic spines. An attempt at an explanation of the neuron connectivity in these synaptic complexes has been made by Réthelyi and Szentágothai (1969) on the basis of combined Golgi and degeneration studies both at the light and the electron microscope level. This arrangement and interpretation is shown diagrammatically in Fig. 15 and might be used as a structural basis for various mechanisms of primary afferent depolarization (Wall, 1962; Schmidt, 1968; Zimmermann, 1968; Jänig and Zimmermann, 1971) or may even serve as basis for speculations on gate control mechanisms that are postulated to exist in the pathway for pain (Melzack and Wall, 1965, see also Wall, Chapter 8).

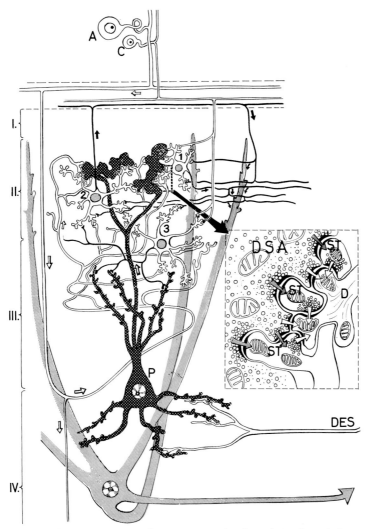

Fig. 15. Diagram illustrating neuronal arrangement in the substantia gelatinosa and the various elements connected in the synaptic complexes (in dashed square EM diagram at right). Lamination of REXED is indicated at left margin. The diagram represents a longitudinal section of the dorsal horn. Two primary sensory afferents are indicated: a large calibered (probably cutaneous afferent A and an unmyelinated small calibered afferent C). They establish contacts with three SG neurons (1–3) two of which belong to lamina II, whereas the third (3) is somewhat larger and is situated (partly) in lamina III. Pyramidal cell (P, cross hatched) situated at the border of lamina III and IV receives contacts from interneuron (3) and possibly also directly from large primary afferent (A). The dorsally directed short axon of the pyramidal neuron participates in the SG synaptic complexes. It is assumed that only A fibers participate in the complexes but this is not certain. Forward conduction from the SG is secured by large lamina IV neuron (hatched), the dendrites of which are embedded into the longitudinal axonal plexus of the SG (in right upper part of diagram; c.f. SZENTÁGOTHAI, 1964). — EM diagram at right shows ultrastructural arrangement in a part of a synaptic complex. Central dense sinuous axon terminal (DSA) is in contact with dendritic ends (D) of substantia gelatinosa neurons and presynaptic to smaller axon terminals (ST) that are mainly primary afferent endings (although some might be also axon terminals of SG neurons). White arrows indicate in this part of the figure ordinary synapses and hatched arrows axo-axonic synapses. Direction of the arrows shows the polarity of the synapse as it would appear from structural criteria. From RÉTHELYI and SZENTÁGOTHAI (1969)

3.2.2 Dorsal Horn Proper. It is difficult to translate into modern architectonic terms (lamination of Rexed, 1954) the classical expressions head (or centre) of the dorsal horn *(nucleus proprius cornus posterioris)*. The difficulty is caused mainly because the cytoarchitectonic borders do not match with those of dendroarchitectonics and neuropil architectonics. The longitudinally oriented axonal plexus — mainly of primary afferent origin (Sterling and Kuypers, 1967a, see also Fig. 3) — corresponds to lamina III, IV and dorsal part of V. Some, although by no means all, of the cells in this region have longitudinally oriented exceedingly long dendrites (Fig. 11). With respect to dendrite orientation the cells of this territory can be subdivided into (i) antenna type neurons, smaller in lamina III (Fig. 14) and large ones in lamina IV (Figs. 7 and 10), with dendrites oriented mainly towards the substantia gelatinosa; (ii) central cells with longitudinally oriented dendrites (Fig. 11); (iii) a third group of cells, mainly in lamina V with transversally oriented dendrites. A considerable number of cells, however, of both laminae IV and V have all the above three types of dendrites in combination (Scheibel and Scheibel, 1966a), so that probably only a limited number of the dorsal horn proper neurons can be classified into one of the above categories. The nucleus of the dorsal horn proper is, therefore, a term corresponding to neuropil architectonics rather than to cytoarchitectonics. One might consider that the neuron population belonging to this nucleus is predominantly related synaptically to the central longitudinal axonal plexus of the dorsal horn. Conversely, it seems more appropriate to exclude from this group large interneuron populations at the base of the dorsal horn especially in its medial and lateral region. These interneuron groups will be included into the general interneuron system of the intermediate region and the ventral horn (paragraph 3.2.4).

The main ascending relay neurons of the dorsal horn proper are the cells of the spinocervical tract (discussed already in 3.1.1). However, a very considerable fraction of the dorsal horn central nucleus neurons are either relatively short propriospinal neurons or even short local interneurons. Very little is known about the dorsal horn propriospinal neurons (Szentágothai, 1951) since it is difficult in degeneration experiments to separate them from the propriospinal neurons at the base of the dorsal horn that have to be considered as belonging to the general interneuron system of the spinal cord. Numerous very short interneurons are present in the central part of the dorsal horn with axons that immediately break up into profuse terminal branches. Whether they can be considered as true Golgi 2nd type neurons is a matter of argument — they are certainly not the same classical Golgi 2nd type neurons as are found in abundance for example in the cerebral cortex — but the richness of the local axonal arborization of such a cell is shown in a photomicrograph in Fig. 16. The abundance of IPSP-s of different origins on various types of interneurons in this region (Hongo et al., 1966) as well as very specific types of inhibitory connexions involved in ascending relays through the dorsal horn would certainly require many and rather specifically arranged inhibitory interneurons. The abundance of various types of synaptic contacts, characterized by different sizes and shapes of synaptic vesicles would favour the assumption that the short axon cells of the type shown in Fig. 16 are indeed inhibitory interneurons.

3.2.3 Clarke's Column. Clarke's column is the only site of ascending relay where the combination of relay (ascending tract) neurons and interneurons

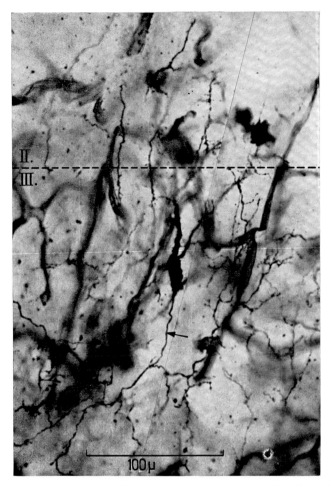

Fig. 16. Short axon cell of lamina III, axonal arborization ascending towards lamina II. Border between lamina II and III is indicated. Axon is indicated by arrow. 7 days old kitten, cervical cord, rapid Golgi procedure

appears to be relatively clear and straight-forward. The two types of neurons: the main dorsal spinocerebellar tract cells (cellules focales) and the smaller border cells (cellules marginales ou limitantes) were clearly described by RAMÓN Y CAJAL (1909). In a recent Golgi study the border cells have been described (RÉTHELYI, 1968) as typical interneurons with few irregular dendrites bearing sparsely distributed but otherwise characteristic spines. The axon, as far as can be traced, arborises within Clarke's column. The accounts given by other recent Golgi studies (BOEHME, 1968; LOEWY, 1970) differ somewhat in minor aspects but not sufficiently to be reviewed here in detail.

The incorporation of interneurons into the relay from primary afferents to dorsal spinocerebellar tract neurons has been considered on the basis of light microscope degeneration studies (SZENTÁGOTHAI and ALBERT, 1955; SZENTÁ-

GOTHAI, 1961 b) but this is now superseded by more detailed electron microscope level information (Réthelyi, 1970). Fig. 17 tries to explain the known facts about synaptic relations, in which the very large (giant) and repeated (climbing type) terminals of primary afferents on the relay cells can be identified clearly. Two types of probably inhibitory interneuron terminals, originating from the border cells, can also be identified. Strangely they may be both presynaptic and postsynaptic according to localization. Excitatory interneuron terminals, of extracolumnar origin, can be found on both the relay and the border cells. There is no convincing evidence about the relation between the primary afferents and the supposedly inhibitory border cells. These structural details appear to be in relatively good agreement with the physiological findings on (i) transmission characteristics from primary afferents to relay neurons (Lloyd and McIntyre, 1950; Jansen et al., 1966; Kuno and Miyahara, 1968), (ii) involvement of excitatory interneurons (Grundfest and Campbell, 1942; Laporte et al., 1956; Holmquist et al., 1956; Eccles et al., 1961 b; Jansen et al., 1966; Kuno and Miyahara, 1968), and (iii) of inhibitory interneurons (Curtis et al., 1958; Jankowska et al., 1964; Hongo and Okada, 1967).

3.2.4 The General Interneuron System of the Intermediate Region and the Ventral Horn. The reasons for lumping together large parts of the grey matter (parts of lamina V, lamina VI and VII and again parts of lamina VIII) are manifold: (i) *cytoarchitectural lamination* (Rexed, 1954), convincing in laminae I–IV, becomes increasingly ambiguous from lamina V onwards; (ii) *neuropil architecture*, although of clear segregation into sagittally oriented sheets in lamina II–III, and exhibiting additionally a conspicuous horizontal lamination in laminae I, II, III, IV and even partly in lamina V, becomes organized into transversally oriented discs (Scheibel and Scheibel, 1968) cutting straight through from V into IX; (iii) *neuropil systematics* (i.e. terminal distribution of axons belonging to various categories) exhibits little if any tendency of laminar distribution (in the sense of Rexed's); (iv) there is no apparent relation between laminar location of cells and destination of their axons, apart from the general rule, that ascending tract axons originating from cells localized dorsally from a horizontal plane passing through the dorsal edge of the central canal are more likely to join the ipsilateral, and those from cells localized ventrally are generally ascending in the contralateral lateroventral funiculi (Oscarsson, 1964).

The main difficulty in evaluation of the possible functional significance of interneuron connections in this part of the spinal grey matter lies in the apparent structural irregularity. In order to understand and to appreciate the spinal grey matter as a neuron network three types of neurons and four aspects of interneuron connectivity have to be considered.

Neuron types: (a) *Relay neurons* giving rise to the long ascending tracts have been discussed already in paragraphs 3.1.2 and 3.1.4. It is likely that the large size cells and probably some, if not all, of the medium size cells, particularly those with axons that join the anterior commissure (Fig. 12) belong to this category. (b) *Medium range propriospinal neurons*, probably mainly small and medium size cells, with both crossed and uncrossed axons. The total distal range of their connections has been found in the lumbar enlargement (Szentágothai, 1951, 1964 b) to be about 5–7 segments. Descending connections appear to be more

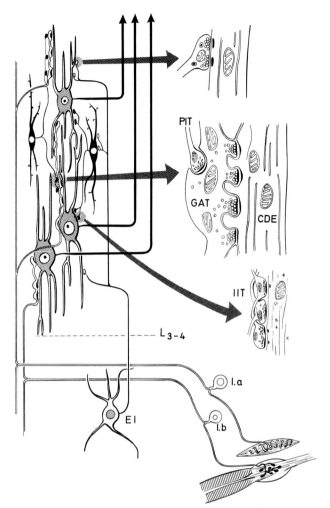

Fig. 17. Neuronal and synaptic arrangement in Clarke's column. The DSCT neurons (stippled) are contacted by very large (giant) climbing type terminals of either Ia or Ib afferents. Excitatory interneurons (EI) situated below the segmental level L_3–L_4 send small contacts containing spheroid vesicles (upper right ultrastructure diagram) to both the DSCT neurons and to smaller so-called border cells of the column. Which are assumed to be inhibitory and are, therefore, drawn in full black. These border cells may either contact the main DSCT neurons directly by small synapses containing flattened vesicles (lower right ultrastructure diagram) or may establish presynaptic inhibitory contacts (PIT) with the large (giant GAT) terminals of the primary (probably mainly Ia) afferents (middle ultrastructural diagram at right; CDE = Clarke DSCT) dendrites. Modified after Réthelyi (1968, 1970)

abundant and longer (3–5 segments) than ascending ones (2–3 segments). They establish synaptic contacts mainly in the intermediate region and in the ventral horn (laminae V–IX). (c) A group of *very short propriospinal interneurons* identified recently by the complete tracing of their axon arborization (Mannen, 1969) are probably the real (general) local interneurons of the spinal cord. The total

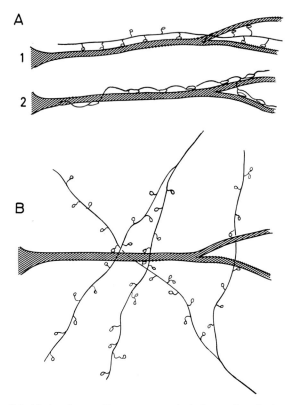

Fig. 18. Two possible kinds of synaptic arrangements between terminal axon branches and dendrites (hatched): A = parallel arrangement that may be either of the "rope-ladder" type (1) or of the true "climbing" type (2); B = "crossing-over" arrangement

range of their axon is a few hundreds of microns; however, one cell of the sample with a total axonal span of 2200 microns might indicate that there are transitions between type (b) and type (c). These cells are probably mainly of the small size group, and their axons or axon branches may repeatedly cross and recross, mainly through the anterior commissure but occasionally also through the posterior.

The important four aspects and/or approaches that have to be considered or used in order to appreciate the neuron connectivity of the general central grey of the spinal cord are as follows: (i) Observation of a single axonal arborization conveys little if any information. In order to appreciate the functional significance of any kind of connection a *population analysis* of similar arborizations has to be made (Figs. 4, 5, 6). This renders it possible to establish the termination focus of this particular type of arborization and to recognize with what group of the neurons the connections are predominantly made. (ii) *The relations between the terminal axon ramifications and the dendrites.* Apart from the dorsal horn and the motor nucleus (SZENTÁGOTHAI, 1964b) axo-somatic synapses seem to be of little significance in the general interneuron system of the spinal cord. It is a very rare observation that any terminal axon branch would be directed specifically to a cell body and would be seen to establish a group of synaptic contacts with the body of the same cell. What has to be considered, therefore, in this central region of the spinal cord are axo-dendritic interrelations. In the geometric relations between axons and dendrites two extreme cases have to be distinguished. Either the preterminal axon branches run in parallel with the dendrites and establish repeated synaptic contacts (Fig. 18A), which may be either of the real "climbing type" or of the "rope-ladder type"; the latter is the more common in the central grey substance of the spinal cord. The other possibility (Fig. 18 B) is that the preterminal fiber crosses the dendrites at random angles and establishes only one or two synaptic contacts with any given neuron. The overwhelming majority of the contacts in the central grey (laminae V–VIII) are of this type. The preterminal branches of the axons cross large parts of the intermediate region and non-motor parts of the ventral horn in remarkably straight course and issue short terminal branches seemingly indiscriminately to whatever dendrite or cell body they come across during their entire course (SZENTÁGOTHAI, 1967b). The only significant exception to this is found in the lateral part of the base of the dorsal horn (lamina V) and in the lateral part of the intermediate region (lamina VI and VII) where horizontally oriented dendrites are in fairly parallel orientation with the preterminal branches of the corticospinal fibers (SCHEIBEL and SCHEIBEL, 1966a, [see their Figs. 3 and 4]). It seems probable on numerous analogies (Clarke's column, cerebellar climbing fibers) that the parallel arrangement corresponds functionally to a very strong, and the crossing arrangement to a very weak contact. (iii) *Neuropil lamination.* The axonal neuropil is not oriented at random but, as pointed out recently by SCHEIBEL and SCHEIBEL (1968, 1969), organized into transversal sheets in the ventral horn and to some extent in the intermediate region (laminae VII, VIII and IX). Although this has been described primarily for the primary afferent collaterals, it applies equally to the collaterals originating from any part of the white matter, i.e. the lateral and the ventral funiculus. As dendritic orientation is predominantly in the transversal plane of the cord in interneurons (SCHEIBEL and SCHEIBEL, 1969) and is assumed to be more longitudinal in the motoneurons, this would mean that there is a higher probability of parallel arrangement between dendrites and preterminal axon branches (with the functional consequences as discussed in [ii]) for interneurons than for motoneurons where the axo-dendritic arrangement would be entirely of the crossing-over type. The important functional consequences were discussed in much detail by SCHEIBEL and SCHEIBEL (1969) and are largely beyond the scope of this review. (iv) *The great abundance and profuse arborization of initial axon collaterals.* A glance at the drawings by RAMÓN Y CAJAL (1909; [see Figs. 141, 143 and 146]) shows convincingly the fundamental importance of initial collaterals in the local connectivity of the spinal interneuron network. The large number and the importance in synaptic connectivity of initial collaterals and/or very short interneurons become apparent also from more recent Golgi (SZENTÁGOTHAI, 1964b, 1967a; MATSUSHITA, 1969; MANNEN, 1969) and degeneration studies (SZENTÁGOTHAI, 1967a and b). It appears, for example, that probably the vast majority of the motoneuron synapses belong to short local connections (SZENTÁGOTHAI, 1967b, see also paragraph 3.3 and Fig. 20). Since initial collaterals are given by both long ascending tract and by medium range propriospinal neurons, the two groups cannot be separated from each other (for the time being) with respect to their role in local connectivity.

3.2.4.1 *Medio-Central Group of the Dorsal Horn Base*, occupying mainly central parts of lamina VI, but protruding somewhat into the two neighbouring laminae (V and VII). Corresponds mainly to the dorsal arborization field of side branches of Ia collaterals (Fig. 4).

3.2.4.2 *Central Field*, in complete overlap with 3.2.4.1, however, extending far beyond in lateral and ventral direction. Corresponds to the arborization of assumed Ib collaterals (Fig. 5), and to massive degeneration field of primary afferent collaterals (SPRAGUE and HA, 1964). Agreement with location of interneurons monosynaptically excited by group I muscle afferents (HONGO et al., 1966) is fairly good, with the exception that some cells localized physiologically are situated more dorsally in laminae IV and V. Congruence between the two territories and the localization of movement receptors by the Wall technique (WALL, 1967; WALL et al., 1967; POMERANZ et al., 1968) is somewhat better than with cytoarchitectonic borders (REXED, 1954). This will be discussed in more detail in Paragraph 4.

3.2.4.3 *Lateral (External) Basilar Region of the Dorsal Horn.* This territory corresponds to the focus of arborization of the corticospinal fibers (SZENTÁGOTHAI-SCHIMERT, 1941b; CHAMBERS and LIU, 1957; NYBERG-HANSEN and BRODAL, 1963; SCHEIBEL and SCHEIBEL, 1966a). Interneurons of this region are assumed to have specific significance in conveying corticospinal impulses to the motor nucleus (VASILENKO and KOSTYUK, 1966; VASILENKO et al., 1967). Indeed abundant connections could be traced from this region to the motor nucleus by degeneration (SZENTÁGOTHAI, 1951, 1964b), and specific short connections of this kind have been shown by MATSUSHITA (1969).

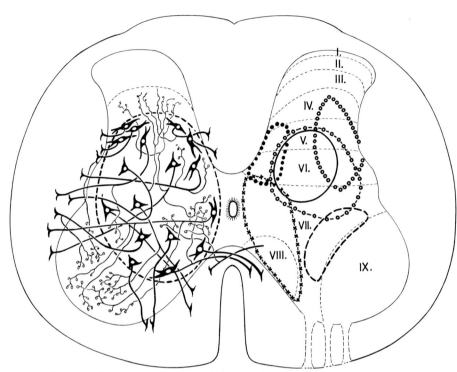

Fig. 19. The general interneuron system of the spinal cord. At left a number of interneurons are assembled from drawings by M. v. Lenhossék (1895), Ramón y Cajal (1909), Szentágothai (1967a), Matsushita (1969) indicating the principal orientation of their axons, and distribution of initial axon collaterals. The coarse dashed line in the left part of the drawing indicates the border of the central interneuron core as illustrated in Fig. 22. — At right an attempt is made at subdividing functional groups of interneurons on the basis of their opportunity to get into abundant contact with certain types of presynaptic elements. The region engulfed by an uninterrupted line corresponds to the dorsal termination territory of nonmotor side branches of Ia afferent collaterals and the region surrounded by dashed line to the ventral arborization territory of non-motor side branches of the same afferents (see Fig. 4B). The region engulfed by the dash-circle-dash line corresponds to the massive arborization on territory of Ib afferents (Fig. 5). The line of open circles engulfs territory of massive termination of pyramidal tract fibers (Scheibel and Scheibel, 1966a), the territory surrounded by dashX-dash line corresponds to arborization region of the medial primary afferent collateral bundle (Fig. 6D). The line of full circles surrounds the medial basilar region (further explanation in 3.2.4.4)

3.2.4.4 Medial Basilar Region of the Dorsal Horn. ("noyau basilaire interne" of Ramón y Cajal, 1909). Well recognizable in regions where Clarke's column is not developed. Axons of the more dorsal cells join the propriospinal tract of the dorsal funiculus, the more ventral cells send their axons to the lateral funiculus (Ramón y Cajal, 1909 [Fig. 146]) and have very numerous initial collaterals to wide areas of the dorsal and ventral horn, including the motor nucleus (Szentágothai, 1967a [Figs. 5 and 6; cells labeled "a"]). Some of the cells are posterior commissural neurons (Matsushita, 1969). The afferents of this region are ill-understood. Most of them appear to arise from the depth of the posterior funiculus, hence, they might be propriospinal. However, this region receives also a great abundance of primary afferents from the segments below (Schimert, 1939; Imai and Kusama, 1969), especially in the upper cervical region where this nucleus is especially well developed.

3.2.4.5 Central and Medial Part of the Ventral Horn. Apart from specific inhibitory inter-neurons to be mentioned briefly in 3.3, it is difficult to subdivide the remaining ventral part of the general interneuron system into separate territories that could be defined by any struc-tural or connection criterion. The medial part of the ventral horn (lamina VIII, and medial regions of VII) receives a special set of medial marginal primary afferent collaterals, and is the focus of termination of vestibulospinal (SCHIMERT, 1938; NYBERG-HANSEN and MASCITTI, 1964) and of the pontine reticulospinal fibers (TORVIK and BRODAL, 1957; NYBERG-HANSEN, 1966). The more central and lateral parts of the ventral horn and the intermediate region (laminae VI and VII) receive the bulk of rubrospinal (SZENTÁGOTHAI-SCHIMERT, 1941b; NYBERG-HANSEN, 1966) tectospinal (STAAL, 1961; NYBERG-HANSEN, 1966) and medullary reticulospinal (NYBERG-HANSEN, 1965) descending systems.

Synaptic architecture on the electron microscope level is only generally known. A number of apparently different types of synaptic terminals can be seen in all parts of this territory (BODIAN, 1966, 1970). Identification of the terminals containing flattened vesicles with inhibitory endings, and those containing spheric vesicles with excitatory endings is still somewhat uncertain. Specific studies on the synaptic architecture in the various fields, mentioned above are urgently needed. Such work has been started recently for the external basilar region (DYACHKOVA et al., 1971).

3.3 Specific Groups of Inhibitory Interneurons

There is ample physiological evidence for the existence of specific inhibitory interneurons in all parts of the spinal grey matter. The occurrence of very short interneurons (MANNEN, 1969) in all parts of the grey matter (Fig. 16), and of synaptic terminals containing flattened synaptic vesicles (BODIAN, 1966; GRAY, 1969; CONRADI, 1969; RÉTHELYI and SZENTÁGOTHAI, 1969; RÉTHELYI, 1970), would support this view from the anatomical side, provided that the UCHIZONO (1965, 1967) concepts of the functional significance of flattened vesicles should be proven correct. The fact that terminals with flattened synaptic vesicles are always of intraspinal origin, and certainly do not occur in the endings of primary afferents (CONRADI, 1969; RÉTHELYI and SZENTÁGOTHAI, 1969; RÉTHELYI, 1970) is in good agreement with the physiological observation (HONGO et al., 1966) that IPSP-s set up from primary afferents on any spinal neuron are invariably disynaptic. ECCLES (1968) enumerates twelve sites in the spinal cord where there is good evidence that inhibitory interneurons are intercalated into postsynaptic inhibitory pathways. Clarification of the inhibitory pathways by step for step cross-corre-lation of physiological and structural data is often complicated by the presence of presynaptic connections (and/or interactions), as has been shown in 3.2.1 for the substantia gelatinosa and in 3.2.3 for Clarke's column.

Two kinds of physiologically well defined (ECCLES et al., 1954a and b) inhibi-tory interneurons appear now at long last (and at least) safely localized:

3.3.1 It was logical to look for the *reciprocal inhibitory interneurons of the Ia monosynaptic reflex pathway* first in the intermediate region (ECCLES et al., 1956; ECCLES et al., 1960) where indeed terminate many sidebranches of the Ia col-laterals (Fig. 4). Only more recently the interneurons were found (HULTBORN et al., 1968) to be localized much more ventrally in lamina VII in the region corresponding to the arborization focus (Fig. 4) of the ventral group of "non-motor" side branches of the Ia collaterals.

3.3.2 The Renshaw Cell Recurrent Inhibition Concept (ECCLES et al., 1954a) has been questioned repeatedly on the basis of Golgi studies (SCHEIBEL and SCHEIBEL, 1964, 1966b) and alternative hypotheses have been offered for the observed phenomena (WEIGHT, 1968; KOELLE, 1969). Experimental anatomical studies (SZENTÁGOTHAI, 1958; and corroborated later on EM level, SZENTÁGOTHAI, 1967c) substantiated the prediction (ECCLES et al., 1954a) that the initial axon collaterals of motoneurons contact small interneurons at the medial border of the motor nucleus. A "population analysis"[8] of the arborization field of the initial collaterals of fifty identified motoneurons (SZENTÁGOTHAI, 1967a) corresponds exactly to the original physiological postulates and with intracellular localization of supposed Renshaw cells by THOMAS and WILSON (1965). Some small cells in this region and slightly mediad on the border of lamina VIII, have been found in Golgi material to contribute most connections to motoneurons (MATSUSHITA, 1969; RÉTHELYI, unpublished). Most recently cells identified as Renshaw cells by intracellular technique have been shown not only to be located as predicted, but to be typical short interneurons (JANKOWSKA, personal communication) The profuse arborizations of their axons could well account for inhibitory terminals to the reciprocal inhibitory interneurons (3.3.1) as inferred from physiological observations (HULTBORN et al., 1968) and for the recurrent disinhibition effects described much earlier (WILSON and BURGESS, 1962).

The structural substrates of these inhibitory effects could be the numerous terminals on motoneurons containing flattened vesicles (BODIAN, 1966; CONRADI, 1969). Interestingly, the synapses persisting on the surface of motoneurons in chronically isolated ventral horn preparations (SZENTÁGOTHAI, 1958) are different in the case if — as judged from the size of the remaining ventral horn fragment — only Renshaw cells have survived besides motoneurons, or if part of the centre of the ventral horn (containing the supposed reciprocal Ia pathway inhibitory interneurons, 3.3.1) remained intact too. In the first case only exceedingly small synaptic terminals remain intact (Fig. 20 upper insets) whereas in the latter ordinary size boutons containing either flattened or spheric vesicles (Fig. 20) are preserved (SZENTÁGOTHAI, 1967c). These might correspond to short (reciprocal) inhibitory and excitatory connections. That such connections may be abundant is quite obvious from Golgi preparations (see [iv] in paragraph 3.2.4). Since the spinal border cells of the ventral horn, giving rise to ventral spinocerebellar tract fibers, cannot be separated from motoneurons in the visual degeneration pictures, or under the electron microscope, everything said in this paragraph on the connections of inhibitory interneurons is equally applicable to these ventral spinocerebellar tract neurons. The new hypothesis of LUNDBERG (1971) of the comparator role of these neurons fully accounts for these possibilities.

---

8 The discrepancy between the observation of SCHEIBEL and SCHEIBEL (1966b) and SZENTÁGOTHAI (1967a) can be explained probably by the different criteria used for identification of motor axons. In the latter study, entrance of the axon into the intraspinal ventral rootlet bundle was considered not sufficient. Only axons being considered as unequivocal motor that could be traced into the extraspinal rootlets (see cell [d] in Fig. 5 of SZENTÁGOTHAI, 1967a).

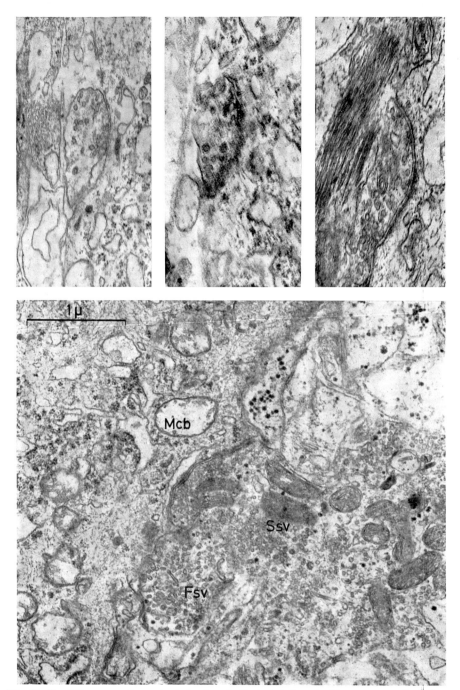

Fig. 20. Persisting synaptic contacts in chronically isolated ventral horn preparation. Upper row of insets from an isolated ventral horn fragment containing only motoneurons and part of the region immediately medially of the motor nucleus where the Renshaw cells are assumed to be located. Only very small axon terminals somewhat impressed into motoneuron body or dendrite surface remained intact. Lower figure shows motoneuron cell body (McB) in contact with two synaptic terminals: one smaller having flattened synaptic vesicles (Fsv) and a larger containing spheroid vesicles (Ssv). This is from a chronically isolated ventral horn preparation, in which part of the ventral horn centre with various types of interneurons was left intact.

(From SZENTÁGOTHAI, 1967c)

3.4 Commissural Systems

3.4.1 The Dorsal Commissural System. The dorsal commissure shows considerable differences in various parts of the spinal cord: it is particularly well-developed in the upper cervical region (Fig. 21) and consists of three distinct bundles in the lower thoracic and upper lumbar segments (Ramón y Cajal, 1909 [Fig. 119]): (a) a dorsal arciform, (b) a middle horizontal, and (c) a ventral arciform bundle. Only a small part of the (more dorsal) commissural fibers are primary sensory in nature (Schimert, 1939; Scheibel and Scheibel, 1969), apart from

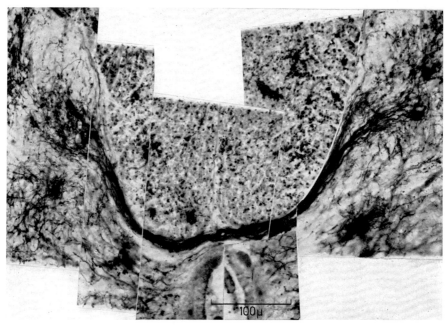

Fig. 21. Dorsal commissure from the upper cervical segments of a young dog. Rapid Golgi procedure. Some of the fibers appear both to arise and to terminate in the substantia gelatinosa (lamina II); certainly from and to lamina III

the caudal part of the spinal cord, where commissural primary afferents are abundant (2.4.5). According to the impression conveyed by Fig. 21 a considerable number of dorsal commissural fibers originates and terminates in the dorsal horn, even some from the substantia gelatinosa (at least from lamina III), (v. Lenhossék, 1895; Szentágothai, 1964a) but this is doubted by Matsushita (1969) who thinks that dorsal commissural axons originate mainly from larger cells at the medial base of the dorsal horn. This is probably correct for the fibers of the middle bundle, while fibers crossing the ventral bundle probably originate from intermediate region cells. Some of the very short neuron axons cross in the posterior commissure (Mannen, 1969). Fibers originating from the dorsal horn and ascending or descending in the lateral funiculus may give collaterals crossing the posterior commissure (Szentágothai, 1951); according to Golgi pictures, collaterals of this type arborize in the intermediate region (Ramón y Cajal, 1909).

3.4.2 The Anterior Commissure. The overwhelming majority of axons crossing in the anterior white commissure are relatively coarse, and hence are obviously long axons of the ascending relay systems. However, all axons upon crossing have both ascending and descending branches. Thus the long ascending neurons obviously have a secondary role in conveying crossed descending short or medium range connections. Their cells of origin have been mapped recently by MATSUSHITA (1970) and his most important summarizing figure is reproduced here in Fig. 12. Also the axons of the very short interneurons traced by MANNEN (1969) cross mainly in the anterior commissure generally immediately after their origin from the cell. Only in one out of the six cells completely traced did a branch of the axon recross through the anterior commissure some 800 microns from the level of the cell body. The same conclusion was reached from degeneration studies, showing that in focal lesions of the spinal grey matter there is abundant degeneration in the anterior commissure in the segment of the lesion but virtually none in neighbouring and more distant segments (SZENTÁGOTHAI, 1951). In this respect the two commissures are radically different. From the long descending systems only the pontine reticulospinal fibers appear to contribute significantly to the anterior commissure (NYBERG-HANSEN, 1966). Probably also the preterminal branches of uncrossed anterior tract pyramidal fibers may cross finally in the anterior commissure but information about this is uncertain.

The initial collaterals of the anterior commissural axons have very characteristic courses and distributions. Collaterals to the ipsilateral grey matter (with reference to the portion of the cell body) are given mainly by cells situated in lamina VIII. They arborize in the most medial parts of the intermediate region (lamina VI and VII). Contralateral collaterals do not, generally, enter the motor nucleus but take a straight course along its dorsomedial border in lamina VII (SZENTÁGOTHAI, 1967a [Fig. 6]). Their short side branches may, of course, contact dendrites of motoneurons, however, they are more likely to have abundant contacts with interneurons of lamina VII.

4. General Structural Concept of the Spinal Segmental Apparatus

After having reviewed in the preceding divisions the numerous, often seemingly unrelated and even controversial, details on how incoming primary sensory impulses might be distributed within a couple of adjacent segments and towards the main lines of ascending relay, it is now appropriate to discuss the spinal segmental apparatus as a whole. An attempt at this has been made already earlier (SZENTÁGOTHAI, 1967b) with more emphasis on the neurogenetic point of view. This side of the whole argument will not be repeated here in detail[9], as it would lead far astray from the original objective of this review. Only certain structural aspects will here be emphasized instead.

---

9 Also in view of the fact that an analysis of the spinal segmental apparatus from the neurogenetic (neuroembryology) point of view will be given soon by Dr. GEORGE SZÉKELY on whose experimental studies most of our (J. Sz.) 1967 reasoning were based (see also an earlier review of SZÉKELY, 1966).

The accumulated body of evidence furnished by behavioral and physiological studies on embryonic transplantation, deplantation and organic recombination experiments with the spinal segmental apparatus (Székely and Szentágothai, 1962a and b; Székely, 1963; Strazniczky, 1963; Szentágothai, 1962) can be summed up for an appraisal of the functional capacities of the spinal segment as follows:

(i) All segments (or groups of segments) of the early medullary tube are equivalent with respect to the capacity of conducting ascending and descending impulses, irrespective how in transplantation experiments the position (sequence) along the neuraxis (or craniocaudal direction) of segments (or segmental groups) had been changed.

(ii) The several segmental groups have strictly determined functional capacities (determination for specific capacities occurs relatively early during embryonic development) enabling them to set into play a limited number of movement patterns — either of reflex or of more complex behavioral character.

(iii) There is a very limited degree of interchangability, for example, between lumbosacral and brachial segments, with the functional results limited to using the "inappropriate" limb according to the inherent movement patterns of the respective segmental group.

(iv) Specific segmental sensory information is non-essential for the production of the basic movement patterns of various segmental groups.

There are also some other general conclusions emerging from such studies, however, as they are irrelevant for this review they will be neglected for the present. As segmental sensory inflow appears to be non-essential for the specific movement patterns of the several segmental groups, it is reasonable to assume that the basic movement patterns are "programmed" in the general (local) interneuron network.

The concepts that will be expounded in the following are based, therefore, on the idea that in looking for the fundamental structuro-functional design of the spinal segmental apparatus the dorsal horn proper, i.e. laminae I–IV on one hand and lamina IX on the other ought to be considered as the dorsal (sensory) and the ventral (motor) appendages and ought to be detached from the real interneuron system, the *central core* of double-cylindric shape. This is shown diagrammatically in Fig. 22 taken over with some minor changes in detail from an earlier paper (Szentágothai, 1967b) in which these concepts were first outlined. The idea was originally developed mainly on the basis of certain differences in synaptic architecture and it was not thought to be an alternative to the laminar cytoarchitectonic concept of Rexed (1954). Most recently, however, the study of perfusion Kopsch-Golgi specimens of the adult spinal cord has revealed dendroarchitectonic pictures that seem to indicate that there is more cytoarchitectonic reality in the concept of a cylindric central core in the spinal grey matter than one might have expected (to be described in detail elsewhere, Réthelyi, 1972). Strangely, the Golgi pictures of new-born or very young animals, in which, for technical reasons, the structure of the spinal cord has always been studied, show little if anything of this characteristic dendritic architecture. It has been mentioned previously that the subdivisions of the grey matter into essentially horizontal (or slightly curved) cytoarchitectonic layers is quite obvious for laminae I–IV, but becomes increasingly unclear in laminae V–VIII. In the illustrations of Rexed (1954) the borders between layers are initially curved, running parallel with the posterior surface of the dorsal horn, but ventrad to lamina IV the borders between lamina IV and V, V and VI, VI and VII become clearly horizontal. This does not at all tally with the observations of Wall and coworkers (Wall, 1967; Wall et al., 1967; Pomeranz et al., 1968) in which the borders between territories having common functional characteristics (apparently corresponding to laminae IV, V and VI) are by no means horizontal but show a distinct convexity in dorsal direction. This would

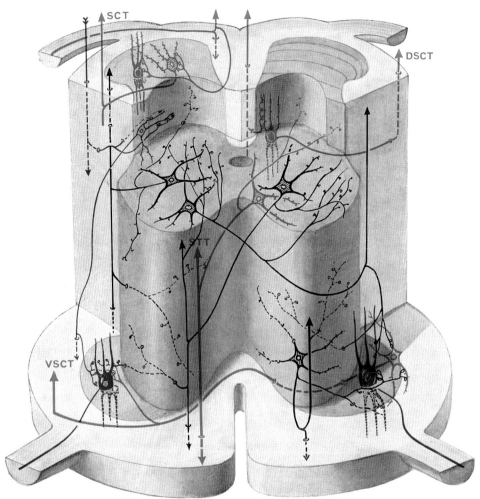

Fig. 22. Stereodiagram illustrating the double-cylinder central core concept of the general spinal interneuron system. Neurons of this system are indicated in black. The secondary ascending tract neurons giving rise to the dorsal spinocerebellar (DSCT), ventral spinocerebellar (VSCT), spinothalamic (STT) and spinocervical (SCT) tracts are drawn in blue. The corticospinal tract and its relay neurons are indicated in red. The relay neurons drawn in colour are generally not — although may act occasionally as — parts of the central core interneuron system. Adapted from an earlier version of Szentágothai (1967b)

certainly agree much better with the assumption of a cylindric organization of the central core of the spinal grey matter, as proposed in Fig. 22.

The central core of the segmental interneuron apparatus would include laminae V–VII of Rexed entirely, and perhaps parts — although not the large antenna neurons — of lamina IV. Whether the medial marginal layer of the ventral horn (lamina VIII) can be included, could be a matter of argument, since the structural organization is somewhat disarranged by the scattered groups of medioventral motoneurons. An attempt was made at indicating, in Fig. 22, the fundamental difference in general synaptic arrangement between the dorsal horn proper and motor nucleus on one hand, and the central core on the other. While synaptic arrangements indicative of a more or less "selective" or "linear" connectivity are predominant in the dorsal horn proper and the motor nucleus (Szentágothai, 1964b) the overwhelming majority of the connection arrangements are established by straight preterminal axon branches crossing large parts of the central core and giving seemingly indiscriminately, short terminal branches with one, or at maximum two, boutons to any cell or dendrite. The functional consequences of this have been discussed in paragraph 3.2.4 (see also Szentágothai, 1964b). Also the dendritic architecture differs somewhat in the central core from that in the dorsal and ventral appendages.

This was first recognized by Leontovich and Zhukova (1963) who gave a very clear account of the characteristic dendro-architectonics in the reticular core of the spinal cord and the brain stem. They termed the dominant cell type of the central core having few dendrites, with indetermined although generally radiate pattern, as "reticular type" cells. The so-called specific cells — more characteristic in the specific nuclei of the brain stem — have dendritic arborization patterns that in one way or the other are more determined in directions, numbers, lengths, branchings etc.; i.e. both in geometry and topology of the dendritic trees. This idea was elaborated upon, and with more emphasis on various types of the "specific" cells of Leontovich and Zhukova (1963), by Ramón-Moliner and Nauta (1966) who distinguished on dendroarchitectonic basis three main cell types in the CNS: "isodendritic" corresponding essentially to the reticular type cell of Leontovich and Zhukova, the "allodendritic" corresponding to the specific cells, and "idiodendritic" as third cell type with dendritic trees still more elaborate and determined both in geometry and topology of the branching pattern. In the spinal cord the differences are often marginal, so that Ramón-Moliner and Nauta (1966) did not classify the spinal cord cells in terms of their new concept. The small neurons of the substantia gelatinosa could be classified as a transitory type of the "allodendritic" and the "idiodendritic" type, while large parts of the dorsal horn neurons and the motoneurons are transitions between the isodendritic and the allodendritic type. It is interesting to note that these concepts with essentially the same functional consequences were developed completely independently from the viewpoint of dendroarchitectonics (Leontovich and Zhukova, 1963; Ramón-Moliner and Nauta, 1966) and from that of synaptic architecture (Szentágothai, 1964b) and the convergence and agreement of the two trends of thought became apparent only much later (Szentágothai, 1966b)[10].

This does not mean, of course, that the "central core" does not contain neurons or synapses corresponding more to the requirements of ascending or descending relay. Clarke's column, for example, although being a part of the central double cylindric core (Réthelyi, 1972), has both allodendritic neurons and a semilinear synaptic arrangement. The ascending relay neurons of the ventral spinocere-

---

10 In fact authors were playing around with such ideas much earlier than that. Rudiments of this way of looking at neural structure can be found already in Ramón y Cajal (1909, 1911). Similar concepts, although still somewhat vague were developed by Bodian (1952) and Szentágothai (1952) but they were perhaps too general in approach and had little influence upon the development of thoughts in neuroanatomy.

bellar tract in the lateral part of lamina V and VI and the Cooper-Sherrington border cells, as well as the crossed anterolateral tract cells mainly in lamina VIII, cannot be classified as belonging to the interneuron system, although they are scattered between the interneurons of the central core. It could also be a matter of argument, whether the cells for the corticospinal relay to motoneurons in the lateral part of the dorsal horn base are relatively specific relay elements or true interneurons.

It would be mistaken to push such arguments, as the categories are not so distinct in reality. Obviously, the same neuron may act as ascending or descending relay neuron with its main axon but at the same time may be part of the local interneuron system by means of its initial collaterals. Also as mentioned in paragraph 3.4.2, the axons of the crossed ascending relay neurons also have descending branches that serve, obviously, some local or intersegmental connection purposes (Fig. 22).

But this does not invalidate the general idea of a structuro-functional division of the spinal segmental apparatus into a general central "computer" with inbuilt functional programs (or subroutines) in the different segmental groups (like the brachial segments for the fore-limb movements and the lumbosacral segments for the hind-limb movements; tail segments for tail movements etc.) and dorsal appendages for reception and processing predominantly of the more specific cutaneous sensory input, and ventral appendages for immediate execution of the movements. The spinal stations for ascending and descending relay appear to have a more dualistic position being at once parts of the central "computer" and have also some independence as links for more or less linear relay.

References

ANDERSSON, S. A.: Projection of different spinal pathways to the second somato sensory area in cat. Acta physiol. scand. **56**, Suppl. 194 (1962).

BODIAN, D.: Introductory survey of neurons. Cold Spr. Harb. Symp. quant. Biol. **17**, 1–13 (1952).

BODIAN, D.: Synaptic types on spinal motoneurons: an electron microscopic study. Bull. Johns Hopk. Hosp. **119**, 16–45 (1966).

BODIAN, D.: An electron microscopic characterization of classes of synaptic vesicles by means of controlled aldehyde fixation. J. Cell Biol. **44**, 115–124 (1970).

BOEHME, C. C.: The neuronal structure of Clarke's nucleus of the spinal cord. J. comp. Neurol. **132**, 445–462 (1968).

BOK, TH.: Das Rückenmark. In: Handbuch der mikroskopischen Anatomie des Menschen, Bd. 4, Teil 1, Nervensystem, pp. 478–578. Ed. by W. MÖLLENDORFF. Berlin: Springer 1928.

BURKE, R. E., LUNDBERG, A., WEIGHT, F.: Spinal border cell, origin of the ventral spinocerebellar tract. Exp. Brain Res. **12**, 283–294 (1971).

CHAMBERS, W. W., LIU, C. N.: Corticospinal tract of the cat. An attempt to correlate the pattern of degeneration with deficits in reflex activity following neocortical lesions. J. comp. Neurol. **108**, 23–55 (1957).

CHRISTENSEN, B. N., PERL, E. R.: Spinal neurons specifically excited by noxious or thermal stimuli: the marginal zone of the dorsal horn. J. Neurophysiol. **33**, 293–307 (1970).

CONRADI, S.: Ultrastructure and distribution of neuronal and glial elements on the motoneuron surface in the lumbosacral spinal cord of the adult cat. Acta physiol. scand. Suppl. **332**, 5–48 (1969).

COOPER, S., SHERRINGTON, C. S.: Gower's tract and spinal border cells. Brain **63**, 123–134 (1940).

CURTIS, D. R., ECCLES, J. C., LUNDBERG, A.: Intracellular recording from cells in Clarke's column. Acta physiol. scand. **43**, 303–314 (1958).

Dyachkova, L.N., Kostyuk, P.G., Pogorelaya, N.Ch.: An electron microscopic analysis of pyramidal tract terminations in the spinal cord of the cat. Exp. Brain Res. **12**, 105–119 (1971).

Earle, K.M.: The tract of Lissauer and its possible relation to the pain pathway. J. comp. Neurol. **96**, 93–111 (1952).

Eccles, J.C.: Postsynaptic inhibition in the central nervous system. In: Structure and Function of Inhibitory Neuronal Mechanisms, pp. 291–308. Ed. by C. von Euler, S. Skoglund and U. Söderberg. Oxford and New York: Pergamon Press 1966/1968.

Eccles, J.C., Eccles, R.M., Lundberg, A.: Types of neurones in and around the intermediate nucleus of the lumbosacral cord. J. Physiol. (Lond.) **154**, 89–114 (1960).

Eccles, J.C., Fatt, P., Koketsu, K.: Cholinergic and inhibitory synapses in a pathway from motor axon collaterals to motor neurons. J. Physiol. (Lond.) **126**, 524–565 (1954a).

Eccles, J.C., Fatt, P., Landgren, S.: The "direct" inhibitory pathway in the spinal cord. Aust. J. Sci. **16**, 130–134 (1954b).

Eccles, J.C., Fatt, P., Landgren, S., Winsbury, G.J.: Spinal cord potentials generated by volleys in the large muscle afferent fibers. J. Physiol. (Lond.) **125**, 590–606 (1954c).

Eccles, J.C., Fatt, P., Landgren, S.: The central pathway for the direct inhibitory action of impulses in the largest afferent nerve fibres to muscles. J. Neurophysiol. **19**, 75–98 (1956).

Eccles, J.C., Hubbard, J.I., Oscarsson, O.: Intracellular recording from cells of the ventral spino-cerebellar tract. J. Physiol. (Lond.) **158**, 486–516 (1961a).

Eccles, J.C., Oscarsson, O., Willis, W.D.: Synaptic action of group I and II afferent fibers of muscle on the cells of the dorsal spinocerebellar tract. J. Physiol. (Lond.) **158**, 517–543 (1961b).

Fink, R.P., Heimer, L.: Two methods for selective silver impregnation of degenerating axons and their synaptic endings in the central nervous system. Brain Res. **4**, 369–374 (1967).

Flechsig, P.: Die Leitungsbahnen in Gehirn und Rückenmark des Menschen. Leipzig, 1876.

Flechsig, P.: Ist die Tabes Dorsalis eine "Systemerkrankung"? Neurol. Zentralbl. **9**, 72–81 (1890).

Foerster, O.: Symptomatologie der Erkrankung des Rückenmarks und seiner Wurzeln. In: Handbuch der Neurologie, vol. 5, pp. 349–358. Ed. by O. Bumke and O. Foerster. Berlin: Springer 1936.

Gray, E.G.: Round and flat synaptic vesicles in the fish central nervous system. In: Cellular Dynapmics of the Neuron, pp. 211–227. Ed. by S.H. Barondes. New York and London: Academic Press 1969.

Grundfest, H., Campbell, B.: Origin, conduction and termination of impulses in the dorsal spinocerebellar tracts of cats. J. Neurophysiol. **5**, 275–294 (1942).

Häggqvist, G.: Analyse der Faserverteilung in einem Rückenmarkquerschnitt (Th 3). Z. mikr.-anat. Forsch. **39**, 1–34 (1936).

Hámori, J., Szentágothai, J.: The "crossing-over" synapse: an electron microscope study of the molecular layer in the cerebellar cortex. Acta biol. Acad. Sci. hung. **15**, 95–117 (1964).

Heimer, L., Wall, P.D.: The dorsal root distribution to the substantia gelatinosa of the rat with a note on the distribution in the cat. Exp. Brain Res. **6**, 89–99 (1968).

Holmqvist, B., Lundberg, A., Oscarsson, O.: Functional organization of the dorsal spinocerebellar tract in the cat. V. Further experiments on convergence of excitatory and inhibitory actions. Acta physiol. scand. **38**, 76–90 (1956).

Hongo, T., Jankowska, E., Lundberg, A.: Convergence of excitatory and inhibitory action on interneurones in the lumbosacral cord. Exp. Brain Res. **1**, 338–358 (1966).

Hongo, T., Jankowska, E., Lundberg, A.: Post-synaptic excitation and inhibition from primary afferents in neurones of the spinocervical tract. J. Physiol. (Lond.) **199**, 569–592 (1968).

Hongo, T., Okada, Y.: Cortically evoked pre- and postsynaptic inhibition of impulse transmission to the dorsal spinocerebellar tract. Exp. Brain Res. **3**, 163–177 (1967).

Hubbard, J.I., Oscarsson, O.: Localization of the cell bodies of the ventral spinocerebellar tract in lumbar segments of the cat. J. comp. Neurol. **118**, 199–204 (1962).

Hultborn, J., Jankowska, E., Lindström, S.: Recurrent inhibition from motor axon collaterals in interneurons monosynaptically activated from Ia afferents. Brain Res. **9**, 367–369 (1968).

Imai, Y., Kusama, T.: Distribution of the dorsal root fibers in the cat. An experimental study with the Nauta method. Brain Res. **13**, 338–359 (1969).

JÄNIG, W., ZIMMERMANN, M.: Presynaptic depolarization of myelinated afferent fibers evoked by stimulation of cutaneous C fibers. J. Physiol. (Lond.) **214**, 29–50 (1971).

JANKOWSKA, E., JUKES, M.G.M., LUND, S.: On the presynaptic inhibition of transmission to the dorsal spinocerebellar tract. J. Physiol. (Lond.) **177**, 19–21 P (1964).

JANKOWSKA, E., LINDSTRÖM, S.: Morphological identification of physiologically defined neurons in the cat spinal cord. Brain Res. **20**, 323–326 (1970).

JANSEN, J.K.S., NICOLAYSEN, K., RUDJORD, T.: Discharge pattern of neurones of the dorsal spinocerebellar tract activated by static extension of primary endings of muscle spindles. J. Neurophysiol. **29**, 1061–1086 (1966).

KAHLER, O.: Faserverlauf in den Hintersträngen des Rückenmarks. Short communication at the 55th Meeting of German biologists and physicians of Eisenach. Berl. klin. Wschr. 640–641 (1882).

KERR, F.W.L.: The ultrastructure of the spinal tract of the trigeminal nerve and the substantia gelatinosa. Exp. Neurol. **16**, 359–376 (1966).

KOELLE, G.B.: Significance of acetylcholinesterase in central synaptic transmission. Fed. Proc. **28**, 95–100 (1969).

KRUGER, L., SIMINOFF, R., WITKOVSKY, P.: Single neuron analysis of dorsal column nuclei and spinal nucleus of trigeminal in cat. J. Neurophysiol. **24**, 333–349 (1961).

KUNO, M., MIYAHARA, T.: Factors responsible for multiple discharge of neurons in Clarke's column. J. Neurophysiol. **31**, 624–638 (1968).

LAPORTE, Y., LUNDBERG, A., OSCARSSON, O.: Functional organization of the dorsal spinocerebellar tract in the cat. II. Single fiber recording in Flechsig's fasciculus on electrical stimulation of various peripheral nerves. Acta physiol. scand. **36**, 187–203 (1956).

LENHOSSÉK, M. v.: Die feinere Bau des Nervensystems im Lichte neuester Forschungen. Eine allgemeine Betrachtung der Strukturprincipien des Nervensystems, nebst einer Darstellung des feineren Baues des Rückenmarkes. p. 409. Berlin: Korfeld 1895.

LEONTOVICH, T.A., ZHUKOVA, G.P.: The specificity of the neuronal structure and topography of the reticular formation in the brain and spinal cord of carnivora. J. comp. Neurol. **121**, 347–380 (1963).

LLOYD, D.P.C., McINTYRE, A.K.: Dorsal column conduction of group I muscle afferent impulses and their relay through Clarke's column. J. Neurophysiol. **13**, 39–54 (1950).

LOEWY, A.: A study of neuronal types in Clarke's column in the adult cat. J. comp. Neurol. **139**, 53–79 (1970).

LUNDBERG, A.: Ascending spinal hindlimb pathways in the cat. In: Physiology of Spinal Neurons. pp. 135–163. Ed. by J.C. ECCLES and J.P. SCHADÉ. Progress in Brain Research, vol. 12. Amsterdam: Elsevier 1964.

LUNDBERG, A.: Function of the ventral spinocerebellar tract. Exp. Brain Res. **12**, 317–330 (1971).

LUNDBERG, A., OSCARSSON, O.: Functional organization of the dorsal spinocerebellar tract in the cat. IV. Synaptic connections of afferents from Golgi tendon organs and muscle spindles. Acta physiol. scand. **38**, 53–75 (1956).

LUNDBERG, A., OSCARSSON, O.: Functional organization of the dorsal spinocerebellar tract in the cat. VII. Identification of units by antidromic activation from the cerebellar cortex with recognition of five functional subdivisions. Acta physiol. scand. **50**, 356–374 (1960).

LUNDBERG, A., OSCARSSON, O.: Three ascending spinal pathways in the dorsal part of the lateral funiculus. Acta physiol. scand. **51**, 1–16 (1961).

LUNDBERG, A., WEIGHT, F.: Functional organizations of the ventral spinocerebellar tract. Exp. Brain Res. **12**, 295–316 (1971).

MANNEN, H.: A new approach for following the total course of the axon of an individual neuron in Golgi stained successive serial sections, Preliminary Report. Proc. of the Japan Acad. vol. **45**, 633–638 (1969).

MARIE, P.: Leçons sur les maladies de la moelle. Paris: Masson, G. 1892.

MATSUSHITA, M.: Some aspects of the interneuronal connections in cat's spinal gray matter. J. comp. Neurol. **136**, 57–80 (1969).

MATSUSHITA, M.: The axonal pathways of spinal neurons in the cat. J. comp. Neurol. **138**, 391–417 (1970).

MELZACK, R., WALL, P.D.: Pain mechanisms: a new theory. Science **150**, 971–979 (1965).

MORIN, F.: A new spinal pathway for cutaneous impulses. Amer. J. Physiol. **183**, 245–252 (1955).

Nansen, F.: The structure and combination of the histological elements of the central nervous system. Bergens Museums Aarsberetning, pp. 24–214, 1886.

Norsell, U., Voorhoeve, P.: Tactile pathway from the hindlimb to the cerebral cortex in cat. Acta physiol. scand. **54**, 9–17 (1962).

Nyberg-Hansen, R.: Sites and mode of termination of reticulo spinal fibers in the cat. An experimental study with silver impregnation methods. J. comp. Neurol. **124**, 71–100 (1965).

Nyberg-Hansen, R.: Functional organization of descending supraspinal fiber systems to the spinal cord. Anatomical observations and physiological correlations. Reviews of Anatomy, Embryology and Cell Biology, vol. **39**. Berlin-Heidelberg-New York: Springer 1966.

Nyberg-Hansen, R., Brodal, A.: Sites of termination of corticospinal fibers in the cat. An experimental study with silver impregnation methods. J. comp. Neurol. **120**, 369–391 (1963).

Nyberg-Hansen, R., Mascitti, T. A.: Sites and mode of termination of fibers of the vestibulo-spinal tract in the cat. An experimental study with silver impregnation methods. J. comp. Neurol. **122**, 369–387 (1964).

Oscarsson, O.: Primary afferent collaterals and spinal relays of the dorsal and ventral spino-cerebellar tracts. Acta physiol. scand. **40**, 222–231 (1957).

Oscarsson, O.: Differential course and organization of uncrossed and crossed long ascending spinal tracts. In: Physiology of Spinal Neurons. pp. 164–178. Ed. by J.C. Eccles and J.P. Schadé. Progress in Brain Research, vol. 12. Amsterdam: Elsevier 1964.

Pomeranz, B., Wall, P. D., Weber, W. V.: Cord cells responding to fine myelinated afferents from viscera, muscle and skin. J. Physiol. (Lond.) **199**, 511–532 (1968).

Ralston, Henry J.: The organization of the substantia gelatinosa Rolandi in the cat lumbo-sacral spinal cord. Z. Zellforsch. **67**, 1–23 (1965).

Ramón y Cajal, S.: Sur l'origine et les ramifications des fibres nerveuses de la moelle embryon-naire. Anat. Anz. 85–95; 111–119, (1890).

Ramón y Cajal, S.: Histologie du Système Nerveux de l'Homme et des Vertébrés. Tome 1–2. Paris: Maloine 1909–1911.

Ramón-Moliner, E., Nauta, W. H. J.: The isodendritic core of the brain stem. J. comp. Neurol. **126**, 311–335 (1966).

Ranson, S. W.: The course within the spinal cord of the non-medullated fibers of the dorsal roots. A study of Lissauer's tract in the cat. J. comp. Neurol. **23**, 259–281 (1913).

Ranson, S. W.: The tract of Lissauer and the substantia gelatinosa Rolandi. Amer. J. Anat. **16**, 97–126 (1914).

Ranson, S. W., Billingsley, P. R.: The conduction of painful impulses in the spinal nerves. Amer. J. Physiol. **40**, 571–589 (1916).

Ranson, S. W., Hess, C. L. v.: The conduction within the spinal cord of afferent impulses producing pain an the vasomotor reflexes. Amer. J. Physiol. **38**, 129–152 (1915).

Réthelyi, M.: The Golgi architecture of Clarke's column. Acta morph. Acad. Sci. hung. **16**, 311–330 (1968).

Réthelyi, M.: Ultrastructural synaptology of Clarke's column. Exp. Brain Res. **11**, 159–174 (1970).

Réthelyi, M.: On the central core of the spinal gray matter. In preparation (1972).

Réthelyi, M., Szentágothai, J.: On a peculiar type of synaptic arrangement in the sub-stantia gelatinosa of Rolando. 8th International Congress of Anatomists, p. 99. Stuttgart: Georg Thieme 1965.

Réthelyi, M., Szentágothai, J.: The large synaptic complexes of the substantia gelatinosa. Exp. Brain Res. **7**, 258–274 (1969).

Rexed, B.: The cytoarchitectonic organization of the spinal cord in the cat. J. comp. Neurol. **96**, 415–495 (1952).

Rexed, B.: A cytoarchitectonic atlas of the spinal cord in the cat. J. comp. Neurol. **100**, 297–379 (1954).

Scheibel, M. E., Scheibel, A. B.: Are there Renshaw cells? Anat. Rec. **148**, 332 (1964).

Scheibel, M. E., Scheibel, A. B.: Terminal axonal patterns in cat spinal cord. I. The lateral corticospinal tract. Brain Res. **2**, 333–350 (1966a).

Scheibel, M. E., Scheibel, A. B.: Spinal motoneurons, interneurons and Renshaw cells. A Golgi study. Arch. ital. Biol. **104**, 328–353 (1966b).

Scheibel, M. E., Scheibel, A. B.: Terminal axonal pattern in cat spinal cord. II. The dorsal horn. Brain Res. **9**, 32–58 (1968).

Scheibel, M. E., Scheibel, A. B.: Terminal patterns in cat spinal cord. III. Primary afferent collaterals. Brain Res. **13**, 417–443 (1969).

Schimert, J.: Die Endigung des Tractus vestibulospinalis. Z. Anat. Entwickl.-Gesch. **108**, 761–767 (1938).

Schimert, J.: Das Verhalten des Hinterwurzelkollateralen im Rückenmark. Z. Anat. Entwickl.-Gesch. **109**, 665–687 (1939).

Schmidt, R. F.: The functional organization of presynaptic inhibition of mechanoreceptor afferents. In: Structure and Function of Inhibitory Neuronal Mechanisms, pp. 227–233. Ed. by C. von Euler, S. Skoglund and U. Söderberg. Oxford: Pergamon Press 1968.

Schultze, F.: Beitrag zur Lehre von der secundären Degeneration im Rückenmarke des Menschen nebst Bemerkungen über die Anatomie der Tabes. Arch. Psychiat. Nervenkr. **14**, 359–390 (1883).

Selzer, M., Spencer, W. A.: Convergence of visceral and cutaneous afferent pathways in the lumbar spinal cord. Brain Res. **14**, 331–348 (1969).

Sprague, J. M.: The distribution of dorsal root fibers on motor cells in the lumbosacral spinal cord of the cat and the site of excitatory and inhibitory terminals in monosynaptic pathways. Proc. roy. Soc. B. **149**, 534–556 (1958).

Sprague, J. M., Ha, H.: The terminal fields of dorsal root fibers in the lumosacral spinal cord of the cat and the dendritic organization of the motor nuclei. In: Organization of the spinal cord, pp. 120–152. Ed. by J. C. Eccles and J. P. Schadé. Progress in Brain Research, vol. 11. Amsterdam: Elsevier 1964.

Staal, A.: Subcortical projections on the spinal grey matter of the cat. Thesis. Leiden: Koninklijke Drukkerijen Lankhout-Immig N.V. S-Gravenhage, 1961.

Sterling, P., Kuypers, H. G. J. M.: Anatomical organization of the brachial spinal cord of the cat. I. The distribution of dorsal root fibers. Brain Res. **4**, 1–15 (1967a).

Sterling, P., Kuypers, H. G. J. M.: Anatomical organization of the brachial spinal cord of the cat. II. The motoneuron plexus. Brain Res. **4**, 16–32 (1967b).

Strazniczky, K.: Function of heterotopic spinal cord segments investigated in the chick. Acta biol. Acad. Sci. hung. **14**, 143–153 (1963).

Székely, G.: Functional specificity of spinal cord segments in the control of limb movements. J. Embryol. exp. Morph. **11**, 431–444 (1963).

Székely, G.: Embryonic determination of neuronal connections. Advanc. Morphogenes. **5**, 181–219 (1966).

Székely, G., Szentágothai, J.: Experiments with "model nervous systems". Acta biol. Acad. Sci. hung. **12**, 253–269 (1962a).

Székely, G., Szentágothai, J.: Reflex and behaviour patterns elicited from supernumerary limbs in the chick. J. Embryol. exp. Morph. **10**, 140–151 (1962b).

Szentágothai, J.: Anatomical considerations of monosynaptic reflex arcs. J. Neurophysiol. **11**, 445–454 (1948).

Szentágothai, J.: Short propriospinal neurons and intrinsic connections of the spinal gray matter. Acta morph. Acad. Sci. hung. **1**, 81–94 (1951).

Szentágothai, J.: Kísérlet az idegrendszer szöveti elemeinek természetes rendszerezésére (An attempt at a "natural systematization" of nervous elements). Magy. Tud. Akad., Biol. orv. Tud. Osztal. Közl. **3**, 365–412 (1952), Hungarian.

Szentágothai, J.: The anatomical basis of synaptic transmission of excitation and inhibition in motoneurons. Acta morph. Acad. Sci. hung. **8**, 287–309 (1958).

Szentágothai, J.: Anatomical aspects of inhibitory pathways and synapses. In: Nervous Inhibitions. pp. 32–46. Ed. by F. Florey. Oxford-London-New York: Pergamon Press 1961a.

Szentágothai, J.: Somatotopic arrangement of primary sensory neurons in Clarke's column. Acta morph. Acad. Sci. hung. **10**, 307–311 (1961b).

Szentágothai, J.: Discussion Remarks in Basic Research in Paraplegia. Ed. by J. D. French and R. W. Porter, pp. 143–150. Springfield, Ill.: Charles C. Thomas 1962.

Szentágothai, J.: Neuronal and synaptic arrangement in the substantia gelatinosa Rolandi. J. comp. Neurol. **122**, 219–240 (1964a).

Szentágothai, J.: Propriospinal pathways and their synapses. In: Organization of the Spinal Cord. pp. 155–177. Ed. by J.C. Eccles and J.P. Schadé. Progress in Brain Research, vol. 11. Amsterdam-New York: Elsevier 1964 b.

Szentágothai, J.: Pathways and subcortical relay mechanisms of visceral afferents. Acta neuroveg. (Wien) **28**, 103–120 (1966 a).

Szentágothai, J.: New anatomical concepts of the brain stem. In: Clinical Experiences in brain stem Disorders. pp. 15–28. Ed. by P. Juhász, Z. Aszalos and R. Walsa. Ac'a 25. Conventus Neuropsychiatrici et EEG Hungarici Budapestini 1966 b.

Szentágothai, J.: Synaptic architecture of the spinal motoneuron pool. In: Recent Advances in Clinical Neurophysiology, Electroenceph. Clin. Neurophysiology, Suppl. 25, pp. 4–19. Ed. by L. Widén. Amsterdam: Elsevier 1967 a.

Szentágothai, J.: The anatomy of complex integrative units in the nervous system. In: Results in Neuroanatomy, Neurohistology, Neuromorphology and Neurophysiology, pp. 9–45. Ed. by K. Lissák. Budapest: Acad. Publ. 1967 b.

Szentágothai, J.: Technical problems in the study of neural networks. Symposium on Neurobiology of Invertebrates, pp. 17–25. Budapest: Acad. Publ. 1967 c.

Szentágothai-Schimert, J.: Die Bedeutung des Faserkalibers und der Markscheidendicke im Zentralnervensystem. Z. Anat. Entwickl.-Gesch. **111**, 201–223 (1941 a).

Szentágothai-Schimert, J.: Die Endigungsweise der absteigenden Rückenmarksbahnen. Z. Anat. Entwickl.-Gesch. **111**, 322–330 (1941 b).

Szentágothai, J., Albert, A.: The synaptology of Clarke's column. Acta morph. Acad. Sci. hung. **5**, 43–51 (1955).

Szentágothai, J., Kiss, T.: Projections of dermatomes on the substantia gelatinosa. Arch. Neurol. Psychiat. (Chic.) **62**, 734–744 (1949).

Szentágothai, J., Székely, G.: Zum Problem der Kreuzung von Nervenbahnen. Acta biol. Acad. Sci. hung. **6**, 215–279 (1956).

Taub, A., Bishop, P.O.: The spinocervical tract: dorsal column linkage: conduction velocity, primary afferent spectrum. Exp. Neurol. **13**, 1–21 (1965).

Thomas, R.C., Wilson, V.J.: Precise localization of Renshaw cells with a new marking technique. Nature (Lond.) **206**, 211–213 (1965)·

Torvik, A., Brodal, A.: The origin of reticulospinal fibers in the cat. An experimental study. Anat. Rec. **128**, 113–138 (1957).

Tower, Sarah S.: Function and structure in the chronically isolated lumbo-sacral spinal cord of the dog. J. comp. Neurol. **67**, 109–131 (1937).

Trepinski, P.: Die embryonalen Fasersysteme in den Hintersträngen und ihre Degeneration bei der Tabes dorsalis. Arch. Psychiat. Nervenkr. 54–81 (1898).

Uchizono, K.: Characteristics of excitatory and inhibitory synapses in the central nervous system of the cat. Nature (Lond.) **207**, 642–643 (1965).

Uchizono, K.: Synaptic organization of the Purkinje cells in the cerebellum of the cat. Exp. Brain Res. **4**, 97–113 (1967).

Vasilenko, D.A., Kostyuk, P.G.: Functional properties of interneurons activated mono-synaptically by the pyramidal tract. Zh. vyssh. nerv. Deyat. Pavlova **16**, 1046–1056 (1966), Russian.

Vasilenko, D.A., Zadorozhny, A.G., Kostyuk, P.G.: Synaptic processes in the spinal neurons, monosynaptically activated by the pyramidal tract. Bull. exp. Biol. Med. **64**, 20–25 (1967), Russian.

Wall, P.D.: The origin of a spinal cord low potential. J. Physiol. (Lond.) **164**, 508–526 (1962).

Wall, P.D.: The laminar organization of dorsal horn and effects of descending impulses. J. Physiol. (Lond.) **188**, 403–424 (1967).

Wall, P.D., Freeman, J., Major, D.: Dorsal horn cells in spinal and in freely moving rats. Exp. Neurol. **19**, 519–529 (1967).

Weight, F.F.: Cholinergic mechanisms in recurrent inhibition of motoneurons. In Public Health Science Publ. **1836**, 69–75 (1968).

Wilson, V.J., Burgess, P.R.: Disinhibition in the cat spinal cord. J. Neurophysiol. **25**, 392–404 (1962).

Zimmermann, M.: Dorsal root potentials after C-fiber stimulation. Science **160**, 896–898 (1968).

Chapter 8

Dorsal Horn Electrophysiology

By

Patrick D. Wall, London (Great Britain)

With 1 Figure

Contents

I. Introduction

The dorsal horn is a nexus of many inputs and outputs. Afferents arrive both from the periphery and from many parts of spinal cord, brain stem and cortex. Efferents pass to the ventral horn, other spinal segments, brain stem, thalamus and cerebellum. In writing on the physiology of such a structure or in assessing an experimental paper or especially in designing an experiment, it is necessary to keep in mind that the scientists' intellectual activities will be based on some conceptual model of the structure. One model sees the dorsal horn as a road inter-section with rotary and flyover systems entered by independent units of traffic which pass through and proceed to their proper destinations except in pathological circumstances of collision, breakdown or collapse. A second analogy is that of the railway marshalling yard where units arrive and leave with their origin and destination labelled but a central control may accelerate or slow them and may dispatch them in mixed trains. My own bias is towards a model which would add to the first two the possibilities of not only controlled collections and dispatch but also of local abstraction, integration, selection and decision. We shall review the available facts on dorsal horn physiology but before doing so it is essential to list the conceptual and technical factors which limit our knowledge.

II. Factors Limiting a Description of Dorsal Horn Physiology

1) *Small cells:* histology shows the existence of small cells in all regions of the dorsal grey matter (Rexed, 1952). These cells either do not produce spikes or do not generate a large enough extracellular field for extracellular recording or cannot survive penetration by intracellular electrodes. As we shall see this problem has so far prevented any knowledge of single cell action within the substantia

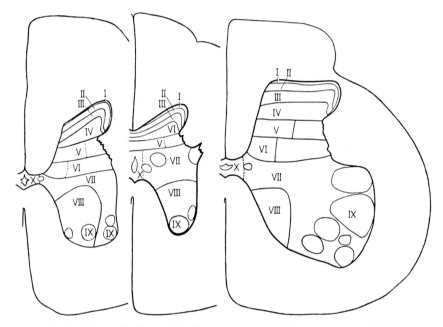

Fig. 1. Left, C5. Middle, T4. Right, L7. Diagrams combined from Rexed's (1952) histological laminar organisation of cat spinal grey matter. Physiological and histological evidence supports this organisation but the lines should not be seen as marking abrupt transitions. The laminae are zones of concentration with intermingled edges

gelatinosa. An indication of what is meant by small is shown in Dilly et al. (1968) who were only just able to record the antidromic spike generated in cells whose axons conducted at 20 m.p.s. or more although there is ample evidence for projection cells with smaller axons. This means that single cell physiology deals with only a fraction of the total and we are free to attribute all sorts of wonderful properties to existing cells whose action cannot at present be observed.

2) *Silent Cells:* extracellular recording in the absence of stimulation depends on cells announcing their presence by spontaneous activity; silent cells can therefore be bypassed. The detection of such cells by extracellular recording depends on stimulation during search and obviously the correct choice of stimulus is crucial.

3) *Stimulus selection:* usually a region is searched during stimulation but since it is not possible to test for all possible locations and types of stimuli, a limited range of stimuli are selected which depend on the particular bias of the experimenter. This is particularly difficult for cells responding to noxious stimuli since the stimuli cannot be exactly repeated because of damage produced by the initial stimulus. A common method of search is to deliver a supramaximal electrical stimulus to some nerve or root and then, when a cell is detected, to search for its receptive field properties. The method has four disadvantages:

A The gross stimulus can produce such massive slow waves as to submerge small amplitude spikes.

B Massive stimuli may inhibit when more discrete stimuli excite.

C The method often fails to reveal pure inhibitory responses.

D Particularly for central projections, pathways are often only revealed if a correct duration and frequency of repetitive stimulation is selected.

4) *Unresponsive State:* any preparation whether anaesthetised, decerebrate, spinal or even freely moving may contain cells in a state of blockade or under strong inhibitory control so that they fail to respond under the particular circumstances of the experiment. As we shall see the degree of convergence of different influences on cells is strongly affected by the activity of control systems.

5) *Inadequate recording:* each type of electrode has its merits but acts as a mechanical or electrical filter excluding recording from some types of structure. For example, high impedance glass fluid-filled-electrodes which are essential for intracellular recording fail to pick up small extracellular fields because of their high inherent noise level.

Almost all known types of peripheral nerve fibres terminate in the dorsal horn. An exception is the group of large myelinated axons in splanchnic nerve which are believed to originate in Pacinian corpuscles. These axons enter the cord and then proceed up the dorsal columns but there are no signs of collaterals entering the dorsal horn since stimulation of the axons fails to produce cord slow waves (WIDEN, 1955) or muscular reflexes (DOWNMAN, 1955) or autonomic reflexes (FRANZ et al., 1966) or interneuron responses (POMERANZ et al., 1968). Dorsal horn also receives inputs from many descending systems including those from other segments of cord, from many brain stem structures and from cortex. It projects to the ventral horn including motoneurons, to other segments of the cord, to the cerebellum, brainstem and thalamus. For many dorsal horn cells, the degree of specialisation depends very much on the circumstances of the experiment and on what is considered by the experimenter to be a relevant manipulation. For example, in cat lumbar dorsal horn, many cells respond to light mechanical stimuli on the ipsilateral leg and are unaffected by similar stimuli to other parts of the body (WALL, 1967). However, if heavy noxious stimuli are applied to the opposite leg, the cells are inhibited (MENDELL, 1966; BROWN and FRANZ, 1969). It is then a question of bias and experimental design whether the cell is described as having a receptive field limited to an area on the ipsilateral leg or on both legs. A more realistic description will have to await much more difficult experiments where the cells are examined in freely moving animals to determine the extent of inhibitory and excitatory convergence with stimuli and conditions which the animal was evolved to handle. A beginning has already been made to such experiments (see POMPEIANO, chapter 12 of this book and WALL, FREEMAN and MAJOR, 1967). In a simpler example of how the choice of stimuli affects the apparent convergence, WALL (1960) recorded cells with discrete pressure sensitive cutaneous receptive fields. Dorsal rootlets were then cut one after the other until the cell under observation failed to respond to any peripheral pressure stimuli. Each cell was apparently completely deafferented for natural stimuli when a microbundle was sectioned within one specific rootlet but, in spite of this, electrical stimuli to distant rootlets or peripheral nerves still elicited monosynaptic responses in the cell. Presumably the synchronous volley produced by electrical stimulation reveals the presence of peripheral afferents which cannot be activated in sufficient numbers at one time by natural stimuli to raise the cell to a firing level. An extreme example of excitatory convergence is shown by WIESENDANGER (1967) who recorded from cord interneurons under chloralose anaesthesia, which responded to visual and auditory stimuli. We have stressed these examples because they show that the description of the physiology of any one dorsal horn cell will depend on a large number of contingencies and restrictions which must be defined and kept in mind. In the following parts of this chapter we will restrict ourselves almost entirely to a description of cells in cat lumbar dorsal horn which are influenced by ipsilateral leg stimuli but since it is important to stress the range of the repertoire of these cells it will be necessary to discuss the interactions of arriving afferents and the descending controls which are discussed separately in other chapters. This chapter will propose four generalisations but will, as usual, have to point to exceptions.

1) *Lamination:* dorsal horn cells are arranged histologically in six laminae, Fig. 1, REXED (1952). Each lamina contains physiologically specialised groups of cells.

2) *Convergence:* the physiology of most of the cells contrasts with those in lemniscal pathways in that each cell is affected by a number of different specific types of peripheral afferents. The extent of convergence increases progressively in cells in more and more ventral laminae.

3) *Interaction:* converging peripheral afferents from different locations and from different specific types of end organ interact by pre- and postsynaptic inhibitory and excitatory mechanisms.

4) *Descending control:* the input-output function of cells may be fundamentally controlled by descending systems.

III. Laminar Organisation of Dorsal Horn

Dorsal horn cells extend from lamina I to VI. They respond to stimuli applied to the ipsilateral leg. The ventral limit of lamina VI, about level with the central canal, is marked physiologically by the appearance of cells characteristic of lamina VII whose receptive fields to light mechanical stimuli extend to both legs. These cells, outside the scope of this chapter, show that the increasing extent of convergence in more ventral cells continues to increase in ventral horn. We shall describe the physiology of the commonly encountered cells within each lamina. One must warn that, with the exception of the anatomically well defined lamina I, all other laminae should be visualised as zones of concentration with intermingled edges rather than as exact laminae with clear edges.

a) *Lamina I:* This zone caps dorsal horn as a thin sheet of flattened cells, usually not more than one cell thick, separating substantia gelatinosa from dorsal columns at the extreme dorsal edge of dorsal horn and extending laterally and then ventrally to curl over the lateral edge of substantia gelatinosa. CHRISTENSEN and PERL (1970) have described the most specific cells yet observed in dorsal horn. They occupy part of the lateral edge of this lamina which covers the dorsolateral extension of the substantia gelatinosa, deep to Lissauer's tract. They describe only those cells which responded to stimulation of peripheral Aδ and unmyelinated afferents. The configuration of the extracellular spikes suggested that they were generated in the somadendritic portions of the neurons. The dendrites of these cells ramify in a dense feltwork within the lamina. One group of cells responded in the spinal animal only to stimulation of high threshold mechanoreceptors requiring strong or frankly noxious stimuli to the skin and whose afferents are of the small myelinated type (BURGESS and PERL, 1967). A second group responded to both myelinated and unmyelinated afferents and were subject to a convergence of both high threshold mechanoreceptors by way of small myelinated afferents and of polymodal high pressure and temperature receptors connected to unmyelinated afferents. A third group was like the second but in addition received unmyelinated afferents responding to innocuous temperature changes. Because of the experimental arrangement only afferents from tail were examined and the receptive fields were all ipsilateral and varied in size from an entire dermatome to 1 cm². All excitatory receptive fields were associated with nearby regions where similar stimuli inhibited the cell. In more medial parts of the lamina, WALL (1968) has recorded from spontaneously active units which have large receptive fields covering up to one third of the leg and which respond to a variety of low threshold mechanical stimuli and some to passive movement of the leg. Nothing is known of the effect of descending impulses on the responses of the cells. It is apparent that even in this, the smallest lamina, a variety of cells exist and there is no reason to think than an exhaustive search has yet been completed.

b) *Laminae II and III:* — No direct physiology exists concerning the activity of cell bodies lying in this region but certain speculative inferences have been made. The zone contains four types of structure 1) Entering afferent fibres. 2) Terminal arborisations of afferents. RALSTON (1968) and others have insisted that peripheral afferents terminated only in lamina 3 the more ventral of the two laminae. However in keeping with the classical view (CAJAL, 1909), HEIMER and WALL (1968) showed that a special set of afferents terminated in lamina 2, the substantia gelatinosa Rolandi, while others terminate in lamina 3 and deeper layers. Sparse terminal degeneration is also observed in this region following section of descending pathways. 3) Dendrites rising from cell bodies in deeper laminae. 4) Small cells of various types as described in the preceding chapter by SZENTÁGOTHAI. I have repeatedly attempted and failed in these laminae to record spike activity which might be attributed to the activity of these small cells. This search was repeated recently following the description by Réthelyi and Szentá-gothai (1969) of a relatively large cell type in lamina III with terminations in lamina II. Five types of electrode, glass fluid filled with impedances of 2–4 MΩ, glass fluid filled with impedances of 40–60 MΩ, platinum, tungsten, and platinum black plated, were used without success. Similarly, attempts have failed to record either compound action potentials or single units in lateral Lissauer's tract which contains axons from the cells of substantia gelatinosa. These negative results do not mean that impulses do not exist; such a statement would have to await the development of superior recording electrodes or a preparation which would allow intracellular recording. In favour of the eventual discovery of spikes within cells in the region is the existence of long running fine unmyelinated axons within the laminae and in Lissauer's tract. The presumed length constant of such structures would not allow electrotonic propagation and would require spike propagation for the cell body to influence distal structures. Rudomin and Muñoz-Martinez (1969) showed that direct microelectrode stimulation still produced slow potentials of the dorsal root potential type when the entire animal was poisoned with tetrodotoxin. The significance of this experiment depends on proving that suffi-cient tetrodotoxin had been introduced to abolish all spike activity and this recording may be beyond present technique although examples are known of terminals completely resistant to tetrodotoxin in much higher concentrations than those used by Rudomin and Muñoz-Martinez. Furthermore, direct stimu-lation may still depolarise terminals normally depolarised by action potentials. Intracellular recordings have been made from cord cells which fail to produce spikes (Somjen, 1970) but these appear to be glia and he proposes that they are responsible for the sustained cord potential but not the DRP.

Wall (1962) suggested, on indirect evidence, that the small cells of substantia gelatinosa were involved in the generation of the large long negative component of the dorsal root potential, DRP. This potential is caused by the prolonged depolarisation of terminals which have carried an afferent volley and of the terminals of their passive neighbours (Barron and Matthews, 1938; Lloyd and McIntyre, 1948; Wall, 1958). This depolarisation is associated with a form of inhibition which might be caused by a block of transmission in the terminals (Howland et al., 1955) or a decrease of transmitter release (Eccles, 1961). It is also associated with the generation of antidromic impulses in those axons whose terminals are strongly depolarised, the dorsal root reflex. It reaches a peak some 20 msec after the arrival of the afferent volley and lasts some 70 msec in unana-esthetised preparations and over 150 msec under anaesthesia. If a source-sink analysis is made, the main sinks, the signs of membrane depolarisation are distributed in the region of substantia gelatinosa (Howland et al., 1955; Wall, 1962). This might be a sign of the depolarisation of the terminals themselves or of activity in either of the other three components of the region. We can eliminate the parent axons as the source because Wall (1958) showed that the amount of depolarisation increased sharply as the terminals were approached as judged by their threshold change measured by microelectrode stimulation. Barron and Matthews (1938) in their original description of the phenomenon suggested that there might be a direct influence of close packed afferent terminals on each other by way of potassium accumulation. Recently Borland et al. (1970) returned to this theme and have suggested that potassium sensitive glia may form the intermediary. In my opinion, glia are unlikely to be responsible for the spread of depolarisation because from what is known of their physiology they buffer rather than exaggerate extracellular ionic changes and their known anatomy does not match the spatial spread of the depolarisation. Certainly some third structure must be responsible for the common depolarisation of both active and passive terminals. The summation of action potentials in deep cells is not a good candidate because barbiturate which shortens the period of repetitive firing actually prolongs the DRP and very heavy concentrations of barbiturate which abolish all detectable spike response to an afferent volley fails to abolish the DRP. Summed EPSP's in the dendrites of deeper cells are so far an unlikely candidate. The reason is that intracellular recording made from the cell bodies whose dendrites rise into the laminae II and III do not show the very prolonged depolarisations after an afferent volley which would be needed if they were to be the cause of the disturbance (HONGO et al., 1968). By exclusion, this tends to point the finger at the other component of the region, the small cells. As we have said direct observation of the physiology of these cells has not been possible but one experiment (WALL, 1962) suggests that Lissauer's tract is involved. If the dorsal root of one segment is stimulated, DRP's exist in the dorsal root of the next segment. A transverse cut was made into dorsal column and dorsal horn until all afferent fibres, which ran from the stimulated root into the rostral segment were cut. A DRP was still present but its onset was delayed. The cut was then extended to section the extreme dorso-lateral white matter and Lissauer's tract and the delayed DRP was completely abolished. This suggests that the fibres of lateral Lissauer's tract which are axons of small cells within laminae 2 and 3 are responsible for the transfer of the disturbance from one segment to another. It must be stressed that this does not prove that these cells are actually responsible for the DRP within a particular segment.

In addition to depolarisation, terminals may also hyperpolarise following the arrival of afferent volleys. The best known example is the hyperpolarisation which follows the depolarisation in unanaesthetised animals and is called DRVI (LLOYD and McINTYRE, 1948). It has also been shown in isolation following partial block of peripheral cutaneous nerve (MENDELL and WALL, 1964; DAWSON et al., 1970) following stimulation of small myelinated fibres from muscle (MENDELL, 1970; BURKE et al., 1971) and in certain trigeminal A delta afferents (DUBNER and SESSLE, 1971). There has been considerable discussion as to the exact circumstances under which these hyperpolarisations arise (see BURKE et al., 1971) and nothing is known of the mechanism. It is not yet known if the hyperpolarisation is produced by an independent mechanism or by the inhibition of a tonic depolarisation.

c) *Lamina IV:* This region contains relatively large cell bodies with dendrites extending dorsally. The activity of the cells can be recorded in the region of the cell bodies but spikes can also be recorded so well in their dendritic arborisation that there is a suspicion that spike activity may occur within dendrites (WALL, 1965). Some of the cells project into the ipsilateral dorsolateral white matter with particularly large diameter axons. Some information about the physiology of cells in this lamina comes from direct extracellular recording in the region of cell bodies

17*

while other information comes from axon recording in the tract. Naturally the tract also contains fibres of quite different origin so that one must be cautious not to consider results from the two recording sites as equivalent (HILLMAN and WALL, 1969).

Cells which have actually been recorded in the region of lamina IV in cat lumbar cord respond to light brushing and to pressure of skin. The excitatory receptive fields are relatively small varying from a fraction of one toe to 8 cm long on the proximal part of the leg. They are somatotopically arranged within the lamina so that medial cells have distal receptive fields and lateral cells tend to have more proximal fields. However this transverse map is distorted by the fact that fibres from one dorsal root and therefore one dermatome begins synapsing laterally close to their entry point and then slant rostrally and medially. Therefore each dermatome is represented with its proximal zone lateral and close to the root entry and its distal zone medial and rostral to the root entry zone.

All of the recordable cells in this zone seem to respond to low level pressure or hair movement. They do not respond to small temperature variations. WALL (1960) measured subcutaneous temperature rather than surface temperature and believed that the cells responded to small temperature rises but BROWN and FRANZ (1969) showed, with proper control, that it was necessary to heat skin surface to 40–45°C before increased firing occurred. The units also respond to the brisk cooling by ethyl chloride but more slowly applied cooling only produces a discharge in some units if the temperature reaches 15–25°C.

The threshold to mechanical disturbance, specificity and spontaneous activity of the units depends on the nature of the preparation. The units are inhibited in the decerebrate animal (WALL, 1967) or under barbiturate anaesthesia (BROWN and FRANZ, 1969) or during pyramidal tract stimulation (FETZ, 1968). In the spinal animal, inhibition is reduced but natural stimulation of the periphery still shows that the excitatory fields of many cells are associated with a nearby inhibitory field. HONGO et al. (1968) have made intracellular recording from cells with lamina IV characteristics and show a post-synaptic inhibition. The time course of the inhibition suggests that it may also have a presynaptic component.

One effect of the cutaneous inhibitory descending system which is active in the decerebrate animal is to appear to increase the specificity of the cells by cutting out less powerful afferents (BROWN and FRANZ, 1969). This system is evidently also active in the intact barbiturate anaesthetised animal because HILLMAN and WALL (1969) found the same type of release from inhibition in these lumbar cells if the cord was cold blocked in the thoracic region. Of 137 cells of the lamina 4 type excited by peripheral stimuli in decerebrate or anaesthetised animals (BROWN and FRANZ, 1969) 17 were stimulated by guard hair movement and by heavy pressure or pinch while 24 were sensitive to tylotrich hair movement alone. However when they examined spinal animals they found no such specificity with respect to which hairs were moved and 33 of 54 cells responded not only to all types of hair movement but to gentle pressure on skin as well. This shows that the degree of convergence in this lamina is under descending control. Furthermore in the decerebrate animals they showed inhibition in the majority of cells produced by light brushing but in the spinal animals heavy pressure or pinching was required in all but one cell. We see therefore in lamina 4 a group of cells responding to light cutaneous stimuli with signs of convergence of a variable number of different types of afferent fibre. The extent of this convergence and the amount of inhibition is affected by descending controls. In addition to these cells which respond to peripheral stimulation there may be others which respond only to descending volleys (ERULKAR et al., 1966).

d) *Lamina V:* is ventral to lamina IV containing large cells occupying the neck of dorsal horn with a lateral region containing bundles of longitudinally running fibres separated from dorso-lateral white matter. Many cells in this lamina are excited by the complete range of peripheral afferent fibres from largest to smallest. The response of the cells to the largest afferents occurs slightly later than the lamina IV cells immediately dorsal to them so that it may be that they are fired by the lamina IV cells. Some cells respond to the smaller myelinated fibres in splanchnic nerve and other to the small myelinated fibres in muscle nerve with a latency consistant with their receiving these axons. Many cells respond to un-myelinated afferents but because of their slow and variable conduction velocity it is not known if the effect is monosynaptic. The commonest cells encountered in this zone also respond to light cutaneous stimulation but show a progression from lamina IV by an exaggeration of the degree of the convergence of peripheral specific fibres and of the complexity of organisation of their receptive fields (WALL, 1967; POMERANZ, WALL and WEBER, 1968; HILLMAN and WALL, 1969). In the decerebrate preparation, the receptive fields are made up of three zones. In the central zone 1, all types of pressure sensitive cutaneous afferents excite the cell from hair movement to those excited by noxious stimulation. Single electrical shocks applied to the skin lead to a more and more prolonged burst of firing as higher and higher threshold axons are recruited. The cells often fire in a complex but repeatable temporal "banding" pattern. Some of these delayed bursts of firing can be attributed to the delayed arrival of impulses in slowly conducting fibres but others must be attributed to some local mechanism for the generation of repetitive discharge (MENDELL, 1966). The cells respond to impulses carried in the three diameter components of a peripheral cutaneous nerve; Aβ, Aδ and C. Following the repetitive burst there follows a period of facilitation which may last for seconds so that if the stimulus is repeated every second the response to each stimulus is greater than the preceding response, "wind up" (MENDELL, 1966). There are also inhibitory mechanisms impinging on these cells. Threshold cutaneous stimuli produce a burst of firing followed by inhibition. Light repeated brushing produces an initial response which habituates. The cell itself is not inhibited during this habituation because it responds normally if the stimulus location is shifted (WALL, 1967). WICKELGREN (1967) showed that the habituation of interneurons in the region mirrors flexor reflex habituation and suggests that post tetanic potentiation of inhibition may be involved. Habituation to light brushing occurs in the decerebrate cat but not in spinal preparations. Light brush habituation occurs in spinal rat but not in spinal cat (WALL, FREEMAN and MAJOR, 1968) and it seems likely that the phenomenon is produced by a segmental inhibitory mechanism which requires a tonic drive from brain stem in the cat. In summary, from zone 1 the cell is excited by low electrical threshold (large diameter) cutaneous afferents after which there is inhibition but if high electrical threshold (small diameter) afferents are active the cell is also excited followed by

facilitation which overwhelms the inhibition associated with low electrical threshold afferents.

In zone 2, which surrounds the first, but extends more in the proximal direction,
light brushing or threshold electrical stimuli inhibit the cells. More intense mechanical or electrical stimulation excites the cells with a longer latency than observed
from zone 1. In an even wider zone, 3, light mechanical or electrical stimulation
inhibits and also heavier stimuli fails to excite. HILLMAN and WALL (1970) have
suggested that the entire organisation of the receptive field is that of three superimposed zones, a small one where light stimuli produce excitation on top of a
larger one where heavy stimuli produce excitation on top of an even larger one
where small stimuli produce inhibition.

Cells of this type are under marked control from brain stem. If the cell is first
examined in the decerebrate animal and then a segment of thoracic cord is cold
blocked the following occurs: spontaneous activity increases, the receptive field for
light brushing expands, habituation disappears, the number of impulses and
amount of facilitation produced by intense mechanical or electrical stimuli
increases and the surround zone 3 from which only inhibition could be elicited
disappears. The descending pathway responsible for this exaggeration of inhibition
lies in the dorsolateral white matter and may be the dorsal reticular spinal system
of ENGBERG et al. (1968). FETZ (1968) has shown that cortico-spinal impulses
affect these cells with a complex of inhibition and excitation and ERULKAR et al.
(1966) have shown cells affected by vestibular nuclei.

This common type of cell is fired both by low and high threshold afferents.
POMERANZ et al. (1968) searched the lamina for cells fired by small myelinated
afferents. In the thoracic cord, cells were located in lamina V which responded,
apparently monosynaptically, to the small myelinated afferents from splanchnic
nerve. All such cells also responded to light brushing of a restricted area of skin.
Furthermore, in the region of termination of a muscle nerve, cells were found
which responded apparently monosynaptically to the Group III afferents from the
muscle but not to the larger diameter muscle afferents. These cells too had a
cutaneous receptive field where light mechanical stimuli excited the cell. These
authors proposed a generalisation about this common type of Lamina V cell which
was that they responded to small myelinated afferents which signalled the state
of tissue, some cells receiving from skin, others from muscle and yet others from
viscera. In addition the cells responded to low level cutaneous stimuli.

Specialised cells also exist in this lamina. EGGER and WALL (1971) traced the
pathway responsible for a cutaneous reflex in deeply anaesthetised animals. The
receptors for the reflex are cutaneous pressure receptors in the plantar cushion.
The afferents are medium size myelinated fibres. Units were located in the extreme
medial edge of lamina IV in L7 monosynaptically activated by stimuli with
receptive fields and thresholds identical to the plantar cushion-toe extension
reflex. These cells fail to respond to light brushing or vibration. Associated with
these monosynaptically activated neurons, there was a second group disynaptically or polysynaptically activated by identical stimuli and lying slightly deeper
mainly in lamina V and slightly more caudal and lateral. Motoneurons were
located on the lateral edge of S1 whose firing pattern showed them to be responsible
for the reflex and whose EPSP latency showed that at most two interneurons could

be interposed between them and the primary afferents. Because no other interneurons with proper characteristics could be found in an extensive search of dorsal
horn, the authors propose that they have located two populations of interneurons
serially linked together to mediate at least the fastest component of this particular
reflex. Under the conditions of this experiment, these cells showed a very much
more specialised input than that seen in the common cells. Other specialised cells
have been located in this lamina. KOSTYUK and VASILENKO (1966) detected cells
in the lateral part of lamina V which are monosynaptically excited by impulses
from the cortico-spinal tract and in turn directly fire motoneurons. Some of these
cells are not influenced by dorsal root stimulation.

e) *Lamina VI:* This region of large cells is observed histologically only in the
cervical and lumbar enlargements. It is the first lamina encountered in the dorsal
ventral progression in which many cells clearly respond to specialised afferents
from muscle and joints. In thoracic cord, where the number of such afferents is
small compared to the numbers arriving from limbs, only a thin layer is detected
physiologically at the base of dorsal horn where cells respond to chest movement.
Clarke's column is a specialised and segmentally restricted medial zone of this
lamina where specialised muscle afferents from hind limb terminate. In cat lumbar
cord, the most commonly encountered cells exhibit a complex convergence of effects
of muscle afferents and effects of cutaneous afferents. The dorsal margin of the zone
is clearly defined by the discovery of cells which respond monosynaptically to
Group I muscle afferents. The ventral border which is at the level of the central
canal is marked by the appearance of lamina VII cells which have widely distributed receptive fields where light stimuli in areas of both legs produce excitation
in the cell. Cells in the lateral part of laminae V, VI and VII have been studied and
shown by HUBBARD and OSCARSSON (1962) to give rise to ventral spino-cerebellar
tract. In the decerebrate cat, WALL (1967) found that most cells responded to both
passive movement of the leg and to cutaneous stimuli. The latency of response to
group I muscle afferent stimulation suggested monosynaptic connection but to
cutaneous stimulation suggested polysynaptic connection. The excitatory cutaneous receptive fields were slightly larger than those found in lamina V. For the
proprioceptive stimuli some cells responded only during movement, others had in
addition a static response when particular joints were moved within part of their
range.

When the spinal cord was cold blocked at segments T13–L1, almost all the
cells examined first in the decerebrate state showed a marked increase of their
excitability to cutaneous stimuli and an increase in the area of their cutaneous
receptive fields. At the same time most cells showed a decrease in their sensitivity
to movement of the leg. In the extreme case, cells were found responsive only to
leg movement in the decerebrate and only to cutaneous stimuli in the spinal
animal, "modality switching", but more commonly there was a shift in balance of
sensitivity away from proprioceptive towards cutaneous responses. Pyramidal
tract stimulation excites many of the cells in this lamina and inhibits a minority
(FETZ, 1968). As in lamina V, the cutaneous responses are inhibited in the decerebrate so that receptive fields are restricted, thresholds raised and habituation is
present. By contrast, in the proprioceptive sphere, movement responses are
enhanced in the decerebrate. The switching of sensitivity from proprioceptive to

cutaneous, matches the overall reflex activity first described by SHERRINGTON and SOWTON (1915) where proprioceptive reflexes dominate the decerebrate animal while they are inhibited in the spinal animal in which cutaneous reflexes predominate.

IV. Gate Control Hypothesis

A. Original Hypothesis

In 1965 MELZACK and WALL proposed the idea of a gate control to bring together the anatomy, physiology and psychology of that time. The intention was to relate the input-output functions of the dorsal horn to known phenomena of sensation with particular emphasis on pain. In brief the suggestion was that the messages transmitted from peripheral nerves to higher centres were the consequence of 1) Convergence of more than one peripheral afferent onto cord cells, 2) Interaction between the effects of arriving impulses, 3) Descending control of dorsal horn excitability.

1) *Convergence:* it was very obvious by that time that afferent fibres exhibited an intensely specific and rigid relationship between their response and the type of physiological stimulus which would evoke that response. The cord cells which had been examined responded to more than one type of peripheral afferent.

2) *Interaction: A:* large diameter afferent cutaneous fibres generally excited cord cells but this excitation was followed by a prolonged inhibition. Smaller diameter myelinated and unmyelinated fibres generally produced excitation followed by prolonged after-discharges and facilitation.

B: In the Melzack-Wall paper, the mechanism of the inhibitions and facilitations was discussed mainly in presynaptic terms. However, it was pointed out that there was no way of knowing if these presynaptic processes were the only, or even the dominant, mechanisms.

C: It was suggested that the substantia gelatinosa was involved in the presynaptic control. This suggestion originated from WALL's finding (1962) that the Lissauer tract, a propriospinal connecting system of substantia gelatinosa, was necessary for the spread of terminal depolarisation from one segment to another.

3) *Descending Control:* It was suggested that impulses descending from cortex and brain stem set the excitability level of both the pre- and post-synaptic mechanisms.

The classical view had been that the messages received from the periphery by the sensorium were almost exactly the messages contained in the individual peripheral fibres. The gate control hypothesis suggested that sensation was abstracted from the messages in peripheral afferents after the messages had passed through a series of gate controls with their three interacting factors. The reason for making this suggestion was not only that it seemed to fit the physiology and anatomy known at that time but also that it might provide a basis for the highly complex relation between stimulus and perceived sensation. Specifically it was hoped that it would provide a model which could be tested experimentally to explain the pains associated with peripheral nerve disease.

B. Subsequent Discoveries which Require Modification of the Gate Control Theory

The least, and perhaps the best, that can be said for the 1965 paper is that it provoked discussion and experiment.

1) *Convergence:* In 1965, one of the paradoxes of peripheral nerve physiology was that very few specific nociceptive fibres had been observed even though it was believed that at least the small myelinated fibres had been adequately sampled (HUNT and McINTYRE, 1960). Since that time as described elsewhere in this volume, other workers particularly IGGO and BURGESS and PERL have shown many such fibres. Furthermore, CHRISTENSEN and PERL (1970) have shown that, among the sparse large cells of lamina 1, there exist some cells which under their conditions appear to respond only to impulses from the peripheral nociceptors. New and important as these findings are, it is important not to assign to them the monopoly of pain. As we wrote, before they had been discovered, "Even if some central cells should be shown unequivocally to respond exclusively to noxious stimuli, their specialised properties still do not make them "pain cells". It is more likely that such cells represent the extreme of a broad distribution of cell thresholds. — Physiological specialisation is a fact which can be retained without acceptance of the psychological assumption that pain is determined entirely by impulses in a straight-through transmission system from the skin to a pain center in the brain". The reasons for this approach are given in MELZACK and WALL (1962 and 1965) and more recent discoveries provide more reasons as we shall show below.

2) *Interaction:* While the emphasis of the 1965 paper was on presynaptic control, the gate control was intended to include both pre- and post-synaptic mechanisms. It was stated "Although there is evidence so far for only presynaptic control, there may also be undetected post-synaptic mechanisms that contribute to the observed input-output functions" (MELZACK and WALL, 1965). Such post-synaptic mechanisms were reported by HONGO, JANKOWSKA and LUNDBERG (1968).

We have discussed above (see III b) the evidence reported by others that either small diameter fibres or specifically nociceptive afferents fail to produce positive dorsal root potentials under the conditions of their experiments. The evidence is reviewed most recently by SCHMIDT (1971). The relative importance of pre- and post-synaptic effects, the conditions under which they appear and the specific afferent fibres responsible for these changes remain to be discovered. Even the mechanism of presynaptic control remains in debate. The two suggested mechanisms are 1) blockade, see WALL (1964) and 2) transmitter release depending on terminal membrane potential, see SCHMIDT (1971). In spite of all these interesting questions, the existance of a balanced inhibition — facilitation mechanism is not questioned. What is questioned is 1) which specific afferents are associated with inhibition and facilitation, 2) how do these controls operate, 3) under what conditions do they operate.

C. Subsequent Discoveries which Support the Gate Control Theory

1) *Convergence.* The extent and the rules of convergence are becoming more apparent. The general plan, as described above, appears to be one of a laminar

organisation with more and more extensive convergence as one passes from dorsal
to ventral laminae (WALL, 1967). This increasing convergence produces not only
larger and larger receptive fields if a single type of stimulus is used, but also cells
which respond to a wider and wider variety of physiologically specific afferents.
Of particular interest as possible candidates for cells feeding information into the
systems which release pain behaviour are the cells of lamina 5. Here we find cells
which respond to small myelinated and unmyelinated afferents. Noxious stimuli
to the cell's receptive field produce intense firing but low level mechanical stimuli
also excite the cell to a low level of firing. POMERANZ, WALL and WEBER (1968)
investigated the origin of the small myelinated afferents which directly or indirectly fired these cells. They found cells responding to small myelinated fibres
either from skin or muscle or viscera. Taking those cells responding to high
threshold visceral afferents as an example, it was also found that these cells
responded to low threshold afferents from skin and this was confirmed in another
region by SELZER and SPENCER (1969a and b). Obviously these cells have properties reminiscent of the phenomenon of referred pain. This type of pain has three
properties. 1) The psychological mislocation of the real origin of the damage.
2) The area to which the pain is referred is tender, that is to say low level pressure
stimuli enchance the pain. 3) Local anaesthesia of the apparently painful region
reduces or abolishes the pain. The matching of the properties for a particular type
of cell and the stimulus-response relationship of a particular type of pain is, of
course, only suggestive that the cell might be involved as an intermediary between
stimulus and response. Within any one lamina cells vary considerably in their
properties even though they form a general family. It is clearly of great importance
to search for the range of convergence within the group rather than to design
experiments which will only demonstrate cells whose input is monopolised by a
specific type of afferent.

2) *Interaction.* The statement in the original paper was that large diameter
cutaneous afferents fed into an inhibitory mechanism while smaller fibres released
facilitation. These conflicting effects had been observed but no biological reason
could be given for why such a balance should occur. We now have an interesting
clue to the reason from stimulus studies on lamina 5 cells (HILLMAN and WALL,
1969). As described above, these cells have complex receptive fields subdivided
into three concentric zones. These receptive fields include an inhibitory surround
dependant on certain large diameter fibres and a second mode for intense stimuli
with facilitations operated by certain smaller afferent fibres.

One of the most specific predictions of the gate control theory was that certain
types of pain were caused by a preferential destruction of the fibres which normally
produce central inhibition. Since larger fibres were implicated as inhibitory and
since such fibres have a low electrical threshold, it was though worth testing the
effects of stimulation of human peripheral nerves by surface electrodes in cases of
severe intractable pain where peripheral nerve damage was suspected. WALL and
SWEET (1967) made such trials in a mixed group of patients and produced relief
of pain in those cases where it was possible to stimulate proximal to the region of
damage and where the patient reported a mild tingling sensation referred to
the peripheral distribution of the stimulated nerve. MEYER and FIELDS (1972)
stimulated peripheral nerves in 10 cases of true causalgia major in military

personnel who had suffered bullet or fragment wounds. If the damaged nerve was stimulated peripheral to the injury, the pain was enhanced. If the damaged peripheral nerve could be stimulated proximal to the injury and if the patient reported paraesthesiae in the distribution of the nerve, the pain and peripheral hypersensitivity disappeared. Stimulation of neighbouring undamaged nerves had no effect on the pain. Surgical sympathectomy is the accepted therapy for causalgia. In one patient the causalgia recurred after sympathectomy but could still be abolished by counterstimulation of the nerve proximal to the injury.

Unfortunately in the great majority of cases of chronic intractable pain produced by partial nerve lesions, it is not possible to stimulate proximal to the injury. One common example is post-herpetic neuralgia where the destruction extends over the entire course of the peripheral nerve and perhaps beyond. Another example is that of root pain following a herniated disc and surgery. Since peripheral stimulation produced encouraging results and since it was known that it was the large fibre component of peripheral nerves which made up the dorsal columns (WALL, 1961) it was an obvious suggestion that dorsal column stimulation might produce the same effect as stimulation of large diameter fibres in peripheral nerves. All known peripheral cutaneous fibres which contribute an axon to dorsal columns also send a collateral into dorsal horn. HILLMAN and WALL (1969) showed that dorsal column stimulation in spinal cat inhibited nociceptive responses in lamina 5 cells. Techniques have been developed to place subdural stimulating electrodes on the surface of dorsal columns in man. The electrodes are connected to a small implanted radio-receiver stimulator which is activated by an external transmitter whose loop antenna is placed on the skin above the buried receiver. SHEALY, MORTIMER and HAGFORS (1970) report on 25 cases, some now followed for up to 4 years with good to excellent results in 12, fair in 8 and failure in one case where they failed to stimulate relevant fibres and in four cases who were shown in preoperative psychological tests to be severely disturbed. NASHOLD and FRIEDMAN (1972) report on 30 cases followed for more than 9 months after dorsal column stimulators had been installed. All had severe chronic pain which had failed to respond to therapy. The results are excellent 9, good 3, and fair 5. Failure occurred in 13 cases who included some with severe preoperative psychiatric disturbances and some failures to stimulated the relevant area.

At present the one explanation for these very encouraging results is that the dorsal column stimulation affects a gate control mechanism in spinal cord but of course there may also be interference mechanisms in the brain.

3) *Descending Control:* The effects of descending control systems are discussed elsewhere in this volume. Some of these affect interneurones which are concerned only with local reflex circuits such as the interneurones described by EGGER and WALL (1971). Others will affect the firing of cells whose axons are in ascending systems which may not intrude on the sensorium. Since the pioneer work of HAGBARTH and KERR (1954), all of the systems which are believed to influence sensation and which have been examined for the effects of descending control have been found to be strongly influenced.

In summary: recent discoveries require a modification of some details of the gate control theory but it still remains a productive model against which to pit both experimental results and therapeutic trials.

References

BARRON, D.H., MATTHEWS, B.H.C.: The interpretation of potential changes in the spinal cord. J. Physiol. (Lond.) **85**, 73–103 (1938).

BORLAND, R.G., MATTHEWS, B.H.C., NICHOLSON, A.N.: Spinal cord and root potentials. J. Physiol. (Lond.) **210**, 166–167P (1970).

BROWN, A.G., FRANZ, D.N.: Responses of spinocervical tract neurones to natural stimulation of identified cutaneous receptors. Exp. Brain Res. **7**, 231–249 (1969).

BURGESS, P.R., PERL, E.R.: Myelinated afferents responding specifically to noxious stimulation of the skin. J. Physiol. (Lond.) **190**, 541–562 (1967).

BURKE, R.F., RUDOMIN, P., VYKLICKÝ, L., ZAJAC, III, F.E.: Primary afferent depolarization and flexion reflexes produced by radiant heat stimulation of the skin. J. Physiol. (Lond.) in press (1971).

CHRISTENSEN, B.N., PERL, E.R.: Spinal neurons specifically excited by noxious or thermal stimuli: Marginal zone of the dorsal horn. J. Neurophysiol. **33**, 293–307 (1970).

DAWSON, G.D., MERRILL, E.G., WALL, P.D.: Dorsal root potentials produced by stimulation of fine afferents. Science **167**, 1385–1387 (1970).

DILLY, P.N., WALL, P.D., WEBSTER, K.E.: Cells of origin of the spinothalamic tract in cat and rat. Exp. Neurol. **21**, 550–562 (1968).

DOWNMAN, C.B.B.: Skeletal muscle reflexes of splanchnic and intercostal origin in acute spinal and decerebrate cats. J. Neurophysiol. **18**, 217–235 (1955).

DOWNMAN, C.B.B., HUSSAIN, A.: Spinal tracts and supraspinal centres influencing visceromotor and allied reflexes in cats. J. Physiol. (Lond.) **141**, 489–499 (1958).

DUBNER, R., SESSLE, B.J.: Presynaptic excitability changes of primary afferent and corticofugal fibres projecting to trigeminal brain stem nuclei. Exp. Neurol. in press (1971).

ECCLES, J.C.: The mechanism of synaptic transmission. Ergebn. Physiol. **51**, 299–430 (1961).

EGGER, D., WALL, P.D.: The plantar cushion reflex circuit: an oligosynaptic cutaneous reflex. J. Physiol. (Lond.) **216**, 483–501 (1971).

ENGBERG, I., LUNDBERG, A., RYALL, R.W.: Reticulospinal inhibition of interneurones. J. Physiol. (Lond.) **194**, 225–236 (1968).

ERULKAR, S.D., SPRAGUE, J.M., WHITSEL, B.L., DOGAN, S., JANETTA, P.J.: Organisation of the vestibular projection to the spinal cord of the cat. J. Neurophysiol. **29**, 626–664 (1966).

FETZ, E.: Pyramidal tract effects on interneurones in the cat lumbar dorsal horn. J. Neurophysiol. **31**, 69–80 (1968).

FRANZ, D.N., EVANS, M.H., PERL, E.R.: Characteristics of viscerosympathetic reflexes in the spinal cat. Amer. J. Physiol. **211**, 1292–1298 (1966).

HAGBARTH, K.E., KERR, D.I.B.: Central influences on spinal afferent conduction. J. Neurophysiol. **17**, 295–307 (1954).

HEIMER, L., WALL, P.D.: The dorsal root distribution to the substantia gelatinosa of the rat with a note on the distribution in the cat. Exp. Brain Res. **6**, 89–99 (1968).

HILLMAN, P., WALL, P.D.: Inhibitory and excitatory factors influencing the receptive fields of lamina 5 spinal cord cells. Exp. Brain Res. **9**, 284–306 (1969).

HONGO, T., JANKOWSKA, E., LUNDBERG, A.: Post-synaptic excitation and inhibition from primary afferents in neurones in the spinocervical tract. J. Physiol. (Lond.) **199**, 569–592 (1968).

HOWLAND, B., LETTVIN, J.Y., McCULLOCH, W.S., PITTS, W.H., WALL, P.D.: Reflex inhibition of dorsal root interaction. J. Neurophysiol. **18**, 1–17 (1955).

HUBBARD, J.I., OSCARSSON, O.: Localisation of cell bodies of the ventral spino-cerebellar tract. J. comp. Neurol. **118**, 199–204 (1962).

HUNT, C.C., McINTYRE, A.K.: An analysis of fibre diameter and receptor characteristics of myelinated cutaneous afferents in cat. J. Physiol. (Lond.) **153**, 99–112 (1960).

KOSTYUK, P.G., VASILENKO, D.A.: Transformation of cortical motor signals in spinal cord. Proc. IEEE **56**, 1049–1058 (1968).

LLOYD, D.P.C., McINTYRE, A.K.: On the origin of dorsal root potentials. J. gen. Physiol. **32**, 409–443 (1948).

MELZACK, R., WALL, P.D.: On the nature of cutaneous sensory mechanisms. Brain **85**, 331–356 (1962).

MELZACK, R., WALL, P.D.: Pain mechanisms: a new theory. Science **150**, 971–979 (1965).

MENDELL, L.M.: Physiological properties of unmyelinated fiber projection to the spinal cord. Exp. Neurol. **16**, 316–332 (1966).

MENDELL, L.M.: Positive dorsal root potentials produced by stimulation of small diameter muscle afferents. Brain Res. **18**, 375–379 (1970).

MENDELL, L.M., WALL, P.D.: Presynaptic hyperpolarization: a role for fine afferent fibres. J. Physiol. (Lond.) **172**, 274–294 (1964).

MEYER, G.A., FIELDS, H.L.: Causalgia treated by selective large fibre stimulation of peripheral nerves. Brain in press (1972).

NASHOLD, B.S., FRIEDMAN, H.: Dorsal column stimulation for pain. A preliminary report on thirty patients. J. Neurosurg. in press (1972).

POMERANZ, B., WALL, P.D., WEBER, W.V.: Cord cells responding to fine myelinated afferents from viscera, muscle and skin. J. Physiol. (Lond.) **199**, 511–532 (1968).

RALSTON, H.J.: Dorsal root projections to dorsal horn neurons. J. comp. Neurol. **132**, 303–329 (1968).

RAMÓN Y CAJAL, S.: Histologie du Système Nerveux de l'Homme et des Vertébrés. Vol. 1. L. AZOULAY (trans.) Paris: Maloine, S. 1909.

RÉTHELYI, M., SZENTÁGOTHAI, J.: The large synaptic complexes of the substantia gelatinosa. Exp. Brain Res. **7**, 258–274 (1969).

REXED, B.: The cytoarchitectonic organisation of the spinal cord of cat. J. comp. Neurol. **96**, 415–495 (1952).

RUDOMIN, P., MUÑOZ-MARTINEZ, J.: A tetrodotoxin resistant primary afferent depolarisation. Exp. Neurol. **25**, 1–17 (1969).

SCHMIDT, R.F.: Presynaptic inhibition in the vertebrate nervous system. Ergebn. Physiol. **63**, 19–101 (1971).

SELZER, M., SPENCER, W.A.: Convergence of visceral and cutaneous afferent pathways in the lumbar spinal cord. Brain Res. **14**, 331–348 (1969a).

SELZER, M., SPENCER, W.A.: Interactions between visceral and cutaneous afferents in the spinal cord: reciprocal primary afferent fibre depolarization. Brain Res. **14**, 349–366 (1969b).

SHEALY, C.N., MORTIMER, J.T., HAGFORS, N.R.: Dorsal column electroanalgesia. J. Neurosurg. **32**, 560–564 (1970).

SHERRINGTON, C.S., SOWTON, S.C.M.: Observations on reflex responses to single break shocks. J. Physiol. (Lond.) **49**, 331–343 (1915).

SOMJEN, G.C.: Evoked sustained focal potentials and membrane potential of neurons and of unresponsive cells of the spinal cord. J. Neurophysiol. **33**, 562–582 (1970).

WALL, P.D.: Excitability changes in afferent fibre terminations and their relation to slow potentials. J. Physiol. (Lond.) **142**, 1–21 (1958).

WALL, P.D.: Repetitive discharge of neurons. J. Neurophysiol. **22**, 303–320 (1959).

WALL, P.D.: Cord cells responding to touch, damage and temperature of the skin. J. Neurophysiol. **23**, 197–210 (1960).

WALL, P.D.: Two transmission systems for skin sensations in sensory communication. pp. 475–496. Ed. by W.A.R. ROSENBLITH. Cambridge: Publ. M.I.T. Press 1961.

WALL, P.D.: The origin of a spinal cord slow potential. J. Physiol. (Lond.) **164**, 508–526 (1962).

WALL, P.D.: Presynaptic control of impulses at the first central synapse in the cutaneous pathway. Progr. Brain Res. **12**, 92–118 (1964).

WALL, P.D.: Impulses recorded in the region of dendrites. J. Physiol. (Lond.) **180**, 116–133 (1965).

WALL, P.D.: The laminar organisation of dorsal horns and effects of descending impulses. J. Physiol. (Lond.) **188**, 403–423 (1967).

WALL, P.D.: The Skin Senses. Ed. by D.R. KENSHALO. Springfield, Ill.: Publ. C.C. Thomas 1968.

WALL, P.D., FREEMAN, J., MAJOR, D.: Dorsal horn cells in spinal and freely moving rats. Exp. Neurol. **19**, 519–529 (1967).

WALL, P.D., SWEET, W.H.: Temporary abolition of pain in man. Science **155**, 108–109 (1967).

WICKELGREN, B.G.: Habituation of spinal interneurons. J. Neurophysiol. **30**, 1404–1423 (1967).

WIDEN, L.: Cerebellar representation of high threshold afferents from splanchnic nerve. Acta physiol. scand. **117**, 1–69 (1955).

WIESENDANGER, M.: Morphological and pathological aspects of interneurones. Electroenceph. clin. Neurophysiol. Suppl. **25**, 47–57 (1967).

Chapter 9

The Trigeminal System

By

Ian Darian-Smith, Baltimore (USA)

With 9 Figures

Contents

A. Introduction

Sensations elicited from the oro-facial region in man and other vertebrates have an importance to the animal beyond those evoked from other somatic tissues. The trigeminal afferent system is organized to serve both the general and the unique somatic sensory functions of this complex area, an area which includes the facial skin and underlying supportive tissues, the cornea, the mucocutaneous junctional tissues bounding the mouth and nostrils, the oral and nasal mucosae, the tongue and teeth, the muscles of mastication, and possibly the extra-ocular muscles. The afferent supply of the meningeal lining of the anterior and middle cranial fossae is also trigeminal, and in primates the facial mimetic muscles may have a trigeminal afferent innervation. Homology within the trigeminal and spinal somatic afferent systems is to be expected only in those neuronal pathways serving similar sensory functions. One aim in the investigation of the trigeminal sensory system is to identify not only those neural mechanisms that have a structural and functional parallel in the spinal somatic sensory system, but also those mechanisms that subserve a special local sensory role.

The predominant sensory function of the trigeminal system, in vertebrates ranging from fish to nonprimates mammals, is that of relaying to the forebrain precise information about the changing environment as the animal enters and explores new territory. This trigeminal input to the central nervous system will normally supplement the visual information obtained simultaneously, but in nocturnal and burrowing animals it may well furnish most of the information about the immediate milieu. Mostly these somatic afferents are excited only by contact, although cutaneous thermoreceptive afferents are sensitive to temperature changes induced by radiant energy. Extreme specialization occurs in the sensory membrane within the facial pit of crotalid snakes, that allows these animals to localize quite small remote sources of infrared radiation. Effective telereception of this type does not occur in mammals, but with the development of vibrissae, unique to this phylum, the animal can actively explore the environment well beyond its facial profile. The elephant's trunk illustrates another evolutionary development, aimed, in part, to extend the sensory space about the head that is monitored by the trigeminal inflow.

The exploratory function of the face and mouth becomes much less important in the higher mammals, particularly in the primates, as the hand evolves and assumes this role. Coincidentally, however, other specialized sensory functions are taken over by the trigeminal system. In amphibia, reptiles and birds the jaws are used to shape and position food in the pharynx ready for swallowing. Deglutition may be reflexly initiated by excitation of lingual mechanoreceptive afferents, but the trigeminal complex plays little further part in the process. In the mammal however, sucking in the newborn, and mastication in the adult normally precede swallowing, and these depend greatly on the trigeminal input to the central nervous system from the lips and intraoral structures, particularly the tongue. This bilateral coordinated sensory-motor activity may be disrupted by the loss of intraoral sensory discriminative capacity.

The most highly developed and most complex function assumed by the trigeminal system is its role in speech in man. The different vowel and consonant sounds require precise, timed variations in a) the vocal tract length, b) its cross-section at different levels, and c) the intraoral pressure (PERKELL, 1969). These modifications of the form of the vocal tract involve both the slowly acting, extrinsic muscles of the tongue, which may alter the position of the larynx within the pharynx, fixate the tongue, and set the angle of the jaw, and also the more rapidly acting intrinsic lingual muscles, that determine the shape of the tongue, and its apposition to teeth, lips and palate. To achieve this precision of motor function, somatosensory feedback from the various intraoral structures via trigeminal afferents is an essential supplement to that provided by auditory cues from the sounds articulated.

The natural history of the trigeminal system during foetal and postnatal development in man reflects a shift in function very similar to that which can be traced in vertebrate phylogeny. Simple jaw and lip movements, together with swallowing, occur spontaneously or reflexly in the foetus. At birth the 'rooting reflex' epitomizes the exploratory function, and sucking is already well developed. Within a few months highly coordinated, largely reflex, chewing movements, and later, masticatory movements are acquired, and finally, a year or more later the learned behavior of speech.

The functional characterization of single neurons has proven to be a powerful tool in the analysis of sensory function. Trigeminal neural mechanisms serving the simpler aspects of sensory discrimination have been studied, and form the basis of this review, but there is little information available about neural mechanisms of the more complex behavior which typifies the oro-facial region. Each of these special functions, such as mastication and speech articulation, requires the continuous integration of sensory information from both sides of the face and mouth. However, bilateral spatial convergence within the specific trigeminal projections, first occurs within the ventrobasal complex of the thalamus and not in the brainstem trigeminal nuclei. No investigation has been made of the functional organization of this convergence.

B. Organization of the Trigeminal Input to the Brainstem

In this section the survey of the sensory innervation of each of the separate tissues supplied by the trigeminal nerve is preceded by a summary of the sensory discriminative behavior associated with this tissue. Most, but not all of the investigations of sensory behavior have been restricted to man, whereas the neurophysiological studies have been mainly in non-primate mammals. Although such a species difference precludes any close comparison of the two sets of data, the psychophysical and behavioral observations supply information about the relative sensitivites of the different trigeminal zones which possibly are valid for species other than man. There are important differences, however, in thermal sensibility between man and non-primate mammals, such as the cat (KENSHALO et al., 1967; see later).

In recent studies of the receptor terminals in somatic tissues, structural similarities rather than the differences have been emphasized. CAUNA (1968), for example, classifies receptors in somatic tissues in two groups: a) *free nerve endings*, which have lost their perineural and myelin sheaths, but remain invested with a layer of Schwann cells and a continuous basement membrane, and b) *corpuscular terminals*, characterized by a well defined structural modification of the fiber terminal, and commonly intimately coupled with specialized epithelial or connective tissue cells. This class includes both the 'expanded nerve endings' such as Merkel's discs, and the 'encapsulated endings' of MILLER, RALSTON and KASAHARA

(1960). This classification provides a useful basis for comparing the receptor terminals found in the various tissues innervated by the trigeminal nerve.

Before considering specific receptors, some general statements can be made about their function. Firstly, with two exceptions (see later), all somatic receptive fibers that have been examined respond preferentially either to some form of mechanical deformation or to heat exchange in the tissue — not to both. This is true not only for those mechanoreceptive and thermoreceptive fibers sensitive to stimuli which evoke touch or thermal sensations in man, but in investigations so far, for myelinated and some unmyelinated receptive afferents responding only to intense noxious stimuli which would evoke pain (Burgess and Perl, 1967; Iggo and Ogawa, 1971). However, unmyelinated cutaneous afferents responding to noxious stimuli of any type have been isolated in the cat (Bessou and Perl, 1969). Secondly, corpuscular endings in skin — Merkel's discs in the epidermis, terminals within the hair follicle, Meissner's corpuscles in the dermis, and the deeply located Pacinian and Golgi-Mazzoni corpuscles — are the terminals of Group II myelinated fibers and are mechanoreceptive in function. The evidence is unequivocal for the Pacinian corpuscle (Hunt and McIntyre, 1960; Sato, 1961; Talbot et al., 1968) and circumstantial but strong for the other types of corpuscular terminal (Iggo, 1963, 1966; Talbot et al., 1968). Terminals of $A\delta$ fibers in the skin have not been identified.

1. Input from Facial Skin

a) **Tactile Sensory Mechanisms.** Common experience of the considerable tactile acuity of facial skin in man is borne out by quantitative measurement. Recently Weinstein (1968) has confirmed some of Weber's early psychophysical observations, demonstrating that the perioral skin is the most sensitive region for detecting contact, that point localization in this area equals that of the finger tips, and that two point discrimination is only slightly less than on the finger tips. Tactile sensitivity falls off on the forehead and scalp.

In the nonprimate, with the exception of the afferent fibers arising from the special vibrissal hair follicles, the sensory innervation of facial skin is structurally and functionally similar to that of other regions of hairy skin. Occasional intraepidermal, and profuse dermal free nerve endings, as well as corpuscular terminals of afferents innervating the different types of hair follicle are found in all areas of the face (Winkelmann, 1960, 1968; Fitzgerald, 1968; Cauna, 1968, 1969; Dixon, 1961). Rapidly adapting mechanoreceptive afferent fibers may be differentiated into Types D, G, and T of Brown and Iggo (1967), innervating down, guard and tylotrich follicles respectively (Darian-Smith, 1970; Rowe, 1968). The terminals of these rapidly adapting afferents are probably those of the cylindrical nerve plexus about the follicle shaft, encapsulated by a condensation of dermal tissue. All these afferents are sensitive to vibratory displacement of the hair or lip of the follicle, being most responsive in the frequency range of 60–300 cps (Rowe, 1968).

Again, if we exclude the vibrissal innervation, two types of slowly adapting mechanoreceptive fiber may be differentiated in subprimate facial skin, comparable with those of other regions of hairy skin. Histological and physiological evidence supports the view that the corpuscular nerve ending-Merkel cell complex of the Haarscheibe of Pinkus (PINKUS, 1904; IGGO, 1963, 1968; IGGO and MUIR, 1969; WERNER and MOUNTCASTLE, 1965; SMITH, 1967) is the terminal of one group of slowly adapting fibers. Its functional properties are described elsewhere in this volume (BURGESS and PERL). STRAILE (1960, 1961) has insisted that the tylotrich follicle and the Haarscheibe are structurally and functionally associated. Many Haarscheiben in facial skin (of the cat) are intimately associated with tylotrich hairs, and commonly surround the mouth of the hair follicle. Deformation of the follicle lip, either by direct contact, or by displacement of the hair, excites the slowly adapting myelinated fibers supplying hair discs of this type; a single nerve fiber may innervate one or several such follicles (ROWE, 1968). Although it is true that the hair disc and the tylotrich follicle are separately innervated by myelinated fibers, which respond differently to mechanical stimulation, it also appears that skin regions devoid of tylotrichs, such as the rabbits pinna, lack both Haarscheiben and slowly adapting mechanoreceptive afferents (MILLER and WEDDELL, 1966; MILLER, 1967; BROWN, IGGO and MILLER, 1967). This correlation is consistent with Strailes' contention.

A second type of slowly adapting mechanoreceptive fiber (Type II of BROWN and IGGO, 1967), most commonly innervating preauricular and supraorbital skin, has a receptive field 3–5 mm in diameter that includes upwards of 10 down hairs. Its dynamic response characteristics are similar to those of other trigeminal slowly adapting afferents with the exception that it responds vigorously to stretching of the skin (DARIAN-SMITH, ROWE and SESSLE, 1968; ROWE, 1968).

The vibrissa. Vibrissae are special sensory hairs found mainly in the perioral region in subprimates mammals; they are uncommon in primates (VINCENT, 1913; WINKELMANN, 1960). In some species such as the whale, in which hair development has regressed, only the vibrissae persist. The heavily innervated vibrissal follicle, with its hair, is a complex tactile exploratory organ, capable of active, rapid and accurate movement in space; the position and form of obstructions to this movement are apparently signalled continuously to the central nervous system. Vibrissal sensory function is probably best developed in mammals with poor vision, such as the rat; in these animals the vibrissal afferent fibers furnish information about the edges of narrow supports, of adjacent vertical obstructions, and helps in the discrimination of inequalities of the path beneath the animal. Each of these activities is impaired if the vibrissae are denervated or cut off (VINCENT). Movements of the vibrissae are controlled by facial motoneurons.

The structure of the vibrissa (see ANDRES, chapter 1) has attracted much attention (VINCENT, 1913; PATRIZI and MUNGER, 1966; ANDRES, 1966). There is no specialized innervation of the region of the follicle lip that is comparable with the Haarscheibe of PINKUS. However, Merkel disc-Merkel cell terminals are uniquely found within the epithelial outer root sheath of vibrissal follicles, and by analogy with the Haarscheibe these may be tentatively considered to be the endings of slowly adapting mechanoreceptive afferents that are excited by displacement of the vibrissa. Other specialized endings of myelinated fibers occur within the extensive cylindrical plexus within the dermal sheath of the follicle, similar to the palisade plexus of simpler hair follicles. These encapsulated endings are likely to be mechanoreceptive and rapidly adapting in character.

18*

About one-third of the myelinated, trigeminal cutaneous afferents innervate the vibrissae in the cat (ROWE, 1968). Each fibre supplies only one follicle, being most readily excited by vibrissal displacement in one particular direction (FITZ-GERALD, 1940; KERR and LYSAK, 1964; ROWE, 1968; ZUCKER and WELKER, 1969). Slowly adapting afferents (about 80 % of the vibrissal afferent population) signal the momentary displacement of the hair relative to the follicle, while the rapidly adapting afferents respond best to the high frequency component of the stimulus (see later). We do not know how the neural signal from a vibrissal follicle is evaluated when the vibrissa itself is being actively swept through the space surrounding the snout.

In man, regardless of sex, the hair follicle density of the facial skin and scalp is 3–4 times greater than in other regions of hairy skin (SZABO, 1958). This hair density, however, is related to the secondary sexual character of facial hair in man rather than to tactile sensory function, since individual hair follicles are much less specialized as sensory organs than are those of vibrissae in nonprimate mammals. The functional properties of mechanoreceptive afferents innervating this skin in monkeys (KERR and LYSAK, 1964) are similar to those innervating hairy skin of the forearm (MERZENICH and HARRINGTON, 1969).

Deep Tissues of the Face. Histological investigation has revealed few corpuscular endings within the deep tissues of the face, although free nerve endings are common (WINKELMANN, 1960; SAKADA and MAEDA, 1967a, b; SAKADA, 1971). Pacinian afferents, readily identified by their unique sensitivity to vibratory stimulation of the skin at 100–300 cps, have not been identified within the trigeminal nerve. However, SAKADA has examined fibers of histologically identified Golgi-Mazzoni corpuscles located in mandibular periostium, and found them to have frequency-response characteristics rather similar to those of Pacinian corpuscles but with more localized receptive fields. SAKADA (1971) also identified myelinated mechanoreceptive fibers with complex unencapsulated endings (? identification) which adapted slowly to steady compression and might well mediate the sense of deep pressure in the face.

b) Thermal Sensory Mechanisms. The evolution of trigeminal sensory function is well illustrated in the phylogeny of thermal sensory capacities. Crotalid snakes have developed specific infrared detecting organs — the facial pit organs — which enables the animal to detect and locate a small heat source (such as a rat) one half metre from the head (NOBLE and SCHMIDT, 1937). Non-primate mammals cannot locate such remote heat sources but they do rely entirely on the thermoreceptive afferents of the face and tongue to detect small increases in the environmental temperature (KENSHALO, DUNCAN and WEYMARK, 1967). In primates the exploratory function of the face and mouth regresses, and coincident with this functional shift, the disparity in the thermal sensitivity between the face and the rest of the body surface largely disappears. Even in man, however, the thermal sensitivity of facial skin is still greater than that of other areas of the body surface (HARDY and OPPEL, 1937).

The facial pit of the rattlesnake is lined by a thin membrane 15 μ thick, at least half being occupied by free nerve endings of the supramaxillary division of trigeminal nerve (BULLOCK and FOX, 1957; BLEICHMAN and DE ROBERTIS, 1962).

The pit organ receptors respond to sudden changes in the membrane temperature of 0.003°C or more, but unlike retinal photoreceptors, which are excited only by electromagnetic energy of certain wavelengths, the pit organ receptors respond to all wavelengths in the proportion that they heat the tissue (BULLOCK and DIECKE, 1956). It is unlikely therefore, that there is a photochemical step (in the infrared) interposed in the excitation sequence leading to receptor discharge; this conclusion applies also to cutaneous thermoreceptive fibers, for similar reasons.

In non-primate mammals the facial skin is much more sensitive to warming and possibly to cooling, than the hairy skin on the trunk and limbs (KENSHALO, 1968; KENSHALO, DUNCAN and WEYMARK, 1967). These sensory differences are at present only partially explicable in terms of the known differences in the thermoreceptive populations innervating each region. All thermoreceptive afferents innervating the hairy skin of the cat's leg are unmyelinated, most of them being 'cold' fibers, but a few 'warm' fibers do occur (IGGO, 1959; HENSEL, IGGO and WITT, 1960; IGGO, 1969). In the same species there are many more 'warm' fibers of unknown diameter in the infraorbital nerve that have receptive fields on the nose (HENSEL and HUOPANIEMI, 1969; HENSEL and KENSHALO, 1969), and in addition Aδ 'cold' afferents are found in this nerve (BOMAN; IRIUCHIJIMA and ZOTTERMAN; IGGO, 1969).

2. Input from the Cornea

Opinions differ concerning the degree of correspondence between the different sensory qualities which the human subject may identify following stimulation of the skin and the cornea (NAFE and WAGONER, 1937; LELE and WEDDELL, 1956; KENSHALO, 1960, 1970). Experiment has shown, however, that mild warming and cooling of the cornea, as well as gentle contact and potentially injurious deformation may be readily differentiated and localized (LELE and WEDDELL, 1956). Localized warming of the cornea by radiant heat is unequivocally identified as such, and sensory dissociation following trigeminal tractotomy is evident not only for ipsilateral facial skin, but also for the cornea (GRANT, GROFF and LEWY, 1940).

Only free nerve endings, often beaded along their course, are found in the cornea (WEDDELL and ZANDER, 1950; ZANDER and WEDDELL, 1951). They can be identified using slip lamp microscopy, following staining with methylene blue, in the living human cornea, but are more clearly demonstrated histologically. No corpuscular terminals have been observed in any animal studied, from fish to primate (ZANDER and WEDDELL, 1951). TOWER (1940) isolated sensitive myelinated, mechanoreceptive afferents in the cat's long ciliary nerve which innervates quite large segments of the cornea. More recently LELE and WEDDELL (1959) recorded from these nerves, reporting excitation of the one fibre by warming, cooling and mechanical stimulation of the cornea. However, in view of the overwhelming evidence of more specific responsiveness of somatic receptors in other tissues, further investigation of corneal afferents is needed.

3. Input from Oral Structures: the Lips, Tongue and Teeth

a) The Oral Mucosa. *Oral Sensory Function.* Tactile sensitivity of the oral mucosa differs considerably in different parts of the mouth. Estimates of the threshold for detection, and two point discrimination, demonstrate a spatial gradation of sensitivity; acuity being greatest near the lips and falling off progressively towards the pharynx (SHERRINGTON, 1917; GROSSMAN, 1967; HENKIN and BANKS, 1967; RINGEL, 1970a, b). This pattern of tactile sensitivity approximates that of the mucosal innervation density (DIXON, 1961). The mobile tongue and soft palate do not entirely conform to this antero-posterior sensory pattern, as each has its own profile of tactile sensitivity related to its special function. The tip of the tongue is especially responsive, the contact threshold (10 mg), two point discrimination (1.70 mm), and textual discrimination all being comparable with similar measures of tactile acuity on the finger tip (RINGEL, 1970a, b, c; HENKIN and BANKS, 1967). However, tactile sensitivity tapers off along the body of the tongue, especially on its ventral surface.

A problem that has attracted attention in recent years is the association of oral sensibility and speech articulation. It might well be anticipated that the continuous monitoring of auditory, and oral somatic sensory information would be essential for normal articulation. However, assessing the respective roles of these different sources of feedback in this complex sensory-motor activity has proven to be difficult. Subjects with severely limited oral tactile sensibility, who discriminate poorly between different solid forms placed in the mouth, may in fact articulate normally (McDONALD and AUNGST, 1970). Even extensive anaesthesia of the lips and tongue, produced by mandibular nerve block may not greatly impair speech in the adult (McCROSKEY, 1958). Possibly this oral sensory feedback is necessary in establishing motor patterns of articulation in the young child, but is no longer essential for well learned motor activity in the adult (COOPER, 1970).

Investigation of oral thermal sensibility has been limited. The tongue, especially at its tip, and the hard palate are more sensitive to cooling and warming than other intraoral structures, but even so, are less responsive than the lips or facial skin (STRUGHOLD, 1925; GROSSMAN and HATTIS, 1967). Although many people ingest near boiling liquids with pleasure, the thermal pain threshold for the hard palate and skin contrary to popular belief, are similar; no pain accompanies this bizarre behavior because the tissue temperature is effectively regulated by a coincident intake of air into the mouth (MARGARIDA, HARDY and HAMMEL, 1962).

Innervation of Oral Mucosa. The distribution of receptor terminals changes at the transition zone between the hairy skin of the lip and the oral mucosa. Free nerve endings in the dermis do not change, but intra-epidermal nerve endings greatly increase in the mucocutaneous junctional region and in the oral mucosa (WINKELMANN, 1968; FITZGERALD, 1968; GROSSMAN and HATTIS, 1967). The corpuscular endings of the hair follicles of the skin of the lip are replaced in the mucocutaneous zone by KRAUSE's end bulbs, formed by the tight intermingling of the unmyelinated terminals of several myelinated fibers. These occur also in the oral and lingual mucosa, and in addition, MEISSNER's corpuscles also become common within the mouth (DIXON, 1957, 1961, 1962, 1963; WILLIAMS and DIXON, 1963; GROSSMAN and HATTIS, 1967). MEISSNER's corpuscles are absent from the mucocutaneous transition zone (WINKELMANN, 1960).

Mechanoreceptive afferents innervating the mucocutaneous zones and the oral mucosa are functionally similar to those of glabrous skin (SAKADA, ITOW and IKE-GAMI, 1966; KERR and LYSAK, 1964; POULOS and LENDE, 1970a). This similarity extends to the sensitivity of slowly adapting fibers to sudden changes in tissue temperature (cf. IGGO, 1969).

'Cold' afferent fibers within the cat's lingual nerve were the first thermoreceptive fibers to be isolated (ZOTTERMAN, 1936) and remained the archetypal thermoreceptor until 'warm' afferents innervating the tongue were isolated in the chorda tympani (DODT and ZOTTERMAN, 1952). Very few 'warm' afferents have been isolated in the lingual nerve since then. The 'warm' afferents in the chorda tympani differed from those isolated more recently in cutaneous nerves (IGGO, 1964, 1969; HENSEL and HUOPANIEMI, 1969; HENSEL and KENSHALO, 1969; DARIAN-SMITH, JOHNSON and LaMOTTE, 1971) in that a) they were myelinated fibers 'somewhat larger in diameter than the cold fibers' (ZOTTERMAN, 1959), and b) their response to warming was small, irregular and bursting in character, unlike the regular rather high frequency discharge of cutaneous 'warm' afferent fibers. Recently it has been shown that some gustatory fibers, the main fibre component of the chorda tympani, are excited by warming of the tongue (NAGAKI et al., 1964; OGAWA et al., 1968), which raises some doubt as to the earlier identification of specific 'warm' afferent fibers in the chorda tympani. If this segregation of 'cold' and 'warm' lingual afferents occurs in man, then trigeminal root section would differentially impair cold sensibility in the tongue, and chorda tympani section would selectively block the detection of warming of this organ. Differential sensory loss of this type has apparently not been reported.

b) The Teeth and Their Supporting Tissues. Extensive reviews of the innervation of the teeth (FEARNHEAD, 1967) and of dental sensory mechanisms (ANDERSON et al., 1970) have been recently published.

Tapping or sustained force applied to the crown of a tooth is readily detected, localized and its line of action identified by the human observer. If the tooth is pulpless this sensory discrimination is only slightly impaired, indicating that most of the relevant mechanoreceptors are external to the tooth (STEWART). On the other hand, in the abnormal situation in which the dentine or pulp is directly excited by mechanical, thermal or chemical stimuli, only pain is elicited. It would be of interest to know if any sensations were elicited from the dental pulp following trigeminal tractotomy in man.

The neural mechanisms accounting for the tactile sensory responses pose no new problems. The relevant receptors are mostly located in the periodontal ligament or adjacent gingiva, and are structurally identical with those found in other regions of oral mucosa (LEWINSKY and STEWART, 1937; KEREBEL, 1965). The receptor sites of single mechanoreceptive afferents are typically localized to one part of the periodontal ligament of a single tooth, and are rarely found on the labial side of the tooth (NESS, 1954). Most of these myelinated afferents (conduction velocities of 25–80 m/sec) are slowly adapting to sustained displacement of the tooth, their discharge frequency is monotonically related to the force applied (PFAFFMAN, 1939a, b; NESS, 1954; YAMADA, 1963), relaying sufficient information to the central nervous system to account for the subjective discriminative behavior.

An unusual aspect of the central projections of these periodontal afferent fibers is that although the cell bodies of some are within the Gasserian ganglion (KERR and LYSAK, 1964; BEAUDREAU and JERGE, 1968), the cell bodies of other apparently similar fibers are located in the trigeminal mesencephalic nucleus (JERGE, 1963a; CORBIN and HARRISON, 1940; SMITH and MARCARIAN, 1968). Those primary afferents entering the trigeminal spinal tract almost certainly project to each nucleus of the brainstem trigeminal complex, as many second order trigeminal neurons have dental receptive fields. The central connections of those afferents in the mesencephalic projection, however, are uncertain (see later).

Free nerve endings and simple expanded terminals are seen within the pulp tissue (HARRIS and GRIFFIN, 1968). The innervation of the dentine, however, is poorly understood. FEARNHEAD (1967) found fine terminals within about 10% of dentinal tubules, but these endings did not extend to the amelodental junction, a highly sensitive area as judged from clinical experience. How these nerve terminals are related to the odontoblast processes within the dentinal tubulus is still controversial 100 years after their first description (ARWILL, 1963; SCOTT, 1966). Because of this limited, or absent, dentinal innervation, BRÄNNSTRÖM (1963) has suggested a 'hydrodynamic' link between the dentinal tubules and receptors within the pulp; any stimulus that displaces the fluid contents of the dentinal tubules (mechanical, thermal or osmotic) would excite the receptor and evoke pain.

The functional characterization of pulp afferent fibers has been less than satisfactory, because of the failure to examine the small myelinated and unmyelinated fiber populations (BROOKHART et al., 1953). The $A\delta$ and C-fiber content of dental nerves (WILSON, 1968) and within the dental pulp (HARRIS and GRIFFIN, 1968) is well documented, as is the correlation between the experience of pain and activity in fibers of this size. The peripheral mechanisms of common toothache will remain unknown however, until the functional characteristics of these small fibers in dental pulp are explored.

4. The Gasserian Ganglion

The fine structure of the Gasserian ganglion is essentially similar to that of the spinal root ganglia (DIXON, 1963b; MAXWELL, 1967; MOSES, 1967; KERR, 1967; PINEDA, MAXWELL and KRUGER, 1967), the rather large cell bodies being entirely surrounded by closely apposed satellite cells. In mammals the axon of the ganglion cell, immediately after it arises from the soma, forms a complex and tortuous intracapsular structure — the glomerulus of CAJAL — before dividing into the peripheral and smaller central branches. Conduction of an impulse along this glomerular segment is slow, about 1.5–2 m/sec (DARIAN-SMITH, MUTTON and PROCTOR, 1965), so that with large myelinated fibers an orthodromically conducted impulse will invade the most remote central terminals of the neuron before depolarization of the soma occurs. This functional isolation of the cell body from the main axon pathway, resulting from the development of the glomerulus, is not seen in lower vertebrates and its relevance is not known. No synaptic junctions have been observed in the several electron microscopic studies of the ganglion, and differences in soma structure, which were the basis for distinguishing different cell populations in some earlier studies, have proven to be artifactual (PINEDA et al., 1967).

A somatotopic organization, based on the peripheral location of the mechanoreceptive field, occurs at all levels in the pathways of primary afferent neurons, including the trigeminal spinal tract. The cell bodies of mechanoreceptive afferents within the ophthalmic division of the nerve are concentrated medially and somewhat anteriorly within the Gasserian ganglion; those of the mandibular division are caudal and lateral within the ganglion. Somas of the maxillary division lie between those of the other divisions (KERR and LYSAK, 1964; DARIAN-SMITH et al., 1965; BEAUDREAU and JERGE, 1968; ZUCKER and WELKER, 1969). KERR and LYSAK, and more recently others, also observed a dorsoventral pattern of projection, with representation of the perioral and oral structures ventrally in the ganglion, and regions remote from the mouth, such as the supraorbital zone in the dorsum of the ganglion. The patterns of distribution of the cell bodies of thermoreceptive and mechanoreceptive neurons within the Gasserian ganglion are probably similar; the cell bodies of lingual mechanoreceptive and thermoreceptive afferents, for example, are located in the same region (POULOS and LENDE, 1970).

Cell bodies of afferent neurons innervating muscle spindles in the masseter, pterygoid and temporalis muscles have not been identified in the Gasserian ganglion, but are found within the uniquely organized mesencephalic trigeminal nucleus, and are discussed later. However, MANNI et al. (1970) have recently located the cell bodies of stretch afferents innervating the extraocular muscles within the ophthalmic projection to the Gasserian ganglion in the sheep and pig; similar cell bodies were not found in the cat and dog.

5. The Trigeminal Spinal Tract

Primary afferent fibres project to the trigeminal nuclear complex mainly through the trigeminal spinal tract, the exception being those fibres which enter the pons within the motor root and project to the mesencephalic nucleus. Unmyelinated fibres enter the spinal tract and, without bifurcating, descend in it to terminate within nucleus caudalis (WINDLE, 1926). Most myelinated fibres in the trigeminal root divide on entering the brainstem, the rostral branch ascending to terminate within the main sensory nucleus, and the caudal branch descending a variable distance within the spinal tract. GERARD (1923) showed that there is a significant falling off in the calibre of myelinated fibers in the trigeminal spinal tract at more caudal levels. In Golgi preparations these descending fibres can be seen to give off collateral branches in the adjacent nuclei, and to continue on as smaller fibres (RAMÓN Y CAJAL, 1909; ASTRÖM, 1953).

Cutaneous mechanoreceptive afferents present at different levels within the trigeminal spinal tract have been analysed using a rather different approach. By recording in the Gasserian ganglion from the somas of individual neurons the functional characteristics of both the peripheral and central axon segments may be determined (DARIAN-SMITH et al., 1965; ROWE, 1968). Each neuron may be discharged orthodromically by appropriate stimulation of the facial skin, or antidromically by electrical stimulation of the spinal tract. It has been shown that in the cat more than 80 % of myelinated fibers project to the rostral pole of nucleus caudalis, and that most of these fibers terminate adjacent to and presumably within this nucleus (DARIAN-SMITH et al., 1965; ROWE, 1968); only about 10% of these fibers project to C2. Conduction of impulses caudally along these fibres slows progressively, indicating thinning, and presumably collateral branching along their course (WALL and TAUB, 1962; DARIAN-SMITH et al., 1965). Direct evidence of this collateral branching within nucleus oralis and nucleus caudalis

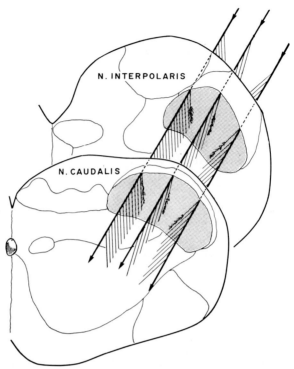

Fig. 1. Diagram illustrating the rostrocaudal 'leaves' formed by the collateral terminals of myelinated trigeminal fibers. Three such radially oriented 'leaves' are shown traversing nucleus interpolaris and nucleus caudalis, but they extend the whole length of the trigeminal tract, and penetrate all trigeminal nuclei (except the mesencephalic nucleus). This pattern of projection ensures that the whole ipsilateral trigeminal receptive sheet is represented at all rostrocaudal levels within the trigeminal complex. This complex is shaded in the figure

has been obtained by recording from single primary afferent terminals within each of these nuclei; each of the mechanoreceptive types recognized in cutaneous nerves was represented in the projection to each of these nuclei (Rowe, 1968). The primary afferent projection to the main sensory nucleus is probably similar, but the input to nucleus interpolaris remains uncertain.

Complementary experimental and clinical studies have shown that the trigeminal spinal tract is somatotopically organized. A laminar projection, with fibres of the ophthalmic, maxillary, and mandibular divisions lying successively more dorsomedial is established for all myelinated fibres, including cutaneous mechanoreceptive afferents (Szentágothai and Kiss, 1949; Torvik, 1956; Kerr, 1963; Darian-Smith and Mayday, 1960; Wall and Taub, 1962), and also for the smaller myelinated and unmyelinated fibres pertinent to the appreciation of thermal and noxious stimuli (Sjöqvist, 1938, 1939; Walker, 1939; Grant et al., 1940; Olivecrona, 1942; Kunc, 1966, 1970). Degeneration studies have also shown that collaterals of these fibres terminate in the underlying trigeminal nucleus at all rostrocaudal levels for myelinated fibres in sharply defined sectors, extending deeply into the nucleus and overlapping neighbouring projections only slightly.

Thus the picture which emerges of the trigeminal projection of myelinated fibres to the brainstem is of a series of stacked terminal 'leaves' which extend the whole length of the trigeminal nuclear complex, each 'leaf' being characterized throughout its length by an identical projection from the periphery (Fig. 1). Such an arrangement implies that the whole ipsilateral trigeminal receptive field is represented at all rostrocaudal levels within the complex. However, this projection may not be identical at each level, as the density of projection in a particular 'leaf' may vary along its axis in different nuclei, or in different parts of the one nucleus. Evidence suggesting that such variations in central representation do occur at different rostrocaudal levels in the brainstem is considered later.

The trigeminal nerve is not the only peripheral input to the trigeminal complex. The analgesic field following trigeminal tractotomy extends beyond that produced by root section in the following regions: tympanic membrane and part of the external auditory canal, mucosa of the posterior third of the tongue, the tonsil and pharynx. Tactile sensibility in these areas is not noticeably altered following the tractotomy (BRODAL, 1947; FALCONER, 1949; KUNC, 1966; TAREN, 1964). Somatic afferent fibres of the facial, glossopharyngeal and vagus nerves supply these same regions, the large myelinated afferents projecting centrally mainly to the nucleus solitarius. Some small fibres, however, join the dorsomedial part of the trigeminal spinal tract, and terminate within nucleus caudalis and the spinal dorsal horn at the levels of C1 and C2 (RAMÓN Y CAJAL, 1909; TORVIK, 1956; KERR, 1962). KERR has also identified terminals within nucleus interpolaris in the cat, which he suggested mediates tactile sensation. TORVIK favors a 'tactile' projection via the nucleus solitarius.

6. The Trigeminal Mesencephalic Nucleus

Most, if not all, neurons in the trigeminal mesencephalic nucleus are unipolar primary afferent cells comparable to sensory ganglion cells. Unlike sensory ganglion cells, however, the somas of these neurons have remained within the central nervous system. They form a column at the edge of the central gray matter that extends from the posterior commissure rostrally, to the level of the trigeminal motor nucleus caudally. Most of these neurons are proprioceptive in function (CORBIN and HARRISON, 1940; JERGE, 1963a), with receptor terminals responding to stretch in the muscles of mastication, and possibly in the extraocular muscles also (COOPER, DANIEL and WHITTERIDGE, 1955). Other mesencephalic neurons innervate the dental supporting tissues (CORBIN and HARRISON, 1940; SZENTÁGOTHAI, 1949; JERGE, 1963a; GABRAWI and TARKHAN, 1967). The central connections of these neurons mainly subserve masticatory reflexes, but there are also projections to the other trigeminal nuclei, which may have a sensory function. BRODAL and SAUGSTAD (1965) report a cerebellar projection.

Feedback control mechanisms of the muscles of mastication, although similar to those of limb muscles, differ in important detail. The masseter, temporalis, and medial pterygoid muscles, with a jaw-closing action, each contain muscle spindles, but the lateral pterygoids have few, if any (FREIMANN, 1954; COOPER, 1960). The Group Ia fibers innervating these muscle spindles enter the brainstem in the trigeminal motor root, and project rostrally into the mesencephalic nuclei, within which their cell bodies are located at various rostrocaudal levels (Corbin and Harrison, 1940; Jerge, 1963a). These neurons have direct axon collateral projections to homonymous trigeminal motoneurons, forming the monosynaptic reflex arc tested by the jaw jerk (Szentágothai, 1949; McIntyre, 1951; McIntyre and Robinson, 1959; Hugelin and Bonvallet, 1957).

Excitatory input from the stretch receptors of the masticatory muscles to trigeminal motoneurons is abolished in man and experimental animals by destruction of the trigeminal mesencephalic nucleus (Hufschmidt and Spuler, 1962), but not if the trigeminal sensory roots is sectioned leaving the motor root intact. In this same operative procedure, however, Group 1b fibers innervating Golgi tendon organs in these same muscles are transected, since their cell bodies are within the Gasserian ganglion and their central projections are within the sensory root. Thus, the Frazier-Spiller operation, in which this selective root section is carried out in man, results in the dissociation of the separate feedback control for muscle length and muscle tension, and a disappearance of the inhibitory effects that characterize the latter (Hufschmidt and Spuler, 1962). The patient, however, suffers no obvious impairment of masticatory function with a unilateral operation.

The action of jaw-closing and jaw-opening muscles on the two sides commonly act in accord; the bilateral projection from each mesencephalic nucleus ensures this paired function (Smith, Marcarian and Niemer, 1967a, b). However, contralateral inhibition of masseteric action following stretching of the ipsilateral muscle does occur (Hufschmidt and Spuler, 1962; Kawamura, 1970), which Kawamura suggests is mediated by a pathway including interneurons within the supratrigeminal nucleus (Jerge, 1963b).

Collaterals of large monopolar neurons within the trigeminal mesencephalic nucleus have been traced to the hypoglossal nucleus and the spinal cervical segments C1 and C2 (Szentágothai, 1949). Szentágothai suggested that these collaterals are part of an inhibitory pathway from the jaw closing muscles to their infrahyoid antagonists. An interneuron is interposed in the reciprocal inhibitory pathways of this type in the spinal cord (Eccles, 1957); corresponding bulbar inhibitory interneurons have not been identified.

The trigeminal mesencephalic nucleus receives no input from the temporomandibular joint (Kawamura and Majima, 1964; Kawamura, 1970), nor from the muscles of the tongue (Corbin and Harrison, 1940; Jerge, 1963a). In the cat there are no muscle spindles in the lingual muscles (Cooper, 1953; Blom, 1960; Porter, 1966) but they are found in the intrinsic muscles of the primate tongue (Cooper, 1953). However, their afferents probably enter the central nervous system in the cervical component of the hypoglossal nerve, and not in the lingual nerve (Engel, Bowman and Combs, 1968).

Although more than 85% of cell bodies within the trigeminal mesencephalic nucleus are those of primary afferents (Dault and Smith, 1969) there are possibly interneurons within the nucleus. The somas of the mesencephalic are varied and some are multipolar (Sheinin, 1930; Pearson, 1949). Further, axosomatic synapses have been described within the nucleus (Ramón y Cajal, 1909; Hinrichsen and Larramendi, 1968), but no identification of the postsynaptic element made.

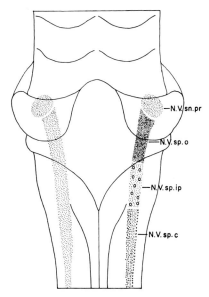

Fig. 2. OLSZEWSKI's figure illustrating on the right side the extent of the different trigeminal nuclei that constitute the spinal trigeminal complex: N.V.sp.c. — caudalis; N.V.sp.ip. — interpolaris; N.V.sp.o. — oralis. The main sensory nucleus is also shown — N.V.sn.pr. The left side of the diagram shows the earlier subdivision into a main sensory nucleus and a spinal trigeminal nucleus. (OLSZEWSKI, 1950)

C. Organization of the Trigeminal Nuclear Complex

Two structurally distinct components of the trigeminal nuclear complex have long been recognized — the main sensory nucleus, and the nucleus of the spinal tract (spinal trigeminal complex of OLSZEWSKI). Three further divisions of the spinal trigeminal complex may be differentiated in the mammal (MEESSEN and OLSZEWSKI, 1949; OLSZEWSKI, 1950; TORVIK, 1956; BRODAL et al., 1956; OLSZEWSKI and BAXTER, 1954; DARIAN-SMITH, 1966a) the nucleus oralis, nucleus interpolaris and nucleus caudalis (Fig. 2). The investigation of trigeminal somatic sensory function is really directed to an analysis of the sensory contributions of these different nuclei, specific questions being: — a) do these structurally distinct nuclei serve different sensory functions; and b) what are the functional homologies in the spinal and trigeminal somatic sensory pathways? Only partial answers can be given to these questions.

The phylogeny of the trigeminal complex reveals certain basic features of organization. In the lower more generalized types of vertebrate, such as cyclostomes, certain fish and tailed amphibia, differentiation of the trigeminal nuclei is slight, but a primordial nucleus caudalis can be recognized (CROSBY and YOSS, 1954). In frogs the trigeminal spinal complex has polarized with a nucleus caudalis being separated from a less differentiated rostral nucleus oralis. The main sensory nucleus can now also be identified. In reptiles and birds the main sensory nucleus increases in size and becomes more distinctive, and nucleus interpolaris, the third component of the trigeminal spinal complex, first appears.

Differentiation of the main sensory nucleus and the three nuclear components of the trigeminal spinal complex is greatest within mammals, but varies somewhat according to behavioral specialization. In monotremes, the main sensory nucleus is very large (ABBIE, 1934), but nucleus interpolaris is poorly differentiated. In higher mammals, and particularly in primates, nucleus oralis is relatively much larger than the main sensory nucleus.

Comparable with the phylogenetic pattern described above is the sequence of differentiation of the trigeminal nuclear subdivision in the human embryo (HUM-PHREY, 1952, 1964, 1970; BROWN, 1956, 1958, 1960, 1962). At 6.5 weeks an undifferentiated cell mass is distinguishable at the site of the future trigeminal nuclear complex; by 7.5 weeks nucleus caudalis has begun to differentiate, and by 9.5 weeks its three subnuclei may be recognized. Differentiation of the rostral part of the alar plate beneath the trigeminal spinal tract does not begin until the 9th week. By the 11th week the main sensory nucleus, as well as nucleus oralis and nucleus interpolaris may be separately identified, but full differentiation is not completed until the 18th week. Reflex behavior in the human fetus, elicited by perioral mechanical stimulation, first occurs at 7.5 weeks (HUMPHREY, 1954, 1964, 1970), at which time nucleus caudalis is recognizable. More localized, reflex activity, evoked by trigeminal stimulation occurs later with the emergence and differentiation of the other trigeminal nuclei.

1. Structure of the Trigeminal Nuclear Complex

a) **The Main Sensory Nucleus.** This forms the most rostral part of the trigeminal nuclear complex (excluding the separate mesencephalic nucleus), enveloping the trigeminal motor nucleus medially and extending a little caudal to the latter. Collaterals of myelinated primary afferent fibers of the trigeminal spinal tract course medially through the nucleus. The neurons seen in Golgi preparations are distributed in clusters, with round or oval cell bodies (10–30 μ), and have a relatively simple bushy pattern of dendritic branching, which, however, may extend across half of the nucleus (RAMÓN Y CAJAL, 1909; TORVIK, 1956, 1957; KUYPERS and TUERK, 1964; GOBEL and DUBNER, 1969). There is no obvious alignment of dendritic branches within the nucleus; dendritic spines are common.

The types of synaptic junction seen within the main sensory nucleus are similar to those in the dorsal column nuclei (WALBERG, 1966). In addition to extensive terminal synapses on the primary dendrites and cell bodies of the relay neurons, characteristic 'glomeruli' have been observed along the intranuclear course of the primary afferent fibers (GOBEL and DUBNER, 1969). Dilatations along the course of these axons constitute the central boutons of such glomeruli, in which synaptic contact is made with small dendritic branches as well as with other axons. GOBEL and DUBNER infer from the ultrastructure of the glomerular synapses that the central bouton of the primary afferent fiber may synaptically activate the dendritic branches or may itself be the post-synaptic element of axo-axonal junctions, which are common within these glomeruli. The axon terminals in the periphery of the glomerous do not degenerate following section of the trigeminal root; whether they arise from cells within the nucleus or beyond is not known (Fig. 3).

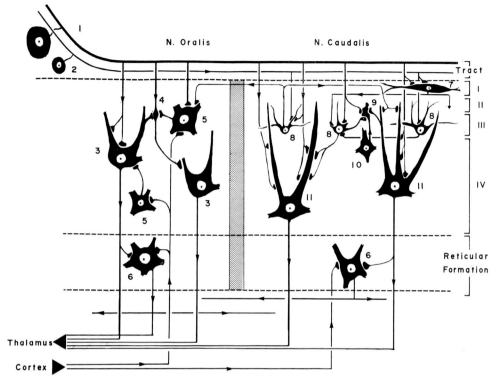

Fig. 3. Diagram illustrating the input, the different cell types, the synaptic linkages and the projections of *nucleus oralis* and *nucleus caudalis*. Large myelinated fibres (1) extend the whole length of the trigeminal complex giving off collaterals to the adjacent nuclei at all levels. Small myelinated fibres and C-fibres (2) project to nucleus caudalis only. *Within nucleus oralis:* large myelinated fibres project to relay neurons (3) and interneurons (5). Their collaterals may form the central boutons of 'glomeruli' (4) within this nucleus (see text). Corticofugal fibres terminate on interneurons (5), and possibly on relay cells (3). The latter (3) have collateral projections on to neurons within the brainstem reticular formation (6). *Within nucleus caudalis:* second order neurons are distributed within 4 laminae (I, II, III and IV). Large myelinated fibres project to subnucleus marginalis (I), to subnucleus gelatinosus (II and III), and to subnucleus magnocellularis (IV). Small myelinated fibres and C-fibres project mainly to the deep part of subnucleus gelatinosus (III), but also to subnucleus marginalis and possibly to subnucleus magnocellularis (IV). Both fibre types project to the cells of Waldeyer (7) and to gelatinosa cells (9 and 10). The larger fibers also terminate on the radially oriented cells of the subnucleus magnocellularis (11). The projections of gelatinosa cells (8) are apparently largely restricted to this region, terminating on other gelatinosa cells, on the apical dendrites of magnocellularis cells, within 'glomeruli' in this region, and possibly within rostral trigeminal nuclei. Some gelatinosa cells (11) project to the thalamus and to the brainstem reticular formation. Neurons (10) are the hypothetical cells of RÉTHELYI and SZENTÁGOTHAI, from which arise the central axon terminals of the glomeruli in this nucleus (see text)

Most neurons within this nucleus project to nucleus ventralis posteromedialis of the thalamus (VPM). These fibers emerge from the ventromedial margin of the main sensory nucleus, and pass to the contralateral brainstem to ascend with the medial lemniscus along its dorsolateral aspect. Neurons in the dorsomedial part of the nucleus with an input from oral structures, however, project to the ipsilateral VPM in a separate and unique pathway — the trigeminal dorsal tract, first described by Wallenberg — which contains no other fibers (Torvik, 1957; Carpenter, 1957). Relay neurons within the main sensory nucleus (most of the cell population) are the only trigeminal cells which undergo degeneration following transsection of the midbrain, and in this respect more nearly resemble neurons of the dorsal column nuclei than other trigeminal cells — they have no collateral terminals within the brainstem reticular formation.

The supratrigeminal nucleus (Lorente de Nó, 1922; Torvik, 1956), an aggregate of loosely packed cells with rather extensive dendritic branching, is located at the dorsomedial angle of the main sensory nucleus. These neurons are internuncials, probably functionally linked with trigeminal motor activity, since proprioceptive afferents project to the nucleus (Jerge, 1963a, b).

b) Nucleus Oralis. This nucleus extends from the rostral pole of the facial nucleus to the rostral third of the inferior olive in the mammal. It is not structurally uniform and its medial border is poorly demarcated from the adjacent reticular nuclei. Rostrally there are some large multipolar cells with the dimensions of a motoneuron, but most of the remaining neurons are small and comparable in size and dendritic pattern with those of the main sensory nucleus. The fine structure of synaptic junctions within this nucleus has not been described, but is presumed to differ little from that of synapses in the main sensory nucleus. The axons of most neurons in this nucleus join the contralateral medial lemniscus and project to VPM (Carpenter and Hanna, 1961; Darian-Smith and Yokota, 1966; Rowe and Sessle, 1968; Sessle, 1968; Eisenman et al., 1963). These neurons differ from relay cells of the main sensory nucleus, however, insofar that there is no ipsilateral projections, and further, that they do not degenerate following section of the medial lemniscus (Torvik, 1957). This probably reflects collateral branching in the brainstem.

c) Nucleus Interpolaris. In mammals this nucleus, continuous with nucleus oralis, extends from the rostral third of the inferior olive to the obex. Astrom has described three cell groups within this nucleus in the mouse: — a) a subnucleus of the marginal plexus consisting of medium to large radially oriented multipolar cells, b) a similar group of cells located dorsomedially, and c) much smaller neurons with rounded somas, and compact dentritic branching, which constitute the remainder of the nucleus. Glomeruli, similar to those seen in the main sensory nucleus, with axodendritic and axo-axonal synapses have been observed within nucleus interpolaris (Westrum and Black), together with separate axo-somatic and axo-dendritic synapses. Surprisingly, no changes were observed within most axo-somatic synapses following trigeminal rhizotomy.

Trigemino-thalamic neurons within this nucleus apparently resemble those of nucleus oralis, but both histological and electro-physiological evidence indicates that they may form only part of the cell population of this nucleus. The thalamic projection is entirely to the contralateral VPM (Carpenter and Hanna, 1961). Terminal degeneration studies in the cat, in which localized lesions were placed in nucleus interpolaris, have demonstrated additional long axon projections to the anterior cerebellar cortex via the inferior cerebellar peduncle, and also the brain-stem reticular formation (CARPENTER and HANNA, 1961).

d) Nucleus Caudalis. This nucleus, extending from the obex to the first cervical root, has long been recognized, and considered an upward extension of the spinal dorsal horn. On passing from the cervical dorsal horn into nucleus caudalis there is considerable structural transformation, and an increase in size, but, nonetheless, the first four cytoarchitectonic laminae of REXED (1952) can be differentiated. OLSZEWSKI (1950) subdivided nucleus caudalis into the following laminar zones: — a) subnucleus marginalis (or zonalis) (lamina I of REXED), b) subnucleus gelatinosus (laminae II and III), and subnucleus magnocellularis, which although much expanded, is probably homologous with REXED's lamina IV (Fig. 3). REXED considered that laminae V and VI do not extend into the medulla, but merge with the brainstem reticular formation.

The primary afferent projection to nucleus caudalis includes both myelinated fibers, 75 % of which are now less than 2 μ in diameter (KERR, 1966), and unmyelinated fibers. Whether trigeminal unmyelinated fibers project only to nucleus caudalis is uncertain. Both groups of fibers penetrate the nucleus from the spinal tract in a spatially ordered radial pattern, contrasting with the terminal projection in the dorsal horn, in which myelinated fibers enter separately from its medial side. As in the more rostral trigeminal nuclei, these intranuclear collaterals of individual primary afferents form 'leaves' extending the rostrocaudal extent of the nucleus (Fig. 1), each 'leaf' being characterized throughout its length by an identical projection from the periphery. The larger fibers terminate mainly within the deep zone of subnucleus gelatinosus (lamina III) (CLARKE and BOWSHER, 1962; KERR, 1963, 1970a, b) and subnucleus magnocellularis (? lamina IV); a few smaller fibers may also be traced to subnucleus marginalis (lamina I), as well as deep into the subjacent reticular formation. As in the dorsal horn (RALSTON, 1965, 1968a, b; SZENTÁGOTHAI, 1964; RÉTHELYI and SZENTÁGOTHAI, 1968; HEIMER and WALL, 1968) there is uncertainty about the occurrence of a primary afferent projection to the outer zone of subnucleus gelatinosus (lamina II), but possibly unmyelinated fibers terminate at this level.

Subnucleus Marginalis. Cells within this region are a) a few moderately large neurons, whose dendritic branches form a flattened but incomplete sheet defining the dorsolateral margin of nucleus caudalis (the marginal cells of WALDEYER in dorsal horn), and b) many smaller cells with a similar 'horizontal' configuration. One input, mainly axo-somatic (KERR, 1966) is from peripheral myelinated fibers. The axons of these cells probably contribute to the fiber projection from nucleus caudalis to rostral trigeminal nuclei.

Subnucleus Gelatinosus. The most characteristic feature of the outer zone of this subnucleus (lamine II) is the profusion of unmyelinated axons, accounting for its pallor in silver stained sections. These are in part replaced by myelinated fibers of exogenous origin in the deeper zone of the subnucleus (lamina III). The neurons in this subnucleus, identical in appearance with those of substantia gelatinosa Rolandi, are small, spindle-shaped, with little cytoplasm, and their dendritic systems are essentially two-dimensional, being aligned rostro-caudally, with the 'leaves' of primary afferent terminals within the nucleus. As in the dorsal horn, these cells appear to be part of an endogenous system; some cells have a local axon projection only, while the axons of others probably constitute the bulk of the rostral projection from this region to nucleus interpolaris, nucleus oralis, and especially the main sensory nucleus (Carpenter and Hanna, 1961; Stewart and King, 1963; Dunn and Matze, 1968).

Most synapses within subnucleus gelatinosus are axo-dendritic or axo-axonal; axo-somatic synapses are rare (Kerr, 1970b; Gruner, 1970b). A specialized synaptic complex is found in subnuclei marginalis and gelatinosus; in this glomerulus a central bouton makes synaptic contact with one or several axons, as well as with small dendrites (Kerr, 1966) (Fig. 3). In comparable glomeruli in the dorsal horn, rhizotomy causes the degeneration of some of the postsynaptic peripherally located axon terminals, but never of the central 'dark sinuous' bouton. Since this central bouton does degenerate following destruction of lamina III, Réthelyi and Szentágothai (1968) have postulated a 'pyramidal' interneuron with its soma in lamina III and axon terminals forming the central boutons of glomeruli. Such a neuron would have connections appropriate to the terminal internuncial in a presynaptic inhibitory pathway modulating cutaneous trigeminal input. Note, however, that this glomerulus and that occurring in the main sensory nucleus are quite differently organized (Fig. 3).

Subnucleus Magnocellularis. This cell group forms the bulk of nucleus caudalis. Like lamina IV of the dorsal horn, it is characterized by medium to large neurons (20–40 μ) whose apical dendritic branches radiate out toward the margin of the nucleus in the form of an inverted cone, extending even to subnucleus marginalis. Myelinated fibres from the spinal tract terminate on the dendrites of these cells both within the deeper zone of subnucleus gelatinosus and in subnucleus magnocellularis; axo-somatic contact also occurs but is less common (Kerr, 1966, 1970b). Axo-axonic synapses are found deep in nucleus caudalis, but are much less frequent than in the outer laminae. Little is known of the terminations of peripheral C-fibres within nucleus caudalis, but they are infrequently seen in subnucleus magnocellularis.

Although the homology of the neuron populations within lamina IV of the dorsal horn and subnucleus magnocellularis is supported by most structural and functional characterization, their long axon projections differ. The major efferent projection of subnucleus magnocellularis is to the posterior thalamus, and is 'spinothalamic' in character (Nauta and Kuypers, 1958; Mehler, Fefferman and Nauta, 1960; Mehler, 1966; Stewart and King, 1963; Rowe and Sessle, 1968). The projection is bilateral, with most fibers ascending within the classical lateral pathways (medial lemniscus and spinothalamic tract). The fibres of some relay neurons, however, ascend through the reticular tegmentum. Like spinothalamic fibres the thalamic projection from nucleus caudalis terminates in: — a) the ventrobasal complex (VPM), b) the magnocellular region of the medial geniculate nucleus, and c) the intralaminar nuclei, with the possible exception of the nucleus centre median (Mehler, 1966). Recent analysis has shown that no fibres of nucleus caudalis join the dorsal trigeminal tract — an ipsilateral projection solely from the main sensory nucleus (Torvik, 1957; Steward and King, 1963). However, spinothalamic fibers in subprimates, with terminal projections in the thalamus similar to those of caudalis cells, apparently do not arise from lamina IV, but probably from laminae V and VI of the dorsal horn (SZENTÁGOTHAI, 1964; SCHEIBEL and SCHEIBEL, 1968; RÉTHELYI and SZENTÁGOTHAI, 1968).

The one identified projection from lamina IV in the cat is the spinocervical projection to the ipsilateral lateral cervical nucleus, which in turn projects to the contralateral ventrobasal complex (REXED and STROM, 1952; TAUB and BISHOP, 1965; BROWN and FRANZ, 1969). The trigeminal homologue of this spinal projection is certainly not obvious.

Nucleus caudalis has an extensive projection to the brainstem reticular formation, particularly to the ipsilateral parvicellular part of the lateral reticular nucleus in the region adjacent to nucleus interpolaris (STEWART and KING, 1963; DUNN and MATZE, 1968). Some fibres originating from nucleus oralis and interpolaris also terminate in the adjacent reticular formation and in the contralateral nucleus reticularis giganto-cellularis, but this projection is small in comparison with that from nucleus caudalis.

Fig. 3 schematizes the known circuitry of nucleus oralis and nucleus caudalis. Connections of the main sensory nucleus differ from those illustrating nucleus oralis in two respects only; trigemino-thalamic axons do not have collaterals terminating in the brainstem reticular formation, and some of these fibers project in the dorsal trigeminal tract to the ipsilateral VPM. The circuitry of nucleus interpolaris has not been included in Fig. 3 because of the limited information available.

2. Functional Organization of the Trigeminal Nuclear Complex: The Effects of Discrete Lesions on Sensory Function

Following occlusion of the posterior inferior cerebellar artery in man, nucleus caudalis and possibly nucleus interpolaris are destroyed; coincidentally, neither painful nor thermal sensations can be elicited from the ipsilateral trigeminal peripheral field, but tactile sensibility is clinically unimpaired (HUN, 1897; GERARD, 1923; SMYTH, 1939). If the peripheral neural input to nucleus caudalis is more specifically blocked by trigeminal tractotomy the same differential sensory loss occurs, indicating that neural mechanisms essential for the appreciation of painful and thermal stimulation of the face or mouth are located within this nucleus. The severity of the sensory loss following tractotomy at the level of the obex is illustrated by the fact that these patients are not able to distinguish test tubes filled with boiling and iced water placed on the ipsilateral cheek (GRANT et al., 1940).

In some patients, following both thrombosis of the posterior inferior cerebellar artery and trigeminal tractotomy (SPILLER, 1915; SMYTH, 1939; GRANT et al., 1940; WEINBERGER and GRANT, 1942; KUNC, 1966, 1970), the thermal sensory loss is less complete than the analgesia. To account for this observation SPILLER (1915) suggested that thermal sensibility may be mediated by trigeminal structures extending somewhat more rostrally than those critical for pain sensation. Such a schema would implicate nucleus interpolaris.

Some tactile sensory loss does result from these lesions, but it is slight or subtle in character, since no impairment of spatial discriminative capacities, such as two point discrimination (SMYTH, 1939) or of the capacity to detect vibratory stimuli occurs. There is, however, a slight loss of sensitivity for detecting light contact on the ipsilateral face (WALKER, 1939; GRANT et al., 1940). A more precise and complete description of the tactile sensory loss in these patients would be of considerable value in assessing the function of the mechanoreceptive neuron population within nucleus caudalis.

The structural similarity of nucleus caudalis and the outer laminae of the spinal dorsal horn has been the basis for considering these regions homologous. The parallel sensory deficits resulting from trigeminal and spinal anteriolateral tractotomies, respectively, certainly supports this view. However, as yet we have an incomplete description of the functional organization of the different neuron populations in these regions that relay information to the forebrain concerning tactile, thermal and noxious stimulation of somatic tissues.

3. Static Functional Properties of Neuron Populations within Trigeminal Nuclei

Our knowledge of the functional characteristics of second order trigeminal sensory neurons is restricted to those responsive to light mechanical stimulation of facial skin, various oral structures and the cornea which we assume relate to tactile sensation. No analysis at the level of the individual neuron of the mechanisms within nucleus caudalis mediating pain and thermal sensation is available. On the one hand specific thermoreceptive neurons within the trigeminal complex have only recently been isolated (POULOS and LENDE, 1970); on the other, although neurons responding only to noxious stimuli have been identified in most trigeminal nuclei (e.g. EISENMAN et al., 1963), their relation to pain sensation is at present uncertain. The recent identification by CHRISTENSEN and PERL (1970), of specific thermoreceptive neurons within lamina I of the cat's dorsal horn, however, provides an important cue for future analysis of nucleus caudalis. These investigators also found neurons within lamina I that respond uniquely to high intensity mechanical and thermal stimulation of the skin, and which might well subserve pain sensation.

a) **Main Sensory Nucleus and Nucleus Oralis.** The functional identity of these two nuclei is established to the extent that they relay to the ventrobasal complex of thalamus similar information about 'tactile' stimuli applied to the face and mouth. This is evident from the similar static and dynamic functional properties of their neuron populations.

Second order neurons within these nuclei functionally resemble the mechanoreceptive afferents that constitute their main input; however, some transformation, even of static functional properties, does occur. Rather surprisingly, trigeminothalamic neurons and internuncials within these nuclei cannot be differentiated by these properties (Fig. 4) (EISENMAN et al., 1963; DARIAN-SMITH et al., 1963a, 1966; DUBNER, 1967; HAMMER, 1968). Most of these cells have small, well-defined excitatory receptive fields, 3–30 times larger than the fields of corresponding primary afferents, indicating a discrete but significant convergence. In the cat, comparable with the primary afferent population, about two-thirds of the cutaneous afferents adapt rapidly to displacement of hairs or of the skin. Their excitatory receptive fields are continuous and except for those neurons with an input from vibrissae, they do not respond selectively to the movement of specific hair types

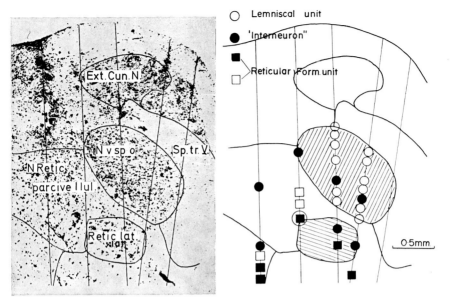

Fig. 4. Transverse section through nucleus oralis of the cat, 5 mm rostral to obex. Electrode tracks indicated by near vertical lines. Position of each neuron identified in this plane shown by the symbols: 'lemniscal' units were specific mechanoreceptive relay neurons; 'interneurons' were similar but did not project to the contralateral thalamus; 'Reticular formation' units had an extensive cutaneous receptive field and were commonly multimodal. Abbreviations: sp.tr.V = trigeminal spinal tract; n.retic.lat. = lateral reticular nucleus; Ext.Cun.N. = external cuneate nucleus; n.Retic.parvicellul. = nucleus reticularis parvicellularis. Reticular neuron surrounded by circle projected to the contralateral thalamus. (DARIAN-SMITH and YOKOTA, 1966 b)

(cf. cutaneous primary afferents). Rather, these neurons are similarly excited by movement of all hairs within the field. Some mystacial neurons may be excited by movement of a single vibrissa only, but usually convergence is less exclusive, from two or more of these hairs (DARIAN-SMITH et al., 1968; ROWE, 1968). The receptive field organization of slowly adapting cutaneous mechanoreceptive neurons is very similar to that of the more common rapidly adapting cells. One difference from the rapidly adapting neurons, however, which first and second order slowly adapting mechanoreceptive neurons share, is their sensitivity to cooling of the skin. However, these neurons usually respond only to sudden changes in the skin temperature; their ongoing activity and dynamic responsiveness to mechanical stimulation is little influenced by quite large shifts in the steady skin temperature (ROWE, 1968). POULOS and LENDE (1970a) have observed a similar thermal sensitivity of slowly adapting lingual mechanoreceptive afferents (their T + M cells).

The static functional properties of neurons with corneal and oral receptive fields are related in a similar way to those of the primary afferents innervating these structures (KRUGER and MICHEL, 1962a, b, c; KERR et al., 1968). The essential specificity of response is retained, such as directional sensitivity of neurons with an input from the periodontal ligament, but some spatial convergence of peripheral input occurs.

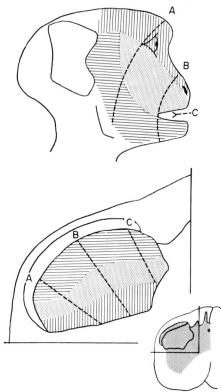

Fig. 5. Diagram of the somatotopic projection of the ipsilateral face and oral structures on to a transverse plane through the trigeminal nuclear complex. Nucleus caudalis is represented, but a similar projection occurs at all rostrocaudal levels. The skin fields of the separate trigeminal divisions are differentiated by shading; their dorso-ventral representation within the nucleus is apparent, with the mandibular division projecting most dorsally. The radial projection of primary fibers also results in an ordered medio-lateral pattern, with the oral structures (C) being represented most medially — the so-called 'onion-skin' organization described by DEJERINE (see text), that is centered about the mouth

Afferent inhibition characterizes the peripheral input to many neurons of the main sensory nucleus and nucleus oralis. The field from which a conditioning mechanical stimulus will inhibit discharge from its excitatory receptive field is usually considerably larger than the latter, and with cutaneous fields, often extends on to the contralateral face; these inhibitory connections have not been identified. This peripheral inhibitory action is probably mainly but not exclusively presynaptic (DARIAN-SMITH, 1965, 1966; DARIAN-SMITH and YOKOTA, 1966a, b; STEWART et al., 1967; SHENDE and KING, 1967). The functional significance of afferent inhibition is discussed elsewhere in this volume (SCHMIDT).

The ipsilateral trigeminal receptor sheet is represented within all transverse planes through these two nuclei, as a consequence of the rostrocaudal organization of the trigeminal spinal tract that was described earlier. This projection to the nuclei is inverted dorsoventrally; in addition, oral and perioral structures are represented medially, and tissues remote from the mouth, such as the preauricular skin, project laterally (Figs. 2 and 3) (DARIAN-SMITH and MAYDAY, 1960; KRUGER and MICHEL, 1962a, b, c; EISENMAN et al., 1963; DARIAN-SMITH et al., 1963b; KERR et al., 1969; ROWE, 1968; NORD, 1967). Relative representation of the peripheral sensory field within this somatotopic projection does not change at different levels in the pons, and is similar to that seen elsewhere in the somatic sensory pathways. Tissues with a high innervation density and tactile sensitivity, such as the perioral skin, have a greater central representation than adjacent less densely innervated tissues. Further, the spatial convergence on second order neurons is more restricted for those receiving an input from the highly sensitive peripheral regions than from other parts of the receptor sheet, as is apparent from their small receptive fields. This somatotopic projection to the rostral trigeminal nuclei is similar in primates, subprimates and in some birds (ZEIGLER and WITKOVSKY, 1968).

Fig. 5 illustrates the somatotopic projection of the face on to a transverse plane in the trigeminal nuclear complex (nucleus caudalis was arbitrarily chosen). The ordered projection of primary afferent fibres is such that a dorsoventral stratified representation of the trigeminal divisions results — a fact familiar to the neurosurgeon. This same patterned projection of primary fibres, however, results in a medio-lateral 'onion-skin' organization centered about the oral projection. Thus, two patterns of sensory loss may result from partial destruction of the trigeminal nucleus. In one, the loss has a divisional distribution, reflecting a vertical intrusion on the nucleus, whereas in the other the sensory deficit is concentric about the mouth, and results from destruction along the medial border, such as was described by DEJERINE (1914) in patients with syringobulbia. Similarly, if the incision made for a tractotomy leaves the dorsomedial part of the trigeminal tract intact, then sensory sparing occurs, centered about the mouth (KUNC, 1966).

In accord with earlier degeneration studies (TORVIK, 1957), most mechanoreceptive neurons within these two nuclei are trigeminothalamic (DARIAN-SMITH et al., 1963a; EISENMAN et al., 1963), projecting specifically to the contralateral VPM (ROWE and SESSLE, 1968; SESSLE, 1968). EISENMAN et al. (1964) have also demonstrated that some cells in the dorsomedial part of the main sensory nucleus, mainly with lingual receptive fields, project to the ipsilateral thalamus. However, both Golgi and physiological single neuron identification studies indicate that interneurons do occur within these trigeminal nuclei.

b) Nucleus Caudalis. A rather surprising finding in the nucleus caudalis of the cat (GORDON et al., 1961) was that mechanoreceptive neurons within subnucleus magnocellularis have static functional properties essentially identical with those of neurons within the main sensory nucleus and nucleus oralis. This has been fully substantiated in the cat (KRUGER et al., 1961; KRUGER and MICHEL, 1962a; DARIAN-SMITH et al., 1963), the rat (NORD, 1967, 1968), and monkey (KERR et al., 1968) (Fig. 6). As in these rostral nuclei, about one-third of the mechanoreceptive population is slowly adapting, cells have circumscribed excitatory receptive fields, and often a 'surround' inhibitory field. Both presynaptic and postsynaptic inhibitory mechanisms contribute to this afferent inhibition; present evidence suggests, however, that the presynaptic inhibitory contribution to afferent inhibition is less within nucleus caudalis than within the rostral trigeminal nuclei (DARIAN-SMITH,

NUCLEUS   CAUDALIS

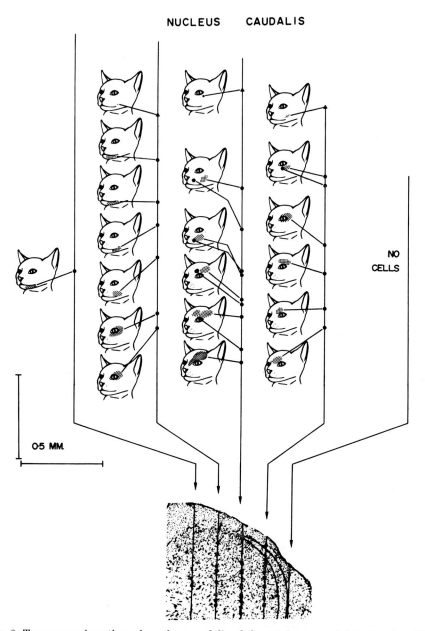

NO
CELLS

0·5 MM.

Fig. 6. Transverse plane through nucleus caudalis of the cat 1 mm caudal to the obex. The vertical lines indicate electrode tracks through the nucleus, and the dots the location of individual second order neurons. The triangles at the top of 3 penetrations indicate the sites of recording from individual primary fibres. The mechanoreceptive receptive fields of the individual neurons are illustrated on the figurines. The pattern of projection of the ipsilateral trigeminal cutaneous field is seen. (Rowe, 1968)

1965). Also, there is a somatotopically organized projection of all parts of the peripheral trigeminal field at all rostrocaudal levels from the obex to Cl that is similar in pattern to that in nucleus oralis. There may be a shift in relative representation along the rostrocaudal axis, with oral and perioral tissues having maximal projections at levels just caudal to the obex, and other trigeminal regions being optimally represented more caudally in the nucleus. However, this has been vigorously denied (KERR et al., 1968; NORD, 1967, 1968). More effective unbiased sampling of these neuron populations in unanesthetized animals will doubtless resolve these topographical details. A similar rostrocaudal arrangement for the projection to nucleus caudalis in man, relevant to pain sensation, has been suggested by several investigators. The analysis of this projection was based on the analgesic effects of trigeminal tractotomy at different levels in the medulla. In the largest and most recent series, KUNC (1966, 1970) has observed that, if the level of complete trigeminal tractotomy is at the rostral pole of nucleus caudalis' then analgesia over the whole ipsilateral trigeminal field is the result. However, if the section is more caudal analgesia is incomplete with sensory sparing occurring in an area centered about the mouth: with more caudal tract incisions this area expands concentrically.

GORDON et al. (1961) first showed that about 40% of mechanoreceptive neurons in nucleus caudalis in the cat project to the contralateral posterior thalamus (Fig. 7); an additional small proportion probably also projects to the ipsilateral thalamus. These trigeminothalamic neurons differ from those in the rostral nuclei in one most important respect; few project to VPM (ROWE and SESSLE, 1968; SESSLE, 1968; STEWART, STOOPS, PILLONE and KING, 1964). Degeneration studies (NAUTA and KUYPERS, 1958; MEHLER et al., 1960; MEHLER, 1966) indicate that many of these neurons project to the magnocellular part of the medial geniculate nucleus and the intralaminar nuclei. It is likely, also, extrapolating from data available concerning the phylogeny of the spinothalamic projection, that the relative projection to these different regions changes greatly in the primates, with a great increase in the projection to VPM. Fresh electrophysiological investigation of this problem in the primate is necessary.

c) **Nucleus Interpolaris.** Earlier histological investigation (CARPENTER and HANNA, 1961) demonstrated that cells within this nucleus project not only to the contralateral VPM, but a significant proportion also project to the anterior lobe of the cerebellum. The cerebellar projection of mechanoreceptive neurons within the nucleus, both directly and via the adjacent lateral reticular nucleus was subsequently demonstrated using single neuron recording methods (DARIAN-SMITH and PHILLIPS, 1964). DARIAN-SMITH and PHILLIPS also reported other differences between the static functional properties of cells in this and the adjacent trigeminal nuclei. Most but not all cutaneous mechanoreceptive neurons within nucleus interpolaris had larger fields than those of nucleus oralis and nucleus caudalis, a condition sufficient to preclude the finely detailed somatotopic organization which typifies these latter nuclei. Few of these cells could be antidromically excited from the contralateral posterior thalamus. In subsequent investigations, however (KERR et al., 1968; NORD, 1967, 1968), somatotopic organization in nucleus interpolaris, quite comparable with that of the adjacent nuclei, was observed in the rat and

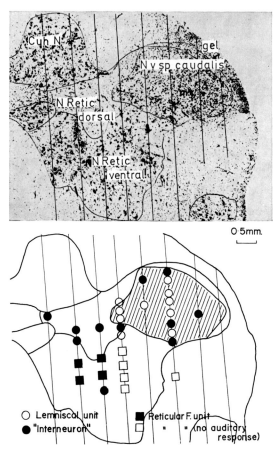

Fig. 7. Transverse section through brainstem of cat 1.5 mm caudal to the obex. The lines define a series of microelectrode tracks. The sites of recording from single neurons is indicated by the symbols in the line drawing. The different cell types are as indicated in the legend of Fig. 4. Additional abbreviations: Cun.N. = cuneate nucleus; gel. = subnucleus gelatinosa; mc. = subnucleus magnocellularis; n.Retic.dorsal., and N.Retic.ventral. subdivisions of the nucleus reticularis medulla oblongata. ■ = neurons in reticular formation responding to both cutaneous and auditory stimuli; □ = cells responding to cutaneous stimulation only. (DARIAN-SMITH and YOKOTA, 1966 b)

monkey. Possibly the anaesthetic status of the experimental animals may account for these disparate findings, since KERR et al. (1968) at no time observed neurons within the adjacent reticular formation which were excited by 'tactile' stimuli from a large cutaneous receptive field; the occurrence of these cells in lightly anesthetized animals is well known (GORDON et al., 1961; EISENMAN et al., 1963; WALL and TAUB, 1962; DARIAN-SMITH and YOKOTA, 1966b — see Figs. 4 and 7.) Further analysis of the function of this nucleus requires a) neuron identification, in which the long axon projections of individual neurons are determined, and b) an examination of the dynamic functional properties of the different neuron types. In view of the significant trigemino-cerebellar linkage, nucleus interpolaris may contribute little to somatic sensation. Whether it has a thermal sensory function, as suggested by some clinical observations, must also be assessed in future investigations.

4. Trigeminal Input to the Brainstem Reticular Formation

The ventromedial border of the various trigeminal nuclei, with the exception of the main sensory nucleus, is poorly demarcated in Golgi and Nissl sections. In this region of transition with the brainstem reticular formation the functional properties of second order neurons change considerably (Figs. 4 and 7). Many neurons still respond to light 'tactile' stimulation of facial skin, but their receptive fields are commonly larger, extending to the contralateral face, to the neck or even to the trunk and limbs; these receptive fields are often discontinuous. The trigeminal input to these reticular neurons is largely relayed through specific trigeminal nuclei, but a direct primary afferent projection also exists (TORVIK, 1956; CLARKE and BOWSHER, 1962; CARPENTER and HANNA, 1961; STEWART and KING, 1963; DUNN and MATZE, 1968). Many of these neurons are excited also by auditory and visual stimuli, reflecting a complex input.

About 30% of these reticular, multimodal neurons project to the contralateral thalamus (DARIAN-SMITH and YOKOTA, 1966b). Reticulothalamic projections have been demonstrated histologically (BRODAL and ROSSI, 1955; RUSSELL, 1954; NAUTA and KUYPERS, 1958; SCHEIBEL and SCHEIBEL, 1957), but these have been mainly from the medial part of the brainstem reticular formation. Russell did, however, observe a significant ipsilateral reticulothalamic projection from the lateral part of the brainstem reticular formation.

A rather differently organized ascending projection arises from the lateral reticular nucleus, an elongate nucleus extending from the rostral pole of the nucleus oralis to the level of the obex (WALBERG, 1952). Tactile stimulation of the face excites many cells within this nucleus from receptive fields that are usually ipsilateral but somewhat larger than those of trigemino-thalamic neurons (DARIAN-SMITH and PHILLIPS, 1964). In the cat about-one-third of these neurons within the lateral reticular nucleus adjacent to nucleus interpolaris share with interpolaris cells a projection to the ipsilateral culmen and declive of the cerebellum (the region of face representation in the anterior lobe). Presumably these neurons have no sensory function.

Some neurons within the brainstem reticular formation adjacent to the trigeminal nuclei lack the divergent sensory input and the long axon projections of the cells described above (Figs. 4 and 7). They are specifically mechanoreceptive, have small receptive fields similar to those of trigeminal relay neurons, but none project to the thalamus (DARIAN-SMITH and YOKATO, 1966b). Their dynamic functional properties are not known.

Unfortunately, no coherent, detailed picture of the sensory function of the brainstem reticular formation emerges from the incomplete investigations of the functional properties of its component neurons. The trigeminal input to the brainstem reticular formation presumably is relevant to sensory function insofar that it may modulate activity in the ascending reticular activating system, and so influence the latter's arousal and alerting functions, but the neuronal mechanisms for this action are unknown.

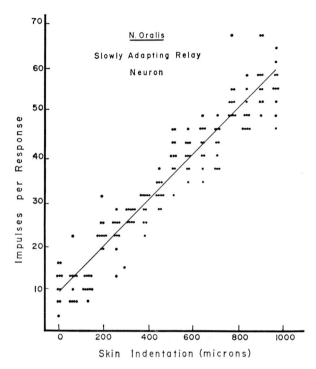

Fig. 8. Stimulus-response curve for a trigemino-thalamic neuron in nucleus oralis in the cat. This slowly adapting mechanoreceptive neuron had a circumscribed receptive field lateral to the outer angle of the eye. The stimulus was a near rectangular deformation of the skin lasting 1000 msec: total stimulus range was 960 microns. The amplitude of each stimulus was one of 16 equal steps across the range of 960 μ, presented in random order. Stimuli presented once every 5 sec. The tip diameter of the stimulus probe was 2 mm. The best fitting linear regression is drawn. (Darian-Smith, Rowe and Sessle, 1968)

5. Dynamic Functional Properties of Neuron Populations within Trigeminal Nuclei

Whole or part of the neuron population within each trigeminal nucleus is mechanoreceptive, with a similar or possibly identical peripheral input to each nucleus. As we have seen, the neuron populations within those nuclei with a thalamic projection have similar static functional properties. Since the morphology and the contribution to tactile sensory function certainly differ considerably for these nuclei, this is unexpected, indicating that within specific somatic sensory pathways the receptive field characteristics and somatotopy are insensitive indices of functional differences. Thus, if the spatial convergent properties of two second-order neuron populations differ, then a functional difference exists, but if their static functional characteristics are similar this does not necessarily demonstrate functional identity.

Neuron populations with similar functional properties, which code the energy form and extensive parameters of the stimulus in a similar way, may however differ profoundly in their capacity to relay information to the forebrain about the intensitytime profile of the stimulus. That is, they may be differentiated and their contribution to sensory function assessed in terms of their dynamic functional characteristics. The results of an investigation in which these dynamic properties were examined suggest that synaptic transmission within the main sensory nucleus and nucleus oralis involves little loss of the information available in the input from cutaneous mechanoreceptive afferents, whereas in nucleus caudalis, with a comparable input, the relay of information about the stimulus is much less (DARIAN-SMITH et al., 1968; ROWE, 1968; DARIAN-SMITH, 1970). This finding, of course, is in accord with the concept of a duality of 'tactile' sensory pathways, a concept with a long history, but one which has been greatly developed in recent years (MOUNTCASTLE, 1961).

Transmission of information by slowly adapting mechanoreceptive neurons within nucleus oralis and nucleus caudalis has been recently examined in the cat (DARIAN-SMITH et al., 1968; ROWE, 1968; DARIAN-SMITH, 1970). The stimulus pattern used was a rectangular indentation of the skin of the receptive field. The average discharge frequency of primary afferents during stimulation charged linearly with the amplitude of indentation, and a similar relationship was observed for trigeminothalamic neurons within nucleus oralis. Furthermore, when the temporal interaction between successive responses was fixed by randomly varying the stimulus amplitude, the variability of response and the slope of the stimulus-response curve for first- and second- order neurons did not differ significantly. This indicates that no important transformation of the neural response resulted from synaptic transfer within nucleus oralis (Fig. 8).

Transmission of information within nucleus caudalis was differently organized. The response discharge frequency of slowly adapting mechanoreceptive relay neurons within this nucleus varied greatly with successive stimuli and only a small component of this variability was accounted for by changes in the stimulus intensity. The 'sensitivity' of these neurons, estimated from the slope of the best fitting linear regression was much less than that of oralis cells.

These stimulus-response curves for the different neuron types provide information about the efficiency of synaptic transmission within the separate nuclei. The application of information theory provides an answer to the following question (GARNER, 1962): how effectively does a single response of a particular neuron define the stimulus which evokes it? In this experimental analysis the upper limit to the amount of information which the neuron can relay concerning the stimulus intensity is estimated — the so-called channel capacity. Fig. 9 illustrates the experimental estimation of the channel capacity for information transmitted about the intensity of indentation of facial skin by a typical slowly adapting mechano-receptive afferent fiber and by trigeminothalamic neurons within nucleus oralis and caudalis respectively. In this analysis the simplest response statistic — the number of impulses during the one second stimulus — was used. Additional information might be coded by the internal pattern of the response but various considerations indicated that this addition would be small. Each response of the primary afferent relayed 2.5 bits of information to the trigeminal nuclei about the stimulus intensity, i.e., each response correctly defined the stimulus as falling into one of five ($2^{2.5} = 5$ approx.) categories equally spaced over the stimulus range: better resolution was not possible. The responses of individual oralis neu-

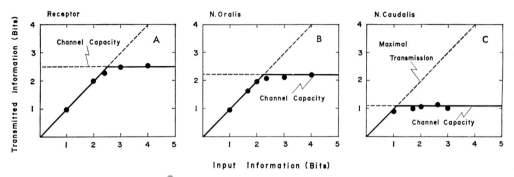

Fig. 9. Estimation of channel capacity for different mechanoreceptive trigeminal neurons with cutaneous receptive fields. These neurons adapted slowly to sustained deformation of the skin. The stimulus was a near-rectangular deformation of the skin lasting 1000 msec; the stimulus range was 960 microns; the stimulus probe tip was 2 mm in diameter. Stimulus repetition rate was 1/5 seconds. Stimulus amplitude was varied in random order. (A). *Afferent fiber.* As the possible values of the stimulus amplitude were increased (an increase in the stimulus uncertainty) by subdividing the stimulus range of 960 microns into 2, 4, 5, 8 and 16 equally spaced categories, the information about the amplitude of a particular stimulus relayed by the number of impulses in the response to that stimulus increased to a limiting value of about 2.5 bits of information the channel capacity. That is, the neural response to a particular stimulus defined its amplitude in a limited way, by signalling which of $2^{2.5}$ (about 5) categories, equally spaced across the stimulus range of 960 microns, encompassed the stimulus. (B). *Slowly adapting relay neurons in nucleus oralis.* Channel capacity equals 2.2 bits, that is 4–5 stimulus categories could be differentiated from the amplitude of a single response. (C). *Slowly adapting neuron in nucleus caudalis.* Channel capacity is 1.1 bits; a binary decision only, whether or not a stimulus had occurred, was possible from the amplitude of a single response of the cell; the neural signal could be unequivocally differentiated from the noise level only when the stimulus was a maximum intensity. It is apparent that little loss of information resulted from transmission across synapses in nucleus oralis, but that a considerable loss of information accompanied synaptic transmission within nucleus caudalis. (Darian-Smith, Rowe and Sessle, 1968)

rons defined the stimulus intensity with little or no additional loss in resolution. On the other hand, cells within nucleus caudalis responded to the stimulus with such variability, that only when the intensity of the stimulus was maximal did the neuron signal to the thalamus unequivocal occurrence (Fig. 9; channel capacity equals 1 bit, that amount of information necessary to determine whether or not the stimulus had occurred). Further evidence suggested that the synaptic basis for this differential transmission of information is that individual primary afferent fibers have a less powerful excitatory synaptic action on caudalis cells than on those cells within nucleus oralis.

The conclusion from this analysis is that although individual, slowly adapting, trigeminothalamic neurons within nucleus oralis and caudalis may code the position of an intense 'tactile' stimulus equally well, only neurons within nucleus oralis signal to the thalamus the occurrence of a weak stimulus, and its amplitude, with an efficiency comparable with that of sensory behavior. Such a finding, in which the trigeminothalamic neurons of nucleus caudalis relay little information about the intensive parameter (a single stimulus dimension), does not necessarily imply that such cells have no 'tactile' sensory function. They may, for example, relay information about multidimensional stimuli, a possibility that has not been explored.

There are also comparable differences in the signalling of vibratory skin movement by the two nuclei (ROWE, 1968; DARIAN-SMITH, 1970). Most rapidly adapting mechanoreceptive afferents innervating the different types of hair follicle in facial skin effectively signal the occurrence of low amplitude sinusoidal skin movement over the range 60–300 cps, discharging once with each cycle. The 'tuning curves' of about 15% of rapidly adapting mechanoreceptive neurons in nucleus oralis are similar to those of the peripheral fibers, but no neurons with these response properties have been isolated in a comparable sample of cells located in nucleus caudalis.

Centrifugal Influences on Synaptic Transmission in the Trigeminal Complex

Several investigations in recent years have focussed on the modulating effects of the cerebral cortex and brainstem reticular formation on synaptic transmission within the trigeminal complex (DARIAN-SMITH and YOKOTA, 1966a, b; DARIAN-SMITH, 1966; STEWART, SCIBETTA and KING, 1967; SHENDE and KING, 1967; WIESENDANGER et al., 1967; WIESENDANGER and FELIX, 1969; HEPP-REYMOND and WIESENDANGER, 1969; DUBNER, 1967, 1970). This subject is considered fully within a more general context elsewhere in this volume (TOWE).

6. Trigeminal Neuralgia

Trigeminal neuralgia, that specific painful affection characterized by recurrent attacks of facial pain, that are localized to the skin field of one or more divisions of the trigeminal nerve, and commonly initiated by touching a localized facial trigger zone, has been the focus of clinical interest in the trigeminal system for most of this century. Additional features which single out this clinical condition are the absence of sensory impairment in the region where the pain occurs, the common absence of any pathological cause for the pain, and the immediate relief given to the patient by trans-section of the trigeminal root, or the trigeminal spinal tract, at or just caudal to the obex. Recently BEAVER et al. (BEAVER, 1967; BEAVER et al., 1965) have reported disorder of structure within the Gasserian ganglion and trigeminal root, which includes vacuole formation within the neuron cell bodies, and segmental demyelination. The segmental demyelination is characterized by both a 'proliferation' of myelin in some areas and a breakdown of the laminar organization of the sheath in adjacent regions. Degenerative changes in axons appear to be secondary to the demyelination. These findings have been substantiated by other investigation (KERR, 1967), but there is doubt concerning the uniqueness of the lesion (GRUNER, 1970a).

Demyelination of the primary afferents suggests the possibility of ephaptic transmission with 'cross-talk' between mechanoreceptive and nociceptive fibers, a mechanism that has been previously proposed to explain the shift in sensory quality between the immediate response to the trigger stimulus and the later painful paroxysm. Although ephaptic transmission may occur at certain synaptic junctions in invertebrates and fish, there is at present no evidence of its occurrence in mammals (GRUNDFEST, 1967). Indeed, several important features of the trigger mechanism are not readily accountable in terms of such a peripheral mechanism. These include the latent period of 5–30 sec between the trigger stimulus and the onset of pain, the temporal and spatial summation which characterizes the pheno-menon, and the refractory state that follows a paroxysm of pain (Kugelberg and Lindblom, 1959). A trigger mechanism, involving transmission in a functionally unstable, multisynaptic, recurrent pathway would on the other hand have these features. We may only surmise how such a functionally unstable pathway may develop. This pathway would almost certainly include cells within nucleus cau-dalis, since trigeminal tractotomy, with differential block of input to this nucleus, immediately relieves the patient.

Pain in the normal subject is evoked by somatic stimulation only if A delta or C-fibers are excited by the stimulus (Landau and Bishop, 1953). It might then be anticipated that stimulation of the trigger zone of a type that would differentially activate these small fibers would be most effective in evoking paroxysmal attacks of pain; in fact the reverse is true. Thermal and noxious stimulation of the trigger zone rarely evoke attacks of pain in these patients, whereas vibratory stimulation or light touch (exciting mainly large myelinated fibers together with unmyelinated fibers) are most effective in precipitating such an attack (Kugelberg and Lind-blom, 1959).

In summary, it appears that only a central disorder of function, probably within nucleus caudalis, can account for all the sensory abnormalities of trigeminal neuralgia. Whether such abnormal central function is accountable in terms of peripheral demyelination remains to be seen. Extensive resumes of the evidence for both a central and a peripheral etiology (King, 1967; Kerr, 1967, 1970; Kaemmerer, 1970) have appeared recently: no firm conclusions are yet possible.

Acknowledgements

The author's research has been supported by grants from the Australian National Health and Medical Research Council, and by Grants NB-06828 and 5 T01 GM00443 of the U.S. Public Health Service.

References

Abbie, A.A.: The brainstem and cerebellum of Echidna aculeata. Phil. Trans. B **224**, 1–69 (1934).

Anderson, D.J., Hannam, A.G., Matthews, B.: Sensory mechanisms in mammalian teeth and their supporting structures. Physiol. Rev. **50**, 171–195 (1970).

Andres, K.H.: Über die Feinstruktur der Rezeptoren und Sinushaare. Z. Zellforsch. **75**, 339–365 (1966).

Arwill, T.: Some morphological aspects of the dentinal innervation. In: Sensory Mechanisms in Dentine. Ed. by D.J. Anderson, pp. 3–14. Oxford: Pergamon Press 1963.

Aström, K.E.: The central course of afferent fibres in the trigeminal, facial, glossopharyngeal, and vagal nerves and their nuclei in the mouse. Acta physiol. scand. **29**, Suppl. 106, 209–320 (1953).

Beaudreau, D.E., Jerge, C.R.: Somatotopic representation in the gasserian of tactile peripheral fields in the cat. Arch. oral Biol. **13**, 247–256 (1968).

Beaver, D.L.: Electron microscopy of the Gasserian ganglion in trigeminal neuralgia. J. Neurosurg. **26**, Suppl. 138–150 (1967).

Beaver, D.L., Moses, H.L., Ganote, C.E.: Electron microscopy of the trigeminal ganglion. III. Trigeminal neuralgia. Arch. Path. **79**, 571–582 (1965).

BESSOU, P., PERL, E.R.: Response of cutaneous sensory units with unmyelated fibers to noxious stimuli. J. Neurophysiol. **32**, 1025–1043 (1969).

BLEICHMAN, H., DEROBERTIS, E.: Submicroscopic morphology of the infrared receptor of pit vipers. Z. Zellforsch. **50**, 748–761 (1962).

BLOM, S.: Afferent influences on tongue muscle activity. Acta physiol. scand. **49**, Suppl. 170 (1960).

BOMAN, K.K.A.: Electrophysiologische Untersuchungen über die Thermoreceptoren der Gesichtshaut. Acta physiol. scand. **44**, Suppl. 149 (1958).

BRÄNNSTRÖM, M.: A hydrodynamic mechanism in the transmission of pain producing stimuli through the dentine. In: Sensory Mechanisms in Dentine. Ed. by D.J. ANDERSON, pp. 73–79. Oxford: Pergamon Press 1963.

BRODAL, A.: Central course of afferent fibers for pain in facialis, glossopharyngeal, and vagus nerves. Clinical observations. Arch. Neurol. Psychiat. (Chic.) **57**, 292–306 (1947).

BRODAL, A., ROSSI, G.F.: Ascending fibers in brain stem reticular formation of cat. Arch. Neurol. Psychiat. (Chic.) **74**, 68–87 (1955).

BRODAL, A., SAUGSTAD, L.F.: Retrograde cellular changes in the mesencephalic trigeminal nucleus in the cat following cerebellular lesions. Acta morph. neerl.-scand. **6**, 147–159 (1965).

BRODAL, A., SZABO, T., TORVIK, A.: Corticofugal fibers to sensory trigeminal nuclei and nucleus of the solitary tract. An experimental study in the cat. J. comp. Neurol. **106**, 527–556 (1956).

BROOKHART, J., LIVINGSTON, W.K., HAUGEN, F.P.: Functional characteristics of afferent fibers from tooth pulp of cat. J. Neurophysiol. **16**, 634–642 (1953).

BROWN, A.G., FRANZ, D.N.: Responses of spinocervical tract neurones to natural stimulation of identified cutaneous receptors. Exp. Brain Res. **7**, 231–249 (1969).

BROWN, A.G., IGGO, A.: A quantitative study of cutaneous receptors and afferent fibres in the cat and rabbit. J. Physiol. (Lond.) **193**, 707–733 (1967).

BROWN, A.G., IGGO, A., MILLER, S.: Myelinated afferent nerve fibers from the skin of the rabbit ear. Exp. Neurol. **18**, 338–349 (1967).

BROWN, J.W.: The development of the nucleus of spinal tract of V in human fetuses. J. comp. Neurol. **106**, 393–424 (1956).

BROWN, J.W.: The development of subnucleus caudalis of the nucleus of the spinal tract of V. J. comp. Neurol. **110**, 105–134 (1958).

BROWN, J.W.: The development of the chief sensory nucleus of V in the human fetus. Anat. Rec. **136**, 171 (1960).

BROWN, J.W.: Differentiation of the human subnucleus interpolaris and subnucleus rostralis of the nucleus of the spinal tract of the trigeminal nerve. J. comp. Neurol. **119**, 55–76 (1962).

BULLOCK, T.H., DIECKE, F.P.J.: Properties of an infrared receptor. J. Physiol. (Lond.) **134**, 47–87 (1956).

BULLOCK, T.H., FOX, W.: The anatomy of the infrared sense organ in the facial pit of pit vipers. Quart. J. micr. Sci. **98**, 219–234 (1957).

BURGESS, P.R., PERL, E.R.: Myelinated afferent fibers responding specifically to noxious stimulation of the skin. J. Physiol. (Lond.) **190**, 541–562 (1967).

CAJAL, S. RAMÓN Y: Histologie du Système Nerveux de l'Homme et des Vertébrés. Paris: Maloine 1909.

CARPENTER, M.B.: The dorsal trigeminal tract in the rhesus monkey. J. Anat. (Lond.) **91**, 82–90 (1957).

CARPENTER, M.B., HANNA, G.R.: Fiber projections from the spinal trigeminal nucleus in the cat. J. comp. Neurol. **117**, 117–132 (1961).

CAUNA, N.: Light and electron microscopal structure of sensory end-organs in skin. In: The Skin Senses. Ed. by D.R. KENSHALO, pp. 15–29. Springfield, Ill.: Thomas 1968.

CHRISTENSEN, B.N., PERL, E.R.: Spinal neurons specifically excited by noxious or thermal stimuli: marginal zone of the dorsal horn. J. Neurophysiol. **33**, 293–307 (1970).

CLARKE, W.B., BOWSHER, D.: Terminal distribution of primary afferent trigeminal fibers in the rat. Exp. Neurol. **6**, 372–383 (1962).

COOPER, F.S.: Comments on Second Symposium on Oral Sensation and Perception. Ed. by J.F. BOSMA, pp. 541–545. Springfield, Ill.: Thomas 1970.

COOPER, S.: Muscle spindles in the intrinsic muscles of the tongue. J. Physiol. (Lond.) **122**, 193–202 (1953).

COOPER, S.: Muscle spindles and other muscle receptors. In: The Structure and Function of Muscles, Vol. I. Ed. by G. H. BOURNE, pp. 381–420. New York: Academic Press 1960.

COOPER, S., DANIEL, P., WHITTERIDGE, D.: Muscle spindles and other sensory endings in the extrinsic eye muscles, the physiology and anatomy of these receptors and their connexions with the brainstem. Brain **78**, 564–583 (1955).

CORBIN, K.B., HARRISON, F.: Function of mesencephalic root of fifth cranial nerve. J. Neurophysiol. **3**, 423–435 (1940).

CROSBY, E.C., YOSS, R.E.: The phylogenetic continuity of neural mechanisms as illustrated by the spinal tract of V and its nucleus. Res. Publ. Ass. nerv. ment. Dis. **33**, 174–208 (1954).

DARIAN-SMITH, I.: Presynaptic component in the afferent inhibition observed within trigeminal brainstem nuclei of the cat. J. Neurophysiol. **28**, 695–709 (1965).

DARIAN-SMITH, I.: Neural mechanisms of facial sensation. Int. Rev. Neurobiol. **9**, 301–395 (1966).

DARIAN-SMITH, I.: Tactile sensory pathways from the face. Trans. Ass. Austral. Neurol. **2**, 27–39 (1966).

DARIAN-SMITH, I.: The neural coding of 'tactile' stimulus parameters in different trigeminal nuclei. In: Trigeminal Neuralgia. Ed. by R. HASSLER and A.E. WALKER. pp. 59–71. Stuttgart: Georg Thieme Verlag 1970.

DARIAN-SMITH, I., DYKES, R.: Peripheral neural mechanisms of thermal sensation. In: Oral-Facial Sensory and Motor Mechanisms. Ed. by R. DUBNER and Y. KAWAMURA, pp. 7–22. New York: Appleton-Century-Croft 1971.

DARIAN-SMITH, I., JOHNSON, K.O., LAMOTTE, C.: Warming and cooling the skin: peripheral neural determinants of perceived changes in skin temperature. In: The Somatic Sensory System. Ed. by H.H. KORNHUBER. In press, 1971.

DARIAN-SMITH, I., MAYDAY, G.: Somatotopic organization within the brainstem trigeminal complex of the cat. Exp. Neurol. **2**, 290–309 (1960).

DARIAN-SMITH, I., MUTTON, P., PROCTOR, R.: Functional organization of tactile cutaneous afferents within the semilunar ganglion and trigeminal tract of the cat. J. Neurophysiol. **28**, 682–694 (1965).

DARIAN-SMITH, I., PHILLIPS, G.: Secondary neurones within a trigemino-cerebellar projection to the anterior lobe of the cerebellum in the cat. J. Physiol. (Lond.) **170**, 53–68 (1964).

DARIAN-SMITH, I., PHILLIPS, G., RYAN, R.D.: Functional organization in the trigeminal main sensory and rostral spinal nuclei of the cat. J. Physiol. (Lond.) **168**, 129–146 (1963).

DARIAN-SMITH, I., PROCTOR, R., RYAN, R.D.: A single-neurone investigation of somatotopic organization within the cat's trigeminal brainstem nuclei. J. Physiol. (Lond.) **168**, 147–157 (1963).

DARIAN-SMITH, I., ROWE, M.J., SESSLE, B.J.: 'Tactile' stimulus intensity: information transmission by relay neurons in different trigeminal nuclei. Science **160**, 791–794 (1968).

DARIAN-SMITH, I., YOKOTA, T.: Cortically evoked depolarization of trigeminal cutaneous afferent fibers in the cat. J. Neurophysiol. **29**, 170–184 (1966).

DARIAN-SMITH, I., YOKOTA, T.: Corticofugal effects on different neuron types within the cat's brainstem activated by tactile stimulation of the face of the cat. J. Neurophysiol. **29**, 185–206 (1966).

DAULT, S.H., SMITH, R.D.: A quantitative study of the nucleus of the mesencephalic tract of the trigeminal nerve of the cat. Anat. Rec. **165**, 79–88 (1969).

DEJERINE, J.: Semiologie des Afferents du Systéme Nerveux, pp. 831–839. Paris: Masson 1914.

DIXON, A.D.: Nerve plexuses in the oral mucosa. J. dent. Res. **36**, 807 (1957).

DIXON, A.D.: The innervation of hair follicles in the mammalian lip. Anat. Rec. **140**, 147–159 (1961).

DIXON, A.D.: Sensory nerve terminations in the oral mucosa. Arch. oral Biol. **5**, 105–114 (1961).

DIXON, A.D.: Fine structure of nerve-cell bodies and satellite cells in the trigeminal ganglion. J. dent. Res. **42**, 990–999 (1963).

DODT, E., ZOTTERMAN, Y.: Mode of action of warm receptors. Acta physiol. scand. **26**, 346–357 (1952).

DUBNER, R.: Interaction of peripheral and central input in the main sensory nucleus of the cat. Exp. Neurol. **17**, 186–202 (1967).

DUBNER, R.: Peripheral and central input to the main sensory nucleus of the cat. In: Second Symposium on Oral Sensation and Perception. Ed. by J.F. BOSMA, pp. 132–147. Springfield, Ill.: Thomas 1970.

DUNN, J., MATZE, H.A.: Efferent fiber connections of the marmoset (Oedipomidas oedipus) trigeminal nucleus caudalis. J. comp. Neurol. **133**, 429–438 (1968).

ECCLES, J.C.: Physiology of Nerve Cells. Baltimore: The Johns Hopkins Press 1957.

EISENMAN, J., LANDGREN, S., NOVIN, D.: Functional organization in the main sensory trigeminal nucleus and in the rostral subdivision of the nucleus of the spinal trigeminal tract in the cat. Acta physiol. scand. **59**, Suppl. 214 (1963).

EISENMAN, J., FROMM, G., LANDGREN, S., NOVIN, D.: The ascending projections of trigeminal neurons in the cat, investigated by antidromic stimulation. Acta physiol. scand. **60**, 337–350 (1964).

ENGEL, R.T., BOWMAN, J.P., COMBS, C.M.: Calibre spectra of the lingual and hypoglossal nerves in the rhesus monkey. J. comp. Neurol. **134**, 163–174 (1968).

FALCONER, M.A.: Intramedullary trigeminal tractotomy and its place in the treatment of facial pain. J. Neurol. Neurosurg. Psychiat. **12**, 297–311 (1949).

FEARNHEAD, R.W.: Innervation of dental tissues. In: Structure and Chemical Organization of Teeth. Vol. I. Ed. by A.E.W. MILES, pp. 247–281. London: Academic Press 1967.

FITZGERALD, M.J.T.: The innervation of the epidermis. In: Skin Senses. Ed. by D.R. KENSHALO, pp. 61–81. Springfield, Ill.: Thomas 1968.

FITZGERALD, O.: Discharges from the sensory organs of the cat's vibrissae and the modification in their activity by ions. J. Physiol. (Lond.) **98**, 163–178 (1940).

FREIMANN, R.: Untersuchung über Zahl und Anordnung der Muskelspindeln in den Kaumuskeln des Menschen. Anat. Anz. **100**, 258–264 (1954).

GABRAWI, A.F., TARKHAN, A.A.: A histological study of the mesencephalic nucleus of the fifth cranial nerve. Acta anat. (Basel) **67**, 361–368 (1967).

GAIRNS, F.W.: The sensory nerve endings of the human gingiva, palate, and tongue. J. dent. Res. **35**, 958 (1956).

GARNER, W.R.: Uncertainty and Structure as Psychological Concepts. New York: Wiley 1962.

GERARD, M.W.: Afferent impulses in the trigeminal nerve. A.M.A. Arch. Neurol. Psychiat. **9**, 306–338 (1923).

GOBEL, S., DUBNER, R.: Fine structural studies of the main sensory nucleus in the cat and rat. J. comp. Neurol. **137**, 459–494 (1969).

GORDON, G., LANDGREN, S., SEED, W.: The functional characteristics of single cells in the caudal part of the spinal nucleus of the trigeminal nerve of the cat. J. Physiol. (Lond.) **158**, 544–559 (1961).

GRANT, F.C., GROFF, R.A., LEWY, F.H.: Section of the descending spinal root of the fifth cranial nerve. A.M.A. Arch. Neurol. Psychiat. 43, 498–509 (1940).

GROSSMAN, R.F.: Methods of determining oral tactile experience. In: Symposium on Oral Sensation and Perception. Ed. by J.F. BOSMA, pp. 161–181. Springfield, Ill.: Thomas 1967.

GROSSMAN, R.F., HATTIS, B.F.: Oral mucosa sensory innervation and sensory experience: a review. In: Symposium on Oral Sensation and Perception. Ed. by J.F. BOSMA, pp. 5–62. Springfield, Ill.: Thomas 1967.

GRUNDFEST, H.: Synaptic and ephaptic transmission. In: The Neurosciences. Ed. by G.C. QUARTON, T. MELNECHUK and F.O. SCHMIDT, pp. 353–372. New York: Rockefeller University 1967.

GRUNER, J.E.: Neuropathology of trigeminal neuralgia. In: Trigeminal Neuralgia. Ed. by R. HASSLER and A.E. WALKER, pp. 7–10. Stuttgart: Georg Thieme Verlag 1970.

GRUNER, J.E.: Concerning the fine structure of the trigeminal root and its connections. In: Trigeminal Neuralgia. Ed. by R. HASSLER and A.E. WALKER, pp. 43–49. Stuttgart: Georg Thieme Verlag 1970.

HAHN, J.F.: Stimulus-response relationships in first order fibres from cat vibrissae. J. Physiol. (Lond.) **213**, 215–226 (1971).

Hammer, B.: Elektrophysiologische Untersuchung von peripheren, corticalen und thalamischen Verbindungen zu Neuronen der bulbären Trigeminuskerne der Katze. Pflügers Arch. ges. Physiol. **299**, 261–284 (1968).

Hardy, J. D., Oppel, T. W.: Studies in temperature sensation. III. The sensitivity of the body to heat and the spatial summation of the endorgan response. J. clin. Invest. **16**, 533–540 (1937).

Harris, R., Griffin, C. J.: Fine structure of nerve endings in the human dental pulp. Arch. oral Biol. **13**, 773–778 (1968).

Heimer, L., Wall, P. D.: The dorsal root distribution to the substantia gelatinosa of the rat with a note on the distribution in the cat. Exp. Brain Res. **6**, 89–99 (1968).

Henkin, R. L., Banks, V.: Tactile perception on the tongue, palate and the hand of normal man. In: Symposium on Oral Sensation and Perception. Ed. by J. F. Bosma, pp. 182–187. Springfield, Ill.: Thomas 1967.

Hensel, H.: Cutane Wärmereceptoren bei Primaten. Pflügers Arch. **313**, 150–152 (1969).

Hensel, H., Boman, K. K. A.: Afferent impulses in cutaneous sensory nerves in human subjects. J. Neurophysiol. **23**, 564–578 (1960).

Hensel, H., Huopaniemi, T.: Static and dynamic properties of warm fibres in the infraorbital nerve. Pflügers Arch. **309**, 1–10 (1969).

Hensel, H., Iggo, A., Witt, I.: A quantitative study of sensitive cutaneous thermoreceptors with C afferent fibres. J. Physiol. (Lond.) **153**, 113–126 (1960).

Hensel, H., Kenshalo, D. R.: Warm receptors in the nasal regions of cats. J. Physiol. (Lond.) **204**, 99–112 (1969).

Hensel, H., Zotterman, Y.: Action potentials of cold fibers and intracutaneous temperature gradient. J. Neurophysiol. **14**, 377–385 (1951).

Hepp-Reymond, M. C., Wiesendanger, M.: Pyramidal influence on the spinal trigeminal nucleus of the cat. Arch. ital. Biol. **107**, 54–66 (1969).

Hinrichsen, C. F. L., Larramendi, L. M.: Synapses and cluster formation of the mouse mesencephalic fifth nucleus. Brain Res. **7**, 296–299 (1968).

Hufschmidt, H.-J., Spuler, H.: Mono- and polysynaptic reflexes of the trigeminal muscles in human beings. J. Neurol. Neurosurg. Psychiat. **25**, 332–335 (1962).

Hugelin, A., Bonvallet, M.: Etude oscillographique d'un reflexe monosynaptique cranien (refléx massetérin). J. Physiol. (Paris) **49**, 210–211 (1957).

Humphrey, T.: The spinal tract of the trigeminal nerve in human embryos between $7^1/_2$ and $8^1/_2$ weeks of menstrual age and its relation to early fetal behavior. J. comp. Neurol. **97**, 143–210 (1952).

Humphrey, T.: The trigeminal nerve in relation to early human fetal activity. Res. Publ. Ass. nerv. ment. Dis. **33**, 127–154 (1954).

Humphrey, T.: Some correlations between the appearance of human fetal reflexes and the development of the nervous system. Progr. Brain Res. **4**, 93–135 (1964).

Humphrey, T.: Reflex activity in the oral and facial area of the human fetus. In: Second Symposium on Oral Sensation and Perception. Ed. by J. F. Bosma, pp. 195–233. Springfield, Ill.: Thomas 1970.

Hun, H.: Analgesia, thermic anaesthesia and ataxia. N. Y. med. J. **65**, 613 (1897).

Hunt, C. C., McIntyre, A. K.: Properties of cutaneous touch receptors in cat. J. Physiol. (Lond.) **153**, 88–98 (1960).

Iggo, A.: Cutaneous heat and cold receptors with slowly conducting (C) afferent fibres. Quart. J. exp. Physiol. **44**, 362–370 (1959).

Iggo, A.: The electrophysiological analysis of afferent fibres in primate skin. Acta neuroveg. (Wien) **24**, 225–240 (1963).

Iggo, A.: Temperature discrimination in the skin. Nature (Lond.) **204**, 481–483 (1964).

Iggo, A.: Cutaneous receptors with a high sensitivity to mechanical displacement. In: Touch, Heat, and Pain. Ed. by A. V. S. de Reuck and J. Knight, pp. 237–255. Boston: Little Brown 1966.

Iggo, A.: Electrophysiological and histological studies of cutaneous mechanoreceptors. In: The Skin Senses. Ed. by D. R. Kenshalo, pp. 84–106. Springfield, Ill.: Thomas 1968.

Iggo, A.: Cutaneous thermoreceptors in primates and subprimates. J. Physiol. (Lond.) **200**, 403–430 (1969).

IGGO, A., MUIR, A.R.: The structure and function of a slowly adapting touch corpuscle in hairy skin. J. Physiol. (Lond.) **200**, 763–796 (1969).

IGGO. A., OGAWA, H.: Primate cutaneous thermal nociceptors. J. Physiol. (Lond.) **216**, 29–30 P (1971).

IRIUCHIJIMA, J., ZOTTERMAN, Y.: The specificity of afferent cutaneous C fibres in mammals. Acta physiol. scand. **49**, 267–278 (1960).

JERGE, C.R.: Organization and function of the trigeminal mesencephalic nucleus. J. Neurophysiol. **26**, 379–392 (1963).

JERGE, C.R.: The function of the nucleus supratrigeminalis. J. Neurophysiol. **26**, 393–402 (1963).

JERGE, C.R.: The neural substratum of oral sensation. In: Symposium on Oral Sensation and Perception. Ed. by J.F. BOSMA, pp. 63–83. Springfield, Ill.: Thomas 1967.

KAEMMERER, E.: A review of the etiologic factors in trigeminal neuralgia. In: Trigeminal Neuralgia. Ed. by R. HASSLER and A.E. WALKER, pp. 175–179. Stuttgart: Georg Thieme Verlag 1970.

KAWAMURA, Y.: A role of afferents for manibular and lingual movements. In: Second Symposium on Oral Sensation and Perception. Ed. by J.F. BOSMA, pp. 170–194. Springfield, Ill.: Thomas 1970.

KAWAMURA, Y., MAJIMA, T.: The role of sensory information from the temporomandibular joint in jaw movement. J. dent. Res. **43**, 813 (1964).

KENSHALO, D.R.: Comparison of the thermal sensitivity of the forehead, lip, conjunctiva and cornea. J. appl. Physiol. **15**, 987–991 (1960).

KENSHALO, D.R.: Behavioral and electrophysiological responses of cats to thermal stimuli. In: The Skin Senses. Ed. by D.R. KENSHALO, pp. 400–418. Springfield, Ill.: Thomas 1968.

KENSHALO, D.R.: Psychophysical studies of temperature sensitivity. In: Contributions to Sensory Physiology, Vol. 4. Ed. by W.D. NEFF, pp. 19–64. New York: Academic Press 1970.

KENSHALO, D.R., DUNCAN, D.G., WEYMARK, C.: Thresholds for thermal stimulation of the inner thigh, footpad and face of cats. J. comp. physiol. Psychol. **63**, 113–138 (1967).

KENSHALO, D.R., GALLEGOS, E.S.: Multiple temperature-sensitive spots innervated by single nerve fibers. Science **158**, 1064–1065 (1967).

KEREBEL, B.: Innervation of human periodontium. Actualités odontostomat. **71**, 289–312 (1965).

KERR, F.W.L.: Facial, vagal and glossopharyngeal nerves in the cat. Arch. Neurol. **6**, 264–281 (1962).

KERR, F.W.L.: The divisional organization of afferent fibers of the trigeminal nerve. Brain **86**, 721–732 (1963).

KERR, F.W.L.: The ultrastructure of the spinal tract of the trigeminal nerve and the substantia gelatinosa. Exp. Neurol. **16**, 359–376 (1966).

KERR, F.W.L.: Correlated light and electron microscopic observations on the normal trigeminal ganglion and sensory root in man. J. Neurosurg. **26**, Suppl. 132–137 (1967).

KERR, F.W.L.: Evidence for a peripheral etiology of trigeminal neuralgia. J. Neurosurg. **26**, Suppl. 168–174 (1967).

KERR, F.W.L.: Fine structure and functional characteristics of the primary trigeminal neuron. In: Trigeminal Neuralgia. Ed. by R. HASSLER and A.E. WALKER, pp. 11–21. Stuttgart: Georg Thieme Verlag 1970.

KERR, F.W.L.: Peripheral versus central factors in trigeminal neuralgia. In: Trigeminal Neuralgia. Ed. by R. HASSLER and A.E. WALKER, pp. 180–190. Stuttgart: Georg Thieme Verlag 1970.

KERR, F.W.L.: Electron microscopic observations on degeneration in the subnucleus caudalis of the trigeminal. In: Oro-Facial Sensory and Motor Mechanisms. Ed. by R. DUBNER. In press. New York: Appleton-Century-Crofts 1970.

KERR, F.W.L., KRUGER, L., SCHWASSMANN, H.O., STERN, R.: Somatotopic organization of mechanoreceptor units in the trigeminal nuclear complex of the macaque. J. comp. Neurol. **134**, 127–144 (1968).

KERR, F.W.L., LYSAK, W.R.: Somatotopic organization of trigeminal ganglion neurons. Arch. Neurol. (Chic.) **11**, 593–602 (1964).

KING, R.B.: Evidence of a central etiology of tic douloureux. J. Neurosurg. **26**, Suppl. 175–180 (1967).

KRUGER, L., MICHEL, F.: A morphological and somatotopic analysis of single unit activity in the trigeminal sensory complex of the cat. Exp. Neurol. **5**, 139–156 (1962).

KRUGER, L., MICHEL, F.: A single neuron analysis of buccal cavity representation in the sensory trigeminal complex of the cat. Arch. oral Biol. **7**, 491–503 (1962).

KRUGER, L., SIMINOFF, R., WITKOVSKY, P.: Single neuron analysis of dorsal column nuclei and spinal nucleus of trigeminal in cat. J. Neurophysiol. **24**, 333–349 (1961).

KUGELBERG, E., LINDBLOM, U.: Studies in the mechanism of pain in trigeminal neuralgia. In: Pain and Itch. Ed. by G.E.W. WOLSTENHOLME and M. O'CONNOR, pp. 98–107. London: Churchill 1960.

KUNC, Z.: Significance of fresh anatomic data on spinal trigeminal tract for possibility of selective tractotomies. In: Pain. Ed. by R.S. KNIGHTON and P.R. DUMKE, pp. 351–363. Boston: Little Brown 1966.

KUNC, Z.: Significant factors pertaining to the results of trigeminal tractotomy. In: Trigeminal Neuralgia. Ed. by R. HASSLER and A.E. WALKER, pp. 90–100. Stuttgart: Georg Thieme Verlag 1970.

KUYPERS, H.G.J.M., TUERK, J.D.: The distribution of the cortical fibres within the nucleus cuneatus and gracilis in the cat. J. Anat. (Lond.) **98**, 143–162 (1964).

LANDAU, W., BISHOP, G.H.: Pain from dermal, periosteal and facial endings from inflammation. Arch. Neurol. Psychiat. (Chic.) **69**, 490 (1953).

LELE, P.P., WEDDELL, G.: The relationship between neurohistology and corneal sensibility. Brain **79**, 119–154 (1956).

LELE, P.P., WEDDELL, G.: Sensory nerves of the cornea and cutaneous sensibility. Exp. Neurol. **1**, 334–359 (1959).

LEWINSKY, W., STEWART, D.: A comparative study of the innervation of the periodontal membrane. Proc. roy. Soc. Med. **30**, 1355–1369 (1937).

LORENTE DE NÓ, R.: Contribution al conocimento del nervio trigemino. Libro en honor RAMÓN Y CAJAL, Vol. 2, p. 13 (1922).

McCROSKEY, R.L.: Some effects of anesthetizing the articulators under conditions of normal and relayed side-tone. Project Nm 001104500. Report No. 65, U.S. Naval School of Aviation Medicine, Naval Air Station, Pensecola, Fla. (1958).

McDONALD, E., AUNGST, L.F.: Apparent independence of oral sensory functions and articulatory efficiency. In: Second Symposium on Oral Sensation and Perception. Ed. by J.F. BOSMA, pp. 391–397. Springfield, Ill.: Thomas 1970.

McINTYRE, A.K.: Afferent limb of the myotatic reflex arc. Nature (Lond.) **168**, 168–169 (1951).

McINTYRE, A.K., ROBINSON, R.G.: Pathway for the jaw-jerk in man. Brain **82**, 468–474 (1959).

MANNI, E., BORTOLAMI, R., DESOLE, C.: Peripheral pathway of eye muscle proprioception. Exp. Neurol. **22**, 1–12 (1968).

MANNI, E., BORTOLAMI, R., DERIU, P.L.: Presence of cell bodies of the afferent from the eye muscles of the semilunar ganglion. Arch. ital. Biol. **108**, 106–120 (1970).

MARGARIDA, R., HARDY, J.D., HAMMEL, H.T.: Measurement of the thermal pain threshold of the hard palate. J. appl. Physiol. **17**, 338–342 (1962).

MAXWELL, D.S.: Fine structure of the normal trigeminal ganglion in the cat and monkey. J. Neurosurg. **26**, Suppl. 127–131 (1967).

MEESSEN, H., OLSZEWSKI, J.: A Cytoarchitectonic Atlas of the Rhombencephalon of the Rabbit. Basel: Karger 1949.

MEHLER, W.R.: Some observations on secondary ascending afferent systems in the central nervous system. In: Pain. Ed. by R.S. KNIGHTON and P.R. DUMKE, pp. 11–32. Boston: Little Brown 1966.

MEHLER, W.R., FEFFERMAN, M.E., NAUTA, W.J.H.: Ascending axon degeneration following anterior cordotomy. An experimental study in the monkey. Brain **83**, 718–750 (1960).

MERZENICH, M.M., HARRINGTON, T.: The sense of flutter vibrations evoked by stimulation of the hairy skin of primates: comparison of human sensory capacity with responses of mechanoreceptive afferents innervating the hairy skin of monkeys. Exp. Brain Res. **9**, 236–260 (1969).

MILLER, M.R., RALSTON, H.J., KASAHARA, M.: The pattern of cutaneous innervation in the human hand, foot, and breast. In: Advances in Biology of Skin, Vol. 1. Cutaneous Innervation. Ed. by W. MONTAGNA, pp. 1–47. New York: Pergamon Press 1960.

MILLER, S.: Excitation of mechanoreceptor units in the skin of the rabbit ear. Arch. ital. Biol. 105, 290–314 (1967).

MILLER, S., WEDDELL, G.: Mechanoreceptors in rabbit ear skin innervated by myelinated nerve fibres. J. Physiol. (Lond.) 187, 291–305 (1966).

MOSES, H.L.: Comparative fine structure of the trigeminal ganglion, including autopsy studies. J. Neurosurg. 26, Suppl. 112–126 (1967).

MOUNTCASTLE, V.B.: Some functional properties of the somatic afferent system. In: Sensory Communication. Ed. by W.A. ROSENBLITH, pp. 403–436. Cambridge, Mass.: M.I.T. Press 1961

NAFE, J.P., WAGONER, K.S.: The insensitivity of the cornea to heat and pain derived from high temperatures. Amer. J. Psychol. 49, 631–635 (1937).

NAGAKI, J., YAMASHITA, S., SATO, M.: Neural response of cat to taste stimuli of varying temperatures. Jap. J. Physiol. 14, 67–89 (1964).

NAUTA, W.J.H., KUYPERS, H.G.J.M.: Some ascending pathways in the brainstem reticular formation. In: Reticular Formation of the Brain. Henry Ford Hospital Symposium. Ed. by H.H. JASPER and L.D. PROCTOR, pp. 3–30. Boston: Little Brown 1958.

NESS, A.R.: The mechanoreceptors of the rabbit mandibular incisor. J. Physiol. (Lond.) 126, 475–493 (1954).

NOBLE, G.K., SCHMIDT, A.: Structure and function of the facial and labial pits of snakes. Proc. Amer. Phil. Soc. 77, 263–288 (1937).

NORD, S.G., KYLER, H.J.: A single unit analysis of trigeminal projections to bulbar reticular nuclei of the rat. J. comp. Neurol. 134, 485–494 (1968).

NORD, S.G.: Somatotopic organization in the spinal trigeminal nucleus, the dorsal column nuclei and related structures in the rat. J. comp. Neurol. 130, 343–356 (1967).

NORD, S.G.: Receptor field characteristics of single cells in the rat spinal trigeminal complex. Exp. Neurol. 21, 236–243 (1968).

OGAWA, H., SATO, M., YAMASHITA, S.: Multiple sensitivity of chorda tympani fibers of the rat and hamster to gustatory and thermal stimuli. J. Physiol. (Lond.) 199, 223–240 (1968).

OLIVECRONA, H.: Tractotomy for relief of trigeminal neuralgia. A.M.A. Arch. Neurol. Psychiat. 47, 544–564 (1942).

OLSZEWSKI, J.: On the anatomical and functional organization of the spinal trigeminal nucleus. J. comp. Neurol. 92, 401–413 (1950).

OLSZEWSKI, J., BAXTER, D.: Cytoarchitecture of the Human Brain Stem. Basel: Karger 1954.

PATRIZI, A., MUNGER, B.: The ultrastructure and innervation of rat vibrissae. J. comp. Neurol. 126, 423–436 (1966).

PEARSON, A.A.: The development and connections of the mesencephalic root of the trigeminal nerve in man. J. comp. Neurol. 90, 1–46 (1949).

PERKELL, J.S.: Physiology of Speech Production: Results and Implications of a Quantitative Cineradiographic Study. pp 104. Cambridge, Mass.: M.I.T. Press 1969.

PFAFFMAN, C.: Afferent impulses from the teeth due to pressure and noxious stimulation. J. Physiol. (Lond.) 97, 207–219 (1939).

PFAFFMAN, C.: Afferent impulses from the teeth resulting from a vibratory stimulation. J. Physiol. (Lond.) 97, 220–232 (1939).

PINEDA, A., MAXWELL, D.S., KRUGER, L.: The fine structure of neurons and satellite cells in the trigeminal ganglion of cat and monkey. Amer. J. Anat. 121, 461–488 (1967).

PINKUS, F.: Über Hautsinnesorgane neben dem menschlichen Haar (Haarscheiben) und ihre vergleichend anatomische Bedeutung. Arch. mikr. Anat. 65, 121–179 (1904).

PORTER, R.: Lingual mechanoreceptors activated by muscle twitch. J. Physiol. (Lond.) 183, 101–111 (1966).

POULOS, D.A., LENDE, R.A.: Response of trigeminal ganglion neurons to thermal stimulation of orofacial regions. I. Steady state response. J. Neurophysiol. 33, 508–517 (1970).

POULOS, D.A., LENDE, R.A.: Response of trigeminal ganglion neurons to thermal stimulation of orofacial regions. II. Temperature change response. J. Neurophysiol. 33, 518–526 (1970).

Ralston, H.J.: The organization of the substantia gelatinosa Rolandi in the cat lumbosacral spinal cord. Z. Zellforsch. **67**, 1–23 (1965).

Ralston, H.J.: The fine structure of neurons in the dorsal horn of the cat spinal cord. J. comp. Neurol. **132**, 275–302 (1968).

Ralston, H.J.: Dorsal root projections to dorsal horn neurons in the cat spinal cord. J. comp. Neurol. **132**, 303–330 (1968).

Réthelyi, M., Szentágothai, J.: The large synaptic complex of the substantia gelatinosa. Exp. Brain Res. **7**, 258–274 (1968).

Rexed, B.: The cytoarchitectonic organization of the spinal cord in the cat. J. comp. Neurol. **96**, 415–495 (1952).

Rexed, B., Strom, G.: Afferent nervous connexions of the lateral cervical nucleus. Acta physiol. scand. **25**, 219–229 (1952).

Ringel, R.L.: Oral region two point discrimination in normal and myopathic subjects. In: Second Symposium on Oral Sensation and Perception. Ed. by J. F. Bosma, pp. 309–322. Springfield, Ill.: Thomas 1970.

Ringel, R.L.: Studies of oral region textural perception. In: Second Symposium on Oral Sensation and Perception. Ed. by J.F. Bosma, pp. 323–331. Springfield Ill.: Thomas 1970.

Rowe, M.J.: Trigeminal neural mechanisms of facial tactile sensation. Thesis. University of New South Wales, Kensington, Australia, 1968.

Rowe, M.J., Sessle, B.J.: Somatic afferent input to posterior thalamic neurones and their axon projection to the cerebral cortex. J. Physiol. (Lond.) **196**, 19–35 (1968).

Russell, G.V.: The dorsal trigemino-thalamic tract in the cat reconsidered as a lateral reticulo-thalamic system of connections. J. comp. Neurol. **101**, 237–262 (1954).

Sakada, S.: Response of Golgi-Mazzoni corpuscles in the cat periostea to mechanical stimuli. In: Oral-Facial Sensory and Motor Mechanisms. Ed. by R. Dubner and Y. Kawamura, pp. 105–122. New York: Appleton-Century-Crofts 1971.

Sakada, S., Itow, H., Ikegami, H.: Comparison of mechanoreceptors for electrophysiological properties in the oral lip of cat. Bull. Tokyo dent. Coll. **7**, 1–20 (1966).

Sakada, S., Maeda, K.: Characteristics of innervation and nerve endings in cat's mandibular periostium. Bull. Tokyo dent. Coll. **8**, 77–94 (1967).

Sakada, S., Maeda, K.: Correlation between histological structure and response to pressure of mechanoreceptors in the cat mandibular periostium. Bull. Tokyo dent. Coll. **8**, 181–196 (1967).

Sato, M.: Response of pacinian corpuscles to sinusoidal vibration. J. Physiol. (Lond.) **159**, 391–401 (1961).

Scheibel, M., Scheibel, A.B.: Terminal axonal patterns in cat spinal cord. II. The dorsal horn. Brain Res. **9**, 32–58 (1968).

Scott, D.: Excitation of the dentinal receptor in the tooth of the cat. In: Touch, Heat and Pain. Ed. by A.V.S. de Reuck and J. Knight, pp. 261–274. Boston: Little Brown 1966.

Sessle, B.J.: Studies of the functional organization of somatic afferent pathways. Ph. D. Thesis. University of New South Wales. Kensington Australia (1968).

Sheinin, J.J.: Typing of the cells of the mesencephalic nucleus of the trigeminal nerve in the dog, based on Nissl-granule arrangement. J. comp. Neurol. **50**, 109–131 (1930).

Shende, M.C., King, R.B.: Excitability changes of trigeminal primary afferent preterminals in brainstem nuclear complex of squirrel monkeys (Saimiri sciureus). J. Neurophysiol. **30**, 949–963 (1967).

Sherrington, C.S.: Reflexes elicitable in the cat from pinna, vibrissae and jaws. J. Physiol. (Lond.) **51**, 404–431 (1917).

Sjöqvist, O.: Studies on pain conduction in the trigeminal nerve. Acta psychiat. (Kbh.) Suppl. **17**, 1–139 (1938).

Sjöqvist, O.: The conduction of pain in the fifth nerve and its bearing on the treatment of trigeminal neuralgia. Yale J. Biol. Med. **11**, 594–600 (1939).

Smith, K.R.: The structure and function of the haarscheibe. J. comp. Neurol. **131**, 459–474 (1967).

Smith, R.D., Marcarian, H.Q.: Centripetal localization of tooth and tongue tension receptors. J. dent. Res. **47**, 616–621 (1968).

Smith, R.D., Marcarian, H.Q., Niemer, W.T.: Bilateral relationships of the trigeminal mesencephalic nuclei and mastication. J. comp. Neurol. **131**, 79–92 (1967).

SMITH, R.D., MARCARIAN, H.Q., NIEMER, W.T.: Direct projections from the masseteric nerve to the mesencephalic nucleus. J. comp. Neurol. **133**, 495–502 (1968).

SMYTH, G.E.: The systemization and central connections of the spinal tract and nucleus of the trigeminal nerve. Brain **62**, 41–87 (1939).

SPILLER, W.G.: Remarks on the central representation of sensation. J. nerv. ment. Dis. **42**, 399–418 (1915).

STEWART, D.: Some aspects of the innervation of the teeth. Proc. roy. Soc. Med. **20**, 1675–1687 (1927).

STEWART, W.A., KING, R.B.: Fiber projections from the nucleus caudalis of the spinal trigeminal nucleus. J. comp. Neurol. **121**, 271–286 (1963).

STEWART, D.H., SCIBETTA, C.J., KING, R.B.: Presynaptic inhibition in the trigeminal relay nuclei. J. Neurophysiol. **30**, 135–153 (1967).

STEWART, W.A., STOOPS, W.L., PILLONE, P.R., KING, R.B.: An electrophysiological study of ascending pathways from nucleus caudalis of the spinal trigeminal complex. J. Neurosurg. **21**, 35–48 (1964).

STRAILE, W.E.: Sensory hair follicles in mammalian skin: The tylotrich follicle. Amer. J. Anat. **106**, 133–147 (1960).

STRAILE, W.E.: The morphology of tylotrich follicles in the skin of the rabbit. Amer. J. Anat. **109**, 1–13 (1961).

STRAILE, W.E.: Encapsulated nerve end-organs in the rabbit, mouse, sheep and man. J. comp. Neurol. **136**, 317–336 (1969).

STRUGHOLD, H.: Die Topographie des Kältesinnes in der Mundhöhle. Z. Biol. **83**, 515–534 (1925).

SZABO, G.: The regional frequency and distribution of hair follicles in human skin. In: The Biology of Hair Growth. Ed. by W. MONTAGNA and R.A. ELLIS, pp. 33–38. New York: Academic Press 1958.

SZENTÁGOTHAI, J.: Neuronal and synaptic arrangement in the substantia gelatinosa Rolandi. J. comp. Neurol. **110**, 219–239 (1964).

SZENTÁGOTHAI, J.: Anatomical considerations of monosynaptic reflex arcs. J. Neurophysiol. **11**, 445–454 (1948).

SZENTÁGOTHAI, J., KISS, T.: Projections of dermatomes in the substantia gelatinosa. Arch. Neurol. (Chic.) **62**, 737–744 (1949).

TALBOT, W.H., DARIAN-SMITH, I., KORNHUBER, H.H., MOUNTCASTLE, V.B.: The sense of flutter-vibrations: comparison of the human capacity with response patterns of mechanoreceptive afferents from the monkey hand. J. Neurophysiol. **31**, 301–334 (1968).

TAREN, J.A.: The positions of the cutaneous components of the facial, glossopharyngeal and vagal nerves in the spinal tract of V. J. comp. Neurol. **122**, 389–397 (1964).

TAUB, A., BISHOP, P.O.: The spinocervical tract: dorsal column linkage, conduction velocity, primary afferent spectrum. Exp. Neurol. **13**, 1–21 (1965).

TORVIK, A.: Afferent connections to the sensory trigeminal nuclei, the nucleus of the solitary tract and adjacent structures. J. comp. Neurol. **106**, 51–141 (1956).

TORVIK, A.: The ascending fibers from the main trigeminal sensory nucleus. Amer. J. Anat. **100**, 1–15 (1957).

TOWER, S.S.: Unit for sensory reception in cornea. J. Neurophysiol. **3**, 486–500 (1940).

VINCENT, S.B.: The tactile hair of the white rat. J. comp. Neurol. **23**, 1–34 (1913).

WALBERG, F.: The lateral reticular nucleus of the medulla oblongata in mammals. A comparative-anatomical study. J. comp. Neurol. **96**, 283–344 (1952).

WALBERG, F.: The fine structure of the cuneate nucleus in normal cats and following interruption of afferent fibers. Exp. Brain Res. **2**, 107–128 (1966).

WALKER, A.E.: Anatomy, physiology and surgical considerations of the spinal tract of the trigeminal nerve. J. Neurophysiol. **2**, 234–248 (1939).

WALL, P.D., TAUB, A.: Four aspects of trigeminal nucleus and a paradox. J. Neurophysiol. **25**, 110–126 (1962).

WEDDELL, G., ZANDER, E.: A critical evaluation of methods used to demonstrate tissue neural elements, illustrated by reference to the cornea. J. Anat. (Lond.) **84**, 168–195 (1950).

WEINBERGER, L.N., GRANT, F.C.: Experiences with intra-medullary tractotomy. III. Studies in sensation. Arch. Neurol. Psychiat. (Chic.) **48**, 355–381 (1942).

WEINSTEIN, S.: Intensive and extensive aspects of tactile sensitivity as a function of body part, sex, and laterality. In: The Skin Senses. Ed. by D. R. KENSHALO, pp. 195–219. Springfield, Ill.: Thomas 1968.

WIESENDANGER, M., FELIX, D.: Pyramidal excitation of lemniscal neurons and fascilitation of sensory transmission in the spinal trigeminal nucleus of the cat. Exp. Neurol. **25**, 1–17 (1969).

WIESENDANGER, M., HAMMER, B., HEPP-REYMOND, M.C.: Corticofugal control mechanisms of somatosensory transmission in the spinal trigeminal nucleus of the cat. In: Trigeminal Neuralgia. Ed. by R. HASSLER and A. E. WALKER, pp. 86–89. Stuttgart: Georg Thieme Verlag 1970.

WERNER, V. B., MOUNTCASTLE, V. B.: Neural activity in mechanoreceptive cutaneous afferents: stimulus-response relations Weber functions, and information transmission. J. Neurophysiol. **28**, 359–397 (1965).

WESTRUM, L. E., BLACK, R. G.: Changes in the synapses of the spinal trigeminal nucleus after ipsilateral rhizotomy. Brain Res. **11**, 706–709 (1968).

WHITE, J.C., SWEET, W.H.: Pain and the Neurosurgeon. Springfield, Ill.: Thomas 1969.

WILLIAMS, T.H., DIXON, A.D.: The intrinsic innervation of the soft palate. J. Anat. (Lond.) **97**, 259–267 (1963).

WILSON, D.J.: The maxillary nerve in the cat: a study in growth and form. Thesis for Doctorate in Dental Science, University of Sydney, Australia (1968).

WINDLE, W.F.: Non-bifurcating nerve fibers of the trigeminal nerve. J. comp. Neurol. **40**, 229–240 (1926).

WINKELMANN, R.K.: Nerve Endings in Normal and Pathologic Skin. Springfield, Ill.: Thomas 1960.

WINKELMANN, R.K.: New methods for the study of nerve endings. In: The Skin Senses. Ed. by D.R. KENSHALO, pp. 38–57. Springfield, Ill.: Thomas 1968.

YAMADA, M.: Electrophysiological studies of excitation of dentine evoked by chemical means. In: Sensory Mechanisms in Dentine. Ed. by D.J. ANDERSON, pp. 47–59. Oxford: Pergamon Press 1963.

ZANDER, E., WEDDELL, G.: Observations on the innervation of the cornea. J. Anat. (Lond.) **85**, 68–99 (1951).

ZEIGLER, H., WITKOVSKY, P.: The main sensory trigeminal nucleus in the pigeon: a single unit analysis. J. comp. Neurol. **134**, 255–264 (1968).

ZOTTERMAN, Y.: Thermal sensation. In: Handbook of Physiology, Section I; Neurophysiology, vol. I. Ed. by H.W. MAGOUN, pp. 431–458. Washington, D.C.: Americ. Physiol. Soc. 1959.

ZOTTERMAN, Y.: Specific action potentials in the lingual nerve of the cat. Scand. Arch. Physiol. **75**, 105–120 (1936).

ZUCKER, E., WELKER, W.I.: Coding of somatic sensory input by vibrissae neurons in the rat's trigeminal ganglion. Brain Res. **12**, 138–156 (1969).

Chapter 10

Ascending and Long Spinal Pathways: Dorsal Columns, Spinocervical Tract and Spinothalamic Tract

By

A.G. Brown[1], Edinburgh (Great Britain)

With 7 Figures

Contents

A. Introduction

The organization of ascending spinal cord pathways concerned with somato-sensory mechanisms is not the same for all mammals. In particular there are differences in the development of the spinocervical and spinothalamic tracts, and also subtle variations in the dorsal column system. Furthermore, the types, proportions and axonal conduction velocities of cutaneous afferent units vary according to species (see chapters 2, 3 and 4). It is obvious, therefore, that extreme caution should be exercised in 1) extrapolating results obtained from one species to another, particularly to man, 2) equating the functions of similar anatomical systems in different species, and 3) equating the functions of differently located ascending systems in different species, e. g. the spinocervical tract of carnivores with the spinothalamic tract of primates.

---

[1] Beit Memorial Research Fellow.

The following review is based mainly on results obtained from cats, since it is in this species that most of the well-controlled physiological work has been done. Comparisons are made with other species where there is sufficient evidence to make such comparisons useful.

B. The Dorsal Columns

Most general accounts of the dorsal columns (posterior funiculi, fasciculus gracilis and fasciculus cuneatus) include some or all of the following assumptions; 1) Dorsal column axons, as they ascend, are arranged in fibre laminae according to their root of origin, so that those from caudal segments are medial and those from rostral segments are lateral. 2) Dorsal column axons are collateral branches of primary afferent nerve fibres. 3) Dorsal column axons arise from nerve fibres that innervate sensitive mechanoreceptors in the skin, subcutaneous tissue and joint capsules. 4) The dorsal columns form part of the fastest and most direct ascending system from skin to the somatosensory cortex. 5) Dorsal column axons all terminate in the dorsal column nuclei (nucleus gracilis and nucleus cuneatus). None of these assumptions can now be accepted unequivocally.

1. Topographical Organization of the Dorsal Columns

Anatomical degeneration studies indicate that dorsal column axons ascend in an orderly way with those from more caudal levels medial to those from more rostral levels (Ferraro and Barrera, 1935, 1936; Walker and Weaver, 1942; Chang and Ruch, 1947; Glees et al., 1951; Shriver et al., 1968; Carpenter et al., 1968). There is, however, extensive overlap, particularly at cervical levels of fasciculus gracilis (Walker and Weaver, 1942; Carpenter et al., 1968).

The arrangement of axons in the dorsal colums of the squirrel monkey has recently been examined in electrophysiological experiments by Werner and Whitsel (1967). The rootlets of each lumbosacral dorsal root, at the entry zone into the spinal cord, contain axons from overlapping but partially shifted portions of the dermatome. This precise arrangement is preserved in fasciculus gracilis at the lumbar level where there is a lamination of fibres running from dorsolateral to ventromedial regions of the fasciculus, the more caudal dorsal root fibres occupying a dorsomedial position and the more rostral fibres a ventrolateral position (Figs. 1A, 2A). This work on the lumbar dorsal columns has been extended to the cervical cord (Whitsel et al., 1970). As the axons from the hindlimb ascend they undergo a resorting process and between lumbar and cervical levels those from non-cutaneous receptors leave the dorsal columns (see below). At cervical levels of fasciculus gracilis the axons are arranged in a series of bands each representing a restricted region of the ipsilateral hindlimb. The bands are arranged so that the tail is represented dorsally, followed by bands for the proximal leg, distal leg, foot, distal leg, proximal leg, and trunk in that order (Figs. 1B, 2B). These results suggest that the characteristic topographical organization of the primary and secondary somatosensory cortical receiving areas, the ventrobasal thalamus and the dorsal column nuclei is already laid down in the cervical dorsal columns and that the sorting process occurs as the axons ascend the cord. It is not known whether there is a similar sorting process for axons in fasciculus cuneatus.

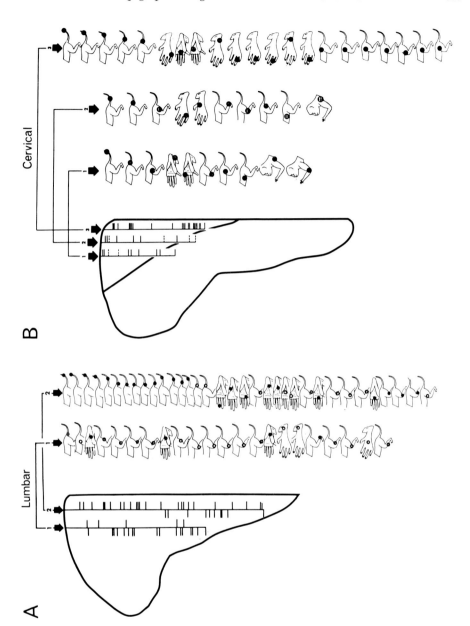

Fig. 1. The arrangement of axons in the dorsal columns of the squirrel monkey. In A two microelectrode penetrations through the lumbar (*L6*) fasciculus gracilis are shown. The sites at which axons were isolated are shown by horizontal lines, to the right for cutaneous units and to the left for deep units. The figurines are arranged in the sequence in which the units were isolated. In B are shown three microelectrode penetrations through the cervical (*C4*) fasciculus gracilis where only cutaneous units were encountered, the unbroken lines representing single unit and the broken lines multi-unit recordings. For *A* and *B* the receptive field centres are plotted on the figurines: ○, single cutaneous units, ⊖ multi-unit cutaneous recordings, ● deep units. (Modified, by permission, from WHITSEL, PETRUCELLI, SAPIRO and HA)

2. Fibre Content of the Dorsal Columns

Most dorsal column fibres are collateral axons of dorsal root fibres. Only 25 %, however, of the myelinated dorsal root fibres which enter the cat's spinal cord at lumbar levels reach the dorsal column nuclei (Glees and Soler, 1951). Group I muscle afferent fibres from the hindlimb do not reach the nuclei (Lloyd and McIntyre, 1950), but the figures of Glees and Soler indicate that most of the cutaneous and joint afferent fibres probably do not reach the nuclei either. Group I muscle afferent fibres from the cat's forelimb ascend in the dorsal columns (Oscarsson and Rosén, 1963; Landgren et al., 1967; Uddenberg, 1968a) and terminate in the main and external cuneate nuclei and in the dorsal horn of the rostral cervical cord (Rosén, 1969).

The projection of cutaneous afferent fibres from the cat's hindlimb through the dorsal columns has been studied in two recent series of experiments (Brown, 1968; Petit and Burgess, 1968). In general the results of these two sets of experiments are in agreement and establish that axons of the following types of cutaneous afferent units project to high cervical levels; hair follicle units Type G and Type T, units with rapidly-adapting mechanoreceptors (including Pacinian corpuscles) in the foot pads, slowly-adapting units Type II, slowly-adapting units with mechanoreceptors in the foot pads and around the base of the claws. Brown reported a few units with high threshold mechanoreceptors that projected whereas Petit and Burgess reported that these units did not project. A further difference between the two sets of results was that Brown reported a few slowly-adapting Type I units projecting whereas Petit and Burgess reported that none of these units projected. There are two possible reasons for these discrepancies, 1) Brown's experiments were not designed to differentiate postsynaptic units in the dorsal columns and in fact the axons of Type I units and high threshold units do excite cells whose axons project through the dorsal columns (see below), 2) there are regional differences in the types of units projecting, e.g. Type I units from the forelimb project (see below) and several of Brown's Type I units had receptive fields on the tail or on the trunk over the pelvis and these Type I units may also project. Other discrepancies between the two sets of results are mainly due to differences in terminology. Petit and Burgess did not recognize Type T hair follicle units, divided their hair follicle units into Types G1 and G2 and also described 'field receptors' which have not been recognized in the cat by other workers (e.g. Hunt and McIntyre, 1960; Brown and Iggo, 1967).

It can be concluded that all types of cutaneous afferent unit with axons conducting at speeds above the Aδ range and with receptors on the cat's hindlimb transmit information through the dorsal columns, either directly or indirectly (see the summary diagram of Fig. 7). The proportions of the different types that project and the reduction in conduction velocity of the axons as they ascend, however, differ according to the type of unit (Brown, 1968; Petit and Burgess, 1968). All Type II units and the majority of hair follicle units Types G and T, slowly-adapting claw and rapidly-adapting foot pad units project (Petit and Burgess, 1968; Brown, unpublished). Very few slowly-adapting foot pad units, high threshold mechanoreceptive units and units with receptors in the subcutaneous tissue have axons that ascend further than the first lumbar segment. Axons of the

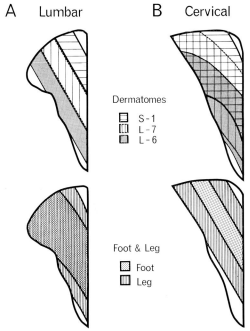

Fig. 2. Diagramatic representation of axonal organization in the dorsal columns. *A* and *B* represent, schematically, the dermatomal and topographical organizations at lumbar and cervical levels respectively. It can be seen that the clear dermatomal organization at lumbar levels becomes obscured at cervical levels. Conversely, the topographical organization is not clear at lumbar levels but is obvious at cervical levels. (Modified, by permission, from WHITSEL, PETRUCELLI, SAPIRO and HA)

Pacinian corpuscles show the least reduction in conduction velocity as they ascend the dorsal columns and are amongst the fastest in the columns, whereas axons of Type G units show the greatest reduction in conduction velocity and are amongst the slowest in the columns (BROWN, 1968 and unpublished). Very few Aδ fibres seem to have collateral axons that ascend the dorsal colums (WALL, 1960b; BROWN, 1968; PETIT and BURGESS, 1968) although PETIT and BURGESS have shown that some Aδ fibres of the plantar nerves do have axons that ascend the columns to high cervical levels. Anatomical studies suggest that the non-myelinated (C) fibres do not have collateral axons that ascend the columns.

The dorsal columns traditionally convey information from the joint receptors. Recent work has severely challenged this long-held belief. BURGESS and CLARK (1969) found, in both cats and squirrel monkeys, that only 8.6% of 468 axons in the posterior articular nerve to the knee joint could be excited from the cervical dorsal columns. Those units that could be excited were all predominantly or exclusively rapidly-adapting, i.e. they were not classical joint units. This paucity of projecting fibres from joint receptors in the hindlimb has been confirmed in the cat (BROWN, unpublished) and the squirrel monkey (WHITSEL et al., 1969). Colateral axons of the joint units leave the dorsal columns at high lumbar levels and information from the joints must ascend in other spinal cord pathways.

Whitsel et al. (1969) have shown that in squirrel monkey there are only rapidly-adapting cutaneous units present in fasciculus gracilis at high cervical levels. Therefore, in addition to the joint units, the slowly-adapting cutaneous units must also have axons that leave the dorsal colums between lumbar and cervical levels. This is a genuine species difference since the cat has several types of slowly-adapting cutaneous units (Type II, claw and foot pad units) whose axons project to high cervical levels.

The input to the dorsal columns from the cat's forelimb has been studied by Uddenberg (1968a, b). In general, the results were similar to those for the hindlimb projection. There was a clear contribution, however, from primary afferent fibres of units with receptive field properties similar to those of Type I slowly-adapting units, which made up about 10% of the sample of 295 axons. Brown et al. (1970) have recorded from axons in the cat's medial lemniscus which are exclusively excited from Type I units and have receptive fields on the forelimb. It seems certain that Type I units from the forelimb project through the dorsal columns. There is no information about the projection of the slowly-adapting carpal tactile hair units (Nilsson and Skoglund, 1965) although Uddenberg (1968a) reported that all of the hair follicle units that he recorded were rapidly-adapting and did not have any resting discharge.

Uddenberg (1968a) has suggested that there is a modality segregation of dorsal column axons at cervical levels in fasciculus cuneatus. Hair follicle units are superficial, slowly-adapting units are deep and Group I muscle afferent units are in between. It is not known how this organization compares with that in funiculus gracilis described by Whitsel et al. (1970).

3. Postsynaptic Units in the Dorsal Columns

Uddenberg (1968b) demonstrated the presence of axons of postsynaptic units in the cervical dorsal columns. The units responded with a rapidly-adapting discharge to hair movement and with a slowly-adapting discharge to pressure on both hairy and hairless skin. An additional discharge was evoked by pinching the skin and by extreme bending of the joints. These results indicate a considerable degree of convergence from different types of primary afferent unit onto the cells. Similar units with receptive fields on the hindlimb have been examined by Petit, Lackner and Burgess (Burgess, personal communication 1970). About 15% of dorsal column units at low thoracic levels were postsynaptic and 55 of 63 of these could be excited from C2 and may therefore project to the dorsal column nuclei. Most of these units responded to hair movement, displacement of cutaneous touch corpuscles (confirmed by Brown, unpublished), mechanically produced skin damage and to heating the skin to 45–47°C. Some units only responded to hair movement and a few only to harmful mechanical stimulation. They responded to electrical stimulation of peripheral Aδ and C fibres in addition to the faster conducting ones. Thus the dorsal columns do not contain only collaterals afferent fibres, nor are they solely concerned with information from sensitive mechanoreceptors. If these results for the cat can be shown to apply to man then the rather unexpected observations (Browder and Gallagher, 1948; Cook and Browder, 1965) that surgical lesions of the dorsal columns can abolish phantom limb pain in human beings might be partly explained.

4. Termination of Dorsal Column Axons

Many axons which enter the dorsal columns at segmental level do not ascend to the dorsal column nuclei through the columns. Group I muscle afferent fibres from the hindlimb and most hindlimb joint afferent fibres leave the cord within a few segments, as do most axons of cutaneous Type I slowly-adapting units, subcutaneous units and units with high thresholds to mechanical stimulation. Axons of most Aδ peripheral nerve fibres also leave the columns soon after their entry. It is usually assumed that axons which ascend to C1 or C2 terminate in the dorsal column nuclei but this is not necessarily so. It would be most useful to know where axons of the postsynaptic units terminate.

As well as the short descending branches of dorsal root fibres in the dorsal columns (CAJAL, 1952) there are other axons which do not belong to the dorsal column-medial lemniscal system. BARILARI and KUYPERS (1969) have described a few propriospinal fibres connecting the spinal enlargements, in both the descending and ascending direction. Furthermore, in rodents a part of the corticospinal tract descends in the dorsal columns (KING, 1910; RANSON, 1913, 1914; REVELEY, 1915; SIMPSON, 1914, 1915a, b; DOUGLAS and BARR, 1950).

It can be seen that many axons in the dorsal columns do not contribute to the ascending dorsal column-medial lemniscal system. It is a mistake to imagine that behavioural changes produced by dorsal column lesions are necessarily due to interference with this system.

C. The Spinocervical Tract

In addition to the dorsal column-medial lemniscal and the spinothalamic pathways there is a third major ascending pathway concerned with somatosensory mechanisms in many mammalian species. This is the pathway described by MORIN (1955) and the spinocervical tract is its spinal part (VAN BEUSEKOM, 1955). It arises from cells in REXED's laminae III, IV and V in the dorsal horn (ECCLES et al., 1960; WALL, 1960a, 1967; FETZ, 1968), ascends in the most medial and superficial part of the ipsilateral dorsolateral funiculus (LUNDBERG and OSCARSSON, 1961; TAUB and BISHOP, 1965) and terminates in the lateral cervical nucleus (REXED and STRÖM, 1952; BRODAL and REXED, 1953; MORIN, 1955; LUNDBERG, 1964; HORROBIN, 1966). Axons from cells of the lateral cervical nucleus cross to the contralateral side at the junction of medulla and cord to run with the medial lemniscus and terminate in the ventrobasal nuclear complex of the thalamus (MORIN, 1955; MORIN and CATALANO, 1955; CATALANO and LAMARCHE, 1957; BUSCH, 1961; GORDON and JUKES, 1963; LANDGREN et al., 1965; HORROBIN, 1966; BOIVIE, 1970). The pathway ultimately projects to the contralateral somatosensory cortical areas SI and SII and to ipsilateral SII (ANDERSSON, 1962; NORRSELL and VOORHOEVE, 1962; NORRSELL and WOLPOW, 1966).

The suggestion that the lateral cervical nucleus receives its input from collateral axons of the dorsal spinocerebellar tract (CAJAL, 1952; MORIN, 1955; MORIN et al., 1963; HA and LIU, 1961, 1962, 1963, 1966) has been refuted (ANDERSSON, 1962; LUNDBERG, 1964; HORROBIN, 1966). HORROBIN's observation that cells of the lateral cervical nucleus cannot be fired by stimulation of the anterior cerebellum is particularly convincing. It remains possible, however, that collateral axons of the dorsal spinocerebellar tract or of other ascending systems could excite an inhibitory system in the lateral cervical nucleus. All cells of the nucleus are not relay cells as Grant and Westman (1969) have shown that cells remain in the nucleus after section of the contralateral medial lemniscus. Fedina et al. (1968) have demonstrated that activity in a crossed ventrolateral ascending pathway leads to inhibitory actions in the lateral cervical nucleus.

A dorsal spino-olivary tract described by Grundfest and Carter (1954) Di Biagio and Grundfest (1954, 1956) and Krieger and Grundfest (1956) may be identical with the spinocervical tract. This spino-olivary tract has a relay in the lateral cervical nucleus (Di Biagio and Grundfest, 1956). It has been shown, both anatomically (Van Beusekom, 1955) and physiologically (Di Biagio and Grundfest, 1956; Horrobin, 1966) that there is a projection from the lateral cervical nucleus to the inferior olive. Horrobin suggests that the fibres to the inferior olive arise as collateral branches of the fibres travelling to the thalamus.

The list of species in which a lateral cervical nucleus has been described continues to grow. This includes cat (Rexed and Ström, 1952), dog (Rexed, 1958; Kitai et al., 1965) sheep, seal and whale (Rexed, 1958), raccoon (Ha et al., 1965), Japanese and owl monkeys (Mizuno et al., 1967), elephant shrew, tree shrew, lemur and several species of monkey (Ha and Morin, 1964). On the one hand Rexed (1958) denies its presence in rat, mouse, guinea-pig and man and Mizuno (1966) states that it is absent in the rabbit. On the other hand Truex et al. (1970) describe it in a rudimentary form in some human material and Gwyn and Waldron (1968, 1969) and Waldron (1969) claim that it is present as a thin lamina of cells extending the whole length of the spinal cord in rat, guinea-pig, rabbit, ferret and hedgehog. It seems obvious that in some of the above examples a certain amount of subjective judgement was involved in deciding what to call a sparse collection of neurones outside the main mass of grey matter. Anatomical observations by themselves do not prove the presence of a functional spinocervical-thalamic system.

1. Electrophysiology of the Spinocervical Tract

The physiological literature on the spinocervical tract is bedevilled by inconsistencies. This is due to two main causes, 1) inadequate evidence on the rostral projections of the units recorded and 2) poor stimulation techniques leading to mixed inputs. In order to ascertain that a particular unit belongs to the spinocervical tract it is necessary to have stimulating electrodes below and above the lateral cervical nucleus and to show that either the rostral pair of electrodes does not excite the unit antidromically or that the conduction velocity of the axon is drastically reduced between the two sets of stimulating electrodes (Lundberg, 1964; Taub and Bishop, 1965; Brown and Franz, 1969). Other controls (Hongo et al., 1968) are 1) monosynaptic excitation from ipsilateral low threshold cutaneous afferent fibres, 2) antidromic invasion from the ipsilateral dorsolateral funiculus at low thoracic levels and 3) location of the cell body in the dorsal horn or intermediate region. None of these latter three controls is sufficient by itself and the first two do not differentiate the spinocervical tract from cutaneous components

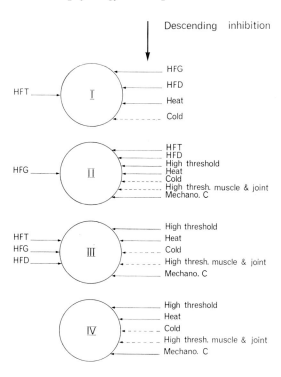

Fig. 3. Schematic classification of spinocervical tract cells according to their excitatory input and the effects of descending inhibition. To the left of the figure are depicted excitatory inputs unaffected by the descending inhibition which is active in the decerebrate cat. To the right those excitatory inputs which are inhibited are shown. The diagram is not intended to indicate the nature of the synaptic linkages, i.e. whether they are mono- or polysynaptic. Key to abbreviations: *HF D*, *G* and *T* — hair follicle afferent units types *D*, *G* and *T* respectively; Heat — units probably with C fibres and which are excited by skin temperatures above 45°C; Cold — units probably with *C* fibres and which are excited by skin temperatures below about 20°C; High thresh. — units with receptors in the skin and subcutaneous tissues that require pressure and pinch to excite them and which have myelinated axons; Mechano. *C* — units excited by mechanical stimulation and which have non-myelinated axons. Dotted lines indicate weak excitatory inputs

of the dorsal spinocerebellar tract. Taken together these three criteria although possibly adequate to exclude non-spinocervical tract units may also exclude spinocervical tract units since some do have long latencies to cutaneous nerve stimulation. It may be assumed, however, that the majority of axons which respond to cutaneous stimulation and which are located in the most superficial and medial parts of the dorsolateral funiculus, particularly at levels caudal to L4, belong to the spinocervical tract. More difficulties of identification are presented when recording from cells in the dorsal horn. According to FETZ (1968) only 43% of recorded cells in lamina IV and only 19% in lamina V have axons which pass into the ipsilateral dorsolateral funiculus. Thus only some 30% of units recorded in these laminae are candidates for the spinocervical tract.

21*

2. Types of Unit in the Spinocervical Tract and Their Descending Control

Careful receptive field analysis, using adequate stimulation of identified receptors, has allowed a classification of spinocervical tract units into several categories (Brown and Franz, 1969). Since the spinocervical tract is under descending control from the brain (Taub, 1964; Wall, 1967; Fetz, 1968) it has also been necessary to determine the equivalence of units in both the spinal and decerebrate preparation (Brown, 1970, 1971). These results are summarized in Fig. 3. Most spinocervical tract units respond to hair movement. In the decerebrate state, however, some respond only to movement of a single type of hair. Thus, Type I units only respond to movement of tylotrichs and Type II only to movement of guard hairs, although these latter units may also respond to pressure and pinch in the decerebrate state unlike Type I units which are never excited by such stimuli. In the spinal state units that respond to hair movement (Types I, II and III) are excited by displacement of all types of hairs in the excitatory receptive field. The descending control, active in the decerebrate animal, in addition to switching off some of the excitatory input from hair follicle afferent units also partially or completely inhibits the excitation produced by moderate or heavy pressure and pinch of the skin and subcutaneous tissues in Types II, III and IV (Fig. 4A). By using well-controlled thermal stimulation the role of the spinocervical tract in handling information from the thermoreceptors has also been clarified (Brown and Franz, 1969). Spinocervical tract units are not excited by the sensitive thermoreceptor afferent units. All *types* of spinocervical tract unit may be excited by heat (above about $45 °C$) and by intense cold (below about $20 °C$) (see Fig. 5). The descending control is also effective in inhibiting these responses to harmful or potentially harmful stimuli. Excitatory input to some spinocervical tract neurones from high threshold muscle and joint afferent fibres has been demonstrated (Lundberg and Oscarsson, 1961; Hongo et al., 1968). It may tentatively be assumed that this polysynaptic input is onto Types II, III and IV units in the above classification.

Some sensitive mechanoreceptive cutaneous afferent units do not excite spinocervical tract cells. These include the rapidly-adapting units from the foot pads, slowly-adapting Type I and Type II units, slowly-adapting foot pad units and the slowly-adapting units with receptors at the base of the claws. Thus the group of neurones in the dorsal horn that are excited by mechanical stimulation of the foot pads (Armett et al., 1961, 1962; Fuller and Gray, 1966; Gray and Lal, 1965) and those excited exclusively by slowly-adapting Type I units (Tapper and Mann, 1968) do not belong to the spinocervical tract. It is not known whether the slowly-adapting carpal tactile hair units (Nilsson and Skoglund, 1965) project onto the spinocervical tract.

Many spinocervical tract units can be excited by C fibre stimulation (Mendell and Wall, 1965; Mendell, 1966). It may be assumed that C fibres are responsible for part of the responses to pressure and pinch and heat and cold.

The spinocervical tract does not show the classical surround inhibition observed for the dorsal column — medial lemniscal system but inhibitory receptive fields on both the ipsilateral and contralateral body surface have been reported (Taub, 1964; Hongo et al., 1968; Brown and Franz, 1969). The descending control

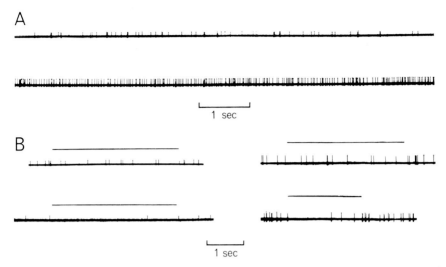

Fig. 4. Effects of descending control on the spinocervical tract. A, Release of excitation to the spinocervical tract from nociceptors on conversion from the decerebrate to the spinal state. In both records the skin of the receptive field was squeezed with a toothed clip. The upper record was obtained in the decerebrate state, the lower record in the spinal state. The spontaneous activity of this unit was 5 imp/sec in the decerebrate state and 10.9 imp/sec in the spinal state. Corresponding figures for the discharge evoked by squeezing were 6.5 and 26.8 imp/sec. The increased evoked activity in the spinal state was therefore genuine and not only a reflection of the increased spontaneous activity. B, Release of inhibition to the spinocervical tract on conversion from the decerebrate to the spinal state. Each pair of records shows the effects of squeezing the skin of the inhibitory receptive field on the spontaneous activity of SCT units in the decerebrate (upper trace) and the spinal (lower traces) preparation. The bar over each record indicates the approximate duration of squeezing. These records were chosen from units for which there was no significant difference between the spontaneous activity, averaged over 10 sec, in either the decerebrate or the spinal state in order to allow direct comparison to be made. On other units in which the rate of spontaneous activity was higher in the spinal state inhibition was always more marked than in the decerebrate state. (Reproduced by permission from BROWN, 1970)

exerts a depressant action on these inhibitory effects (Fig. 4B) which are predominant on Types II, III and IV units (BROWN, 1970, 1971). HILLMAN and WALL (1969) have suggested that cells in lamina V, which may include some spinocervical tract neurones, have overlapping excitatory and inhibitory fields. In HILLMAN and WALL's experiments inhibition was most marked in the decerebrate state which is in contrast to the situation reported by BROWN. The interesting suggestion (HONGO et al., 1968) that inhibitory fields situated close to excitatory fields may form the substrate for directional sensitivity has not been substantiated. No directional sensitivity apart from that due to the alignment of the hairs in the receptive field, can be observed in the discharges of spinocervical tract units (BROWN, unpublished).

The descending control of the spinocervical tract acts to impart a degree of selectivity to movement of particular types of hairs. It also inhibits excitatory actions from mechanoreceptors responding to moderate or heavy pressure and

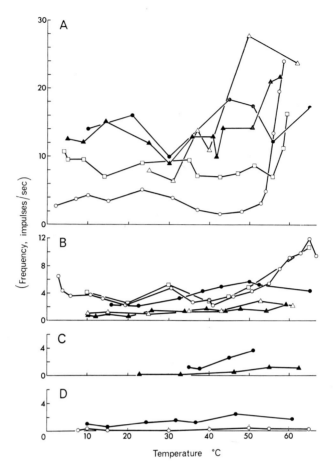

Fig. 5. Graphs of the responses of spinocervical tract units to thermal stimulation of the receptive fields. Each point is the mean frequency calculated from records of 1–10 sec duration. A) Spinal cats, units responding to hair movement (○ □ △); units responding to hair movement and skin pressure (● ▲). B) Decerebrate (○ □ △) and anaesthetized (● ▲) cats; units responding to movement of all three types of hairs. C) Anaesthetized cats; units responding to movement of guard hairs. D) Decerebrate (○) and anaesthetized (●) cats; units responding to movement of tylotrichs. (From Brown and Franz, 1969)

pinch and from heat receptors, thereby inhibiting actions from various nociceptors. At the same time the descending influences release the spinocervical tract from inhibitory actions at the segmental level.

The site of origin of the descending system or systems and the mode of action remain uncertain. Taub (1964) demonstrated that both spontaneous and evoked discharges could be inhibited by electrical stimulation of cerebellar nuclei, the mesencephalic tegmentum and a central pontobulbar region. Fetz (1968) has shown that pyramidal tract activation may inhibit lamina IV cells, although earlier reports (Lundberg et al., 1963; Wall, 1967) failed to show any effects of stimulating either the sensorimotor cortex or the pyramidal tract respectively.

Electrical stimulation at several sites in the cervical spinal cord suppressed transmission through the spinocervical tract of unanaesthetized spinal cats (BROWN et al., 1972). The sites, which were bilateral, were in the dorsal columns, the dorsolateral funiculi and the most medial and ventral parts of the ventral funiculi. Inhibition was produced from the cervical dorsal columns even though the dorsal columns at low thoracic and first lumbar levels had been removed. Presumably this inhibition from the dorsal columns indicates activation of a propriospinal pathway through collateral axons of dorsal root fibres. More recent experiments (BROWN and MARTIN, 1972) have demonstrated how some, at least, of these descending systems may be activated. In decerebrate unanaesthetized cats stimulation of either the cervical dorsal columns in an ascending direction, or the dorsal column nuclei, leads to inhibition of transmission through the spinocervical tract. This inhibition is reduced, but not abolished, by cerebellectomy. It is abolished by transection of the brain stem just rostral to the dorsal column nuclei. Activity ascending the dorsal columns and relaying through the dorsal column nuclei can, therefore, lead to activation of descending pathways that control transmission through the spinocervical tract. The central parts of the pathway include the brain stem and the cerebellum.

TAUB (1964) suggested that part of the inhibitory action of descending systems was due to presynaptic mechanisms. It has been shown that both the descending (BROWN et al., 1972) and segmental (BROWN and KIRK, unpublished) inhibition has a time course of 150–200 msec, with a maximal action at 20–40 msec which supports TAUB's suggestion. Both descending and segmental inhibition act preferentially on polysynaptic and small fibre inputs to the spinocervical tract (BROWN, 1971; BROWN et al., 1972) and occlusion can be demonstrated between the two sets of inhibitory inputs (BROWN and MARTIN, unpublished). These results suggest that there is convergence onto common interneurones in the inhibitory pathways and that the release from segmental inhibition produced by descending activity is an occlusion phenomenon.

3. Conduction Velocities of Spinocervical Tract Axons

The conduction velocity range of spinocervical tract axons is greater than that of dorsal columns axons. At the upper end, velocities over 100 m/sec for nearly the whole length of the tract have been observed in Type I and III units (BROWN and FRANZ, 1969) compared with up to 70 m/sec for dorsal column axons of rapidly-adapting foot pad receptors (Pacinian corpuscles) (BROWN, 1968) which do not excite the spinocervical tract. At the lower end, velocities down to 15 m/sec have been observed whereas dorsal column axons conduct down to about 10 m/sec (BROWN, 1968; PETIT and BURGESS, 1968). Most low velocity axons in the spinocervical tract belong to Type II units which, as a group, have statistically lower velocities than any other (BROWN and FRANZ, 1969; BROWN, 1970, 1971). Because of the differential slowing of dorsal column axons (see pp. 318–319) activity from tylotrich follicle receptors reaches high cervical levels (and possibly the cerebral cortex, see NORRSELL and VOORHOEVE, 1962; NORRSELL and WOLPOW, 1966) earlier through the spinocervical system than through the dorsal column system. One possibly important function of the spinocervical system is to speed up information transmission from hair follicle receptors (the 'short distance receptors') to

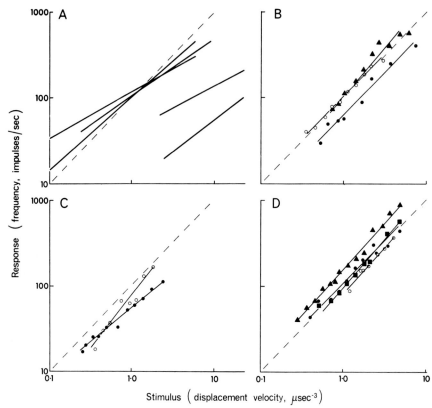

Fig. 6. Stimulus-response relationships to hair movement. A) Primary hair follicle afferent units, taken from the paper of BROWN and IGGO (1967) for comparison with the spinocervical tract units. B) Spinocervical tract units in spinal cats. C) Spinocervical tract units excited by movement of tylotrichs in anaesthetized (○) and decerebrate (●) cats. D) Spinocervical tract units excited by movement of all three types of hairs in anaesthetized (○) and decerebrate (● ▲ ■) cats. The dashed reference line in each figure has a slope of unity. (From BROWN and FRANZ, 1969)

the brain. Whether this rapid conduction serves to alert the animal with subsequent activation of descending systems as suggested by TAUB (1964) remains to be seen. It is intriguing to speculate that the spinocervical tract may act to open or close other ascending pathways including the dorsal column-medial lemniscal system. Indeed, DART and GORDON (1970) have shown that relay cells in the dorsal column nuclei may be excited by electrical stimulation of the ipsilateral dorsolateral funiculus (see also DAVIDSON and SMITH, 1970; TOMASULO and EMMERS, 1970).

4. Transmission of Information through the Spinocervical Tract

Information transmission about the rate of hair movement is accurately coded in the spinocervical tract. The precise relationship between impulse frequency and rate of hair movement observed in primary hair follicle afferent units (BROWN and IGGO, 1967) is maintained through the spinocervical tract (Fig. 6). The main difference being an increase in sensitivity as shown by the increased slopes of the lines (higher exponent of the power function). Some of this increase may be a peripheral effect due to the innervation of single hairs by more than one primary afferent fibre and to overlapping of receptive fields of primary afferent units that converge onto a single spinocervical tract cell. Some of the increase may occur at the spinocervical tract cell itself.

Since many spinocervical tract cells transmit information from a number of different receptor types there is the possibility of stimulus modality coding. A start in the investigation of this has been made by BROWN and FRANZ (1970). Separate spinocervical tract neurones of the same type may exhibit markedly different discharge patterns to the same kind of natural stimulation. Furthermore, unrelated kinds of maintained stimulation may produce distinctly different patterns of discharge in an individual spinocervical tract neurone without necessarily altering the mean frequency of the discharge. These observations suggest that dissimilar modalities of sensory information may be transmitted in the output of individual spinocervical tract cells.

5. Comparison of the Dorsal Columns and the Spinocervical Tract

Sufficient evidence is now available to allow useful comparisons to be made between the inputs to these two systems and to attempt to explain some of the behavioural results that have been obtained after selective spinal cord lesions. Figs. 3 and 7 summarize the physiological data on the input and organization of the two systems. Between them, they carry information from all receptor types known to be present in the skin and subcutaneous tissue of the cat's hindlimb with the exception of the sensitive thermoreceptors. Notable points are 1) the projection of Pacinian corpuscle units, slowly-adapting Types I and II units, pad and claw units through the dorsal columns and not the spinocervical tract, 2) the high incidence of spinocervical tract units conveying information from the ubiquitous, very sensitive down hair follicle receptors and 3) the presence in both systems of units carrying information about harmful or potentially harmful stimuli.

There have been several recent reports on the supposed functions of these two systems as revealed by spinal cord lesions. The general conclusion that can be drawn from these experiments is that it is very difficult to observe any behavioural deficits after such lesions. As the electrophysiological evidence accumulates the reasons for this and for the various discrepancies in the behavioural work become clearer. It is increasingly difficult to consider the two systems in isolation, since each carries information that is also handled by the other. Furthermore, the identification of dorsal column postsynaptic units that transmit information from nociceptors, the virtual absence of input from joint receptors in the dorsal columns and particularly the recent observations of non-dorsal column input to the dorsal column nuclei, possibly from the spinocervical tract itself, emphasize these difficulties. Any behavioural work should be based on the anatomical and physiological evidence available. At present, the cat is probably the only animal for which the background knowledge is sufficient for behavioural experiments.

KENNARD (1954) noted that section of the dorsal quadrant of the spinal cord led to some modification in the response of cats to harmful stimulation and suggest-

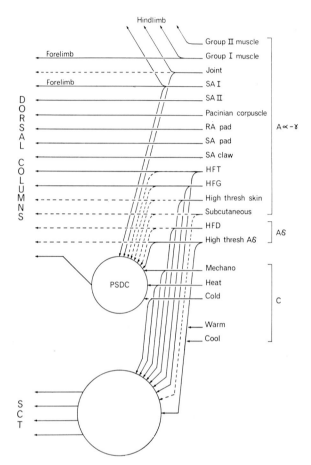

Fig. 7. The distribution of afferent fibres to the dorsal columns and spinocervical tract. The afferent fibres are arranged according to their conduction velocity and the receptors they innervate. Projections that are weak or about which the evidence is not decisive are indicated by dotted lines. Key to the abbreviations: SA I, II, pad and claw — Slowly-adapting units Type I, II, with receptors in the foot pads and at the claw bases respectively; RA pad — rapidly-adapting units with receptors in the foot pads, including Pacinian corpuscles; HF D, G and T — hair follicle units Type D, G and T respectively; High thresh. skin — units with receptors that need strong mechanical stimulation to excite them; Mechano. — units with C fibres excited by mechanical stimulation; Heat, Cold — units probably with C fibres and which are excited by skin temperatures above 45°C and below 20°C respectively; Warm, cool — the sensitive thermoreceptive units; PSDC — postsynaptic dorsal column system (which may require further subdivision); SCT — spinocervical tract

ed that fibres essential for recognition of painful stimuli ascend in this part of the cord. This has been amply confirmed by electrophysiological work. Kitai and Weinberg (1968) trained cats, whose eyes had been enucleated, in a rough-smooth discrimination test. After dorsal column section at C1 there was recovery to 90% of control levels within three weeks, whereas after a midline myelotomy from the lower medulla to C3 (which should transect axons of the lateral cervical nuclei) or after midline myelotomy plus dorsal column section there was recovery only to 35–70% of the control levels. NORRSELL (1966) concluded that in the dog the spinocervical tract was the main afferent pathway necessary for conditioned reflexes to light tactile stimuli and that the dorsal columns were of secondary importance. The stimuli were effective if applied to either the fore or hindlimbs and even after removal of the cortical somatosensory receiving areas (NORRSELL, 1967). These findings are of interest since WHITEHORN et al. (1969) have shown that cortical evoked potentials produced by forepaw stimulation in the cat are relayed through the dorsal columns but not through the spinocervical tract. TAPPER (1970) using an avoidance-conditioning procedure trained cats to respond to mechanical stimulation of cutaneous touch corpuscles. Dorsal column section had little effect (one cat even performed better after this!) whereas lesions of the dorsolateral funiculus, which always included part of the dorsal columns, produced some loss. Since electrophysiological experiments (BROWN and FRANZ, 1969) show that stimulation of individual touch corpuscles does not evoke a discharge in spinocervical tract cells any different from that evoked by similar stimulation of adjacent hairy skin it may be concluded that the changes observed by TAPPER were not due to transmission of information from touch corpuscles through the spinocervical tract.

The above behavioural experiments seem to show in most instances that the information necessary for the responses is transmitted through the spinocervical tract. That this conclusion is most probably an over-simplification is emphasized by the work of DENAVIT and KORSINSKI (1968). These authors have shown that a localized area of the subthalamus (nucleus of the field of Forel) receives input from the spinocervical — thalamic system but not from the dorsal column — medial lemniscal system. This area seems to have something to do with attention and wakefulness, since localized cooling of the area leads to slowing of cortical activity (EEG) and behavioural sleep (NAQUET et al., 1966). Loss of behavioural responses after spinocervical tract sections may therefore by due to inattentiveness and not to the spinocervical tract carrying the information necessary for the response.

D. The Spinothalamic Tract

The spinothalamic tracts are the classical ventral spinal cord pathways relaying information from the skin. Two tracts are described on each side, the ventral or anterior and the lateral spinothalamic tracts. Direct spinothalamic connexions have been demonstrated in man and some other primate species (EDINGER, 1889; MOTT, 1895; COLLIER and BUZZARD, 1903; GOLDSTEIN, 1910; WALKER, 1940; WEAVER and WALKER, 1941; BOWSHER, 1961). The spinothalamic tract is said to arise from large cells of the dorsal horn, cross the cord in the anterior commissure and ascend in the ventral column with the fibres from the more caudal segments being pushed laterally by the fibres from more rostral segments. The termination of the tract, according to BOWSHER (1961) who used the Nauta and Glees methods for demonstrating preterminal and terminal degeneration, is in N. ventralis posterolateralis, N. parafascicularis and N. centralis lateralis of the thalamus. The spinothalamic system is supposed to subserve touch, itch, pain and temperature sensations (Kroll, 1930; Foerster and Gagel, 1932; Walker, 1942; Drake and McKenzie, 1953).

The general agreement on the presence of a spinothalamic tract in primate species is not carried over to other mammals. In the rabbit Marchi degeneration studies have indicated the presence of a spinothalamic tract (Wallenberg, 1896, 1900; Kohnstamm, 1900). Furthermore, a tract in the ventral spinal cord of the rabbit, with monosynaptic excitatory connexions from contralateral cutaneous nerves has been described (Magni and Oscarsson, 1962). There has been no evidence yet, however, that the tract described by Magni and Oscarsson terminates in the thalamus.

In the cat the situation is complicated by the presence of a well developed spinocervical tract. Experiments on cats in which the dorsal columns were sectioned and evoked responses recorded in the thalamus (Gaze and Gordon, 1955; Whitlock and Perl, 1959; Perl and Whitlock, 1961) do not necessarily indicate that the activity ascended in the ventral cord, since the spinocervical tract ascends in the dorsolateral funiculus. The spinocervical-thalamic system terminates in N. ventralis posterolateralis, the posterior nuclear complex and in the magnocellular part of the medial geniculate body (Landgren et al., 1965; Boivie, 1970) and this partly invalidates the finding of preterminal degeneration in thalamic nuclei after lesions that section axons of the lateral cervical nuclei (Getz, 1952; Anderson and Berry, 1959) as a demonstration of the presence of a spinothalamic tract in the cat. After cord section at T1, however, degeneration has been observed in N. ventralis posterolateralis (Anderson and Berry, 1959).

Large fibred tracts in the cat's ventral spinal cord, the contralateral and the bilateral flexor reflex tracts (Lundberg and Oscarsson, 1962), receive polysynaptic excitation from cutaneous afferent fibres. They have been shown to project to the inferior olive and the lateral reticular nuclei respectively (Grant and Oscarsson, 1966; Grant et al., 1966). Whether there is any projection from these latter structures to the thalamus is uncertain, but van Beusekom (1955) assumes such a projection from the lateral reticular nuclei. These tracts, therefore, may be part of a pathway from cutaneous receptors to the thalamus.

It appears that there may be a direct spinothalamic tract in the cat (see below). No such system could be demonstrated by the Marchi or Haggqvist methods (Morin and Thomas, 1955; van Beusekom, 1955) and this suggests that most of the axons would be of small diameter. Any spinothalamic projection in the cat is likely to be mainly polysynaptic. This is the view of van Beusekom (1955) who states that all ascending fibres in the ventral spinal cord except those of the ventral spinocerebellar tract terminate in the lateral reticular nucleus or the ventrolateral substance of the medulla. More recently, however, the problem has been re-opened by Boivie (1971) who states that there are direct spinothalamic fibres with a wide area of termination ipsilateral to the course of the axons in the ventral spinal cord.

That there is a pathway from cutaneous receptors and high threshold muscle afferent fibres to the cerebral cortex ascending in the ventral spinal cord has been shown by Norrsell and Wolpow (1966). Moreover, Dilly et al. (1968) and Trevino et al. (1972) have observed cells in the cervical dorsal horn and, mainly, the lumbar laminae VII and VIII, respectively, that can be excited antidromically from the contralateral medial lemniscus.

Physiological knowledge about spinothalamic connexions is almost non-existent. With the exception of the experiments of DILLY et al. (1968) and TRE-VINO et al. (1972) no recordings have been made from spinal cord neurones with axons that have been shown to project in the contralateral medial lemniscus. Furthermore, these two groups of workers have not reported in detail how these neurones responded to natural stimulation of the skin. It is therefore not possible to define the physiological properties of the system. There is a need for a well-controlled electrophysiological study of the spinothalamic system in primate species.

The results of anterolateral cordotomy in human beings, performed usually in an attempt to relieve intractable pain, have led to the belief that the spinothalamic tracts subserve touch, itch, pain and temperature sensations. Most of the cordotomy material was not subjected to histological control after the death of the patient and the sensory testing performed after the operation was usually crude, e.g. testing the ability to differentiate the sharp from the blunt end of a pin. It is, perhaps, not surprising that the results of anterolateral cordotomy are very variable. There is usually some alteration in pain and temperature sensation below the lesion on the contralateral side, and in some cases analgesia and thermana-esthesia may be complete, presumably depending on the extent of the section and the cause of the original pain. There is a need for more experimental work on both the extent of development of spinothalamic connexions in various primate species including man, and the function of this system using both physiological and beha-vioural methods with well-controlled stimulation techniques.

References

ANDERSON, F. D., BERRY, C. M.: Degeneration studies of long ascending fiber systems in the cat's brain stem. J. comp. Neurol. 111, 195–231 (1959).

ANDERSSON, S. A.: Projection of different spinal pathways to the second somatosensory area in the cat. Acta physiol. scand. 56, Suppl. 194 (1962).

ARMETT, C. J., GRAY, J. A. B., HUNSPERGER, R. W., LAL, S.: The transmission of information in primary receptor neurones and second order neurones of a phasic system. J. Physiol. (Lond.) 164, 395–421 (1962).

ARMETT, C. J., GRAY, J. A. B., PALMER, J. F.: A group of neurones in the dorsal horn associated with cutaneous mechanoreceptors. J. Physiol. (Lond.) 156, 611–622 (1961).

BARILARI, M. G., KUYPERS, H. G. J. M.: Propriospinal fibers interconnecting the spinal enlarge-ments in the cat. Brain Res. 14, 321–330 (1969).

BOIVIE, J.: The termination of the cervicothalamic tract in the cat. An experimental study with silver impregnation methods. Brain Res. 19, 333–360 (1970).

BOIVIE, J.: The termination of the spinothalamic tract in the cat. An experimental study with silver impregnation methods. Exp. Brain Res. 12, 331–353 (1971).

BOWSHER, D.: The termination of secondary somatosensory neurones within the thalamus of M. mulatta. An experimental degeneration study. J. comp. Neurol. 117, 213–228 (1961).

BRODAL, A., REXED, B.: Spinal afferents to the lateral cervical nucleus in the cat. An experi-mental study. J. comp. Neurol. 98, 179–213 (1953).

BROWDER, J., GALLAGHER, J. P.: Dorsal cordotomy for painful phantom limb. Ann. Surg. 128, 456–469 (1948).

BROWN, A. G.: Cutaneous afferent fibre collaterals in the dorsal columns of the cat. Exp. Brain Res. 5, 293–305 (1968).

BROWN, A. G.: Descending control of the spinocervical tract in decerebrate cats. Brain Res. 17, 152–155 (1970).

Brown, A.G.: Effects of descending impulses on transmission through the spinocervical tract. J. Physiol. (Lond.) **219**, 103–125 (1971).

Brown, A.G., Franz, D.N.: Responses of spinocervical tract neurones to natural stimulation of identified cutaneous receptors. Exp. Brain Res. **7**, 231–249 (1969).

Brown, A.G., Franz, D.N.: Patterns of response in spinocervical tract neurones to different stimuli of long duration. Brain Res. **17**, 156–160 (1970).

Brown, A.G., Gordon, G., Kay, R.H.: Cutaneous receptive properties of single fibres in the cat's medial lemniscus. J. Physiol. (Lond.) **211**, 37–39 P (1970).

Brown, A.G., Iggo, A.: A quantitative study of cutaneous receptors and afferent fibres in the cat and rabbit. J. Physiol. (Lond.) **193**, 707–733 (1967).

Brown, A.G., Kirk, E.J., Martin III, H.F.: The actions and locations in the spinal cord of descending pathways that inhibit transmission through the spinocervical tract. J. Physiol. (Lond.) **223**, 27–28 P (1972).

Brown, A.G., Martin III, H.F.: Effects on transmission through the spinocervical tract evoked from the dorsal columns and the dorsal column nuclei. J. Physiol. (Lond.) **224**, 34–35 P (1972).

Burgess, P.R., Clark, F.J.: Dorsal column projection of fibres from the cat knee joint. J. Physiol. (Lond.) **203**, 301–315 (1969).

Busch, H.F.M.: An anatomical analysis of the white matter in the brain stem of the cat. Doctoral Thesis, Leiden: van Gorcum 1961.

Cajal, S. Ramón y: Histologie du système nerveux de l'homme et des vertébrés. Vol. I. Madrid: Consejo superior de investigationes cientificas 1952.

Carpenter, M.B., Stein, B.M., Shriver, J.E.: Central projections of spinal dorsal roots in the monkey. II. Lower thoracic, lumbosacral and coccygeal dorsal roots. Amer. J. Anat. **123**, 75–118 (1968).

Catalano, J.V., Lamarche, G.: Central pathway for cutaneous impulses in the cat. Amer. J. Physiol. **189**, 141–144 (1957).

Chang, H.T., Ruch, T.C.: Organization of the dorsal columns of the spinal cord and their nuclei in the spider monkey. J. Anat. (Lond.) **81**, 140–149 (1947).

Collier, J., Buzzard, E.F.: The degeneration resulting from lesions of posterior nerve roots and from transverse lesions of the spinal cord in man. A study of twenty cases. Brain **26**, 559–591 (1903).

Cook, A.W., Browder, E.J.: Function of the posterior columns in man. Arch. Neurol. **12**, 72–79 (1965).

Dart, A.M., Gordon, G.: Excitatory and inhibitory afferent inputs to the dorsal column nuclei not involving the dorsal columns. J. Physiol. (Lond.) **211**, 36–37 P (1970).

Davidson, N., Smith, C.A.: Second-order neurone inhibition in the rat cuneate nucleus evoked from the contralateral periphery. J. Physiol. (Lond.) **210**, 60–61 P (1970).

Denavit, M., Korsinski, E.: Somatic afferents to the cat subthalamus. Arch. ital. Biol. **106**, 391–411 (1968).

Di Biagio, F., Grundfest, H.: Afferent relations of inferior olivary nucleus. II. Site of relay from hind limb afferents into dorsal spino-olivary tract in cat. J. Neurophysiol. **18**, 299–304 (1954).

Di Biagio, F., Grundfest, H.: Afferent relations of inferior olivary nucleus. IV. Lateral cervical nucleus as site of final relay to inferior olive in cat. J. Neurophysiol. **19**, 10–20 (1956).

Dilly, P.N., Wall, P.D., Webster, K.E.: Cells of origin of the spinothalamic tract in the cat and rat. Exp. Neurol. **21**, 550–562 (1968).

Douglas, A.S., Barr, M.L.: The course of the pyramidal tract in rodents. Rev. canad. Biol. **9**, 118–122 (1950).

Drake, C.G., McKenzie, K.G.: Mesencephalic tractotomy for pain. J. Neurosurg. **10**, 457–462 (1953).

Eccles, J.C., Eccles, R.M., Lundberg, A.: Types of neurone in and around the intermediate nucleus of the lumbosacral cord. J. Physiol. (Lond.) **154**, 89–114 (1960).

Edinger, L.: Vergleichend-entwicklungsgeschichtliche und anatomische Studien im Bereiche des Zentralnervensystems: II. Über die Fortsetzung der hinteren Rückenmarkswurzeln zum Gehirn. Anat. Anz. **4**, 121–128 (1889).

FEDINA, L., GORDON, G., LUNDBERG, A.: The source and mechanisms of inhibition in the lateral cervical nucleus of the cat. Brain Res. **11**, 694–696 (1968).

FERRARO, A., BARRERA, S.E.: Posterior column fibers and their termination in Macacus rhesus. J. comp. Neurol. **62**, 507–530 (1935).

FERRARO, A., BARRERA, S.E.: Lamination of the medial lemniscus in Macacus rhesus. J. comp. Neurol. **64**, 313–324 (1936).

FETZ, E.E.: Pyramidal tract effects on interneurones in the cat lumbar dorsal horn. J. Neurophysiol. **31**, 69–80 (1968).

FOERSTER, O., GAGEL, O.: Die Vorderseitenstrangdurchschneidung beim Menschen. Z. ges. Neurol. Psychiat. **138**, 1–92 (1932).

FULLER, D.R.G., GRAY, J.A.B.: The relation between mechanical displacements applied to a cat's pad and the resultant impulse patterns. J. Physiol. (Lond.) **182**, 465–483 (1966).

GAZE, R.M., GORDON, G.: Some observations on the central pathways for cutaneous impulses in the cat. Quart. J. exp. Physiol. **40**, 187–194 (1955).

GETZ, B.: The termination of spinothalamic fibres in the cat as studied by the method of terminal degeneration. Acta anat. (Basel) **16**, 271–290 (1952).

GLEES, P., LIVINGSTON, R.B., SOLER, J.: Der intraspinale Verlauf und die Endigungen der sensorischen Wurzeln in den Nucleus Gracilis und Cuneatus. Arch. Psychiat. Nervenkr. **187**, 190–204 (1951).

GLEES, P., SOLER, J.: Fibre content of the posterior column and synaptic connections of nucleus gracilis. Z. Zellforsch. **36**, 381–400 (1951).

GOLDSTEIN, K.: Über die aufsteigende Degeneration nach Querschnittsunterbrechung des Rückenmarkes (Tractus spino-cerebellaris posterior, Tractus spino-olivaris, Tractus spino-thalamicus). Neurol. Centralbl. **29**, 898–911 (1910).

GORDON, G., JUKES, M.G.M.: An investigation of cells in the lateral cervical nucleus of the cat which respond to stimulation of the skin. J. Physiol. (Lond.) **169**, 28–29P (1963).

GRANT, G., OSCARSSON, O.: Mass discharges evoked in the olivocerebellar tract on stimulation of muscle and skin nerves. Exp. Brain Res. **1**, 329–337 (1966).

GRANT, G., OSCARSSON, O., ROSÉN, I.: Functional organization of the spino-reticulocerebellar path with identification of its spinal component. Exp. Brain Res. **1**, 306–319 (1966).

GRANT, G., WESTMAN, J.: The lateral cervical nucleus in the cat. IV. A light and electron microscopical study after midbrain lesions with demonstration of indirect Wallerian degeneration at the ultrastructural level. Exp. Brain Res. **7**, 51–67 (1969).

GRAY, J.A.B., LAL, S.: Effects of mechanical and thermal stimulation of cat's pads on the excitability of dorsal horn neurones. J. Physiol. (Lond.) **179**, 154–162 (1965).

GRUNDFEST, H., CARTER, W.: Afferent relations of inferior olivary nucleus. I. Electrophysiological demonstration of dorsal spino-olivary tract in cat. J. Neurophysiol. **17**, 72–91 (1954).

GWYN, D.G., WALDRON, H.A.: A nucleus in the dorsolateral funiculus of the spinal cord of the rat. Brain Res. **10**, 342–351 (1968).

GWYN, D.G., WALDRON, H.A.: Observations on the morphology of a nucleus in the dorsolateral funiculus of the spinal cord of the Guinea-pig, rabbit, ferret and cat. J. comp. Neurol. **136**, 233–236 (1969).

HA, H., KITAI, S.T., MORIN, F.: The lateral cervical nucleus of the racoon. Exp. Neurol. **11**, 441–450 (1965).

HA, H., LIU, C.-N.: An anatomical investigation on the lateral cervical nucleus of the cat. Anat. Rec. **139**, 234 (1961).

HA, H., LIU, C.-N.: Spinal afferents to the lateral cervical nucleus and their terminals. Anat. Rec. **142**, 237–238 (1962).

HA, H., LIU, C.-N.: Synaptology of spinal afferents in the lateral cervical nucleus of the cat. Exp. Neurol. **8**, 318–327 (1963).

HA, H., LIU, C.-N.: Organization of the spino-cervico-thalamic system. J. comp. Neurol. **127**, 445–470 (1966).

HA, H., MORIN, F.: Comparative anatomical observations of the cervical nucleus, N. cervicalis lateralis. Anat. Rec. **148**, 374–375 (1964).

HILLMAN, P., WALL, P.D.: Inhibitory and excitatory factors influencing the receptive fields of lamina 5 spinal cord cells. Exp. Brain Res. **9**, 284–306 (1969).

Hongo, T., Jankowska, E., Lundberg, A.: Postsynaptic excitation and inhibition from primary afferents in neurones of the spinocervical tract. J. Physiol. (Lond.) **199**, 569–592 (1968).

Horrobin, D.F.: The lateral cervical nucleus of the cat; an electrophysiological study. Quart. J. exp. Physiol. **51**, 351–371 (1966).

Hunt, C.C., McIntyre, A.K.: An analysis of fibre diameter and receptor characteristics of myelinated cutaneous afferent fibres in cat. J. Physiol. (Lond.) **153**, 99–112 (1960).

Kennard, M.A.: The course of ascending fibers in the spinal cord of the cat essential to the recognition of painful stimuli. J. comp. Neurol. **100**, 511–524 (1954).

King, J.L.: The corticospinal tract of the rat. Anat. Rec. **4**, 245–252 (1910).

Kitai, S.T., Ha, H., Morin, F.: Lateral cervical nucleus of the dog: anatomical and microelectrode studies. Amer. J. Physiol. **209**, 307–311 (1965).

Kitai, S.T., Weinberg, J.: Tactile discrimination study of the dorsal column-medial lemniscal system and spino-cervico-thalamic tract in cats. Exp. Brain Res. **6**, 234–246 (1968).

Kohnstamm, O.: Über die gekreuzt-aufsteigende Spinalbahn und ihre Beziehung zum Gowerschen Strang. Neurol. Centralbl. **19**, 242–249 (1900).

Krieger, H., Grundfest, H.: Afferent relations of inferior olivary nucleus. III. Electrophysiological demonstration of a second relay in dorsal spino-olivary pathway in cat. J. Neurophysiol. **19**, 1–9 (1956).

Kroll, F.W.: Schwellenuntersuchungen bei Läsionen der afferenten Leitungsbahnen. Z. ges. Neurol. Psychiat. **128**, 751–776 (1930).

Landgren, S., Nordwall, A., Wengström, C.: The location of the thalamic relay in the spino-cervical-lemniscal pathway. Acta physiol. scand. **65**, 164–175 (1965).

Landgren, S., Silfvenius, H., Wolsk, D.: Somato-sensory paths to the second cortical projection areas of the group I muscle afferents. J. Physiol. (Lond.) **191**, 543–559 (1967).

Lloyd, D.P.C., McIntyre, A.K.: Dorsal column conduction of Group I muscle afferent impulses and their relay through Clarke's column. J. Neurophysiol. **13**, 39–54 (1950).

Lundberg, A.: Ascending spinal hindlimb pathways in the cat. In: Progress in Brain Research, Vol. 12. Ed. by J.C. Eccles and J.P. Schadé. Amsterdam-London-New York: Elsevier 1964.

Lundberg, A., Norrsell, U., Voorhoeve, P.: Effects from the sensorimotor cortex on ascending spinal pathways. Acta physiol. scand. **59**, 462–473 (1963).

Lundberg, A., Oscarsson, O.: Three ascending spinal pathways in the dorsal part of the lateral funiculus. Acta physiol. scand. **51**, 1–16 (1961).

Lundberg, A., Oscarsson, O.: Two ascending spinal pathways in the ventral part of the cord. Acta physiol. scand. **54**, 270–286 (1962).

Magni, F., Oscarsson, O.: Principal organization of coarse-fibred ascending spinal tracts in phalanger, rabbit and cat. Acta physiol. scand. **54**, 53–64 (1962).

Mendell, L.M.: Physiological properties of unmyelinated fiber projection to the spinal cord Exp. Neurol. **16**, 316–332 (1966).

Mendell, L.M., Wall, P.D.: Responses of single dorsal cord cells to peripheral cutaneous unmyelinated fibres. Nature (Lond.) **206**, 97–99 (1965).

Mizuno, N.: An experimental study of the spino-olivary fibers in the rabbit and cat. J. comp. Neurol. **127**, 267–292 (1966).

Mizuno, N., Nakano, K., Imaizumi, M., Okamoto, M.: The lateral cervical nucleus of the Japanese monkey (Macaca fuscata). J. comp. Neurol. **129**, 375–381 (1967).

Morin, F.: A new spinal pathway for cutaneous impulses. Amer. J. Physiol. **183**, 245–252 (1955).

Morin, F., Catalano, J.V.: Central connections of a cervical nucleus (Nucleus cervicalis lateralis of the cat). J. comp. Neurol. **103**, 17–32 (1955).

Morin, F., Kitai, S.T., Portnov, H., Demirijan, C.: Afferent projections to the lateral cervical nucleus: A microelectrode study. Amer. J. Physiol. **204**, 667–672 (1963).

Morin, F., Thomas, L.M.: Spinothalamic fibers and tactile pathways in the cat. Anat. Rec. **121**, 344 (1955).

Mott, F.W.: Experimental enquiry upon the afferent tracts of the central nervous system of the monkey. Brain **18**, 1–20 (1895).

NAQUET, R., DENAVIT, M., ALBE-FESSARD, D.: Comparaison entre le rôle du subthalamus et celui des afferentes structures bulbomésencephaliques dans le maintien de la vigilance. Electroenceph. clin. Neurophysiol. **20**, 149–164 (1966).

NILSSON, B.Y., SKOGLUND, C.R.: The tactile hairs on the cat's foreleg. Acta physiol. scand. **65**, 364–369 (1965).

NORRSELL, U.: The spinal afferent pathways of conditioned reflexes to cutaneous stimuli in the dog. Exp. Brain Res. **2**, 269–282 (1966).

NORRSELL, U.: A conditioned reflex study of sensory defects caused by cortical somatosensory ablations. Physiol. Behav. **2**, 75–81 (1967).

NORRSELL, U., VOORHOEVE, P.: Tactile pathways from the hindlimb to the cerebral cortex in cat. Acta physiol. scand. **54**, 9–17 (1962).

NORRSELL, U., WOLPOW, E.R.: An evoked potential study of different pathways from the hindlimb to the somatosensory areas in the cat. Acta physiol. scand. **66**, 19–33 (1966).

OSCARSSON, O., ROSÉN, I.: Projection to cerebral cortex of large muscle-spindle afferents in forelimb nerves of the cat. J. Physiol. (Lond.) **169**, 924–945 (1963).

PERL, E.R., WHITLOCK, D.G.: Somatic stimuli exciting spinothalamic projections to thalamic neurons in cat and monkey. Exp. Neurol. **3**, 256–296 (1961).

PETIT, D., BURGESS, P.R.: Dorsal column projection of receptors in cat hairy skin supplied by myelinated fibers. J. Neurophysiol. **31**, 849–855 (1968).

RANSON, S.W.: The fasciculus cerebro-spinalis in the albino rat. Amer. J. Anat. **14**, 411–424 (1913).

RANSON, S.W.: A note on the degeneration of the fasciculus cerebro-spinalis in the albino rat. J. comp. Neurol. **24**, 503–507 (1914).

REVELEY, I.L.: The pyramidal tract of the Guinea-pig (Cavia aperea). Anat. Rec. **9**, 297–305 (1915).

REXED, B.: Personal communication in: J. JANSEN and A. BRODAL: Handbuch der mikroskopischen Anatomie des Menschen, IV/8. Das Kleinhirn. p. 241. Berlin-Göttingen-Heidelberg: Springer 1958.

REXED, B., STRÖM, G.: Afferent nervous connection of the lateral cervical nucleus. Acta physiol. scand. **25**, 219–229 (1952).

ROSÉN, I.: Afferent connexions of Group I activated cells in the main cuneate nucleus of the cat. J. Physiol. (Lond.) **205**, 209–236 (1969).

SHRIVER, J.E., STEIN, B.M., CARPENTER, M.B.: Central projection of spinal dorsal roots in the monkey. I. Cervical and upper thoracic dorsal roots. Amer. J. Anat. **123**, 27–74 (1968).

SIMPSON, S.: The pyramidal tract in the red squirrel (Sciurus hudsonius) and chipmunk (Tamius striatus lipteris). J. comp. Neurol. **24**, 137–160 (1914).

SIMPSON, S.: The motor areas and pyramidal tract in the Canadian porcupine (Erethrizon dorsatus Linn.). Quart. J. exp. Physiol. **8**, 79–102 (1915a).

SIMPSON, S.: The pyramidal tract in the striped gopher. Quart. J. exp. Physiol. **8**, 383–390 (1915b).

TAPPER, D.N.: Behavioural evaluation of the tactile pad receptor system in hairy skin of the cat. Exp. Neurol. **26**, 447–459 (1970).

TAPPER, D.N., MANN, M.D.: Single presynaptic impulse evokes postsynaptic discharge. Brain Res. **11**, 688–690 (1968).

TAUB, A.: Local, segmental and supraspinal interactions with a dorsolateral spinal cutaneous afferent system. Exp. Neurol. **10**, 357–374 (1964).

TAUB, A., BISHOP, P.O.: The spinocervical tract: Dorsal column linkage, conduction velocity, primary afferent spectrum. Exp. Neurol. **13**, 1–21 (1965).

TOMASULO, K.C., EMMERS, R.: Spinal afferents to SI and SII of the rat thalamus. Exp. Neurol. **26**, 482–497 (1970).

TREVINO, D.L., MAUNZ, R.A., BRYAN, R.N., WILLIS, W.D.: Location of cells of origin of the spinothalamic tract in the lumbar enlargement of cat. Exp. Neurol. **34**, 64–77 (1972).

TRUEX, R.C., TAYLOR, M.J., SMYTHE, M.Q., GILDENBERG, P.L.: The lateral cervical nucleus of cat, dog and man. J. comp. Neurol. **139**, 93–104 (1970).

UDDENBERG, N.: Differential organization in dorsal funiculi of fibres originating from different receptors. Exp. Brain Res. **4**, 367–376 (1968a).

Uddenberg, N.: Functional organization of long, second-order afferents in the dorsal funiculi. Exp. Brain Res. **4**, 377–382 (1968b).

Van Beusekom, G.T.: Fibre analysis of the anterior and lateral funiculi of the cord in the cat. Doctoral Thesis, Leiden: E. Ijdo, N.V. 1955.

Waldron, H.A.: The morphology of the lateral cervical nucleus in the hedgehog. Brain Res. **16**, 301–306 (1969).

Walker, A.E.: The spinothalamic tract in man. Arch. Neurol. Psychiat. (Chic.) **43**, 284–298 (1940).

Walker, A.E.: Somatotopic localization of spinothalamic and sensory trigeminal tracts in mesencephalon. Arch. Neurol. Psychiat. (Chic.) **48**, 885–889 (1942).

Walker, A.E., Weaver, T.A.: The topical organization of the fibers of the posterior columns in M. mulatta. J. comp. Neurol. **76**, 145–158 (1942).

Wall, P.D.: Cord cells responding to touch, damage and temperature of skin. J. Neurophysiol. **23**, 197–210 (1960a).

Wall, P.D.: Two transmission systems for the skin senses. In: Sensory Communication. Ed. by W.A. Rosenblith. New York: Wiley 1960b.

Wall, P.D.: The laminar organization of dorsal horn and effects of descending impulses. J. Physiol. (Lond.) **188**, 403–424 (1967).

Wallenberg, A.: Die sekundäre Bahn des sensiblen Trigeminus. Anat. Anz. **12**, 95–110 (1896).

Wallenberg, A.: Secundäre sensible Bahnen im Gehirnstamm des Kaninchens. Anat. Anz. **18**, 81–105 (1900).

Weaver, T.A., Walker, A.E.: Topical arrangement within the spinothalamic tract of the monkey. Arch. Neurol. Psychiat. (Chic.) **46**, 877–887 (1941).

Werner, G., Whitsel, B.L.: The topology of dermatomal projections in the medial lemniscal system. J. Physiol. (Lond.) **192**, 123–144 (1967).

Whitehorn, D., Morse, R.W., Towe, A.L.: Role of the spinocervical tract in production of the primary cortical response evoked by forepaw stimulation. Exp. Neurol. **25**, 349–364 (1969).

Whitlock, D.G., Perl, E.R.: Afferent projections through ventrolateral funiculi to thalamus of cat. J. Neurophysiol. **22**, 133–148 (1959).

Whitsel, B.L., Petrucelli, L.M., Sapiro, G.: Modality representation in the lumbar and cervical fasciculus gracilis of squirrel monkey. Brain Res. **15**, 67–78 (1969).

Whitsel, B.L., Petrucelli, L.M., Sapiro, G., Ha, H.: Fiber sorting in the fasciculus gracilis of squirrel monkey. Exp. Neurol. **29**, 227–242 (1970).

Chapter 11

Functional Organization of Spinocerebellar Paths

By

Olov Oscarsson, Lund (Sweden)

With 11 Figures

Contents

A. Introduction

Recent anatomical and physiological investigations have supplied a basic knowledge of the organization of the cerebellar cortex and its efferent paths (Eccles, Ito and Szentágothai, 1967). Understanding of cerebellar function requires also knowledge of the afferent paths and the information carried by them. This chapter surveys the present knowledge about the spinocerebellar paths activated by somatic afferents. These paths are better known than those activated by visceral afferents (Dow and Moruzzi, 1958; Newman and Paul, 1969) and the afferent paths from higher brain centres (Jansen and Brodal, 1958; Evarts and Thach, 1969).

Twelve spinocerebellar paths have been identified in physiological investigations and there are scattered observations (Jansen and Brodal, 1958; Larson, Miller and Oscarsson, 1969a; Bloedel and Burton, 1970) indicating that more exist. The identified paths and their abbreviations are given in Table 1. They consist of two main groups which terminate in the cerebellar cortex as mossy fibres and climbing fibres respectively (p. 371). The mossy fibre paths can be divided into *direct* and *indirect*. The former include the spino- and cuneocerebellar tracts which reach the cortex uninterrupted by additional relays in the brain stem. The DSCT and CCT both consist of proprioceptive and exteroceptive components which should be regarded as separate tracts. The indirect paths are relayed in the cord and brain stem. They include paths interrupted in reticular and pontine nuclei (Jansen and Brodal, 1958) but only one of them (LRN–SRCP) has been investigated in detail with physiological techniques. The spinocerebellar paths terminating as climbing fibres presumably all relay in the inferior olive (Eccles et al., 1967).

The peripheral input to the spinocerebellar paths is indicated in Table 1. Proprioceptive information permitting good spatial discrimination is carried by components in the DSCT and CCT. Spatially discriminative information from exteroceptors is carried by other components in these tracts and by one of the climbing fibre paths (DLF–SOCP). The remaining paths receive their main input from the flexor reflex afferents (FRA, see below). The information carried by these paths can not be classified as either proprioceptive or exteroceptive. It lacks modality specificity and permits only very crude spatial discrimination. These paths offer a challenge to future research and might provide essential clues for the understanding of cerebellar function.

Degeneration experiments and investigations with evoked potential technique indicate that the spinocerebellar paths terminate mainly in the anterior lobe, paramedian lobules, and pyramis (Dow and Moruzzi, 1958; Jansen and Brodal, 1958; Grant, 1962b; Brodal, 1967). The physiological investigations have, with few exceptions, been concerned with paths terminating in the anterior lobe. However, there is evidence that some paths terminate in all the projection areas (Jansen and Brodal, 1958; Grant, 1962b) and that the multiple termination in some cases is effected by branching of mossy and climbing fibres (Oscarsson and Uddenberg, 1964; Armstrong, Harvey and Schild, 1971; Cooke, Larson, Oscarsson and Sjölund, 1971a). Almost all physiological investigations have been performed on the cat. The only comparative studies have been concerned with the group I activated components of the dorsal and ventral spinocerebellar tracts and demonstrate that these components have a similar organization in many different mammals (MAGNI and OSCARSSON, 1962a; OSCARSSON, ROSÉN and UDDENBERG, 1963, 1964).

In addition to the paths terminating in the cerebellar cortex there are paths to the efferent relay nuclei of the cerebellum: the intracerebellar and vestibular

Table 1. *Spinocerebellar paths: classification, main peripheral input, maximum conduction velocity of spinal tract, and cortical latency (arrival time of afferent volley) on nerve stimulation* (LUNDBERG and OSCARSSON, 1960, 1962a; HOLMQVIST et al., 1963a; OSCARSSON and UDDENBERG, 1964; GRANT et al., 1966; LARSON et al., 1969a; and unpublished data). FRA, flexor reflex afferents

Paths and abbreviations	Main peripheral input	Conduction velocity (m/sec)	Latency (msec) Hindlimb	Forelimb
Direct mossy fibre paths				
Proprioceptive component of dorsal spinocerebellar tract, DSCT	Group I afferents Joint afferents	110	5	—
Proprioceptive component of cuneocerebellar tract, CCT	Group I afferents (Joint afferents ?)	—	—	3
Exteroceptive component of DSCT	Cutaneous afferents	110	5	—
Exteroceptive component of CCT	Cutaneous afferents	—	—	4
Ventral spinocerebellar tract, VSCT	FRA	120	5	—
Rostral spinocerebellar tract, RSCT	FRA	95	—	3
Indirect mossy fibre path				
Spinoreticulocerebellar path relayed through lateral reticular nucleus, LRN–SRCP	FRA	120	10	8
Climbing fibre paths				
Dorsal spino-olivocerebellar path, DF–SOCP	FRA	—	18	10
Dorsolateral spino-olivocerebellar path, DLF–SOCP	Cutaneous afferents	70	21	17
Ventral spino-olivocerebellar path, VF–SOCP	FRA	40	22	20
Lateral climbing fibre-spinocerebellar path, LF–CF–SCP	FRA	?	25	19
Ventral climbing fibre-spinocerebellar path, VF–CF–SCP	FRA	30	25	28

nuclei (JANSEN and BRODAL, 1958; ECCLES et al., 1967; ITO, KAWAI, UDO and MANO, 1969; ITO, YOSHIDA, OBATA, KAWAI and UDO, 1970; MATSUSHITA and IKEDA, 1970a, b). The information carried by these paths is unknown but they are partly formed by collaterals of mossy and climbing fibres. The functional significance of the sparsely occurring cerebellar afferents which contain monoamines is also unknown (HÖKFELT and FUXE, 1969; BLOOM, HOFFER and SIGGINS, 1971; HOFFER, SIGGINS, WOODWARD and BLOOM, 1971; OLSON and FUXE, 1971).

B. Information Forwarded

It is usually assumed that ascending spinal paths forward information about peripheral events. This is presumably the case with the DSCT and CCT which carry modality and space specific information from proprioceptors and extero-ceptors. However, the organization of many ascending paths suggests that they monitor activity in lower motor centres rather than peripheral events. These paths include the many spinocerebellar paths which receive their main peripheral input from the *flexor reflex afferents (FRA)*. It is convenient, in order to avoid repetition, to discuss at this stage the organization and possible function of these paths.

The FRA are defined as those myelinated afferents which evoke the flexion reflex in the spinal preparation. They include low and high threshold cutaneous afferents, groups II and III muscle afferents, and high threshold joint afferents (Eccles and Lundberg, 1959; Holmqvist and Lundberg, 1961). It is not certain if all the afferents in these groups contribute to the FRA and it is possible that unmyelinated afferents should be included (Carpenter, Engberg, Funken-stein and Lundberg, 1963; Franz and Iggo, 1968; Vyklický, Rudomin, Zajac and Burke, 1969).

Ascending paths activated or inhibited by *all* the components of the FRA have been denoted *ascending FRA paths*. They have the following characteristics in common:

1. The information from the periphery is without modality specificity since excitation and inhibition is evoked by all the components of the FRA.

2. The receptive fields are large and may include one or several limbs. They sometimes consist of excitatory and inhibitory areas but permit only very crude spatial discrimination.

3. The FRA effects on the ascending paths are mediated by pools of interneu-rones in the spinal cord and brain stem.

4. These interneurones are strongly excited and inhibited by descending tracts.

There are remarkable similarities in the organization of the ascending FRA paths and the reflexes evoked by the FRA (Lundberg, 1959, 1964; Oscarsson, 1967; Miller and Oscarsson, 1970). In both cases the same combination of afferents is involved, the receptive fields are large, and the synaptic actions are mediated by interneurones. Furthermore, the interneurones are in both cases under similar supraspinal control: for example, they are excited by the pyramidal tract and inhibited by reticulospinal paths (Holmqvist, Lundberg and Oscars-son, 1960a; Magni and Oscarsson, 1961; Lundberg, Norrsell and Voor-hoeve, 1963; Carpenter, Engberg and Lundberg, 1965).

The diffuse afferent organization of the ascending FRA paths would seem to make them unsuitable as channels for specific information about peripheral events. On the other hand, the characteristics of these paths can be explained if they are assumed to carry information about the activity in pools of interneurones that are, at the same time, reflex centers and links in descending motor paths, as suggested in Fig. 1 (Lundberg, 1959, 1964; Oscarsson, 1967, 1968; Miller and Oscarsson, 1970). It is unknown if the interneurones should be regarded primarily as reflex centres which are controlled by descending motor paths or primarily as links in descending motor paths which are modulated by the peripheral input.

However, such a distinction might be meaningless: there is evidence that motor performance partly depends on mobilization and inhibition of reflex arcs by higher centers (LUNDBERG, 1966; HONGO, JANKOWSKA and LUNDBERG, 1969a, b). It is possible that the activity of the interneurones in many cases is determined primarily by signals in the descending tracts as many ascending FRA paths are only weakly influenced by natural stimulation of receptors (see below). It is interesting that many interneurones in the cord are discretely activated from small areas in the sensorimotor cortex, perhaps even from single cortical cell columns, and diffusely activated by peripheral nerves from wide receptive fields (ASANUMA, STONEY and THOMPSON, 1971). These interneurones are presumably links in motor paths and are possible candidates for the interneurones mediating FRA effects on ascending paths.

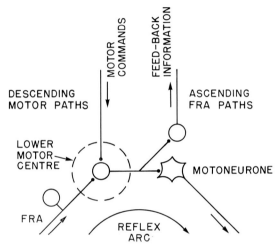

Fig. 1. Suggested function of ascending paths influenced from the flexor reflex afferents (FRA). It is assumed that these paths monitor activity in lower motor centres represented by pools of interneurones that are, at the same time, reflex arcs and links in descending motor paths

The FRA are presumably involved in many kinds of motor mechanisms as indicated by the diverse reflex actions which can be evoked from them (ECCLES and LUNDBERG, 1959; HOLMQVIST, 1961; LUNDBERG, 1966; GRILLNER, 1969). If each of these mechanisms is monitored separately an explanation would be given for the large number of ascending FRA paths. The possible significance of these paths for cerebellar motor control will be discussed later.

C. The Direct Paths: The Spino- and Cuneocerebellar Tracts

These paths reach the cerebellar cortex after only one relay which is situated in the cord or brain stem. The single relay and the fast conduction velocity of the tract fibres allow these paths to carry proprioceptive and exteroceptive information to the cerebellum with very little delay (Table 1). An interesting parallel is offered by the fast conducting proprioceptive and exteroceptive paths to the cerebral motor cortex (Oscarsson and Rosén, 1966a). It might be essential that these paths are fast in order to serve as efficient feed-back channels in the control of movement exerted by the cerebellum and motor cortex.

Four direct pathways to the cerebellum have been distinguished on anatomical and physiological grounds. Information from the hindlimbs is carried by the dorsal and ventral spinocerebellar tracts (DSCT and VSCT) and information from the forelimbs by the cuneocerebellar and rostral spinocerebellar tracts (CCT and RSCT) (Holmqvist, Oscarsson and Rosén, 1963a; Holmqvist, Oscarsson and Uddenberg, 1963b; Oscarsson and Uddenberg, 1964). The DSCT and CCT are activated by group I muscle afferents and cutaneous afferents and provide relatively simple paths for proprioceptive and exteroceptive information. Many neurones in the VSCT and RSCT are activated by group I afferents and these tracts have therefore been assumed to carry proprioceptive information. However, these tracts are strongly influenced by the FRA and descending tracts and their main function may be to monitor activity in lower motor centres. Corresponding hindlimb and forelimb paths are anatomically distinct but their functional organization is similar, although not identical. It is not known why the information from hindlimbs and forelimbs is carried by different tracts. It has been suggested that they have developed independently and therefore represent analogous rather than serially homologous structures (Oscarsson, 1965b; Oscarsson and Uddenberg, 1965).

The course of the tracts and their termination in Larsell's lobules IV and V of the anterior lobe are shown in Fig. 2. There are conspicuous differences in the termination of the DSCT and CCT on the one hand and of the VSCT and RSCT on the other (Lundberg and Oscarsson, 1960, 1962a; Grant, 1962a, b; Oscarsson and Uddenberg, 1964; Voogd, Broere and van Rossum, 1969; Cooke et al., 1971a; Burke, Lundberg and Weight, 1971). The termination of the DSCT and CCT is ipsilateral and largely restricted to the pars intermedia. Antidromic stimulation experiments suggest that the individual fibres terminate in relatively restricted cortical areas. The DSCT terminates in lobule IV and further rostrally and the CCT in lobule V. These regions correspond to the classical hindlimb and forelimb areas delimited with evoked potential technique (see Dow and Moruzzi, 1958).

The VSCT and RSCT terminate in bilateral zones which cover most of the mediolateral extent of the anterior lobe. The axons of these tracts often send one branch to each side of the anterior lobe, although the densest termination is ipsilateral to the tract cell bodies and to the main afferent input. The main branches arborize to innervate relatively large cortical areas. The VSCT terminates rostrally in the hindlimb region of the anterior lobe, whereas the RSCT terminates in both hindlimb and forelimb regions.

The information from the mossy fibres is dispersed in the medial and lateral directions by the parallel fibres which extend for up to 1.5 mm in each direction. This would presumably increase the projection areas of the tracts as indicated by the stippled regions in Fig. 2.

The DSCT and CCT also send many fibres to the pyramis and the ipsilateral paramedian lobule (Grant, 1962a, b; Cooke et al., 1971a). The VSCT and RSCT terminate only sparsely in these parts of the cerebellum (Grant, 1962b; Oscarsson and Uddenberg, 1964). The anterior and posterior projection areas are presumably innervated by branches of the same mossy fibres as demonstrated for the CCT, VSCT and RSCT.

The DSCT and CCT consist of two major components, proprioceptive and exteroceptive, which are activated by group I muscle afferents and cutaneous afferents, respectively (Table 1). The proprioceptive and exteroceptive components of the DSCT originate from cells in different parts of the same nucleus, Clarke's column (Lindström and Takata, 1971 b), whereas the proprioceptive and exteroceptive components of the CCT originate from cells in different nuclei,

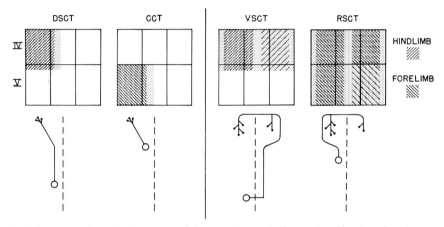

Fig. 2. Course and projection areas of direct spinocerebellar paths. The dorsal and ventral spinocerebellar tracts (DSCT and VSCT) carry information from the hindlimbs, whereas the cuneocerebellar and rostral spinocerebellar tracts (CCT and RSCT) carry information from the forelimbs. Upper diagrams represent Larsell's lobules IV and V of the anterior lobe. Vertical lines indicate borders between intermediate parts and vermis. Hatching indicates projection areas of tracts activated from left side. Sparse hatching indicates sparse termination. Stippling indicates expanded projection areas due to spread of information through the parallel fibres.
Degree of branching and general course of tract axons are shown in lower diagrams

the external cuneate nucleus and the rostral part of the main cuneate nucleus, respectively (Cooke et al., 1971 a). The proprioceptive components terminate predominantly in the depth of the cerebellar sulci and the exteroceptive components at the apex of the folia (Körlin and Larson, 1970; Ekerot and Larson, 1972). The nomenclature in relation to the DSCT and CCT is not satisfactory. The hindlimb and forelimb tracts carry information which is similar and they can be regarded as belonging to the same system. On the other hand, the proprioceptive and exteroceptive components of the DSCT and CCT should be regarded as separate tracts as they have different origin, termination, and function.

The VSCT and possibly the RSCT consist of several functional components (see below). The differences between these components may be less fundamental than in the DSCT and CCT and there is at present no need to regard them as separate tracts.

1. Proprioceptive Component of DSCT

It has recently been demonstrated that some DSCT neurones in Clarke's column are monosynaptically activated by joint afferents originating from Ruffini endings (LINDSTRÖM and TAKATA, 1971a). However, the following description refers to those DSCT neurones that receive monosynaptic excitation from group I muscle afferents. They constitute the majority of the neurones in the proprioceptive component and have been extensively investigated.

a) **Synaptic Connections.** The monosynaptic excitation of DSCT neurones by group I muscle afferents was established in early investigations (GRUNDFEST and CAMPBELL, 1942; LLOYD and McINTYRE, 1950; LAPORTE, LUNDBERG and OSCARSSON, 1956a, b). It was later demonstrated that muscle spindle and tendon organ afferents activate different neurones (LUNDBERG and OSCARSSON, 1956, LUNDBERG and WINSBURY, 1960; JANSEN and RUDJORD, 1965). The observations suggesting that occasional tract cells receive excitation from both Ia and Ib afferents (LUNDBERG and OSCARSSON, 1956; ECCLES, OSCARSSON and WILLIS, 1961b) are of doubtful significance but might relate to aberrant connections. Many of the neurones receive additional monosynaptic excitation from group II muscle afferents (LAPORTE et al., 1956b; ECCLES et al., 1961b). It might represent a highly specific convergence of primary and secondary muscle spindle afferents to the same tract neurones and has also been observed in the cuneocerebellar tract and in the forelimb group I projection to the cerebral cortex (ROSÉN, 1969b; COOKE et al., 1971b).

The efficacy of the transmission from group I afferents to the tract neurones is high and presynaptic volleys can be transmitted faithfully at frequencies as high as 500 impulses or more per second. Contributing factors are large synaptic potentials, lack of recurrent inhibition, and a small and short lasting after-hyperpolarization (ECCLES et al., 1961b; KUNO and MIYAHARA, 1968; EIDE, FEDINA, JANSEN, LUNDBERG and VYKLICKÝ, 1969a, b). The synaptic potentials evoked by group I afferents have been studied in detail. About 15 group I afferents converge on to each DSCT neurone. The unitary EPSPs are large, up to 5 mV in amplitude, with an estimated content of transmitter quanta as high as 50–100. The large EPSPs are presumably generated by the giant end bulbs described by SZENTÁGOTHAI and ALBERT (1955). Two or three unitary EPSPs are sufficient to evoke a discharge. The EPSPs decay with a fast time constant (about 3–5 msec) suggesting that there is no long lasting transmitter action. However, the response to a single volley in group I afferents is sometimes repetitive in the DSCT neurones and frequently repetitive with as many as six action potentials in the corresponding CCT neurones (HOLMQVIST et al., 1963a). The possibility that the repetitive discharge is due to a re-excitation of the discharge zone by action potentials conducted out into the dendrites should be considered.

The tract neurones are often disynaptically inhibited from group I afferents (CURTIS, ECCLES and LUNDBERG, 1958; ECCLES et al., 1961b). Presynaptic inhibition of Ia and Ib afferents from both Ib afferents and the FRA has been demonstrated (ECCLES, SCHMIDT and WILLIS, 1963; JANKOWSKA, JUKES and LUND, 1965).

In many neurones weak excitation or inhibition is evoked by volleys in the FRA presumably through polysynaptic connections (LUNDBERG and OSCARSSON,

1960; HONGO and OKADA, 1967; KOSTYUK, 1969). The DSCT neurones are spontaneously active in the spinal state even when there is no input from the group I afferents. This activity, which is often remarkably regular, might be due to excitation from interneurones (HOLMQVIST, LUNDBERG and OSCARSSON, 1956) or to an intrinsic pacemaker function (WALLÖE, JANSEN and NYGAARD, 1969).

Although recurrent collaterals from DSCT axons have been reported to terminate in Clarke's column (RÉTHELYI, 1968; but see LOEWY, 1970) there is no evidence for recurrent inhibition (HONGO and OKADA, 1967; KUNO and MYIAHARA, 1968; EIDE et al., 1969a) and observations suggesting recurrent facilitation require confirmation (KOSTYUK, 1969).

b) Functional Organization. On natural stimulation of muscle receptors the tract neurones respond as if activated from either primary endings in muscle spindles or from tendon organs (LUNDBERG and OSCARSSON, 1956; LUNDBERG and WINSBURY, 1960; JANSEN and RUDJORD, 1965). Some DSCT neurones are activated by both primary and secondary muscle spindle afferents but the contribution from the secondary endings has so far not been distinguished in experiments with receptor stimulation.

The transmission of information from group I afferents to the tract neurones has been studied in some detail (JANSEN, NICOLAYSEN and RUDJORD, 1966; WALLÖE, 1968; KOSTYUK, 1969; JANSEN and WALLÖE, 1970). The discharge frequency of the tract neurones is linearly related to muscle length and is similar to that in the primary afferents. However, the regular activity in the primary afferents is converted into an irregular discharge. The loss of information entailed in this process may be partly offset by the serial dependency of the interspike intervals (WALLÖE, 1968). The transfer of information about muscle length through individual Ia activated DSCT neurones has a peak value with observation times near 100 msec. With such observation times the firing pattern conveys enough information to distinguish four different muscle lengths if the signal is read in a frequency code. This would seem to be a low rate of transmission of information but it might be improved by the utilization of many parallel lines in the DSCT.

The excitatory actions from group I afferents usually arise from a single muscle or a few synergists but inhibitory actions are often supplied by several muscles, particularly the antagonists (HOLMQVIST et al., 1956; JANSEN, NICOLAYSEN and WALLÖE, 1967). The inhibition seems to be specifically related to one receptor system: neurones activated by Ia afferents from toe extensors are probably inhibited by the Ia afferents from synergistic ankle extensors, and neurones activated by Ia afferents from ankle and toe flexors are probably inhibited by the Ib afferents in antagonistic ankle extensors. It is not known to what extent these convergence patterns represent more general patterns of interaction between afferents from synergists and antagonists. Obviously these DSCT neurones carry information which is a complex function of length, velocity and tension in a number of interrelated muscles. It is possible that other groups of tract neurones constitute more simple channels of information from one receptor type (spindles or tendon organs) in one muscle.

The significance of the relatively weak connections from the FRA is unknown. Even intense stimulation of cutaneous receptors is without effect on the group I activated neurones in the spinal preparation (Oscarsson, 1957b). The FRA effects can be inhibited by reticulospinal paths tonically active in the decerebrate preparation, and facilitated by the pyramidal tract (p. 342).

Stimulation of the pyramidal tract seems to influence the group I activated DSCT neurones through several mechanisms (Hongo and Okada, 1967; Hongo, Okada and Sato, 1967; Jansen, Nicolaysen and Wallöe, 1969). Excitation and inhibition can be evoked through the facilitation of FRA interneurones mentioned above. The dominant pyramidal effect on the tract neurones is, however, inhibition. This may be partly due to facilitation of the interneurones which mediate inhibition from the FRA and group I afferents, and partly due to excitation of a more independent group of segmental interneurones. Stimulation of the pyramidal tract presumably causes presynaptic inhibition of the Ib, but not Ia, path to the Clarke's column. The significance of these various actions exerted by the pyramidal tract is unknown.

c) **Comparative Aspects.** The group I activated component of the DSCT has similar properties in all mammalian species investigated: phalanger, rabbit, cat, dog and monkey (Magni and Oscarsson, 1962a; Oscarsson et al., 1964). It receives monosynaptic excitation from Ia as well as Ib afferents, which presumably activate different groups of neurones, and the response to a single volley is often repetitive. There is sometimes additional excitation from group II muscle afferents but no, or only weak, effects from group III muscle afferents and cutaneous afferents. There is little convergence of excitation from different muscle nerves to the same neurone. Observations on the duck suggest that the DSCT either does not exist in birds or has an organization different from that in mammals (Oscarsson et al., 1963; cf. Matsushita, 1968; Akker, 1970).

2. Proprioceptive Component of CCT
(Holmqvist et al., 1963a; Cooke et al., 1971a, b; Rosén and Sjölund, 1972a, b)

Most of the neurones in this component are monosynaptically activated by group I muscle afferents. The cell bodies lie in the external cuneate nucleus, where forelimb muscles are somatotopically represented (Johnson, Welker and Pubols, 1968; Rosén, 1969a; Cooke et al., 1971a). Muscle spindles and tendon organs activate different groups of neurones. Some of these receive additional excitation from group II muscle afferents. The majority of the neurones are activated from one muscle only but occasionally there is convergence of excitation from close synergists. Disynaptic inhibition from group I afferents is common from muscles not supplying excitation and might provide an inhibitory surround. It can be concluded that the group I activated CCT neurones have an organization that is similar to that of the corresponding DSCT neurones, but the receptive fields in the CCT tend to be smaller.

Some CCT neurones in the external cuneate nucleus are activated mainly or exclusively from group II muscle afferents and may constitute a specific path for information from spindle secondaries (Cooke et al., 1971b; Rosén and Sjölund, 1972a). It is unknown if the CCT like the DSCT contains an additional group of neurones activated by joint afferents.

3. Exteroceptive Components of DSCT and CCT

(LUNDBERG and OSCARSSON, 1960; HOLMQVIST et al., 1963a; HONGO and OKADA, 1967; HONGO et al., 1967; COOKE et al., 1971a, b; MANN, 1971)

The neurones of the exteroceptive components receive excitation from cutaneous afferents which is monosynaptic in the DSCT and disynaptic in the CCT. The cell bodies of the DSCT neurones lie in Clarke's column (LINDSTRÖM and TAKATA, 1971b), whereas those of the CCT lie intermingled with lemniscal neurones in the rostral part of the main cuneate nucleus (COOKE et al., 1971a). The site of the interneurones which mediate the excitation from primary afferents to CCT neurones is not known but it is likely that they occur in the main cuneate nucleus.

The afferent organization of the exteroceptive components in the DSCT and CCT is similar, although the receptive fields, which vary from less than 1 to more than 100 square cm, tend to be smaller in the CCT (HOLMQVIST et al., 1963a). Observations on natural stimulation of cutaneous receptors indicate that the exteroceptive components of the two tracts contain similar subdivisions for information from different receptors (LUNDBERG and OSCARSSON, 1960; HOLMQVIST et al., 1963a; COOKE et al., 1971b; MANN, 1971). The most common type of neurone is activated from fast adapting hair receptors as well as from slowly adapting touch receptors. A second group of neurones is activated from fast adapting hair receptors only, and a third group from slowly adapting pressure receptors in foot pads. Presumably a fourth group of neurones is activated exclusively from slowly adapting touch receptors in hairy skin.

Many neurones in the exteroceptive components of the DSCT and CCT receive additional excitation from high threshold muscle afferents. In the CCT it has been demonstrated that these afferents originate mainly from rapidly adapting receptors activated by pressure against deep structures and not to any appreciable extent from slowly adapting receptors in muscle (spindle secondaries) (COOKE et al., 1971b). It is possible that the high threshold muscle afferents contribute excitation from deeply situated exteroceptors that is subsidiary to the excitation from the cutaneous receptors.

4. Ventral Spinocerebellar Tract (VSCT)

Most of the cell bodies of the VSCT seem to occur in the third to sixth lumbar segments (OSCARSSON, 1957a; HUBBARD and OSCARSSON, 1962; BURKE et al., 1971). The axons of these cells immediately cross the midline of the cord, ascend ventral to the DSCT and reach the cerebellum through the brachium conjunctivum. They terminate bilaterally in the anterior lobe (Fig. 2).

All VSCT neurones receive strong polysynaptic actions from the ipsilateral FRA. In the vast majority of the neurones these actions are predominantly inhibitory. Monosynaptic excitation and disynaptic inhibition from ipsilateral group I afferents occur in many neurones. Two groups of VSCT cells have been described. One group receives strong monosynaptic excitation from tendon organ (Ib) afferents and will be denoted the Ib–VSCT. The cell bodies of this group occupy a relatively dorsal position in the grey matter: most of them are situated in the lateral part of Rexed's layers V–VII. The other group of VSCT neurones originates

from the spinal border cells of Cooper and Sherrington (1940) and will be denoted
the SBC–VSCT (Burke et al., 1971). The spinal border cells occur along the ventrolateral border of the ventral horn. Many of these neurones receive weak excitation from primary muscle spindle (Ia) afferents but others are not excited from
any group I afferents. The separation of the Ib–VSCT and SBC–VSCT is presumably artificial but at present expedient as the two groups have been studied under
different conditions in separate investigations. Among the dorsally located
Ib–VSCT neurones there are presumably also some VSCT neurones which do not
receive group I excitation (Eccles, Hubbard and Oscarsson, 1961a) and some Ib
activated cells occur ventrally among the SBC–VSCT neurones.

   a) Ib–VSCT (Oscarsson, 1956, 1957b, 1960, 1965a, b; Eccles et al., 1961a;
Lundberg and Oscarsson, 1962a; Oscarsson and Uddenberg, 1964). The
Ib–VSCT neurones are by definition monosynaptically excited by tendon organ
afferents. An afferent volley evokes a single discharge in the tract neurones, but
not a repetitive one as often found in the DSCT and CCT. The transmission can
occur at very high frequencies (up to more than 500/sec) and is strongly potentiated at frequencies between 50 and 80 impulses per second. Many Ib afferents
from the same nerve converge on to one VSCT neurone and there is no evidence
for large unitary EPSPs like those occurring in the DSCT neurones. There is no
recurrent inhibition and the after-hyperpolarization is relatively small.

   The convergence of monosynaptic excitation from muscle nerves to single
tract neurones is extensive: many neurones are activated from one synergistic
muscle group at each of the hip, knee, ankle and toe joints. Most of the neurones
belong to one of two groups: (1) neurones activated from hip extensors, knee
flexors, and ankle and toe extensors; (2) neurones activated from knee, ankle
and toe extensors and sometimes also from hip extensors. Presumably each group
is activated from muscles that contract together in the execution of a certain
movement or the maintenance of a certain posture.

   Convergence of inhibition from group I afferents appears less extensive than
the convergence of excitation. Disynaptic inhibition is mainly produced by Ia
afferents. In general it is uncommon, though it is almost always evoked by the
quadriceps nerve in neurones of group (1). Since these cells are excited from the
antagonistic muscles, there would appear to be a reciprocal organization. However,
disynaptic inhibition does not occur from other antagonistic muscles and the
inhibition from the quadriceps nerve sometimes occurs also in neurones of group
(2) which are activated from the same muscle, the quadriceps. Inhibition from Ib
afferents is found in some neurones and is then usually tri- or polysynaptic. There
is no indication that it is organized in a reciprocal pattern.

   Polysynaptic actions from the FRA reach the tract neurones from all the limbs
and sometimes also from the trunk. The effects from the ipsilateral hindlimb are
strong, those from the other limbs weaker. In most neurones inhibitory actions
from the ipsilateral hindlimb predominate. The main inhibitory area usually
comprises the entire ipsilateral hindlimb but is sometimes smaller and is then
distally situated, particularly for the neurones of group (2) described above. The
inhibitory area is usually surrounded by an excitatory area which often includes
the contralateral hindlimb. The FRA actions from the forelimbs may be excitatory
or inhibitory in various combinations. On natural stimulation the FRA effects

can be evoked from skin by light touch (bending of hairs), pressure and pinching, and from muscle by stretch and contraction.

The Ib–VSCT neurones are strongly influenced by descending pathways (OSCARSSON, 1960; MAGNI and OSCARSSON, 1961; ECCLES et al., 1961a; LUND-BERG and OSCARSSON, 1962b; CARPENTER et al., 1965). Fig. 3A shows a tentative diagram of the descending connections as described by MAGNI and OSCARSSON (1961). The transmission from the FRA is facilitated by the pyramidal tract and inhibited by reticulospinal paths, as is also found with other pathways activated by the FRA. A weak monosynaptic excitation is evoked in many neurones on stimulation of fibres descending in the ipsilateral ventral quadrant (VQ in Fig. 3A). The origin of these fibres is unknown but is possibly similar to that of the ventral fibres exciting the SBC–VSCT neurones (see below). Stimulation of the cerebral

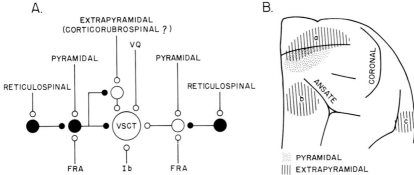

Fig. 3. Supraspinal control of transmission to Ib–VSCT as suggested by MAGNI and OSCARS-SON (1961). A. Segmental arrangement of ascending and descending connections to VSCT neurones. Inhibitory neurones black. FRA, flexor reflex afferents; Ib, tendon organ afferents; VQ, tract descending in ventral quadrant of cord. The excitatory connection from the FRA is usually much weaker than the inhibitory connection. B. Dorsolateral aspect of rostral pole of cerebral hemisphere. VSCT neurones receive extrapyramidal facilitation on stimulation of the hatched areas and pyramidal inhibition on stimulation of the stippled area

cortex in the hatched areas of Fig. 3B facilitates the Ib–VSCT neurones through an extrapyramidal pathway which descends through the dorsal part of the lateral funiculus. The effect from the rostral area, a, has a latency of about 6.5 msec indicating that the efferent path consists of not more than two or three neurones. It has been suggested that a corticorubrospinal system is involved. The facilitation from areas b and c has a longer latency and is presumably exerted through indirect paths. Volleys in either the FRA or pyramidal tract very effectively depress the cortical facilitation mediated by the extrapyramidal system. The mechanism suggested by MAGNI and OSCARSSON (1961) is shown in Fig. 3A and assumes inter-calation of a segmental interneurone on the extrapyramidal pathway. The inter-connections between the descending pathways might be mechanisms through which one system may gain dominance by suppressing the other. In the present case inhibition from the pyramidal tract might suppress facilitation from the extrapyramidal pathway, whereas the reticulospinal paths might suppress all effects exerted by the pyramidal tract.

b) SBC-VSCT. These neurones have only recently been identified and investigated (Burke et al., 1971; Lundberg and Weight, 1971). Most of the SBC–VSCT neurones were not spontaneously active in the preparations used and a peculiar feature was the usual lack of spike discharge on stimulation of nerves. The synaptic effects have been studied by intracellular recording.

Monosynaptic excitation from group I afferents does not occur in about 30% of the neurones. The majority of the remaining cells receive monosynaptic excitation from Ia afferents and a few receive Ib excitation. A small group of neurones appears to receive di- or polysynaptic group I excitation. The group I excitation is almost always subliminal which explains why it was overlooked in previous investigations based on evoked spike discharges. Convergence of Ia excitation from muscle groups acting at different joints is uncommon. The largest group of neurones is activated mainly or exclusively from knee extensors and a smaller group from knee flexors.

Disynaptic inhibition from group I afferents occurs in about 50% of the neurones and is evoked from Ia afferents in about half of these. As in the Ib–VSCT, Ia inhibition is most common from the quadriceps nerve. It occurs often in neurones receiving Ia excitation from the same nerve. In a few cases reciprocal patterns of Ia actions from knee extensors and flexors have been observed. Ia inhibition seems to be uncommon from distal muscles.

Ib disynaptic inhibition is supplied by various muscle groups including distal ones. Convergence of inhibitory actions from several muscle groups seems to be more common with Ib than with Ia inhibition. Tri- and polysynaptic inhibition from group I afferents may occur relatively often but has not been investigated in detail. Some neurones receive neither excitation nor inhibition from group I afferents.

All cells receive strong polysynaptic inhibition from the FRA. However, excitatory effects from the FRA are more common in the SBC–VSCT than in the Ib–VSCT. As in the latter path inhibition dominates from ipsilateral nerves and there is often predominant excitation from contralateral nerves. Presumably the general pattern of FRA actions is similar to that in the Ib–VSCT.

The complex and varying organization of the SBC–VSCT neurones is also demonstrated by the effects evoked on stimulation at the thoracic level of ipsilateral fibres in the lateral and ventral funiculi of the cord. Some neurones receive no monosynaptic actions from these fibres, whereas others receive monosynaptic excitation, or monosynaptic inhibition, or both. The observations of Baldissera and Weight (1969) indicate that the vestibulospinal tract originating from Deiters' nucleus is responsible for some of the EPSPs. Stimulation of the medial longitudinal fascicle, probably activating fibres from the lower pontine region, produces monosynaptic EPSPs in some neurones and monosynaptic IPSPs in others. Baldissera and Ten Bruggencate (1969) have demonstrated that some SBC–VSCT neurones receive monosynaptic excitation and (or) polysynaptic excitation and inhibition from the rubrospinal tract.

c) Information Forwarded. All VSCT neurones receive polysynaptic actions from the ipsilateral FRA but many subgroups can be distinguished on the basis of the connections from Ia and Ib afferents and from rubrospinal, reticulospinal, and vestibulospinal tracts. Only one or a few of these paths activate a given subgroup of VSCT neurones. An important question is whether all these subgroups carry basically the same kind of information.

The VSCT neurones receive polysynaptic actions from the FRA of large receptive fields. The transmission from the FRA is facilitated by the pyramidal tract and, in the decerebrate preparation, tonically inhibited by reticulospinal paths. Ascending paths with these characteristics have been assumed to carry information about activity in lower motor centers (p. 342). This hypothesis is supported by recent observations made in I.M. GELFAND's department in Moscow (personal communication). The activity in DSCT and VSCT neurones was recorded during the stepping movements that can be elicited in the mesencephalic cat (see SHIK, 1971). Both kinds of neurones discharged rhythmically in phase with the hindlimb

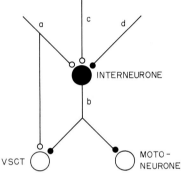

Fig. 4. Information carried by VSCT according to hypothesis of LUNDBERG (1971). VSCT neurones are assumed to carry information about the transmittability through inhibitory interneurones (black) which are parts of reflex arcs and also links in descending motor paths. VSCT neurones would signal when the transmission from a given path, *a*, through a group of interneurones, *b*, is modified by activity in convergent paths, *c* and *d*. See text

movements. After hindlimb deafferentation which did not prevent the stepping movements, the DSCT neurones ceased to be active but the VSCT neurones continued to discharge rhythmically.

LUNDBERG (1971) has recently suggested a hypothesis which would give a common explanation of the varying and convergent actions to the VSCT neurones. He assumes that the VSCT carries information about the transmittability of inhibitory interneurones which are the final links in segmental reflex arcs and descending motor paths. In the simplest case the VSCT neurone would receive axon collaterals (*b* in Fig. 4) from the inhibitory interneurones as well as axon collaterals from one of the paths to these interneurones (*a* in Fig. 4). The synaptic actions from these two paths (*a* and *b*) to the VSCT neurone would largely cancel each other and the VSCT neurone would signal when the transmission from path *a* through the interneurone is modified by activity in other convergent paths (*c* and *d* in Fig. 4). The subgroups of the VSCT activated by Ia or Ib afferents or by one of the descending tracts would assess the efficacy of each of these paths in controlling a group of inhibitory interneurones. The reader is referred to the original paper for a detailed discussion of this hypothesis and modifications thereof. Further experiments are needed to demonstrate if monosynaptic excitation and disy-

naptic inhibition from the same system is common in VSCT neurones, as would be
required by the hypothesis. One puzzling implication is that there would be a
specific pathway for information about the transmittability through inhibitory,
but not excitatory, interneurones. It is uncertain if the hypothesis can be adapted
to explain the organization of the forelimb equivalent of the VSCT, the RSCT,
which receives predominant excitation from the FRA.

The excitatory and inhibitory actions exerted by group I afferents on VSCT
neurones might indicate that the VSCT also carries proprioceptive information,
although other interpretations are possible (see Lundberg, 1971). It has been
suggested that the characteristic convergence of Ib excitation from often one
synergistic muscle group at each joint indicates that the Ib–VSCT neurones signal
movements (or position) involving the whole limb (Oscarsson, 1960). The Ia
excitation in SBC–VSCT neurones is usually limited to either flexors or extensors
of the knee and might signal movement at this joint. The inhibition from group I
afferents which occurs in many VSCT neurones might help to specify the movements.

d) Comparative Aspects. The mass discharge evoked in the VSCT and recorded
at the spinal level has been studied in the phalanger, rabbit, cat, dog, and monkey
(Magni and Oscarsson, 1962a; Oscarsson et al., 1964). In all these species the
mass discharge is evoked monosynaptically by high threshold group I muscle
afferents, which presumably originate from tendon organs. The discharge is relatively large in the phalanger, rabbit and cat but small in the dog and monkey.
The effect of a conditioning volley in the ipsilateral FRA on the mass discharge is
strong inhibition in the cat and phalanger, moderate inhibition in the rabbit and
monkey, and facilitation in the dog. The latter species differences might only
indicate that the relative number of VSCT units receiving predominantly excitation and predominantly inhibition from the FRA varies in the different animals.

It can be concluded that a Ib activated and FRA influenced component is a
basic feature of the VSCT in mammals. Presumably a component corresponding
to the SBC–VSCT exists also in other mammals than the cat as suggested by anatomical observations on spinal border cells in the monkey (Cooper and Sherrington, 1940; Morin, Schwartz and O'Leary, 1951; Sprague, 1953). The duck
has a crossed pathway activated from group I afferents in the leg which might
correspond to the VSCT in mammals (Oscarsson et al., 1963).

5. Rostral Spinocerebellar Tract
(Oscarsson and Uddenberg, 1964, 1965; Oscarsson, 1965a)

The RSCT originates from cell bodies located rostral to Clarke's column and
ascends uncrossed in the lateral funiculus. It reaches the cerebellum partly through
the brachium conjunctivum and partly through the restiform body to terminate
bilaterally in the anterior lobe (Fig. 2). The tract receives monosynaptic excitation
from group I afferents and polysynaptic excitation from the FRA. The receptive
fields are ipsilateral and related to the forelimb.

The discharge evoked in the RSCT on stimulation of group I muscle afferents is
probably mainly or exclusively due to tendon organ afferents. The convergence of
group I excitation to individual neurones is extensive: there is usually excitation
from synergistic muscle groups at several joints and sometimes from one muscle

group at each of the shoulder, elbow, wrist and toe joints. Presumably each neurone is activated from the muscles that contract together in the execution of a certain movement or the maintenance of a certain posture. It is possible that the RSCT like the VSCT contains a component which is not activated by group I volleys (cf. OSCARSSON and UDDENBERG, 1964).

The convergence of polysynaptic excitation from cutaneous afferents and high threshold muscle afferents is often extensive and not obviously related to the group I receptive field. Stretch of muscle supplying FRA excitation usually evokes a slowly adapting response in the RSCT neurones which may be due to impulses from secondary muscle spindle afferents. The effects of stimulation of cutaneous receptors have been weak and sometimes missing in the preparations investigated.

a) Comparison of VSCT and RSCT. The RSCT is a forelimb equivalent of the VSCT. This is demonstrated by the general similarity of the afferent connections and the similar mode of termination in the anterior lobe. However, there are important differences in the anatomical and functional organization and it has been suggested that the two tracts have developed independently along converging lines of organization (OSCARSSON and UDDENBERG, 1965). The RSCT is uncrossed and the VSCT crossed at the segmental level. Uncrossed and crossed ascending tracts seem to differ in fundamental respects (MAGNI and OSCARSSON, 1962b; HOLMQVIST and OSCARSSON, 1963; OSCARSSON, 1964; SZENTÁGOTHAI, 1964; MATSUSHITA, 1969, 1970). Uncrossed tracts ascend in the dorsal part of the lateral funiculus and originate from cell bodies in the dorsomedial part of the spinal grey matter, whereas crossed tracts ascend in the ventral part of the cord and originate from cell bodies in the ventrolateral part of the grey matter. Uncrossed tracts receive polysynaptic excitation and inhibition from ipsilateral receptive fields and crossed tracts from bilateral fields (OSCARSSON, 1964).

The FRA exert a predominantly excitatory action on the RSCT and a predominantly inhibitory action on the VSCT. However, it should be recalled that some VSCT units in the cat receive mainly excitation from the FRA and that excitation is the dominant effect in the VSCT of the dog. There are conspicuous differences in synaptic linkage between the Ib afferents and the two groups of tract neurones. In the VSCT the monosynaptic EPSP evoked from Ib afferents is markedly potentiated on repetitive stimulation and the transmission consequently improved. In the RSCT the ability to transmit impulses decreases at increasing frequencies just as with the transmission from group I afferents to DSCT and CCT neurones. Furthermore, group I excitation to RSCT neurones has a marked temporal spread, possibly because of additional di- and polysynaptic connections, whereas group I excitation to VSCT neurones usually is exclusively monosynaptic and of short duration (ECCLES et al., 1961a; LUNDBERG and WEIGHT, 1971).

D. Spinoreticulocerebellar Path Relayed through Lateral Reticular Nucleus (LRN-SRCP)

a) Anatomical Aspects (JANSEN and BRODAL, 1958; BRODAL, MARSALA and BRODAL, 1967). All axons of cells in the lateral reticular nucleus (LRN) probably terminate in the cerebellum as suggested by the total cell loss after cerebellectomy. The axons ascend through the restiform body to end in all parts of the ipsilateral half of the cerebellum. The LRN receives afferents from the cerebral cortex, red nucleus, fastigial nucleus, and spinal cord. Each of the four contingents of afferents has a separate termination area within the nucleus, although there is ample overlapping between the regions (Brodal et al., 1967). Anatomical investigations indicate that spinal afferents originate from all levels of the cord, ascend through the ventral part of the lateral funiculus, and terminate mainly in the ventrolateral region of the LRN: the parvicellular part and adjoining area of the magnocellular part (Brodal, 1949, 1957). Some observations suggest that the spinal fibres in addition terminate sparsely in wide areas of the magnocellular part (Morin, Kennedy and Gardner, 1966). The parvicellular part and adjoining magnocellular part of the LRN project to the vermis which would be the main termination area for the LRN–SRCP. However, electrophysiological investigations indicate that neurones activated from the spinal cord occur in all parts of the magnocellular and parvicellular regions of the LRN which would suggest that information from the cord reaches wide areas of the cerebellar cortex (Kitai, Kennedy, Morin and Gardner, 1967; Bruckmoser, Hepp-Reymond and Wiesendanger, 1970 b).

b) Ascending Connections. The LRN-SRCP has been investigated by extracellular recording from neurones in the reticular nucleus (Crichlow and Kennedy, 1967; Kitai et al., 1967; Bruckmoser et al., 1970a, b) and by recording from reticulocerebellar axons at the level of the restiform body (Grant, Oscarsson and Rosén, 1966; Oscarsson and Rosén, 1966 b). Only a few units recorded in the region of the LRN were identified by antidromic activation from the cerebellar cortex and it cannot be excluded that some of the units were passing fibres or neurones not projecting to the cerebellum. The responses recorded from the restiform body were studied in preparations with the cord transected in the cervical region sparing only the ipsilateral ventral quadrant. This would eliminate most other spinocerebellar paths reaching the cerebellum through the restiform body. The sampling of units would be contaminated by some RSCT fibres and possibly by some fibres from the gigantocellular reticular nucleus. The former are readily distinguished but the latter seem to have properties similar to the LRN-SRCP units (Avanzino, Hösli and Wolstencroft, 1966). The results from three of the investigations demonstrate that the LRN-SRCP is activated by the FRA from very wide receptive fields (Grant et al., 1966; Oscarsson and Rosén, 1966 b; Crichlow and Kennedy, 1967; Bruckmoser et al., 1970a, b). The observations in the remaining study might suggest that the path also contains units with a more restricted input with regard to both modality and receptive field (Kitai et al., 1967).

Fig. 5 shows the organization of the LRN–SRCP as described by Grant, Oscarsson and Rosén (1966). The spinoreticular tract has been identified as the 'bilateral ventral flexor reflex tract' (bVFRT) of Lundberg and Oscarsson (1962b). This tract originates from cell bodies located ventromedially in the spinal grey matter (Grillner, personal communication). The axons have conduction velocities between 50 and 120 m/sec. They cross the midline of the cord close to their segmental origin, ascend in the ventral part of the lateral funiculus, and terminate at the level of the LRN. The bVFRT receives polysynaptic excitation and inhibition from the FRA and the responses evoked from ipsilateral and contralateral nerves are of equal intensity and latency. Most of the LRN neurones are activated and inhibited from receptive fields including three or four limbs. It

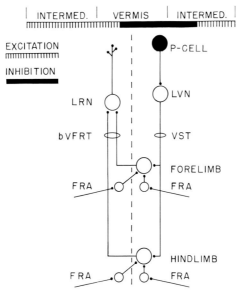

Fig. 5. Connections of the spinoreticulocerebellar path, LRN–SRCP. The neurones of the lateral reticular nucleus (LRN) send their axons to the ipsilateral cerebellar cortex and are activated by the bilateral ventral flexor reflex tract (bVFRT). This tract is polysynaptically activated and inhibited by the flexor reflex afferents (FRA) of bilateral receptive fields and monosynaptically activated by the vestibulospinal tract (VST) originating from the lateral vestibular nucleus (LVN). The bVFRT receives strong inhibition and excitation on stimulation of the longitudinal zones in the anterior lobe that are indicated (see key). The inhibition is due to the inhibitory action exerted by Purkinje cells (P-cell) on the VST. The excitation is mediated by complex and unknown paths presumably activating the VST. Intermed. = pars intermedia. Midline of neuraxis indicated by interrupted line

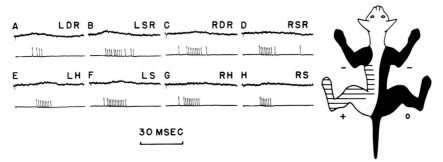

Fig. 6. Peripheral input to reticulocerebellar unit. Mass discharge recorded from dissected left restiform body (upper beam) and unit response recorded from axon in left restiform body (lower beam) on single shock stimulation of left and right (L and R) deep radial (DR), superficial radial (SR), hamstring (H) and sural (S) nerves. The cat diagram shows excitatory (hatched) and inhibitory (black) areas delimited by stimulation of cutaneous receptors. The effect of repetitive stimulation of nerves is indicated by + (excitation) and — (inhibition) at the appropriate limb. No effect (0) was obtained from the right hindlimb suggesting a balance between excitatory and inhibitory actions. Decerebrate and decerebellate preparation with spinal cord transected in upper cervical region sparing only left ventral quadrant. Modified from OSCARSSON and ROSÉN (1966b)

is unknown if the convergence from forelimb and hindlimb levels occurs mainly in the LRN, as shown in Fig. 5, or in the cord.

Fig. 6 illustrates, for a typical LRN unit, the responses evoked by nerve stimulation and the receptive fields determined by stimulation of cutaneous receptors. The reticulocerebellar neurones respond with trains of action potentials on single shock stimulation of the FRA. The trains evoked from forelimb nerves may have a latency as short as 8 msec and those evoked from hindlimb nerves as short as 10 msec, but much longer latencies (up to 50 msec) are found in some units. Many nerves supply mainly or exclusively inhibitory actions which can be displayed against the usually high background activity. The same nerve often supplies both excitatory and inhibitory actions. For example, the unit in Fig. 6 responded with trains of action potentials on single shock stimulation of all tested nerves but inhibition was demonstrated on repetitive stimulation of some nerves and on stimulation of cutaneous receptors in a large part of the receptive field.

The effects on natural stimulation of receptors are often weak, sometimes absent, despite strong effects on nerve stimulation. Presumably synchronous volleys are more readily transmitted than the asynchronous barrage evoked by natural stimulation. Responses can be obtained from the skin on pressure and pinching and from deep structures (Oscarsson and Rosén, 1966b; Crichlow and Kennedy, 1967; Kitai et al., 1967). The efficacy of the peripheral stimulation and the size of the receptive field depend on the anaesthetic and type of preparation. The receptive fields are more restricted under pentobarbitone anaesthesia than under chloralose anaesthesia and in unanaesthetized preparations (Crichlow and Kennedy, 1967). The FRA effects can be almost completely suppressed by the tonic inhibition exerted from bulbar centres in the decerebrate preparation (Holmqvist et al., 1960a).

c) **Descending Connections.** The LRN-SRCP is similar to other FRA paths in that the segmental interneurones mediating the FRA effects are inhibited by reticulospinal paths tonically active in the decerebrate preparation and facilitated by the pyramidal tract (Holmqvist et al., 1960a; Magni and Oscarsson, 1961; Lundberg et al., 1963; Carpenter et al., 1965) (Fig. 7). Recent observations suggest that these interneurones are facilitated also by the rubrospinal tract (see Hongo et al., 1969b).

The bVFRT neurones terminating in the LRN are monosynaptically excited by the vestibulospinal tract originating in Deiters' nucleus (Holmqvist et al., 1960b; Lundberg and Oscarsson, 1962b; Grant et al., 1966; Grillner, Hongo and Lund, 1968). These bVFRT neurones are strongly excited and inhibited on electrical stimulation of the longitudinal zones in the anterior lobe that are indicated in Fig. 5. The inhibition which has a very short latency, can be attributed to the inhibitory action exerted by Purkinje cells on vestibulospinal neurones (Fig. 5). The excitation, which has a long latency, is mediated by complex and unknown paths presumably activating the vestibulospinal tract.

Recent observations demonstrate similarities between the connections made by descending ventral fibre systems to motoneurones and to bVFRT neurones. Motoneurones receive monosynaptic excitation and disynaptic inhibition from two groups of ventral fibres: vestibulospinal originating from Deiters' nucleus and reticulospinal originating from pontine reticular nuclei and descending through the medial longitudinal fasciculus (Grillner and Lund, 1968; Grillner, 1969; Grillner, Hongo and Lund, 1970). The vestibulospinal fibres

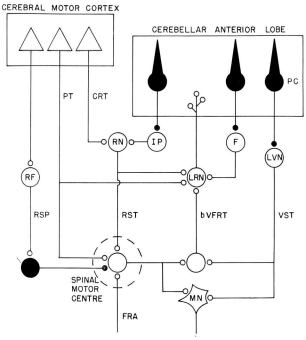

Fig. 7. Ascending and descending connections of LRN–SRCP. Some connections are hypothetical (see text). It is suggested that the LRN–SRCP carries information about command signals reaching the motoneurones (MN) from pyramidal and extrapyramidal paths via segmental interneurones (spinal motor centres) as well as about signals reaching the motoneurones directly from the vestibulospinal tract (VST). The LRN–SRCP is influenced by the pyramidal tract (PT) and rubrospinal tract (RST) not only at the segmental level but also at the brain stem level which might permit a comparison of the command signals in these tracts with the effects these signals evoke at the segmental level. PC, Purkinje cell; RN, red nucleus; IP, interpositus nucleus; F, fastigial nucleus; LVN, lateral vestibular nucleus; LRN, lateral reticular nucleus; RF, reticular formation; RSP, reticulospinal paths; CRT, corticorubral tract; bVFRT, bilateral ventral flexor reflex tract; FRA, flexor reflex afferents. Inhibitory neurones black

excite knee and ankle extensors and the reticulospinal fibres knee and ankle flexors as well as hip and some toe extensors. Disynaptic inhibition is reciprocally organized and has been demonstrated in knee and ankle extensors from the reticulospinal tract and in knee flexors from the vestibulospinal tract. Similar observations have been made on bVFRT neurones (GRILLNER et al., 1968). Many of these are monosynaptically activated by vestibulospinal fibres. However, some receive monosynaptic excitation on stimulation of the medial longitudinal fascicle and disynaptic inhibition from the vestibulospinal tract. The bVFRT seems to differ from the motoneurones in that monosynaptic excitation is supplied also from a group of propriospinal fibres descending in the ventral quadrant. It is not known if the propriospinal tract converges on to the same bVFRT neurones that are activated from the vestibulospinal and reticulospinal tracts and if all these categories of bVFRT neurones terminate in the LRN.

The majority of the LRN neurones are activated not only from the spinal cord but also by stimulation of the contralateral pericruciate cortex, contralateral red nucleus, and ipsilateral fastigial nucleus (BRUCKMOSER et al., 1970a, b). The latencies of the responses evoked from the supraspinal structures are often so short as to indicate monosynaptic excitation by direct fibres (Fig. 7). It is unclear to what extent the monosynaptic excitation from different supraspinal structures converges on to the same neurones.

d) Information Forwarded. The possible significance of the ascending and descending connections to the LRN–SRCP will be discussed in relation to the hypothetical diagram in Fig. 7. It is unknown if the collaterals to bVFRT neurones and motoneurones are branches of the same axons as indicated in the figure and if the pyramidal and rubral excitation of the spinal interneurones and of the LRN cells are exerted by the same group of fibres as is also indicated. Experimental observations suggest that the LRN–SRCP can be effectively controlled from the cerebral motor cortex and the anterior lobe of the cerebellum, both areas of paramount importance in the control of movement. The motor cortex exerts its effects through the pyramidal tract and presumably also through extrapyramidal paths via the red nucleus and reticular formation. The anterior lobe exerts its effects through the vestibulospinal tract. The connections suggested in Fig. 7 would indicate that the LRN–SRCP carries information about signals reaching the motoneurones from pyramidal and extrapyramidal paths via segmental interneurones (spinal motor centres) as well as about signals reaching the motoneurones directly from the vestibulospinal tract.

The LRN–SRCP is influenced by the cerebral cortex and red nucleus not only at the segmental level but also at the brain stem level. This might permit a correlation or comparison of command signals from the motor cortex with the effects these signals evoke at segmental levels which are also controlled by other descending paths and by afferents from the periphery (Bruckmoser et al., 1970a).

Besides carrying information about segmental motor control the LRN–SRCP may have other important functions. Stimulation of the bVFRT has been demonstrated to evoke cerebral arousal (Andersson, Norrsell and Wolpow, 1964; Andersson, 1967). It is not excluded that a loop through the cerebellum is involved. The LRN–SRCP projects mainly to the vermis which participates in the regulation of EEG and sleep-wakefulness patterns (see Evarts and Thach, 1969; Giannazzo, Manzoni, Raffaele, Sapienza and Urbano, 1969). The LRN-SRCP might be important in determining the background activity in the vermal cortex (Oscarsson and Rosén, 1966b). In this connection it is interesting that the mossy fibres of the LRN terminate on superficial granule cells which make synaptic contacts with the superficial branches of the Purkinje dendrites. In contrast, the mossy fibres of the DSCT and VSCT terminate on deep granule cells which make contacts with the proximal dendrites (Szentágothai, 1962; but see Sasaki and Strata, 1967). This organization seems to parallel the termination of specific and unspecific thalamic afferents in the cerebral cortex. The former, forwarding space and modality specific information, terminate mainly in cortical layer IV close to the cell bodies, whereas the unspecific afferents, presumably related to cortical arousal, seem to generate synaptic potentials predominantly in the distal branches of the dendrites (Lorente de Nó, 1949; Jasper, 1960; Nacimiento et al., 1964).

E. Climbing Fibre Paths

a) Origin and Course of Climbing Fibres. In 1959 Szentágothai and Rajkovits demonstrated, with anatomical technique, that the axons of the inferior olive terminate as climbing fibres in the cerebellar cortex. This has been corroborated by physiological investigations (Armstrong and Harvey, 1966, 1968; Eccles, Llinás and Sasaki, 1966; Bell and Grimm, 1969; Crill, 1970). Anatomical and physiological investigations indicate that in mammals the other known pathways to the cerebellar cortex terminate as mossy fibres (Jansen and Brodal, 1958; Szentágothai, 1964; Brodal, 1967; Eccles et al., 1967; Sasaki and Strata, 1967; Sasaki, Kawaguchi, Shimono and Yoneda, 1969). However, the possibility that some climbing fibres may originate from non-olivary structures should be kept in mind (Szentágothai and Rajkovits, 1959; Sousa-Pinto and Brodal, 1969; Batini and Pumain, 1971). In amphibians some vestibular fibres terminate as climbing fibres (Llinás, Precht and Kitai, 1967).

The axons of the olive cross the midline, ascend through the restiform body, and terminate in all parts of the cerebellar cortex (Brodal, 1940). Each part of the olive projects in an orderly way to a particular area of the cortex. Recent anatomical and physiological investigations indicate that the cerebellar projections from the olive are longitudinally organized: each small olivary region projects to a narrow sagittal strip of the cerebellar cortex (Oscarsson, 1969b; Voogd, 1969). Each Purkinje cell receives, with very few exceptions, only one climbing fibre (Eccles et al., 1967). At least some of the climbing fibres branch to innervate several Purkinje cells (Fox, Andrade and Schwyn, 1969). It has been shown that Purkinje cells in the anterior lobe and paramedian lobule can be activated by the same fibres (Armstrong et al., 1971) and this applies also to Purkinje cells arranged sagittally in adjacent folia of the anterior vermis (Faber and Murphy, 1969). If it is assumed that the inferior olive is the exclusive source of climbing fibres in mammals, a comparison of the number of olivary neurones and Purkinje cells would indicate that each olivary neurone innervates on the average 10–15 Purkinje cells (Moatamed, 1966; Escobar, Sampedro and Dow, 1968; Eccles, 1969).

b) Characteristics of Olivary Relay. The activity of the olivary neurones shows a number of characteristic features.

1. The responses consist of a single action potential or a burst of usually two to three potentials (Armstrong and Harvey, 1966, 1968; Eccles et al., 1966; Crill, 1970).

2. The background activity is usually only 0.2–2 discharges per second and similar in different species and preparations (Bell and Grimm, 1969; Miller and Oscarsson, 1970).

3. Each response is followed by a profound inhibition lasting 50–150 msec. This inhibition is sometimes followed by a rebound excitation (Armstrong and Harvey, 1966, 1968; Crill, 1970).

4. Slow fluctuations in the transmittability occur especially at stimulus frequencies of 2–20/second. Periods of responsiveness alternate with periods of refractoriness. The total cycle length may be as long as 30 seconds. The fluctuations are synchronous in large groups of olivary neurones indicating some synchronizing mechanism (Carrea, Guevara, Epstein and Folino, 1964; Miller and Oscarsson, 1970).

Some of the properties of the olivary neurones have been studied with intracellular recording technique (Crill and Kennedy, 1967; Armstrong, Eccles,

Harvey and Matthews, 1968; Crill, 1970). Antidromic, orthodromic, and direct electrical stimulation of olivary neurones evokes an initial action potential followed by a large depolarization lasting 10–15 msec. One or two spikes are often superposed on this depolarization which explains the short burst of activity characterizing the olivary responses, the depolarization is presumably caused mainly by action currents produced by spikes propagating out into the dendrites. However, some observations suggest that the repetitive discharge in olivary neurones partly depends on excitation mediated by recurrent collaterals (Eccles et al., 1966).

The excitation of olivary neurones is followed by a long lasting hyperpolarization which can be graded and presumably represents recurrent inhibition. The hyperpolarization is followed by a rebound depolarization after 100–150 msec. There is no explanation for the slow fluctuations in transmittability described above but the synchronization of these fluctuations might be due to spread of recurrent inhibition and recurrent excitation.

c) **Climbing Fibre Responses in Cerebellar Cortex.** The climbing fibre responses evoked in Purkinje cells are readily recognized either by recording from single cells or by recording the mass activity at the cerebellar surface or in the molecular layer of the cortex. The responses recorded from the Purkinje cells have an all-or-nothing character and consist of short bursts of impulses. The repetitive discharge is partly due to the large EPSP evoked in the Purkinje cell by a single action potential in the climbing fibre, and partly due to the burst discharge of olivary neurones. The mass activity in the Purkinje cells can be recorded as a positive potential at the cortical surface and as a negative field in the molecular layer (Eccles et al., 1966; Oscarsson and Uddenberg, 1966; Armstrong and Harvey, 1968; Eccles, Provini, Strata and Táboříková, 1968a; Miller and Oscarsson, 1970). The climbing fibre responses recorded from the cerebellar surface usually have a larger amplitude and longer latency than the mossy fibre responses (Table 1) and can usually be recognized by the slow fluctuations in amplitude referred to above. The characteristic features of these potentials allow them to be recognized in publications which appeared before their identification as climbing fibre responses. They correspond to potential III of Grundfest and Campbell (1942) and to potential y of Morin, Catalano and Lamarche (1957).

The impulses in climbing fibres evoke not only excitation in Purkinje cells but also inhibition (Bloedel and Roberts, 1971; Latham and Paul, 1971; Murphy and Sabah, 1971). The inhibition can be graded and may produce a pause in the background activity which lasts for up to 800 msec. The inhibition depends partly on activation of inhibitory interneurones in the cerebellar cortex by the climbing fibre collaterals (cf. Eccles et al., 1967).

d) **Spino-Olivocerebellar Paths.** The inferior olive receives afferents from several spinal pathways and supra-olivary structures (Brodal, Walberg and Blackstad, 1950; Walberg, 1956; Jansen and Brodal, 1958; Fox and Williams, 1968; Oscarsson, 1968, 1969a, b; Larson et al., 1969a, b; Sousa-Pinto and Brodal, 1969). The spino-olivocerebellar paths terminate in the anterior lobe, paramedian lobules and pyramis (Lamarche and Morin, 1957; Jansen and Brodal, 1958; Miller and Oscarsson, 1970; Armstrong et al., 1971).

Five spinal paths terminating as climbing fibres in the anterior lobe have been described and there are scattered observations which indicate that there are addi-

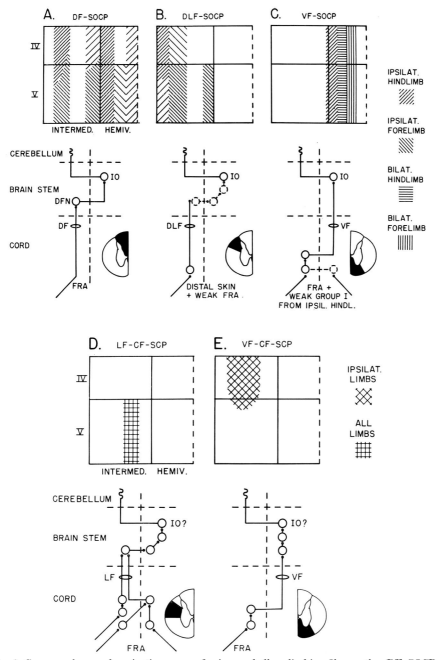

Fig. 8. Course, relays and projection areas of spinocerebellar climbing fibre paths: DF–SOCP, DLF–SOCP, VF–SOCP, LF–CF–SCP and VF–CF–SCP. The projection areas in Larsell's lobules IV and V are indicated by hatching (see key) in upper diagrams. Sparse hatching indicates areas with small or inconstant responses. The course and relays of the paths are shown in lower diagrams. The kinds of afferents supplying excitation are indicated. Interrupted vertical line indicates midline of neuraxis. The sectors of the cord containing the paths at the level of the third cervical segment are indicated by black areas in the cord diagrams. Intermed., pars intermedia; Hemiv., hemivermis; Ipsilat., ipsilateral; Bilat., bilateral; IO, inferior olive; DFN, dorsal funiculus nuclei; DF, dorsal funiculus; DLF, dorsolateral funiculus; LF, lateral funiculus; VF, ventral funiculus; FRA, flexor reflex afferents

tional paths (Oscarsson, 1968, 1969a; Larson et al., 1969a, b). The classification and some properties of the five paths are given in Table 1. The organization of the paths and their projection areas in lobules IV and V of the anterior lobe are shown in Fig. 8. Three of the paths have been identified as spino-olivocerebellar paths, SOCPs. The other two paths are almost certainly relayed through the inferior olive but this has so far not been demonstrated. They are denoted climbing fibre-spinocerebellar paths, CF–SCPs. The characteristics of the paths have been determined by recording climbing fibre responses evoked in Purkinje cells after spinal lesions interrupting all spino-olivary paths except one or two (Oscarsson and Uddenberg, 1966; Oscarsson, 1968, 1969a; Larson et al., 1969a, b). Climbing fibre and olivary responses recorded in preparations with intact spinal cord (Morin, Lamarche and Ostrowsky, 1957; Armstrong et al., 1968; Eccles et al., 1968a, b; Kitai, Táboříková, Tsukahara and Eccles, 1969) agree in a general way with those to be expected from the observations on the different climbing fibre paths. However, the detailed characteristics of these paths are obscured by their simultaneous activation (cf. Larson et al., 1969a).

1. Ventral Spino-Olivocerebellar Path
(Oscarsson and Uddenberg, 1966; Oscarsson, 1968)

The ventral path was identified anatomically by Brodal, Walberg and Blackstad in 1950. Recent investigations with electrophysiological technique have confirmed and extended some of their observations. The course and termination of the VF–SOCP is shown in Fig. 8C. The primary afferents activate the spino-olivary tract through interneurones (Oscarsson, unpublished). The tract neurones send their axons across the midline to ascend in the ventral funiculus, where the hindlimb component occupies a lateral position and the forelimb component a medial position. The spinal tract terminates in certain parts of the dorsal and medial accessory olives. These parts send their axons across the midline to terminate in the vermis, contralaterally to the olive and spinal tract, but ipsilateral to the main afferent input. The projection area in the anterior lobe has a somatotopical organization (Fig. 8C). The fibres terminating in the lateral part of the vermis are activated exclusively from ipsilateral hindlimb nerves, those terminating in the adjacent more medial zone from ipsilateral and contralateral hindlimb nerves, and those terminating in the most medial zone from ipsilateral and contralateral forelimb nerves. Fibres terminating in a zone transitional between the last two are often activated from all four limbs.

The VF–SOCP is activated by the FRA. Ipsilateral nerves supply strong excitation and contralateral nerves weak, or no, excitation. Weak additional excitation is evoked by group I muscle afferents but, remarkably enough, only from the nerves in the ipsilateral hindlimb. This excitation is mainly or exclusively from tendon organ afferents in some nerves but presumably also from spindle afferents in the quadriceps nerve. The group I afferents and the FRA activate the same neurones. Excitatory convergence is extensive: most units can be activated from all the nerves in one or more limbs.

Excitatory and inhibitory effects on natural stimulation are remarkably weak. Only half of the units can be influenced at all. The effects are almost always excitatory and can only be evoked by moderate or strong pressure against deep structures. Bending of joints, vibration, and even intense stimulation of the skin are ineffective. Evidently the asynchronous barrage of impulses evoked by natural stimulation is much less effective than the synchronous volleys evoked by nerve stimulation. The receptive fields delimited by natural stimulation are diffuse and include most of an ipsilateral limb, although the effects are usually stronger from distal parts.

2. Dorsal Spino-Olivocerebellar Path (OSCARSSON, 1969a)

The responses evoked through the dorsal path in the anterior lobe are as large as these evoked from the VF–SOCP but occur more extensively and it would seem that the dorsal path activates larger regions of the olive (Fig. 8A). In the spinal cord the path is located in the dorsal funiculus and consists of primary afferents which terminate in the dorsal funiculus nuclei. Anatomical studies indicate that the relay is in the rostral parts of the nuclei, which send axons to the contralateral accessory olives (HAND and LIU, 1966; EBBESON, 1968). The olivocerebellar path recrosses the midline and terminates both in the vermis and intermediate part of the anterior lobe. In the vermis the hindlimb and forelimb components terminate in different sagittal zones overlapping those of the VF–SOCP. In the pars intermedia the termination is also in sagittal zones. However, the zones representing the forelimb are mainly limited to lobule V and the zones representing the hindlimb are mainly limited to lobule IV and further rostrally.

The dorsal path is activated exclusively by the FRA. The neurones are usually activated from all the nerves in the ipsilateral limb that constitutes the receptive field. On natural stimulation of receptors effects can be demonstrated in about half of the units. They are almost always excitatory and best elicited by pressure against deep structures and by tapping against the paw. The receptive fields delimited by natural stimulation are usually large and with indistinct borders.

3. Dorsolateral Spino-Olivocerebellar Path (LARSON et al., 1969a)

The responses evoked through this path in the anterior lobe are often smaller than those evoked through the VF–SOCP. The spinal tract is almost certainly monosynaptically activated by primary afferents (Fig. 8B). It occupies a lateral position in the lumbar cord and a dorsolateral position in the cervical cord. The DLF–SOCP is interrupted by at least three or four synapses in the lower brain stem. It relays partly in the same areas of the olive that are activated by the DF–SOCP. It terminates in sagittal zones in the pars intermedia, ipsilateral to the afferent input.

The DLF–SOCP is strongly excited by stimulation of cutaneous nerves from the paws and receives weak additional excitation from the FRA, especially in distal nerves. The effects on natural stimulation are best elicited by tapping against the plantar surface of the paws. The receptive field is limited to the foot and sometimes restricted to part of the plantar surface. Different parts of the plantar surface seem to be represented in different patches of the cerebellar cortex but without any obvious somatotopical organization.

4. Ventral Climbing Fibre-Spinocerebellar Path (Oscarsson, 1968)

The course and termination of this path is tentatively shown in Fig. 8E. It ascends through the ventral funiculus and has presumably a similar segmental organization as the VF–SOCP. The input is, however, exclusively from the ipsilateral side. The long latency of the cerebellar responses both on nerve stimulation and on direct stimulation of the spinal tract (Oscarsson, unpublished) suggests that interneurones are interpolated in the brain stem. The VF–CF–SCP is activated from the FRA in hindlimb nerves and terminates in lobule IV and further rostrally in the pars intermedia. Stimulation of ipsilateral forelimb nerves sometimes evokes responses in approximately the same cortical area. These responses are presumably mediated by a much more complex path as they have a longer latency than the hindlimb responses (Table 1). The responses evoked in the VF–CF–SCP on natural stimulation of receptors are weak and also similar in other respects to those evoked through the VF–SOCP.

5. Lateral Climbing Fibre-Spinocerebellar Path (Larson et al., 1969 b)

The termination of the lateral path and a tentative diagram of its anatomical organization are shown in Fig. 8D. The responses evoked through this path have, like those of the VF–CF–SCP, not been observed in all preparations presumably because of inhibition or lack of facilitation from supraspinal structures. At the spinal level the LF–CF–SCP seems to consist of one more dorsally located tract with ipsilateral receptive fields and one more ventrally located tract with bilateral receptive fields. The latter path is possibly identical with the bVFRT. The LF–CF–SCP is interrupted by several synapses in the brain stem and terminates in a narrow strip in the pars intermedia of lobule V. This strip occupies the gap between the forelimb zones of the DF–SOCP and DLF–SOCP.

The LF–CF–SCP is activated by the FRA in all four limbs. The majority of the neurones receive equally strong excitation from all the limbs. The responses on natural stimulation of receptors are evoked by strong pressure against deep structures.

a) Supraspinal Control. No systematic studies have been made of the supraspinal control of transmission through the spinocerebellar climbing fibre paths. The four paths strongly activated by the FRA would be expected to receive facilitation from the pyramidal tract and inhibition from reticulospinal paths as in other pathways influenced from the FRA. Grant and Oscarsson (1966) showed that stimulation of fibres in the dorsolateral funiculus evoked intense activity in the VF–SOCP. Presumably pyramidal tract fibres were at least partly responsible. It is possible that the pyramidal tract also activates the DF–SOCP relay in the dorsal funiculus nuclei. This relay is situated in the region which receives many fibres from the cerebral cortex (Walberg, 1957; Kuypers and Tuerk, 1964). The discharge in ascending spinal paths activated by the FRA can be almost completely suppressed by the tonic inhibition in decerebrate animals (Holmqvist et al., 1960a). As these paths include the spinal tracts of the VF–SOCP, LF–CF–SCP and VF–CF–SCP it can be assumed that also these paths are under inhibitory control. The observations of Carli, Diete-Spiff and Pompeiano (1967) suggest that the DF–SOCP and VF–SOCP are heavily depressed during orienting reactions and during periods of rapid eye movements in desynchronized sleep (cf. Miller and Oscarsson, 1970).

b) Integration in Inferior Olive. A complex integration of information from different paths occurs in the inferior olive. The olivary neurones which project to the anterior lobe are usually activated from one or two spinal pathways as well as from the cerebral motor cortex (CRILL and KENNEDY, 1967; MILLER, NEZLINA and OSCARSSON, 1969).

The majority of the olivary neurones projecting to the lateral vermis belong to both the DF–SOCP and VF–SOCP demonstrating convergence at the olivary level. The forelimb zones of the DF–SOCP and DLF–SOCP overlap in the pars intermedia and it has been demonstrated that almost all neurones projecting to these zones are shared by the two paths. It is not known why the hindlimb components of the DF–SOCP and DLF–SOCP do not show the same convergence.

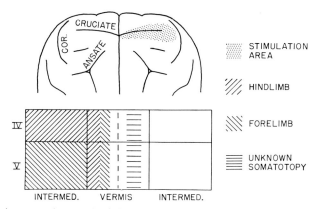

Fig. 9. Projection areas in anterior lobe of climbing fibre paths from cerebral motor cortex. Optimal stimulation area indicated by stippling in upper diagram. Projection areas in Larsell's lobules IV and V are indicated by hatching (see key) in lower diagram. See text. Cor. = coronal sulcus; Intermed. = pars intermedia

Stimulation of the motor area of the cerebral cortex evokes climbing fibre responses in the parts of the anterior lobe indicated by hatching in Fig. 9 (MILLER et al., 1969). The latency of the contralateral responses is about 12 msec or slightly longer and the latency of the ipsilateral responses 16–20 msec. The contralateral responses are presumably mediated by slowly conducting pyramidal tract fibres (KITAI, OSHIMA, PROVINI and TSUKAHARA, 1969). The ipsilateral responses, which are limited to the vermis, are presumably mediated by an indirect pathway. Recent anatomical observations (SOUSA-PINTO and BRODAL, 1969) suggesting that the cortical fibres terminate mainly in the contralateral olive, which projects to the ipsilateral cerebellum, are not supported by physiological observations. A comparison of Figs. 8 and 9 demonstrates that the somatotopy of the cortical projection is roughly similar to that of the combined projections of the spinocerebellar climbing fibre paths (PROVINI, REDMAN and STRATA, 1968).

The olivary neurones belonging to the DF–SOCP, DLF–SOCP and VF–SOCP are almost always effectively activated from the cerebral cortex (MILLER et al., 1969). The climbing fibre neurones belonging to the LF–CF–SCP and VF–CF–SCP presumably receive a similar excitation from the cerebral cortex but this has not been demonstrated.

c) **Information Carried by Climbing Fibre Paths.** In the following discussion it will be assumed that the CF–SCPs relay in the inferior olive, although this is unimportant for the arguments and conclusions. The following features must be taken into account when considering the possible kind of information carried by the climbing fibre paths:

1. Four of the paths are activated by the FRA from wide receptive fields. The information lacks modality specificity and permits only very crude spatial discrimination.

2. The fifth climbing fibre path, the DLF–SOCP, is activated by cutaneous afferents from restricted areas of the plantar surface of the paws.

3. In all five pathways only weak effects are evoked by natural stimulation of receptors.

4. With all pathways there are pre-olivary relays in the cord and brain stem which presumably are controlled by higher centres.

5. The olivary neurones are activated both from the spinal paths and the motor cortex.

These characteristics of the climbing fibre paths as well as other considerations suggest that they forward information about activity in motor centres rather than about peripheral events (OSCARSSON, 1967, 1968, 1969a, b; LARSON et al., 1969a, b; MILLER and OSCARSSON, 1970). It is assumed that the ascending paths to the olive carry information about the activity in pools of interneurones which represent motor centres in the cord and brain stem. These interneurones would be links in descending motor paths as well as parts of segmental and suprasegmental reflex arcs. The weak effects on natural stimulation might suggest that the activity of the interneurones is determined primarily by the command signals in the descending paths. The four climbing fibre paths activated by the FRA would be related to some of the many reflex arcs activated by these afferents (see p. 343). The DLF–SOCP might be related to reflex arcs activated specifically from the plantar surface of the foot such as the magnet reaction (RADEMAKER, 1931) and the extension reflex described by ENGBERG (1964). The VF–SOCP would monitor activity in spinal motor centres and the DLF–SOCP activity in brain stem centres. The LF–CF–SCP and VF–CF–SCP might be related to both spinal and medullary motor centres and concerned with integrative actions between bulbar and segmental reflex arcs. It is possible that the DF–SOCP carries information related to a brain stem reflex involving the rostral parts of the dorsal funiculus nuclei, where this pathway relays. These rostral parts project not only to the thalamus but also to a number of brain stem nuclei (HAND and LIU, 1966) which may have a motor function. For example, the FRA ascending through the dorsal funiculi are known to activate the red nuclei (MASSION and URBANO, 1968).

The motor functions represented by the various reflex arcs and assumed to be monitored by the climbing fibre paths have not been identified. Possible clues might be obtained by considering the functions of the termination areas of the climbing fibre paths in the anterior lobe. The ablation studies of CHAMBERS and SPRAGUE (1955a, b) indicate that the vermis is concerned with posture, locomotion and equilibrium of the entire body, whereas each pars intermedia is concerned with spatially organized and skilled movements in the ipsilateral limbs. Observations made by LAWRENCE and KUYPERS (1968) suggest that the former functions are controlled by a descending ventromedial brain-stem system and the latter functions by a descending lateral brain-stem system. The ventromedial and lateral systems terminate in different parts of the spinal grey matter presumably to exert their control through separate motor centres. It is possible that the climbing fibre paths terminating in the vermis and pars intermedia, respectively, carry information about the activity in these two descending systems and corresponding spinal centres. The vermis and pars intermedia are each divided into several sagittal zones by the climbing fibre projection areas suggesting that different aspects of the motor functions subserved by the vermis and pars intermedia are represented in each zone.

Olivary neurones are activated not only from the various spinal paths but also from the motor cortex and it has therefore been suggested that the olive acts as a comparator (MILLER and OSCARSSON, 1970). Command signals issued from higher motor centres would be compared with the effects these commands evoke in lower motor centres which are influenced by the pyramidal tract, extrapyramidal paths, and segmental afferents. The results of such a comparison might be used in the cerebellar integration of higher motor activity and reflex activity.

Unfortunately, observations on Purkinje cells in the anterior lobe have thrown little light on the adequate conditions for evoking climbing fibre responses. Natural stimulation of receptors is remarkably ineffective. In the anaesthetized cat many Purkinje cells do not respond with climbing fibre responses even on pinching or squeezing the skin and deeper tissues and the remaining cells respond with only one or a few responses (see above and THACH, 1967). In the unanaesthetized monkey, active hand movements presumably causing an intense barrage of impulses in exteroceptive and proprioceptive afferents usually resulted in no response (THACH, 1968, 1970). Only when the animal responded with a hand movement to a given signal was a climbing fibre response evoked in some cells. In these cases a single climbing fibre response appeared either before or after the initiation of the movement. The scarcity of positive observations might be partly explained by inadequate sampling. The recording site would be highly critical if a climbing fibre response is evoked only in connection with a particular motor function, different for different sagittal zones. Furthermore, the small degree of divergence and convergence in the connections between climbing fibres and Purkinje cells (Fig. 11, D) would make sense if each climbing fibre carries highly specific, perhaps unique, information. If so, one would expect a climbing fibre response to be elicited only under highly specific conditions set both by the peripheral input and by the activity in motor centres.

F. Functional Significance

The many hypotheses of how the cerebellum performs its motor control remain conjectural despite recent advances in cerebellar anatomy and physiology (cf. ECCLES et al., 1967; ECCLES, 1969; EVARTS and THACH, 1969; MARR, 1969; OSCARSSON, 1969b). It is sometimes assumed that the cerebellum corrects errors in motor performance on the basis of a comparison between the motor commands issued from higher centres and the evolving movement. The corrections might be required in order to compensate for unexpected peripheral events, for example changes in load or resistance, and in order to compensate for reflex actions at

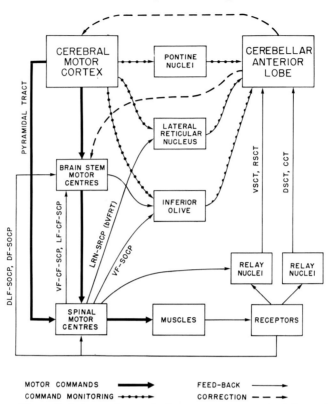

Fig. 10. Some of the paths between the cerebral motor cortex, anterior lobe, and lower motor centres with an interpretation of the function of these paths. The anterior lobe is assumed to correct errors in motor activity elicited from the cerebral cortex and carried out by command signals through pyramidal and extrapyramidal paths. The command signals are assumed to be monitored by the anterior lobe through paths relayed in the inferior olive and pontine and reticular nuclei. The spinocerebellar paths are assumed to serve as feed-back channels which monitor the activity in lower motor centres and the evolving movement. See text. Abbreviations of paths given in Table 1

lower levels. The latter might be particularly important since motor activity evoked from higher centres partly depends on facilitation and inhibition of reflex arcs (Lundberg, 1966; Hongo et al., 1969a, b). Recent observations on the afferent paths to the anterior lobe are consistent with the possibility that this part of the cerebellum operates as a comparator. It is particularly relevant that the cerebellar projections from the motor cortex and spinal cord overlap in both the vermis and pars intermedia of the anterior lobe (Provini et al., 1968; Miller et al., 1969) and that many of the spinal paths presumably monitor activity in lower motor centres rather than peripheral events.

Fig. 10 shows some of the paths between the cerebral motor cortex, anterior lobe, and lower motor centres, and suggests possible functions for these paths (Oscarsson, 1971). It is postulated that the anterior lobe is important for correcting errors in motor activity elicited from the cerebral cortex and carried out by command signals through pyramidal and extrapyramidal paths. The command signals may be monitored by the anterior lobe through cerebrocerebellar paths relayed in the pontine nuclei, the lateral reticular nucleus, and inferior olive (cf. EVARTS and THACH, 1969). The spinocerebellar paths can be regarded as feedback paths which monitor the effects of the command signals on the activity in lower motor centres and on the evolving movement. The majority of these paths would carry information about the modifications of the command signals that occur at lower motor levels due to the peripheral input (cf. Fig. 1). The evolving movement would be monitored by the proprioceptive and exteroceptive paths in the DSCT and CCT and possibly partly by the VSCT and RSCT.

The activity in lower motor centres would be compared with the original command signals in the anterior lobe and in the precerebellar nuclei (cf. Fig. 7). On the basis of this comparison corrections might already have begun before the initiation of the movement. The evolving movement would be compared with the original commands and with the activity in lower motor centres and the results of the comparison used for corrections during the movement. The corrections would be carried out through the well known efferent paths to the motor cortex and brain stem. These suggestions are not inconsistent with the observations made by THACH (1968, 1970) on unanaesthetized monkeys performing hand movements in response to visual signals. Many Purkinje cells in the anterior lobe showed changes in their activity immediately before and after the initiation of the movement. These changes depended mainly on alterations in the mossy fibre input but occasionally a climbing fibre response was observed either before or after the beginning of the movement. The changes in activity occurring before the movement might be due to signals either from the motor cortex or from lower motor centres. The changes occurring after the initiation of the movement might be due to a proprioceptive and exteroceptive feedback.

The generalized diagram in Fig. 10 does not take into account the differences in termination of the climbing fibre and mossy fibre paths. Some of the excitatory connections established in the cerebellum by the two systems are illustrated in Fig. 11, D. The small degree of divergence and convergence in the connections between the climbing fibres and Purkinje cells contrasts with the enormous divergence and convergence in the mossy fibre paths. The differences in mode of termination demonstrate that the information from climbing fibres and mossy fibres is processed in entirely different ways and may suggest that the two systems convey different kinds of information. This is also suggested by the difference in the organization of the projection areas formed by the climbing fibre and mossy fibre paths (OSCARSSON, 1969b; VOOGD, 1969). The former project to narrow sagittal zones with a width of about one mm. Seven main zones can be recognized in the anterior lobe, as shown in Fig. 11, A. Each zone receives one or two climbing fibre paths (cf. Fig. 8). In contrast, the mossy fibre paths have projections areas that extend widely in the transverse plane, as shown for the spino- and cuneocerebellar tracts in Fig. 11, B and C. The projection area of the LRN–SRCP is not known in detail but recent observations indicate that it extends over wide areas of the anterior lobe (cf. p. 356).

It has been suggested that each sagittal zone (Fig. 11, A) represents a functional unit integrating nervous activity related to a certain motor function, different for the different zones (OSCARSSON, 1969b). Recent anatomical investiga-

24*

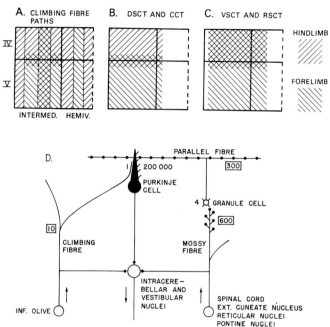

Fig. 11. Differences in mode of termination of climbing fibres and mossy fibres. A–C. Projection areas (hatched) of climbing fibre paths (A) and mossy fibre paths (B and C) in Larsell's lobules IV and V of cerebellar anterior lobe. Intermed., pars intermedia; hemiv., hemivermis. Areas receiving information from hindlimbs and forelimbs, respectively, are indicated by different hatching (see key). The projection areas of the climbing fibre paths form narrow sagittal zones (cf. Fig. 8), whereas those of the mossy fibre paths, represented by the spino- and cuneocerebellar tracts, form areas extending widely in the transverse plane (cf. Fig. 2). D. Main excitatory connections established by climbing fibres and mossy fibres. Approximative degree of divergence (figures in boxes) and convergence (other figures) between various neurones is indicated (Eccles, 1969). See text

tions indicate that each zone has specific efferent connections (Jansen, 1969; Korneliussen, 1969; Voogd, 1969) through which the appropriate motor function could be controlled. The climbing fibre path(s) terminating in a certain zone would monitor nervous activity related to the particular motor function this zone is concerned with. They would carry information about command signals controlling this motor function as well as about modifications of these signals at lower motor levels. The mossy fibre paths, which terminate widely in the transverse plane to reach many sagittal zones, would carry more general information. Each sagittal zone would require information about the evolving movement as signalled by proprioceptors and exteroceptors. This information is mainly supplied by the DSCT and CCT. In addition, each zone would require information not only about nervous activity related to the motor function it is particularly concerned with, but also about nervous activity related to other motor functions. This latter information would be supplied by the VSCT and RSCT as well as the LRN–SRCP. It has been demonstrated that the VSCT and LRN–SRCP carry information about activity in the major motor paths: the pyramidal, rubrospinal, vestibulospinal and reticulospinal tracts. The information carried by the VSCT, RSCT and LRN–SRCP might relate to the sum total of the motor effects exerted at the segmental level by descending tracts and spinal afferents.

This work was supported by the Swedish Medical Research Council. Project Nr B71-14X-1013-07C. I would like to thank my colleagues D. J. COOKE, B. LARSON and I. ROSÉN for reading and criticizing the manuscript.

References

AKKER, VAN DEN, L. M.: An anatomical outline of the spinal cord of the pigeon. (Thesis.) Assen: van Gorcum & Comp. 1970.

ANDERSSON, S. A.: Suppression of cortical spontaneous barbiturate spindles via specific and unspecific projection spinal pathways. Acta physiol. scand. **69**, 191–202 (1967).

ANDERSSON, S. A., NORRSELL, U., WOLPOW, E. R.: Cortical synchronization and desynchronization via spinal pathways. Acta physiol. scand. **61**, 144–158 (1964).

ARMSTRONG, D. M., ECCLES, J. C., HARVEY, R. J., MATTHEWS, P. B. C.: Responses in the dorsal accessory olive of the cat to stimulation of hind limb afferents. J. Physiol. (Lond.) **194**, 125–145 (1968).

ARMSTRONG, D. M., HARVEY, R. J.: Responses in the inferior olive to stimulation of the cerebellar and cerebral cortices in the cat. J. Physiol. (Lond.) **187**, 553–574 (1966).

ARMSTRONG, D. M., HARVEY, R. J., SCHILD, R. F.: Distribution in the anterior lobe of the cerebellum of branches from climbing fibres to the paramedian lobule. Brain Res. **25**, 203–206 (1971).

ASANUMA, H., STONEY, S. D., JR., THOMPSON, W. D.: Characteristics of cervical interneurones which mediate cortical motor outflow to distal forelimb muscles of cats. Brain Res. **27**, 79–95 (1971).

AVANZINO, G. L., HÖSLI, L., WOLSTENCROFT, J. H.: Identification of cerebellar projecting neurones in nucleus reticularis gigantocellularis. Brain Res. **3**, 201–203 (1966).

BALDISSERA, F., BRUGGENCATE, G. TEN: Rubrospinal effects on spinal border cells. Acta physiol. scand. Suppl. **330**, 119 (1969).

BALDISSERA, F., WEIGHT, F.: Descending monosynaptic connexions to spinal border cells. Acta physiol. scand. **76**, 28A–29A (1969).

BATINI, C., PUMAIN, R.: Données électrophysiologiques sur l'origine des fibres grimpantes. Arch. ital. Biol. **109**, 189–209 (1971).

BELL, C. C., GRIMM, R. J.: Discharge properties of Purkinje cells recorded on single and double microelectrodes. J. Neurophysiol. **32**, 1044–1055 (1969).

BLOEDEL, J. R., BURTON, E. J.: Electrophysiological evidence for a mossy fiber input to the cerebellar cortex activated indirectly by collaterals of spinocerebellar pathways. J. Neurophysiol. **33**, 308–321 (1970).

BLOEDEL, J. R., ROBERTS, W. J.: Action of climbing fibers in cerebellar cortex of the cat. J. Neurophysiol. **34**, 17–31 (1971).

BLOOM, F. E., HOFFER, B. J., SIGGINS, G. R.: Studies on norepinephrine-containing afferents to Purkinje cells of rat cerebellum. I. Localization of the fibers and their synapses. Brain Res. **25**, 501–521 (1971).

BRODAL, A.: Experimentelle Untersuchungen über die olivo-cerebellare Lokalisation. Z. ges. Neurol. Psychiat. **169**, 1–153 (1940).

BRODAL, A.: Die Verbindungen des Nucleus cuneatus externus mit dem Kleinhirn beim Kaninchen und bei der Katze. Experimentelle Untersuchungen. Z. ges. Neurol. Psychiat. **171**, 167–199 (1941).

BRODAL, A.: Spinal afferents to the lateral reticular nucleus of the medulla oblongata in the cat. J. comp. Neurol. **91**, 259–295 (1949).

BRODAL, A.: The Reticular Formation of the Brain Stem. Anatomical Aspects and Functional Correlations. Edinburgh: Oliver & Boyd 1957. 87 pp.

BRODAL, A.: Anatomical studies of cerebellar fibre connections with special reference to problems of functional localization. In: The Cerebellum. Ed. by C. A. FOX and R. S. SNIDER. Progress in Brain Research **25**, 135–173 (1967). Amsterdam-New York: Elsevier Publishing Company.

BRODAL, A., WALBERG, F., BLACKSTAD, T.: Termination of spinal afferents to inferior olive in cat. J. Neurophysiol. **13**, 431–454 (1950).

BRODAL, P., MARSALA, J., BRODAL, A.: The cerebral cortical projection to the lateral reticular nucleus in the cat, with special reference to the sensorimotor cortical areas. Brain Res. **6**, 252–274 (1967).

BRUCKMOSER, P., HEPP-REYMOND, M.C., WIESENDANGER, M.: Cortical influence on single neurons of the lateral reticular nucleus of the cat. Exp. Neurol. **26**, 239–252 (1970a).

BRUCKMOSER, P., HEPP-REYMOND, M.C., WIESENDANGER, M.: Effects of peripheral, rubral, and fastigal stimulation on neurons of the lateral reticular nucleus of the cat. Exp. Neurol. **27**, 388–398 (1970b).

BURKE, R.E., LUNDBERG, A., WEIGHT, F.: Spinal border cell origin of the ventral spinocerebellar tract. Exp. Brain Res. **12**, 283–294 (1971).

CARLI, G., DIETE-SPIFF, K., POMPEIANO, O.: Cerebellar responses evoked by somatic afferent volleys during sleep and waking. Arch. ital. Biol. **105**, 499–528 (1967).

CARPENTER, D., ENGBERG, I., FUNKENSTEIN, H., LUNDBERG, A.: Decerebrate control of reflexes to primary afferents. Acta physiol. scand. **59**, 424–437 (1963).

CARPENTER, D., ENGBERG, I., LUNDBERG, A.: Differential supraspinal control of inhibitory and excitatory actions from the FRA to ascending spinal pathways. Acta physiol. scand. **63**, 103–110 (1965).

CARREA, R., GUEVARA, J.A., EPSTEIN, R., FOLINO, J.C.: Periodic variations of cerebellar electrocortical activity in the cat. Acta neurol. lat.-amer. **10**, 189–229 (1964).

CHAMBERS, W.W., SPRAGUE, J.M.: Functional localization in the cerebellum. I. Organization in longitudinal corticonuclear zones and their contribution to the control of posture, both extrapyramidal and pyramidal. J. comp. Neurol. **103**, 105–129 (1955a).

CHAMBERS, W.W., SPRAGUE, J.M.: Functional localization in the cerebellum. II. Somatotopic organization in cortex and nuclei. Arch. Neurol. Psychiat. (Chic.) **74**, 653–680 (1955b).

COOKE, J.D., LARSON, B., OSCARSSON, O., SJÖLUND, B.: Origin and termination of cuneocerebellar tract. Exp. Brain Res. **13**, 339–358 (1971a).

COOKE, J.D., LARSON, B., OSCARSSON, O., SJÖLUND, B.: Organization of afferent connections to cuneocerebellar tract. Exp. Brain Res. **13**, 359–377 (1971b).

COOPER, S., SHERRINGTON, C.S.: Gower's tract and spinal border cells. Brain **63**, 123–134 (1940).

CRICHLOW, E.C., KENNEDY, T.T.: Functional characteristics of neurons in the lateral reticular nucleus with reference to localized cerebellar potentials. Exp. Neurol. **18**, 141–153 (1967).

CRILL, W.E.: Unitary multiple-spiked responses in cat inferior olive nucleus. J. Neurophysiol. **33**, 199–209 (1970).

CRILL, W.E., KENNEDY, T.T.: Inferior olive of the cat: intracellular recording. Science **157**, 716–718 (1967).

CURTIS, D.R., ECCLES, J.C., LUNDBERG, A.: Intracellular recording from cells in Clarke's column. Acta physiol. scand. **43**, 303–314 (1958).

DOW, R.S., MORUZZI, G.: The physiology and pathology of the cerebellum. Minneapolis: The University of Minnesota Press 1958.

EBBESSON, S.O.E.: A connection between the dorsal column nuclei and the dorsal accessory olive. Brain Res. **8**, 393–397 (1968).

ECCLES, J.C.: The dynamic loop hypothesis of movement control. In: Information Processing in the Nervous System, pp. 245–269. Ed. by K.N. LEIBOVIC. Berlin-Heidelberg-New York: Springer 1969.

ECCLES, J.C., HUBBARD, J.I., OSCARSSON, O.: Intracellular recording from cells of the ventral spinocerebellar tract. J. Physiol. (Lond.) **158**, 486–516 (1961a).

ECCLES, J.C., ITO, M., SZENTÁGOTHAI, J.: The Cerebellum as a Neuronal Machine. Berlin-Heidelberg-New York: Springer 1967.

ECCLES, J.C., LLINÁS, R., SASAKI, K.: The excitatory synaptic action of climbing fibres on the Purkinje cells of the cerebellum. J. Physiol. (Lond.) **182**, 268–296 (1966).

ECCLES, J.C., OSCARSSON, O., WILLIS, W.D.: Synaptic action of group I and II afferent fibres of muscle on the cells of the dorsal spinocerebellar tract. J. Physiol. (Lond.) **158**, 517–543 (1961b).

ECCLES, J.C., PROVINI, L., STRATA, P., TÁBOŘÍKOVÁ, H.: Analysis of electrical potentials evoked in the cerebellar anterior lobe by stimulation of hindlimb and forelimb nerves. Exp. Brain Res. **6**, 171–194 (1968a).

ECCLES, J.C., PROVINI, L., STRATA, P., TÁBOŘÍKOVÁ, H.: Topographical investigations on the climbing fiber inputs from forelimb and hindlimb afferents to the cerebellar anterior lobe. Exp. Brain Res. **6**, 195–215 (1968b).

ECCLES, J.C., SCHMIDT, R.F., WILLIS, W.D.: Inhibition of discharges into the dorsal and ventral spinocerebellar tracts. J. Neurophysiol. **26**, 635–645 (1963).

ECCLES, R.M., LUNDBERG, A.: Synaptic actions in motoneurones by afferents which may evoke the flexion reflex. Arch. ital. Biol. **97**, 199–221 (1959).

EIDE, E., FEDINA, L., JANSEN, J., LUNDBERG, A., VYKLICKÝ, L.: Properties of Clarke's column neurones. Acta physiol. scand. **77**, 125–144 (1969a).

EIDE, E., FEDINA, L., JANSEN, J.K.S., LUNDBERG, A., VYKLICKÝ, L.: Unitary components in the activation of Clarke's column neurones. Acta physiol. scand. **77**, 145–158 (1969b).

EKEROT, C.F., LARSON, B.: Differential termination of the exteroceptive and proprioceptive components of the cuneocerebellar tract. Brain Res. **36**, 420–424 (1972).

ENGBERG, I.: Reflexes to foot muscles in the cat. Acta physiol. scand. **62**, Suppl. 235 (1964).

ESCOBAR, A., SAMPEDRO, E.D., DOW, R.S.: Quantitative data on the inferior olivary nucleus in man, cat and vampire bat. J. comp. Neurol. **132**, 397–404 (1968).

EVARTS, E.V., THACH, W.T.: Motor mechanisms of the CNS: Cerebro-cerebellar interrelations. A. Rev. Physiol. **31**, 451–498 (1969).

FABER, D.S., MURPHY, J.T.: Axonal branching in the climbing fiber pathway to the cerebellum. Brain Res. **15**, 262–267 (1969).

FERRARO, A., BARRERA, S.E.: The nuclei of the posterior funiculi in Macacus rhesus. An anatomical and experimental investigation. Arch. Neurol. Psychiat. (Chic.) **33**, 262–275 (1935).

FOX, C.A., ANDRADE, A., SCHWYN, R.C.: Climbing fiber branching in the granular layer. In: Neurobiology of Cerebellar Evolution and Development, pp. 603–611. Ed. by R. LLINÁS. Chicago: American Medical Association 1969.

FOX, M., WILLIAMS, T.D.: Responses evoked in the cerebellar cortex by stimulation of the caudate nucleus in the cat. J. Physiol. (Lond.) **198**, 435–450 (1968).

FRANZ, D.N., IGGO, A.: Dorsal root potentials and ventral root reflexes evoked by nonmyelinated fibers. Science **162**, 1140–1142 (1968).

GIANNAZZO, E., MANZONI, T., RAFFAELE, R., SAPIENZA, S., URBANO, A.: Effects of chronic fastigal lesions on the sleep-wakefulness rhythm in the cat. Arch. ital. Biol. **107**, 1–18 (1969).

GRANT, G.: Projection of the external cuneate nucleus onto the cerebellum in the cat: An experimental study using silver methods. Exp. Neurol. **5**, 179–195 (1962a).

GRANT, G.: Spinal course and somatotopically localized termination of the spinocerebellar tracts. An experimental study in the cat. Acta physiol. scand. **56**, Suppl. 193 (1962b).

GRANT, G., OSCARSSON, O.: Mass discharges evoked in the olivocerebellar tract on stimulation of muscle and skin nerves. Exp. Brain Res. **1**, 329–337 (1966).

GRANT, G., OSCARSSON, O., ROSÉN, I.: Functional organization of the spinoreticulocerebellar path with identification of its spinal component. Exp. Brain Res. **1**, 306–319 (1966).

GRILLNER, S.: Supraspinal and segmental control of static and dynamic γ-motoneurones in the cat. Acta physiol. scand. Suppl. **327**, 1–34 (1969).

GRILLNER, S., HONGO, T., LUND, S.: The origin of descending fibres monosynaptically activating spinoreticular neurones. Brain Res. **10**, 259–262 (1968).

GRILLNER, S., HONGO, T., LUND, S.: The vestibulospinal tract. Effects on alpha-motoneurones in the lumbosacral spinal cord in the cat. Exp. Brain Res. **10**, 94–120 (1970).

GRILLNER, S., LUND, S.: The origin of a descending pathway with monosynaptic action on flexor motoneurones. Acta physiol. scand. **74**, 274–284 (1968).

GRUNDFEST, H., CAMPBELL, B.: Origin, conduction and termination of impulses in the dorsal spinocerebellar tracts of cats. J. Neurophysiol. **5**, 275–294 (1942).

HAND, P., LIU, C.N.: Efferent projections of the nucleus gracilis. Anat. Rec. **154**, 353–354 (1966).

HÖKFELT, T., FUXE, K.: Cerebellar monoamine nerve terminals, a new type of afferent fibers to the cortex cerebelli. Exp. Brain Res. **9**, 63–72 (1969).

HOFFER, B.J., SIGGINS, G.R., WOODWARD, D.J., BLOOM, F.E.: Spontaneous discharge of Purkinje neurons after destruction of catecholamine-containing afferents by 6-hydroxydopamine. Brain Res. **30**, 425–430 (1971).

HOLMQVIST, B.: Crossed spinal reflex actions evoked by volleys in somatic afferents. Acta physiol. scand. **52**, Suppl. 181 (1961).

Holmqvist, B., Lundberg, A.: Differential supraspinal control of synaptic actions evoked by volleys in the flexion reflex afferents in alpha motoneurones. Acta physiol. scand. 54, Suppl. 186 (1961).

Holmqvist, B., Lundberg, A., Oscarsson, O.: Functional organization of the dorsal spinocerebellar tract in the cat. V. Further experiments on convergence of excitatory and inhibitory actions. Acta physiol. scand. 38, 76–90 (1956).

Holmqvist, B., Lundberg, A., Oscarsson, O.: Supraspinal inhibitory control of transmission to three ascending spinal pathways influenced by the flexion reflex afferents. Arch. ital. Biol. 98, 60–80 (1960a).

Holmqvist, B., Lundberg, A., Oscarsson, O.: A supraspinal control system monosynaptically connected with an ascending spinal pathway. Arch. ital. Biol. 98, 402–422 (1960b).

Holmqvist, B., Oscarsson, O.: Location, course, and characteristics of uncrossed and crossed ascending spinal tracts in the cat. Acta physiol. scand. 58, 57–67 (1963).

Holmqvist, B., Oscarsson, O., Rosén, I.: Functional organization of the cuneocerebellar tract in the cat. Acta physiol. scand. 58, 216–235 (1963a).

Holmqvist, B., Oscarsson, O., Uddenberg, N.: Organization of ascending spinal tracts activated from forelimb afferents in the cat. Acta physiol. scand. 58, 68–76 (1963b).

Hongo, T., Jankowska, E., Lundberg, A.: The rubrospinal tract. I. Effects on alpha-motoneurones innervating hindlimb muscles in cats. Exp. Brain Res. 7, 344–364 (1969a).

Hongo, T., Jankowska, E., Lundberg, A.: The rubrospinal tract. II. Facilitation of interneuronal transmission in reflex paths to motoneurones. Exp. Brain Res. 7, 365–391 (1969b).

Hongo, T., Okada, Y.: Cortically evoked pre- and postsynaptic inhibition of impulse transmission to the dorsal spinocerebellar tract. Exp. Brain Res. 3, 163–177 (1967).

Hongo, T., Okada, Y., Sato, M.: Corticofugal influences on transmission to the dorsal spinocerebellar tract from hindlimb primary afferents. Exp. Brain Res. 3, 135–149 (1967).

Hubbard, J.I., Oscarsson, O.: Localization of the cell bodies of the ventral spinocerebellar tract in lumbar segments of the cat. J. comp. Neurol. 118, 199–204 (1962).

Ito, M., Kawai, N., Udo, M., Mano, N.: Axon reflex activation of Deiters neurones from the cerebellar cortex through collaterals of the cerebellar afferents. Exp. Brain Res. 8, 249–268 (1969).

Ito, M., Yoshida, M., Obata, K., Kawai, N., Udo, M.: Inhibitory control of intracerebellar nuclei by the Purkinje cell axons. Exp. Brain Res. 10, 64–80 (1970).

Jankowska, E., Jukes, M.G.M., Lund, S.: The pattern of presynaptic inhibition of transmission to the dorsal spinocerebellar tract of the cat. J. Physiol. (Lond.) 178, 17–18P (1965).

Jansen, J.: On cerebellar evolution and organization from the point of view of a morphologist. In: Neurobiology of Cerebellar Evolution and Development, pp. 881–893. Ed. by R. Llinás. Chicago: American Medical Association 1969.

Jansen, J., Brodal, A.: Handbuch der mikroskopischen Anatomie des Menschen, IV/8, Das Kleinhirn. Berlin-Göttingen-Heidelberg: Springer 1958.

Jansen, J.K.S., Nicolaysen, K., Rudjord, T.: Discharge pattern of neurons of the dorsal spinocerebellar tract activated by static extension of primary endings of muscle spindles. J. Neurophysiol. 29, 1061–1086 (1966).

Jansen, J.K.S., Nicolaysen, K., Wallöe, L.: On the inhibition of transmission to the dorsal spinocerebellar tract by stretch of various ankle muscles of the cat. Acta physiol. scand. 70, 362–368 (1967).

Jansen, J.K.S., Nicolaysen, K., Wallöe, L.: The firing pattern of dorsal spinocerebellar tract neurones during inhibition. Acta physiol. scand. 77, 68–84 (1969).

Jansen, J.K.S., Rudjord, T.: Dorsal spinocerebellar tract: response pattern of nerve fibres to muscle stretch. Science 149, 1109–1111 (1965).

Jansen, J.K.S., Wallöe, L.: Transmission of signals from muscle stretch receptors to the dorsal spinocerebellar tract. In: The Cerebellum in Health and Disease, pp. 143–171. Ed. by W.S. Fields and W.D. Willis. St. Louis: Warren H. Green 1970.

Jasper, H.H.: Unspecific thalamocortical relations. Chapter 53 in Handbook of Physiology. Section 1: Neurophysiology. 2. 1307–1321. Washington, D.C.: American Physiological Society 1960.

Johnson, J.I., Jr., Welker, W.I., Pubols, B.H. Jr.: Somatotopic organization of raccoon dorsal column nuclei. J. comp. Neurol. 132, 1–44 (1968).

KITAI, S.T., KENNEDY, D.T., MORIN, F., GARDNER, E.: The lateral reticular nucleus of the medulla oblongata of the cat. Exp. Neurol. **17**, 65–73 (1967).

KITAI, S.T., OSHIMA, T., PROVINI, L., TSUKAHARA, N.: Cerebro-cerebellar connections mediated by fast and slow conducting pyramidal tract fibres of the cat. Brain Res. **15**, 267–271 (1969).

KITAI, S.T., TÁBOŘÍKOVÁ, H., TSUKAHARA, N., ECCLES, J.C.: The distribution to the cerebellar anterior lobe of the climbing and mossy fiber inputs from the plantar and palmar cutaneous afferents. Exp. Brain Res. **7**, 1–10 (1969).

KÖRLIN, D., LARSON, B.: Differences in cerebellar potentials evoked by the group I and cutaneous components of the cuneocerebellar tract. Fifth International Meeting of Neurobiologists. Excitatory Synaptic Mechanisms, pp. 237–241. Ed. by P. ANDERSEN and J. JANSEN 1970.

KORNELIUSSEN, H.K.: Cerebellar organization in the light of cerebellar nuclear morphology and cerebellar corticogenesis. In: Neurobiology of Cerebellar Evolution and Development, pp. 515–523. Ed. by R. LLINÁS. Chicago: American Medical Association 1969.

KOSTYUK, P.G.: On the functions of dorsal spino-cerebellar tract in cat. In: Neurobiology of Cerebellar Evolution and Development, pp. 539–548. Ed. by R. LLINÁS. Chicago: American Medical Association 1969.

KUNO, M., MIYAHARA, J.T.: Factors responsible for multiple discharge of neurons in Clarke's column. J. Neurophysiol. **31**, 624–638 (1968).

KUYPERS, H.G.J.M., TUERK, J.D.: The distribution of the cortical fibres within the nuclei cuneatus and gracilis in the cat. J. Anat. (Lond.) **98**, 143–162 (1964).

LAMARCHE, G., MORIN, F.: Latencies and pathways for cutaneous projections to posterior cerebellar lobe. J. Neurophysiol. **20**, 275–285 (1957).

LAPORTE, Y., LUNDBERG, A., OSCARSSON, O.: Functional organization of the dorsal spinocerebellar tract in the cat. I. Recording of mass discharge in dissected Flechsig's fasciculus. Acta physiol. scand. **36**, 175–187 (1956a).

LAPORTE, Y., LUNDBERG, A., OSCARSSON, O.: Functional organization of the dorsal spinol cerebellar tract in the cat. II. Single fibre recording in Flechsig's fasciculus on electricastimulation of various peripheral nerves. Acta physiol. scand. **36**, 188–203 (1956b).

LARSON, B., MILLER, S., OSCARSSON, O.: Termination and functional organization of the dorsolateral spino-olivocerebellar path. J. Physiol. (Lond.) **203**, 611–640 (1969a).

LARSON, B., MILLER, S., OSCARSSON, O.: A spinocerebellar climbing fibre path activated by the flexor reflex afferents from all four limbs. J. Physiol. (Lond.) **203**, 641–649 (1969b).

LATHAM, A., PAUL, D.H.: Spontaneous activity of cerebellar Purkinje cells and their responses to impulses in climbing fibres. J. Physiol. (Lond.) **213**, 135–156 (1971).

LAWRENCE, D.G., KUYPERS, H.G.J.M.: The functional organization of the motor system in the monkey. II. The effects of lesions of the descending brain-stem pathways. Brain **91**, 15–36 (1968).

LINDSTRÖM, S., TAKATA, M.: Monosynaptic excitation of dorsal spinocerebellar tract neurones by low threshold joint afferents. Abstracts of Volunteer Papers, XXV Int. Physiol. Congr. Munich 1971. p. 347.

LINDSTRÖM, S., TAKATA, M.: Manuscript under preparation (1971b).

LLINÁS, R., PRECHT, W., KITAI, S.T.: Climbing fibre activation of Purkinje cell following primary vestibular afferent stimulation in the frog. Brain Res. **6**, 371–375 (1967).

LLOYD, D.P.C., McINTYRE, A.K.: Dorsal column conduction of group I muscle afferent impulses and their relay through Clarke's column. J. Neurophysiol. **13**, 39–54 (1950).

LOEWY, A.D.: A study of neuronal types in Clarke's column in the adult cat. J. comp. Neurol. **139**, 53–79 (1970).

LORENTE DE NÓ, R.: Cerebral cortex: Architecture, intracortical connections, motor projections. In: Physiology of the Nervous System, pp. 288–315. (3rd ed.) by J.F. FULTON. New York: Oxford Univ. Press 1949.

LUNDBERG, A.: Integrative significance of patterns of connections made by muscle afferents in the spinal cord. Symposia and Special Lectures, XXI. Int. physiol. Congr. Buenos Aires 1959. pp. 100–105.

LUNDBERG, A.: Ascending spinal hindlimb pathways in the cat. In: Physiology of Spinal Neurons. Ed. by J.C. ECCLES and J.P. SCHADÉ. Progress in Brain Research **12**, 135–163 (1964). Amsterdam-New York: Elsevier Publishing Company.

Lundberg, A.: Integration in the reflex pathway. In: Nobel Symposium. I. Muscular Afferents and Motor Control, pp. 275–305. Ed. by R. Granit. Stockholm: Almqvist & Wiksell 1966.

Lundberg, A.: Function of the ventral spinocerebellar tract. A new hypothesis. Exp. Brain Res. **12**, 317–330 (1971).

Lundberg, A., Norrsell, U., Voorhoeve, P.: Effects from the sensorimotor cortex on ascending spinal pathways. Acta physiol. scand. **59**, 462–473 (1963).

Lundberg, A., Oscarsson, O.: Functional organization of the dorsal spino-cerebellar tract in the cat. IV. Synaptic connections of afferents from Golgi tendon organs and muscle spindles. Acta physiol. scand. **38**, 53–75 (1956).

Lundberg, A., Oscarsson, O.: Functional organization of the dorsal spino-cerebellar tract in the cat. VII. Identification of units by antidromic activation from the cerebellar cortex with recognition of five functional subdivisions. Acta physiol. scand. **50**, 356–374 (1960).

Lundberg, A., Oscarsson, O.: Functional organization of the ventral spino-cerebellar tract in the cat. IV. Identification of units by antidromic activation from the cerebellar cortex. Acta physiol. scand. **54**, 252–269 (1962a).

Lundberg, A., Oscarsson, O.: Two ascending spinal pathways in the ventral part of the cord. Acta physiol. scand. **54**, 270–286 (1962b).

Lundberg, A., Weight, F.: Functional organization of connexions to the ventral spinocerebellar tract. Exp. Brain Res. **12**, 295–316 (1971).

Lundberg, A., Winsbury, G.: Functional organization of the dorsal spino-cerebellar tract. VI. Further experiments on excitation from tendon organ and muscle spindle afferents. Acta physiol. scand. **49**, 165–170 (1960).

Magni, F., Oscarsson, O.: Cerebral control of transmission to the ventral spinocerebellar tract. Arch. ital. Biol. **99**, 369–396 (1961).

Magni, F., Oscarsson, O.: Comparison of ascending spinal tracts activated by group I muscle afferents in the phalanger, rabbit, and cat. Acta physiol. scand. **54**, 37–52 (1962a).

Magni, F., Oscarsson, O.: Principal organization of coarse-fibred ascending spinal tracts in phalanger, rabbit, and cat. Acta physiol. scand. **54**, 53–64 (1962b).

Mann, M.D.: Axons of dorsal spinocerebellar tract which respond to activity in cutaneous receptors. J. Neurophysiol. **34**, 1035—1050 (1971).

Marr, D.: A theory of cerebellar cortex. J. Physiol. (Lond.) **202**, 437–470 (1969).

Massion, J., Urbano, A.: Projections sur le noyau rouge par les colonnes dorsales. Arch. ital. Biol. **106**, 297–309 (1968).

Matsushita, M.: Zur Zytoarchitektonik des Hühnerrückenmarkes nach Silberimprägnation. Acta anat. (Basel) **70**, 238–259 (1968).

Matsushita, M.: Some aspects of the interneuronal connections in cat's spinal gray matter. J. comp. Neurol. **136**, 57–79 (1969).

Matsushita, M.: The axonal pathways of spinal neurons in the cat. J. comp. Neurol. **138**, 391–417 (1970).

Matsushita, M., Ikeda, M.: Olivary projections to the cerebellar nuclei in the cat. Exp. Brain Res. **10**, 488–500 (1970a).

Matsushita, M., Ikeda, M.: Spinal projections to the cerebellar nuclei in the cat. Exp. Brain Res. **10**, 501–511 (1970b).

Miller, S., Nezlina, N., Oscarsson, O.: Projection and convergence patterns in climbing fibre paths to the cerebellar anterior lobe activated from the cerebral cortex and the spinal cord. Brain Res. **14**, 230–233 (1969).

Miller, S., Oscarsson, O.: Termination and functional organization of spino-olivocerebellar paths. In: The Cerebellum in Health and Disease, pp. 172–200. Ed. by W.S. Fields and W.D. Willis. St. Louis: Warren H. Green 1970.

Moatamed, F.: Cell frequencies in the human inferior olivary nuclear complex. J. comp. Neurol. **128**, 109–116 (1966).

Morin, F., Catalano, J.V., Lamarche, G.: Wave form of cerebellar evoked potentials. Amer. J. Physiol. **188**, 263–273 (1957).

Morin, F., Kennedy, D.T., Gardner, E.: Spinal afferents to the lateral reticular nucleus. I. An histological study. J. comp. Neurol. **126**, 511–522 (1966).

MORIN, F., LAMARCHE, G., OSTROWSKI, A. Z.: Responses of the inferior olive to peripheral stimuli and the spinal pathways involved. Amer. J. Physiol. **189**, 401–406 (1957).

MORIN, F., SCHWARTZ, H. G., O'LEARY, J. L.: Experimental study of the spinothalamic and related tracts. Acta psychiat. (Kbh.) **26**, 371–396 (1951).

MURPHY, J. T., SABAH, N. H.: Cerebellar Purkinje cell responses to afferent inputs. I. Climbing fiber activation. Brain Res. **25**, 449–467 (1971).

NACIMIENTO, A. C., LUX, H. D., CREUTZFELDT, O. D.: Postsynaptische Potentiale von Nerven-zellen des motorischen Cortex nach elektrischer Reizung spezifischer und unspezifischer Thalamuskerne. Pflügers Arch. ges. Physiol. **281**, 152–169 (1964).

NEWMAN, P. P., PAUL, D. H.: The projection of splanchnic afferents on the cerebellum of the cat. J. Physiol. (Lond.) **202**, 223–237 (1969).

OLSON, L., FUXE, K.: On the projections from the locus coeruleus noradrenaline neurons: The cerebellar innervation. Brain Res. **28**, 165–171 (1971).

OSCARSSON, O.: Functional organization of the ventral spino-cerebellar tract in the cat. I. Electrophysiological identification of the tract. Acta physiol. scand. **38**, 145–165 (1956).

OSCARSSON, O.: Primary afferent collaterals and spinal relays of the dorsal and ventral spino-cerebellar tracts. Acta physiol. scand. **40**, 222–231 (1957 a).

OSCARSSON, O.: Functional organization of the ventral spino-cerebellar tract in the cat. II. Connections with muscle, joint, and skin nerve afferents and effects on adequate stimulation of various receptors. Acta physiol. scand. **42**, Suppl. 146 (1957 b).

OSCARSSON, O.: Functional organization of the ventral spino-cerebellar tract in the cat. III. Supraspinal control of VSCT units of I-type. Acta physiol. scand. **49**, 171–183 (1960).

OSCARSSON, O.: Differential course and organization of uncrossed and crossed long ascending spinal tracts. In: Physiology of Spinal Neurones. Ed. by J. C. ECCLES and J. P. SCHADÉ. Progress in Brain Research **12**, 164–176 (1964). Amsterdam-New York: Elsevier Publishing Company.

OSCARSSON, O.: Integrative organization of the rostral spinocerebellar tract in the cat. Acta physiol. scand. **64**, 154–166 (1965 a).

OSCARSSON, O.: Functional organization of the spino- and cuneocerebellar tract. Physiol. Rev. **45**, 495–522 (1965 b).

OSCARSSON, O.: Functional significance of information channels from the spinal cord to the cerebellum. In: Neurophysiological Basis of Normal and Abnormal Motor Activities. 3rd Symposium of the Parkinson's Disease Information and Research Center, pp. 93–117. Ed. by M. D. YAHR and D. P. PURPURA. Hewlett, N. Y.: Raven Press 1967.

OSCARSSON, O.: Termination and functional organization of the ventral spino-olivocerebellar path. J. Physiol. (Lond.) **196**, 453–478 (1968).

OSCARSSON, O.: Termination and functional organization of the dorsal spino-olivocerebellar path. J. Physiol. (Lond.) **200**, 129–149 (1969 a).

OSCARSSON, O.: The sagittal organization of the cerebellar anterior lobe as revealed by the projection patterns of the climbing fiber system. In: Neurobiology of Cerebellar Evolution and Development, pp. 525–537. Ed. by R. LLINÁS. Chicago: American Medical Association 1969 b.

OSCARSSON, O.: Note in 'Central Control of Movement'. Ed. by E. V. EVARTS, E. BIZZI, R. E. BURKE, M. DELONG and W. T. THACH. Neurosci. Res. Progr. Bull. **9**, No 1, 97–103 (1971).

OSCARSSON, O., ROSÉN, I.: Short-latency projections to the cat's cerebral cortex from skin and muscle afferents in the contralateral forelimb. J. Physiol. (Lond.) **182**, 164–184 (1966 a).

OSCARSSON, O., ROSÉN, I.: Response characteristics of reticulo-cerebellar neurones activated from spinal afferents. Exp. Brain Res. **1**, 320–328 (1966 b).

OSCARSSON, O., ROSÉN, I., UDDENBERG, N.: Organization of ascending tracts in the spinal cord of the duck. Acta physiol. scand. **59**, 143–153 (1963).

OSCARSSON, O., ROSÉN, I., UDDENBERG, N.: A comparative study of ascending spinal tracts activated from hindlimb afferents in monkey and dog. Arch. ital. Biol. **102**, 137–155 (1964).

OSCARSSON, O., UDDENBERG, N.: Identification of a spinocerebellar tract activated from forelimb afferents in the cat. Acta physiol. scand. **62**, 125–136 (1964).

OSCARSSON, O., UDDENBERG, N.: Properties of afferent connections to the rostral spinocere-bellar tract in the cat. Acta physiol. scand. **64**, 143–153 (1965).

Oscarsson, O., Uddenberg, N.: Somatotopic termination of spino-olivocerebellar path. Brain Res. **3**, 204–207 (1966).

Provini, L., Redman, S., Strata, P.: Mossy and climbing fibre organization on the anterior lobe of the cerebellum activated by forelimb and hindlimb areas of the sensorimotor cortex. Exp. Brain Res. **6**, 216–233 (1968).

Rademaker, G.G.J.: Das Stehen. Monographien a. d. ges. geb. Neurologie u. Psychiatrie **59**, 1–476 (1931). Berlin: Springer.

Réthelyi, M.: The Golgi architecture of Clarke's column. Acta morph. hung. **16**, 311–330 (1968).

Rosén, I.: Localization in caudal brain stem and cervical spinal cord of neurones activated from forelimb group I afferents in the cat. Brain Res. **16**, 55–71 (1969a).

Rosén, I.: Afferent connexions to group I activated cells in the main cuneate nucleus of the cat. J. Physiol. (Lond.) **205**, 209–236 (1969b).

Rosén, I., Sjölund, B.: Organization of group I activated cells in main and external cuneate nuclei: I. Identification of muscle receptors. Exp. Brain Res. (in press) (1972a).

Rosén, I., Sjölund, B.: Organization of group I activated cells in main and external cuneate nuclei: II. Convergence patterns demonstrated by natural stimulation. Exp. Brain Res. (in press) (1972b).

Sasaki, K., Kawaguchi, S., Shimono, T., Yoneda, Y.: Responses evoked in the cerebellar cortex by the pontine stimulation. Jap. J. Physiol. **19**, 95–109 (1969).

Sasaki, K., Strata, P.: Responses evoked in the cerebellar cortex by stimulating mossy fibre pathways to the cerebellum. Exp. Brain Res. **3**, 95–110 (1967).

Shik, M.L.: The controlled locomotion of the mesencephalic cat. Abstracts of Lectures and Symposia, XXV Int. Physiol. Congr. Munich 1971. Vol. 8. pp. 104–105.

Sousa-Pinto, A., Brodal, A.: Demonstration of a somatotopical pattern in the cortico-olivary projection in the cat. An experimental anatomical study. Exp. Brain Res. **8**, 364–386 (1969).

Sprague, J.M.: Spinal "border cells" and their role in postural mechanism (Schiff-Sherrington phenomenon). J. Neurophysiol. **16**, 464–474 (1953).

Szentágothai, J.: Anatomical aspects of junctional transformation. In: Information Processing in the Nervous System. Ed. by R.W. Gerard. Excerpta Medica 119–136. Amsterdam 1962.

Szentágothai, J., Albert, A.: The synaptology of Clarke's column. Acta morph. hung. **5**, 43–51 (1955).

Szentágothai, J., Rajkovits, K.: Über den Ursprung der Kletterfasern des Kleinhirns. Z. Anat. Entwickl.-Gesch. **121**, 130–141 (1959).

Thach, W.T.: Somatosensory receptive fields of single units in cat cerebellar cortex. J. Neurophysiol. **30**, 675–696 (1967).

Thach, W.T.: Discharge of Purkinje and cerebellar nuclear neurons during rapidly alternating arm movements in the monkey. J. Neurophysiol. **31**, 785–797 (1968).

Thach, W.T.: Discharge of cerebellar neurons related to two maintained postures and two prompt movements. II. Purkinje cell output and input. J. Neurophysiol. **33**, 537–547 (1970).

Voogd, J.: The importance of fiber connections in the comparative anatomy of the mammalian cerebellum. In: Neurobiology of Cerebellar Evolution and Development, pp. 493–514. Ed. by R. Llinás. Chicago: American Medical Association 1969.

Voogd, J., Broere, G., van Rossum, J.: The medio-lateral distribution of the spinocerebellar projection in the anterior lobe and the simple lobule in the cat and a comparison with some other afferent fibre systems. Psychiat. Neurol. Neurochir. (Amst.) **72**, 137–151 (1969).

Vyklický, L., Rudomin, P., Zajac III, F.E., Burke, R.E.: Primary afferent depolarization evoked by a painful stimulus. Science **165**, 184–186 (1969).

Walberg, F.: Descending connections to the inferior olive. An experimental study in the cat. J. comp. Neurol. **104**, 77–173 (1956).

Walberg, F.: Corticofugal fibres to the nuclei of the dorsal columns. An experimental study in the cat. Brain **80**, 273–287 (1957).

Wallöe, L.: Transfer of signals through a second order sensory neuron. (Thesis.) Inst. of Physiol., Oslo University 1968.

Wallöe, L., Jansen, J.K.S., Nygaard, K.: A computer simulated model of a second order sensory neurone. Kybernetik **6**, 130–140 (1969).

Chapter 12

Reticular Formation

By

Ottavio Pompeiano, Pisa (Italy)*

With 26 Figures

Contents

* This work was supported by Public Health Service Research Grant NS 07685-04 from the National Institute of Neurological Diseases and Blindness, N.I.H., Public Health Service, USA and by a research grant from the Consiglio Nazionale delle Ricerche, Italy.

I. Introduction

The term reticular formation (RF) has been used by most anatomists to indicate those neurones of different size, scattered within the core of the medulla, pons and mesencephalon and surrounded by a rich and complex network of fibres (see CAJAL, 1909–1911). On the basis of physiological studies, however, there has been the tendency to extend the term to include various diencephalic structures. This tendency has been followed also by several anatomists who studied the specificity of the neuronal structure and the topography of the RF in the brain (see LEONTOVICH and ZHUKOVA, 1963). Since in this way the concept "reticular formation" loses its original precision, we like to follow the definition of the RF given by previous authors (see BRODAL, 1957, 1965, 1966; ROSSI and ZANCHETTI, 1957) who exclude the diencephalic structures from this term.

The observation made by the old anatomists that long ascending and descending projections arise from the RF has been essential for the physiologists, who found that the sphere of influence of the brain stem RF is much broader in scope than was hitherto suspected. It is well known that the RF may influence not only vegetative functions, such as respiration, cardiovascular activity etc., but also somatic functions. The classical observation of MAGOUN (1944) that posture and movements are influenced by reticular stimulation and that of MORUZZI and MAGOUN (1949) that ascending reticular volleys are responsible for the so-called arousal reaction, indicate that the reticular structures are concerned with the control of lower activities in the spinal cord such as the regulation of posture and movements, as well as with the control of high activities in the brain such as wakefulness and sleep. It should finally be mentioned that the RF may also control the sensory communication to the brain by operating at each level of different sensory pathways not only during wakefulness (see HERNÁNDEZ-PÉON, 1961), but also during sleep (see POMPEIANO, 1967 b, 1970). The RF may thus contribute to the processing of sensory information during wakefulness, thus playing a considerable part in the integrated work of the brain, involved in perceptual attention, learning and memory (HERNÁNDEZ-PÉON, 1961). It may also represent the source for the endogenous sensory volleys leading to the oniric activity during desynchronized sleep (POMPEIANO, 1967 b, 1970).

The main aim of this review is to illustrate the role played by the RF in the elaboration and transmission through both ascending and descending reticular projections of the somatosensory volleys originating from both cutaneous and muscular receptors. For this reason it will be essential to survey the anatomical organization i) of those reticular structures, which contribute with their efferent axons to the ascending and descending reticular projections, and ii) of the spinal afferent projection impinging upon the RF. The anatomical and functional organization of the connections between the cerebral cortex and the brain stem reticular structures, as well as the anatomical and functional organization of those reticular nuclei which are specifically related to the cerebellum (namely the paramedian reticular nucleus, the lateral reticular nucleus or nucleus funiculi lateralis, and the nucleus reticularis tegmenti pontis: see BRODAL, 1957) will not be considered here.

II. Anatomy of the Brain Stem Reticular Formation

1. Cytoarchitecture and Synaptology

The RF represents an aggregation of several discrete anatomical units, whose cytoarchitecture has been carefully investigated by OLSZEWSKI and his collaborators in the rabbit (MEESSEN and OLSZEWSKI, 1949) and man (OLSZEWSKI, 1954; OLSZEWSKI and BAXTER, 1954). The main nuclear groups distinguished by these authors have been identified in several mammals both by light microscopy (BRODAL, 1957; ROSSI and ZANCHETTI, 1957; SCHEIBEL and SCHEIBEL, 1958; MANNEN, 1960, 1966a, b; MEHLER et al., 1960; TABER, 1961; VALVERDE, 1962; LEONTOVICH and ZHUKOVA, 1963; PETROVICKY, 1966; RAMÓN-MOLINER and NAUTA, 1966; GRANTYNE, 1967; RAMÓN-MOLINER, 1968) as well as electron microscopy (WESTMAN et al., 1968; BOWSHER and WESTMAN, 1970).

Figure 1 is a diagrammatic map of the RF of the cat, where together with other structures the following reticular nuclei have been outlined respectively in the medulla (nucleus reticularis ventralis, nucleus reticularis lateralis, nucleus reticularis parvicellularis, nucleus reticularis gigantocellularis), the pons (nucleus reticularis pontis caudalis and oralis), and the midbrain (reticular formation of the mesencephalon). Among these reticular structures one may distinguish two main regions, the lateral one-third, composed of small and medium sized cells, and the medial two-thirds, where large and even giant size cells are also present. This distribution is clear-cut in the medulla and pons where the large-sized cells make up the nucleus reticularis gigantocellularis and the nucleus reticularis pontis caudalis, but is less evident in the mesencephalon. However different types of neurones can be found also within the same reticular nuclear region (BRODAL, 1957), for example, the magnocellular region of the bulbar RF, where large polydendritic and smaller oligodendritic neurones can be found (WESTMAN et al., 1968; BOWSHER and WESTMAN, 1970). The dendritic trees of the reticular neurones are highly developed (SCHEIBEL and SCHEIBEL, 1958; VALVERDE, 1961a; MANNEN, 1965a, b) and appear to be oriented chiefly in a plane perpendicular to the long axis of the brain (SCHEIBEL, 1951; SCHEIBEL and SCHEIBEL, 1958), however differences may exist in the patterns of dendritic distribution within the medial and the lateral regions of the RF.

Both axosomatic and axodendritic synapses made by passing axons are widely distributed in the RF. Such an arrangement of synapses ensures the rapid spread of impulses to a large number of neurones in the RF. The observation that axoaxonal synapses, which are the morphological substrate of presynaptic inhibition, can be found among the axodendritic synapses, indicates that the processes occurring in these parts of the brain are capable of coordination and directional control (BOGOLEPOV, 1966).

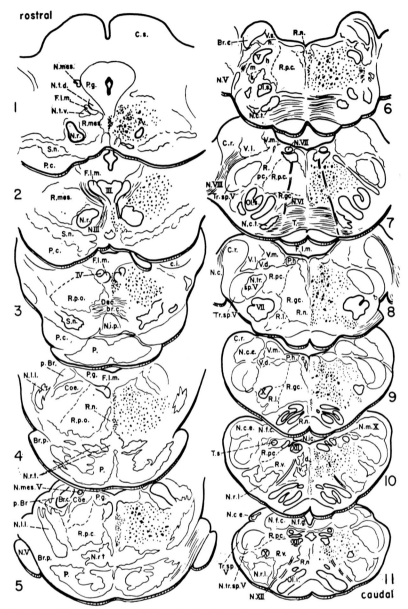

Fig. 1. A cytoarchitectonic map of the reticular formation of the brain stem of the cat. In a series of equally spaced transverse sections are plotted the various cellular groups and their composition of small, medium sized and large cells (Brodal, 1957). Some abbreviations: a, d, and v: Subdivisions of the paramedian reticular nucleus. N.r.: Red nucleus. N.r.l.: Lateral reticular nucleus (nucleus of lateral funiculus). N.r.p.: Nucleus reticularis paramedianus. N.r.t.: Nucleus reticularis tegmenti pontis. R.gc.: Nucleus reticularis gigantocellularis. R.l.: Nucleus reticularis lateralis (Meessen and Olszewski). R.mes.: Reticular formation of the mesencephalon. R.n.: Nucleus of the raphe. R.p.c.: Nucleus reticularis pontis caudalis. R.pc.: Nucleus reticularis parvicellularis. R.p.o.: Nucleus reticularis pontis oralis. R.v.: Nucleus reticularis ventralis. S.c.: Nucleus subcoeruleus. T.s.: Tractus solitarius surrounded by nucleus of solitary tract

As to the synaptic density, it has been calculated that the average density of synapses on dendrites in the gigantocellular region corresponds to about 20% of the total area (KOSITZYN, 1964; BOWSHER and WESTMAN, 1970) and that if we apply these figures for synaptic density to the estimated total neuronal surface (MANNEN, 1966b; BOWSHER and WESTMAN, 1970) we arrive at the figure of 7560 as the total number of synapses in contact with the average polydendritic neurone.

2. Efferent Connections from the Reticular Formation

The different cytoarchitectonic structure of the various nuclei of the RF suggests that they are not functionally equivalent. This hypothesis is supported by investigations on the efferent connections of the various nuclei. We will not consider here the detailed projections of those reticular nuclei which are directed to the cerebellum (see Introduction), but we will devote our attention to the remaining reticular structures of the brain stem. There is a difference in the contribution of the medial two thirds and the lateral one third of these structures to the ascending and descending reticular connections. By studying with the modified Gudden method (BRODAL, 1940) the distribution of cells in the RF showing retrograde changes following transection of the spinal cord or the brain stem rostral to the midbrain, it was found that long ascending and descending fibres arise only in the medial two thirds of the RF (BRODAL and ROSSI, 1955; TORVIK and BRODAL, 1957, respectively). This was confirmed with the Golgi method (SCHEIBEL and SCHEIBEL, 1958, 1961; VALVERDE, 1960, 1961a)[1]. On the contrary the lateral part, composed of small cells, does not give rise to long axons (NAUTA and KUYPERS, 1958; SCHEIBEL and SCHEIBEL, 1958; VALVERDE, 1961b).

Ascending Reticular Projections. The long ascending fibres arise mainly from two fairly well circumscribed regions in the medial RF (BRODAL and ROSSI, 1955). One is in the medulla and covers the caudal part of the nucleus reticularis gigantocellularis and the rostral part of the nucleus reticularis ventralis. The other is in the pons and comprises the caudal part of the nucleus reticularis pontis caudalis (Fig. 2A).

Experimental studies of the termination of the ascending fibres meet serious difficulties, because any lesion of the RF may interrupt fibres ascending from more caudal levels. However observations made with silver impregnation techniques (NAUTA and KUYPERS, 1958; BOWSHER, 1961, 1966, 1967) and the Golgi method (SCHEIBEL and SCHEIBEL, 1958) agree that the fibres coming from pontine and medullary levels reach several non-specific thalamic structures and the subthalamus, chiefly ipsilaterally, while some do not pass beyond the mesencephalic RF. The fibres arising from the mesencephalic tegmentum appear to ascend further than those from the pontine and medullary RF and have been traced chiefly to the ipsilateral hypothalamus, the preoptic area, the septal nuclei and, to a lesser extent, even to the basal ganglia.

Reticulospinal Projections. Interruption of direct reticulospinal fibres leads to retrograde changes in the RF. In particular, reticulospinal fibres appear to arise

---

1 Recent physiological studies (AVANZINO et al., 1966; HÖSLI and WOLSTENCROFT, 1967; AVANZINO and WOLSTENCROFT, 1970) have lead to the identification of neurones in nucleus reticularis gigantocellularis and pontis caudalis which project not only rostrally and/or to the spinal cord, but also to the cerebellum (cf. also ITO et al., 1970).

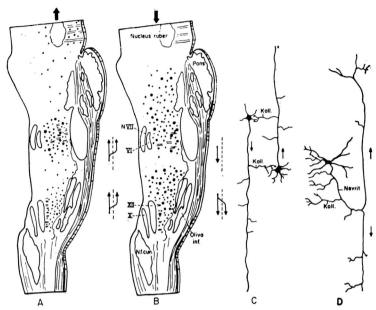

Fig. 2. *A* and *B*: Diagrams showing the distribution of cells of the reticular formation of the cat having long axons ascending beyond the mesencephalon (*A*) and of cells sending long axons to the spinal cord (*B*) plotted on parasagittal sections of the brain stem. Large dots indicate giant cells. Note maximal regions of origin, and that the caudally projecting regions are situated rostral to the rostrally projecting ones. *C:* Diagram showing that by way of collaterals long ascending fibres may act on neurones projecting caudally and *vice versa. D:* Simplified drawing of a reticular neurone whose axon divides into an ascending and a descending branch, illustrating that a single cell may act on the spinal cord and also on levels above the mesencephalon. (BRODAL, 1966)

in the medulla and pons (KOHNSTAMM, 1899; GEHUCHTEN, 1903; LEWANDOWSKY, 1904; PITTS, 1940; BODIAN, 1946; NIEMER, 1948) and perhaps in the mesencephalon (BODIAN, 1946). TORVIK and BRODAL (1957) have shown that in the medulla the somata of the reticulospinal neurones were located in the entire nucleus reticularis gigantocellularis, the rostral part of the nucleus reticularis ventralis and the medial part of the nucleus reticularis lateralis. While in the pons the somata of the reticulospinal neurones were located in the rostral part of the nucleus reticularis pontis caudalis and the caudal part of the nucleus reticularis pontis oralis (Fig. 2 B).

The two medullary and pontine regions projecting to the spinal cord (Fig. 2 B), although partially overlapping those giving-off long ascending fibres (Fig. 2 A) are situated more rostrally. A very close relationship however exists between ascending and descending reticular pathways (BRODAL, 1957, 1966). This is shown by the fact that long ascending and descending axons give off collaterals during their course, the rostral regions having large opportunity for influencing the caudal regions and *vice versa* (Fig. 2 C). Moreover there are cells in the medial third of the RF, whose axons dichotomize, shortly beyond their origin, into long ascending and long descending branches (Fig. 2 D) (HELD, 1893; CAJAL, 1909–1911; SCHEIBEL, 1955 b; SCHEIBEL and SCHEIBEL, 1958).

RETICULO-SPINAL FIBERS

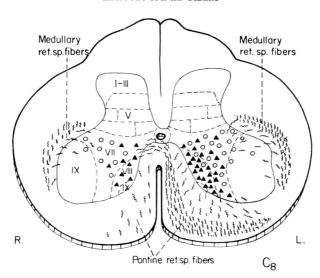

▲ Sites of termination of pontine ret. sp. fibers
○ Sites of termination of medullary ret. sp. fibers

Fig. 3. Diagram showing the sites of termination and the course within the spinal cord of the cat of reticulospinal fibres coming from the pontine and the medullary region of origin, respectively (Fig. 2B). Note difference in distribution of the two components. Roman numbers refer to Rexed's laminae of the cord. (NYBERG-HANSEN, 1965)

The descending reticular fibres course along the ventral funiculus and the ventral part of the lateral funiculus (PAPEZ, 1926; PITTS, 1940; BODIAN, 1946; BEUSEKOM, 1955; TORVIK and BRODAL, 1957; BUSCH, 1964; VERHAART, 1964). While the fibres coming from the pons which course in the medial part of the ventral funiculus are strictly ipsilateral, those arising in the medulla are placed more laterally and are present on both sides of the cord, though chiefly ipsilaterally. These different components of the reticulospinal pathway have also been identified physiologically (ITO et al., 1970).

It was considered doubtful whether the reticulospinal fibres descend below L1, because lesions at more caudal levels did not result in clear-cut retrograde changes in the RF (BODIAN, 1946; TORVIK and BRODAL, 1957). It was then suggested that at caudal levels of the spinal cord the descending reticular pathways are continued by propriospinal fibres (BEUSEKOM, 1955). However, in recent anatomical studies lesions were made in the regions of origin of the reticulospinal fibres, and the degenerating fibres were traced caudally. In this way it could be shown that reticulospinal fibres pass to the lowermost levels of the cord. The explanation for the failure of retrograde degeneration studies to show these fibres may be that the presence of cervical collaterals (BODIAN, 1946; VALVERDE, 1961a) enables reticulospinal neurones to resist chromatolysis following low cord lesions. FOULKES and ROBINSON (1968) introduced [14C]-leucine into the medulla of rat and looked for axonal migration of labelled protein to the spinal cord. They failed to demonstrate reticulospinal fibres with this method. However, electrophysiological experiments have recently shown the existence of reticulospinal neurons in the rat (Fox, 1970). The termination in the grey matter of the cord of the two groups of reticulospinal fibres originating from the medulla and the pons is illustrated in Fig. 3 (NYBERG-HANSEN, 1965, 1966).

Both in cat and monkey, the supraspinal descending pathways can be grouped in two anatomical systems, on the basis of their terminal distribution in the spinal grey matter (SCHIMERT, 1938; SZENTÁGOTHAI-SCHIMERT, 1941; KENNARD and FULTON, 1942; KUYPERS, 1960, 1963, 1964, 1966; KUYPERS et al., 1960, 1962; BUSCH, 1961; STAAL, 1961; NYBERG-HANSEN, 1966; PETRAS, 1967; LAWRENCE and KUYPERS, 1968). The *ventromedial system*, which descends in the ventral, the ventromedial and ventrolateral part of the lateral funiculi, originates in part at least from the medial pontine and medullary RF (and the vestibular nuclei) and terminates preferentially in the ventromedial part of the internuncial zone, namely in the ventromedial parts of laminae VII–VIII (NYBERG-HANSEN and MASCITTI, 1963; NYBERG-HANSEN, 1964, 1965). The *lateral system*, which descends into the lateral funiculus, derives from the sensorymotor cortex and the red nucleus and terminates preferentially in the dorsolateral part of the internuncial zone, namely in the lateral part of laminae V–VII (NYBERG-HANSEN and BRODAL, 1963, 1964).

Interneurones located primarily in the ventral and medial parts of the internuncial zone lead to proximal motor neurones such as those of axial and girdle muscles including extremity extensors, while those located primarily in the dorsal and lateral parts of the internuncial zone lead to distal motor neurones including those of extremity flexors (LLOYD, 1941; BERNHARD and REXED, 1945; APPELBERG, 1962; cf. KUYPERS, 1966; STERLING and KUYPERS, 1968). Physiological observations seem to support this conclusion (KUYPERS, 1963; LAWRENCE and KUYPERS, 1965). It should be mentioned, however, that while the corticospinal and rubrospinal axons have somatotopically organized origins (CHAMBERS and LIU, 1957; POMPEIANO and BRODAL, 1957b; NYBERG-HANSEN and BRODAL, 1963), the medially descending pathways such as the pontine and medullary reticulospinal tracts apparently do not have somatotopically organized origins (BRODAL, 1957; TORVIK and BRODAL, 1957; KUYPERS et al., 1962).

3. Spinal Afferent Connections to the Reticular Formation

The spinoreticular fibres course along the ventrolateral funiculi. Ascending spinoreticular fibres end exclusively within the RF (PROBST, 1902; COLLIER and BUZZARD, 1903; KOHNSTAMM and QUENSEL, 1908; MORIN et al., 1951; JOHNSON, 1954; BEUSEKOM, 1955; MEHLER et al., 1956, 1960; ROSSI and BRODAL, 1957; NAUTA and KUYPERS, 1958). Fibres terminating in the RF may also be provided by collaterals of other ascending systems as the spinothalamic (CAJAL, 1909–1911; MORIN et al., 1951; GLEES, 1952; SCHEIBEL, 1955a; MEHLER et al., 1956, 1960; ROSSI and BRODAL, 1957; NAUTA and KUYPERS, 1958; SCHEIBEL and SCHEIBEL, 1958; MEHLER, 1966), the ventral (COLLIER and BUZZARD, 1903; BLAKELSEE et al., 1938; BEUSEKOM, 1955) and the dorsal spinocerebellar tracts (THIELE and HORSLEY, 1901; COLLIER and BUZZARD, 1903; BEUSEKOM, 1955).

In Golgi studies (CAJAL, 1909–1911; SCHEIBEL, 1955a; SCHEIBEL and SCHEIBEL, 1958, 1961) it appears that the collaterals to the RF given off by the spinotha-

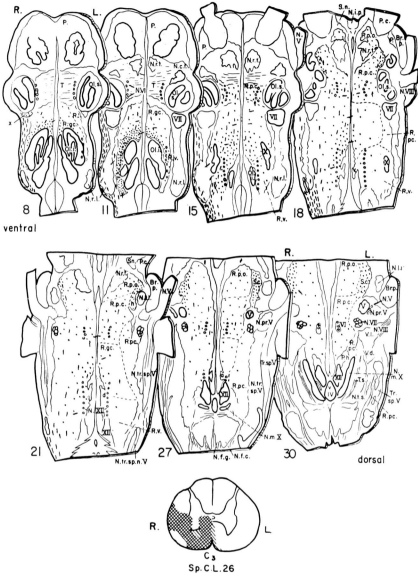

Fig. 4. Diagram showing the distribution within the brain stem reticular formation of ascending fibres from the cord that are degenerating as a consequence of an extensive lesion of the ventro-lateral funiculus of the cord at C_3 (below) in the cat. Sites of termination are indicated by dots, degenerating fibres by waves lines. Note two preferential areas of termination, one in the pons, another in the medulla. In addition fibres end in the nucleus subcoeruleus. The borders of the nuclei are shown, labelled as in Fig. 1. (ROSSI and BRODAL, 1957)

lamic and other long sensory tracts leave the parent fibre with a direction approximately perpendicular to its course. There is therefore a similarity between the orientation of the afferent sensory fibres impinging onto the RF and that of the reticular dendrites, which were reported to be arranged on parallel planes (Schei-bel, 1951; Scheibel and Scheibel, 1958).

The course and termination of the spinoreticular fibres has been investigated in different mammals and in man with the Marchi technique, as well as with the Häggqvist method (see Brodal, 1957; Rossi and Zanchetti, 1957 for references). A more detailed study of the preterminal degeneration of the spinoreticular fibres following spinal cord lesions has been made with silver techniques (Glees and Nauta-Gygax methods) (Johnson, 1954; Mehler et al., 1956, 1960; Mehler, 1957; Rossi and Brodal, 1957; Nauta and Kuypers, 1958).

Johnson (1954) and Mehler et al. (1956, 1960) working in the cat and monkey respectively, showed that most of the reticular subdivisions of the medulla oblong-ata and the pons received spinal afferents, while in the midbrain only the peri-aqueductal grey seemed to have such connections. According to Rossi and Bro-dal (1957) some of the spinoreticular fibres penetrate the lateral regions of the medulla, together with the spinothalamic and ventral spinocerebellar tracts and reach the RF bending medially together with collaterals from these tracts. Other fibres course medially to the lateral reticular nucleus, and can be followed more rostrally, although progressively decreasing in number throughout the medulla and pons (Fig. 4). Thus the spinoreticular fibres are seen to terminate in practically all regions of the bulbar and pontine RF. These fibres terminate chiefly ipsilater-ally within the medulla, whereas an almost equal number of degenerated endings is found on both sides of the pons. Their maximal density is in the medulla, par-ticularly in the ventral part of the nucleus reticularis ventralis and the ventro-caudal part of the nucleus reticularis gigantocellularis (cf. also Bowsher, 1957, 1961; Mehler et al., 1960). The terminations of spinoreticular fibres are rather scanty in the rostral medulla, but again clearly present in the pons, particularly in the nucleus reticularis pontis caudalis and, to a less extent, in the rostralmost part of the nucleus reticularis pontis oralis. Their maximal concentration in the pontine RF is found in the dorsolateral region called nucleus subcoeruleus (cf. also Mehler et al., 1956, 1960; Mehler, 1962) No spinoreticular endings have been found in the mesencephalic RF. It appears also that the spinoreticular projection is not somatotopically organized. These results of Rossi and Brodal (1957) have been confirmed by Nauta and Kuypers (1958) and Anderson and Berry (1959) in cats with the Nauta-Gygax method. According to all these workers, however, some spinal fibres terminate in the lateral regions of the periaqueductal grey and in the mesencephalic tegmentum. Direct spinal afferent fibres to the midbrain RF have been demonstrated also in monkey (Mehler et al., 1960) and man (Bowsher, 1962)[2].

Phylogenetic studies on the course and terminations of the spinoreticular fibres have been performed by Mehler (1957, 1959, 1962, 1966, 1969) and Mehler et al. (1956, 1960). Comparison of the resulting patterns of terminal degeneration in the brain stem of the different species immediately indicated a marked simi-larity of the connections made by the ascending, degenerating spinal fibres. These

---

2 The spinoreticular fibres are rather slender (Johnson, 1954; Rossi and Brodal, 1957; Anderson and Berry, 1959; Busch, 1964; Verhaart, 1964) in contrast with the reticulo-spinal tract which contains a large number of coarse fibres (Torvik and Brodal, 1957; Busch, 1961; Verhaart, 1964; Nyberg-Hansen, 1965).

findings also basically agree with the description given by previous authors (BOWSHER, 1957; ROSSI and BRODAL, 1957). The only differences which can be noticed concern the identification of the reticular nuclei in the pons and the distribution of the spinoreticular fibres on these reticular structures.

An interesting finding which arises from the phylogenetic studies is that the termination of spinal fibres in the upper brain stem is well pronounced only in the higher species. In particular in the nonprimates the spino-mesencephalic fibres chiefly follow widely scattered courses through the more central midbrain tegmentum. In the opossum only a few fibres ascend in the dorsolateral tegmentum. In the rat and cat respectively, increasing numbers of ascending fibres appear in this region and the density of fibres ascending in the dorsolateral tegmentum is almost equal to the density of fibres ascending in the central tegmental region. In the primate species, however, all of the ascending fibres at mesencephalic level are incorporated into one compact, dorsolateral tegmental fibre group corresponding to the position of the "classical" spinothalamic tract of human anatomy (*i.e.*, the neospinothalamic tract). Apparently the mesencephalic connections of these fibres do not change, but there is an apparent phyletic shift in the region of passage of the "palaeospinothalamic" projections (HERRICK and BISHOP, 1958; BISHOP, 1959) from the central to the dorsolateral tegmentum. Although the terminal connections with the mesencephalon and diencephalon do not change, the apparent phyletic shift in the region of passage of the palaeospinothalamic fibre projections might explain some of the interspecific differences encountered in functional studies of the system in question (cf. DELGADO, 1955; MELZACK et al., 1958; LALONDE and POIRIER, 1959; DENNIS and KERR, 1961).

BOWSHER et al. (1968 b, and BOWSHER and WESTMAN (1970) have studied the spinal afferent degeneration to the gigantocellularis reticular region of cat at both light and electron microscope. Degenerating presynaptic terminals of spinal origin were seen in contact with both soma and dendrites of both types of neurones, polydendritic and oligodendritic. Spinal afferents to polydendritic (and oligodendritic) neurones are extremely scattered in their distribution on the neurone surface, varying from distal dendrites to soma. Rough counts in silver impregnated sections from hemichordotomized animals suggest that each side of the spinal cord contributes something of the order of 100 boutons to every $10^6 \mu^2$ of the gigantocellular area. Further calculations suggest that only one in 1000, at the most, of presynaptic endings on polydendritic neurones are of direct spinal origin. It was suggested that such a minute proportion of presynaptic endings could not alone fire gigantocellular neurones from the periphery without assuming the existence of a relay in the caudalmost part of the bulbar RF intercalated between the spinal cord and the gigantocellular region. It appears however from a further study (WESTMAN and BOWSHER, 1971) that the spinal afferents in the caudal medullary reticular area terminate in the same way as in the gigantocellular region. Synaptic contacts are thus made with both oligodendritic and polydendritic cells, but the amount of terminal degeneration after spinal hemisection seems to be very low on each individual neurone.

The terminal distribution of the spinoreticular fibres is largely coincident with those parts of the RF which are the main site of origin of the long fibres ascending to the thalamus and the subthalamus (BRODAL, 1957; ROSSI and BRODAL, 1957).

This distinction however should not be taken too strictly, as they synapse also with reticulospinal neurones. There is in fact physiological evidence indicating that somatic afferent volleys may trigger not only ascending but also descending reticular neurones (see Sections V, VI and VII).

The possibility that reticular elements may receive sensory information not only by way of collaterals or terminals of sensory reticulopetal fibres, but also by sending the dendritic branches outside the reticular structures, mainly to the sensory nuclei and the sensory tracts themselves, has been clearly documented in Golgi studies (Scheibel, 1951). However, there is no positive evidence that fibres from the medial lemniscus enter the RF (Torvik, 1956; Bowsher, 1958; Valverde, 1961 a).

A final comment concerns the possibility that primary spinal afferents terminate directly on the brain stem RF. It appears that following lumbosacral dorsal rhizotomies (L1, L5, L6 and S1) degenerating fibres from all roots, excepting S1, terminate not only in the spinal trigeminal complex, but also in the nucleus reticularis parvicellularis bilaterally (Hand, 1966). The pathway from the dorsal roots to the nucleus reticularis parvicellularis was not determined in this study. Preliminary findings, however, suggested that the dorsal root projection to the spinal trigeminal complex and nucleus reticularis parvicellularis ascend the dorsal funiculus and shift laterally at higher cord levels (thoracic or cervical) into the spinal trigeminal tracts. At levels rostral to the obex, sparse degenerating fibres pass bilaterally from the ventral region of the tractus spinalis trigemini into the ventral regions of the spinal trigeminal complex and the nucleus reticularis parvicellularis (Hand, 1966).

In summary both the projections descending to the spinal cord (cf. Torvik and Brodal, 1957) and those ascending to the thalamus, the subthalamus, the hypothalamus and the basal ganglia (cf. Brodal and Rossi, 1955; Nauta and Kuypers, 1958) arise from cells lying within the medial RF. Although some degree of overlapping is constantly present between the two neuronal populations, the cells giving rise to the fibres descending to the spinal cord are mostly located in the rostral medulla and in the middle pons (Torvik and Brodal, 1957), while those sending their axons to rostral brain structures are concentrated in the caudal medulla and the caudal pons (Brodal and Rossi, 1955; Nauta and Kuypers, 1958). Furthermore ascending fibres originate in the midbrain also, while the descending projections arise only in the medulla and in the pons. From these considerations on the efferent connections of the RF it is clear that the view that this structure is diffusely organized can hardly be maintained (Brodal, 1957). One may conclude that the RF is an assembly of different units having different efferent projections and presumably different functions.

These units however should not be considered as mutually independent as shown also by the Golgi studies which have furnished the anatomical basis for a rich interplay between the various "units" (Scheibel, 1951, 1955a, b; Scheibel and Scheibel, 1958; Valverde, 1961a, b; 1962). *First*, there is a partial overlapping in the medial region between the sites of origin of the descending and the ascending fibres (Torvik and Brodal, 1957). *Second*, many reticular units dichotomize into a rostrally and caudally projecting branch (Held, 1893; Cajal, 1909–1911; Scheibel, 1955b; Scheibel and Scheibel, 1958). *Third*, the long neurites arising from cells belonging to the medial parts of the RF, which are characterized by a longitudinal course, establish connections with other levels of the brain stem, which are sometimes placed at a considerable distance (SCHEIBEL, 1955b; SCHEIBEL et al., 1955; BRODAL, 1966). *Fourth*, reticular axons send collaterals not only to these remote structures in the brain, but also to motor and sensory nuclei of the cranial nerves (SCHEIBEL and SCHEIBEL, 1958) and also to neighbouring regions of the RF. This is the case for the neurones of the lateral RF, whose axons project mainly onto neighbouring medial regions approximately at the same level of the brain stem.

If we consider now the organization of the afferent fibres to the RF which originate from the spinal cord, it appears that most of these afferent fibres are mainly ditributed within the medial rather than the lateral reticular regions. Moreover the spinoreticular path ends mostly within the caudal parts of the medulla and pons (ROSSI and BRODAL, 1957), *i.e.*, in those regions which give rise mainly to fibres ascending to the thalamus and the subthalamus. However, even reticulospinal neurons may receive spinal afferents.

These observations should be correlated with the finding that the direct cortico-reticular fibres, which originate chiefly from the sensorimotor cortex, end in groups of reticular cells which are placed rostrally to those receiving spinal projections (see ROSSI and BRODAL, 1956), *i.e.*, in those regions which give rise to reticulospinal fibres. However, some of the direct corticoreticular fibres end also in the more caudal part of those regions which receive spinal afferents and send long ascending fibres (ROSSI and BRODAL, 1956; BRODAL, 1957, 1965).

The relative specificity of different regions of the RF is also suggested by the fact that the reticulopetal projections arising from the basal ganglia, the hypothalamus and the epithalamus go to the midbrain reticular formation (see BRODAL, 1957; ROSSI and ZANCHETTI, 1957 for references), which in turn project to the hypothalamus and to the basal ganglia. On the contrary, the mesencephalic reticular structures receive very few, if any cortical and spinal fibres.

All these findings, together with the observations made on the cytoarchitecture and the synaptology of these structures indicate that the RF cannot be regarded as a homogeneous structure, but rather as an extremely complex aggregate of cell groups, sometimes interconnected, but certainly having their own functional significance.

III. Ascending Reticular Influences Induced by Somatic Afferent Volleys in the Intact, Free-Moving Animal

1. EEG and Behavioural Effects Induced by Cutaneous Afferent Volleys

Sensory stimulation in mammals causes arousal associated with the orienting reflex. The desynchronization of the electroencephalogram (EEG) associated with the arousal reaction is attributed to excitation of the ascending reticular activating system (MORUZZI and MAGOUN, 1949) and the mechanisms involved have been reported in detail in several review articles (MAGOUN, 1950, 1954, 1958; ROSSI and ZANCHETTI, 1957; MORUZZI, 1958). It appears in particular that this effect

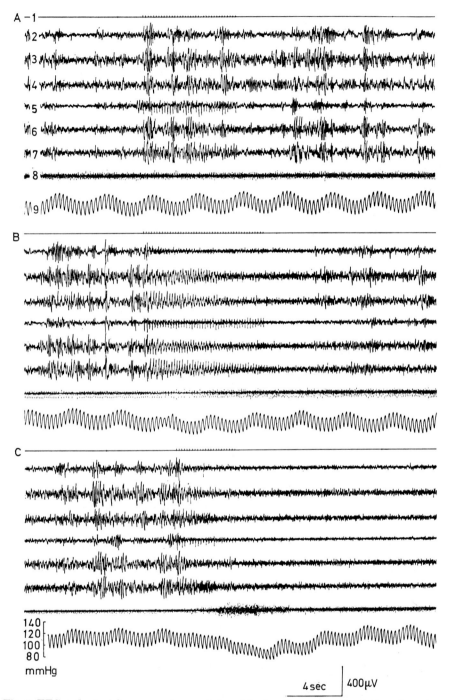

Fig. 5. EEG and arterial pressure changes induced by low frequency stimulation of a cutaneous nerve with increasing stimulus intensities. Intact unanaesthetized cat. Experiment made
36 hours after implantation of the electrodes and cannulation of the left femoral artery. Stimulation of the left superficial radial nerve with rectangular pulses at 5/sec, 0.5 msec pulse dura-

is mediated via the unspecific thalamocortical system (JASPER, 1960). On the other hand section of the spinal cord at C_1 may produce EEG synchronization (HODES, 1963; D'ANNA and BONVALLET, 1966). An interesting problem is to know whether sensory stimulation under particular conditions can induce a synchronized cortical activity and behavioral signs of sleep.

The attempt to produce sleep by applying given patterns of afferent stimulation in well-controlled conditions originates from the experiments of the Pavlov's school (PAVLOV, 1932; cf. MORUZZI, 1960, 1964). Behavioral and/or EEG manifestations of sleep have been obtained by natural stimulation (KOCH, 1932a, b; SCHWEITZER, 1937; KREINDLER, 1946; BONVALLET et al., 1954; NAKAO et al., 1956; MAZZELLA et al., 1957; GLUCK and ROLAND, 1959; MANCIA et al., 1959; TAKAGI et al., 1959; ARDUINI and HIRAO, 1960; OSWALD, 1960; WEISS, 1961; VAN REETH and CAPON, 1962; CAPON and VAN REETH, 1963; KUMAZAWA, 1963), and by electrical stimulation of receptors or sensory organs (GRASTYÁN et al., 1952; MAZZELLA et al., 1957; BONVALLET and SIGG, 1958; OSWALD, 1960; ROITBAK, 1960; WEISS, 1961; MARILLAUD et al., 1966).

Among the different kinds of afferent systems which were able to induce EEG and behavioral signs of sleep, was included the spinal afferent system (TAKAGI et al., 1959; ROITBAK, 1960; WEISS, 1961; KUMAZAWA, 1963). Intense exteroceptive stimulation even produced sleep in normal humans although the stimuli were considered unpleasant (OSWALD, 1960). These findings are not in agreement with the observations of COLLE and GYBELS (1957), who demonstrated that, in the curarized cat, high or low frequency of stimulation at various intensities of a peripheral nerve caused arousal.

POMPEIANO and SWETT (1961a, b, c; 1962a, b) devised experiments for testing the conditions under which EEG synchronization or arousal could be elicited by peripheral nerve stimulation. A preliminary requirement for this type of investigations is to apply well controlled patterns of sensory stimulation in the unanaesthetized, unrestrained animal. By using this approach it became clear that EEG and behavioural effects of sleep or wakefulness appeared with carefully controlled cutaneous nerve stimulation. Moreover, the stimulus response characteristics proved to be precise and repeatable and could be correlated with known afferent

---

tion. Bipolar records. I: stimulus marker; 2: left fronto-frontal; 3: left parieto-temporal; 4: left temporo-occipital; 5: right fronto-frontal; 6: right parieto-temporal; 7: right temporo-occipital; 8: left neck EMG; 9: arterial pressure recorded from the left femoral artery. A: stimulation with 0.30 V causes a generalized EEG synchronization outlasting the stimulus. Note waxing and waning of the response. There is a slight tendency for the synchronization to follow the rate of stimulation; note the primary evoked potentials recorded from the right postcentral gyrus (record 5). No changes in arterial pressure are observed. B: stimulation with 0.37 V causes EEG synchronization in parietal, temporal and occipital leads which gives way to arousal. The rhythm of synchronization follows the rate of stimulation. Note the effectiveness of the arousal in the frontal leads and the slight reduction in amplitude of the primary evoked potentials compared with A. During arousal there is a slight drop in arterial pressure. C: stimulation with 0.50 V causes strong EEG and EMG signs of arousal. There is a marked fall of arterial pressure and a slight increase of the heart rate. In this preparation the threshold for the primary evoked potential was 0.17 V, the threshold for EEG synchronization 0.19 V, and that for arousal 0.37 V. (POMPEIANO and SWETT, 1962b)

fibre groups in terminal experiments, when an analysis of the conduction velocities was made with those stimulus intensities yielding EEG synchronization or desynchronization (see Pompeiano, 1963, 1965).

The EEG and the EMG were recorded in the cat with chronically implanted electrodes, while stimulating electrodes were applied to cutaneous nerves (Pompeiano and Swett, 1961a, b; 1962a). Provided that the general EEG background was not strongly activated, it was always possible to produce EEG synchronization and behavioral sleep with low rate stimulation of low threshold cutaneous fibres. Particularly trains of low rate (3–8/sec), low intensity rectangular pulses applied to the superficial radial nerve produced rhythmic, high voltage, low frequency oscillations over wide regions of the cortex (Fig. 5A). Induced EEG synchronization was bilateral and best developed in the parietal, temporal and occipital cortices. This pattern of synchronization was accompanied by closure of the eyes at the onset of the stimulus and by reduction of the EMG activity of the skeletal musculature (Section V). The waxing and waning of the large cortical waves, so often seen when the EEG is spontaneously synchronized, was often observed during induced synchronization. This phenomenon had the tendency to outlast the duration of the stimulus (Fig. 5A). With increased intensities of stimulation the EEG synchronization became more pronounced. With additional increases of stimulus intensity, however, a point was reached which brought about temporary EEG desynchronization and abolition of the synchronizing influences (Fig. 5B). Stronger stimuli caused a generalized and longer lasting pattern of EEG desynchronization (Fig. 5C). A strong arousal reaction was accompanied by opening of the eyes and a marked increase in the tonic EMG activity.

The effects of changing not only the stimulus intensity but also the stimulus frequency applied to the cutaneous nerve were also investigated. The frequency of the synchronous waves followed that of the electrical pulses, provided the rate of stimulation was lower than 8/sec; above 8/sec there was a gradual reduction in the amplitude of the synchronized EEG patterns. When rates of stimulation higher than 12–16/sec were used, only EEG and behavioral arousal was obtained. Thus the same low threshold cutaneous afferents can elicit EEG synchronization or arousal depending on the rate of stimulation. The higher threshold cutaneous fibres cause arousal at either low or high stimulus frequencies.

The optimum stimulus parameters for obtaining EEG synchronization were ineffective when applied on an EEG background of low voltage, fast activity, either during behavioral arousal or during desynchronized sleep. Furthermore, the threshold for induced arousal on low rate stimulation of the cutaneous afferents increased during transition from quiet wakefulness to synchronized or light sleep and reached its highest values during desynchronized or deep sleep.

An analysis of the primary evoked potentials elicited by cutaneous nerve stimulation during the different EEG backgrounds indicated that during arousal the primary responses were small. They increased in amplitude during synchronized sleep, while during desynchronized sleep they were always equal to or greater than the responses observed in synchronous state. It appears therefore that the primary evoked potentials undergo a steady increase in size with increasing depths of sleep, while the pattern of induced synchronization becomes prominent only during light sleep.

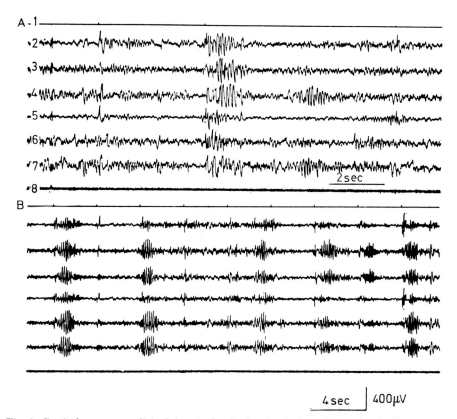

Fig. 6. Cortical responses elicited by single shock stimulation of low threshold cutaneous afferents. Unrestrained, unanaesthetized cat. Experiment made 3 days after the implantation of the electrodes. Stimulation of the right superficial radial nerve with 0.13 V, 0.5 msec pulse duration. Bipolar records taken at different speeds. 1: stimulus marker; 2: left fronto-parietal; 3: left parieto-temporal; 4: left temporo-occipital; 5: right fronto-parietal; 6: right parieto-temporal; 7: right temporo-occipital; 8: EMG of the posterior cervical muscles. The generalized cortical responses elicited by single shock stimulation of low threshold cutaneous afferents is composed of an early and a late component. The early component usually has the characteristic of a diphasic positive-negative deflection and a latency of 20–30 msec as observed at the C.R.O. with monopolar recording. It is often followed by a burst of rhythmic waves, similar to "tripped" spindle bursts. (POMPEIANO, 1965)

When the frequency of stimulation applied on a background of drowsiness was reduced to 1/sec, while the stimulus intensity was maintained at low levels, a generalized response was evident in the dorsal aspect of the neocortex, which was generally made up of two components (Fig. 6). The early component, a diphasic positive-negative potential, had a latency of 20–30 msec (range 15–60 msec) while the late component was a prolonged burst of rhythmic waves. The early component had the same characteristics as the secondary evoked potentials recorded from the associative areas of the cortex in unanaesthetized cats and resulted from spinal activation of the nonspecific thalamic structures including the thalamic *centre median* (MAGOUN and MCKINLEY, 1942; STARZL et al., 1951a; FRENCH et

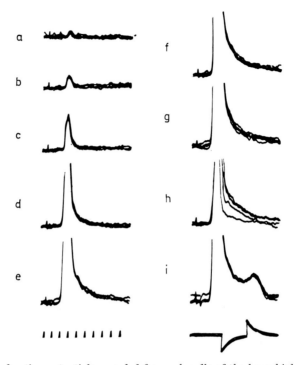

Fig. 7. Compound action potentials recorded from a bundle of the branchial plexus initiated by electrical stimulation of the superficial radial nerve. Cat under Nembutal anaesthesia. Monopolar recording. Stimulation of the right superficial radial nerve with rectangular pulses 0.6 msec duration, and increasing voltages. Five superimposed sweeps for each record (except for h). Nerve length 138 mm. Time: 1000/sec. Voltage calibration: 100 μV. For each record the voltage of stimulation and the lowest conduction velocity of the compound action potential are the following: a: 0.08 V, corresponding to the threshold for the primary evoked potential (48 m/sec); b: 0.09 V, corresponding to the threshold for synchronization at 4/sec (46 m/sec); c: 0.13 V (38 m/sec); d: 0.19 V (29 m/sec); e: 0.22 V corresponding to the threshold for arousal at 4/sec (19 m/sec); f: 0.25 V (16 m/sec); g: 0.31 V (16 m/sec); h: 4 superimposed sweeps, obtained by increasing stimulus strengths (respectively 0.19–0.22–0.25–0.31 V) showing the additional activation of fibres conducting at rates lower than 38 m/sec when the threshold for arousal is reached; i: 1.17 V (16 m/sec) showing full activation of group III fibres (peak at 20 m/sec). Comparison of the neurograms corresponding to the threshold for EEG synchronization or arousal shows that group II fibres are responsible for EEG synchronization; however, when the threshold for arousal is reached the most important change of the neurogram is the widening of the wave due to activation of slower conducting fibres belonging to group III. The highest conduction velocity in this case was 81 m/sec. (POMPEIANO and SWETT, 1962b)

al., 1952; BUSER and BORENSTEIN, 1955, 1956, 1957, 1959; BUSER, 1957; ALBE-FESSARD and ROUGEUL, 1958; ALBE-FESSARD et al., 1959; KRUGER and ALBE-FESSARD, 1960; ALBE-FESSARD and FESSARD, 1963). The late component was similar to the slow after-discharge or "tripped" spindle bursts which had been shown to occur when stimulating certain thalamic structures (MORISON and DEMPSEY, 1942; JASPER, 1949, 1960; BREMER and BONNET, 1950). Similarly to the induced EEG synchronization elicited by repetitive stimulation of the cutaneous nerve, the secondary evoked responses and the following "tripped" spindles became prominent only during light sleep.

The nature of the cutaneous afferent volleys causing generalized EEG synchronization was analyzed by POMPEIANO and SWETT (1961c, 1962b). After careful control of the thresholds for induced EEG synchronization and arousal, the cats were anaesthetized with Nembutal, and the neurogram of the superficial radial nerve was recorded from the posterior division of the brachial plexus (Fig. 7). Group II cutaneous fibres which conducted at rates above 36 m/sec, were found to be responsible for the EEG synchronization when low rate of stimulation was used. On the other hand, high rate stimulation of group II cutaneous afferents as well as low and high stimulation of group III afferents, constantly produced EEG and behavioural arousal.

It is known that different modalities of cutaneous sensation cannot be strictly referred to definite fibre sizes (see BURGESS and PERL, Chapter 2). It seems, however, that touch receptors are essentially confined to the group II range, hair and pressure receptors account for a large proportion of both group II and III cutaneous afferent groups, while fibres belonging to temperature-sensitive and pain receptors appear to be restricted to the group III range of the myelinated fibres and group IV fibres (see POMPEIANO and SWETT, 1962b for references). It may be inferred from these findings that stimulation of touch, pressure and hair receptors, producing low rate synchronous volleys in group II cutaneous afferents should be capable of producing cortical synchronization. This conclusion fits the common observation that cats tend to relax and show a sleeping behavior when their fur is gently and rhythmically stroked. Strong stimulation of the same cutaneous modalities, such as wrong way stroking of the hairs which would produce higher rates of discharges in a higher number of receptors, or stimulation of receptors innervated by group III fibres, which are partially nociceptive in nature, should be capable of producing arousal.

Concerning the pathways responsible for these ascending effects, stimulation (MAGNES et al., 1961) and lesion experiments (POMPEIANO and SWETT, 1962b) indicate that the dorsal column system is not critically responsible for the induced pattern of EEG synchronization; nor is this pathway involved in the induced arousal (cf. also ANDERSSON, 1962a, 1967; ANDERSSON et al., 1964). Moreover both EEG synchronization and arousal could still be obtained after cerebellectomy. Hence, the ascending volleys responsible for both these effects are likely to be mediated by fibres ascending along the ventral and lateral funiculi. When the spinal cord section also affected the dorsal part of the lateral funiculi, there was a tendency of the animal to show the desynchronized EEG pattern typical of the waking state (cf. also GIAQUINTO et al., 1964b; D'ANNA and BONVALLET, 1966)[3]. Moreover the threshold for both the flexion reflex and the arousal reaction was decreased after this transection (GIAQUINTO et al., 1964b; ANDERSSON, 1967; cf. D'ANNA and BONVALLET, 1966). These effects can be referred to interruption of supraspinal descending pathways exerting a tonic inhibitory control on the central transmission of cutaneous afferent volleys to both flexor motoneurones and ascend-

---

3 Similar effect was also observed after injection of novocaine to one side of the spinal cord at C_1 (HODES, 1964).

ing spinoreticular pathway (Section X). However, even in this condition both the arousing as well as the synchronizing effects of the somatic volleys could still be elicited.

This finding should be correlated with the observation that tracts ascending in the cat's ventral and lateral funiculi other than the spinocerebellar tracts are activated not only by group III cutaneous fibres (Collins and O'Leary, 1954; Collins and Randt, 1956), but also by low threshold cutaneous afferents (cf. Oscarsson, 1958; Lundberg and Oscarsson, 1961, 1962 b). Additional interruption of the dorsolateral funiculus and of its ascending pathways, leaving only the ventral columns and the ventral part of the lateral columns intact, also permits transmission of group II and III cutaneous volleys, which thus ascend the cord via the ventral quadrants of the spinal cord to reach structures of the brain stem RF where EEG synchronizing (or arousing) effects may be brought into play.

The observation that group II and III cutaneous afferents produced EEG synchronization or arousal respectively when stimulated at low rates indicate the existence of two entirely different ascending mechanisms exerting on the EEG, and possibly on the animal behaviour, opposite influences (see Moruzzi, 1960, 1964; Bonvallet and Block, 1961). It is of interest that even in the brain stem reticular formation there are regions which upon stimulation at low rates may elicit either EEG synchronization (Magnes et al., 1961; Favale et al., 1961) or EEG arousal (Magnes et al., 1961). However, since reticular neurones do not have the intrinsic property of producing regular rhythmic bursts of unit discharge in such a relation to thalamic spindles as to suggest an intimate functional relationship (Junge and Sveen, 1968), one may suggest that the reticular influences on the cortical rhythm mentioned above most likely reflect changes in the temporal pattern of ascending volleys impinging on the thalamic pacemaker mechanism.

It will be shown later (Section VII, 5) that stimulation of group II cutaneous afferents influences preferentially the caudalmost part of the brain stem, particularly the nucleus reticularis gigantocellularis, while stimulation of the higher threshold cutaneous afferents activates also neurones of the mesencephalic and pontine reticular formation (Pompeiano and Swett, 1963a).

It may be asked how these different regions of the brain stem reticular formation can produce opposite EEG effects when impinged upon by group II and group III cutaneous volleys. The early component of the synchronizing EEG response elicited by single shock stimulation of group II cutaneous afferents, similar to that elicited by single shock stimulation of brain stem structures including the reticular formation (Moruzzi and Magoun, 1949; Rossi and Zanchetti, 1957; Magnes et al., 1961), can be attributed to active driving of the nonspecific thalamic structures including the *centre median* (see page 397). Indeed the same type of activity can also be obtained by electrical stimulation of thalamic nuclei (for references see Spencer and Brookhart, 1961). The arrival of synchronous volleys at these nuclei is made possible by the fact that the nucleus reticularis gigantocellularis activates the thalamic structures either directly or through an oligosynaptic chain of ascending reticular neurones (Albe-Fessard et al., 1962; Albe-Fessard and Mallart, 1962; Bowsher et al., 1963; Petit and Mallart, 1964; Albe-Fessard and Bowsher, 1965; Bowsher, 1966; Bowsher and Petit, 1966; Bowsher et al., 1968a). On the other hand the late component of the EEG response, represented by a series of rhythmic waves similar to a "tripped" spindle burst, is probably the consequence of autochthonus activity of the thalamic pacemaker in response to the arrival of synchronous impulses (BREMER and BONNET, 1950; JASPER, 1960; PURPURA and YAHR, 1966; ANDERSEN and ANDERSSON, 1968).

It should be pointed out that the EEG synchronization induced by low rate stimulation of cutaneous nerves may outlast the end of the stimulus by several seconds. Since the pattern of EEG synchronization is, in itself, generally regarded as the expression of a decrease in tonic activity of the ascending reticular activating system, it may be postulated that the synchronous response which outlasts the stimulus signifies a reduction or removal of tonic EEG desynchronizing influences arising from the reticular activating system (cf. also MORUZZI, 1960, 1964; DELL et al., 1961). There is no evidence, however, that neurones belonging to the ascending reticular activating system are *directly* inhibited by the synchronous sensory volleys (POMPEIANO and SWETT, 1963a).

So far we have considered the effects produced by low rate stimulation of group II cutaneous afferents. Group III cutaneous volleys may also influence the synchronizing mechanisms of the thalamus; and indeed there is evidence that group II and III volleys converge on the thalamic structures, which are considered responsible for the associative responses (KRUGER and ALBE-FESSARD, 1960; MALLART, 1960, 1961). However, when the higher threshold cutaneous afferent volleys are activated, there is also an activation of the ascending reticular system (MORUZZI and MAGOUN, 1949), which overwhelms the synchronizing response. The desynchronization of the EEG in spite of the low rate stimulation of the group III cutaneous afferents is probably due to asynchronous bombardement of the aspecific thalamic nuclei by a polysynaptic chain of ascending reticular neurones.

In summary, the opposite EEG reactions, namely the synchronization and the arousal elicited respectively by selective low frequency stimulation of group II and III cutaneous fibres, are apparently due to activation of different reticular pathways, made by oligosynaptic and polysynaptic chains of ascending reticular neurones.

It should finally be recalled that high frequency stimulation of group II cutaneous afferents also produced arousal, whereas at low frequency it induced EEG synchronization. Therefore, the same ascending pathway can exert different EEG effects depending on its temporal pattern of discharge. It is of interest that an EEG arousal can also be obtained with high frequency stimulation of brain stem structures which elicited EEG synchronization if stimulated at low rates (MAGNES et al., 1961; FAVALE et al., 1961).

2. EEG and Behavioural Effects Induced by Muscular Afferent Volleys

Low rate stimulation of hindlimb muscular nerves performed in unrestrained, unanaesthetized cats, elicited EEG synchronization with stimulus intensities at or above threshold for muscular contraction (POMPEIANO and SWETT, 1962a). A stronger stimulus caused a marked arousal. The higher the frequency of stimulation, the lower was the threshold for arousal. However, when muscular contraction was prevented by ligature of the nerve distally to the stimulating electrodes, induced EEG synchronization was abolished, but the arousal reaction could still be elicited, particularly when high stimulus strengths were applied to the muscle nerves.

Analysis of the muscle nerve fibres conducting the volleys responsible for the EEG arousal was carried out by utilizing animals whose threshold for arousal was well substantiated in several trials (Pompeiano and Swett, 1962b). As a terminal experiment the cats were anaesthetized with Nembutal, and the neurogram of the hamstring or the gastrocnemius nerve was recorded from L7–S1 dorsal roots.

Group I muscular afferents, which originate from primary endings of muscle spindles and Golgi tendon organs, were entirely without influence on both behaviour and EEG, while the arousal reaction occurred with low frequency stimulation of group III muscular afferents, which originate apparently from pressure-pain receptors. For high stimulus rates, high threshold group II muscular afferents may have contributed to the production of arousal.[4] These results were obtained by stimulating hindlimb muscular nerves on a background of drowsiness or synchronized sleep. Similar to the finding obtained by stimulating cutaneous nerve, even the arousal threshold obtained by muscular nerve stimulation increased with increasing depth of sleep (Pompeiano and Swett, 1962a). In desynchronized sleep particularly, the threshold for behavioral arousal was higher than during synchronized EEG backgrounds, thus duplicating the findings obtained by stimulating brain stem structures under the same conditions (Rossi et al., 1961). The activation of the ascending reticular activating system by the group II and III muscular afferent volleys is mediated by pathways ascending along the ventral quadrants (Pompeiano and Swett, 1962b).

Since forelimb may be more effective than hindlimb muscle nerves, a second series of experiments was performed in unrestrained, unanaesthetized animals to compare the effects of fore- and hindlimb muscular nerve stimulation during stages of synchronized sleep and wakefulness (Giaquinto et al. 1962, 1963b). It was found that high rate stimulation (200/sec) of the group I afferent fibres in both fore- and hindlimb muscular nerves did not produce any detectable EEG or behavioral change in awake or sleeping cats. Both the mechanisms of spatial and temporal summation of group I impulses were ineffective in producing arousal. In fact, simultaneous stimulation at high rates of the deep radial nerve of both sides produced an arousal reaction only at stimulus intensities above the group II threshold. Contrary to the group I volleys, group II afferent volleys from the hamstring nerve provoked weak behavioral arousal only when the EEG patterns were those of relaxed wakefulness. During synchronized sleep, arousal could usually be obtained at stimulus intensities near threshold for group III activation. Group II afferent volleys from the deep radial nerve had more powerful arousing actions than those from the hamstring nerve. Strong arousal could in fact be obtained with group II volleys either during synchronized sleep or wakefulness. The quantitative difference between the arousal thresholds obtained with hindlimb

---

4 Although the majority of group II fibres come from secondary endings in muscle spindles (cf. Hunt, 1954), the presence of fibres of this diameter innervating other receptors has been shown by Paintal (1960), Barker (1962) and Barker et al. (1962). Thus the presence of "group II effects" does not necessarily imply that they are caused by secondary endings from the spindles.

and forelimb muscular nerve stimulation can be referred to several factors. It has been postulated in particular that differences in central actions of muscular afferent volleys originating from various deep nerves depend primarily upon differences in their afferent fibre constituents (McINTYRE, 1962a, b; GIAQUINTO et al., 1963b). It has also been suggested that the forelimb muscular afferents may have a more intense projection into the brain stem reticular formation compared with hindlimb projection (GIAQUINTO et al., 1963b).

In summary, no EEG synchronization could be obtained in unrestrained cats with low rate stimulation of muscular afferents, provided that muscular contraction was prevented by ligature of the nerve distally to the stimulating electrodes. The only EEG effect observed by stimulating a muscular nerve was the arousal reaction. This effect occurred with low frequency stimulation of group III fibres, which are assumed to innervate pressure-pain receptors. For higher stimulus rates, high threshold group II muscular afferents, which originate from the secondary endings of muscle spindles, may contribute to the production of arousal. In any case, however, high rate stimulation of group I afferent fibres in fore- and hindlimb muscular nerves was unable to produce any EEG change in awake or sleeping cats.

More recently experiments were performed in which the EEG was recorded together with spinal reflexes induced by muscular afferent volleys in unrestrained, unanaesthetized cats (GIAQUINTO et al., 1963a, 1964a). It is known that the motoneurones of the lateral gastrocnemius muscle, which is extensor in function, are monosynaptically activated by group Ia afferent volleys coursing in the medial gastrocnemius nerve, but are inhibited by group Ib, II and III fibres of same nerve. The high threshold muscular afferents of this nerve also excite polysynaptically the flexor motoneurones, including those innervating the tibialis anterior muscle. GIAQUINTO et al. (1963a, 1964a, b) have recorded EMG responses of the lateral gastrocnemius and of the tibialis anterior to graded electrical stimulation of the medial gastrocnemius nerve. Repetitive stimulation (at 100/sec for 2 sec) of the low threshold muscular afferents capable of activating only the heteronymous monosynaptic reflex pathway, never produced an arousal reaction (Fig. 8A). The threshold for an arousal reaction was reached only when the high threshold muscular afferents were stimulated, as shown by the typical occurrence of the flexion reflex pattern (Fig. 8B–D). This fact gives further support to the claim that the group Ia afferent volleys do not exert any particular influence on the ascending reticular activating system.

It was assumed for years that the somatic afferent sources impinging upon the reticular formation include low threshold stretch sensitive afferents from muscles. The observation that afferent volleys confined to the group I spectrum of both fore- and hindlimb muscular nerves failed to elicit any observable EEG and behavioral changes (POMPEIANO and SWETT, 1962b; GIAQUINTO et al., 1963b) indicate that volleys originating from the primary endings of muscle spindles and the Golgi tendon organs, do not have any detectable influence upon the ascending reticular activating system. It may be questioned therefore, whether the arousal produced by activation of the spindle receptors after injection of succinylcholine (MOTOKIZAWA and FUJIMORI, 1964) can be referred to group Ia afferent volleys, and whether the decrease of such impulses during muscle relaxation plays an

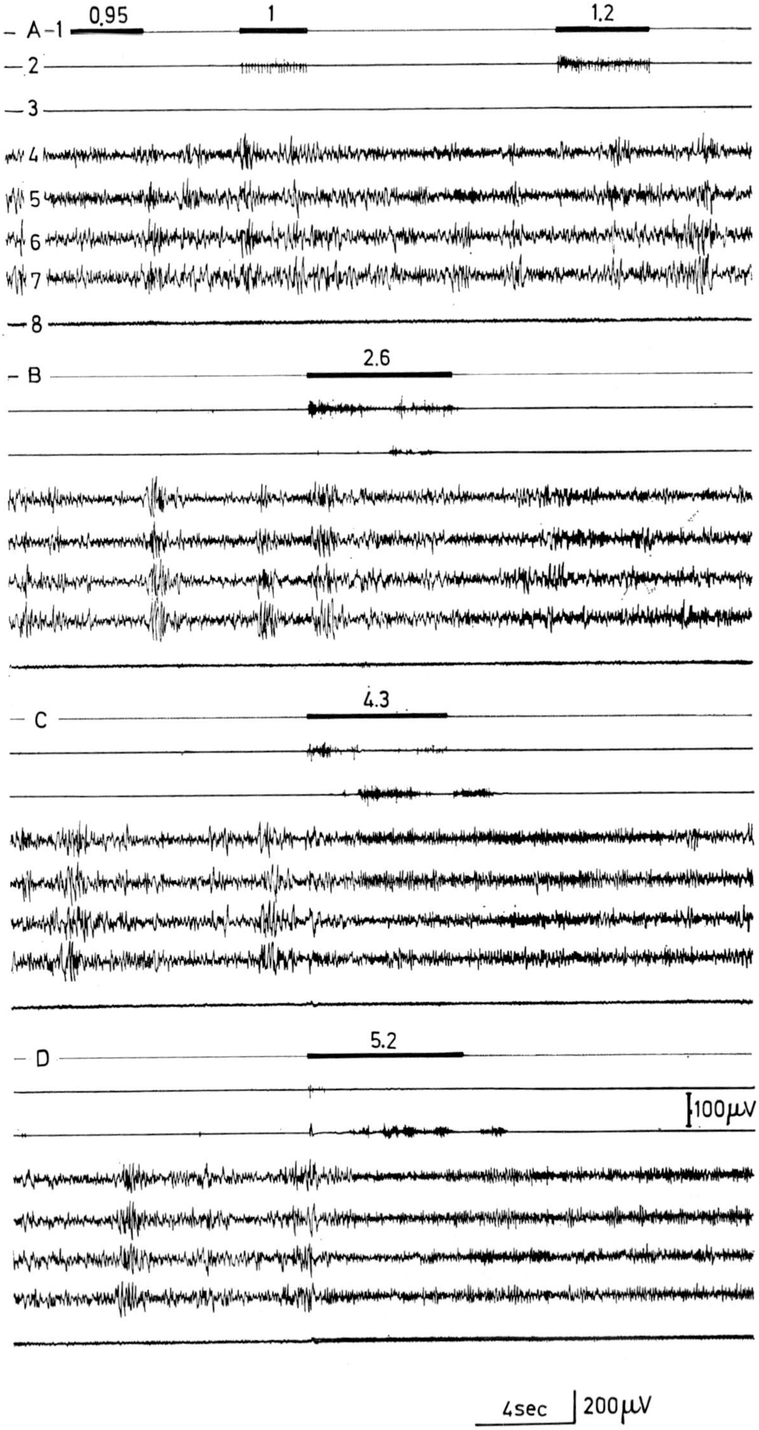

Fig. 8

important role in precipitating sleep (KLEITMAN, 1929, 1939; GAY and GELLHORN, 1949; GELLHORN, 1958; HODES, 1962; LISSÁK et al., 1962; BLOCH, 1965; BLOCH et al., 1965). In both groups of experiments, the described effects can actually be referred to activation or inactivation of the secondary endings of the muscle spindles. Moreover the arousal reaction elicited by passive movements of the limbs (BERNHAUT et al., 1953) can be attributed to stimulation of receptors other than the muscle spindles.

The findings reported above should be correlated with the observation made in decerebrate, cerebellectomized animals indicating that group II and group III muscular afferents are able to influence the activity of brain stem reticular units, recorded either extracellularly or intracellularly (POMPEIANO and SWETT, 1963a, b; MAGNI and WILLIS, 1964b; LIMANSKII, 1966; BARNES and POMPEIANO, 1971a; POMPEIANO and BARNES, 1971). Some units, however, could also be influenced by Ib muscle afferents, but not by Ia afferents (POMPEIANO and BARNES, 1971). There is also evidence that the associative nuclei of the thalamus do not receive either group I and II muscular afferents volleys, but only group III afferent volleys (MALLART, 1960, 1961).

3. Sensory Discrimination with Cutaneous and Muscular Nerve Volleys

Animals can be easily trained to discriminate between relatively gross somaesthetic cues (ALLEN, 1947; STAMM and SPERRY, 1957), but little has been done in the past to establish a clear relationship between a somaesthetic discrimination threshold and the requisite amount of peripheral nerve activity (ZUBEK, 1952).

The number of fibres activated can be rigidly controlled by direct electrical stimulation of peripheral nerve bundles, first achieved in human studies (HEINBECKER et al., 1933; PRATTLE and WEDDELL, 1948; COLLINS et al., 1960; SHAGASS and SCHWARTZ, 1961, 1963; DEBECKER and DESMEDT, 1964; GIBLIN, 1964; UTTAL and COOK, 1964; DEBECKER et al., 1965), and recently in experimental animals by implanting an electrode around a peripheral nerve. In particular, the method of indwelling peripheral nerve-stimulating electrodes in chronic animals, devel-

Fig. 8. Thresholds for the monosynaptic and polysynaptic reflexes as well as for the arousal measured on an EEG background of synchronization in an unrestrained, unanaesthetized cat with spinal cord intact. Stimulation of the left medial gastrocnemius nerve at 100/sec, 0.05 msec pulse duration. Bipolar records. 1: stimulus marker; 2: EMG of the left lateral gastrocnemius muscle; 3: EMG of the left tibialis anterior muscle; 4: left parieto-temporal; 5: left temporo-occipital; 6: right parieto-temporal; 7: right temporo-occipital; 8: EMG of the posterior cervical muscles. A: monosynaptic reflex (MR) obtained at progressively increasing stimulus intensities. These are expressed in multiples of the threshold for the heteronymous MR elicited on a background of wakefulness. Note the complete absence of any EEG arousal by stimulating the nerve for stimulus intensities capable of eliciting only the MR. B: stimulation of the nerve with stimulus intensity at threshold for the ipsilateral flexion reflex. The threshold for the inhibition of the MR was 1.72 T (not shown). C,D: a further increase in the stimulus intensity is followed by an enhancement of the segmental effects elicited by stimulating the FRA (i.e., inhibition of the extensor and facilitation of the flexor muscle) and by marked arousal reaction. Actually, the threshold for the arousal was 3.4 T during synchronized sleep, but increased up to 5.5 T on a background of desynchronized sleep. (GIAQUINTO et al., 1964b)

oped by POMPEIANO and SWETT (1962a, b), has been later used by BOURASSA and SWETT (1966, 1967), SWETT and BOURASSA (1967b), SWETT et al. (1964) in behavioral discrimination responses. Cats were trained to bar-press for food rewards in response to sensory cues produced by direct stimulation of cutaneous and muscle nerves. By varying stimulus intensity, sensory discrimination thresholds from a cutaneous nerve were compared with the reactions produced by muscle nerve volleys. This approach incidentally provided a test to reveal whether or not afferent discharges from stretch receptors in mammalian striated muscle play an important role in sensory perception.

The sensory discrimination threshold to superficial radial nerve volleys occurred at essentially the same stimulus intensity that produced a threshold response in the peripheral nerve and the contralateral cerebral cortex (SWETT et al., 1964; BOURASSA and SWETT, 1966, 1967), thus confirming results in humans (HEINBECKER et al., 1933; PRATTLE and WEDDELL, 1948; COLLINS et al., 1960; HENSEL and BOMAN, 1960; SHAGASS and SCHWARTZ, 1961, 1963; DEBECKER and DESMEDT, 1964; GIBLIN, 1964; DEBECKER et al., 1965). It was postulated that only a very small number of cutaneous afferent fibres need be activated to permit sensory discrimination in the cat, in agreement with experiments on man from which it was inferred that a single sensory receptor of the skin, when activated may affect conscious experience (HENSEL and BOMAN, 1960; MELZACK and WALL, 1962).

The results also support the statement by MOUNTCASTLE and POWELL (1959b) "... that the threshold for cortical response, which is assumed to lead to perception of the peripheral event, is set by the threshold of the sensory receptors in the periphery". However an evoked cortical response is not necessarily associated with perception (GIBLIN, 1964), particularly when a muscular nerve is stimulated (see page 407).

It has already been mentioned in Section III, 2 that no EEG changes could be elicited by direct stimulation of muscle nerves at group I intensities in the cat (POMPEIANO and SWETT, 1962a, b; GIAQUINTO et al., 1963b). The evidence that afferent discharges from muscle stretch receptors give rise to conscious experience in man is contradictory. On the basis of introspective and clinical evidence, early experimenters suggested that conscious sensations from muscle, if present at all, were extremely weak, and could play no direct role in kinaesthesis, which was assumed to be mediated primarily by joint afferents (cf. PROVINS, 1958; MOUNTCASTLE and POWELL, 1959a; ROSE and MOUNTCASTLE, 1959). There was not always complete agreement (WINTER, 1912; CLEGHORN and DARCUS, 1952; GOODWIN et al., 1972), though several investigations tend to confirm this view (SARNOFF and ARROWOOD, 1947; COHEN, 1952; BROWNE et al., 1954; PROVINS, 1958; DAY and SINGER, 1964; MERTON, 1964; CARTER and GELFAN, 1965; GELFAN and CARTER, 1967). Moreover, stretch receptors in the extraocular eye muscles of man may fail to give rise to conscious sensations (IRVINE and LUDVIGH, 1936; LUDVIGH, 1952; BRINDLEY and MERTON, 1960; MERTON, 1961).

More direct evidence in the cat that these afferent volleys are unable to produce a sensory cue for triggering a behavioural response was given by BOURASSA and SWETT (1966), SWETT and BOURASSA (1967b) and SWETT et al. (1964). In these preparations the sensory discrimination threshold to cutaneous nerve volleys occurred at stimulus intensity which produced threshold activation of the peripheral nerve, but they responded to deep radial nerve volleys only when the stimulus intensity was at or above group II afferent fibre threshold. Sensory discrimination thresholds with hamstring nerve volleys occurred at stimulus intensities approaching group III afferent fibre threshold.

Spatial and temporal facilitation of group I afferent volleys was also ineffective in exposing any latent ability of the subject to discriminate group I volleys (cf. GIAQUINTO et al., 1963 b).

The observation that subjects could not discriminate group I hamstring nerve volleys (SWETT and BOURASSA, 1967 b) would have been easy to understand on the basis of early studies indicating that information from primary endings of hindlimb muscle spindles does not reach to sensorimotor cortex (MOUNTCASTLE et al., 1952; GARDNER and HADDAD, 1953; McINTYRE, 1953, 1962 a, b; KRUGER, 1956; MOUNTCASTLE and POWELL, 1959 a; ROSE and MOUNTCASTLE, 1959; MALLART, 1960, 1961; ANDERSSON, 1962 b; NORRSELL and WOLPOW, 1966). Recent experiments, however, indicate that group I afferents from the hindlimb may influence the cerebral cortex in both primates (ALBE-FESSARD and LIEBESKIND, 1964, 1966; ALBE-FESSARD et al., 1964, 1965, 1966; LAMARRE and LIEBESKIND, 1965; LIEBESKIND et al., 1965), and cats (LANDGREN and SILFVENIUS, 1968 a, b, 1969 a; LANDGREN, 1969). Group I volleys from the forelimb, particularly from the deep radial nerve, also failed to produce discrimination in cats (SWETT and BOURASSA, 1967 b) in spite of the large-amplitude evoked response which can be recorded from the contralateral posterior sigmoid gyrus in a small zone anterior to the postcruciate dimple (AMASSIAN and BERLIN, 1958 a, b; OSCARSSON and ROSÉN, 1963, 1966; OSCARSSON, 1964 b, 1966; ANDERSSON et al., 1966; BOURASSA and SWETT, 1966; OSCARSSON et al., 1966; SWETT and BOURASSA, 1966, 1967 a, b; GRAMPP and OSCARSSON, 1968; OSCARSSON et al., 1969; LANDGREN, 1969).[5]

Similar considerations have been applied to secondary spindle afferents. The central projections of these group II afferents are little known, but in view of the inability of the cat to discriminate group II hamstring volleys, it has been postulated that secondary spindle afferents of the forelimb also do not contribute to discrimination (SWETT and BOURASSA, 1967 b). The fact that the subjects responded to deep radial nerve volleys at intensities near group II afferent fibre threshold was attributed to activation of joint afferents, which are absent from the hamstring nerve at the site of stimulation.

The inability of the subject to discriminate forelimb group I volleys and the observation that the area of the cerebral cortex influenced by these volleys is anterior to the postcruciate dimple have led to the conclusion that supraspinal group I actions are engaged in motor functions (OSCARSSON, 1964 b; SWETT and BOURASSA, 1967 a, b). This hypothesis is apparently supported by the fact that pyramidal tract cells can be activated by group I afferent volleys (SWETT and

---

5 The group I volleys from cat's forelimb apparently influence other cortical regions in addition to the area near the dimple (ANDERSSON et al., 1966; LANDGREN and WOLSK, 1966; LANDGREN et al., 1967; SILFVENIUS, 1968; LANDGREN, 1969). There is also evidence that low threshold muscle afferents of hand and forearm project to part of the first somatic sensory area of baboon's cortex (PHILLIPS et al., 1971).

BOURASSA, 1966, 1967a). According to OSCARSSON et al. (1966) the extensive and widespread convergence in the group I projection path to the motor cortex suggests that the modality of information carried concerns changes in muscle tone, rather than stages of movements and position. Direct experiments are reguired to test this hypothesis.

It is particularly interesting that ascending group I volleys from forelimb muscles ascend in the dorsal funiculus (HOLMQVIST et al., 1963; OSCARSSON and ROSÉN, 1963) to relay in the dorsal column nuclei and the ventrobasal complex (OSCARSSON and ROSÉN, 1963, 1966; MALLART, 1964a, b, 1968; OSCARSSON, 1964b, 1966; ANDERSSON et al., 1966; SWETT and BOURASSA, 1966, 1967a; ROSÉN, 1967, 1968a, b, 1969a, b, c, 1970; LANDGREN, 1969; ROSÉN and SJÖLUND, 1969) before reaching the cerebral cortex, thus paralleling the primary cutaneous sensory pathway in the dorsal column-medial lemniscal system. The group I path from the hindlimb ascends in the dorsolateral funiculus of the spinal cord, with the medullary relay in nucleus z of BRODAL and POMPEIANO (1957), as shown recently (LANDGREN, 1969; LANDGREN and SILFVENIUS, 1969b, 1971; SEGUIN et al., 1972), while the thalamic relay is located in a restrict region of nucleus ventralis postero-lateralis (BOIVIE et al., 1970; LANDGREN and SILFVENIUS, 1970).

Group I and cutaneous primary relay systems may interact at the level of the thalamus and cortex (ANDERSSON et al., 1966; OSCARSSON et al., 1966; LANDGREN and SILFVENIUS, 1968a). Low threshold cutaneous and group I volleys also have powerful converging excitatory action on pyramidal tract and non-pyramidal tract cells in the cortical group I projection zone (OSCARSSON et al., 1966; SWETT and BOURASSA, 1966, 1967a). SWETT and BOURASSA (1967a, b) suggest that the neurones influenced by group I afferent volleys are not a part of the neuronal systems involved in the discriminative process. The same cells, when influenced by cutaneous volleys, also may not be involved in the discriminative process. Consequently, discrimination to weak cutaneous volleys may have resulted from activation of neurones that were not within the sphere of influence of the group I afferent systems. Many regions of the brain stem reticular formation, thalamus and cerebral cortex that are powerfully influenced by cutaneous volleys do not appear to receive any significant group Ia action (MALLART, 1960, 1961; POMPEIANO and SWETT, 1963a, b; MAGNI and WILLIS, 1964b; LIMANSKII, 1966; BARNES and POMPEIANO, 1971a; POMPEIANO and BARNES, 1971).

IV. Ascending Reticular Influences Induced by Somatic Afferent Volleys in the Acute, Thalamic Animal

The observation by POMPEIANO and SWETT (1962a, b) that electrical stimulation of a cutaneous nerve may precipitate a pattern of sleep or wakefulness according to the parameters of stimulation applied to the different groups of cutaneous afferents led CARLI et al. (1964) to find out whether the same volleys may also be able to modify the sham-range behaviour in acute thalamic cats, which occurs spontaneously, i.e., in the absence of purposeful stimulation (CANNON and

BRITTON, 1925; BARD, 1928). This behaviour which results from release of hypo-thalamic, subthalamic and tegmental structures (BARD, 1928; CARLI et al., 1966), can also be elicited reflexly by weak peripheral stimuli, in which case the sham-rage is attributed to reflex stimulation of the ascending reticular activating system, whose volleys impinge upon the hypothalamus (MALLIANI et al., 1963). CARLI et al. (1964) have applied a bipolar collar-type electrode carrier on the superficial radial nerve of hypothalamic cats. Low frequency stimulation (at 4–8/sec) of the group II cutaneous fibres was unable to inhibit the sham-rage behaviour, whereas low frequency stimulation of group III cutaneous afferents or high frequency repetitive stimulation of group II afferents generally produced rage outbursts. In the most excitable preparations repetitive electrical stimulation of the superficial radial nerve (at 100–300/sec) produced attacks of sham-rage at a threshold stimulus intensity corresponding to 1.2–1.5 times the threshold for the most excitable group II afferents and also by light tactile stimulation.

Thalamic transection releases the diencephalic mechanisms from forebrain inhibition, thus leading to a very high degree of excitability of these mechanisms and this experimental situation may explain why low rate stimulation of group II cutaneous afferents, which induces an EEG and behavioral pattern of light sleep in the intact preparation, is unable to depress the sham-rage behaviour in the decorticate animals.

It may be asked now whether high rate electrical stimulation of the group I fibres, which is unable to induce electrocorticographic or behavioural arousal in intact unrestrained cats (POMPEIANO and SWETT, 1962a, b; GIAQUINTO et al., 1963b), can produce behavioural effects when the excitability background of the preparation is increased. MALLIANI et al. (1968) have tested electrical stimulation of low threshold muscle afferents in the acute thalamic cat using the hamstring nerve. Sham-rage outbursts were elicited by high frequency stimulation of the hamstring nerve at intensities ranging from 1.36 to 2.88 T with a mean value of 1.72 T. These effects persisted in some experiments even after cerebellectomy. Since the threshold for the group II fibres evaluated at dorsal root level in 10 of these experiments ranged from 1.70 to 2.12 T it appears that a least in some experiments, the induced sham rage was due to stimulation of group II muscle afferents. In the remaining experiments, however, sham-range outbursts were induced reflexly by stimulation of high threshold group I muscular afferents.

The results of MALLIANI et al. (1968) indicate that electrical stimulation of the hamstring nerve is capable of activating the diencephalic mechanisms of rage behavior at an average threshold (1.72 T) lower than that obtained for the arousal reaction tested on a background of quiet wakefulness in the intact preparation (2.64 T in the experiments of GIAQUINTO et al., 1963b). This lower value may result from an increased responsiveness of the ascending reticular neurones in the hypothalamic preparation due to descending facilitatory influences from the subthalamus (ADEY and LINDSLEY, 1959) and other rostrally placed structures. It appears also that the high threshold group I muscular afferents, probably origi-nating from Golgi tendon organs, are capable of activating the diencephalic mechanisms of rage behavior after they are released by decortication or thalamic transection.

We conclude this section by mentioning that vegetative changes can be elicited by selective stimulation of different groups of cutaneous and muscular afferents in different types of preparation other than the decorticate animal. The effects of cutaneous afferent volleys were tested in anaesthetized preparations (Molina et al., 1953; Laporte and Montastruc, 1957), unanaesthetized curarized (Colle and Gybels, 1957) or free-moving animals (Pompeiano and Swett, 1962b), and in decerebrate preparations (Laporte and Montastruc, 1957). Differences in the results obtained may be attributed to differences in the experimental preparations used.

The reflex changes in blood pressure elicited by repetitive stimulation of the different groups of muscular afferents have been investigated by Laporte et al. (1960, 1962) in cats decerebrated at an intercollicular level or anaesthetized with chloralose. All these experiments were performed under artificial respiration following curarization in order to abolish the circulatory changes due to somatic and respiratory reflexes. Repetitive stimulation of group I fibres, innervating the primary endings of the muscle spindles and the Golgi tendon organs, was not followed by any reflex change in general blood pressure (cf. also Skoglund, 1960; Johansson, 1962; Malliani et al., 1968). Stimulation of group II muscle afferents innervating the secondary endings of the muscle spindles was unable to produce any effect at low rates, while a moderate increase in blood pressure occurred at high frequencies of stimulation (200/sec). Stimulation of group III muscular afferents produced hypotension at low frequencies of stimulation, and hypertension when high frequencies of stimulation were used. In any case high frequency stimulation of unmyelinated group IV fibres produced large hypertension.

V. Descending Reticular Influences Induced by Somatic Afferent Volleys in the Intact, Free-Moving Animal

Low rate stimulation of group II cutaneous afferents, performed in unrestrained, unanaesthetized cats, produces EEG synchronization over the entire dorsal aspect of the neocortex and behavioural sleep (see Section III, 1). High rate stimulation (above 12–16/sec) of group II and low or high rate stimulation of group III cutaneous afferents produces EEG desynchronization and behavioural arousal (Pompeiano and Swett, 1962a, b). Experiments were performed to find out whether, in the same preparations, stimulation of cutaneous afferents is also able to produce changes in postural tonus and spinal reflexes (Giaquinto and Pompeiano, 1963a, b, 1964).

Low rate stimulation (from 1 to 10/sec, 0.05 msec pulse duration) of the superficial radial nerve, at stimulus intensities capable of activating only the group II cutaneous afferents, did not produce any change in postural tonus when performed on a background of strong arousal, whereas on a background of relaxed wakefulness or synchronized sleep the same stimulation was followed by a decrease of the postural tonus of the neck musculature and of the lateral gastrocnemius (antigravitary muscles). The spontaneous activity of the tibialis anterior (flexor muscle) was also depressed by the low threshold cutaneous afferent volleys.

The effects increased in intensity and occurred earlier when the rate of stimulation was increased from 1 to 10/sec; at 20/sec the initial decrease in the tonus of the neck muscles was followed by marked enhancement, while at 100/sec only an increase of the electromyographic activity of neck muscles was observed.

Low rate stimulation of group II cutaneous afferents also reduced or abolished the heteronymous monosynaptic reflex produced by stimulating the medial gastrocnemius nerve at 100/sec with stimulus intensities ranging from 1.0 to 1.2 times the threshold for the monosynaptic reflex (Fig. 9). The reflexly-induced depression of the monosynaptic response was i) increased by raising from 1 to 10/sec the rate of stimulation of the superficial radial nerve (Fig. 9) as well as its intensity, provided the stimulus remained subliminal for group III cutaneous afferents, and ii) little evident in the aroused state, but prominent in the stages of relaxed wakefulness or synchronized sleep, i.e., when the central excitatory state decreased.

The abolition of the heteronymous monosynaptic reflex produced by low rate stimulation of group II cutaneous afferents was a consequence of an inhibitory process which did not depend upon mechanisms of reciprocal innervation, since i) it was observed by stimulating both the ipsilateral and the contralateral superficial radial nerve; ii) the reduction of the tonus and the decrease of the monosynaptic response of the antigravity muscles were not accompanied by reciprocal effects on the antagonistic flexor muscles. Actually, when not only the monosynaptic reflex but also the polysynaptic reflex were elicited by appropriate stimulation of the medial gastrocnemius nerve, low rate stimulation of cutaneous group II fibres inhibited both reflexes.

In summary, low rate stimulation of group II cutaneous afferents, performed in the unrestrained, unanaesthetized cat produced a striking inhibition of both spontaneous and reflex muscular activities. This phenomenon was generalized, and affected both the extensor and flexor muscles, as well as the heteronymous monosynaptic extensor and the polysynaptic flexor reflex produced by repetitive stimulation of the medial gastrocnemius nerve.

The depression of the somatic activities induced by group II cutaneous afferent volleys is reminiscent of the depression of the spinal motility, particularly of the spinal reflexes, observed when the pressure was increased within the carotid sinus or following electrical stimulation of the Hering nerve or of vagal afferents (see GIAQUINTO and POMPEIANO, 1964 for references). Although in several instances the depression of the somatic activities might have been related to the fall of blood pressure, in other cases this cause of error was eliminated or found to be unimportant. Even in these experiments, behavioral manifestations of sleep and/or EEG synchronization were obtained by natural stimulation (KOCH, 1932a, b; SCHWEITZER, 1937; KREINDLER, 1946; BONVALLET et al., 1954; NAKAO et al., 1956; MAZZELLA et al., 1957; VAN REETH and CAPON, 1962; CAPON and VAN REETH, 1963) and by electrical stimulation (GRASTYÁN et al., 1952; MAZZELLA et al., 1957; BONVALLET and SIGG, 1958) of baroceptive and vagal afferents.

The depression of the spinal reflex activity induced by cutaneous nerve stimulation is usually accompanied by an electrocortical synchronization; however, this

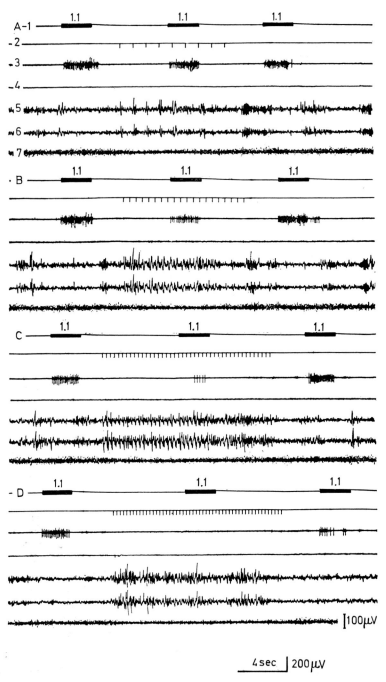

Fig. 9. Effects of different frequencies of stimulation of the group II cutaneous afferents on the monosynaptic extensor reflex. Unrestrained, unanaesthetized cat. Experiment made 4 days after implantation of the electrodes. 1: stimulus marker relative to the left medial gastrocnemius nerve, crushed and tied distally to the stimulating electrode; 2: stimulus marker

depression does not necessarily depend on it (POMPEIANO and SWETT, 1962a, b). The EEG synchronizing effect of cutaneous nerve stimulations is observed only when low rate stimulation of group II fibres is applied in a background of drowsiness and is missed altogether when the animal shows EEG and behavioral patterns of arousal (POMPEIANO and SWETT, 1962a). In this experimental condition, however, the inhibition of the spinal reflexes may still be observed.

The depression of spinal reflexes elicited by group II cutaneous afferent volleys is stronger than the slight reduction which appears spontaneously in the unrestrained unanaesthetized cat, during transition from wakefulness to synchronized sleep (GIAQUINTO et al., 1964a), thus resembling that which occurs during desynchronized sleep (GIAQUINTO et al., 1964a). The slight depression of spinal reflexes during synchronized sleep is generally attributed to reduction of the descending facilitatory influences impinging upon both a- and γ-motoneurones. There is evidence for this in the fact that fusimotor activity is reduced during synchronized sleep (EULER and SÖDERBERG, 1956; BUCHWALD and ELDRED, 1961; HONGO et al., 1962, 1963; SHIMAZU et al., 1962a, b; GASSEL and POMPEIANO, 1965). On the other hand, stimulation of group II cutaneous afferents, besides influencing the ascending mechanisms which lead to the occurrence of EEG synchronization — a condition which *per se* would produce only a very slight depression of the spinal reflexes — may also produce a much greater reduction of spinal activities, possibly by activating neural mechanisms which come spontaneously to light during the physiological episodes of desynchronized sleep. It has been demonstrated that the abolition of spinal reflexes occurring spontaneously during desynchronized sleep is due to excitation of supraspinal inhibitory structures probably localized in the medullary and pontine reticular formation (GIAQUINTO et al., 1964b).

The lack of regular effects of the group II volleys on the brain stem centres responsible for the ascending and descending manifestations of desynchronized sleep may arise because spatial and temporal summation of the group II cutaneous volleys is required to exert a complete activation of the brain stem inhibitory structures. When high rate stimulation of the group II cutaneous afferents is performed or when higher threshold group III cutaneous afferents are activated, there is also a specific excitation of the neurones of the mesencephalic and pontine reticular formation, where the ascending and descending activating systems are located (AMASSIAN and DEVITO, 1954; COLLINS and O'LEARY, 1954; COLLINS and RANDT, 1960, 1961; POMPEIANO and SWETT, 1963a). In this case the costimulation of the ascending activating system, as well as of the facilitatory reticulospinal system, counteracts the triggering action exerted by low threshold cutaneous

---

relative to the left superficial radial nerve; 3: EMG of the left lateral gastrocnemius muscle; 4: EMG of the left tibialis anterior muscle; 5: left fronto-temporal; 6: right fronto-temporal; 7: EMG of the left posterior cervical muscles. A: stimulation of the left superficial radial nerve at 0.95/sec, 0.05 msec pulse duration, 0.34 V does not affect the monosynaptic reflex. B, C, D: stimulation of the same nerve at the same voltage but at 2/sec, 3.1/sec and 3.75/sec respectively, gradually reduces and abolishes the monosynaptic reflex. (GIAQUINTO and POMPEIANO, 1964)

afferent volleys on the supraspinal descending inhibitory structures which become spontaneously active during desynchronized sleep.

Because of the localization of these structures in the lower brain stem one might expect that the mechanisms responsible for the somatic aspects of desynchronized sleep would be present also in the decerebrate animal. Indeed the relaxation of the postural tonus typical of desynchronized sleep in unrestrained animals (JOUVET, 1962) appears also during the cataleptic periods that have been observed in the chronic decerebrate preparation (RIOCH, 1952, 1954; BARD and MACHT, 1958; JOUVET, 1962, 1967).

It will be shown in Section VI that the circuits transmitting somatic impulses to supraspinal descending inhibitory mechanisms may still be operative even in the absence of the forebrain.

Hypnosis. When a rabbit is placed on its back and prevented from moving for a few seconds it becomes motionless for a fairly long time. This type of behaviour, called animal hypnosis, may be observed in several animal species (cf. CARLI, 1969 for references). During hypnosis the main behavioral symptoms are immobility, absence of righting reflexes and hypotonia (CATE, 1928; RIJLANT, 1933; GILMAN and MAROUSE, 1949; TAKAGI, 1957; SVORAD, 1957; VAN REETH, 1963; KLEMM, 1966; VOLGYESI, 1966; CARLI, 1969). Using the same technique described by POMPEIANO and SWETT (1962a) to stimulate peripheral nerves and to elicit extensor and flexor muscle reflexes in unanaesthetized, free-moving animals (GIAQUINTO et al., 1964a), CARLI (1969) has shown that rabbit hypnosis is also characterized by a tonic depression of both the heteronymous monosynaptic extensor and the polysynaptic flexor reflexes, similar to that observed during desynchronized sleep (GIAQUINTO et al., 1964a). Previous studies had already shown that the polysynaptic reflex is depressed during hypnosis in humans (HERNÁNDEZ-PÉON et al., 1960), but not in guinea pig (ECKSTEIN, 1919). During rabbit hypnosis the animal's EEG may be either synchronized or desynchronized. However, contrary to the response obtained in synchronized sleep where arousal is always a generalized phenomenon, sensory stimulation of the animal under synchronized hypnosis may produce EEG arousal and pupillary dilation, without interrupting the trance. Moreover contrary to desynchronized sleep, the pupils are dilated during hypnosis while the phasic events typical of this phase of sleep such as the rapid eye movements and the clonic twitches are absent (cf. CARLI, 1969 for references). It appears therefore that the motor mechanisms are selectively affected during hypnosis (KLEMM, 1966), a condition which is similar to human catalepsy.

Somatic stimulation may precipitate the behavioral signs of hypnosis, namely absence of righting reflexes and immobility, not only in intact preparations but also in decorticate (VERWORN, 1897; SZYMANSKY, 1912; BERITOFF, 1927, 1929; SIMINOV, 1963), hypothalamic (CARLI, 1971) and precollicular decerebrate animals (SPIEGEL and GOLDBLOOM, 1925; CARLI, 1971) and even after cerebellectomy. It has been suggested that the supraspinal mechanisms responsible for the hypnotic akinesia take place at the brain stem reticular level (GEREBTZOFF, 1941; SVORAD, 1957; KLEMM, 1966, 1969; BUSER and VIALA, 1968; KLEMM et al., 1968; McBRIDE and KLEMM, 1969).

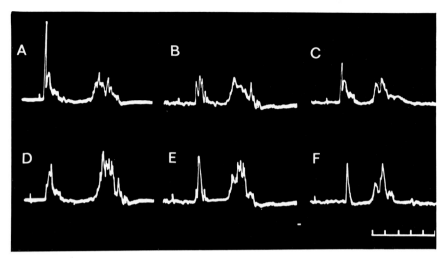

Fig. 10. "Initial" and "delayed" segmental reflex responses at lumbar, thoracic, and cervical levels. Decerebrate cat. Responses were recorded from ventral root L_7 following ipsilateral stimulation of DRL_7 (A) and sural nerve (D). Responses were recorded from one branch of the intercostal nerve at T_6 following stimulation of DRT_6 (B) and the other branch of intercostal nerve at T_6 (E). Responses were recorded from deep branch of radial nerve following stimulation of DRC_6 (C), and superficial branch of radial nerve (F). Time scale 5 msec intervals. (SHIMAMURA and LIVINGSTON, 1963)

VI. Descending Reticular Influences Induced by Somatic Afferent Volleys in the Decerebrate or Anaesthetized Animal

1. Propriospinal and Spino-Bulbo-Spinal Reflexes

Appropriate stimulation of any spinal afferent nerve can initiate motor responses throughout many segments of the spinal cord. However, besides the descending (LLOYD, 1942) and the ascending propriospinal systems (GERNANDT and MEGIRIAN, 1961) there is another system which contributes to a longitudinal coordination between different spinal cord segments (GERNANDT and SHIMAMURA, 1961; SHIMAMURA and LIVINGSTON, 1963; SHIMAMURA et al., 1964; SHIMAMURA and AKERT, 1964; SHIMAMURA et al., 1967a); the resulting reflex effect is commonly known as the spino-bulbo-spinal (SBS) reflex, which depends upon relay through the bulbar reticular formation and recurrent projection to spinal motoneurones in decerebrate cats and also in dogs, monkeys and men.

Fig. 10 shows that in decerebrate cats, responses to dorsal root stimulation recorded from corresponding ventral root or peripheral nerve consist of classical segmental monosynaptic and polysynaptic reflexes followed, after a period of little or no ventral root activity, by additional reflex discharges. If stimulation is applied to a muscle nerve, the late reflex discharges are weak and inconstant; if applied to a purely cutaneous nerve the late reflex discharges are larger in amplitude. Flexor rather than extensor motor units are involved in these late reflex discharges. Moreover, both the early and the late polysynaptic reflex responses can be recorded from ipsilateral and contralateral ventral roots all along the spinal cord following stimulation of a given dorsal root or peripheral nerve.

The observation that latencies for the early polysynaptic response became steadily longer in both directions along the spinal cord away from the site of stimulation indicated the propriospinal origin of this reflex response (effective central transmission velocity of 20 ± 5 m/sec and 23 ± 5 m/sec for the ascending and descending propriospinal projections). On the contrary, the latencies for the late polysynaptic response become steadily shorter as one records from segments closer to the medulla, indicating that the late polysynaptic reflex response is due to a volley of impulses descending the spinal cord (ascending transmission velocity of 60 ± 7 m/sec and descending transmission velocity from the medulla to the spinal motor outflows of 33 ± 4 m/sec).

The supraspinal localization of the relay for the SBS reflex is indicated by the fact that while decerebration at the intercollicular level does not modify the late reflex responses, transection of the spinal cord at C_1 eliminates them (GERNANDT and SHIMAMURA, 1961). Moreover asphyxia and Nembutal anaesthesia affect SBS responses promptly and eliminate them long before propriospinal responses show any signs of deterioration (SHIMAMURA and AKERT, 1965). SHIMAMURA and LI-VINGSTON (1963) indicate that the relay for the SBS reflex system is located in the caudal part of the medulla oblongata, a region including the medullary reticular formation.

In summary, while propriospinal reflex pathways activated by stimulation of lumbosacral dorsal roots spread out along the spinal cord from their level of entry, reaching the nearest motor response systems first, the SBS reflex patterns activated by similar stimulation do not evoke motor responses until they have reached the medulla, relayed there and re-entered the spinal cord from above downward. The reflex effects thus initiated have a centrifugal pattern of motor response, successively affecting forelimb, intercostal and hindlimb motor systems.

2. Effects of Spino-Bulbo-Spinal Reflex Volleys on Extensor Motoneurones

A first attempt has been made to analyze the effects of the SBS reflex volleys onto the extensor motoneurones (SHIMAMURA et al., 1967b). In particular, a conditioning volley was applied to the ipsilateral sural nerve, while the extensor monosynaptic reflex (MR) in VR L7 or S1 following stimulation of the gastrocnemius-soleus (GS) nerve was the test response. When the interval between conditioning and testing shocks was increased gradually, the test MRs showed slight initial changes in their amplitude (Fig. 11, I and II) followed by two marked depressions, an early and a late one, which lasted 20 and 25 msec respectively (Fig. 11, III and IV). The early interaction resulted from the direct action by the cutaneous afferents and was not affected by spinal transection. On the other hand, the late interaction still persisted after decerebration or cerebellectomy, but it was eliminated after spinal transection at the C_1 level together with SBS reflex (Fig. 11, dashed line). This implies that the late effect on the MR is concerned with long reflex activities which engages supraspinal mechanisms.

In addition to these findings single shock stimulation of the sural nerve yielded initial changes of membrane potential in ipsilateral GS motoneurones followed by an early hyperpolarization and a late depolarization. For the same conditioning stimulus there was also an early and a late depression of the monosynaptic EPSP recorded from the ipsilateral GS motoneurons. Since this late depression appeared in the absence of IPSP in motoneurons, it was postulated that a presynaptic mechanism contributed to this interaction. Indeed stimulation of the ipsilateral sural nerve produced an early and a late dorsal root potential (DRP), which were

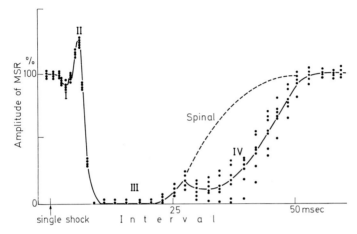

Fig. 11. Effects of sural nerve stimulation on the monosynaptic reflex of the gastrocnemius-soleus muscle. In chloralose-anaesthetized cats the ratio of amplitude variations of the monosynaptic reflex response induced by stimulation of nerves to the gastrocnemius-soleus muscle relative to the control (= 100%) is plotted against time, when conditioned by single shock to the ipsilateral sural nerve at increasing intervals, before (solid line) and after (dashed line) high spinalization. (SHIMAMURA et al., 1967b)

attributed by the authors to primary afferent depolarization (PAD) in the group Ia fibres of the GS muscle. The demonstration that the late effects persisted after precollicular decerebration, but were eliminated following spinal transection at the C_1 level, indicated that the delayed depolarization in the group Ia fibres from the GS muscle following sural nerve stimulation was due to a SBS reflex mechanism.

In summary it is concluded that cutaneous afferents, while they yielded the SBS reflex in flexor motoneurones (SHIMAMURA and LIVINGSTON, 1963; SHIMAMURA and AKERT, 1965), are unable to induce any SBS reflex in extensor motor nerves. In contrast the descending volleys of the SBS reflex appear to have an inhibitory influence on the extensor motoneurones, which is attributed to presynaptic mechanism. Although PAD in the Ia pathway will certainly lead to a diminution in amount of excitatory transmitter released by the primary afferent terminals, we would not exclude the possibility that the depression of the MR was also due in part at least to postsynaptic inhibition, which was obscured by concomitant EPSPs developed at the motoneurones.

3. Effects of Spino-Bulbo-Spinal Reflex Volleys on Flexor Motoneurones

The effects of the SBS volleys on the flexor motoneurones have also been analyzed (SHIMAMURA and AOKI, 1969).

Effects of Stimulation of the Cutaneous Nerve on the Monosynaptic and the Polysynaptic Flexor Reflexes. Conditioning stimulation of the sural nerve produced profound changes of the monosynaptic (MR) and the polysynaptic flexor reflex (PR) recorded from the VR L7 on single shock stimulation of the nerve to the anterior tibial muscle. The test MR was augmented at stimulus intervals over the range of 3–300 msec. During the initial part of the augmentation there were two phases, early and late, which corresponded in time to the conditioning PR and SBS reflex responses. The late phase of the augmentation peaked at 25 msec interval between two stimuli; after a rapid drop from this peak it diminished more gradually but persisted for 150–300 msec (prolonged augmentation). The test PR evoked by anterior tibial nerve stimulation was also augmented during an interval of 1–20 msec by conditioning stimulation of the sural nerve. Even here there were two phases of augmentation, early and late, which corresponded to the time of occurrence of the conditioning PR and SBS reflexes. However, the augmentation of the PR was followed by a prolonged diminution in response, beginning at stimulus intervals of 20–25 msec and continuing through intervals of 150–300 msec. These changes were similar to those of the PR elicited by single shock stimulation of the sural nerve following conditioning stimulation of the same cutaneous nerve. All these signs of interaction except the early phase of augmentation were completely abolished by spinal transection at C_1 level. The prolonged changes in the MR and PR responses recorded from ventral root L7 following conditioning stimulation of the sural nerve were paralleled by similar changes in MR and PR EPSP amplitudes recorded from tibialis anterior motoneurones covering the same time periods.

Intracellular Potentials of Flexor Motoneurones Induced by Sural Nerve Stimulation. Single shock stimulation of the ipsilateral sural nerve elicited in some anterior tibial motoneurones initial depolarization (EPSP), early and late, which corresponded to the time of occurrence of the PR and SBS reflex responses. On the other hand the prolonged augmentation of the MR and prolonged diminution of PR in the anterior tibial motoneurones could be associated with different types of membrane potential changes (slight depolarization or hyperpolarization). These changes however could be detected only in 22% of the tested motoneurones. When the SBS reflex pathway was interrupted by spinal transection at C_1 level, the late EPSP and the prolonged membrane potential changes were completely abolished, while the early EPSP still persisted.

Primary Afferent Depolarization in the Group Ia Fibres Following Sural Nerve Stimulation. Stimulation of the sural nerve yielded two types of depolarization, early and late, in the group Ia fibres of the anterior tibial muscle and in the primary afferent fibres of the sural nerve. The early potential, which began with a delay of about 5 msec, corresponded in time to the local segmental PR response from the ventral root. The late wave of depolarization began about 25 msec after the stimulation and had a total duration in excess of 300 msec. Simultaneously there was also a parallel increase in excitability of the terminals of afferent fibres from the sural nerve and from the anterior tibial muscle. The time course of the increased amplitude of the response exactly matched the time course of the PAD in fibres of the cutaneous and muscle nerves. The test antidromic volley in the group Ia fibres in the anterior tibial nerve showed changes, that were in all respect like those characterizing responses to cutaneous nerve recording.[6]

The early depolarization was generated by volleys of cutaneous afferents at spinal levels since high spinal transection did not modify them. In contrast the late depolarization of primary afferents in cutaneous and tibialis anterior muscle nerves depended on intact pathways to supraspinal centres, since spinal transection at the C_1 level eliminated them completely.

In summary, stimulation of the sural nerve induced augmentation, early and late, of flexor reflexes, both mono- and polysynaptic (MR and PR). The early augmentation resulted from direct action of the cutaneous afferents and was unaffected by spinal transection. In contrast, the late augmentation was abolished by spinal transection at C_1 level.

Intracellular recordings from flexor motoneurones exhibited EPSP at a time corresponding to the PR and the SBS reflexes in the spinal ventral root. This implies that the augmentation, both early and late, of the MR and PR are the results of postsynaptic depolarization (EPSP) induced by the arrival of PR and later by SBS reflex volleys, both being evoked by stimulation of the sural nerve.

The prolonged diminution of the flexor PR can be attributed only in part to postsynaptic events (involving IPSP and disfacilitation) since only few motoneurones showed prolonged hyperpolarization after the SBS reflex response. The prolonged diminution of the flexor PR can therefore be attributed either to presynaptic inhibition in the cutaneous afferents or to postsynaptic inhibition of the spinal interneurones intercalated in the PR pathway.

On the other hand the prolonged augmentation of the flexor MR can be attributed only in part to motoneuronal depolarization following the SBS reflex, since this appeared only in relatively few motoneurones. The prolonged augmentation of the flexor MR may therefore be attributed to presynaptic inhibition leading to reduced input to inhibitory interneurones to the flexor motoneurones (disinhibition). An alternative possibility could be that prolonged facilitation or disinhibition from the supraspinal structures affected the spinal interneurones, in which case membrane potential changes would not be observed in motoneurones.

4. Cholinergic Properties of Spino-Bulbo-Spinal Reflex Inhibition

Histochemical techniques (SHUTE and LEWIS, 1963, 1965; HOLMES and WOLSTENCROFT, 1964; PAVLIN, 1965) have shown the existence of acetylcholinesterase in reticular neurones some of them being localized in nuclei such as the nucleus gigantocellularis, nucleus pontis caudalis and pontis oralis, which contribute to the reticulospinal projection. Moreover physiological experiments have shown the existence of cholinoceptive neurones in the medullary and pontine reticular forma-

---

6 Recent observations also indicate that cutaneous afferent volleys are able to evoke centrifugal cutaneous nerve discharges in the posterior limb of the decerebrate marsupial phalanger *Trichosurus vulpecola*. These discharges are abolished by spinal cord transection (MEGIRIAN, 1970a, b).

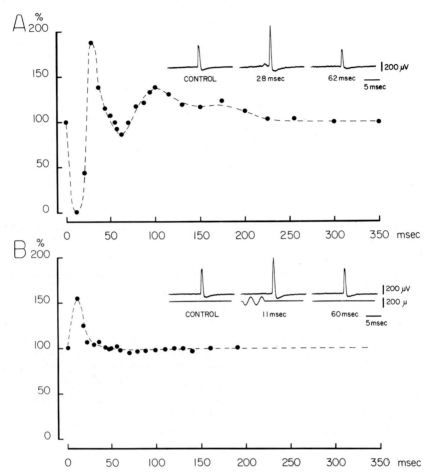

Fig. 12. Effects of conditioning electrical stimulation of a lumbar dorsal root or sinusoidal stretch of the gastrocnemius-soleus muscle on the ipsilateral monosynaptic extensor reflex before intravenous injection of eserine. Precollicular decerebrate cat. A: Conditioning stimulation of the left dorsal root L6 with two 0.05 msec rectangular pulses delivered at the interval of 1.4 msec, 10 times the threshold for the segmental polysynaptic reflex recorded from ipsilateral ventral root L7. Testing stimulation applied to the left Pl-FDHL nerves with single pulses of 0.1 msec in duration, 2.0 times the threshold for the monosynaptic reflex. B: conditioning mechanical stimulation with 2 cycles at 280/sec, 178 μ peak-to-peak amplitude, applied to the Achilles tendon. Testing stimulation as in A. (THODEN et al., 1971a)

tion (BRADLEY and MOLLICA, 1958; BRADLEY and WOLSTENCROFT, 1962, 1964, 1965, 1967; SALMOIRAGHI and STEINER, 1963; BRADLEY et al., 1964, 1966; KRUG et al., 1970).

Several lines of evidence indicate the existence of a cholinergic system in the brain stem which exerts descending inhibitory influences on the lumbar cord. It is known for instance that the postural atonia, as well as the depression of the spinal reflexes which occurs in the intact preparation during desynchronized sleep, is due to supraspinal descending inhibitory volleys (POMPEIANO, 1967a). Recent studies indicate that this phase of sleep, including the collapse of the postural activity, can be produced by eserine sulphate in decerebrate cats (MATSUZAKI and KASA-HARA, 1966; MATSUZAKI et al., 1967, 1968; MATSUZAKI, 1968, 1969). It has been postulated that this medullary inhibitory centre is triggered by a pontine reticular structure which becomes active during desynchronized sleep (JOUVET, 1967). Eserine probably acts on the pontine reticular neurones by facilitating the medullary inhibitory region.

Additional evidence of a brain stem cholinergic inhibitory system has been reported by BARNES (1970), BARNES and POMPEIANO (1970d, 1971) and THODEN et al. (1971a, b), who found that the inhibitory phase of the SBS reflex, performed in decerebrate cats, was augmented by the i.v. administration of a small dose of eserine sulphate (Figs. 12A and 13A).

5. Peripheral Afferent Volleys Responsible for the Spino-Bulbo-Spinal Reflex Effects

A detailed analysis of the afferent sources responsible for the different components of the SBS reflex can be performed in precollicular decerebrate cats.

SHIMAMURA and AKERT (1965) have shown that stimulation of the sural nerve elicited the long latency SBS response when only the low threshold cutaneous afferents were excited (conduction velocity 50–80 m/sec). Conversely the short latency propriospinal response appeared only with higher stimulus intensities. SBS reflexes could also be elicited by mechanical stimulation of the skin ipsilaterally and contralaterally.

Stimulation of the gastrocnemius nerve elicited segmental monosynaptic and polysynaptic reflexes from VR S1. Long latency SBS response may appear occasionally and without consistency at a higher intensity, i.e., when group II and III muscular afferent fibres are involved.

THODEN et al. (1971a, b) have studied whether the proprioceptive volleys originating from muscle spindles are able to trigger the brain stem reticular structures exerting an inhibitory control on spinal reflexes. It is known that small amplitude sinusoidal stretch of a de-efferented muscle provides a powerful stimulus for the primary endings of the muscle spindles, while it has less effect in exciting secondary endings (see Section VII, 8).

Conditioning stimulation of the GS muscle with two sinusoidal stretches (at 250–300/sec, 50–200 μ amplitude) elicited an early facilitation of heteronymous monosynaptic extensor reflexes (Fig. 12B). However, no further changes of the test reflex were observed at the appropriate interval (of about 60 msec) at which electrical stimulation of the ipsilateral dorsal root L6 elicited SBS inhibition (Fig. 12A). Sinusoidal stretch of the GS muscle was unable to produce inhibition of the test reflex even after i.v. injection of eserine sulphate (Fig. 13B), at a dose which greatly potentiated the inhibitory phase of the SBS reflex elicited by dorsal root stimulation in the same preparation (Fig. 13A). It appears therefore that natural stimulation of the primary endings of the muscle spindles is unable to trigger the supraspinal descending reticular mechanism responsible for the inhibitory component of the SBS reflex. Negative results were also obtained by natural stimulation of Golgi tendon organs or by stimulating both primary and secondary endings of muscle spindles during dynamic muscle stretch (MAGHERINI et al., 1972).

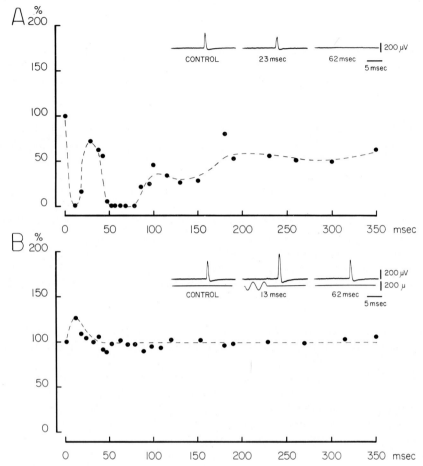

Fig. 13. Effects of conditioning electrical stimulation of a lumbar dorsal root or of sinusoidal stretch of the gastrocnemius-soleus muscle on the ipsilateral monosynaptic extensor reflex after intravenous injection of eserine. Same experiment as in Fig. 12. A, same experimental condition as for Fig. 12A, 5 min after i.v. injection of eserine sulphate (0.1 mg/kg). B, same as in Fig. 12B, 17 min after injection of the drug. (THODEN et al., 1971a)

VII. Responses of the Brain Stem Reticular Formation to Somatic Afferent Volleys

1. General Properties of Reticular Neurones

No accurate information can be obtained on the background of spontaneous firing of the reticular neurones by macroelectrode recording. The most appropriate method for this purpose is to record the spontaneous activity of single reticular units either extracellularly or intracellularly.

Activity of single neurones has been recorded from the medullary (MOLLICA et al., 1953; BAUMGARTEN and MOLLICA, 1954; BAUMGARTEN et al., 1954; MORUZZI,

1954, 1956; SCHEIBEL et al., 1955; GAUTHIER et al., 1956; HUTTENLOCHER, 1961; WOLSTENCROFT, 1961, 1962, 1964; ALBE-FESSARD et al., 1962; BACH-Y-RITA, 1962a, b, 1964; BENJAMIN, 1962; POMPEIANO and SWETT, 1962c–f, 1963a, b; SCHEIBEL and SCHEIBEL, 1963a, 1965a, b; BOWSHER and PETIT, 1966; BOWSHER et al., 1968a; CASEY, 1968; BOWSHER, 1969, 1970), pontine (PALESTINI et al., 1957; BACH-Y-RITA, 1962a, b, 1964; POMPEIANO and SWETT, 1962c–f, 1963a, b; SCHEIBEL and SCHEIBEL, 1963a, 1965a; HAYASHI and YOSHII, 1966; KRUG et al., 1968), and mesencephalic reticular formation (AMASSIAN and DE VITO, 1954; HÉRNANDEZ-PÉON and HAGBARTH, 1955; MACHNE et al., 1955; SCHEIBEL et al., 1955; AMASSIAN et al., 1956, 1961; MANCIA et al., 1957; AMASSIAN and WALLER, 1958; BACH-Y-RITA, 1962a, b, 1964; POMPEIANO and SWETT, 1962c, d, 1963a; BELL et al., 1963, 1964; WAGMAN and MCMILLAN, 1968; MCMILLAN and WAGMAN, 1971). Units were also recorded in the tecto-tegmental region (POMPEIANO and SWETT, 1963a; BELL et al., 1963, 1964; HILL and HORN, 1964; HORN and HILL, 1966) including the nucleus of the posterior commissure (BOWSHER and PETIT, 1969, 1970).

In all these studies the unit discharge was recorded extracellularly. The activity of the reticular units occurred "spontaneously", *i.e.*, in the absence of any intentional stimulation of sensory receptors or of central structures. However, silent units could also be encountered, which became active only after peripheral stimulation.

Many reticular units could fire spontaneously even in the mesencephalic slab, *i.e.*, when all reticulopetal influences had been abolished by premammillary and pretrigeminal transections (BONVALLET et al., 1956).

Reticular neurones in different unanaesthetized animals, can fire spontaneously according to the following patterns: i) low frequency irregular discharge; ii) continuous discharge occurring regularly at higher frequencies (50–100/sec); iii) bursts of unit discharges varying from 50–70/sec (MOLLICA et al., 1953; MORUZZI, 1954, 1956) up to 500/sec, sometimes separated by silent intervals (SCHEIBEL et al., 1955; GAUTHIER et al., 1956; MANCIA et al., 1957).

A more detailed analysis of the properties of the reticular neurones originates from observations made with intracellular recordings (LIMANSKII, 1961, 1962, 1963, 1965, 1966; MAGNI and WILLIS, 1963a, b; 1964a, b, c, 1965; WILLIS and MAGNI, 1964; SEGUNDO et al., 1967a, b; ITO et al., 1970; UDO and MANO, 1970). Most of these neurones were recorded from the bulbar reticular formation of cerebellectomized cats, either anaesthetized or unanaesthetized; the resting potentials ranged from —40 to —90 mV. Some of the impaled neurones (20% according to SEGUNDO et al., 1967a; 48% according to MAGNI and WILLIS, 1964b; 60% according to LIMANSKII, 1963) showed spontaneous hyperpolarizing and depolarizing subthreshold oscillations of the transmembrane potential (IPSPs and EPSPs) while the remaining neurones did not show PSP activity.

Certain reticular neurones showed a constant rhythmical activity quite apart from the advent of any afferent impulse activity controlled by the experimenter (cf. LIMANSKII, 1962, 1963, 1965; SEGUNDO et al., 1967a), either irregular activity or with regular intervals between spike potentials (LIMANSKII, 1965). The essential difference between the two types of rhythmic activity lies in the nature of the slow changes in the resting potential preceding action potentials. In the first type, the action potential developed on a background of "synaptic noise" characterized by the irregular occurrence of slow EPSPs and IPSPs. In neurones with regular rhythmic activity the action potentials were preceded by a smooth, slowly increasing depolarization very like a generator potential or the "pacemaker potential" of cells particularly capable of generating rhythmic impulses; they have been termed "prepotentials" since they precede the generation of action potentials. These slow prepotentials, which are distinct from postsynaptic potentials, represent therefore a process of slow steadily increasing depolarization, which undergoes transition to the action potential when values of 2–10 mV are reached in neurones with persistent rhythmic activity. The slow prepotential rate and, consequently, the action potential rate varied in different neurones from 20 to 150/sec according to LI-MANSKII (1965) and from 40 to 100/sec according to SEGUNDO et al. (1967a). This slow prepotential thus reflects a special form of excitatory process which is the basis of the autogenous rhythmic activity of reticular neurones.

All neurones showed sharp all-or-nothing action potentials with fast ascent and decay. In some instances the action potential took off from a depolarizing wave which was either an EPSP or a pacemaker drift. In other instances the action potential took off at close to right angles from a nondepolarized level (cf. HAAPANEN et al., 1958; KOSTYUK, 1961; LIMANSKII, 1963; SEGUNDO et al., 1967a). This was observed in some cells with PSPSs and of course in all cells with neither PSP nor pacemaker activity. In the latter cases recording was probably made from axons (see MAGNI and WILLIS, 1963a, b, 1965; WILLIS and MAGNI, 1964).

2. Identification of Reticular Neurones

The problem of identification of reticular neurones represents one of the crucial problems of reticular physiology (MORUZZI, 1956, 1958). In fact any information that can be obtained by recording the response of reticular units to somatic afferent volleys can hardly be evaluated unless the pathways to which the RF units belong are identified and the excitatory or the inhibitory nature of the recorded neurones is determined. A first approach was to correlate the firing pattern of a reticular unit with the extensor rigidity in the decerebrate preparation, or with the EEG patterns in the *encéphale isolé* or curarized cat, but the results obtained are fragmentary and inconclusive (cf. ROSSI and ZANCHETTI, 1957).

A second approach was utilized by PALESTINI et al. (1957). It has already been pointed out in the anatomical section that the RF is not structurally homogeneous. Microelectrode recordings from two pontine regions, one characterized by the predominance of rostrally projecting neurones and the other by caudally projecting neurones showed identical patterns of resting discharge in both populations, similar proportions of unresponsive neurones, and the same extent of sensory convergence. Quantitative differences however were found between medial and lateral reticular regions. It is known that the medial pontine reticular regions give rise to either rostral or caudal projections, while the lateral reticular areas are almost devoid of neurones with long projections and appear basically composed of short axon cells (see Section II, 2). From lateral pontine reticular areas, units were recorded less frequently, and most of them were uninfluenced at all or influenced only by a single kind of afferent, mostly trigeminal. Only a limited number of units showing convergence was found. It is clear that even with the approach used by PALESTINI et al. (1957), a knowledge of the position of an electrode tip within a given region of the RF is of little use in indicating cell type.

A third approach provides a means of determining whether reticular neurones belong to a descending or to an ascending pathway. The direction in which the axons of reticular neurones projected was first proved by recording extracellularly the antidromically conducted impulses that resulted from stimulation of the axons at levels caudal or rostral to the cell bodies of the neurones (WOLSTENCROFT, 1961, 1962, 1964; FOX, 1970; POMPEIANO and BARNES, 1971; PETERSON and FELPEL,

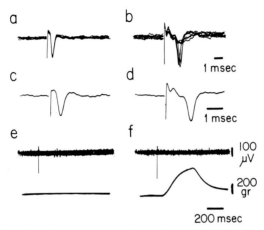

Fig. 14. Identification of a reticular neurone. Decerebrate cat with ventral roots intact. Micro-electrode recording from a brain stem reticular neuron on the right side. In these records, downward deflection indicates negativity at the microelectrode and the first downward deflection in *a–d* indicates the stimulation artifact. *a,b:* superimposed responses of the reticular neurone to bipolar stimulation at 10/sec, 0.1 msec pulse duration, 10 V of the descending (*a*) and the ascending (*b*) MLF. *c,d:* same as *a,b*, but at higher sweep speed. Note the short latency antidromic response of the reticular neurone to stimulation of the descending MLF and the monosynaptic activation of the same neurone to stimulation of the ascending MLF. *e,f:* low-frequency discharge of the reticular neurone with the left GS muscle at 6 mm of initial exten-sion (*e*) and no effect during vibration of this muscle at 200/sec, 250 *μ* peak-to-peak amplitude, for 330 msec (*f*). (POMPEIANO and BARNES, 1971)

1971; PETERSON et al., 1971). Reticular units were identified by antidromic stimu-lation of their axons in the ascending medial longitudinal fasciculus (MLF) at mesodiencephalic level (POMPEIANO and BARNES, 1971) and in the descending MLF at lower medullary level (POMPEIANO and BARNES, 1971) or in the spinal cord (WOLSTENCROFT, 1961, 1962, 1964; FOX, 1970; PETERSON and FELPEL, 1971, PETERSON et al., 1971). The criteria used to distinguish antidromic excitation have been reported in detail in these original papers.

Fig. 14 shows that the same unit was activated antidromically by stimulation of the descending MLF (*a, c*) and orthodromically by stimulation of the ascending MLF (*b, d*). While the latency to antidromic stimulation was 0.36 msec (*c*) and was constant with repetition at the same stimulus strength (*a*), the latency to orthodromic stimulation was longer (1.18 msec), allowing time for one synaptic delay (d); moreover, the latency of the response shifted slightly with repetition of the stimulus (b). The reticular unit was able to respond antidromically to each stimulus at rates of stimulation of 10/sec (a), however, the same unit was unable to follow the same rate on orthodromic stimulation (b).

Fig. 14b, d allows also an analysis of the focal potentials recorded from the reticular structures after stimulation of the ascending MLF. These potentials consisted of an early positive (or positive-negative) wave due to arrival of afferent impulses at the terminals, followed by a sharp negative spike, which appeared 0.66 msec after the arrival of afferent impulses at the terminal (d). On high frequency stimulation of the MLF the spike was sometimes abolished and replaced by a slow negative wave of small amplitude, which may be partly a synaptic potential of the reticular neurone (b).

Most of the units located in the medial RF of the medulla and pons could be activated antidromically by stimulating either the descending or the ascending MLF. In some instances antidromic activation did not occur, although the same unit could be activated orthodromically by stimulating either one or both the ascending and the descending MLF. Moreover, single units could be activated antidromically by stimulation of both the ascending and the descending MLF. These cells apparently have axons that dichotomize in both ascending and descending directions (HELD, 1893; CAJAL, 1909–1911; SCHEIBEL and SCHEIBEL, 1958; cf. BRODAL and ROSSI, 1955; BRODAL, 1957; TORVIK and BRODAL, 1957).

Neurones of the medullary and pontine RF (MAGNI and WILLIS, 1963a, b, 1965; WILLIS and MAGNI, 1964; ITO et al., 1970) have also been identified by intracellular recording of the antidromically conducting action potentials that resulted from stimulation of their axons at either mesencephalic or spinal cord levels.

In most of the antidromically invaded units recorded by ITO et al. (1970) the spike showed a clear inflection at about the midpoint of the rising phase as shown also with extracellular recording (Fig. 14b) and was followed by an after-hyperpolarization of several mV in amplitude that lasted for about 100 msec. Other units exhibited full-sized spikes which, however, resembled those of axons in having no visible inflection on their rising phase and in being followed by a very small after-hyperpolarization. We believe that the axon-like spikes were common among reticular units sampled by some authors (MAGNI and WILLIS, 1963b; cf. SEGUNDO et al., 1967a). As a matter of fact almost all the so-called reticular neurones recorded by MAGNI and WILLIS (1963b) were impaled within the region of the MLF, where ascending and descending fibres of both reticular and vestibular origin course.

According to MAGNI and WILLIS (1963b) among the 520 recorded units 417 were reticulospinal neurones (conduction velocity 90–130 m/sec), while 86 neurones with axons ascending rostrally and 17 neurones with axons projecting both to the spinal cord and rostrally. According to ITO et al. (1970) 126 cells of 209 (60%) were invaded antidromically from C_2 or C_3 and/or from the spinobulbar junction. Antidromic invasion from the midbrain tegmentum occurred in 20 cells of 162 examined (12%), and in 11 of these 20 cells activated from the midbrain, antidromic invasion was caused also from C_2–C_3 levels.

The demonstration that more than half of the pontomedullary reticular units project into the spinal cord is in accordance with the histological observations (TORVIK and BRODAL, 1957). These descending fibres course along the ventral quadrant ipsilaterally or contralaterally (ITO et al., 1970; FOX, 1970) and may project even to the lumbosacral segments of the cord (MAGNI and WILLIS, 1963b; WOLSTENCROFT, 1964; FOX, 1970). It is of interest that the reticulospinal cells are dispersed over the pontomedullary RF in both rostrocaudal and ventrodorsal directions (ITO et al., 1970; UDO and MANO, 1970). Most of their neurones located in the dorsocranial areas project to the medial portion of the ventral funiculi, while most of the neurones located in the ventrocaudal portions of the pontome-dullary RF project ipsilaterally through the ventrolateral part of the cord. The conduction velocity of the reticulospinal fibres showed wide variations: 20–138 m/sec according to WOLSTENCROFT (1964) (cf. also SHIMAMURA and LIVINGSTON, 1963; FOX, 1970; ITO et al., 1970).

As to the ascending reticular neurones it appears that the proportion of the cells invaded antidromically from the midbrain is reduced significantly as the recording electrode is shifted from the rostral to the caudal area (ITO et al., 1970). This is in agreement with the histological data indicating a difference in the ori-gins of ascending axons from pontine and medullary RF, since from the former more than half of the giant cells issue ascending axons, whereas from the latter only relatively small sized cells project cranially (BRODAL and Rossi, 1955; TORVIK and BRODAL, 1957).

Once the reticular neurones have been identified by antidromic stimulation of their axons, it would be of interest to know whether these neurones are excitatory or inhibitory in function. There is no direct method so far to know whether the impaled neurones are excitatory or inhibitory. The observation recently made by ITO et al. (1970) who found that the antidromic activation of the pontomedullary reticular neurones both from the cervical cord and from the mesencephalon, evoked monosynaptic IPSPs or EPSPs in them, suggests the existence of both inhibitory and excitatory reticular neurones.

3. Evoked Potentials Elicited by Somatic Afferent Volleys

Evoked potentials have been recorded with macroelectrodes from the medul-lary, pontine and mesencephalic RF following stimulation of either the trunk or limbs or of their sensory cutaneous and/or muscular fibres (STARZL et al., 1951b; FRENCH et al., 1952, 1953a; MORIN, 1953; COLLINS and O'LEARY, 1954; HER-NÁNDEZ-PÉON and HAGBARTH, 1955; ROSSI and ZANCHETTI, 1957; FRENCH, 1960; HARA et al., 1961; LINDSLEY and ADEY, 1961; MORILLO and BAYLOR, 1963; BOWSHER and PETIT, 1966; HAYASHI and YOSHII, 1966; BONVALLET and NEW-MAN-TAYLOR, 1967; BOWSHER et al., 1968a; BOWSHER, 1969, 1970). These poten-tials were characterized by an initial positive component followed by a slow nega-tive one. In contrast with the features exibited by the classical lemniscal respon-ses, the reticular responses evoked by somatic afferent stimulation displayed a slower rise and fall and had a longer latency. In particular it was shown (FRENCH et al., 1953a) that sciatic potentials reached the pontine and mesencephalic teg-mentum and the midline portion of the thalamus in 13 to 23 msec, i.e., with an increase of 7 to 14 msec over lemniscal times. Moreover the responses in the direct pathways were not modified by relatively high rates of stimulation, whereas the reticular potentials were greatly depressed and even disappeared when the stimuli were delivered in rapid succession (Starzl et al., 1951 b; French et al., 1952, 1953 a; Bowsher et al., 1968 a).

The evoked potentials recorded from the RF persisted even after cerebellectomy or bilateral ablation of the primary sensory areas of the cortex as well as after decerebration. Moreover bilateral lesion of the lemniscal sensory paths (Starzl et al., 1951 b) or section of the dorsal columns in the spinal cord had no effect on these evoked potentials (cf. however Collins and Kendrick, 1966), while a bilateral section of the anterolateral funiculi of the cord abolished them. These findings exclude the possibility that the potentials evoked from the RF are due to collateral fibres arising from the lemniscal sensory path below its interruption, as suggested by Starzl et al. (1951 b) and indicate that such responses are mediated through direct spinoreticular projections.

4. Responses of Reticular Neurones to Somatic Afferent Volleys

Sensory Modalities. The most effective form of cutaneous stimulation to influence brain stem reticular units localized in the bulbar and pontine RF was represented by deep pressure, brusque tapping of the body, and pinching of the skin over most of the body surface such as the trunk head, neck, tail and four limbs (Baumgarten and Mollica, 1954; Scheibel et al., 1955; Palestini et al., 1957; Wolstencroft, 1961, 1962, 1964; Scheibel and Scheibel, 1965 a, b; Bowsher and Petit, 1966; Bowsher et al., 1968 a; Casey, 1968). Mechanical stimuli of this type have been found necessary to activate also all non-specific thalamic centres (Bowsher and Albe-Fessard, 1962; Albe-Fessard and Fessard, 1963; for reviews see Albe-Fessard, 1965, and Chapter 13), probably acting through cutaneous nociceptive afferents. Some of the units, however, responded to brusque but not necessarily noxious stimuli. Both pressure and taps may still be effective after removal of the skin (Wolstencroft, 1964).

In addition to strong stimuli, light cutaneous stimuli are also able to influence the reticular units. Units in the bulbar and pontine RF may be influenced by light and brief touch, blowing air through a narrow tube onto the skin, displacing or pulling one or more hairs (Wolstencroft, 1961, 1962, 1964; Bach-y-Rita, 1962 a, b, 1964; Segundo et al., 1967 b; Casey, 1968 and others) in unanaesthetized preparations, i.e., in decerebrate cats (Wolstencroft, 1961, 1962, 1964; Casey, 1968) or in cats immobilized with gallamine tri-ethiodide (Segundo et al., 1967 b; Bach-y-Rita, 1962 a, b, 1964), as well as in anaesthetized (chloralose) preparations (Bach-y-Rita, 1962 a, b, 1964).

These observations contrast with those made by Bowsher et al. (1968 a) and Bowsher and Petit (1966) who found that light touch and air movement did not affect bulbar RF units recorded in cats anaesthetized with chloralose. The reticular structures, in contrast to the specific projections, are greatly susceptible to anaesthetic drugs, owing in part at least to their multisynaptic organization (French et al., 1953 b; Arduini and Arduini, 1954). Some of the differences mentioned above can be due in part at least to the use of anaesthesia. The effects of selective stimulation of different groups of cutaneous afferents on reticular neurones will be reported in Section VII, 5 and 6.

Cutaneous stimuli affect not only the bulbar and pontine reticular units but also units recorded from the mesencephalic RF; low threshold units, including those responsive to phasic hair movements (blowing), occur dorsally in the mid-brain at the tecto-tegmental transitional zone (AMASSIAN and DE VITO, 1954; BELL et al., 1964), i.e., in that region which includes the nucleus of the posterior commissure (BOWSHER and PETIT, 1969, 1970).

In addition to exteroceptive impulses, proprioceptive impulses could also influence the activity of the brain stem reticular formation (see DELL and BON-VALLET, 1956; MORUZZI, 1956). Examination of the methods employed, however, revealed that when natural proprioceptive stimulation was able to affect reticular neurones, stimuli such as passive movements of the limbs, tapping the limbs and squeezing or stretching of muscles had been used (MORIN, 1953; AMASSIAN and DE VITO, 1954; SCHEIBEL et al., 1955; GAUTHIER et al., 1956; MANCIA et al., 1957; PALESTINI et al., 1957; WOLSTENCROFT, 1964; CASEY, 1968). With these forms of stimulation, it is sometimes difficult to avoid costimulation of joint and cutaneous receptors, which are known to affect reticular structures. Moreover when manual extension or flexion of limbs or muscle stretch was able to influence reticular neurones (WOLSTENCROFT, 1961, 1962, 1964) the response was quickly adapting, thus suggesting that it depended upon stimulation of joint and deep Pacinian receptors, rather than of muscle spindle receptors. It should be finally mentioned that brain stem reticular neurones also responded to stretch of the extraocular muscles (COOPER et al., 1953). The responses of reticular neurones to selective stimulation of different groups of muscular afferents and of the corresponding muscle receptors will be reported in Section VII, 7 and 8.

Pattern of Response. The majority of reticular neurones were excited by natural or electrical stimulation of cutaneous and/or muscular afferents, while a minority of units were inhibited. Unresponsive units were also found. A complex pattern of response of reticular neurones to somatic afferent volleys consisting of an initial short latency discharge, followed by a silent period and a late discharge was found either in unanaesthetized preparations or in cats anaesthetized with chloralose (AMASSIAN and DE VITO, 1954; BAUMGARTEN and MOLLICA, 1954; MACHNE et al., 1955; SCHEIBEL et al., 1955; MANCIA et al., 1957; PALESTINI et al., 1957; AMASSIAN and WALLER, 1958; SCHLAG, 1959; BACH-Y-RITA, 1962a, b, 1964; POMPEIANO and SWETT, 1962f, 1963b; WOLSTENCROFT, 1964; HAYASHI and YOSHII, 1966; SEGUNDO et al., 1967b; BOWSHER et al., 1968a; PETERSON and FELPEL, 1971; PETERSON et al., 1971). This pattern of response, however, was obtained particularly in reticular neurones which displayed a steady rhythmic activity (cf. also LIMANSKII, 1961, 1963). In fact, any inhibitory component of the reticular unit response could hardly be detected in the absence of any steady rhythmic discharge, at least when extracellular recording of unit activity was used. When reticular units were silent, their responsiveness to somatic afferent volleys was indicated only by the appearance of more or less short lived bursts of spikes (BAUMGARTEN et al., 1954; GAUTHIER et al., 1956; ROSSI and ZANCHETTI, 1957; LIMANSKII, 1961, 1963; POMPEIANO and SWETT, 1963a, b).

Complex responses characterized by excitation followed by inhibition were found more frequently in preparations with the cerebellum intact. The inhibition was sometimes followed by a late discharge (POMPEIANO and SWETT, 1963a, b; WOLSTENCROFT, 1964). It is postulated that the early excitation is due to activation of the spinoreticular pathway, while the late inhibition followed by a late discharge can be attributed to activation followed by inhibition of the cerebellar efferent inhibitory pathways.

Experiments employing intracellular recording from bulbar reticular units in anaesthetized and unanaesthetized preparations indicate that somatic afferent volleys elicited in the responsive neurones either a depolarizing wave or more rarely a hyperpolarizing wave or an alternatingly de- and hyperpolarizing oscillation (LIMANSKII, 1961, 1963, 1966; MAGNI and WILLIS, 1964a, b, c, 1965; SEGUNDO et al., 1967a). Depolarizing PSPs create conditions favouring acceleration of rhythmic frequency on the active reticular neurones and discharges of action potentials of varying duration in the inactive neurones and conversely for the hyperpolarizing PSP. Complex sequence of short-lasting IPSP and EPSP could also be elicited by individual sensory stimuli in cerebellectomized preparations (MAGNI and WILLIS, 1964b, c). This finding suggests the staggered activation of many excitatory and/or inhibitory synaptic inputs even in the absence of cerebellar circuits. The events can be detected also with extracellular recordings of reticular neurones in chloralose-anaesthetized, cerebellectomized animals (PETERSON and FELPEL, 1971; PETERSON et al., 1971).

It is of interest that stimuli applied to different parts of the field produce the same type of response. There are neurones however which are accelerated from one area and slowed from another (POMPEIANO, and SWETT, 1963a; BELL et al., 1964; SEGUNDO et al., 1967a). The type of response elicited from a given area was generally consistent throughout the experiment (cf. however HERNÁNDEZ-PÉON and HAGBARTH, 1955).

The consistency of the type and pattern of response of a reticular neurone to a somatic afferent volley is supported by the work of AMASSIAN et al. (AMASSIAN et al., 1956; AMASSIAN and WALLER, 1958). SEGUNDO et al. (1967a) report that the consistency and specificity noted by AMASSIAN and his group in the "locus-spike timing" relation results from consistency and specificity in the "locus-PSP profile" relation. The latter probably results from the fact that stimulation of each "locus" triggers, in a characteristic sequence, a characteristic set of presynaptic terminals.

Convergence. Convergence is the ability of units to respond to stimulation of two more different inputs; originating either from different types of receptor organs (heterosensory convergence) or from different topographical regions of the same sensory system (heterotopic convergence). The existence of heterosensory convergence on single reticular neurones has been reviewed (cf. ROSSI and ZANCHETTI, 1957; POTTHOFF et al., 1967) and will not be considered here. Heterotopic convergence occurs when units respond to stimulation of two or more limbs, in anaesthetized (chloralose) and in unanaesthetized cats (AMASSIAN and DE VITO, 1954; MORUZZI, 1954, 1956; WOLSTENCROFT, 1954; SCHEIBEL et al., 1955; MANCIA et al., 1957; PALESTINI et al., 1957; AMASSIAN and WALLER, 1958; ALBE-FESSARD et al., 1962; BACH-Y-RITA, 1962a, b, 1964; BELL et al., 1963, 1964; POMPEIANO and SWETT, 1963a, b; SEGUNDO et al., 1967b; BOWSHER et al., 1968a; CASEY, 1968; BOWSHER, 1969, 1970; BOWSHER and PETIT, 1969, 1970). In cats anaesthetized with chloralose, 77% of the caudal bulbar reticular units responded to single shocks applied to all four limbs (BOWSHER, 1969, 1970), 95% of the units in the nucleus reticularis gigantocellularis (BOWSHER et al., 1968a) and 87.3% of the units in the nucleus of the posterior commissure (BOWSHER and PETIT, 1970). The problem of convergence needs to be investigated systematically with intracellular recording, since reticular neurones described as "silent" elements or neurones with limited convergence, may actually react to afferent impulses with subliminal PSP (LIMANSKII, 1963).

Detailed and systematic investigations on the receptive fields of medullary (bulbar) and mesencephalic reticular units have been made respectively by SEGUNDO et al. (1967) and BELL et al. (1963, 1964), either in cerebellectomized cats immobilized with gallamine tri-ethiodide (SEGUNDO et al., 1967b) or in anaesthetized (chloralose) or unanaesthetized cats with the cerebellum intact (BELL et al., 1963, 1964). The fields were mapped in 175 responsive units from the bulbar reticular formation (SEGUNDO et al., 1967b). In 149 units localized in the rostral bulbar RF, 39%, 22% and 39% had widespread, restricted and highly restricted field respectively, while in 26 units in the caudal bulbar RF proportions were 3.8%, 42% and 54% respectively.

From the point of view of the bulbar RF representation the body was separated in three main regions; i) the ipsilateral face, whose representation includes a large contingent of cells with "highly restricted fields". The preponderant and special role of the trigeminal input was analyzed by several authors (PALESTINI et al., 1957; LAMARCHE et al., 1958, 1960; GORDON et al., 1961; KRUGER and MICHEL, 1962; LAMARCHE and LANGLOIS, 1962; LANGLOIS and LAMARCHE, 1962; DARIAN-SMITH et al., 1963a, b; BELL et al., 1964; DARIAN-SMITH and PHILLIPS, 1964; DARIAN-SMITH and YOKOTA, 1966; SEGUNDO et al., 1967b; BURTON, 1968); ii) the ipsilateral and contralateral forelimbs, whose representation includes a substantial contingent of cells with "highly restricted" or "restricted" fields; iii) the rest of the body including the contralateral face, whose representation is predominantly formed by cells with "widespread" fields.

The bulbar RF units differed from their mesencephalic counter parts in terms of field laterality, size and face involvement. Unilateral fields were usually ipsilateral (84% in the rostral bulbar RF), "widespread" and "highly restricted" fields were equally frequent (39%) and the face contained the great majority of "highly restricted" fields (79%) (SEGUNDO et al., 1967b; cf. also BURTON, 1968).

At midbrain level, however, BELL et al. (1963, 1964) reported that unilateral fields were usually contralateral (97%), "widespread" fields predominated (52%) (cf. also AMASSIAN and DE VITO, 1954; BOWSHER and PETIT, 1969, 1970), and the face contained a smaller proportion of "highly restricted" fields (41%). The different lateralities are explained by the respective distributions of spinoreticular fibres.

The occurrence of widespread fields in the RF contrasts with highly restricted fields in the principal somatic pathway (ROSE and MOUNTCASTLE, 1959; PERL et al., 1962; PERL, 1963; POGGIO and MOUNTCASTLE, 1963) as well as in the trigeminal nucleus (GORDON et al., 1961; KRUGER and MICHEL, 1962; DARIAN-SMITH et al.,

1963 a, b, 1965; Darian-Smith and Phillips, 1964; Darian-Smith and Yokota, 1966). Hence the RF response specificity is poor in comparison with that in the somatic pathway, and in addition there is no somatotopia in the brain stem RF (Amassian and Waller, 1958; French, 1960; Pompeiano and Swett, 1963 a and others). This finding is thus in agreement with the anatomical observations.

Latency. The latency of the responses of single reticular units to somatic afferent volleys could be evaluated by applying single shocks to both fore- and hindlimb nerves, and varied from 10–15 msec to 30–60 msec in the different preparations.

The results obtained by Bowsher et al. (1968a), Bowsher (1969, 1970), Bowsher and Petit (1970), in cats anaesthetized with chloralose allow a comparison of the mean latencies of the responses of reticular units recorded from different levels of the brain stem RF to supramaximal electrical stimuli delivered through needle electrodes inserted in the skin of each of the four limbs

	ipsilateral forelimb msec	contralateral forelimb msec	ipsilateral hindlimb msec	contralateral hindlimb msec
caudal bulbar reticular formation (Bowsher, 1969, 1970)	16.8	17.2	22.8	22.8
nucleus reticularis gigantocellularis (Bowsher et al., 1968a)	18.2 ± 1.3	18.1 ± 1.1	25.7 ± 1.3	26.0 ± 1.5
mesencephalic region (nucleus of the posterior commissure) (Bowsher and Petit, 1970)	22.0 ± 1.8	20.5 ± 1.5	28.4 ± 2.3	27.3 ± 1.8

In conclusion, analysis of discrete areas of the RF shows marked differences in functional organization. These differences, overlapping as they do in time, may make possible a differential input analysis by the organism as a whole which permit it to carry out appropriate integrated reaction at subcortical level according to the stimulus site.

In addition to the short-latency responses indicated above, some reticular units responded to somatic afferent volleys with long-latencies in both anaesthetized and unanaesthetized preparations. The presence of long-latencies units discharge in brain stem cells was first noted by Cooper et al. (1953) in goats. Long-latency responses from less than 300 msec up to more than 3 sec were noted in the medullary (Albe-Fessard et al., 1962; Pompeiano and Swett, 1963a; Bowsher et al., 1968a; Bowsher, 1969, 1970), pontine (Bach-y-Rita, 1962a, 1964) and mesencephalic reticular formation (Amassian and De Vito, 1954). These responses generally consisted of a burst of spikes followed by a silent period and a certain time later, by a late burst of spikes. The extremely long latencies described above are not due to activation of slow conducting fibres, since the late response could also be obtained by stimulation of low threshold cutaneous afferents (Amassian and

DE VITO, 1954; BACH-Y-RITA, 1962a, 1964). Analogous responses have been recorded in the centrum medianum (ALBE-FESSARD and KRUGER, 1962).

The presence of late discharge in units studied after precollicular decerebration allows the conclusion that areas rostral to the section are not essential in the elaboration of the late response. After cerebellectomy no response of more than about 350 msec was observed (BACH-Y-RITA, 1962a, 1964). Latencies of responses as long as 875 msec, however, could still be observed in unanaesthetized decerebrate cats after cerebellectomy (POMPEIANO and SWETT, 1963a).

BACH-Y-RITA (1964) suggested that the latencies observed (up to more than 3 sec) are sufficiently long to consider the possible involvement of a neurohumoral mechanism. Long-latency effects of reticular activity on cortical EEG have been noted (BONVALLET et al., 1954) even on isolated cortical slab (INGVAR, 1955) and delayed arousal has been described in cats with intact RF, but with the direct pathways sectioned (LINDSLEY et al., 1950). Further experiments are required to investigate the origin of these late responses.

Following Frequencies, Attenuation, Learning. Reticular evoked potentials are greatly depressed and even disappear when the stimuli are delivered in rapid succession (STARZL et al., 1951b; FRENCH et al., 1952, 1953a; BOWSHER et al., 1968a), as are reticular units responses (AMASSIAN and DE VITO, 1954; HUTTENLOCHER, 1961; SCHEIBEL and SCHEIBEL, 1963a, 1965a, b; BELL et al., 1964; SEGUNDO et al., 1967b; BOWSHER et al., 1968; BOWSHER and PETIT, 1970). There is a progressive decline in the proportion of effective stimuli and/or in the amplitude of each response as a train of repetitive stimuli are continued, a phenomenon referred to as "attenuation". This term is used here descriptively, and should be preferred to others such as "accommodation", "adaptation" and "habituation" which convey implications to be avoided. Modality, location and intensity of the stimulus influence the following frequency. In all instances however the low following frequencies contrast with higher sustained rates reported in principal sensory pathways (HUNT and KUNO, 1959; CREUTZFELDT, 1961; POGGIO and MOUNTCASTLE, 1963).

The low following capacity and attenuation may be due to the multisynaptic character of the chain, since the likelihood of failure increases with each successive synaptic linkage intercalated in the pathway. However the lack of clear correlation between following frequency and latency suggests that the number of synapses may not be the only important factor (BELL et al., 1964). BELL et al. (1964) proposed that the failure depends upon the activation of an inhibitory loop, or the development of a synaptic transmission block (Wedensky inhibition, etc.). The low following capacity of some reticular units may also relate to the small area of postsynaptic membrane covered by any one of the multiple afferents to each reticular cell or the diffuse type of axonal ending, which contrasts sharply with the "bushy arbor" terminations found in the principal pathway (SCHEIBEL and SCHEIBEL, 1963b). Intracellular recording from reticular neurones showed that repetitive sensory stimulation became less effective simply because PSPs became smaller, and SEGUNDO et al. (1967b) proposed that attenuation is determined at intrareticular junctions, where activity is followed by prolonged subnormality of the presynaptic terminal. A reticular unit which ceased to respond to repetitive stimulation of one limb, could be reactivated by changing the site of stimulation

to another limb while continuing to stimulate at the same frequency (BELL et al., 1964;
SCHEIBEL and SCHEIBEL, 1965a; BOWSHER et al., 1968a), which suggests that the
fatiguability of these units following repetitive stimulation of a single peripheral
locus appears at synapses in the afferent pathway below the point of heterotopic
convergence. Finally, RF units may be conditioned to respond after several trials;
mesencephalic RF units may become sensitive to previously ineffective stimuli
by association of the latter with effective ones (YOSHII and OGURA, 1960; KAMI-
KAWA et al., 1963; BUREŠOVÁ and BUREŠ, 1965; BUREŠ and BUREŠOVÁ, 1967; cf.
BUREŠ, 1965).

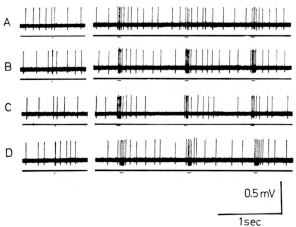

Fig. 15. Type A unit in mesencephalic reticular formation facilitated by superficial radial
nerve volleys in a decerebrate, cerebellectomized cat. Left column shows effects at 1/sec
stimulation and the right column effects at 100/sec. Duration of stimulus train at 100/sec,
50 msec. A,B: stimulation of the ipsilateral superficial radial nerve at 1.76 and 2.35 T, respectively. C,D: stimulation of the contralateral superficial radial nerve at 1.33 and 2,66 T respectively. The threshold values for these unit responses at 1/sec and 100/sec were, respectively,
the following: ipsilateral radial nerve 1.76 T and 1.53 T; contralateral radial nerve 1.33 T and
1.20 T. The same unit was also facilitated by high rate stimulation (100/sec) of the ipsilateral
and contralateral hamstring nerves at threshold values of 7.2 and 6.5 T, respectively. No effect
at 1/sec. (POMPEIANO and SWETT, 1963a)

5. Effects of Stimulation of Myelinated Cutaneous Afferents

It has been shown in Sections III, 1 and V that low rate stimulation of group
II cutaneous afferents elicited EEG synchronization in the normal cat as well as
a generalized inhibition of spontaneous and reflex muscular activity, due to spinal
activation of bulbospinal inhibitory mechanisms; conversely, high rate stimulation
of group II fibres, as well as low and high rate stimulation of group III cutaneous
fibres caused EEG and behavioural arousal. These findings indicate that both
group II and III cutaneous volleys reach the brain stem RF (cf. also AMASSIAN
and DE VITO, 1954; COLLINS and O'LEARY, 1954; COLLINS and RANDT, 1961).
POMPEIANO and SWETT (1962c, 1963a) analyzed the response patterns of reticular
units to group II and group III cutaneous afferent volleys elicited by controlled

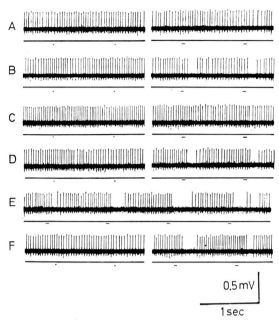

Fig. 16. Type B unit in mesencephalic reticular formation inhibited by cutaneous and muscular nerve volleys. The same experiment as in Fig. 15. Left column shows effects at 1/sec, right column and E effects at 100/sec. A, B: stimulation of the ipsilateral superficial radial nerve at 6.0 and 7.05 T, respectively. C, D, E: stimulation of the contralateral superficial radial nerve at 4.0, 5.3 and 8.0 T, respectively. F: stimulation of the ipsilateral hamstring nerve at 8.0 T. Similar effects were obtained from contralateral hamstring (not illustrated). No effects were observed when stimulating both the superficial radial nerves and the hamstring nerves up to 16.0 T at 1/sec. Threshold for inhibitory unit response at 100/sec are as follows: ipsilateral radial 7.05 T, contralateral radial 4.5 T, ipsilateral hamstring 5.1 T, contralateral hamstring 4.5 T. (POMPEIANO and SWETT, 1963a)

stimulation of the superficial radial nerves in precollicular decerebrate animals. Since the cerebellum provides additional pathways from the periphery to the brain stem, a complete cerebellectomy was performed in order that reticular responses could be attributed solely to direct spinoreticular influences.

The electrical activity of 551 brain stem units in response to graded volleys at 1/sec and 100/sec from the superficial radial nerves of both forelimbs was examined; 337 (61.1% of the total) were not influenced, 185 (33.6%) were facilitated, and 25 (4.6%) were inhibited. This finding is in agreement with previous observations indicating that the inhibitory responses are apparently outnumbered by facilitatory ones at all levels of the brain stem (see Section VII, 4). Only 4 units (0.7%) were influenced in a reciprocal manner, *i.e.*, ipsilateral facilitation and contralateral inhibition or *vice versa*. A unit was classified as negative if failed to respond to cutaneous volleys volleys up to 20T with low or high rate stimulation.

Unit response patterns, a rise or fall of the spontaneous discharge, were apparently simple in configuration and relatively constant at a given stimulus intensity (Figs. 15 and 16). Increases in rate or intensity of stimulation always intensified the original response, whether facilitatory or inhibitory, and invariably reduced the latency of the responses.

The unit responses were also classified into types A or B in relation to the type of cutaneous volleys which were effective. Whenever the intensity of the electrical pulses was kept below 3.5T, the stimulation was limited to group II fibres.

Type A units were influenced by stimulus intensities below 3.5T at 1/sec, which closely approximated stimulating conditions required for eliciting EEG synchronization in the normal animal.

Type B units were influenced by stimulus intensities above 3.5T at 1/sec, i.e., above threshold for group III afferent fibres. B unit thresholds were equivalent to stimulation above arousal threshold in the normal animal. The response thresholds of the same units at 100/sec were lower than those obtained with 1/sec stimulation both for A and B units; the stimulus intensities responsible for unit responses of type A were always below the threshold for group III fibres, independently of the stimulus rate. Those B units, which were not influenced at 1/sec rates, responded to 100/sec rates above 3.5T, but many B units, which were affected by group III afferent volleys at 1/sec, could be influenced at 100/sec rates at intensities below 3.5T.

The majority of the brain stem units influenced by cutaneous nerve stimulation (194 out of 214) were classified as A or B units. Only 16 units were classified separately as A–B or "mixed" units since they responded at 1/sec to low threshold volleys on one side (type A) and high threshold on the other (type B). The A–B units showed facilitatory responses. The 4 remaining units responded in a reciprocal fashion, i.e., inhibition from one side and facilitation from the other.

Although the two functionally different groups of units were found spatially intermixed at all levels of the brain stem, a segregation was observed. In particular type A units represented respectively 62.5 and 56.1% of the responding units at the border between pons and medulla or within the medulla itself, whereas only 24.1 and 26.3% were in the midbrain or in the pons. Low rate group II cutaneous volleys were shown to influence particularly the nucleus reticularis gigantocellularis. This finding has been recently confirmed by LIMANSKII (1966). On the other hand the periaqueductal central grey, the midbrain reticular formation and the nucleus reticularis pontis oralis and caudalis were preferentially influenced by low rate stimulation of both group II and III cutaneous fibres and high rate group II cutaneous volleys.

Summing up, units facilitated by single shock stimulation of group II and III cutaneous afferents were not distributed uniformly throughout the reticular core. Low threshold cutaneous volleys influenced approximately 60% of the total number of the affected units in the medulla and caudal pons, whereas in the pons and midbrain, group II cutaneous afferents affected only 25% of the units. Thus 40% of the units in the medulla and lower pons and 75% in the pons and midbrain responded to cutaneous volleys suprathreshold for group III activation.

The predominance of higher threshold responses in the midbrain and pons suggests that they both play an important role in the arousal response, in agreement with other work indicating that high threshold cutaneous afferent volleys impinge upon the mesencephalic reticular substance (AMASSIAN and DE VITO, 1954; COLLINS and O'LEARY, 1954; COLLINS and RANDT, 1960, 1961; WAGMAN and MCMILLAN, 1968), and the periaqueductal grey (cf. also ABRAHMS et al., 1962). Both these structures therefore may contribute to the arousal reaction elicited by low rate stimulation of the group III cutaneous afferents, which probably depends upon activation of polysynaptic ascending reticular pathways. The lower brain stem can, however, also be affected by arousing stimuli, such as high rate stimulation of group II cutaneous fibres or low and high rate stimulation of group III cutaneous afferents (cf. also CASEY, 1968).

The preferential distribution of group II cutaneous facilitatory influences on the caudalmost part of the brain stem should now be considered. The bulbo-pontine structures, which receive the majority of the group II actions, are certainly involved in the EEG synchronization induced by low rate stimulation of the group II cutaneous afferents. The hypothesis that this pattern of EEG synchronization is due to a direct inhibitory influence of cutaneous group II afferent volleys on the mesencephalic reticular activating system (cf. BONVALLET and BLOCK, 1961) was not confirmed in our study. Only a limited number of midbrain reticular units were inhibited when group II cutaneous afferents were stimulated at electrical parameters required for producing EEG synchronization in normal animals. An inhibition of the activating reticular system by group II cutaneous volleys mediated by structures lying above the level of decerebration is not excluded by these experiments.

An alternative explanation of the induced EEG synchronization is that low rate group II cutaneous volleys exert a rhythmic excitatory influence on the diencephalic synchronizing system. The production of synchronous constant latency responses at cortical levels (POMPEIANO and SWETT, 1962a, b) implies that group II cutaneous volleys reach thalamic areas via ascending oligosynaptic paths, including the nucleus reticularis gigantocellularis. Indeed there is evidence that the somatic afferent volleys responsible for the so-called associative cortical evoked potentials in unrestrained animals (BUSER, 1957; BUSER and BORENSTEIN, 1957, 1959; ALBE-FESSARD and FESSARD, 1963) ascend to the centrum medianum and related nuclei via the nucleus reticularis gigantocellularis (ALBE-FESSARD et al., 1962) and experiments have been made indicating that EEG synchronization can also be elicited by low rate stimulation of medullary structures (FAVALE et al., 1961; MAGNES et al., 1961). The nucleus reticularis gigantocellularis, which receives numerous spinal afferents, gives off long ascending axons, many of which terminate in the centrum medianum-parafascicular complex (NAUTA and KUYPERS, 1958). This ascending pathway is also open to group III cutaneous volleys since they reach the nucleus reticularis gigantocellularis, and contribute to the cortical associative responses. However other ascending reticular pathways, probably polysynaptic in nature, are activated by low rate group III cutaneous volleys (as well as by high rate stimulation of group II cutaneous afferents) thus leading to the disruption of the induced EEG synchronization.

6. Effects of Stimulation of Unmyelinated Cutaneous Afferents

There has been speculation as to whether specific regions in the brain stem RF represent the relay station in the pain pathway to higher levels (cf. NACHMANSOHN and MERRITT, 1956; HERRICK and BISHOP, 1958; MEHLER, 1962, 1966).

Classical neurology assigns to anterolateral spinal pathways the role of conducting impulses which give rise to the conscious sensation of pain (cf. Bowsher, 1963; Albe-Fessard and Bowsher, 1968). Indeed experimental evidence indicates that the ventrolateral funiculus includes a major nociceptive pathway synaptically activated by dorsal root afferents (Manfredi, 1970). Stimulation of cutaneous or mixed nerves can elicit postsynaptic activity in both the contralateral and ipsilateral anterolateral column of the spinal cord, not only when large and small myelinated fibres are stimulated (group II and group III corresponding to A-beta and A-delta fibres respectively) but also when non-myelinated group IV (C fibres) are selectively excited (Manfredi, 1970). The main problem now is to find out the specific pathways in the spinal cord and the relay stations in the brain stem which are responsible for disagreeable sensation.

The fibres which course along the ventrolateral funicles are: 1) the spinoreticular fibres studied both in cat and man (Section II, 3), which project via the RF to the centre median-parafascicular complex of the thalamus (Bowsher and Albe-Fessard, 1962; Albe-Fessard and Fessard, 1963; Albe-Fessard, 1965; Bowsher et al., 1968a); and 2) the spinothalamic fibres described in monkey and man (Collier and Buzzard, 1903; Mehler, 1957; Bowsher, 1961). The area of termination of these fibres corresponds exactly to that obtained in cat and monkey with electrophysiological techniques (Whitlock and Perl, 1961).

Mehler (1957) divides the spinothalamic fibres in two groups: the neospinothalamic and the palaeospinothalamic. The neospinothalamic fibres, which join the fibres originating from the dorsal column nuclei, project to the contralateral VPL nucleus where they make mainly, but not exclusively, axodendritic synapses (Bowsher, 1961). Destruction of the VPL does not abolish pain, and electrical stimulation of this nucleus in the awaken man does not elicit pain (Ervin and Mark, 1960; Guiot et al., 1962). The palaeospinothalamic fibres terminate in the intralaminar complex (i.e., in the centre median-parafascicular complex, in the nucleus centralis lateralis) and in the reticular nucleus of the thalamus (cf. Bowsher, 1961; Bowsher and Albe-Fessard, 1962). This projection is bilateral and the synapses of these fibres are only axosomatic (Bowsher, 1961). Section of the ventrolateral funiculus abolishes pain probably because it interrupts all the extralemniscal afferents originating from regions situated below the section, which include both the spino-reticulo-thalamic and the palaeospinothalamic pathways. On the contrary, a lateral section made at the level of the brain stem and affecting the classical neospinothalamic fibres does not suppress pain because the majority of the extralemniscal fibres have reached a medial position and therefore are not involved by the lesion (cf. Bowsher, 1963).

Myelinated group III cutaneous afferents may reach different regions of the brain stem RF (see Section VII, 5) and it is well known that nociceptive afferents are included among this population of fibres. Selective stimulation of unmyelinated C fibres performed in cats (Collins and Randt, 1958, 1960) and monkeys (Wagman and McMillan, 1968; McMillan and Wagman, 1971) may influence (either increase or decrease) the neuronal activity of the medullary (Collins and Randt, 1958) and the mesencephalic RF (Collins and Randt, 1960; Wagman and McMillan, 1968; McMillan and Wagman, 1971). The regions affected by these afferent volleys were rather discrete and corresponded to a small paramedian reticular area in the caudal medulla (COLLINS and RANDT, 1958) and to the ventral tegmentum in the midbrain of cats (COLLINS and RANDT, 1960) as well as to the parvicellular region of the mesencephalic RF in monkeys (WAGMAN and McMILLAN 1968). Nociceptive stimuli (such as pricking, burning or crushing the skin in rats), which quite certainly involved C fibres, were able to influence reticular neurones concentrated in a 1 mm cube of the ventromedial RF of the caudal medulla (BEN-JAMIN, 1962). This small medullary region affected by C afferent volleys, strikingly corresponds to that region which upon direct stimulation produced a strong arousal reaction in the *encéphale isolé* preparation (MAGNES et al., 1961). This effect was obtained not only with high rate but also with low rate stimulations, indicating that ascending projection from this area is polysynaptic in nature thus preventing the arrival of synchronous volleys to the non-specific thalamic nuclei.

Repetitive stimuli to the unmyelinated fibres were generally required to elicit reticular responses (COLLINS and RANDT, 1958, 1960; WAGMAN and McMILLAN, 1968; McMILLAN and WAGMAN, 1971). The medullary responses elicited in cats by selective stimulation of C fibres in either a forelimb (superficial radial nerve) or a hindlimb nerve (saphenous nerve) occurred at latencies of 380 and 560 msec respectively (COLLINS and RANDT, 1958). Longer latencies were also obtained from the mesencephalic RF by selective stimulation of the C fibres in the contralateral superficial radial nerve (550–600 msec) and the contralateral peroneal nerve (850–930 msec) in the same species (COLLINS and RANDT, 1960). In monkeys the latencies were generally longer than 450 msec (WAGMAN and McMILLAN, 1968). Control experiments excluded that these responses were related to the blood pressure rise seen after the stimulation (COLLINS and RANDT, 1958). Reticular units responding to C fibres also responded to the group III (δ) fibres, indicating that myelinated and unmyelinated afferents converge on brain stem units.

One may therefore conclude that the reticular neurones influenced by the C fibres constitute part of a pain system ascending the central core of the brain stem. Much more work is required to find out the area of termination of C afferents in the RF and the interaction (occlusion, inhibition) which may be elicited at this level by low threshold somatic afferent volleys as well as by descending cortical and subcortical mechanisms. The possibility, however, that in addition to the RF other structures such as the central grey matter play a role in the transmission of afferent patterns subserving pain perception should also be considered (KERR et al., 1955; HUNSPERGER, 1956; MELZACK et al., 1958; FAVALE et al., 1960; MEHLER, 1966).

7. Effects of Stimulation of Myelinated Muscular Afferents

Since low or high rate stimulation of muscular nerves in normal animals failed to elicit any detectable EEG and behavioural reactions when only group I muscular afferents were stimulated (POMPEIANO and SWETT, 1962b; GIAQUINTO et al., 1963b; see Section III, 2) the influence of fore- and hindlimb muscular afferents on the brain stem unit activity was also investigated, to find out whether there is any influence of group I volleys on reticular neurones, in decerebrate, cerebellectomized cats (POMPEIANO and SWETT, 1962d, 1963a), as well as in decerebrate animals with the cerebellum intact (POMPEIANO and SWETT, 1962e, f, 1963b).

In the first group of experiments performed in decerebrate, cerebellectomized cats, Pompeiano and Swett (1963a) studied the effects of hamstring and deep radial nerve afferent volleys on 455 spontaneously firing units localized in the brain stem from the midbrain to the medulla. Only 90 of these units responded to muscular afferent volleys at 100 or 200/sec rates at stimulus intensities up to 20T. Units influenced by hindlimb muscular volleys also responded to forelimb muscular volleys. Considering fore- and hindlimb muscular effects together, 74 units were apparently facilitated and 16 inhibited. All units affected by hindlimb muscular volleys also responded to forelimb cutaneous volleys, demonstrating widespread convergence of different sensory modalities on these neurones.

Preliminary observations indicated that group I was maximally activated at about 2.0T, 1.0T being the threshold for the most excitable fibres belonging to group I; group II afferent threshold apparently occurred between 1.75–2.25T, thereby overlapping with the higher threshold group I fibres. Total activation of group II was not defined, but it is likely to occur above group III threshold. Group III afferents did not make their appearance until about 5–7T.

Table 1. *Threshold values of brain stem unit responses to fore- and hindlimb muscle nerve stimulation at 200/sec*

Nerve	Side	Total number of units	Threshold values Range–Average		Number of units influenced at 2 T and below
Deep radial	ipsilateral	55	1.50–6.0	2.54	21
nerve	contralateral	45	1.71–7.90	2.91	11
Hamstring	ipsilateral	20	1.87–11.0	4.28	4
nerve	contralateral	17	1.71–11.0	4.50	4

Threshold responses of brain stem units were always considerably higher for the hindlimb than the forelimb muscular volleys, thus confirming the finding that threshold for arousal reaction in the normal cat was higher with hamstring volleys than for deep nerve volleys (Giaquinto et al., 1963b). The threshold for arousal during light sleep was close to threshold activation of group III muscular afferents with hamstring nerve volleys, whereas the arousal threshold value was close to group II threshold when the deep radial nerve was stimulated. Unit responses were obtained at lower intensities than were required for arousal. No unit was affected by hamstring nerve volleys below 2.30T, *i.e.*, at stimulus intensities below group II threshold. Most units were affected at stimulus values in the vicinity of group III threshold.

In contrast to hamstring nerve actions, deep radial nerve volleys evoked a small number of unit responses with high threshold group I volleys above 1.60 to 1.75T. Simultaneous stimulation of the deep radial nerve of both sides may lower the threshold of response of a reticular unit due to spatial summation. The effect was very weak, however, and no response could be observed with combined stimulation of both the nerves at stimulus intensities below 1.56T.

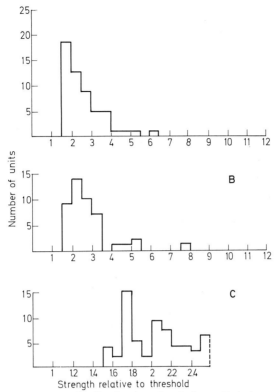

Fig. 17. Histograms illustrating the distribution of reticular units in terms of response thresholds to stimulation of the deep radial nerves at 200/sec stimulus rates in decerebrate cats with the cerebellum intact. A: distribution of 55 units and their threshold responses to stimulation of the ipsilateral nerve. B: distribution of 45 out of the 55 units shown in A with stimulation of the contralateral nerve. C: expanded base line showing the distribution of those unit responses plotted in A and B at 2.5 T and below. (POMPEIANO and SWETT, 1963b)

When considering the differences in central actions of muscular afferent volleys originating from the deep radial nerve and the hamstring nerve, it may be postulated that they depend primarily upon differences in their afferent fibre constituents (McINTYRE, 1962b; GIAQUINTO et al., 1963b). It is of interest, however, that the low threshold group I muscle afferents which originate from the primary endings of muscle spindles are apparently unable to influence the reticular neurones. This finding has been confirmed with intracellular recording techniques in both pyramidal and decerebrate cats, all cerebellectomized (MAGNI and WILLIS, 1964b).

The question now arises whether a group I influence on brain stem reticular units can be detected in the classical decerebrate preparation, *i.e.*, when the cerebellum is intact. Since group I volleys impinge on the cerebellum where they can also modify the activity of Purkinje neurones (see IOSIF et al., 1972 and POMPEIANO, 1972 for references), experiments were performed in decerebrate cats with cerebellum intact (POMPEIANO and SWETT, 1963b) to test for group I effects on units localized in the pontine and medullary reticular formation (mainly the nucleus reticularis pontis oralis, caudalis and gigantocellularis) (Table 1).

In these experiments many reticular units responded to high rate stimulation (200/sec) of the deep radial nerves only for stimulus intensities above 2.0 T, *i.e.*, supraliminal for group II activation (Fig. 17 A and B). Some units were influenced by stimulus intensities below 2.0 T, the lower limits ranging from 1.50 for the ipsilateral nerve to 1.71 T for the contralateral nerve (Fig. 17 C). In these cases at least 50% of the group I component were activated before reticular units were affected.

Reticular units influenced by deep radial nerve volleys were also affected by hamstring volleys, a higher threshold to hamstring volleys than for the deep radial nerves. Most thresholds were above 2.0 T. The lower limits ranged from 1.71 T for the contralateral nerve to 1.87 T for the ipsilateral nerve. These effects were due to higher threshold group I muscular afferents or to low threshold group II afferents. At these intensities 70–98% of the group I fibres can be activated.

The effects elicited by muscular nerve stimulation at near threshold values were characterized by a weak facilitation or, in some instances, inhibition. Stimulus intensities higher than 2.0 T increased the intensity of the response, shortened the latency and brought out more complicated response patterns (Fig. 18). These were generally characterized by an initial burst of spikes, followed by a pause and a late discharge, which were attributed to inhibitory and facilitatory influences.

The absence of low threshold group I influences on reticular units cannot be attributed to an increase in threshold of the unit response due to the removal of the forebrain, since cutaneous volleys were capable of influencing the same units at far lower thresholds. For instances, a group of reticular units which was influenced with an average stimulus intensity of 1.78 T from the deep radial nerves, was influenced at very low stimulus intensities (average 1.07–1.08 T) from the superficial radial nerves. At these latter intensities only 5% of the group II cutaneous afferents was activated.

Group I volleys from both fore- and hindlimb nerves reach the cerebellum through several ascending spinal pathways (cf. Oscarsson, 1972); nevertheless the response of reticular units to group I volleys was poor, though not always entirely absent, when the cerebellum is intact.

Since no effect from the deep radial nerve was ever observed with intensities below 1.50–1.71 T, it was concluded that total activation of group Ia fibres was apparently unable to influence reticular units. The effects elicited in the high threshold group I range were probably due to I b afferents (from Golgi tendon organs) and/or to activation of large diameter afferent fibres originating from deep receptors other than muscle spindles and Golgi tendon organs (see discussion in Giaquinto et al., 1963 b).

The results obtained by Pompeiano and Swett (1963 b) with extracellular recording have been basically confirmed by Limanskii (1966) who studied the effects of stimulation of afferent fibres from muscle nerves (quadriceps) on reticular units recorded intracellularly from the nucleus reticularis gigantocellularis in cats anaesthetized with chloralose and Nembutal and with the cerebellum intact. In all instances the threshold excitation of the reticular neurones during stimulation of muscle nerves was always higher than that obtained by stimulation of cutaneous nerves.

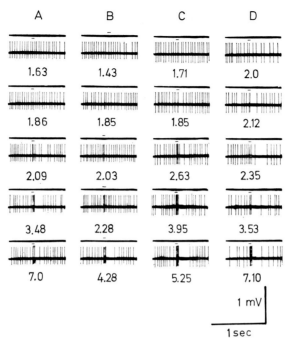

Fig. 18. Effects of fore- and hindlimb muscular afferent volleys on a medullary reticular unit in a decerebrate cat with the cerebellum intact. In this figure all nerves were stimulated at 200/ sec, 0.1 msec pulse duration. The stimulus train duration was 50 msec. Stimulus intensities relative to nerve threshold are indicated under each record. A: stimulation of the ipsilateral deep radial nerve. The threshold was 1.79 T (not shown). B: contralateral deep radial nerve. Threshold 1.71 T (not shown). C: ipsilateral hamstring nerve. Threshold 1.71 T. D: contra-lateral hamstring nerve. Threshold 2.12 T. For supraliminal stimuli a strong facilitatory response was followed by a silent period in all cases. No clear rebound effect occurred after the pause. In A the duration of the pause was shortened at higher stimulus intensities. (POM-PEIANO and SWETT, 1963b)

The results described above confirm previous findings, namely that a consider-able difference exists between the connections of the proprioceptive and cutaneous afferents to the reticular neurones (POMPEIANO and SWETT, 1963a, b). Whereas threshold stimulation of cutaneous nerves activated a large number of reticular neurones, proprioceptive stimulation elicited unit responses when group II and III muscle afferents are stimulated; on the contrary excitation of the group I fibres rarely produced an effect.

8. Effects of Mechanical Stimulation of Muscle Receptors

The technique of graded electrical stimulation may give ambiguous results, since there is some overlapping within the group I diameter range of the group Ia fibres which have been related with primary spindle afferents and the group Ib fibres related with Golgi tendon organs (BRADLEY and ECCLES, 1953; HUNT, 1954; ECCLES et al., 1957a; LAPORTE and BESSOU, 1957; McINTYRE, 1965). Moreover, contamination of the group I volley by group II impulses may occur, since the upper range of excitability of group I fibres overlaps with that of the group II afferents (ECCLES et al., 1957b; ECCLES and LUNDBERG, 1959b). The group I diameter range may include fibres from pressure-pain receptors (HUNT and McIN-TYRE, 1960; PAINTAL, 1960); moreover, group II diameter range includes not only secondary spindle afferents (MATTHEWS, 1933; BARKER, 1948; MERTON, 1953;

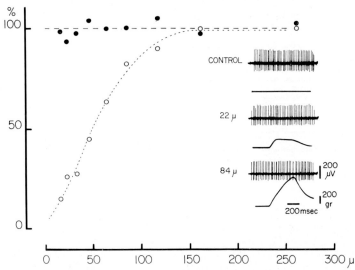

Fig. 19. Activity of a reticular unit during reflex contraction of the gastrocnemius-soleus (GS) muscle elicited by a series of vibrations of increasing amplitudes applied to the Achilles tendon. Decerebrate cat with ventral roots intact, GS muscle at 6 mm of initial extension. In each group of records the upper traces represent the discharge recorded from a brain stem reticular unit on the right side; the lower traces represent the reflex contraction of the left GS muscle elicited by vibrations applied to the Achilles tendon for 350 msec, at 200/sec and increasing peak-to-peak amplitudes, as indicated near the records. The reticular unit was activated antidromically by single-shock stimulation of the ascending MLF and disynaptically by stimulation of the descending MLF. Responses partially shown on the right have been plotted diagrammatically. Changes in frequency of unit discharge relative to the control values (dots) as well as changes in amplitude of the induced tension (circles) are plotted as a function of the amplitude of vibration. The mean frequency of the unit discharge in the absence of vibration (control) corresponded to 29.5/sec. In this experiment and in that represented by Fig. 22, 10 controls and 10 responses for each value of vibration were recorded. (POMPEIANO and BARNES, 1971)

HUNT, 1954), but also fibres supplying tendon organs, pressure-pain receptors and vascular afferents (HUNT, 1954; HUNT and McINTYRE, 1960; PAINTAL, 1960; BARKER, 1962; BARKER et al., 1962).

WOLSTENCROFT (1964) in cerebellectomized cats has shown that reticulospinal units may respond to ventral root stimulation after extrafusal paralysis by gallamine triethiodide. These results indicate that some muscle afferent fibres relay to reticulospinal neurones. It is not known, however, from this study whether these effects are due to activation of the primary or the secondary endings of the muscle spindles.

Vibration of a muscle provides a powerful stimulus for the primary endings of the muscle spindles, while it has less effect in exciting secondary endings of the spindles (BIANCONI and VAN DER MEULEN, 1963; BROWN et al., 1967; STUART et al., 1970). The resulting contraction of the vibrated muscle is due to monosynaptic reflex excitation of the corresponding motoneurones (MATTHEWS, 1966; BARNES and POMPEIANO, 1970a, b). BROWN et al. (1967) have shown that amplitudes of vibration up to 50 μ applied longitudinally to a non-contracting muscle produce driving of nearly all primary endings without any significant increase of firing of secondary endings or Golgi tendon organs (cf. STUART et al., 1970).

POMPEIANO and BARNES (1971) used small sinusoidal changes of length, applied longitudinally to the gastrocnemius-soleus (GS) muscle, as a specific stimulus to the primary endings of muscle spindles to study the central effects of group Ia volleys on the unit discharge recorded from the brain stem reticular formation in precollicular decerebrate cats, with the cerebellum intact; not only in normal preparations, but also when the contraction of the GS muscle from reflex excitation of motoneurones was abolished after section of ventral roots or after injection of Flaxedil, which leads to paralysis of the extrafusal muscle end-plates. The primary endings of muscle spindles could then be activated selectively without costimulation of Golgi tendon organs induced by reflex muscle contraction.

We will summarize first the results of the *experiments performed in decerebrate preparations with ventral roots intact* (POMPEIANO and BARNES, 1971).

The effects of muscle vibration on decerebrate cats with ventral roots intact were tested on 83 units recorded from the brain stem reticular formation at medullary and lower pontine level following the method described by MORELLI et al. (1970). Fig. 19 shows both the progressive increase in reflex contraction amplitude upon increasing the amplitude of the vibration (at 200/sec) from 15 μ to 150 μ and also the stabilization of these reflex contractions for amplitudes up to 250 to 300 μ. The same figure shows that in spite of the reflex contraction of the GS muscle, neither the frequency nor the pattern of discharge of a reticular unit was modified (cf. also Fig. 14e, f). If the reflex contraction of the GS muscle is due to stimulation of primary endings from muscle spindles, and activation of Golgi tendon organs is likely to appear as a result of the reflexly induced tension, it may be concluded that both types of muscle receptors are ineffective in the reticular unit illustrated. It appears now that 61 out of 83 units were not affected by muscle vibration. However 22 out of 83 units were influenced by muscle vibration. Most of these units were influenced at threshold amplitudes of vibration responsible for the induced reflex tension and the maximum effect was generally elicited by amplitudes of vibration of less than 100–150 μ. In most instances (17 units) a facilitation was induced by muscle vibration. Only in a few instances (5 units) were the units inhibited.

Fig. 20 shows the effects of changing amplitude (A) and frequency of vibration (B), as well as changing initial muscle length (C), on the unit discharge. The unit discharge appears on the rising phase of the reflex muscle tension and the magnitude of the response depends upon the amplitude of the contraction induced by muscle vibration.

Although the reflex contraction of the GS muscle elicited by vibration is due to stimulation of primary endings from muscle spindles, it is possible that the

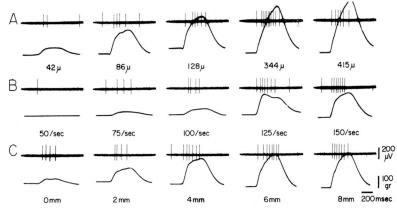

Fig. 20. Excitation of a reticular unit during reflex contraction of the GS muscle elicited by vibrations applied to the Achilles tendon. Decerebrate cat with ventral roots intact. In each group of records the upper traces represent the discharge recorded from a brain stem reticular unit on the left side; the lower traces represent the reflex contraction of the GS muscle elicited by vibration applied to the Achilles tendon. A,B: GS muscle at 6 mm of initial extension. In A vibrations at 200/sec and increasing peak-to-peak amplitudes, as indicated at the bottom of the records. In B, vibrations at 172 μ amplitude and increasing frequencies, as indicated at the bottom of the records. C: vibrations, 172 μ at 200/sec applied at different initial muscle length.
(Pompeiano and Barnes, 1971)

unit responses were due to activation of Golgi tendon organs as a result of the reflexly-induced tension.

　　None of the recorded units which responded to muscle vibration at 200/sec (in some instances 300/sec) at amplitudes lower than 100–150 μ were influenced by the same parameters of vibration after injection of Flaxedil, which abolished the induced reflex contraction. These units either became unresponsive to muscle vibration or responded to amplitudes of vibration above those values (Fig. 21).

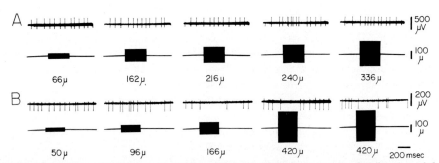

Fig. 21. Excitation or inhibition of reticular units induced by large amplitude vibration of the GS muscle in decerebrate cats with ventral roots intact, immobilized with Flaxedil. Microelectrode recording from two reticular units located on the left side. Left GS muscle at 6 mm of initial extension. A: unit accelerated by vibration of the GS at 200/sec and increasing peak-to-peak amplitudes, as indicated at the bottom of the records. The threshold for the facilitation of this reticular unit corresponds to 240 μ. B: unit inhibited by vibration of the GS muscle at 200/sec. Inhibition of the unit discharge occurs first at 166 μ. (Pompeiano and Barnes, unpublished figure)

The fact that these units responded to amplitudes of vibration larger than those required to elicit a maximum reflex contraction of the GS muscle excludes the possibility that the effect is due to proprioceptive afferent volleys originating from primary endings of muscle spindles. These responses have been attributed to stimulation of secondary endings of muscle spindles.

The effects of vibration of the GS muscle in de-efferented preparations (POM-PEIANO and BARNES, 1971).

Vibration of the de-efferented GS muscle for 200–400 msec at 200–300/sec, at amplitudes up to 350–400 μ, did not change the frequency and the pattern of discharge in 65 out of 71 reticular units (*e.g.*, Fig. 22 A).

In these experiments a motoneuronal discharge occurred synchronously with each wave of vibration. The synchrony as well as the short latency of these discharges suggests that the discharges are monosynaptic in origin (cf. also BARNES and POMPEIANO, 1970a, b).

There was a powerful activation of the primary endings of muscle spindles by vibration of the GS muscle and strong central effects of the induced group Ia volleys on heteronymous extensor motoneurones (Fig. 22 B). These positive results elicited at segmental level contrasted with the negative results obtained in the same experiment on the reticular unit during vibration of similar amplitudes applied to the GS muscle stretched at comparable initial muscle extension.

Only 6 out of 71 reticular units responded to muscle vibration in the de-efferented animal. Three of them were facilitated and three were inhibited. Only in one of these 6 units could the responses be attributed with certainty to group Ia afferent volleys. On the contrary, the remaining 5 units were influenced by amplitudes of vibration larger than 100 μ, which is required to produce maximal activation of the primary endings of muscle spindles. The secondary endings of muscle spindles were probably responsible for the effect in these 5 units.

The units recorded during muscle vibration both in the intact as well as in the de-efferented preparation were located particularly in the nucleus reticularis pontis caudalis, gigantocellularis, parvicellularis, reticularis ventralis and reticularis lateralis both ipsilaterally and contralaterally to the side of stimulation. Moreover some of these units could be activated antidromically by stimulating either the ascending or the descending MLF (Fig. 14).

Units which were unresponsive to longitudinal vibration of the GS muscle both in the intact and in the de-efferented preparation could be excited by cutaneous stimulation applied to the ipsilateral and/or the contralateral limbs. Fore- or hindlimbs were found most effective. Reticular units generally responded to stimulation of hair receptors, touch receptors, pressure receptors or joint receptors.

In summary, the main result of these experiments was the demonstration that longitudinal vibration of the ankle extensor muscles at 200–300/sec performed in the de-efferented preparation did not affect the frequency or the pattern of discharge of most of the brain stem reticular units. Only one of the 71 units recorded in de-efferented animals showed changes in its activity during vibration of the GS muscle at amplitudes lower than 100μ. The same vibration was effective at spinal cord level, as shown by the fact that in all these experiments a short latency motoneuronal discharge could be recorded from ventral roots during each cycle of vibration, indicating the monosynaptic origin of the response (BARNES and

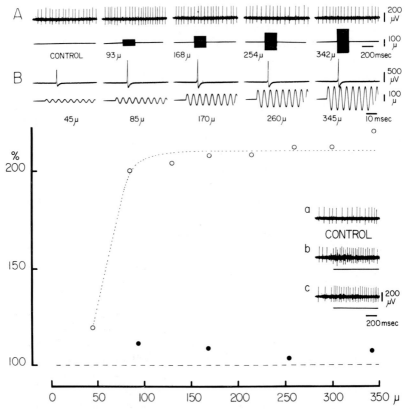

Fig. 22. Effects of changing amplitudes of vibration of the lateral gastrocnemius-soleus (LGS) muscle on the discharge of a reticular unit and the medial gastrocnemius (MG) monosynaptic reflex in a de-efferented preparation. Decerebrate cat with ventral roots L6–S2 of the left side completely cut. Left LGS muscle at 6 mm of initial extension. In each group of records above the diagram, the upper traces represent (A) the discharge recorded from a brain stem reticular unit on the right side, or (B) the monosynaptic reflex recorded from ventral root L7 on single-shock stimulation of the MG nerve (0.1 msec rectangular pulse at 2.0 T). The lower traces represent the output of the photoelectric length meter. Vibrations applied for 210 msec, at 200/sec and increasing peak-to-peak amplitudes, as indicated at the bottom of records. Responses partially shown above have been plotted diagrammatically. Changes in frequency of unit discharge relative to the control values (dots) are plotted as a function of the amplitude of vibration. The mean frequency of the unit discharge in the absence of vibration (control) corresponded to 17.9/sec and was not affected by muscle vibration. Circles indicate the percentage facilitation of the MG monosynaptic reflex during vibrations of the LGS muscle at increasing amplitudes. An acceleration of the spontaneous discharge of the same unit (a) was elicited by tactile stimulation applied to the left (b) and the right (c) forelimb. (Pompeiano and Barnes, 1971)

Pompeiano, 1970b). There is apparently no proprioceptive control from the primary endings of muscle spindles on the brain stem reticular formation.

It is well known that contraction is a very effective means of exciting Golgi tendon organs (Matthews, 1933; Hunt and Kuffler, 1951; Jansen and Rud-jord, 1964). When the muscle is contracting reflexly during vibration, the Golgi tendon organs become appreciably more sensitive to vibration, while the sensitivity of primary endings to vibration is reduced by muscle contraction (BROWN et al., 1967). That the unit responses in these instances were due to activation of Golgi tendon organs was shown by the fact that none of the recorded units which responded to amplitudes of vibration lower than 100 μ were influenced by the same parameters of vibration after injection of Flaxedil, which abolished the induced reflex contraction. On the other hand the reticular unit responses elicited by threshold amplitudes of vibration higher than 100–150 μ, both in the intact or in the de-efferented preparation could be attributed to stimulation of the secondary sensory endings (cf. STUART et al., 1970).

It has already been mentioned that most of the recorded reticular neurones unresponsive to muscle vibration could be activated antidromically by stimulating either the ascending or the descending MLF. Stimulation of the primary endings of muscle spindles was apparently unable to affect brain stem reticular units, which had either an ascending or a descending axon. This finding gives support to observations summarized in previous sections, which indicate that both ascending and descending influences exerted by the brain stem reticular formation escape proprioceptive control by the primary endings of muscle spindles.

We are now confronted with the problem of explaining why group I afferent volleys to the cerebellum (cf. OSCARSSON, 1972) are apparently unable to change the pattern of discharge of reticular units, while such marked effects are obtained with group II and III muscular and cutaneous afferents. Observations reported elsewhere (see IOSIF et al., 1972 and POMPEIANO, 1972 for references) indicate that if there is any postsynaptic influence on Purkinje cells when only group I volleys reach the cerebellar cortex, the effect is quite small in size.

VIII. Reticular Control of Transmission in Reflex Paths to Motoneurones

It is well known that reticulospinal volleys coursing in the ventral quadrants of the spinal cord may either excite or inhibit postsynaptically the a (MAGOUN and RHINES, 1946; RHINES and MAGOUN, 1946; MAGOUN, 1950) as well as the γ motoneurones (GRANIT and KAADA, 1952). The excitability of the a motoneurones may thus be modified either directly or indirectly through the well-known efferent γ-control of the muscle spindles (LEKSELL, 1945; GRANIT, 1955). In addition to these pathways there are also other descending reticular paths which affect transmission from primary afferents to motoneurones.

1. The Dorsal Reticulospinal System

Lesion experiments. Experiments performed in decerebrate cats indicate that both the excitatory and the inhibitory component of the flexion reflex (SHERRINGTON and SOWTON, 1915; FORBES et al., 1923; BALLIF et al., 1925; FULTON, 1926; LIDDELL et al., 1932; JOB, 1953; DOWNMAN and HUSSEIN, 1958) increase markedly

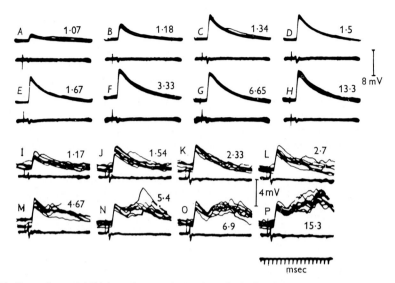

Fig. 23. Decerebrate inhibition of transmission from high threshold muscle afferents to motoneuron. Intracellular recording (upper traces) was performed from many PBST motoneurones
in a decerebrate cat before and after a spinal transection. Lower traces are from the dorsal root
entry zone. The PBSt nerve was stimulated and the strengths are indicated in the records in
multiples of threshold strengths from the nerve. Records A–H were obtained before transection of the spinal cord and volleys in high threshold muscle afferents do not evoke an EPSP
(F–H). Records I–P were obtained from another PBSt motoneurone after transection of the
cord and illustrate the characteristic excitatory action evoked from high threshold afferents
in the spinal state (L–P). (Eccles and Lundberg, 1959a)

after transection of the spinal cord. The release was attributed by Fulton (1926)
to disappearance of inhibitory action on interneurones mediating the reflex.

Lundberg and his group compared synaptic actions in motoneurones of
decerebrate and spinal cats (see Lundberg, 1964b, 1966, 1967); tonic inhibition
was found in the decerebrate state of polysynaptic transmission to motoneurones
from the cutaneous and the high threshold muscle afferents (Eccles and Lundberg, 1959a), i.e., from those afferents which give rise to the flexion reflex (FRA)
(Eccles and Lundberg, 1959b; Lundberg, 1959). Both the excitatory (Fig. 23)
and the inhibitory actions from the FRA are effectively inhibited in the decerebrate state. A similar tonic inhibition is also exerted on the Ib excitatory and
inhibitory pathways but not on the Ia inhibitory pathway. These findings were
confirmed by Kuno and Perl (1960).

Experiments with spinal cord lesions indicate that the responsible paths
descend along the dorsal part of the lateral funicle. Since the tonic control is
maintained as long as either funicle is intact (Holmqvist and Lundberg, 1959),
it is suggested that the effect is bilateral. The centres responsible for this control
are restricted to the ventromedial part of the medullary and lower pontine brain
stem (Holmqvist, 1961; Holmqvist and Lundberg, 1961). A low pontine lesion
gives a release of the inhibitory path from the FRA, while the excitatory path is
released only after a more caudal medullary lesion. It will be shown later that in

the decerebrate preparation the tonic control on the FRA pathway to motoneurones is paralleled by a tonic inhibition of transmission in the FRA pathway to
primary afferents (CARPENTER et al., 1963) and to ascending pathways (HOLMQVIST
et al., 1960a).

Stimulation experiments. Depression of reflex transmission to motoneurones
has also been demonstrated with electrical stimulation of the RF under conditions
when the effect could not be due to inhibition of motoneurones (AUSTIN, 1952;
HUGELIN, 1955; KLEYNTJENS et al., 1955; LINDBLOM and OTTOSSON, 1955;
KOIZUMI et al., 1959; HUGELIN and DUMONT, 1960).

ENGBERG et al. (1965, 1968a; cf. also LUNDBERG, 1966, 1967) studied the
descending inhibition coursing along the dorsolateral funiculus uncomplicated by
effects on motoneurones and on primary afferents. In order to prove inhibition of
interneurones it is necessary to employ stimuli that do not evoke primary afferent
depolarization (PAD). Furthermore, if actions on transmission to motoneurones
are investigated, it is difficult to judge the effect on interneuronal transmission
of such reticular stimuli that evoke postsynaptic inhibition. Large IPSPs can be
evoked in motoneurones from the same brain stem region (LLINÁS and TERZUOLO,
1964; JANKOWSKA et al., 1964, 1968). In order to prevent this reticulospinal postsynaptic inhibition of motoneurones, the experiments were performed in decerebrate and cerebellectomized cats after transection of the ventral quadrants which
mediate the inhibitory effect (JANKOWSKA et al., 1964, 1968). In these preparations
ENGBERG et al. (1965, 1968a) have shown that stimulation of the ventromedial
part of the caudal brain stem that does not evoke IPSP in motoneurones or PAD,
may selectively depress the excitatory and inhibitory synaptic actions on motoneurones evoked from the FRA and the Ib afferents. The effects described above were
evoked from a region within the area of MAGOUN's inhibitory centre (MAGOUN and
RHINES, 1946), but from a somewhat more rostral and ventral region than the one
from which postsynaptic inhibition can be evoked in motoneurones at low strength
of stimulation (JANKOWSKA et al., 1964, 1968). Moreover the effect was mediated
by axons with a conduction velocity of at least 20 m/sec.

Evidence that stimulation of the brain stem may evoke inhibition at an
interneuronal level is shown by more direct experiments in which the effects of
brain stem stimulation were investigated on interneurones in the dorsal horn and
intermediate region after partial transection of the spinal cord (ENGBERG et al.,
1966, 1968b). Stimulation of the brain stem that depresses the reflex transmission
without giving PAD, inhibits the discharge evoked from the FRA in interneurones.
Brain stem stimulation did not give postsynaptic potentials in the great majority
of interneurones, but effectively depressed the EPSPs and IPSPs evoked from
the FRAs in these interneurones. It has been suggested that a dorsal reticulospinal
system inhibits reflex transmission by producing postsynaptic inhibition in first
order interneurones.

The dorsal reticulospinal system is well defined with respect to its origin in the
brain stem and the location of the descending pathway in the dorsal part of the
lateral funiculus, but it cannot at present be identified with any anatomically
established descending tract. With retrograde degeneration technique TORVIK
and BRODAL (1957) failed to demonstrate a reticulospinal tract in the dorsal part
of the lateral funiculus. Similar results have also been reported by authors using

the method of orthograde degeneration following small lesions in the reticular formation (cf. NYBERG-HANSEN, 1965). Some findings reported as a result of larger lesions (PAPEZ, 1926; KURU et al., 1959) have been attributed by ENGBERG et al. (1968a) to concomitant degeneration of rubrospinal axons. It appears therefore that the effects are not mediated by a continuous tract but are relayed in the upper part of the spinal cord and conducted in a propriospinal tract (see KUYPERS 1964).

2. Descending Monoaminergic Pathways

The dorsal reticulospinal system is probably not the only pathway responsible for the inhibition of spinal interneurones. Recent studies (ANDÉN et al., 1964a, 1966a, b; ENGBERG and RYALL, 1965, 1966; RYALL, 1965; cf. LUNDBERG, 1966; ENGBERG et al., 1968c) have provided evidence for the existence of one noradrenergic and one 5-hydroxytryptaminergic pathway with inhibitory effect on transmission of single volleys from the FRA and Ib afferents. Both the excitatory and the inhibitory actions from the FRA to motoneurones and ascending pathways as well as transmission to primary afferent terminals are inhibited by these pathways.

It would be of interest to know whether activity in these monoaminergic descending pathways contributes to the tonic decerebrate inhibition of transmission from the FRA. Experiments therefore were performed to find out if 5-HT and NA antagonists release reflex pathways from this tonic control (LUNDBERG, 1966; ENGBERG et al., 1968d). There was no indication that the noradrenaline pathway contributes to this mechanism. Administration of 5-HT antagonists, however, can give some release of reflex transmission from the tonic decerebrate control. There are some functional differences between the effects mediated by the monoaminergic pathway and those of the dorsal reticulospinal system and the tonic decerebrate control (ANDÉN et al., 1964b)[7]. In addition the dorsal reticulospinal system originates from the brain stem reticular formation, whereas the 5HT neurones giving rise to descending pathways are located mainly in the raphe nuclei (DAHLSTRÖM and FUXE, 1964, 1965; FUXE, 1965). The axons of some of the raphe nuclei descend in the dorsolateral funiculus (BRODAL et al., 1960). Moreover, while the axons of the dorsal reticulospinal system have a conduction velocity of at least 20 m/sec, the axons of the descending monoaminergic pathways in the spinal cord are unmyelinated with a diameter of about 0.5–1 μ (CARLSSON et al., 1964; DAHLSTRÖM and FUXE, 1965; FUXE, 1965). It is also of interest that the tonic inhibition of transmission from the FRA can be partially maintained after complete destruction of the medullary and pontine raphe nuclei (ENGBERG et al., 1968d), so that this descending inhibition does not come exclusively from the raphe nuclei. It is more likely that this decerebrate effect on reflex transmission is caused mainly by activity in the dorsal reticulospinal tract discussed above.

---

7 The organization of the reflex pathways influenced by these monoaminergic descending fibres has been investigated in detail and will not be treated here (ANDÉN et al., 1966c; BERGMANS and GRILLNER, 1967; JANKOWSKA et al., 1967a, b; GRILLNER, 1969; cf. LUNDBERG, 1965, 1966).

IX. Reticular Control of Transmission in Reflex Paths to Primary Afferents

The brain stem reticular formation may influence spinal reflexes by producing primary afferent depolarization (PAD) and thereby presynaptic inhibition (FRANK and FUORTES, 1957; ECCLES et al., 1961; cf. ECCLES, 1964a, b). Moreover brain stem reticular structures may affect transmission from primary afferents to the primary afferents. These two aspects of the problem will be discussed below.

1. Primary Afferent Depolarization Evoked from the Brain Stem

In precollicular decerebrate cats, submitted to cerebellectomy, negative DRPs can be evoked by repetitive stimulation of wide areas of the brain stem (CARPENTER et al., 1962, 1966; cf. LUNDBERG, 1964b, 1967). In particular a short-latency DRP was evoked by stimulation of the dorsal region of the brain stem, either on the midline or 2 mm on the left of the midline, but not on the right side of the brain stem (contralateral to the side tested in the spinal cord). Mapping in the rostro-caudal direction revealed that the short latency DRP could only be evoked from the caudal brain stem, i.e., from the medulla and the caudal pons. This area seems to be more rostral than that giving postsynaptic inhibition on motoneurones (JANKOWSKA et al., 1968). The short latency DRP is mediated via ventral spinal pathways as shown by a complete disappearance of the short latency effect after transection of the ventral quadrants.

DRPs were also evoked from more ventral regions of the brain stem at the same low threshold as those from the dorsal part, but they had longer latency than those evoked with the electrode in a more dorsal position. Long latency DRPs are not only evoked from the medial regions but also from the whole lateral extent of the brain stem, including not only the medulla and pons (CARPENTER et al., 1966) but also the mesencephalic reticular formation (MORRISON and POMPEIANO, 1965). These DRPs can be evoked after transection of either the ventral or dorsal quadrants of the spinal cord (CARPENTER et al., 1966).

Experiments with excitability measurements from the terminals of different types of afferents following the WALL's method (1958) revealed that there is a depolarization in Ia (Fig. 24) and Ib afferents and in cutaneous afferents (CARPENTER et al., 1966). The region from which a depolarization can be evoked in Ia afferents corresponds reasonably well to that from which the short-latency DRP is evoked. Equally strong effects were found to Ia afferents of a flexor and an extensor. The effects in Fig. 24 are produced through a pathway descending in the ventral quadrant of the spinal cord.

Stimulation in more ventral region of the brain stem evoked PAD in Ib and cutaneous afferents but not in Ia afferents, by pathways descending in dorsal as well as ventral parts in the ventrolateral funicles. It seems likely therefore that PAD can be evoked from at least two neuronal systems.

The demonstration that PAD in Ia, Ib and cutaneous afferents can be evoked from the dorsal region of the brain stem particularly at midline level indicates that the pathway responsible for this effect is the MLF, the descending fibres of which originate in part from the medial vestibular nucleus.

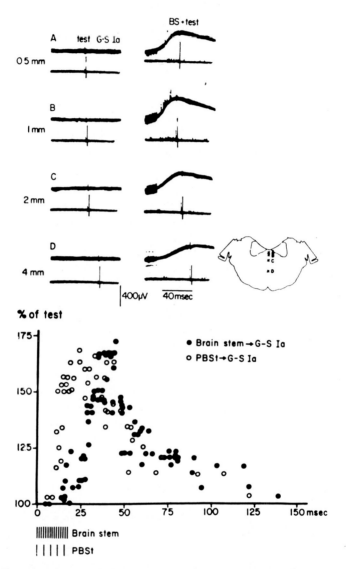

Fig. 24. PAD evoked from the brain stem in Ia afferent nerve fibres. The upper traces are DRPs recorded from the most caudal dorsal rootlet in L6. The change in excitability in Ia afferents is judged from the lower traces in which the terminals of Ia afferents are stimulated through a microelectrode inserted in the GS motor nucleus and the test discharge recorded peripherally in the GS nerve. Brain stem stimulation gives an increased excitability at a depth of 0.5 and 1 mm from the 4th ventricle but not in C and D at a depth of 2 and 4 mm respectively. The time course of the increased excitability is shown in the curve (●) and for comparison is shown the effect of a train of group I volleys in the PBSt nerve (o). Calibration below D refers to the dorsal root potential. All records consist of superimposed traces. (Carpenter et al., 1966)

cutaneous afferents, and reaching mainly cutaneous afferents. This path is apparently not subject to decerebrate inhibition. Component II, on the other hand, is part of the flexor reflex actions and this path from the FRA to the FRA is subject to a very effective tonic inhibitory control in the decerebrate state.

It is concluded that there is a tonic inhibition in the decerebrate state of transmission from the FRA to the FRA, but there is neither inhibition of the short latency path from cutaneous afferents to cutaneous afferents nor of the path from group I muscle afferents to Ia, Ib and cutaneous afferents.

The release after spinal cord transection of the DRPs evoked from the FRA is comparable with the release of actions from the FRA to motoneurones and it is likely to be mediated by the same dorsal reticulospinal system.

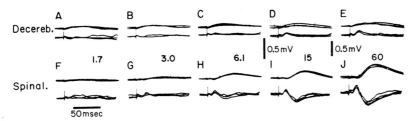

Fig. 25. Dorsal root potentials evoked from high threshold muscle afferents in decerebrate and spinal cats. The upper traces were recorded from the most caudal dorsal rootlet in L6 and the lower traces from the dorsal root entry zone in L7. Single stimuli were given to the gastrocnemius-soleus nerve before and after spinal transection. Corresponding records in the upper and lower row were obtained at the same stimulus strength, which is indicated between corresponding records and expressed in multiples of threshold strengths. (CARPENTER et al., 1963)

The centres responsible for the tonic control of transmission from the FRA to motoneurones are located in the medial brain stem (HOLMQVIST and LUNDBERG, 1959); a low pontine lesion gives an almost complete release of the inhibitory path to extensor motor nuclei from decerebrate control, without any release of the excitatory path to flexor nuclei, which is released only after a more caudal lesion (HOLMQVIST and LUNDBERG, 1961; HOLMQVIST, 1961). The release of actions from the FRA to primary afferents parallels the release of the excitatory path to flexor motoneurones in its occurrence with a caudal medullary lesion.

Stimulation experiments. ENGBERG et al. (1968a) studied the effects of brain stem stimulation on transmission of reflexes to primary afferents, in decerebrate cerebellectomized cats after transection of the ventral quadrants. As with transmission to motoneurones, conditioning stimulation in the brain stem may depress DRP evoked from peripheral nerves without producing any DRP in itself. The DRPs evoked by single or tetanic stimulation of group I muscle afferents are not reduced by the brain stem stimulation. On the other hand the large DRP elicited by stronger stimulation of muscle nerves, activating high threshold muscle afferents, is very effectively depressed. DRPs evoked from skin nerves were found less affected by the brain stem stimulation.

It has already been shown in the previous section that component I of the DRPs evoked from skin nerves is identical in decerebrate and spinal cats, whereas component II which is assumed to be an FRA effect (being recruited by stronger stimuli) only appears after spinal transection; only the latter was reduced by the brain stem stimulation.

The Ventral Reticulospinal System. Stimulation of the brain stem may decrease the DRP evoked from various afferent sources, probably by inhibition at an interneuronal level of reflex transmission to primary afferents (LUNDBERG and VYKLICKÝ, 1963, 1966; cf. LUNDBERG, 1964b, 1966, 1967). These experiments were made on decerebrate, decerebellate cats with the spinal cord transected in the lower thoracic region, except for the ventral quadrant ipsilateral to the side tested on the lumbosacral region. Stimulation of the caudal brain stem at fairly low frequencies which does not evoke any DRP is able to depress the DRPs evoked from cutaneous and high threshold muscle afferents (FRA). These DRPs represent the PAD in the FRA afferents (ECCLES et al., 1962b). The effects are evoked from the ventral medial region of the caudal brain stem and mediated by ventral spinal pathways.

The inhibitory action from the brain stem is not confined to the DRP evoked from the FRA. There is also a depression of the DRP evoked from group Ia muscle afferents. This DRP represents the PAD in Ia afferents (ECCLES et al., 1961, 1962c) and the results indicate that the pathway from Ia to Ia afferents can also be inhibited. A similar depression is also found of the DRP evoked by volleys in group Ib afferents which give PAD to Ib afferents and to cutaneous afferents (ECCLES et al., 1963a, b). Also the depression of the DRPs from group Ia and Ib is mediated by pathways descending in the ipsilateral ventral quadrant. The effective region corresponds to the medial part of the medulla, where reticulospinal neurones are located.

In summary, these experiments indicate that the DRPs evoked from different primary afferent systems can be inhibited by brain stem stimuli that do not evoke any DRP. Hence this inhibition cannot be due to a PAD and it is postulated that the action is exerted at an interneuronal level. The inhibition is evoked from the caudal medial reticular formation and is probably a reticulospinal action. This represents another example of descending inhibition of interneurones of spinal reflex pathways.

Attempts have been made to find out whether this descending control system also inhibits transmission in reflex paths to motoneurones as shown for the dorsal reticulospinal system (JANKOWSKA et al., 1968). Stimulation of the medullary reticular formation in preparations with the ventral spinal cord intact generally produces very large IPSPs in both extensor and flexor motoneurones (JANKOWSKA et al., 1964, 1968). The conductance change associated with the IPSPs (LLINÁS and TERZUOLO, 1964; JANKOWSKA et al., 1964, 1968) will decrease the synaptic potentials in the motoneurones and it is therefore not easy to disclose an inhibitory effect on transmission of the synaptic actions in the path to the motoneurones. In some instances however a depression of polysynaptic PSPs was observed in a few motoneurones in which the reticular stimuli did not evoke an IPSP (JANKOWSKA et al., 1968). It was then postulated that there is an inhibition also of transmission to motoneurones. This inhibitory effect was observed with respect to transmission from the FRA, but we do not know whether or not interneuronal transmission from Ia or Ib afferents is also influenced. The comparison of effects on interneuronal transmission to primary afferent terminals and to motoneurones suggests that the same neuronal system is responsible. This system can then be differentiated from the dorsal reticulospinal system not only by the different location of descending axons in the spinal cord, but also by the fact that it inhibits transmission from Ia and Ib to primary afferent terminals (LUNDBERG and VYKLICKY, 1966), whereas the dorsal reticulospinal system has no effect on transmission from Ia and Ib afferents to primary afferent terminals (ENGBERG et al., 1968).

X. Reticular Control of Transmission to Ascending Spinal Pathways

A mass discharge can be recorded from the ventral quadrant of the spinal cord on stimulation of ipsilateral and contralateral hindlimb nerves (OSCARSSON, 1958, 1964a; HOLMQVIST et al., 1959; LUNDBERG and OSCARSSON, 1962b; MAGNI and OSCARSSON, 1962; HOLMQVIST and OSCARSSON, 1963; LUNDBERG, 1964a; OSCARSSON et al., 1964). These discharges result on stimulation of group II and III muscle afferents, the high threshold joint fibres and the cutaneous afferents but not of the group I volleys. The receptive field from which the neurones of this ascending path draw their excitation is bilateral (OSCARSSON, 1958; LUNDBERG and OSCARSSON, (1962b) including many muscles and large areas of skin. The axons of these neurones have a mean conduction velocity of 84 m/sec, ranging from 50 to 120 m/sec. Lower conduction velocities have been found by UDO and MANO (1970).

The ventral spinobulbar tract has no monosynaptic connections, but only polysynaptic connections from the periphery. This explains why the neurones of this pathway show a train of impulses on electrical stimulation of cutaneous and muscular hindlimb nerves. The interneurones transmitting effects from the FRA to ascending pathways are similar to those which transmit information from the FRA to motoneurones. For this reason the ventral pathway activated from them has been designated as the bilateral ventral flexion reflex tract or bVFRT (LUNDBERG and OSCARSSON, 1962b). This ascending spinal pathway may carry information regarding flexor reflex pattern (ECCLES and LUNDBERG, 1959b; LUNDBERG, 1959, 1964b).

Cell bodies of the bVFRT are probably located in the ventromedial part of the grey matter, while their axons reach the brain stem. This tract seems to correspond to the spinoreticular pathway (LUNDBERG and OSCARSSON, 1962b; LUNDBERG, 1964a; cf. BOHM, 1953).

Neurones of the bVFRT predominantly receive excitation from the FRA. Excitation of these neurones also occurs on adequate activation from muscle and skin such as touch, pressure and pinching. It is also possible to inhibit this pathway from the periphery. All adequate stimuli of muscle and skin that give excitation, can also give inhibition to this pathway and there is often inhibition and excitation to the same cells from different regions and sometimes even from the same region of the receptive field (LUNDBERG and OSCARSSON, 1962b). These findings parallel those obtained at segmentary level showing the existence of excitatory and inhibitory reflex paths from the FRA (Eccles and Lundberg, 1959a, b; Holmqvist and Lundberg, 1961; Carpenter et al., 1963).

There are three main supraspinal control systems which are able to influence the transmission to the neurones giving rise to the so-called bVFRT.

The *first* supraspinal control system originating in the brain stem and descending along the ipsilateral ventral quadrant, exerts monosynaptic excitatory influences on these neurones of the bVFRT (Holmqvist et al., 1960b). This pathway originates in part at least from the Deiters' nucleus (Grillner et al., 1968). The *second* system is represented by the corticospinal tract which exerts an excitatory action on interneurones transmitting effects from cutaneous and high threshold muscular afferents to the neurones of the ventral ascending pathways (Magni and Oscarsson, 1961; Lundberg et al., 1963; Hongo and Okada, 1967; Hongo et al., 1967). These effects are similar to the facilitatory effects exerted by the corticospinal tract on interneurones from the FRA to motoneurones (Lundberg and Voorhoeve, 1962; Lundberg et al., 1962). The *third* system finally is a reticulospinal pathway, which exerts a tonic inhibitory influence on transmission from cutaneous and high threshold muscular afferents to the neurones of the ventral ascending spinal pathways (Holmqvist et al., 1960a; Carpenter et al., 1965; cf. also Hagbarth and Kerr, 1954; Oscarsson, 1958). The descending pathways responsible for this effect are located in the dorsal part of the lateral funicle and from each side a bilateral effect is exerted (Holmqvist et al., 1960a). This is shown in Fig. 26, where the left hamstring nerve was stimulated at two different strengths and recording was made from the right spinal half. With intact left spinal half the late mass discharge is small (A, B). Section of the dorsal half of the spinal cord gives a large release (C, D), which does not further increase with complete transection of the cord (E, F). Not only the excitatory but also the inhibitory effects from the FRA to the bVFRT can be depressed by the control pathway described here. The centres responsible for this control appear to be located in the medial ventral part of the medullary and lower pontine reticular formation (Holmqvist et al., 1960a; Carpenter et al., 1965) and there is actually a differential supraspinal control of inhibitory and excitatory actions from the FRA to ascending pathways. Carpenter et al. (1965) have shown in fact that after a low pontine lesion there is release of the inhibitory paths to ascending pathways, but for release of the corresponding excitatory paths a more caudal medullary lesion is required. These observations parallel those obtained by previous authors indicating the existence of a differential control from the brain stem of the inhibitory and excitatory FRA paths to motoneurones (Section VIII, 1). A low pontine lesion gives release from the tonic decerebrate control of the inhibitory paths from the FRA to motoneurones, whereas release of the excitatory paths only occurs after a more caudal medullary lesion (Holmqvist and Lundberg, 1959, 1961; Holmqvist, 1961).

It has been suggested that the descending inhibition is exerted at an interneuronal level and that there are separate descending systems controlling the inhibitory and excitatory reflex paths from the FRA. These findings also suggest that the inhibitory and excitatory actions from the FRA to ascending pathways are informative of inhibitory and excitatory reflex paths to motoneurones respectively.

Recently a further similarity in the transmission from the FRA to ascending paths and to motoneurones was demonstrated by POMPEIANO et al. In both cases the transmission is heavily depressed during the periods of rapid eye movements (REM) occurring in desynchronized sleep and during orienting reactions (GASSEL and POMPEIANO, 1967; POMPEIANO et al., 1967; LENZI et al., 1968). A depression of tactile and nociceptive spinal evoked potentials in the cat has also been described during attentive behavior (HERNÁNDEZ-PÉON and BRUST-CARMONA, 1961; cf. WALL, 1967, 1968; WALL et al., 1967).

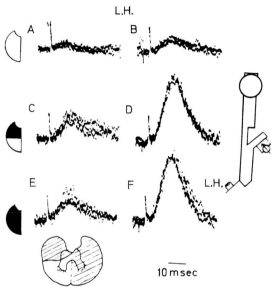

Fig. 26. Control of transmission to a ventrally located pathway by a descending system in the dorsal part of the other spinal half. Experimental conditions as shown in the schematic drawing with recording from the right spinal half on stimulation of the left hamstring nerve, in A, C, E at about 10 and in B, D, F at about 50 times threshold for the nerve. Decerebrate unanaesthetized cat. A and B were recorded with the left spinal half intact, C and D after section of the dorsal half of the left lateral funicle (histological control indicated in the drawing), E and F, finally after complete division of the cord. (HOLMQVIST et al., 1960a)

It is of interest that the same supraspinal mechanism exerting a tonic inhibitory influence on transmission from the FRA to the ascending spino-bulbar pathway also exerts a tonic inhibition on the interneurones mediating excitatory action from the FRA to the DSCT (HOLMQVIST et al., 1956, 1960a) and on those mediating inhibitory action to the VSCT neurones in the decerebrate preparation (OSCARSSON, 1960; HOLMQVIST et al., 1960a; LUNDBERG and OSCARSSON, 1962a; cf. MAGNI and OSCARSSON, 1961).

The existence of a supraspinal descending control mechanism inhibiting transmission from the FRA volleys to ascending spinal hindlimb pathways was shown not only by lesion but also by stimulation experiments (LUNDBERG and OSCARSSON, 1962b; ENGBERG et al., 1968a).

It has been concluded that transmission of the FRA messages to ascending pathways could be informative of flexion reflex events in the spinal cord (Lund-berg, 1959; Eccles and Lundberg, 1959b; Holmqvist et al., 1960a). This possibility is supported by the fact that transmissions of FRA volleys to motoneu-rones and to bVFRT neurones respectively are controlled in much the same way by supraspinal descending mechanisms. The arrival of flexion reflex afferents to the brain stem reticular formation would certainly be required in motor regulation. Relevant in this connection is the demonstration that both the excitatory and the inhibitory components of the SBS reflex are triggered by cutaneous and high threshold muscle afferents (Section VI, 5).

It should be pointed out however that this cannot be the exclusive function of the bVFRT. It has been shown anatomically that the spinoreticular pathway constitutes an important afferent input not only to reticulospinal neurones but also to ascending reticular neurones. Moreover it has been proved that repetitive acti-vation of this tract by impulses which segmentally give rise to the flexion reflex elicit generalized electroencephalographic synchronization or behavioral arousal according to the pattern of stimulation (Pompeiano and Swett, 1962a, b).

XI. Summary

Attempts have been made to integrate the best known anatomical and phy-siological facts dealing with the following subjects: i) somatic influences on ascend-ing reticular systems, ii) somatic influences on descending reticular systems, iii) somatic influences on brain stem reticular neurones, iv) descending reticular con-trol on somato-sensory transmission to motoneurones and ascending spinoreticular pathway.

It is rather difficult at the present time to draw a complete picture of the anatomical and functional organization of the ascending and descending reticular systems and on their responses to different somatic inputs. However, contrary to the original idea that changes in reticular activity lead only to widespread effects, both anatomical and physiological experiments point to the existence of a frac-tional organization of both the ascending and descending reticular systems. Expe-rimental data also indicate that the both these systems may be able to discrimi-nate between spinal afferent impulses and that their efferent discharge may selectively influence different mechanisms in the forebrain and the spinal cord.

References

Abrahms, V.C., Hilton, S.M., Malcolm, J.L.: Sensory connexions to the hypothalamus and midbrain, and their role in the reflex activation of the defence reaction. J. Physiol. (Lond.) **164**, 1–16 (1962).

Adey, W.R., Lindsley, D.F.: On the role of subthalamic areas in the maintenance of brain-stem reticular excitability. Exp. Neurol. **1**, 407–426 (1959).

Albe-Fessard, D.: Organisation of somatic central projections. In: W.D. Neff (Ed.). Con-tributions to sensory physiology. New York: Academic Press, 2, 101–167 (1965).

Albe-Fessard, D., Bowsher, D.: Responses of monkey thalamus to somatic stimuli under chloralose anaesthesia. E.E.G. clin. Neurophysiol. **19**, 1–15 (1965).

ALBE-FESSARD, D., BOWSHER, D.: Central pathways for painful messages. Proc. XXIV int. Congr. physiol. Sci., Washington, D.C., **6**, 241–242 (1968).

ALBE-FESSARD, D., BOWSHER, D., MALLART, A.: Réponses évoquées dans la formation reticulée bulbaire au niveau du noyau gigantocellularis d'Olszewski. Role de ce noyau dans la transmission vers le centre médian du thalamus des afférences somatiques. J. Physiol. (Paris) **54**, 271 (1962).

ALBE-FESSARD, D., FESSARD, A.: Thalamic integrations and their consequences at telencephalic level. In: G. MORUZZI, A. FESSARD and H. H. JASPER (Eds.). Progress in Brain Research. Vol. **1**. Brain mechanisms. Amsterdam: Elsevier Publ. Co., 115–148 (1963).

ALBE-FESSARD, D., KRUGER, L.: Duality of unit discharges from cat centrum medianum in response to natural and electrical stimulation. J. Neurophysiol. **25**, 3–20 (1962).

ALBE-FESSARD, D., LAMARRE, Y., PIMPENEAU, A.: Sur l'origine fusoriale de certaines afférences somatiques atteignant le cortéx moteur du Singe. J. Physiol. (Paris) **58**, 443–444 (1966).

ALBE-FESSARD, D., LIEBESKIND, J.: Comparaison entre les propriétés des cortex prés- et postrolandiques chez le Macaque. J. Physiol. (Paris) **56**, 271 (1964).

ALBE-FESSARD, D., LIEBESKIND, J.: Origine des messages somato-sensitifs activant les cellules du cortex moteur chez le singe. Exp. Brain Res. **1**, 127–146 (1966).

ALBE-FESSARD, D., LIEBESKIND, J., LAMARRE, Y.: Projection au niveau du cortex somatomoteur du singe d'afférences provenant des récepteurs musculaires. C. R. Acad. Sci. (Paris) **261**, 3891–3894 (1965).

ALBE-FESSARD, D., LIEBESKIND, J., MALLART, A.: Stimulation naturelles provoquant l'activation des cellules du cortex moteur chez le singe. J. Physiol. (Paris) **56**, 525–526 (1964).

ALBE-FESSARD, D., MALLART, A.: Réponses évoquées dans la formation réticulée bulbaire au niveau de noyau giganto cellularis d'Olszewski. Rôle de ce noyau dans la transmission vers le centre médian du thalamus des afférences somatiques. J. Physiol. (Paris) **54**, 271 (1962).

ALBE-FESSARD, D., ROCHA-MIRANDA, C., OSWALDO-CRUZ, E.: Activités d'origines somesthésiques évoquées au niveau du cortex non-specifique et du centre médian du thalamus chez le singe anesthésié au chloralose. E.E.G. clin. Neurophysiol. **11**, 777–787 (1959).

ALBE-FESSARD, D., ROUGEUL, A.: Activités d'origine somesthésique évoqués sur le cortex non-spécifique du Chat anesthésié au chloralose: rôle du centre médian du thalamus. E.E.G. clin. Neurophysiol. **10**, 131–152 (1958).

ALLEN, W.F.: Effect of partial and complete destruction of the tactile cerebral cortex on correct conditioned differential foreleg responses from cutaneous stimulation. Amer. J. Physiol. **151**, 325–337 (1947).

AMASSIAN, V.E., BERLIN, L.: Early cortical projection of group I afferents in forelimb muscle nerves of cat. J. Physiol. (Lond.) **143**, 61 P (1958a).

AMASSIAN, V.E., BERLIN, L.: Early projection of large muscle afferents from forelimb of cat to somatosensory cortex. Fed. Proc. **17**, 3 (1958b).

AMASSIAN, V.E., DE VITO, R.V.: Unit activity in reticular formation and nearby structures. J. Neurophysiol. **17**, 575–603 (1954).

AMASSIAN, V.E., MACY, J., WALLER, H.J.: Patterns of activity of simultaneously recorded neurons in midbrain reticular formation. Ann. N.Y. Acad. Sci. **89**, 883–895 (1961).

AMASSIAN, V.E., TOWE, A.L., WALLER, H.J.: Representation of the periphery in cerebral cortex and reticular formation. Abstr. Comm. XX int. physiol. Congr., Bruxelles, 24–25 (1956).

AMASSIAN, V.E., WALLER, H.J.: Spatiotemporal patterns of activity in individual reticular neurons. In: H.H. JASPER et al. (Eds.). Reticular formation of the brain. Henry Ford Hospital International Symposium. Boston-Toronto: Little, Brown and Co., 69–108, 1958.

ANDÉN, N.-E., JUKES, M.G.M., LUNDBERG, A.: Spinal reflexes and monoamine liberation. Nature (Lond.) **202**, 1222–1223 (1964a).

ANDÉN, N.-E., JUKES, M.G.M., LUNDBERG, A.: The effect of DOPA on the spinal cord. 2. A pharmacological analysis. Acta physiol. scand. **67**, 387–397 (1966a).

ANDÉN, N.-E., JUKES, M.G.M., LUNDBERG, A., VYKLICKÝ, L.: A new spinal flexor reflex. Nature (Lond.) **202**, 1344–1345 (1964b).

ANDÉN, N.-E., JUKES, M.G.M., LUNDBERG, A., VYKLICKÝ, L.: The effect of DOPA on the spinal cord. 1. Influence on transmission from primary afferents. Acta physiol. scand. **67**, 373–386 (1966b).

ANDÉN, N.-E., JUKES, M.G.M., LUNDBERG, A., VYKLICKÝ, L.: The effect of DOPA on the spinal cord. 3. Depolarization evoked in the central terminals of ipsilateral Ia afferents by volleys in the flexor reflex afferents. Acta physiol. scand. **68**, 322–336 (1966c).

ANDERSEN, P., ANDERSSON, S.A.: Physiological basis of the alpha rhythm. New York: Appleton-Century-Crofts, VII–235 pp., 1968.

ANDERSON, F.D., BERRY, C.M.: Degeneration studies of long ascending fiber systems in the cat brain stem. J. comp. Neurol. **111**, 195–229 (1959).

ANDERSSON, S.A.: Cortical effects by activity in a ventral ascending spinal pathway. Med. Exp. **6**, 25–28 (1962a).

ANDERSSON, S.A.: Projection of different spinal pathways to the second somatic sensory area in cat. Acta physiol. scand. **56**, Suppl. 194, 1–74 (1962b).

ANDERSSON, S.A.: Suppression of cortical spontaneous barbiturate spindles via specific and unspecific projection spinal pathways. Acta physiol. scand. **69**, 191–202 (1967).

ANDERSSON, S.A., LANDGREN, S., WOLSK, D.: The thalamic relay and cortical projection of Group I muscle afferents from the forelimb of the cat. J. Physiol. (Lond.) **183**, 576–591 (1966).

ANDERSSON, S.A., NORRSELL, U., WOLPOW, E.R.: Cortical synchronization and desynchronization via spinal pathways. Acta physiol. scand. **61**, 144–158 (1964).

APPELBERG, B.: The effect of electrical stimulation of nucleus ruber on the gamma motor system. Acta physiol. scand. **55**, 150–159 (1962).

ARDUINI, A., ARDUINI, M.G.: Effect of drugs and metabolic alterations on brain stem arousal mechanism. J. Pharmacol. (Kyoto) **110**, 76–85 (1954).

ARDUINI, A., HIRAO, T.: EEG synchronization elicited by light. Arch. ital. Biol. **98**, 275–292 (1960).

AUSTIN, G.M.: Suprabulbar mechanisms of facilitation and inhibition of cord reflexes. Res. Publ. Ass. nerv. ment. Dis. **30**, 196–222 (1952).

AVANZINO, G.L., HÖSLI, L., WOLSTENCROFT, J.H.: Identification of cerebellar projecting neurones in nucleus reticularis gigantocellularis. Brain Res. **3**, 201–203 (1966).

AVANZINO, G.L., WOLSTENCROFT, J.H.: Delimitazione delle aree du proiezione di neuroni del nucleo reticolare gigantocellulare al lobo anteriore del cervelletto. Arch. Fisiol. **68**, 33–34 (1970).

BACH-Y-RITA, P.: Caractéristiques des réponses évoquées dans la formation réticulée pontique chez le Chat. C.R. Soc. Biol. (Paris) **156**, 1228–1230 (1962a).

BACH-Y-RITA, P.: Caractéristiques des activités evoquées dans divers régions de la réticulée bulbaire et mésencéphalique. J. Physiol. (Paris) **54**, 283–284 (1962b).

BACH-Y-RITA, P.: Convergent and long-latency unit responses in the reticular formation of the cat. Exp. Neurol. **9**, 327–344 (1964).

BALLIF, L., FULTON, J.F., LIDDELL, E.G.T.: Observations on spinal and decerebrate knee-jerks with special reference to their inhibition by single break-shocks. Proc. roy. Soc. B **98**, 589–607 (1925).

BARD, P.: A diencephalic mechanism for the expression of rage with special reference to the sympathetic nervous system. Amer. J. Physiol. **84**, 490–515 (1928).

BARD, P., MACHT, M.B.: The behavior of chronically decerebrate cats. In: G.E.W. WOLSTENHOLME and C.M. O'CONNOR (Eds.). Neurological basis of behavior. Ciba Foundation Symposium. London: J. and A. Churchill, 55–71, 1958.

BARKER, D.: The innervation of the muscle-spindles. Quart. J. micr. Sci. **89**, 143–186 (1948).

BARKER, D.: The structure and distribution of muscle receptors. In: D. BARKER (Ed.). Symposium on muscle receptors. Hong Kong: Hong Kong University Press, 227–240, 1962.

BARKER, D., IP, M.C., ADAI, M.N.: A correlation between the receptor population of the cat's soleus muscle and the afferent fibre-diameter spectrum of the nerve supplying it. In: D. BARKER (Ed.). Symposium on muscle receptors. Hong Kong: Hong Kong University Press, 257–261, 1962.

BARNES, C.D.: Cholinergic properties of spino-bulbo-spinal reflex inhibition. Neuropharmacology **9**, 185–190 (1970).

BARNES, C.D., POMPEIANO, O.: Effects of muscle vibration on the pre- and postsynaptic components of the extensor monosynaptic reflex. Brain Res. **18**, 384–388 (1970a).

BARNES, C.D., POMPEIANO, O.: Presynaptic and postsynaptic effects in the monosynaptic reflex pathway to extensor motoneurons following vibration of synergic muscles. Arch. ital. Biol. 108, 259–294 (1970b).

BARNES, C.D., POMPEIANO, O.: Dissociation of presynaptic and postsynaptic effects produced in the lumbar cord by vestibular volleys. Arch. ital. Biol. 108, 295–324 (1970c).

BARNES, C.D., POMPEIANO, O.: A brain stem cholinergic system activated by vestibular volleys. Neuropharmacology 9, 391–394 (1970d).

BARNES, C.D., POMPEIANO, O.: Effects of muscle afferents on brain stem reticular and vestibular units. Brain Res. 25, 179–183 (1971a).

BARNES, C.D., POMPEIANO, O.: Vestibular nerve activation of a brain stem cholinergic system influencing the spinal cord. Neuropharmacology 10, 425–436 (1971b).

BAUMGARTEN, R. v., MOLLICA, A.: Der Einfluß sensibler Reizung auf die Entladungsfrequenz kleinhirnabhängiger Reticulariszellen. Pflügers Arch. ges. Physiol. 259, 79–96 (1954).

BAUMGARTEN, R., v., MOLLICA, A., MORUZZI, G.: Modulierung der Entladungsfrequenz einzelner Zellen der Substantia reticularis durch corticofugale and cerebellare Impulse. Pflügers Arch. ges. Physiol. 259, 56–78 (1954).

BELL, C., BUENDIA, N., SIERRA, G., SEGUNDO, J.P.: Mesencephalic reticular responses to natural and to repeated sensory stimuli. Experientia (Basel) 19, 308–312 (1963).

BELL, C., SIERRA, G., BUENDIA, N., SEGUNDO, J.P.: Sensory properties of neurones in the mesencephalic reticular formation. J. Neurophysiol. 27, 961–981 (1964).

BENJAMIN, R.M.: Single neurons in the rat medulla responsive to nociceptive stimulation. Proc. XXII int. Congr. physiol. Sci, Leiden, II, n. 1039 (1962).

BERGMANS, J., GRILLNER, S.: Reflex activation and regulation of spontaneous activity in static and dynamic γ-motoneurones. Brain Res. 5, 114–117 (1967).

BERITOFF, J.: Über die individuell-erworbene Tätigkeit des Zentralnervensystems. J. Psychol. Neurol. (Lpz.) 33, 113–335 (1927).

BERITOFF, J.: Über die Entstehung der tierischen Hypnose. Z. Biol. 89, 77–82 (1929).

BERNHAUT, M., GELLHORN, E., RASMUSSEN, A.T.: Experimental contribution to problem of consciousness. J. Neurophysiol. 16, 21–35 (1953).

BERNHARD, C.G.: The spinal cord potentials in leads from the cord dorsum in relation to peripheral source of afferent stimulation. Acta physiol. scand. 29, Suppl. 106, 1–29 (1953).

BERNHARD, C.G., REXED, B.: The localization of the premotor interneuron discharging through the peroneal nerve. J. Neurophysiol. 8, 387–392 (1945).

BEUSEKOM, G.T. van: Fibre analysis of the anterior and lateral funiculi of the cord in the cat. Thesis, Leiden: E. Ijdo N.V., 143 pp., 1955.

BIANCONI, R., VAN DER MEULEN, J.F.: The response to vibration of the end-organs of mammalian muscle spindles. J. Neurophysiol. 26, 177–190 (1963).

BISHOP, G.H.: The relation between nerve fiber size and sensory modality: phylogenetic implications of the afferent innervation of cortex. J. nerv. ment. Dis. 128, 89–114 (1959).

BLAKELSEE, G.A., FREIMAN, J.S., BARRERA, S.E.: The nucleus lateralis medullae. An experimental study of its anatomic connections in Macacus rhesus. Arch. Neurol. Psychiat. (Chic.) 39, 687–704 (1938).

BLOCH, V.: Le contrôle central de l'activité électrodermale. J. Physiol. (Paris) 57, Suppl. XIII, 134 pp. (1965).

BLOCH, V., VALAT, M., ROY, J.-C.: Influences des afférences musculaires sur le tonus réticulaire. J. Physiol. (Paris) 57, 561–562 (1965).

BODIAN, D.: Spinal projections of brainstem in rhesus monkey deduced from retrograde chromatolysis. Anat. Rec. 94, 512 (1946).

BOGOLEPOV, N.N.: Structure of synapses in brain-stem reticular formation. Fed. Proc. Transl., Suppl. 25, 919–923 (1966).

BOHM, E.: An electro-physiological study of the ascending spinal anterolateral fibre system connected to coarse cutaneous afferents. Acta physiol. scand. 29, Suppl. 106, 106–137 (1953).

BOIVIE, J., GRANT, G., SILFVENIUS, H.: A projection from nucleus z to the ventral nuclear complex of the thalamus in the cat. Acta physiol. scand. 80, 11A (1970).

BONVALLET, M., BLOCK, V.: Bulbar control of cortical arousal. Science 133, 1133–1134 (1961).

BONVALLET, M., DELL, P., HIEBEL, G.: Tonus sympathique et activité électrique corticale. E.E.G. clin. Neurophysiol. **6**, 119–144 (1954).

BONVALLET, M., HUGELIN, A., DELL, P.: Milieu intérieur et activité automatique des cellules réticulaires mésencéphaliques. J. Physiol. (Paris) **48**, 403–406 (1956).

BONVALLET, M., NEWMAN-TAYLOR, A.: Neurophysiological evidence for a differential organization of the mesencephalic reticular formation. E.E.G. clin. Neurophysiol. **22**, 54–73 (1967).

BONVALLET, M., SIGG, B.: Étude électrophysiologique des afférences vagales au niveau de leur pénétration dans le bulbe. J. Physiol. (Paris) **50**, 63–74 (1958).

BOURASSA, C.M., SWETT, J.E.: Cortical evoked potentials and detection of somatic sensory volleys in awake cats. Proc. Ann. Conv. Amer. Psychol. Assoc., 74th., New York City, 103–104, 1966.

BOURASSA, C.M., SWETT, J.E.: Sensory discrimination thresholds with cutaneous nerve volleys in the cat. J. Neurophysiol. **30**, 515–529 (1967).

BOWSHER, D.: Termination of the central pain pathway in man: the conscious appreciation of pain. Brain **80**, 606–621 (1957).

BOWSHER, D.: Projection of the gracile and cuneate nuclei in *Macaca mulatta*. An experimental degeneration study. J. comp. Neurol. **110**, 135–155 (1958).

BOWSHER, D.: The termination of secondary somatosensory neurones within the thalamus of *Macaca mulatta*. An experimental degeneration study. J. comp. Neurol. **117**, 213–228 (1961).

BOWSHER, D.: The topographical projection fibres from the anterolateral quadrant of the spinal cord to the sub-diencephalic brain stem in man. Mschr. Psychiat. Neurol. **143**, 75–99 (1962).

BOWSHER, D.: Les relais des sensibilités somesthésique et douloureuse au niveau du tronc cérébrale et du thalamus. Toulouse méd. **64**, 965–984 (1963).

BOWSHER, D.: Some afferent and efferent connections of the parafascicular-center median complex. In: D.P. PURPURA (Ed.). Thalamic integration of sensory and motor activities. New York: Columbia University Press, 99–108, 1966.

BOWSHER, D.: Étude comparée des projections thalamiques de deux zones localisées des formations réticulées bulbaires et mésencéphaliques. C.R. Acad. Sci. (Paris) **265** D, 340–342 (1967).

BOWSHER, D.: Propriétés sensorielles de la formation reticulée du bulbe caudal chez le chat. J. Physiol. (Paris) **61**, 234 (1969).

BOWSHER, D.: Place and modality analysis in caudal reticular formation. J. Physiol. (Lond.) **209**, 473–486 (1970).

BOWSHER, D., ALBE-FESSARD, D.: Patterns of somatosensory organization within the central nervous system. In: C.A. KEELE and R. SMITH (Eds.). U.F.A.W. Symposium on the assessment of pain in man and animals. London: J. and A. Churchill, 107–122, 1962.

BOWSHER, D., ALBE-FESSARD, D., MALLART, A.: Central extralemniscal afferents. J. Anat. (Lond.) **97**, 151–152 (1963).

BOWSHER, D., MALLART, A., PETIT, D., ALBE-FESSARD, D.: A bulbar relay to the centre median. J. Neurophysiol. **31**, 288–300 (1968 a).

BOWSHER, D., PETIT, D.: Single unit analysis of ventromedial medullary reticular formation in cat. J. Physiol. (Lond.) **186**, 117–118P (1966).

BOWSHER, D., PETIT, D.: Single unit analysis of dorsal mesencephalic reticular responses in chloralosed cat. J. Physiol. (Lond.) **201**, 24–25P (1969).

BOWSHER, D., PETIT, D.: Place and modality analysis in nucleus of posterior commissure. J. Physiol. (Lond.) **206**, 663–675 (1970).

BOWSHER, D., WESTMAN, J.: The gigantocellular reticular region and its spinal afferents: a light and electron microscope study in the cat. J. Anat. (Lond.) **106**, 23–36 (1970).

BOWSHER, D., WESTMAN, J., GRANT, G.: Electron microscopic study of spinal afferent distribution to gigantocellular formation in cat. J. Anat. (Lond.) **103**, 192 (1968 b).

BRADLEY, K., ECCLES, J.C.: Analysis of the fast afferent impulses from thigh muscles. J. Physiol. (Lond.) **122**, 462–473 (1953).

BRADLEY, P.B., DHAWAN, B.N., WOLSTENCROFT, J.H.: Some pharmacological properties of cholinoceptive neurones in the medulla and pons of the cat. J. Physiol. (Lond.) **170**, 59–60P (1964).

BRADLEY, P.B., DHAWAN, B.N., WOLSTENCROFT, J.H.: Pharmacological properties of cholino-ceptive neurones in the medulla and pons of the cat. J. Physiol. (Lond.) **183**, 658–674 (1966).

BRADLEY, P.B., MOLLICA, A.: The effect of adrenaline and acetylcholine on single unit activity in the reticular formation of the decerebrate cat. Arch. ital. Biol. **96**, 168–186 (1958).

BRADLEY, P.B., WOLSTENCROFT, J.H.: Excitation and inhibition of brain-stem neurones by noradrenaline and acetylcholine. Nature (Lond.) **196**, 840, 873 (1962).

BRADLEY, P.B., WOLSTENCROFT, J.H.: The action of drugs on single neurones in the brain stem. In: P.B. BRADLEY, F. FLÜGEL and P. HOCH (Eds.). Neuropsychopharmacology. Amsterdam: Elsevier Publ. Co., **3**, 237–240 (1964).

BRADLEY, P.B., WOLSTENCROFT, J.H.: Actions of drugs on single neurones in the brainstem. Brit. med. Bull. **20**, 8–15 (1965).

BRADLEY, P.B., WOLSTENCROFT, J.H.: Effects of acetylcholine, nicotine and muscarine on brainstem neurons. Ann. N.Y. Acad. Sci. **142**, 15–20 (1967).

BREMER, F., BONNET, V.: Interprétation des réactions rythmiques prolongées des aires sensorielles de l'écorce cérébrale. E.E.G. clin. Neurophysiol. **2**, 389–400 (1950).

BRINDLEY, G.S., MERTON, P.A.: The absence of position sense in the human eye. J. Physiol. (Lond.) **153**, 127–130 (1960).

BRODAL, A.: Modification of Gudden method for study of cerebral localization. Arch. Neurol. Psychiat. (Chic.) **43**, 46–58 (1940).

BRODAL, A.: The reticular formation of the brain stem. Anatomical aspects and functional correlations. Edinburgh-London: Oliver and Boyd, VII–87 pp., 1957.

BRODAL, A.: Anatomical points of view on the alleged morphological basis of consciousness. Acta neurochir. (Wien) **12**, 166–186 (1965).

BRODAL, A.: Some points of view on the anatomy of the brain stem, with particular reference to the reticular formation. Proc. IIIrd int. Congr. neurol. Surgery, Copenhagen, 23–28 August 1965. Excerpta Medica int. Congr. Series, Amst., no. **110**, 449–460 (1966).

BRODAL, A., POMPEIANO: O.: The vestibular nuclei in the cat. J. Anat. (Lond.) **91**, 438–454 (1957).

BRODAL, A., POMPEIANO, O., WALBERG, F.: The vestibular nuclei and their connections. Anatomy and functional correlations. Edinburgh-London: Oliver and Boyd, VIII–193 pp., 1962.

BRODAL, A., ROSSI, G.F.: Ascending fibers in brain stem reticular formation of cat. Arch. Neurol. Psychiat. (Chic.) **74**, 68–87 (1955).

BRODAL, A., TABER, E., WALBERG, F.: The raphe nuclei of the brain stem in the cat. II. Efferent connections. J. comp. Neurol. **114**, 239–259 (1960).

BROWN, M.C., ENGBERG, I., MATTHEWS, P.B.C.: The relative sensitivity to vibration of muscle receptors of the cat. J. Physiol. (Lond.) **192**, 773–780 (1967).

BROWNE, K., LEE,J., RING, P.A.: The sensation of passive movement at the metatarso-phalangeal joint of the great toe in man. J. Physiol. (Lond.) **126**, 448–458 (1954).

BUCHWALD, J.S., ELDRED, E.: Relations between gamma efferent discharge and cortical activity. E.E.G. clin. Neurophysiol. **13**, 243–247 (1961).

BUREŠ, J.: Comment. In: P. KIMBLE (Ed.). The anatomy of memory. Palo Alto, California: Science and Behavior Books, 365, 1965.

BUREŠ, J., BUREŠOVÁ, O.: Plastic changes of unit activity based on reinforcing properties of extracellular stimulation of single neurones. J. Neurophysiol. **30**, 98–113 (1967).

BUREŠOVÁ, O., BUREŠ, J.: Classical conditioning and reticular units. Acta physiol. Acad. Sci. hung. **26**, 53–57 (1965).

BURTON, H.: Somatic sensory properties of caudal bulbar reticular neurons in the cat (Felis domestica). Brain Res. **11**, 357–372 (1968).

BUSCH, H.F.M.: An anatomical analysis of the white matter in the brain stem of the cat. Thesis, Leiden: Te Assen Bij Van Gorcum and Comp. N.V., 116 pp., 1961.

BUSCH, H.F.M.: Anatomical aspects of the anterior and lateral funiculi at the spinobulbar junction. In: J.C. ECCLES and J.P. SCHADÉ (Eds.). Progress in Brain Research. Vol. 11. Organization of the spinal cord. Amsterdam: Elsevier Publ. Co., 223–237, 1964.

BUSER, P.: Activités de projection et d'association de néocortex cérébral des mammifères. Deuxième partie. Activités d'association et d'élaboration; projections non spécifiques. J. Physiol. (Paris) **49**, 589–656 (1957).

Buser, P., Borenstein, P.: Recherches sur les réponses "secondaires" recueillies au niveau du cortex cérébral du Chat lors d'une stimulation somesthésique, ou visuelle, ou auditive. C.R. Soc. Biol. (Paris) **149**, 1342–1347 (1955).

Buser, P., Borenstein, P.: Données sur la répartition des réponses sensorielles corticales (somesthésiques, visuelles, auditives) chez le Chat curarisé non anesthésié. J. Physiol. (Paris) **48**, 419–421 (1956).

Buser, P., Borenstein, P.: Réponses corticales "secondaires" a la stimulation sensorielle chez le chat curarizé non anesthésié. E.E.G. clin. Neurophysiol. Suppl. **6**, 89–108 (1957).

Buser, P., Borenstein, P.: Réponses somesthésiques, visuelles et auditives, recuillies au niveau du cortex "associative" suprasylvian chez le chat curarisé non anesthésié. E.E.G. clin. Neurophysiol. **11**, 285–304 (1959).

Buser, P., Viala, G.: Analyse du mécanisme de l'akinésie induite "hypnotique" chez le lapin. Actualités neurophysiol. **8**, 179–196 (1968).

Cajal, S., Ramón y: Histologie du système nerveux de l'homme et des vertébrés. Paris: A. Maloine, vol. I, XV–986 pp., 1909; vol. II, 933 pp., 1911.

Cangiano, A., Cook, W.A., Jr., Pompeiano, O.: Primary afferent depolarization in the lumbar cord evoked from the fastigial nucleus. Arch. ital. Biol. **107**, 321–340 (1969a).

Cangiano, A., Cook, W.A., Jr., Pompeiano, O.: Cerebellar inhibitory control of the vestibular reflex pathways to primary afferents. Arch. ital. Biol. **107**, 341–364 (1969b).

Cannon, W.B., Britton, S.W.: Studies on the conditions of activity in endocrine glands. XV. Pseudaffective medulliadrenal secretion. Amer. J. Physiol. **72**, 283–294 (1925).

Capon, A., Reeth, P.C. van: Effect hypnogénique des stimulations laryngées chez le lapin. J. Physiol. (Paris) **55**, 216 (1963).

Carli, G.: Dissociation of electrocortical activity and somatic reflexes during rabbit hypnosis. Arch. ital. Biol. **107**, 219–234 (1969).

Carli, G.: Sub-cortical mechanisms of rabbit hypnosis. Arch. ital. Biol. **109**, 15–26 (1971).

Carli, G., Malliani, A., Zanchetti, A.: Stimolazione a varia cadenza di diversi gruppi di fibre cutanee, nel gatto talamico acuto. Boll. Soc. ital. Biol. sper. **40**, 2158–2161 (1964).

Carli, G., Malliani, A., Zanchetti, A.: Lesioni selettive di varie strutture ipotalamiche e comportamento spontaneo e provocato di falsa rabbia del gatto decorticato acuto. Boll. Soc. ital. Biol. sper. **42**, 291–294 (1966).

Carlsson, A., Falck, B., Fuxe, K., Hillarp, N.-Å.: Cellular localization of monoamines in the spinal cord. Acta physiol. scand. **60**, 112–119 (1964).

Carpenter, D., Engberg, I., Funkenstein, H., Lundberg, A.: Decerebrate control of reflexes to primary afferents. Acta physiol. scand. **59**, 424–437 (1963).

Carpenter, D., Engberg, I., Lundberg, A.: Presynaptic inhibition in the lumbar cord evoked from the brain stem. Experientia (Basel) **18**, 450–451 (1962).

Carpenter, D., Engberg, I., Lundberg, A.: Differential supraspinal control of inhibitory and excitatory actions from the FRA to ascending spinal pathways. Acta physiol. scand. **63**, 103–110 (1965).

Carpenter, D., Engberg, I., Lundberg, A.: Primary afferent depolarization evoked from the brain stem and the cerebellum. Arch. ital. Biol. **104**, 73–85 (1966).

Carter, S.J., Gelfan, S.: On "muscle sense" in man. Physiologist 8, 129 (1965).

Casey, K.L.: Sensory responses of medial medullary reticular neurons: natural stimuli and fiber spectrum. Proc. XXIV int. Congr. physiol. Sci., Washington, DC, VII, 77, n. 231 (1968).

Cate, J. ten: Zur Frage nach dem Entstehen der Zustände der sog. tierischen Hypnose. Biol. Zbl. **48**, 664–679 (1928).

Chambers, W.W., Liu, C.N.: Corticospinal tract of the cat. An attempt to correlate the pattern of degeneration with the deficits in the reflex activity following neocortical lesions. J. comp. Neurol. **108**, 23–55 (1957).

Chan, S.H.H., Barnes, C.D.: Brain stem reticular formation evoked DRP and PAD in the lumbar cord. Fed. Proc. **30**, 213 Abs. (1971).

Cleghorn, T.E., Darcus, H.D.: The sensibility to passive movement of the human elbow joint. Quart. J. exp. Psychol. **4**, 66–77 (1952).

COHEN, L.A.: Contributions of tactile musculo-tendinous and joint mechanisms to position sense in human shoulder. J. Neurophysiol. **21**, 563–568 (1952).

COLLE, J., GYBELS, J.: Étude des réactions tensionnelles, respiratoires et corticales produites par l'excitation électrique des fibres afférents d'un nerf somatique. Arch. int. Physiol. **65**, 547–567 (1957).

COLLIER, J., BUZZARD, E.F.: The degeneration resulting from lesions of posterior nerve roots and from transverse lesions of the spinal cord in man. A study of twenty cases. Brain **26**, 559–591 (1903).

COLLINS, W.F., KENDRICK, J.F.: Spinal afferent pathways to mid-brain reticular core of cat: dorsal column. Fed. Proc. **25**, 395, n. 1162 (1966).

COLLINS, W.F., NULSEN, F.E., RANDT, C.T.: Relation of peripheral nerve fiber size and sensation in man. Arch. Neurol. (Chic.) **3**, 381–385 (1960).

COLLINS, W.F., O'LEARY, J.L.: Study of a somatic evoked response of midbrain reticular substance. E.E.G. clin. Neurophysiol. **6**, 619–628 (1954).

COLLINS, W.F., RANDT, C.T.: An electrophysiolocal study of small myelinated axons in anterolateral column in cat. J. Neurophysiol. **19**, 438–445 (1956).

COLLINS, W.F., RANDT, C.T.: Evoked central nervous system activity relating to peripheral unmyelinated or "C" fibers in cat. J. Neurophysiol. **21**, 345–352 (1958).

COLLINS, W.F., RANDT, C.T.: Midbrain evoked response relating to peripheral unmyelinated or "C" fibers in cat. J. Neurophysiol. **23**, 47–53 (1960).

COLLINS, W.F., RANDT, C.T.: Fiber size and organization of afferent pathways. Arch. Neurol. (Chic.) **5**, 202–209 (1961).

COOK, W.A., JR., CANGIANO, A., POMPEIANO, O.: Dorsal root potentials in the lumbar cord evoked from the vestibular system. Arch. ital. Biol. **107**, 275–295 (1969a).

COOK, W.A., JR., CANGIANO, A., POMPEIANO, O.: Vestibular control of transmission in primary afferents to the lumbar spinal cord. Arch. ital. Biol. **107**, 296–320 (1969b).

COOMBS, J.S., CURTIS, D.R., ECCLES, J.C.: The interpretation of spike potentials of motoneurons. J. Physiol. (Lond.) **139**, 198–231 (1957).

COOPER, S., DANIEL, P.M., WHITTERIDGE, D.: Nerve impulses in the brain-stem of the goat. Responses with long latencies obtained by stretching the extrinsic eye muscles. J. Physiol. (Lond.) **120**, 491–513 (1953).

CREUTZFELDT, O.D.: General physiology of cortical neurons and neuronal information in the visual system. In: M.A.B. BRAZIER (Ed.). Brain and behavior. Washington, D.C.: Amer. Inst. Biol. Sci. **1**, 299–358 (1961).

DAHLSTRÖM, A., FUXE, K.: Evidence for the existence of monoamine neurons in the central nervous system. I. Demonstration of monoamines in the cell bodies of brain stem neurons. Acta physiol. scand. **62**, Suppl. 232, 1–55 (1964).

DAHLSTRÖM, A., FUXE, K.: Evidence for the existence of monoamine neurons in the central nervous system. II. Experimentally induced changes in the intraneuronal amine levels of bulbospinal neuron systems. Acta physiol. scand. **64**, Suppl. 247, 1–36 (1965).

D'ANNA, L., BONVALLET, M.: Modifications de l'activité réticulaire consécutive à l'interruption de différentes voies de conduction spinales. Arch. ital. Biol. **104**, 263–279 (1966).

DARIAN-SMITH, I., MUTTON, P., PROCTOR, R.: Functional organization of tactile cutaneous afferents within the semilunar ganglion and trigeminal spinal tract of the cat. J. Neurophysiol. **28**, 682–694 (1965).

DARIAN-SMITH, I., PHILLIPS, G.: Secondary neurones within a trigemino-cerebellar projection to the anterior lobe of the cerebellum in the cat. J. Physiol. (Lond.) **170**, 53–68 (1964).

DARIAN-SMITH, I., PHILLIPS, G., RYAN, R.D.: Functional organization in the trigeminal main sensory and rostral spinal nuclei of the cat. J. Physiol. (Lond.) **168**, 129–146 (1963a).

DARIAN-SMITH, I., PROCTOR, R., REGAN, R.D.: A single neurone investigation of somatotopic organization within the cat's trigeminal brain-stem nuclei. J. Physiol. (Lond.) **168**, 147–157 (1963b).

DARIAN-SMITH, I., YOKOTA, T.: Corticofugal effects on different neuron types within the cat's brain stem activated by tactile stimulation of the face. J. Neurophysiol. **29**, 185–206 (1966).

DAY, R.H., SINGER, G.: The relationship between kinesthetic spatial aftereffect and variations in muscular involvement during stimulation. Aust. J. Psychol. **16**, 200–208 (1964).

Debecker, J., Desmedt, J.E.: Les potentiels évoqués cerebraux et les potentiels du nerf sensible chez l'homme. Acta neurol. belg. **64**, 1212–1248 (1964).

Debecker, J., Desmedt, J.E., Manil, J.: Sur la relation entre la seuil de perception tactile et les potentiels évoqués de l'écorce cérébrale somato-sensible chez l'homme. C.R. Acad. Sci. (Paris) **260**, 687–689 (1965).

Delgado, J.M.R.: Cerebral structures involved in transmission and elaboration of noxious stimulation. J. Neurophysiol. **18**, 261–275 (1955).

Dell, P., Bonvallet, M.: Mise en jeu des effects de l'activité réticulaire par le milieu extérieur et le milieu intérieur. Abstr. Rev. XX int. physiol. Congr., Bruxelles, 286–306 (1956).

Dell, P., Bonvallet, M., Hugelin, A.: Mechanisms of reticular deactivation. In: G.E.W. Wolstenholme and M. O'Connor (Eds.). The nature of sleep. Ciba Foundation Symposium. London: J. and A. Churchill, 86–107, 1961.

Dennis, B.J., Kerr, D.I.B.: Somaesthetic pathways in the marsupial phalanges, Trichosurus vulpecula. Abstr. J. exp. Biol. med. Sci. **39**, 29 (1961).

Downman, C.B.B., Hussein, A.: Spinal tracts and supraspinal centres influencing visceromotor and allied reflexes in cats. J. Physiol. (Lond.) **141**, 489–499 (1958).

Eccles, J.C.: The physiology of synapses. Berlin-Göttingen-Heidelberg-New York: Springer, 316 pp., 1964a.

Eccles, J.C.: Presynaptic inhibition in the spinal cord. In: J.C. Eccles and J.P. Schadé (Eds.). Progress in Brain Research. Vol. 12. Physiology of spinal neurons. Amsterdam: Elsevier Publ. Co., 65–91, 1964b.

Eccles, J.C., Eccles, R.M., Lundberg, A.: Synaptic actions on motoneurones in relation to the two components of the group I muscle afferent volley. J. Physiol. (Lond.) **136**, 527–546 (1957a).

Eccles, J.C., Eccles, R.M., Lundberg, A.: Synaptic actions on motoneurones caused by impulses in Golgi tendon organ afferents. J. Physiol. (Lond.) **138**, 227–252 (1957b).

Eccles, J.C., Eccles, R.M., Magni, F.: Central inhibitory action attributable to presynaptic depolarization produced by muscle afferent volleys. J. Physiol. (Lond.) **159**, 147–166 (1961).

Eccles, J.C., Kostyuk, P.G., Schmidt, R.F.: Central pathways responsible for depolarization of primary afferent fibres. J. Physiol. (Lond.) **161**, 237–257 (1962a).

Eccles, J.C., Kostyuk, P.G., Schmidt, R.F.: Presynaptic inhibition of the central actions of flexor reflex afferents. J. Physiol. (Lond.) **161**, 258–281 (1962b).

Eccles, J.C., Magni, F., Willis, W.D.: Depolarization of central terminals of Group I afferent fibres from muscle. J. Physiol. (Lond.) **160**, 62–93 (1962c).

Eccles, J.C., Schmidt, R.F., Willis, W.D.: Depolarization of central terminals of group Ib afferent fibres of muscle. J. Neurophysiol. **26**, 1–27 (1963a).

Eccles, J.C., Schmidt, R.F., Willis, W.D.: Depolarization of the central terminals of cutaneous afferent fibers. J. Neurophysiol. **26**, 646–661 (1963b).

Eccles, R.M., Lundberg, A.: Supraspinal control of interneurones mediating spinal reflexes. J. Physiol. (Lond.) **147**, 565–584 (1959a).

Eccles, R.M., Lundberg, A.: Synaptic actions in motoneurones by afferents which may evoke the flexion reflex. Arch. ital. Biol. **97**, 199–221 (1959b).

Eckstein, A.: Weitere Untersuchungen zur tierischen Hypnose. Pflügers Arch. ges. Physiol. **177**, 38–56 (1919).

Engberg, I., Lundberg, A., Ryall, R.W.: Reticulospinal inhibition of transmission through interneurones of spinal reflex pathways. Experientia (Basel) **21**, 612–613 (1965).

Engberg, I., Lundberg, A., Ryall, R.W.: Reticulospinal inhibition of interneurones in the lumbar cord. J. Physiol. (Lond.) **187**, 41–42P (1966).

Engberg, I., Lundberg, A., Ryall, R.W.: Reticulospinal inhibition of transmission in reflex pathways. J. Physiol. (Lond.) **194**, 201–223 (1968a).

Engberg, I., Lundberg, A., Ryall, R.W.: Reticulospinal inhibition of interneurones. J. Physiol. (Lond.). **194**, 225–236 (1968b).

Engberg, I., Lundberg, A., Ryall, R.W.: The effect of reserpine on transmission in the spinal cord. Acta physiol. scand. **72**, 115–122 (1968c).

Engberg, I., Lundberg, A., Ryall, R.W.: Is the tonic decerebrate inhibition of reflex paths mediated by monoaminergic pathways? Acta physiol. scand. **72**, 123–133 (1968d).

ENGBERG, I., RYALL, R. W.: The actions of mono-amines upon spinal neurones. Life Sci. **4**, 2223–2227 (1965).

ENGBERG, I., RYALL, R. W.: The inhibitory action of noradrenaline and other monoamines on spinal neurones. J. Physiol. (Lond.) **185**, 298–322 (1966).

ERVIN, F. R., MARK, V. H.: Stereotactic thalamotomy in the human. Arch. Neurol. (Chic.) **3**, 368–380 (1960).

EULER, C., V., SÖDERBERG, U.: The relation between gamma motor activity and the electro-encephalogram. Experientia (Basel) **12**, 278 (1956).

FAVALE, F., LOEB, C., PARMA, M., ROSSI, G. F., SACCO, G.: Effects de la stimulation de structures du tronc cerebral sur le comportement du chat. Neuro-chirurgie **6**, 89–91 (1960).

FAVALE, E., LOEB, C., ROSSI, G. F., SACCO, G.: EEG synchronization and behavioral signs of sleep following low frequency stimulation of the brain stem reticular formation. Arch. ital. Biol. **99**, 1–22 (1961).

FORBES, A., COBB, S., CATTELL, H.: Electrical studies in mammalian reflexes. III. Immediate changes in the flexion reflex after spinal transection. Amer. J. Physiol. **63**, 30–44 (1923).

FOULKES, J. A., ROBINSON, N.: [^{14}C] Leucine incorporation of axoplasmic flow in the rat brainstem reticular formation. Brain Res. **11**, 638–647 (1968).

FOX, J. E.: Reticulospinal neurones in the rat. Brain Res. **23**, 35–40 (1970).

FRANK, K., FUORTES, M. G. F.: Presynaptic and postsynaptic inhibition of monosynaptic reflexes. Fed. Proc. **16**, 39–40 (1957).

FRENCH, J. D.: The reticular formation. In: H. W. MAGOUN (Ed.). Handbook of Physiology. Section I. Neurophysiology. Washington, D. C.: American Physiological Society, II, 1281–1305, 1960.

FRENCH, J. D., AMERONGEN, F. K. V., MAGOUN, H. W.: An activating system in brain stem of monkey. Arch. Neurol. Psychiat. (Chic.) **68**, 577–590 (1952).

FRENCH, J. D., VERZEANO, M., MAGOUN, H. W.: An extralemniscal sensory system in the brain. Arch. Neurol. Psychiat. (Chic.) **69**, 505–518 (1953a).

FRENCH, J. D., VERZEANO, M., MAGOUN, H. W.: A neural basis of the anesthetic state. Arch. Neurol. Psychiat. (Chic.) **69**, 519–529 (1953b).

FULTON, J. F.: Muscular contraction and the reflex control of movement. Baltimore: Williams and Wilkins Co., 644 pp., 1926.

FUXE, K.: Evidence for the existence of monoamine neurons in the central nervous system. IV. Distribution of monoamine nerve terminals in the central nervous system. Acta physiol. scand. **64**, Suppl. 247, 37–85 (1965).

GARDNER, E., HADDAD, B.: Pathways to the cerebral cortex for afferent fibers from the hindleg of the cat. Amer. J. Physiol. **172**, 475–482 (1953).

GASSEL, M. M., POMPEIANO, O.: Fusimotor function during sleep in unrestrained cats. Arch. ital. Biol. **103**, 347–368 (1965).

GASSEL, M. M., POMPEIANO, O.: Tonic and phasic changes in threshold of arousal during desynchronized sleep. Arch. ital. Biol. **105**, 480–498 (1967).

GAUTHIER, C., MOLLICA, A., MORUZZI, G.: Physiological evidence of localized cerebellar projections to bulbar reticular formation. J. Neurophysiol. **19**, 468–483 (1956).

GAY, J. R., GELLHORN, E.: Cortical projection of proprioception in the cat and monkey. Proc. Soc. exp. Biol. (N.Y.) **70**, 711–718 (1949).

GEHUCHTEN, A. VAN: La dégénérescence dite rétrograde. IV. Fibres réticulo-spinales ventrales. Névraxe **5**, 88–107 (1903).

GELFAN, S., CARTER, S.: Muscle sense in man. Exp. Neurol. **18**, 469–473 (1967).

GELLHORN, E.: The influence of curare on hypothalamic excitability and the electroencephalogram. E.E.G. clin. Neurophysiol. **10**, 697–703 (1958).

GEREBETZOFF, M. A.: État fonctionnel de l'écorce cérébrale au cours de l'hypnose animale. Arch. int. Physiol. **51**, 365–378 (1941).

GERNANDT, B. E., MEGIRIAN, D.: Ascending propriospinal mechanisms. J. Neurophysiol. **24**, 364–376 (1961).

GERNANDT, B. E., SHIMAMURA, M.: Mechanisms of interlimb reflexes in cat. J. Neurophysiol. **24**, 665–676 (1961).

Giaquinto, S., Pompeiano, O.: Inibizione del tono posturale e di riflessi spinali prodotti dalla stimolazione appropriata di nervi cutanei in gatti integri non anestetizzati. Boll. Soc. ital. Biol. sper. **39**, 1258–1261 (1963a).

Giaquinto, S., Pompeiano, O.: Generalized inhibition of spinal reflexes induced by cutaneous nerve stimulation in unrestrained cats. Experientia (Basel) **19**, 653–654 (1963b).

Giaquinto, S., Pompeiano, O.: Inhibition of proprioceptive spinal reflexes induced by cutaneous afferent volleys in unrestrained cats. Arch. ital. Biol. **102**, 393–417 (1964).

Giaquinto, S., Pompeiano, O., Somogyi, I.: Ulteriori ricerche comprovanti l'assenza di una reazione elettroencefalografica di risveglio stimolando le fibre afferenti muscolari del gruppo I. Rend. Accad. naz. Lincei, Cl. Sci. fis., mat. nat., Ser. VIII, **34**, 449–451 (1963a).

Giaquinto, S., Pompeiano, O., Somogyi, I.: Supraspinal modulation of monosynaptic and of polysynaptic spinal reflexes during natural sleep and wakefulness. Arch. ital. Biol. **102**, 245–281 (1964a).

Giaquinto, S., Pompeiano, O., Somogyi, I.: Descending inhibitory influences on spinal reflexes during natural sleep. Arch. ital. Biol. **102**, 282–307 (1964b).

Giaquinto, S., Pompeiano, O., Swett, J.E.: Sulla diversa efficacia delle afferenze propriocettive di alcuni nervi muscolari nel produrre il risveglio elettrico corticale. Boll. Soc. ital. Biol. sper. **38**, 940–942 (1962).

Giaquinto, S., Pompeiano, O., Swett, J.E.: EEG and behavioral effects of fore- and hind-limb muscular afferent volleys in unrestrained cats. Arch. ital. Biol. **101**, 133–148 (1963b).

Giblin, D.R.: Somatosensory evoked potentials in healthy subjects and in patients with lesions of the nervous system. Ann. N.Y. Acad. Sci. **112**, 93–142 (1964).

Gilman, T.T., Marcuse, F.L.: Animal hypnosis. Psychol. Bull. **46**, 151–165 (1949).

Glees, P.: Der Verlauf und die Endigung des Tractus spinothalamicus und der medialen Schleife, nach Beobachtungen beim Menschen und Affen. Verh. anat. Ges. (Jena) **50**, 48–49 (1952).

Gluck, M., Roland, V.: Defensive conditioning of electrographic arousal with delayed and differentiated auditory stimuli. E.E.G. clin. Neurophysiol. **11**, 485–496 (1959).

Goodwin, G.M., McCloskey, D.I., Matthews, P.B.C.: A systematic distorsion of position sense produced by muscle vibration. J. Physiol. (Lond.) **221**, 8–9P (1972).

Gordon, G., Landgren, S., Seed, W.A.: The functional characteristics of single cells in the caudal part of the spinal nucleus of the trigeminal nerve of the cat. J. Physiol. (Lond.) **158**, 544–559 (1961).

Grampp, W., Oscarsson, O.: Inhibitory neurons in the group I projection area of the cat's cerebral cortex. In: C. von Euler, S. Skoglund and U. Söderberg (Eds.). Structure and functions of inhibitory neuronal mechanisms. Oxford: Pergamon Press, 351–356, 1968.

Granit, R.: Receptors and sensory perception. New Haven: Yale University Press, XI–366 pp., 1955.

Granit, R., Kaada, B.R.: Influence of stimulation of central nervous structures on muscle spindles in cat. Acta physiol. scand. **27**, 130–160 (1952).

Grantyne, A.A.: Morphology, topography and connections of the medulla oblongata and the pons of the cat. In: A.V. Valdman (Ed.). Progress in Brain Research. Vol. 20. Pharmacology and physiology of the reticular formation. Amsterdam: Elsevier Publ. Co., 128–147, 1967.

Grastyán, E., Hasznos, T., Lissák, K., Molnár, L., Ruzsonyi, Z.: Activation of the brain stem activating system by vegetative afferents. Acta physiol. hung. **3**, 103–122 (1952).

Grillner, S.: Supraspinal and segmental control of static and dynamic γ-motoneurones in the cat. Acta physiol. scand. **77**, Suppl. 327, 1–34 (1969).

Grillner, S., Hongo, T., Lund, S.: The origin of descending fibres monosynaptically activating spinoreticular neurones. Brain Res. **10**, 259–262 (1968).

Guiot, G., Albe-Fessard, D., Arfel, G., Hertzog, E., Vourc'h, G., Hardy, J., Derome, P., Aléonard, P.: Interprétation des effects de la stimulation du thalamus de l'homme par chocs isolés. C.R. Acad. Sci. (Paris) **254**, 3581–3583 (1962).

Haapanen, J., Kolmoden, G.M., Skoglund, C.R.: Membrane and action potentials of spinal interneurones in the cat. Acta physiol. scand. **43**, 315–348 (1958).

Hagbarth, K.-E.: Centrifugal mechanisms of sensory control. Ergebn. Biol. **22**, 47–66 (1960).

HAGBARTH, K.-E., KERR, D.I.B.: Central influences on spinal afferent conduction. J. Neurophysiol. **17**, 295–307 (1954).

HAND, P.J.: Lumbosacral dorsal root termination in the nucleus gracilis of the cat. Some observations on terminal degeneration in other medullary sensory nuclei. J. comp. Neurol. **126**, 137–156 (1966).

HARA, T., FAVALE, E., ROSSI, G.F., SACCO, G.: Responses in mesencephalic reticular formation and central grey matter evoked by somatic peripheral stimuli. Exp. Neurol. **4**, 297–309 (1961).

HAYASHI, Y., YOSHII, N.: Mesencephalic reticular influence on electrical activities of the pontine reticular formation. Jap. J. Physiol. **16**, 335–353 (1966).

HEINBECKER, P., BISHOP, G.H., O'LEARY, J.L.: Pain and touch fibers in peripheral nerves. Arch. Neurol. Psychiat. (Chic.) **29**, 771–789 (1933).

HELD, H.: Beiträge zur feineren Anatomie des Kleinhirns und Hirnstammes. Arch. Anat. Physiol. (Lpz.) Anat. Abt., 435–446 (1893).

HENSEL, H., BOMAN, K.K.A.: Afferent impulses in cutaneous sensory nerves in human subjects. J. Neurophysiol. **23**, 564–578 (1960).

HERNÁNDEZ-PÉON, R.: Reticular mechanisms of sensory control. In: W.A. ROSENBLITH (Ed.) Sensory communication. Cambridge, Mass.: M.I.T. Press, 497–520, 1961.

HERNÁNDEZ-PÉON, R., BRUST-CARMONA, H.: Inhibition of tactile and nociceptive spinal evoked potentials in the cat during distraction. Acta neurol. lat.-amer. **7**, 289–298 (1961).

HERNÁNDEZ-PÉON, R., DITTBORN, J., BORLONE, M., DAVIDOVICH, A.: Modifications of a forearm skin reflex during hypnotically induced anesthesia and hyperesthesia. Acta neurol. lat.-amer. **6**, 32–42 (1960).

HERNÁNDEZ-PÉON, R., HAGBARTH, K.-E.: Interaction between afferent and cortically induced reticular responses. J. Neurophysiol. **18**, 44–55 (1955).

HERNÁNDEZ-PÉON, R., SCHERRER, H., VELASCO, M.: Central influences on afferent conduction in the somatic and visual pathways. Acta neurol. lat.-amer. **2**, 8–22 (1956).

HERRICK, C.J., BISHOP, G.H.: A comparative survey of the spinal lemniscus systems. In: H.H. JASPER et al. (Eds.). Reticular formation of the brain. Henry Ford Hospital International Symposium. Boston: Little, Brown and Co., 353–364, 1958.

HILL, R.M., HORN, G.: Responsiveness to sensory stimulation of cells in the rabbit midbrain. J. Physiol. (Lond.) **175**, 40–41P (1964).

HODES, R.: Electrocortical synchronization resulting from reduced proprioceptive drive cauded by neuromuscular blocking agents. E.E.G. clin. Neurophysiol. **14**, 220–232 (1962).

HODES, R.: Electrocortical synchronization produced by unilateral intervention at the cervical cord level. E.E.G. clin. Neurophysiol. **15**, 651–659 (1963).

HODES, R.: Electrocortical desynchronization resulting from spinal block: evidence for synchronizing influences in the cervical cord. Arch. ital. Biol. **102**, 183–196 (1964).

HÖSLI, L., WOLSTENCROFT, J.H.: Rostral, spinal and cerebellar projections of reticular neurons determined by neurophysiological method. J. Anat. (Lond.) **101**, 603 (1967).

HOLMES, R.L., WOLSTENCROFT, J.H.: Cholinesterase in the medulla and pons of the cat. J. Physiol. (Lond.) **175**, 55–56P (1964).

HOLMQVIST, B.: Crossed spinal reflex actions evoked by volleys in somatic afferents. Acta physiol. scand. **52**, Suppl. 181, 1–67 (1961).

HOLMQVIST, B., LUNDBERG, A.: On the organization of the supraspinal inhibitory control of interneurones of various spinal reflex arcs. Arch. ital. Biol. **97**, 340–356 (1959).

HOLMQVIST, B., LUNDBERG, A.: Differential supraspinal control of synaptic actions evoked by volleys in the flexion reflex afferents in alpha motoneurones. Acta physiol. scand. **54**, Suppl. 186, 1–51 (1961).

HOLMQVIST, B., LUNDBERG, A., OSCARSSON, O.: Functional organization of the dorsal spinocerebellar tract in the cat. V. Further experiments on convergence of excitatory and inhibitory actions. Acta physiol. scand. **38**, 76–90 (1956).

HOLMQVIST, B., LUNDBERG, A., OSCARSSON, O.: The relationship between the flexion reflex and certain ascending spinal pathways. Experientia (Basel) **15**, 195 (1959).

HOLMQVIST, B., LUNDBERG, A., OSCARSSON, O.: Supraspinal inhibitory control of transmission to three ascending pathways influenced by the flexion reflex afferents. Arch. ital. Biol. **98**, 60–80 (1960a).

Holmqvist, B., Lundberg, A., Oscarsson, O. A supraspinal control system monosynaptical-
    ly connected with an ascending spinal pathway. Arch. ital. Biol. **98**, 402–422 (1960b).
Holmqvist, B., Oscarsson, O.: Location, course, and characteristics of uncrossed and crossed
    ascending spinal tracts in the cat. Acta physiol. scand. **58**, 57–67 (1963).
Holmqvist, B., Oscarsson, O., Rosén, R.: Functional organization of the cuneocerebellar
    tract in the cat. Acta physiol. scand. **58**, 216–235 (1963).
Hongo, T., Kubota, K., Shimazu, H.: EEG spindle and depression of gamma motor activity.
    J. Neurophysiol. **26**, 568–580 (1963).
Hongo, T., Okada, Y.: Cortically evoked pre- and postsynaptic inhibition of impulse trans-
    mission to the dorsal spinocerebellar tract. Exp. Brain Res. **3**, 135–149 (1967).
Hongo, T., Okada, Y., Sato, M.: Corticofugal influences on transmission to the dorsal spino-
    cerebellar tract from hindlimb primary afferents. Exp. Brain Res. **3**, 135–149 (1967).
Hongo, T., Shimazu, H., Kubota, K.: A supraspinal inhibitory action on the gamma motor
    system. In: D. Barker (Ed.). Symposium on muscle receptors. Hong-Kong: Hong-Kong
    University Press, 59–65, 1962.
Horn, G., Hill, R.M.: Responsiveness to sensory stimulation of units in the superior collicu-
    lus and subjacent tectotegmental regions of the rabbit. Exp. Neurol. **14**, 199–223 (1966).
Hugelin, A.: Analyse de l'inhibition d'un réflexe nociceptif (réflexe linguo-maxillaire) lors de
    l'activation du système réticulo-spinal dit "facilitateur". C.R. Soc. Biol. (Paris) **149**,
    1893–1898 (1955).
Hugelin, A., Dumont, S.: Controle réticulaire du réflexe linguo-maxillaire et des afférences
    somesthésiques. J. Physiol. (Paris) **52**, 119–120 (1960).
Hunsperger, R.W.: Affektreaktionen auf elektrische Reizung im Hirnstamm der Katze.
    Helv. physiol Acta **14**, 70–92 (1956).
Hunt, C.C.: Relation of function to diameter in afferent fibers of muscle nerves. J. gen. Physiol.
    38, 117–131 (1954).
Hunt, C.C., Kuno, M.: Background discharge and evoked responses of spinal interneurones.
    J. Physiol. (Lond.) **147**, 364–384 (1959).
Hunt, C.C., Kuffler, S.W.: Stretch receptor discharges during muscle contraction. J. Phy-
    siol. (Lond.) **113**, 298–315 (1951).
Hunt, C.C., McIntyre, A.K.: Characteristics of responses from the flexor longus digitorum
    muscle and the adjoining interosseous region of the cat. J. Physiol. (Lond.) **153**, 74–87 (1960).
Huttenlocher, P.R.: Evoked and spontaneous activity in single units of medial brain stem
    during natural sleep and waking. J. Neurophysiol. **24**, 451–468 (1961).
Ingvar, D.H.: Extraneuronal influences upon the electrical activity of isolated cortex follow-
    ing stimulation of the reticular activating system. Acta physiol. scand. **33**, 169–193 (1955).
Iosif, G., Pompeiano, O., Strata, P., Thoden, U.: The effect of stimulation of spindle
    receptors and Golgi tendon organs on the cerebellar anterior lobe. Arch. ital. Biol. **110**,
    476–501, 502–542, (1972).
Irvine, S.R., Ludvigh, E.J.: Is ocular proprioceptive sense concerned in vision? Arch.
    Ophtal. (N.Y.) **15**, 1037–1049 (1936).
Ito, M., Hongo, T., Yoshida, M., Okada, Y., Obata, K.: Antidromic and transsynaptic
    activation of Deiters' neurons during stimulation of the spinal cord. Jap. J. Physiol. **14**,
    638–658 (1964).
Ito, M., Udo, M., Mano, N.: Long inhibitory and excitatory pathways converging onto cat
    reticular and Deiters' neurons and their relevance to reticulofugal axons. J. Neurophysiol.
    33, 210–226 (1970).
Jankowska, E., Jukes, M.G.M., Lund, S., Lundberg, A.: The effect of DOPA on the spinal
    cord. 5. Reciprocal organization of pathways transmitting excitatory action to alpha moto-
    neurones of flexors and extensors. Acta physiol. scand. **70**, 369–388 (1967a).
Jankowska, E., Jukes, M.G.M., Lund, S., Lundberg, A.: The effect of DOPA on the spinal
    cord. 6. Half-centre organization of interneurones transmitting effects from the flexor
    reflex afferents. Acta physiol. scand. **70**, 389–402 (1967b).
Jankowska, E., Lund, S., Lundberg, A., Pompeiano, O.: Postsynaptic inhibition in moto-
    neurones evoked from the lower reticular formation. Experientia (Basel) **20**, 701–702 (1964).
Jankowska, E., Lund, S., Lundberg, A., Pompeiano, O.: Inhibitory effects evoked through
    ventral reticulospinal pathways. Arch. ital. Biol. **106**, 124–140 (1968).

JANSEN, J.K.S., RUDJORD, T.: On the silent period and Golgi tendon organs of the soleus muscle of the cat. Acta physiol. scand. **62**, 364–379 (1964).

JASPER, H.H.: Diffuse projection systems: the integrative action of the thalamic reticular system. E.E.G. clin. Neurophysiol. **1**, 405–420 (1949).

JASPER, H.H.: Unspecific thalamocortical relations. In: J. FIELD, H.W. MAGOUN and V.E. HALL (Eds.), Handbook of Physiology. Section I. Neurophysiology. Washington, D.C.: American Physiological Society, II, 1307–1321, 1960.

JOB, C.: Über autogene Inhibition und Reflexumkehr bei spinalisierten und decerebrierten Katzen. Pflügers Arch. ges. Physiol. **256**, 406–418 (1953).

JOHANSSON, B.: Circulatory responses to stimulation of somatic afferents with special reference to depressor effects from muscle nerves. Acta physiol. scand. **57**, Suppl. 198, 1–91 (1962).

JOHNSON, F.H.: Experimental study of spino-reticular connections in the cat. Anat. Rec. **118**, 316 (1954).

JOUVET, M.: Recherches sur les structures nerveuses et les mecanismes responsables des differentes phases du sommeil physiologique. Arch. ital. Biol. **100**, 125–206 (1962).

JOUVET M.: Neurophysiology of the states of sleep. Physiol. Rev. **47**, 117–177 (1967).

JUNGE, K., SVEEN, O.: Exclusive thalamic location of subcortical spontaneous barbiturate spindles. Acta physiol. scand. **73**, 22–31 (1968).

KAMIKAWA, K., McILWAIN, J.T., ADEY, W.R.: Subcortical unit firing patterns during classical conditioning. Fed. Proc. **22**, 1423 (1963).

KENNARD, M.A., FULTON, J.F.: Corticostriatal interrelations in monkey and chimpanzee. Res. Publ. Ass. nerv. ment. Dis. **21**, 228–245 (1942).

KERR, D.I.B., HAUGEN, F.P., MELZACK, R.: Responses evoked in the brain stem by tooth stimulation. Amer. J. Physiol. **183**, 253–258 (1955).

KLEITMAN, N.: Sleep. Physiol. Rev. **9**, 624–665 (1929).

KLEITMAN, N.: Sleep and wakefulness. Chicago, Ill.: The University of Chicago Press, XII–638 pp., 1939.

KLEMM, W.R.: Electroencephalographic-behavioral dissociations during animal hypnosis. E.E.G. clin. Neurophysiol. **21**, 365–372 (1966).

KLEMM, W.R.: Mechanisms of the immobility reflex (animal hypnosis). II. EEG and multiple units correlates in the brain stem. Comm. Behav. Biol. **3**, 43–52 (1969).

KLEMM, W.R., McBRIDE, R.L., McGRAW, C.P.: Brain systems controlling the motor inhibition of animal hypnosis. Fed. Proc. **27**, 374 (1968).

KLEYNTJENS, F., KOIZUMI, K., BROOKS, C.McC.: Stimulation of suprabulbar reticular formation. Arch. Neurol. Psychiat. (Chic.) **73**, 425–438 (1955).

KOCH, E.: Die Irradiation der pressoreceptorischen Kreislaufreflexe. Klin. Wschr. **11**, 225–227 (1932a).

KOCH, E.: Irradiation der pressorezeptorischen Kreislaufreflexe auf das animale Nervensystem. Z. Kreisl.-Forsch. **24**, 251–258 (1932b).

KOHNSTAMM, O.: Über Ursprungskerne spinaler Bahnen im Hirnstamm speciell über das Atemcentrum. Arch. Psychiat. Nervenkr. **32**, 681–684 (1899).

KOHNSTAMM, O., QUENSEL, F.: Das Centrum receptorium (sensorium) der Formatio reticularis. Neurol. Zbl. **27**, 1046–1047 (1908).

KOIZUMI, K., USHIYAMA, J., BROOKS, C.McC.: A study of reticular formation action on spinal interneurons and motoneurons. Jap. J. Physiol. **9**, 282–303 (1959).

KOSITZYN, N.S.: Axo-dendritic relations in the brain stem reticular formation. J. comp. Neurol. **122**, 9–17 (1964).

KOSTYUK, P.G.: The nature of excitation and inhibition in single internuncial neurons of the spinal cord. Sechenov Physiol. J. U.S.S.R. **47**, 1241–1253 (1961).

KREINDLER, A.: Recherches expérimentales sur les relations entre la sinus carotidien et le système nerveux central. Bull. Soc. Sci. Acad. roumaine **28**, 448–481 (1946).

KRUG, M., SCHMIDT, J., MATTHIES, H.: Impulsintervallanalyse von spontan tätigen Neuronen der pontinen Formation reticularis der Ratte. Acta biol. med. germ. **21**, 811–825 (1968).

KRUG, M., SCHMIDT, J., MATTHIES, H.: Beeinflussung des Impulsmusters von spontan tätigen Neuronen der pontine Formatio reticularis der Ratte durch Noradrenalin, Serotonin und Azetylcholin. Acta biol. med. germ. **25**, 455–467 (1970).

KRUGER, L.: Characteristics of the somatic afferent projection to the percentral cortex in the monkey. Amer. J. Physiol. **186**, 475–482 (1956).

KRUGER, L., ALBE-FESSARD, D.: Distribution of responses to somatic afferent stimuli in the diencephalon of the cat under chloralose anesthesia. Exp. Neurol. **2**, 442–467 (1960).

KRUGER, L., MICHEL, F.: Reinterpretation of the representation of pain based on physiological excitation of single neurons in the trigeminal sensory complex. Exp. Neurol. **5**, 157–178 (1962).

KUMAZAWA, T.: "Deactivation" of the rabbit's brain by pressure application to the skin. E.E.G. clin. Neurophysiol. **15**, 660–671 (1963).

KUNO, M., PERL, E.R.: Alteration of spinal reflexes by interaction with suprasegmental and dorsal root activity. J. Psysiol. (Lond.) **151**, 103–122 (1960).

KURU, M., KURATI, T., KOYAMA, Y.: The bulbar vesico-constrictor center and the bulbo-sacral connections arising from it. A study of the function of the lateral reticulospinal tract. J. comp. Neurol. **113**, 365–388 (1959).

KUYPERS, H.G.J.M.: Central cortical projections to motor and somato-sensory cell groups. Brain **83**, 161–184 (1960).

KUYPERS, H.G.J.M.: The organization of the "motor system". Int. J. Neurol. (Montevideo) **4**, 78–91 (1963).

KUYPERS, H.G.J.M.: The descending pathways to the spinal cord, their anatomy and function. In: J.C. ECCLES and J.P. SCHADÉ (Eds.). Progress in Brain Research. Vol. 11. Organization of the spinal cord. Amsterdam: Elsevier Publ. Co., 178–202, 1964.

KUYPERS, H.G.J.M.: The descending pathways of the spinal cord. J. Neurosurg., Suppl. part. II, 200–202 (1966).

KUYPERS, H.G.J.M., FLEMING, W.R., FARINHOLT, J.W.: Descending projections to spinal motor and sensory cell groups in the monkey: cortex versus subcortex. Science **132**, 38–40 (1960).

KUYPERS, H.G.J.M., FLEMING, W.R., FARINHOLT, J.W.: Subcorticospinal projections in the rhesus monkey. J. comp. Neurol. **118**, 107–137 (1962).

LALONDE, J.-L., POIRIER, L.J. Study of various modalities of pain sensation in the monkey. J. comp. Neurol. **112**, 185–201 (1959).

LAMARCHE, G., HÉON, M., MORIN, F.: Activités unitaires et modalités réactionnelles de la formation réticulée et de quelques noyaux bulbaires secondaires à des influx sensitifs. Laval méd. **26**, 644–654 (1958).

LAMARCHE, G., LANGLOIS, J.M.: Les neurones de la formation réticulaire ponto-bulbaire et la stimulation trigéminale. Canad. J. Biochem. **40**, 261–271 (1962).

LAMARCHE, G., LANGLOIS, J.M., HÉON, M.: Unit study of the trigeminal projections in the reticular formation of the medulla oblongata in the cat. Canad. J. Biochem. **38**, 1163–1166 (1960).

LAMARRE, Y., LIEBESKIND, J.C.: Projections des afférences d'origine musculaire au niveau de cortex sensori-moteur chez le singe. J. Physiol. (Paris) **57**, 259 (1965).

LANDGREN, S.: Projection of group I muscle afferents to the cerebral cortex. Acta physiol. scand. **77**, Suppl. 330, 35, n. 40 (1969).

LANDGREN, S., SILFVENIUS, H.: Cortical projections of group IA muscle afferents from the hindlimb. Proc. XXIV int. Congr. physiol. Sci., Washington, D.C., VII, 253, n. 758 (1968a).

LANDGREN, S., SILFVENIUS, H.: Cortical projections of Group I muscle afferents from the hindlimb. Acta. physiol. scand. **73**, 14–15A (1968b).

LANDGREN, S., SILFVENIUS, H.: Projection to cerebral cortex of group I muscle afferents from the cat's hind limb. J. Physiol. (Lond.) **200**, 353–372 (1969a).

LANDGREN, S., SILFVENIUS, H.: The medullary relay in the path from hindlimb muscle spindles to the cerebral cortex of the cat. Acta physiol. scand. **77**, Suppl. 330, 119, n. 190 (1969b).

LANDGREN, S., SILFVENIUS, H.: The projection of Group I muscle afferents from the hindlimb to the contralateral thalamus of the cat. Acta physiol. scand. **80**, 10A (1970).

LANDGREN, S., SILFVENIUS, H.: Nucleus z, the medullary relay in the projection path to the cerebral cortex of group I muscle afferents from the cat's hind limb. J. Physiol. (Lond.) **218**, 551–571 (1971).

LANDGREN, S., SILFVENIUS, H., WOLSK, D.: Somatosensory paths to the second cortical projection area of the group I muscle afferents. J. Physiol. (Lond.) **191**, 543–559 (1967).

Landgren, S., Wolsk, D.: A new cortical area receiving input from Group I muscle afferents. Life Sci. 5, 75–79 (1966).

Langlois, J.M., Lamarche, G.: Trigeminal projections in the reticular formation of the pons in the cat. Canad. J. Biochem. 40, 7–12 (1962).

Laporte, Y., Bessou, P.: Distribution dans les sous-groups rapide et lent du groupe I des fibres Ia d'origine fusoriale et des fibres Ib d'origine golgienne. C.R. Soc. Biol. (Paris) 151, 178–182 (1957).

Laporte, Y., Bessou, P., Bouisset, S.: Action réflexe des différents types de fibres afférents d'origine musculaire sur la pression sanguine. Arch. ital. Biol. 98, 206–221 (1960).

Laporte, Y., Leitner, L.-M., Pagès, B.: Absence d'effets réflexes circulatoires des fibres afférentes du groupe I. C.R. Soc. Biol. (Paris) 156, 2130–2133 (1962).

Laporte, Y., Montastruc, P.: Rôle des différents types de fibres afférentes dans les réflexes circulatoires généraux d'origine cutanée. J. Physiol. (Paris) 49, 1039–1049 (1957).

Lawrence, D.G., Kuypers, H.G.J.M.: Pyramidal and non-pyramidal pathways in monkeys: anatomical and functional correlation. Science 148, 973–975 (1965).

Lawrence, D.G., Kuypers, H.G.J.M.: The functional organization of the motor system in the monkey. II. The effects of lesions of the descending brain-stem pathways. Brain 91, 15–36 (1968).

Leksell, L.: The action potential and excitatory effects of the small ventral root fibres to skeletal muscle. Acta physiol. scand. 10, Suppl. 31, 1–84 (1945).

Lenzi, G.L., Pompeiano, O., Rabin, B.: Supraspinal control of transmission in the polysynaptic reflex pathway to motoneurones during sleep. Pflügers Arch. ges. Physiol. 301, 311–319 (1968).

Leontovich, T.A., Zhukova, G.P.: The specificity of the neuronal structure and topography of the reticular formation in the brain and spinal cord of carnivora. J. comp. Neurol. 121, 347–379 (1963).

Lewandowsky, M.: Untersuchungen über die Leitungsbahnen des Truncus cerebri und ihren Zusammenhang mit denen der Medulla spinalis und des Cortex cerebri. Neurobiol. Arb., Zweite Serie, Weitere Beiträge zur Hirnanatomie. Jena: G. Fischer, 1, 63–147 (1904).

Liddell, E.G.T., Matthes, K., Oldberg, E., Ruch, T.C.: Reflex release of flexor muscles by spinal section. Brain 55, 239–246 (1932).

Liebeskind, J., Lamarre, Y., Albe-Fessard, D.: Studies of somatic projections to macaque motor cortex. Proc. XXIII int. Congr. physiol. Sci., Tokyo V, 394, n. 927 (1965).

Limanskii, Y.P.: Intracellular derivation of the action potentials of individual neurons in the reticular formation of the medulla. Sechenov physiol. J. U.S.S.R. 47, 671–677 (1961).

Limanskii, Y.P.: Synaptic modifications of the resting potential of individual neurones in the medulla oblongata reticular formation. Sechenov physiol. J. U.S.S.R. 48, 126–133 (1962).

Limanskii, Y.P.: Characteristics of afferent convergence on neurons of the medullary reticular formation. Fed. Proc., Transl. Suppl. 22, 1090–1093T (1963).

Limanskii, Y.P.: Slow and fast prepotentials in neurons of medullary reticular formation. Fed. Proc., Transl. Suppl. 24, 1008–1010T (1965).

Limanskii, Y.P.: Responses of neurons of the medullary reticular formation to afferent impulses from cutaneous and muscle nerves. Fed. Proc., Transl. Suppl. 25, 15–17 (1966).

Lindblom, U.F., Ottosson, J.O.: Bulbar influence on spinal cord dorsum potentials and ventral root reflexes. Acta physiol. scand. 35, 203–214 (1955).

Lindsley, D.B., Schreiner, L.H., Knowles, W.B., Magoun, H.W.: Behavioral and EEG changes following chronic brain stem lesions in the cat. E.E.G. clin. Neurophysiol. 2, 483–498 (1950).

Lindsley, D.F., Adey, W.R.: Availability of peripheral input to the midbrain reticular formation. Exp. Neurol. 4, 358–376 (1961).

Lissák, K., Karmos, G., Grastyán, E.: The importance of muscular relaxation in the organization of the "paradoxical phase" of sleep. Proc. XXII int. Congr. physiol. Sci., Leiden II, n. 932 (1962).

Llinás, R., Terzuolo, C.A.: Mechanisms of supraspinal actions upon spinal cord activities. Reticular inhibitory mechanisms on alpha-extensor motoneurons. J. Neurophysiol. 27, 579–591 (1964).

Llinás, R., Terzuolo, C.A.: Mechanisms of supraspinal actions upon spinal cord activities. Reticular inhibitory mechanisms upon flexor motoneurons. J. Neurophysiol. **28**, 413–422 (1965).

Lloyd, D.P.C.: Activity in neurons of the bulbospinal correlation system. J. Neurophysiol. **4**, 115–134 (1941).

Lloyd, D.P.C.: Mediation of descending long spinal reflex activity. J. Neurophysiol. **5**, 435–458 (1942).

Ludvigh, E.J.: Possible role of proprioception in the extraocular muscles. Arch. Ophthal. **48**, 436–441 (1952).

Lundberg, A.: Integrative significance of patterns of connections made by muscle afferents in the spinal cord. Symp. XXI int. Congr. physiol. Sci., Buenos Aires, 100–105 (1959).

Lundberg, A.: Ascending spinal hindlimb pathways in the cat. In: J.C. Eccles and J.P. Schadé (Eds.). Progress in Brain Research. Vol. 12. Physiology of spinal neurons. Amsterdam: Elsevier Publ. Co., 135–163, 1964a.

Lundberg, A.: Supraspinal control of transmission in reflex path to motoneurones and primary afferents. In: J.C. Eccles and J.P. Schadé (Eds.). Progress in Brain Research. Vol. 12. Physiology of spinal neurons. Amsterdam: Elsevier Publ. Co., 196–221, 1964b.

Lundberg, A.: Interaction entre voies réflexes spinales. Actualités neurophysiol., sixième série, 121–137 (1965).

Lundberg, A.: Integration in the reflex pathway. In: R. Granit (Ed.). Nobel Symposium I: Muscular afferents and motor control. Stockholm: Almqvist and Wiksell, 275–305, 1966.

Lundberg, A.: The supraspinal control of transmission in spinal reflex pathways. In: L. Widén (Ed.). Recent advances in clinical neurophysiology. E.E.G. clin. Neurophysiol. Suppl. **25**, 35–46 (1967).

Lundberg, A., Norrsell, U., Voorhoeve, P.: Pyramidal effects on lumbosacral interneurones activated by somatic afferents. Acta physiol. scand. **56**, 220–229 (1962).

Lundberg, A., Norrsell, U., Voorhoeve, P.: Effects from the sensorimotor cortex on ascending spinal pathways. Acta physiol. scand. **59**, 462–473 (1963).

Lundberg, A., Oscarsson, O.: Three ascending spinal pathways in the dorsal part of the lateral funiculus. Acta physiol. scand. **51**, 1–16 (1961).

Lundberg, A., Oscarsson, O.: Functional organization of the ventral spinocerebellar tract in the cat. IV. Identification of units by antidromic activation from the cerebellar cortex. Acta physiol. scand. **54**, 252–269 (1962a).

Lundberg, A., Oscarsson, O.: Two ascending pathways in the central part of the cord. Acta physiol. scand. **54**, 270–286 (1962b).

Lundberg, A., Voorhoeve, P.: Effects from the pyramidal tract on spinal reflex arcs. Acta physiol. scand. **56**, 201–219 (1962).

Lundberg, A., Vyklický, L.: Brain stem control of reflex paths to primary afferents. Acta physiol. scand. **59**, Suppl. 213, 91 (1963).

Lundberg, A., Vyklický, L.: Inhibition of transmission to primary afferents by electrical stimulation of the brain stem. Arch. ital. Biol. **104**, 86–97 (1966).

Machne, X., Calma, I., Magoun, H.W.: Unit activity of central cephalic brain stem in EEG arousal. J. Neurophysiol. **18**, 547–558 (1955).

Magherini, P.C., Pompeiano, O., Seguin, J.J.: The effect of stimulation of Golgi tendon organs and spindle receptors from hindlimb extensor muscles on supraspinal descending inhibitory mechanisms. Arch. ital. Biol. **111**, 24–57 (1973).

Magnes, J., Moruzzi, G., Pompeiano, O.: Synchronization of the EEG produced by low-frequency electrical stimulation of the region of the solitary tract. Arch. ital. Biol. **99**, 33–67 (1961).

Magni, F., Oscarsson, O.: Cerebral control of transmission of the ventral spino-cerebellar tract. Arch. ital. Biol. **99**, 369–396 (1961).

Magni, F., Oscarsson, O.: Principal organization of coarse-fibred ascending spinal tracts in phalanger, rabbit, and cat. Acta physiol. scand. **54**, 53–64 (1962).

Magni, F., Willis, W.D.: Antidromic activation of neurons of the reticular formation. Nature (Lond.) **198**, 592–594 (1963a).

Magni, F., Willis, W.D.: Identification of reticular formation neurons by intracellular recording. Arch. ital. Biol. **101**, 681–702 (1963b).

MAGNI, F., WILLIS, W.D.: Cortical control of brain stem reticular neurons. Arch. ital. Biol. **102**, 418–433 (1964a).

MAGNI, F., WILLIS, W.D.: Subcortical and peripheral control of brain stem reticular neurons. Arch. ital. Biol. **102**, 434–448 (1964b).

MAGNI, F., WILLIS, W.D.: Afferent connections to reticulo-spinal neurons. In: J.C. ECCLES and J.P. SCHADÉ (Eds.). Progress in Brain Research. Vol. 12. Physiology of spinal neurons. Amsterdam: Elsevier Publ. Co., 246–258, 1964c.

MAGNI, F., WILLIS, W.D.: Intracellular recording from neurones of the reticular formation. In: D.R. CURTIS and A.K. McINTYRE (Eds.). Studies in physiology. Berlin-Heidelberg-New York: Springer, 206–214, 1965.

MAGOUN, H.W.: Bulbar inhibition and facilitation of motor activity. Science **100**, 549–550 (1944).

MAGOUN, H.W.: Caudal and cephalic influences of the brain stem reticular formation. Physiol. Rev. **30**, 459–474 (1950).

MAGOUN, H.W.: The ascending reticular system and wakefulness. In: E.D. ADRIAN, B. BREMER and H.H. JASPER (Eds.). Brain mechanisms and consciousness. Oxford: Blackwell Sci. Publ., 1–15, 1954.

MAGOUN, H.W.: The waking brain. Springfield, Ill.: C.C. Thomas, VIII–188 pp., 1958.

MAGOUN, H.W., McKINLEY, W.A.: The termination of ascending trigeminal and spinal tracts in the thalamus of the cat. Amer. J. Physiol. **137**, 409–416 (1942).

MAGOUN, H.W., RHINES, R.: An inhibitory mechanism in the bulbar reticular formation. J. Neurophysiol. **9**, 165–171 (1946).

MALLART, A.: Données sur le type de fibres conduisant dans les nerf périphérique les influx afférents d'origine somatique vers les relais primaires et associatifs du thalamus. J. Physiol. (Paris) **52**, 159–160 (1960).

MALLART, A.: Données sur les types de fibres conduisant les afférences somatiques au noyau centre médiane du thalamus. J. Physiol. (Paris) **53**, 422–423 (1961).

MALLART, A.: Projections des afferences musculaires de la parte anterieure au niveau du thalamus chez le chat. C.R. Acad. Sci. (Paris) **259**, 1215–1218 (1964a).

MALLART, A.: Projection thalamique des afferences musculaires de la patte anterieur chez le chat. J. Physiol. (Paris) **56**, 399 (1964b).

MALLART, M.A.: Thalamic projection of muscle nerve afferents in the cat. J. Physiol. (Lond.) **194**, 337–353 (1968).

MALLIANI, A., BIZZI, E., APELBAUM, J., ZANCHETTI, A.: Ascending afferent mechanisms maintaining sham rage behavior in the acute thalamic cat. Arch. ital. Biol. **101**, 632–647 (1963).

MALLIANI, A., CARLI, G., MANCIA, G., ZANCHETTI, A.: Behavioral effects of electrical stimulation of group I muscle afferents in acute thalamic cats. J. Neurophysiol. **31**, 210–220 (1968).

MANCIA, M., MECHELSE, K., MOLLICA, A.: Microelectrode recording from midbrain reticular formation in the decerebrate cat. Arch. ital. Biol. **95**, 110–119 (1957).

MANCIA, M., MEULDERS, M., SANTIBAÑEZ-H., G.: Synchronization de l'électroencéphalogramme provoquée par la stimulation visuelle répétitive chez le chat "médiopontin prétrigéminal". Arch. int. Physiol. **67**, 661–670 (1959).

MANFREDI, M.: Modulation of sensory projections in anterolateral column of cat spinal cord by peripheral afferents of different size. Arch. ital. Biol. **108**, 72–105 (1970).

MANNEN, H.: Noyau fermé et noyau ouvert. Arch. ital. Biol. **98**, 333–350 (1960).

MANNEN, H.: Contribution to the quantitative study of the nervous tissue. A new method for measurement of the volume and surface area of neurons. J. comp. Neurol. **126**, 75–90 (1966a).

MANNEN, H.: Contribution to the morphological study of dendritic arborisation in the brain stem. In: T. TOKIZANE and J.P. SCHADÉ (Eds.). Progress in Brain Research. Vol. 21A. Correlative neurosciences. Fundamental mechanisms. Amsterdam: Elsevier Publ. Co., 131–162, 1966b.

MARILLAUD, A., GAHERY, Y., DELL, P.: Diamètre et nature des fibres responsables de l'endormement vago-aortique. J. Physiol. (Paris) **58**, 251 (1966).

MATSUZAKI, M.: Differential effects of Na-butyrate and physostigmine on brain stem activities of para-sleep. Brain Res. **11**, 251–255 (1968).

Matsuzaki, M.: Differential effects of sodium butyrate and physostigmine upon the activities of para-sleep in acute brain stem preparations. Brain Res. 13, 247–265 (1969).

Matsuzaki, M., Kasahara, M.: Induction of para-sleep by cholinesterase inhibitors in the mesencephalic cat. Proc. Jap. Acad. 42, 989–993 (1966).

Matsuzaki, M., Okada, Y., Shuto, S.: Cholinergic actions related to paradoxical sleep induction in the mesencephalic cat. Experientia (Basel) 23, 1029–1030 (1967).

Matsuzaki, M., Okada, Y., Shuto, S.: Cholinergic agents related to para-sleep state in acute brain stem preparations. Brain Res. 9, 253–267 (1968).

Matthews, B.H.C.: Nerve endings in mammalian muscle. J. Physiol. (Lond.) 78, 1–53 (1933).

Matthews, P.B.C.: The reflex excitation of the soleus muscle of the decerebrate cat caused by vibration applied to its tendon. J. Physiol. (Lond.) 184, 450–472 (1966).

Mazzella, H., García Mullin, R., García Austt, E.: Effect of carotid sinus stimulation in the EEG. Acta neurol. lat.-amer. 3, 361–364 (1957).

McBride, R.L., Klemm, W.R.: Mechanisms of the immobility reflex (animal hypnosis). I. Influences of repetition of induction, restriction of auditory visual input and destruction of brain areas. Comm. Behav. Biol. 3, 33–41 (1969).

McIntyre, A.K.: Cortical projection of afferent impulses in muscle nerves. Proc. Univ. Otago med. Sch. 31, 5–6 (1953).

McIntyre, A.K.: Cortical projection of impulses in the interosseous nerve of the cat's hind limb. J. Physiol. (Lond.) 163, 46–60 (1962a).

McIntyre, A.K.: Central projection of impulses from receptors activated by muscle stretch. In: D. Barker (Ed.). Symposium on muscle receptors. Hong Kong: Hong Kong University Press, 19–30, 1962b.

McIntyre, A.K.: Some applications of input-output technique. In: D.R. Curtis and A.K. McIntyre (Eds.). Studies in physiology. Berlin-Heidelberg-NewYork: Springer, 199–206, 1965.

McMillan, J.A., Wagman, I.H.: Activity in midbrain monkey related to C fiber stimulation. Fed. Proc. 30, 664 Abs., n. 2622 (1971).

Meessen, H., Olszewski, J.: A cytoarchitectonic atlas of the rhombencephalon of the rabbit. Basel-New York: Karger, 52 pp., 1949.

Megirian, D.: Centrifugal cutaneous nerve discharges in the decerebrate phalanger, Trichosurus vulpecula. Arch. ital. Biol. 108, 388–399 (1970a).

Megirian, D.: Longitudinal conducting system serving centrifugal cutaneous nerve discharges in the decerebrate-decerebellate phalanger, Trichosurus vulpecula. Arch. ital. Biol. 108, 577–590 (1970b).

Mehler, W.R.: The mammalian "pain tract" in phylogeny. Anat. Rec. 127, 332 (1957).

Mehler, W.R.: The mammalian "pain tract" in phylogeny. Ph. D. Thesis, University of Maryland, 1959.

Mehler, W.R.: The anatomy of the so-called "pain tract" in man: an analysis of the course and distribution of the ascending fibers of the fasciculus anterolateralis. In: J.D. French and R.W. Borter (Eds.). Basic research in paraplegia. Springfield, Ill.: C.C. Thomas, 26–55, 1962.

Mehler, W.R.: Some observations on secondary ascending afferent systems in the central nervous system. In: R.S. Knighton and H.H. Dumke (Eds.). Pain. Boston, Mass.: Little, Brown and Co., 11–32, 1966.

Mehler, W.R.: Some neurological species differences — a posteriori. Ann. N.Y. Acad. Sci. 167, 424–468 (1969).

Mehler, W.R., Feferman, M.E., Nauta, W.J.H.: Ascending axon degeneration following anterolateral chordotomy in the monkey. Anat. Rec. 124, 332–333 (1956).

Mehler, W.R., Feferman, M.E., Nauta, W.J.H.: Ascending axon degeneration following anterolateral chordotomy. An experimental study in the monkey. Brain 83, 718–750 (1960).

Melzack, R., Stotler, W.A., Livingston, W.K.: Effects of discrete brain stem lesions in cats on perception of noxious stimulation. J. Neurophysiol. 21, 353–367 (1958).

Melzack, R., Wall, P.D.: On the nature of cutaneous sensory mechanisms. Brain 85, 331–356 (1962).

Merton, P.A.: Slowly conducting muscle spindles afferents. Acta physiol. scand. 29, 87–88 (1953).

MERTON, P.A.: The accuracy of directing the eyes and the hand in the dark. J. Physiol. (Lond.) **156**, 555–557 (1961).

MERTON, P.A.: Human position sense and sense of effort. Symp. Soc. exp. Biol. **18**, 387–400 (1964).

MOLINA, F. DE, ACHARD, O., WYSS, O.A.M.: Respiratory and vasomotor responses to stimulation of afferent fibres in somatic nerves. Helv. physiol. Acta **11**, 1–19 (1953).

MOLLICA, A., MORUZZI, G., NAQUET, R.: Décharges réticulaires induites par la polarisation du cervelet: leurs rapports avec le tonus postural et la réaction d'eveil. E.E.G. clin. Neurophysiol. **5**, 571–584 (1953).

MORELLI, M., NICOTRA, L., BARNES, C.D., CANGIANO, A., COOK, W.A., JR., POMPEIANO, O.: An apparatus for producing small-amplitude high-frequency sinusoidal stretching of the muscle. Arch. ital. Biol. **108**, 222–232 (1970).

MORILLO, A., BAYLOR, D.: Electrophysiological investigation of lemniscal and paralemniscal input to the midbrain reticular formation. E.E.G. clin. Neurophysiol. **15**, 455–464 (1963).

MORIN, F.: Afferent projections to the midbrain tegmentum and their spinal course. Amer. J. Physiol. **172**, 483–496 (1953).

MORIN, F., SCHWARTZ, H.G., O'LEARY, J.L.: Experimental study of the spinothalamic and related tracts. Acta psychiat. scand. **26**, 371–396 (1951).

MORISON, R.S., DEMPSEY, E.W.: A study of thalamo-cortical relations. Amer. J. Physiol. **135**, 281–292 (1942).

MORRISON, A.R., POMPEIANO, O.: Pyramidal discharge from somatosensory cortex and cortical control of primary afferents during sleep. Arch. ital. Biol. **103**, 538–568 (1965).

MORUZZI, G.: The physiological properties of the brain stem reticular system. In: E.D. ADRIAN F. BREMER and H.H. JASPER (Eds.). Brain mechanisms and consciousness. Oxford: Blackwell Sci. Publ., 21–48, 1954.

MORUZZI, G.: Spontaneous and evoked electrical activity in the brain stem reticular formation. Abstr. Rev. XX int. Physiol. Congr., Bruxelles, 269–286, 1956.

MORUZZI, G.: The functional significance of the ascending reticular system. Arch. ital. Biol. **96**, 17–28 (1958).

MORUZZI, G.: Synchronizing influences of the brain stem and the inhibitory mechanisms underlying the production of sleep by sensory stimulation. E.E.G. clin. Neurophysiol. Suppl. **13**, 231–256 (1960).

MORUZZI, G.: Reticular influence on the EEG. E.E.G. clin. Neurophysiol. **16**, 2–17 (1964).

MORUZZI, G., MAGOUN, H.W.: Brain stem reticular formation and activation of the EEG. E.E.G. clin. Neurophysiol. **1**, 455–473 (1949).

MOTOKIZAWA, F., FUJIMORI, B.: Arousal effect of afferent discharges from muscle spindles upon electroencephalograms in cats. J. Physiol. (Lond.) **14**, 344–353 (1964).

MOUNTCASTLE, V.B., COVIAN, M.R., HARRISON, C.R.: The central representation of some forms of deep sensitivity. Res. Publ. Ass. nerv. ment. Dis. **30**, 339–370 (1952).

MOUNTCASTLE, V.B., POWELL, T.P.S.: Central nervous mechanisms subserving position sense and kinesthesis. Johns Hopk. Hosp. Bull. **105**, 173–200 (1959a).

MOUNTCASTLE, V.B., POWELL, T.P.S.: Neural mechanism subserving cutaneous sensibility with special reference to the role of afferent inhibition in sensory perception and discrimination. Johns Hopk. Hosp. Bull. **105**, 201–232 (1959b).

NACHMANSOHN, D., MERRITT, H.H.: Nerve impulse. New York: Josiah Macy Jr. Foundation, 256 pp., 1956.

NAKAO, H., BALLIM, H.M., GELLHORN, E.: The role of sinoaortic receptors on the action of adrenaline, nor-adrenaline and acetylcholine on the cerebral cortex. E.E.G. clin. Neurophysiol. **8**, 413–420 (1956).

NAUTA, W.J.H., KUYPERS, H.G.J.M.: Some ascending pathways in the brain stem reticular formation. In: H.H. JASPER et al. (Eds.). Reticular formation of the brain. Henry Ford Hospital International Symposium. Boston-Toronto: Little, Brown and Co., 3–30, 1958.

NIEMER, T.: Connections of the brainstem reticular formation. Anat. Rec. **100**, 699–700 (1948).

NORSELL, V., WOLPOW, E.R.: An evoked potential study of different pathways from the hindlimb to the somatosensory areas in the cat. Acta physiol. scand. **66**, 19–33 (1966).

Nyberg-Hansen, R.: Origin and termination of fibers from the vestibular nuclei descending in the medial longitudinal fasciculus. An experimental study with silver impregnation methods in the cat. J. comp. Neurol. **122**, 355–368 (1964).

Nyberg-Hansen, R.: Sites and mode of termination of reticulo-spinal fibers in the cat. An experimental study with silver impregnation methods. J. comp. Neurol. **124**, 71–100 (1965).

Nyberg-Hansen, R.: Functional organization of descending supraspinal fibre systems to the spinal cord. Anatomical observations and physiological correlations. Ergebn. Anat. Entwickl.-Gesch. **39**, n. 2, 1–48 (1966).

Nyberg-Hansen, R., Brodal, A.: Sites of termination of corticospinal fibers in the cat. An experimental study with silver impregnation methods J. comp. Neurol. **120**, 369–392 (1963).

Nyberg-Hansen, R., Brodal, A.: Sites and modes of termination of rubrospinal fibers in the cat. An experimental study with silver impregnation methods. J. Anat. (Lond.) **98**, 235–253 (1964).

Nyberg-Hansen, R., Mascitti, T. A.: Sites and mode of termination of fibers of the vestibulospinal tract in the cat. An experimental study with silver impregnation methods. J. comp. Neurol. **122**, 369–387 (1963).

Olszewski, J.: The cytoarchitecture of the human reticular formation. In: E.D. Adrian, F. Bremer and H.H. Jasper (Eds.). Brain mechanisms and consciousness. Oxford: Blackwell Sci. Publ., 54–76, 1954.

Olszewski, J., Baxter, D.: Cytoarchitecture of the human brain stem. Basel-New York: Karger, 199 pp., 1954.

Oscarsson, O.: Further observations on ascending spinal tracts activated from muscle, joint and skin nerves. Arch. ital. Biol. **96**, 199–215 (1958).

Oscarsson, O.: Functional organization of the ventral spino-cerebellar tract in the cat. III. Supraspinal control of VSCT units of I-type. Acta physiol. scand. **49**, 171–183 (1960).

Oscarsson, O.: Differential course and organization of increased and crossed long ascending spinal tracts. In: J.C. Eccles and J.P. Schadé (Eds.). Progress in brain research. Vol. 12. Physiology of spinal neurons. Amsterdam: Elsevier Publ. Co., 164–178, 1964a.

Oscarsson, O.: Three ascending tracts activated from group I afferents in forelimb nerves of the cat. In: J.C. Eccles and J.P. Schadé (Eds.). Progress in Brain Research. Vol. 12. Physiology of spinal neurons. Amsterdam: Elsevier Publ. Co., 179–196, 1964b.

Oscarsson, O.: The projection of Group I muscle afferents to the cat cerebral cortex. In: R. Granit (Ed.). Nobel Symposium I. Muscular afferents and motor control. Stockholm: Almqvist and Wiksell, 307–316, 1966.

Oscarsson, O.: Functional organization of spinocerebellar paths. In: A. Iggo. Handbook of sensory physiology. Vol. II. Somatosensory system. Berlin-Heidelberg-New York: Springer, 1972, in press.

Oscarsson, O., Rosén, I.: Projection to cerebral cortex of large muscle spindle afferents in forelimb nerves of the cat. J. Physiol. (Lond.) **169**, 924–945 (1963).

Oscarsson, O., Rosén, I.: Stort-latency projections to the cat's cerebral cortex from skin and muscle afferents in the contralateral forelimb. J. Physiol. (Lond.) **182**, 164–184 (1966).

Oscarsson, O., Rosén, I., Sjölund, B.: Information carried by the forelimb group I path to the cerebral cortex. Acta physiol. scand. **77**, Suppl. 330, 37 (1969).

Oscarsson, O., Rosén, I., Sulg, I.: Organization of neurones in the cat cerebral cortex that are influenced from group I muscle afferents. J. Physiol. (Lond.) **183**, 189–210 (1966).

Oscarsson, O., Rosén, I., Uddenberg, N.: A comparative study of ascending spinal tracts activated from hindlimb afferents in monkey and dog. Arch. ital. Biol. **102**, 137–155 (1964).

Oswald, F.: Falling asleep open-eyed during intense rhythmic stimulation. Brit. med. J. **1**, 1450–1455 (1960).

Paintal, A.S.: Functional analysis of group III afferent fibres of mammalian muscles. J. Physiol. (Lond.) **152**, 250–270 (1960).

Palestini, M., Rossi, G.F., Zanchetti, A.: An electrophysiological analysis of pontine reticular regions showing different anatomical organization. Arch. ital. Biol. **95**, 97–109 (1957).

Papez, J.W.: Reticulo-spinal tracts in the cat. Marchi method. J. comp. Neurol. **41**, 365–399 (1926).

Pavlin, R.: Cholinesterases in reticular nerve cells. J. Neurochem. **12**, 515–518 (1965).

PAVLOV, I.P.: Les réflexes conditionnels. Paris: Librairie F. Alcan, 379 pp., 1932.

PERL, E.R.: Somatosensory mechanisms. Ann. Rev. Physiol. **25**, 459–492 (1963).

PERL, E.R., WHITLOCK, D.G., GENTRY, J.R.: Cutaneous projection to second order neurons of the dorsal column system. J. Neurophysiol. **25**, 337–358 (1962).

PETERSON, B.W., FELPEL, L.P.: Excitation and inhibition of reticulospinal neurons by vestibular, cortical and cutaneous stimulation. Brain Res. **27**, 373–376 (1971).

PETERSON, B.W., FELPEL, L.P., WILSON, V.J., ANDERSON, M.E.: Excitation and inhibition of reticular neurons and reticular system. Proc. XXV int. Congr. physiol. Sci., Munich, IX, 449, n. 1334 (1971).

PETIT, D., MALLART, A.: Voies spinales afférents vers le noyau centre médian du thalamus chez le chat. J. Physiol. (Paris) **56**, 423–424 (1964).

PETRAS, J.M.: Cortical, tectal and tegmental fiber connections in the spinal cord of the cat. Brain Res. **6**, 275–324 (1967).

PETROVICKY, P.: A comparative study of the reticular formation of the guinea pig. J. comp. Neurol. **128**, 85–108 (1966).

PHILLIPS, C.G., POWELL, T.P.S., WIESENDANGER, M.: Projection from low-threshold muscle afferents of hand and forearm to area 3a of baboon's cortex. J. Physiol. (Lond.) **217**, 419–446 (1971).

PITTS, R.F.: The respiratory center and its descending pathways. J. comp. Neurol. **72**, 605–625 (1940).

POGGIO, G.F., MOUNTCASTLE, V.B.: The functional properties of ventrobasal thalamic neurons studied in unanesthetized monkeys. J. Neurophysiol. **26**, 775–806 (1963).

POMPEIANO, O.: EEG synchronization induced by peripheral nerve stimulation. In: G. MORUZZI, A. FESSARD and H.H. JASPER (Eds.). Progress in Brain Research. Vol. 1. Brain mechanisms. Amsterdam: Elsevier Publ. Co., 429–443, 1963.

POMPEIANO, O.: Ascending and descending influences of somatic afferent volleys in unrestrained cats: supraspinal inhibitory control of spinal reflexes during natural and reflexly induced sleep. In: Aspects anatomo-fonctionnels de la physiologie du sommeil. Paris: Editions du C.N.R.S., 309–395, 1965.

POMPEIANO, O.: The neurophysiological mechanisms of the postural and motor events during desynchronized sleep. Res. Publ. Ass. nerv. ment. Dis. 45, 351–423 (1967a).

POMPEIANO, O.: Sensory inhibition during motor activity in sleep. Pp. 323–375. In: D.P. PURPURA and M.D. YAHR (Eds.). Neurophysiological basis of normal and abnormal motor activities. Hewlett, New York: Raven Press, 323–375, 1967b.

POMPEIANO, O.: Mechanisms of sensorimotor integration during sleep. In: E. STELLAR and J.M. SPRAGUE (Eds.). Progress in Physiological Psychology. New York-London: Academic Press **3**, 1–179 (1970).

POMPEIANO, O.: Spinovestibular relations: anatomical and physiological aspects. In: A. BRODAL and O. POMPEIANO (Eds.). Progress in Brain Research. Vol. 37. Basic aspects of central vestibular mechanisms. Amsterdam: Elsevier Publ. Co., 263–296, 1972.

POMPEIANO, O., BARNES, C.D.: Response of brain stem reticular neurons to muscle vibration in the decerebrate cat. J. Neurophysiol. **34**, 709–724 (1971).

POMPEIANO, O., BRODAL, A.: The origin of vestibulospinal fibres in the cat. An experimental-anatomical study, with comments on the descending medial longitudinal fasciculus. Arch. ital. Biol. **95**, 166–195 (1957a).

POMPEIANO, O., BRODAL, A.: Experimental demonstration of a somatotopical origin of rubrospinal fibers in the cat. J. comp. Neurol. **108**, 225–251 (1957b).

POMPEIANO, O., CARLI, G., KAWAMURA, H.: Transmission of sensory information through ascending spinal hindlimb pathways during sleep and wakefulness. Arch. ital. Biol. **105**, 529–572 (1967).

POMPEIANO, O., MORRISON, A.R.: Vestibular influences during sleep. III. Dissociation of the tonic and phasic inhibition of spinal reflexes during desynchronized sleep following vestibular lesions. Arch. ital. Biol. **104**, 231–246 (1966).

POMPEIANO, O., SWETT, J.E.: EEG synchronization produced by peripheral nerve stimulation. Experientia (Basel) **17**, 323–325 (1961a).

POMPEIANO, O., SWETT, J.E.: Sincronizzazione elettrica corticale prodotta da stimoli periferici. Boll. Soc. ital. Biol. sper. **37**, 432–435 (1961b).

Pompeiano, O., Swett, J.E.: Analisi delle fibre afferenti responsabili della sincronizzazione e del risveglio elettrico corticale prodotti da stimoli periferici. Boll. Soc. ital. Biol. sper. 37, 913–915 (1961c).

Pompeiano, O., Swett, J.E.: EEG and behavioral manifestations of sleep induced by cutaneous nerve stimulation in normal cats. Arch. ital. Biol. 100, 311–342 (1962a).

Pompeiano, O., Swett, J.E.: Identification of cutaneous and muscular afferent fibers producing EEG synchronization or arousal in normal cats. Arch. ital. Biol. 100, 343–380 (1962b).

Pompeiano, O., Swett, J.E.: Azione dei vari gruppi di fibre cutanee mieliniche su unità del tronco dell'encefalo in animali decerebrati e cerebellectomizzati. Boll. Soc. ital. Biol. sper. 38, 942–945 (1962c).

Pompeiano, O., Swett, J.E.: Assenza di risposta di unità reticolari a stimolazione delle fibre afferenti propriocettive a più bassa soglia in animali decerebrati e cerebellectomizzati. Boll. Soc. ital. Biol. sper. 38, 945–947 (1962d).

Pompeiano, O., Swett, J.E.: Sull'azione esercitata dai diversi gruppi di fibre afferenti muscolari su unità reticolari in animali decerebrati a cervelletto integro. Boll. Soc. ital. Biol. sper. 38, 948–951 (1962e).

Pompeiano, O., Swett, J.E.: Componenti eccitatrici ed inibitrici della risposta di singoli neuroni reticolari a stimolazione graduata di nervi somatici. Boll. Soc. ital. Biol. sper. 38, 951–954 (1962f).

Pompeiano, O., Swett, J.E.: Actions of graded cutaneous and muscular afferent volleys on brain stem units in the decerebrate, cerebellectomized cat. Arch. ital. Biol. 101, 552–583 (1963a).

Pompeiano, O., Swett, J.E.: Cerebellar potentials and responses of reticular units evoked by muscular afferent volleys in the decerebrate cat. Arch. ital. Biol. 101, 584–613 (1963b).

Potthoff, P.C., Richter, H.P., Burandt, H.-R.: Multisensorische Konvergenzen an Hirnstammneuronen der Katze. Arch. Psychiat. u. Z. ges. Neurol. 210, 36–60 (1967).

Prattle, R.E., Weddell, G.: Observations on electrical stimulation of pain fibers in an exposed human nerve. J. Neurophysiol. 11, 83–98 (1948).

Probst, M.: Zur Kenntnis der Schleifenschicht und über centripetale Rückenmarksfasern zum Deiters'schen Kern, zum Sehhügel und zur Substantia reticularis. Mschr. Psychiat. Neurol. 11, 3–12 (1902a).

Provins, K.A.: The effect of peripheral nerve block on the appreciation and execution of finger movements. J. Physiol. (Lond.) 143, 55–67 (1958).

Purpura, D.P., Yahr, M.D.: The thalamus. New York-London: Columbia Univ. Press, IX–438 pp., 1966.

Ramón-Moliner, E.: The morphology of dendrites. In: G.H. Bourne (Ed.). The structure and function of nervous system. New York-London: Academic Press, I, 205–267 (1968).

Ramón-Moliner, E., Nauta, W.J.H.: The isodendritic core of the brain stem. J. comp. Neurol. 126, 311–336 (1966).

Rhines, R., Magoun, H.W.: Brain stem facilitation of cortical motor response. J. Neurophysiol. 9, 219–229 (1946).

Rijlant, P.: Le tonus musculaire chez un mammifère en état d'hypnose. C.R. Soc. Biol. (Paris) 113, 421–424 (1933).

Rioch, D.McK.: Summary. The EEG in relation to psychiatry. E.E.G. clin. Neurophysiol. 4, 457–462 (1952).

Rioch, D.McK.: In: E.D. Adrian, F. Bremer and H.H. Jasper (Eds.). Brain mechanisms and consciousness. Oxford: Blackwell Sci. Publ., 133–134, 1954.

Roitbak, A.I.: Electrical phenomena in the cerebral cortex during the extinction of orientation and conditioned reflexes. E.E.G. clin. Neurophysiol. Suppl. 13, 91–100 (1960).

Rose, J.E., Mountcastle, V.B.: Touch and kinesthesis. In: Handbook of Physiology. Section I. Neurophysiology. Washington, D.C.: American Physiological Society, I, 387–429, 1959.

Rosén, I.: Functional organization of group I activated neurones in the cuneate nucleus of the cat. Brain Res. 6, 770–772 (1967).

Rosén, I.: Patterns of convergence at different levels of the group I afferent pathway to the cat cerebral cortex. Acta physiol. scand. 73, Suppl. 310, 13–14A (1968a).

Rosén, I.: Patterns of convergence at different levels of the group I afferent pathway to the cat cerebral cortex. Proc. XXIV int. Congr. Physiol. Sci., Washington, D.C., VII, 373, n. 1117 (1968b).

Rosén, I.: Afferent connexions to group I activated cells in the main cuneate nucleus of the cat. J. Physiol. (Lond.) **205**, 209–236 (1969a).

Rosén, I.: Excitation of group I activated thalamocortical relay neurones in the cat. J. Physiol. (Lond.) **205**, 237–255 (1969b).

Rosén, I.: Localization in caudal brain stem and cervical spinal cord of neurones activated from forelimb group I afferents in the cat. Brain Res. **16**, 55–71 (1969c).

Rosén, I.: Projection of forelimb group I muscle afferents to the cat cerebral cortex. Thesis, Lund, 32 pp., 1970.

Rosén, I., Sjölund, B.: Natural stimulation of group I activated cells in the cuneate nuclei of the cat. Acta physiol. scand. **77**, Suppl. **330**, 118, n. 189 (1969).

Rossi, G.F., Brodal, A.: Corticofugal fibers to the brain-stem reticular formation. An experimental study in the cat. J. Anat. (Lond.) **90**, 42–62 (1956).

Rossi, G.F., Brodal, A.: Terminal distribution of spinoreticular fibers in the cat. Arch. Neurol. Psychiat. (Chic.) **78**, 438–453 (1957).

Rossi, G.F., Favale, E., Hara, T., Giussani, A., Sacco, G.: Researches on the nervous mechanisms underlying deep sleep in the cat. Arch. ital. Biol. **99**, 270–292 (1961).

Rossi, G.F., Zanchetti, A.: The brain stem reticular formation. Anatomy and physiology. Arch. ital. Biol. **95**, 199–435 (1957).

Ryall, R.W.: The physiological release and action of monoamines in the spinal cord. In: U.S. von Euler, S. Russell and B. Uvnäs (Eds.). Mechanisms of release of biogenic amines. Oxford: Pergamon Press, 355–356, 1966.

Salmoiraghi, G.C., Steiner, F.A.: Acetylcholine sensitivity of cats medullary neurons. J. Neurophysiol. **26**, 581–597 (1963).

Sarnoff, S.J., Arrowood, J.G.: Differential spinal block. III. The block of cutaneous and stretch reflexes in the presence of unimpaired position sense. J. Neurophysiol. **10**, 205–210 (1947).

Scheibel, A.B.: On detailed connections of the medullary and pontine reticular formation. Anat. Rec. **109**, 345–346 (1951).

Scheibel, A.B.: Axonal afferent patterns in the bulbar reticular formation. Anat. Rec. **121**, 361–362 (1955a).

Scheibel, M.E.: Axonal efferent patterns in the bulbar reticular formation. Anat. Rec. **121**, 362 (1955b).

Scheibel, M.E., Scheibel, A.B.: Structural substrates for integrative patterns in the brain stem reticular core. In: H.H. Jasper et al., (Eds.) Reticular formation of the brain. Henry Ford Hospital Int. Symposium. Boston-Toronto: Little, Brown and Co., 31–55, 1958.

Scheibel, M.E., Scheibel, A.B.: On circuit patterns of the brain stem reticular core. Ann. N.Y. Acad. Sci. **89**, 857–865 (1961).

Scheibel, M.E., Scheibel, A.B.: Adaptation of reticular units to repetitive stimulation. Anat. Rec. **145**, 348 (1963a).

Scheibel, M.E., Scheibel, A.B.: Representational systems and bushy arbor termini in the neuraxis. Anat. Rec. **145**, 349 (1963b).

Scheibel, M.E., Scheibel, A.B.: The response of reticular units to repetitive stimuli. Arch. ital. Biol. **103**, 279–299 (1965a).

Scheibel, M.E., Scheibel, A.B.: Periodic sensory non-responsiveness in reticular neurones. Arch. ital. Biol. **103**, 300–316 (1965b).

Scheibel, M.E., Scheibel, A.B., Mollica, A., Moruzzi, G.: Convergence and interaction of afferent impulses on single units of reticular formation. J. Neurophysiol. **18**, 309–331 (1955).

Schimert, J.S.: Die Endigungsweise des Tractus vestibulospinalis. Z. Anat. Entwickl.-Gesch. **108**, 761–767 (1938).

Schlag, J.: L'activité spontanée des cellules du système nerveaux central. Bruxelles: Éditions Arscia S.A., 192 pp., 1959.

Schweitzer, A.: Die Irradiationen autonomer Reflexe. Untersuchungen zur Funktion des autonomen Nervensystems. Basel: S. Karger, VIII–376 pp., 1937.

SEGUIN, J.J., MAGHERINI, P.C., POMPEIANO, O.: The response of neurones in the nucleus Z to vibration of cat's hindlimb muscle. Arch. Fisiol. **68**, 341–342 (1972).

SEGUNDO, J.P., TAKENAKA, T., ENCABO, H.: Electrophysiology of bulbar reticular neurons. J. Neurophysiol. **30**, 1194–1220 (1967a).

SEGUNDO, J.P., TAKENAKA, T., ENCABO, H.: Somatic sensory properties of bulbar reticular neurons. J. Neurophysiol. **30**, 1221–1238 (1967b).

SHAGASS, C., SCHWARTZ, M.: Evoked cortical potentials and sensation in man. J. Neuropsychiat. **2**, 262–270 (1961).

SHAGASS, C., SCHWARTZ, M.: Cerebral responsivenes in psychiatric patients. Arch. gen. Psychiat. **8**, 177–189 (1963).

SHERRINGTON, C.S., SOWTON, S.C.M.: Observations on reflex responses to single break-shocks. J. Physiol. (Lond.) **49**, 331–348 (1915).

SHIMAMURA, J., AKERT, K.: Peripheral nervous relations of propriospinal and spino-bulbospinal reflex systems. Jap. J. Physiol. **15**, 638–647 (1965).

SHIMAMURA, M., AOKI, M.: Effects of spino-bulbo-spinal reflex volleys on flexor motoneurons of hindlimb in the cat. Brain Res. **16**, 333–349 (1969).

SHIMAMURA, M., LIVINGSTON, R.B.: Longitudinal conduction systems serving spinal and brain-stem coordination. J. Neurophysiol. **26**, 258–272 (1963).

SHIMAMURA, M., MORI, S., MATSUSHIMA, S., FUJIMORI, B.: On the spino-bulbo-spinal reflex in dogs, monkeys and man. J. Physiol. (Lond.) **14**, 411–421 (1964).

SHIMAMURA, M., MORI, S., YAMAUCHI, T.: Interactions of spino-bulbo-spinal reflexes with cortically evoked pyramidal and extrapyramidal activities. Brain Res. **4**, 93–102 (1967a).

SHIMAMURA, M., MORI, S., YAMAUCHI, T.: Effects of spino-bulbo-spinal reflex volleys on extensor motoneurons of hindlimb in cats. J. Neurophysiol. **30**, 319–332 (1967b).

SHIMAZU, H., HONGO, T., KUBOTA, K.: Two types of central influences on gamma motor system. J. Neurophysiol. **25**, 309–323 (1962a).

SHIMAZU, H., HONGO, T., KUBOTA, K.: Nature of central regulation of muscle-spindle activity. In: BARKER D. (Ed.). Symposium on muscle receptors. Hong Kong: Hong Kong University Press, 49–57, 1962b.

SHUTE, C.C.D., LEWIS, P.R.: Cholinesterase-containing systems of the brain of the rat. Nature (Lond.) **199**, 1160–1164 (1963).

SHUTE, C.C.D., LEWIS, P.R.: Cholinesterase-containing pathways of the hindbrain: afferent cerebellar and centrifugal cochlear fibres. Nature (Lond.) **205**, 242–246 (1965).

SILFVENIUS, H.: Cortical projections of large muscle afferents from the cat's forelimb. Acta physiol. scand. **74**, 25–26A (1968).

SIMONOV, P.V.: Complex motor unconditioned reflexes in decerebrate rabbits. In: E. SUTMAN and P. HNIK (Eds.). Central and peripheral mechanisms of motor functions. Prague: Czechoslovak Academy of Sciences, 44–51, 1963.

SKOGLUND, C.R.: Vasomotor reflexes from muscle. Acta physiol. scand. **50**, 311–327 (1960).

SPENCER, W.A., BROOKHART, J.M.: Electrical patterns of augmenting and recruiting waves in depths of sensorimotor cortex of cat. J. Neurophysiol. **24**, 26–49 (1961).

SPIEGEL, E.A., GOLDBLOOM, A.A.: Die Innervation der Körperhaltung im Zustande der sogenannten Hypnose bei Säugetieren. Pflügers Arch. ges. Physiol. **207**, 361–369 (1925).

STAAL, A.: Subcortical projections on the spinal grey matter of the cat. Thesis. Leiden: Koninklijke Drukkerijen Lankhout-Immig N.V.-S-Gravenhage, 164 pp., 1961.

STAMM, J.S., SPERRY, R.W.: Function of corpus callosum in contralateral transfer of somesthetic discrimination in cats. J. comp. physiol. Psychol. **50**, 138–143 (1957).

STARZL, T.E., TAYLOR, C.W., MAGOUN, H.W.: Ascending conduction in reticular activating system, with special reference to the diencephalon. J. Neurophysiol. **14**, 469–477 (1951a).

STARZL, T.E., TAYLOR, C.W., MAGOUN, H.W.: Collateral afferent excitation of reticular formation of brain stem. J. Neurophysiol. **14**, 479–496 (1951b).

STERLING, P., KUYPERS, H.G.J.M.: Anatomical organization of the brachial spinal cord of the cat. III. The propriospinal connections. Brain Res. **7**, 419–443 (1968).

STUART, D.G., MOSHER, C.G., GERLACH, R.L., REINKING, R.M.: Selective activation of Ia afferents by transient muscle stretch. Exp. Brain Res. **10**, 477–487 (1970).

SVORAD, D.: Reticular activating system of brain stem and "animal hypnosis". Science **125**, 156 (1957).

SWETT, J.E., BOURASSA, C.M.: Activation of corticospinal tract fibers by group I afferent volleys. Physiologist 9, 301 (1966).

SWETT, J.E., BOURASSA, C.M.: Short latency activation of pyramidal tract cells by Group I afferent volleys in the cat. J. Physiol. (Lond.) 189, 101–117 (1967a).

SWETT, J.E., BOURASSA, C.M.: Comparison of sensory discrimination thresholds with muscle and cutaneous nerve volleys in the cat. J. Neurophysiol. 30, 530–545 (1967b).

SWETT, J.E., BOURASSA, C.M., INOUE, S.: Effects of cutaneous and muscle sensory nerve volleys in awake cats: a study in perception. Science 145, 1071–1073 (1964).

SZENTÁGOTHAI-SCHIMERT, J.: Die Endigungsweise der absteigenden Rückenmarksbahnen. Z. Anat. Entwickl.-Gesch. 111, 322–330 (1941).

SZYMANSKĬ, J.S.: Über künstliche Modifikationen des sogenannten hypnotischen Zustandes bei Tieren. Pflügers Arch. ges. Physiol. 148, 111–140 (1912).

TABER, E.: The cytoarchitecture of the brain stem of the cat. I. Brain stem nuclei of cat. J. comp. Neurol. 116, 27–70 (1961).

TAKAGI, K.: Über den Einfluß des mechanischen Hautdruckes auf die vegetativen Funktionen. Acta neuroveg. (Wien) 16, 439–446 (1957).

TAKAGI, K., NAKAYAMA, T., NAGASAKA, T.: Skin pressure reflex and the EEG inhibitory response. E.E.G. clin. Neurophysiol. Suppl. 18, 3–5 (1959).

TASAKI, I.: Nervous transmission. Springfield, Ill.: C.C. Thomas, X–164 pp., 1953.

THIELE, F.H., HORSLEY, V.: A study of the degenerations observed in the central nervous system in a case of fracture of the spine. Brain 24, 519–531 (1901).

THODEN, U., MAGHERINI, P.C., POMPEIANO, O.: Effects of muscle afferents on supraspinal descending inhibitory mechanisms. Brain Res. 29, 339–342 (1971a).

THODEN, U., MAGHERINI, P.C., POMPEIANO, O.: Proprioceptive control of supraspinal descending inhibitory mechanisms. Arch. ital. Biol. 109, 130–151 (1971b).

TORVIK, A.: Afferent connections to the sensory trigeminal nuclei, the nucles of the solitary tract and adjacent structures. An experimental study in the rat. J. comp. Neurol. 106, 51–142 (1956).

TORVIK, A., BRODAL, A.: The origin of reticulospinal fibers in the cat. An experimental study. Anat. Rec. 128, 113–138 (1957).

UDO, M., MANO, N.: Discrimination of different spinal monosynaptic pathways converging onto reticular neurons. J. Neurophysiol. 33, 227–238 (1970).

UTTAL, W.R., COOK, L.: Systematics of the evoked somatosensory cortical potential: A psychophysical-electrophysiological comparison. Ann. N.Y. Acad. Sci. 112, 60–80 (1964).

VALVERDE, F.: Contributión al conocimiento de la estructura sináptica en la formación reticular pontobulbar. Ann. Anat. Univ. Zaragoza 9, 569–581 (1960).

VALVERDE, F.: Reticular formation of the pons and medulla oblongata. A Golgi study. J. comp. Neurol. 116, 71–99 (1961a).

VALVERDE, F.: A new type of cell in the lateral reticular formation of the brain stem. J. comp. Neurol. 117, 189–196 (1961b).

VALVERDE, F.: Reticular formation of the albino rat's brain stem. Cytoarchitecture and corticofugal connections. J. comp. Neurol. 119, 25–53 (1962).

VAN REETH, P.C.: Analysis électrophysiologique et comportementale de l'hypnose animale. J. Physiol. (Paris) 55, 354 (1963).

VAN REETH, P.C., CAPON, A.: Sommeil provoqué chez le lapin par des stimulations profondes, céphaliques et cervicales. C.R. Acad. Sci. (Paris) 225, 3050–3052 (1962).

VERHAART, W.J.C.: A stereotaxic atlas of the brain stem of the cat. Assen, The Netherlands: Van Gorcum, 1964.

VERWORN, M.: Allgemeine Physiologie. Jena: G. Fischer, XI–606 pp., 1897.

VOLGYESI, F.A.: Hypnosis of man and animals. London: Ballière, Tindall and Cassel, XIV–216 pp., 1966.

WAGMAN, I.H., McMILLAN, J.A.: Responses of single brain stem units to stimulation of peripheral myelinated and amyelinated cutaneous fibers in M. Mulatta. Proc. XXIV int. Congr. physiol. Sci., Washington, D.C., VII, 456, n. 1368 (1968).

WALL, P.D.: Excitability changes in afferent fibre terminations and their relation to slow potentials. J. Physiol. (Lond.) 142, 1–21 (1958).

WALL, P.D.: The laminar organization of dorsal horn and effects of descending impulses. J. Physiol. (Lond.) **188**, 403–423 (1967).

WALL, P.D.: Organization of cord cells with transmit sensory cutaneous information. In: D.R. KENSHALO (Ed.). The skin senses. Springfield, Ill.: C.C. Thomas, 6, 512–533, 1968.

WALL, P.D., FREEMAN, J., MAJOR, D.: Dorsal horn cells in spinal and freely moving rats. Exp. Neurol. **19**, 519–529 (1967).

WEISS, T.: Changes in the sleeping and waking electrocorticogram in the rat produced by external stimuli. Physiol. bohemoslov. **10**, 21–26 (1961).

WESTMAN, J., BOWSHER, D.: Ultrastructural observations on the degenerations of spinal afferents to the nucleus medullae oblongatae centralis (pars caudalis) of the cat. Brain Res. **26**, 395–398 (1971).

WESTMAN, J., BOWSHER, D., GRANT, G.: Ultrastructure of giganto-cellular region of bulbar reticular formation in cat. J. Anat. (Lond.) **103**, 192–193 (1968).

WHITLOCK, D.G., PERL, E.R.: Thalamic projections of spinothalamic pathways in monkey. Exp. Neurol. **3**, 240–255 (1961).

WILLIS, W.D., MAGNI, F.: The properties of reticulo-spinal neurons. In: J.C. ECCLES and J.P. SCHADÉ (Eds.). Progress in Brain Res. Vol. 12. Physiology of spinal neurons. Amsterdam: Elsevier Publ. Co. **4**, 56–64, 1964.

WINTER, J.E.: The sensation of movement. Psychol. Rev. **19**, 374–385 (1912).

WOLSTENCROFT, J.H.: Effects of afferent stimulation on reticulo-spinal neurones. J. Physiol. (Lond.) **157**, 26P (1961).

WOLSTENCROFT, J.H.: Activation of reticular neurones by muscle afferents. Proc. XXII int. Congr. physiol. Sci., Leiden, II, n. 931 (1962).

WOLSTENCROFT, J.H.: Reticulospinal neurones. J. Physiol. (Lond.) **174**, 91–108 (1964).

YOSHII, N., OGURA, H.: Studies on the unit discharge in the brainstem reticular formation in the cat. I. Changes in reticular unit discharge following conditioning procedure. Med. J. Osaka Univ. **11**, 1–17 (1960).

ZUBEK, J.P.: Studies in somesthesis. II. Role of somatic sensory areas I and II in roughness discrimination in cat. J. Neurophysiol. **15**, 401–408 (1952).

Chapter 13

Convergent Thalamic and Cortical Projections — The Non-Specific System

By

Denise Albe-Fessard and J. M. Besson, Paris (France)

With 40 Figures

Contents

A. Introduction

The central projections of the sensory systems are far more complex than was thought 40 years ago when the first work on primary evoked potentials appeared.

Since that time the majority of studies has been devoted to looking for the thalamic somatic, visual and auditory primary relays, their organisation and their cortical projections. Only a few studies have dealt with the search for regions that lack the topographic and specific organization of these primary systems. They have resulted in the recognition, at different levels, of structures that received convergent inputs from one or even three of the main specific sensory systems and where therefore the specificity and local sign were poorly represented.

The first cortical regions that were described having afferent convergent properties were the second somatic area (Bremer et al., 1954), the anterior marginal cortex (Amassian, 1954) and the precruciate and suprasylvian gyri (Albe-Fessard and Rougeul, 1955). In the deep structures, convergent zones were described in the reticular formation (Scheibel et al., 1955) and at the thalamic level (Magoun and MacKinley, 1942; French et al., 1953a; Albe-Fessard and Rougeul, 1958). We shall leave aside in this paper the convergence that appears in cerebellum and which would deserve a paper in itself.

We shall deal here essentially with the different diencephalic and telencephalic convergent systems, referring only to reticular formation convergent areas when messages to thalamus are relayed at this level.

We shall successively examine:

I – The localization of thalamic zones which are known to receive convergent impulses.

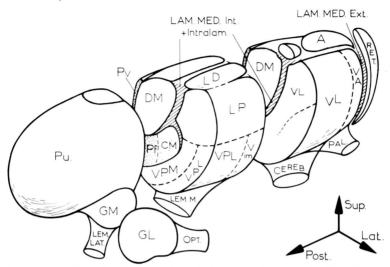

Fig. 1. Superoposterolateral schematic view of the right thalamus showing the respective positions of the different nuclei (orientation is indicated by arrows). Sections have been made in order to make apparent the relative position of the main structures mentioned in this paper

A	anterior
CEREB	brachium conjonctivum (cerebellar afferences)
CM	nucleus "centre median"
DM	Dorsalis medialis (or medialis)
GL	nucleus geniculatus lateralis
GM	nucleus geniculatus medialis
Intralam.	nuclei intralaminares
LAM. MED. Ext.	lamina medullaris externa
LAM. MED. Int.	lamina medullaris interna
LD	nucleus lateralis dorsalis
LEM. M.	lemniscus medialis
LEM. LAT.	lemniscus lateralis
LP	nucleus lateralis posterior
OPT	tractus opticus
PAL	pallidal afferences
Pf	nucleus parafascicularis
Pu	nucleus pulvinaris
Pv	nuclei paraventriculares
RET	nucleus reticularis
VA	nucleus ventralis anterior
Vim	nucleus ventralis intermedius
VL	nucleus ventralis lateralis
VPL	nucleus ventralis posterior lateralis
VPM	nucleus ventralis posterior medialis

II – The pathways that mediate impulses to the different thalamic zones and the central controls exerted on the relays of these pathways.

III – The telencephalic areas that present convergent properties and the mesencephalic thalamic and cortico-cortical connections of these areas.

IV – The possible functional role played by the different types of convergent systems.

B. Thalamic Zones Receiving Convergent Impulses

1. Note on Anatomical Nomenclature

The thalamus is a paired structure, each thalamus being subdivided into three nuclear masses, anterior, medial and lateral (Fig. 1). These masses are recognized as entities because they are separated by a lamina of white matter, called the internal medullary lamina. Fibres from the internal medullary lamina separate medial and lateral groups of nuclei. In the superior anterior part, this lamina bifurcates and gives rise to two branches that contain the anterior nucleus. In the posterior inferior part, a less clear bifurcation separates the medial dorsal nucleus from a group of nuclei called n. Parafascicularis and Centrum Medianum.

In the lamina itself, groups of cells have developed which are called intra-laminar systems and comprise nuclei centralis lateralis (n CL), paracentralis (n Pc) and centralis medialis (n C med). In addition, surrounding all the lateral wall of the thalamus, lies the reticular thalamic nucleus, the dimension of which undergoes large interspecies variations. We shall here make use of these subdivisions and nomenclature mainly based on a schematic proposal of WALKER (1938). For more knowledge on these points, see BRODAL (1969).

Discrepancies in nomenclature have been very important for two nuclei of which we will have to speak very often in this article: the nuclei centrum media-num and ventralis lateralis.

The n. centrum medianum is a nucleus which manifests a great development through the phylogenetic scale. Quite non existent in rats, small in carnivores, it becomes large in primates. In primates (MEHLER, 1966b), it consists of a ventro-lateral region having small cells and a dorso-medial region with larger ones. There is evidence that only the former region should be considered as the equivalent of the centrum medianum of Luys, well developed in humans only and that the region of large cells is derived from the parafascicular nucleus. The development of this large cell region changes less through phylogeny than does the small cell region.

This observation partly explains the discrepancies which can be noticed in the literature between results of the neurophysiological and anatomical workers. We will ourselves speak here of the centrum medianum-parafascicular complex (CM-Pf), accepting that the small cell portion (true CM for MEHLER, 1966b; PERCHERON, 1966) is not involved in this grouping.

The region designated as VL in monkeys (WALKER, 1938) and cats (JASPER and AJMONE-MARSAN, 1954) is not really a single homogeneous nucleus. Schematically in Man, two parts are recognized in the ventralis oralis (homologue of a part of the VL) posterior and anterior part (Vop and Voa). The ventralis intermedius nucleus (Vim) separates ventralis posterior from ventralis oralis posterior (HASS-LER, 1959). Approximately the same divisions are made by OLSZEWSKI (1952) in monkeys, Vim however being called in his atlas Vplo. We will speak here of VL in general, differentiating in some cases the different parts, and making special reference to the intermediate zone (Vim or Vplo).

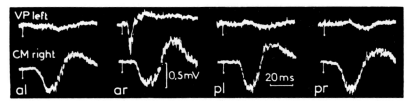

Fig. 2. Macaca under chloralose anaesthesia. Responses recorded in ventralis posterior and centrum medianum (CM). Stimulation of the four limbs left (1) and right (r). *General Remarks on all Figures.* Downward deflection denotes positivity (negativity upward). Type of stimulation is usually indicated at the bottom of the tracings. The anterior limbs are marked a (contralateral ca, ipsilateral ia), the posterior limbs p (contralateral cp, ipsilateral ip). For macroelectrodes in deep structures, recordings were normally obtained by means of concentric bipolar electrodes. Surface macroelectrodes were monopolar, the reference electrode being in the frontal sinus. For microelectrode recordings, micropipettes filled with 3M KCl were used

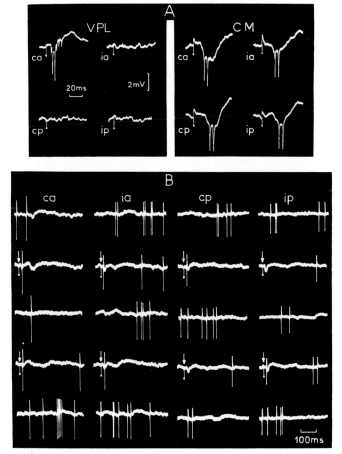

Fig. 3. A: Cat under chloralose anaesthesia; responses recorded in VP and CM, electrical stimulations of four limbs. B: Cat under local analgesia; a unit spontaneously active in CM is driven by electrical stimulation of the 4 limbs (arrows). In each column, spontaneous and stimulation traces are presented successively

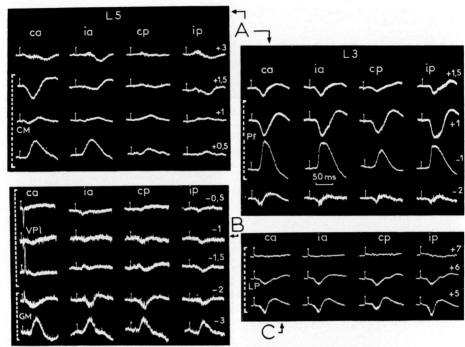

Fig. 4. Four examples of convergent type II responses recorded in three monkeys under chloralose anaesthesia during progressive lowering of electrodes (depth at right) and stimulation of the four limbs. A: 2 electrodes in the same monkey were placed in same anterior plane at two lateralities (L_3, L_5). Note the totally heterotopic responses observed in Pf, and the partial convergence in CM. B: In another plane, specific responses recorded in VP, then convergent ones in magno-cellularis part of medial geniculate. C: Responses in lateralis posterior. (Modified from Bowsher and Albe-Fessard, 1965)

2. Thalamic Regions Presenting Heterotopic Convergent Responses

In lemniscal relays (ventralis posterior pars lateralis and pars medialis, VPl and VPm, in the nomenclature we are using), a topographic organization exists relating specific peripheral and central points according to an exact plan (Mount-castle and Henneman, 1949, 1952; Rose and Mountcastle, 1952; Gaze and Gordon, 1954; Poggio and Mountcastle, 1960 etc...). By contrast, other thalamic regions exist which present evoked responses without topographic organization to stimulation applied to peripheral areas that may be very distant from each other (Fig. 2).

This property is due to the fact that each individual cell (Fig. 3) of this region has a very large peripheral field which can be as large as the entire body surface, or occasionally one half of the body, two posterior or two anterior limbs. Even when the peripheral field is restricted (Fig. 4), it is always larger than the one observed at different levels of the specific system.

This sort of thalamic region is said to receive heterotopic convergent messages and is called a "convergent", "non-specific" or "non-primary" zone, even an "association" area when the cortical convergent zones are described.

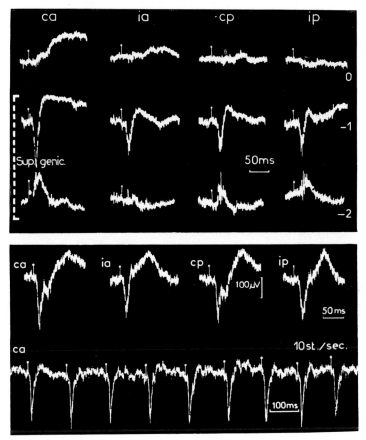

Fig. 5. Example of responses in type I convergent areas, in animals under chloralose ana-esthesia. Above: Suprageniculate responses recorded in a macaca. Below: Responses of the n. subparafascicularis recorded in a cat under local analgesia. Note in this case the relatively high rate that can be followed. (From DENAVIT, 1968)

We shall ourselves use the general term of convergent non-specific zones in which we will differentiate between the convergent thalamic nuclei which receive non-organized heterosensory afferents (called by BUSER and BIGNALL, 1967, non-specific Type II) and the regions which are not specific in the accepted meaning of the term but which do not receive the same general heterosensory inflow. We will call these latter regions non-specific Type I, using the classification of BUSER and BIGNALL with a slightly larger meaning.

a) Type II Thalamic Nuclei. The first place where evoked responses produced by heterotopic stimulation were described was in the CM-Pf of non-anaesthetized monkeys (FRENCH et al., 1953a). Similar properties were observed under chlora-lose anaesthesia in homologous regions of the cat thalamus (ALBE-FESSARD and ROUGEUL, 1958) (Figs. 2, 3).

A systematic macrophysiological exploration, made under the same conditions of chloralose anaesthesia in the cat (KRUGER and ALBE-FESSARD, 1960) and in

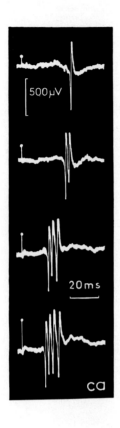

the monkey (Albe-Fessard and Bowsher, 1965), has shown (Fig. 4) that this sort of convergent heterotopic response can be recorded not only in the CM-Pf complex (see definition page 492), but also in the intralaminar nuclei (n. CL, n. PC, n. c. med), in a part of n. lateralis posterior, a small part of dorsalis medialis (Feltz et al., 1967), in n. Reticularis, in a large region of VL nucleus including a part of VA (Massion et al., 1965a) and in the magnocellularis part of the medial geniculate (GMmc).

Large regions of convergence exist also in the hypothalamus (Feldman and Porter, 1960), but those will not be considered.

b) Type I Thalamic Nuclei. A special type of convergence appears in regions just adjacent anteriorly and superiorly to VPl (Vim, Vplo) (Landgren et al., 1965) and posteriorly in the suprageniculate nucleus (Fig. 5) The suprageniculate is a part of a complex region called posterior group by Rose and Mountcastle (1960),

Fig. 6. Responses recorded in CM-Pf of a cat under chloralose anaesthesia during the increase of an electrical stimulation applied to the forepaw. Note the large variation of the latency

Poggio and Mountcastle (1960) which in the cat comprises portions of medial geniculate, posterior and suprageniculate nuclei. A similar sort of convergence appears in the n. sub-parafascicularis and in the subthalamus in regions of the zona incerta in cats (Denavit, 1968; Denavit and Kosinski, 1968) and monkeys.

Thus the property of heterotopic convergence is not unique to the region that has been called the diffuse thalamic system (essentially made up of CM, Pf, n. CL, Reticularis and VA), a region recognized as a whole on the basis of the effect of its repetitive stimulation giving rise to rhythmic cortical activities resembling sleep spindling (see Jasper, 1960; Roitback and Eristavi, 1966). The convergent thalamus is comprised of more nuclei than the diffuse thalamic system.

3. Characteristics of Non-Specific Type II Thalamic Nuclei Responses to Somatic Stimulation

a) Duration and Latency of Responses. When macroelectrode recordings are made in these thalamic regions, positive evoked potentials appear. They are approximately 50 msec in duration and have a latency a little longer than the corresponding primary responses (for example, in Fig. 3, CM-Pf, responses for the

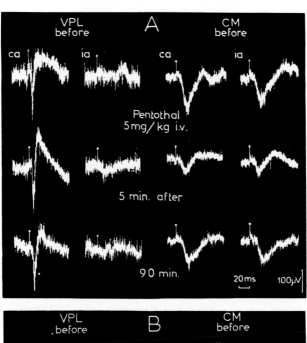

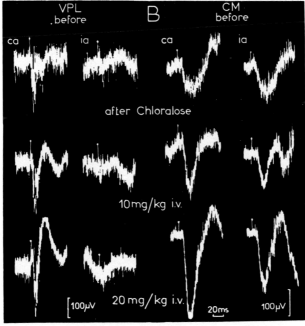

Fig. 7. In two cats under local analgesia two electrodes were placed, one in VP, the other in CM-Pf. Anterior stimulations only. End-tidal CO_2 was maintained at 4%. Intravenous injections were made, in A of pentothal, in B of chloralose. Note the opposite variation of amplitude of CM responses obtained under either conditions. (Modified from ALBE-FESSARD et al., 1970a, as are also Figs. 8, 10 and 11)

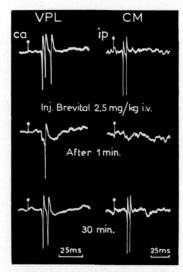

Fig. 8. Example in two units or cells of the effects on the evoked responses in VP and CM of intravenous injections of Brevital. Note that response disappears in CM, is only reduced in VP

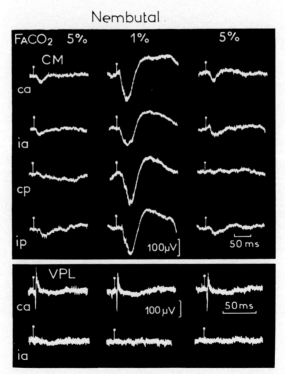

Fig. 9. Cat under light nembutal anaesthesia. End-tidal CO_2 is measured ($FACO_2$). Note that reduction in $FACO_2$ causes a convergent response to appear in CM-Pf. VP response is not modified

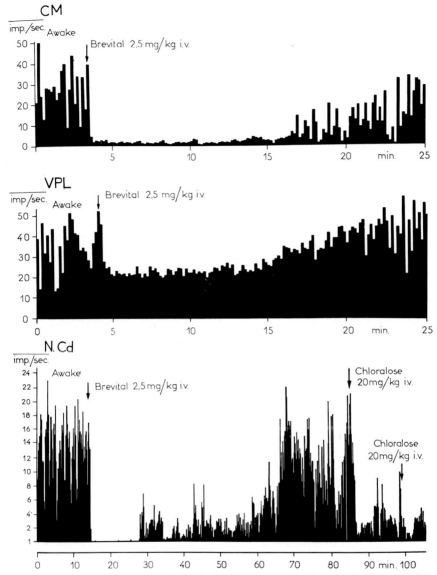

Fig. 10. Cats under local analgesia. Evolution of the spontaneous impulse frequencies of three cells. One in CM and one in VPl after injection of same dose of Brevital. One in Caudate (N Cd) after an injection of Brevital followed, after recovery, by injections of Chloralose

hand stimulation appear after 11 msec while the latency in VP for the same stimulation is of 7.5 msec). In monopolar recordings, this positive phase might be followed by a negative one. During microelectrode recording a short burst of spikes is observed corresponding in position to the positive wave in macroelectrode recordings. When stimulus intensity is increased, the number of spikes increases and the latency of the burst decreases in the same way as in the primary relays

32*

(Fig. 6). However the change in latency is more marked in the non-specific nuclei, and is attributable to the low safety factor existing in this system (see page 515).

b) Effect of Anaesthetics. In cats as well as in monkeys, no matter which anaesthetic or analgesic drugs are employed, responses in specific nuclei are present and only slightly modified in amplitude. On the contrary, convergent responses are dependent upon the type of anaesthetic used.

In experiments where a comparison was made between specific and non-specific responses under different modes of anaesthesia, it was shown that the

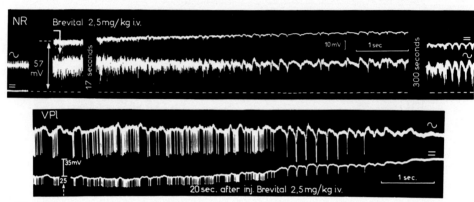

Fig. 11. Cats under local analgesia. Hyperpolarizations obtained after injections of Brevital during intracellular recordings. For the two tracings simultaneous Dc ($=$) and Ac ($\sim$) recordings at different sensitivities. NR: Cell of nucleus ruber before and after penetration followed by intravenous brevital injection. VPl: Intracellular recording observed 20 sec after intravenous injection of brevital

amplitude of evoked responses undergoes opposite variations when chloralose or barbiturates are used (see Fig. 7A and B and 8) (Albe-Fessard et al., 1970a). Complementary experiments have shown afterwards that another anaesthetic (hydroxydione) has effects similar to chloralose and that volatile anaesthetic agents (halothane, nitrous oxyde, ether) have effects similar to the barbiturates.

These facts explain why the majority of the systematic acute experiments in non-specific thalamus were done under chloralose anaesthesia. It explains also why, for a time, convergent thalamic responses were considered, by workers accustomed to barbiturate anaesthesia, to be artefacts due to the chloralose anaesthesia employed.

These criticisms were however eliminated when it was shown that responses could be recorded in CM-Pf in normal awake cats (Figs. 3, 7, 8), in awake acutely decorticated preparations (Meulders et al., 1963), in chronically implanted cats (Albe-Fessard et al., 1961; Guilbaud, 1968, 1970; see Fig. 12) and in animals anaesthetized with barbiturates but under abnormal respiratory conditions (low level of end tidal CO_2, Fig. 9) (references in Albe-Fessard, 1967). It is important to note that an effect of anaesthetics similar to the one observed in non-specific thalamus can be seen in reticular formation. This observation has two consequences:

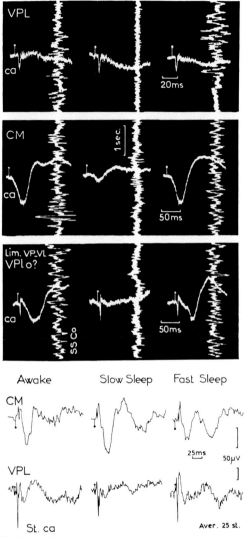

Fig. 12. *Upper part:* Horizontally, responses recorded in chronic implanted cats in VPl, CM and at the limit of VL and VP, after stimulation of superficial radial nerve. Vertical tracings correspond to the spontaneous cortical activities recorded on suprasylvian gyrus. Note that in CM, the large evoked potential appears only when cortical slow waves are recorded. In VP on the contrary, the response is only slightly affected by the state of alertness of the animal. At the limit of VP and VL, two responses appear in succession. Only the long latency slow wave varies like the CM response. *Lower part:* Averaged responses from a chronic animal during wakefulness and the two stages of sleep (slow wave and fast wave sleep)

1. The common effect of all anaesthetics was considered after the first work of FRENCH et al. (1953 b) to be *a reduction* of evoked responses recorded in reticular formation or in non-specific thalamus. The fact that some anaesthetics increase and others reduce these responses obliges one to reconsider this assertion.

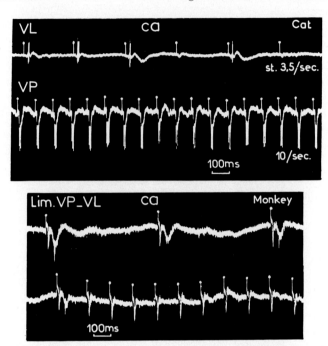

Fig. 13. Comparison of the effect of repetitive stimulation on convergent type II responses and primary activities. *Cat:* responses are recorded in VL (upper tracing) and in VP (lower one). *Monkey:* a double response is recorded at the limit of VP and VL. The two responses appear when a low frequency of stimulation is used. During rapid repetition (lower tracing) the second one disappeared except at the beginning

2. Searching for a common effect of all anaesthetics, it was shown that a hyperpolarization of the membrane is observed in the specific nuclei as well as in the convergent regions when chloralose as well as barbiturates are intravenously injected (Albe-Fessard et al., 1970a). This fact was indirectly demonstrated extracellularly by reduction of spiking observed in both structures (Fig. 10) and by increase in amplitude of slow waves and spikes. Moreover, in a few cases where membrane potentials were recorded intracellularly in different nuclei (Fig. 11), it was shown that the intravenous injection of a short-acting barbiturate produced a hyperpolarization which disappeared after the drug was eliminated.

These results have shown that the differential action of the two types of anaesthetics is not due to differential effects on the membranes of the cells of specific and non-specific brain areas, but has to be attributed to a modification of the afferent messages received by both systems; we shall discuss afterwards the different characteristics of these afferents messages and the effects of anaesthetics on their transmission (section 4a V).

c) **Behavioral Characteristics.** In chronically implanted cats, responses evoked in VP and in CM-Pf undergo opposite kinds of modifications when the animal's state of alertness changes.

As it is shown in Fig. 12 B, this opposition is even clearer when the two types of sleep are considered. The amplitude of the VP responses, which is only slightly

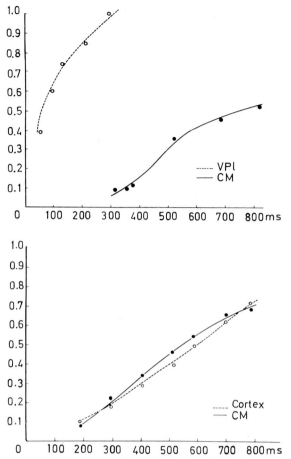

Fig. 14. Recovery curves obtained during a double shock procedure. *Upper curves:* responses recorded in VP and CM of the same animal. *Lower curves:* responses recorded in CM and a convergent type II cortical zone. (From ALBE-FESSARD and ROUGEUL, 1958)

modified during the change from a state of alertness to sleep with slow cortical waves, becomes large during the fast phase of sleep. The amplitude of responses recorded in CM-Pf regions changes in the opposite direction: large during slow phase of sleep, it becomes small during wakefulness and fast phase of sleep.

The same observation was made for other regions with convergent type II properties (LP and anterior VL) (GUILBAUD, 1970). This property is thus a general rule for the non-specific type II nuclei. This rule seems to fail only for posterior VL nucleus. This region receives descending projections from the primary cortex (STRATFORD, 1954; DORMONT and MASSION, 1965; NAKAMURA and SCHLAG, 1968). The increase of reactivity of primary cortical areas during fast sleep makes a new responses appear in the non-specific nucleus during this phase. Responses of posterior VL become typical of type II structures during sleep, only when the somatic primary area is ablated (GUILBAUD, 1970).

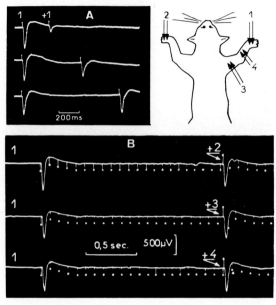

Fig. 15. A: Recovery of CM responses during a double shock procedure. B: Repetitive stimul-ations applied to same peripheral area (1 on the figurine) give rise to a response for the first shock only. The inhibition that is developed by this repetitive stimulation does not prevent stimulation applied to another area (2, 3, 4) from provoking a response

d) Recovery Cycles. In animals under chloralose anaesthesia with a stimulus repetition rate higher than 3 per second, cell responses rapidly disappear in con-vergent type II structures. On the other hand, in VP, units are often able to follow a stimulus presented at rates exceeding 10 per second (Fig. 13). A similar fact is demonstrated by the long recovery period observed in convergent struc-tures compared to that observed in VP (Figs. 13 and 14). The high fatiguability of convergent structures seems to be due to effects appearing at two different levels (Massion et al., 1965a). If shocks are given at two different peripheral places, or at the same place, they must be separated in time in order to obtain a double response (Fig. 15A). However, when a five per second stimulation is given at a localized point (1 in Fig. 15) and the response is recorded in CM-Pf (or in VL), only the first stimulus gives rise to a response. After this response, an inhibitory effect is developed by the repetitive stimulation and, even if stimulation is pursued during a long period, a response never reappears (Fig. 15B).

However the inhibition developed by stimulating a localized point is acting only on afferents coming from the level where the repetitive stimulus is applied, and a response is easy to evoke during this inhibition by applying a stimulus elsewhere on the body surface with a delay due to the characteristic of the central convergent areas under exploration (determined by the heterotopic double shock procedure, Fig. 15A). Thus this first inhibition is acting before the convergence of afferents coming from different dermatomes has taken place, i.e. certainly at a spinal level (see section 4a).

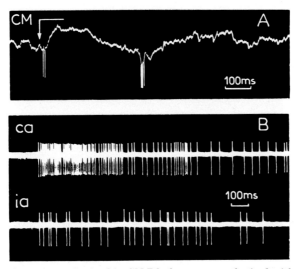

Fig. 16. A: Typical responses obtained in CM-Pf of a cat anaesthetized with chloralose for a natural stimulation (short tap) applied to any point of the peripheral field. Note the duality of the response. (From ALBE-FESSARD and KRUGER, 1962). B: Animal under local analgesia. CM-Pf recording. In this type of preparation, responses similar to that in A are in general recorded. However, on some occasions, convergent responses can be recorded after a puff of air is applied to different hairy skin regions; here an example of this type of convergent response is given

e) Natural Stimuli Evoking Heterotopic Convergent Type II Responses. Given the difficulty of recording from this type of structure in animals under barbiturate, systematic studies, using microelectrodes to search for natural stimuli evoking convergent thalamic responses, have been made only in chloralose anaesthetized animals (ALBE-FESSARD and KRUGER, 1962). A few observations have also been obtained from locally anaesthetized preparations.

Peripheral Receptors Involved. As is well known, a great number of different peripheral manipulations of the tissues are able to evoke impulses in the specific somatic pathway. Light touch (including movement of hair or slight stroking of glabrous areas), as well as superficial or deep pressure, joint rotation, pinching of deep tissues, deformation of muscles, are all effective in driving unit activity in different areas of VP.

On the contrary, somatic stimuli that produce unitary responses in convergent nuclei are all very similar. They consist of light, but sharply applied, stimuli, rapidly applied pressure, taps or pin pricks (Fig. 16 A), the rapidity of the onset being the most important characteristic of this effective stimulus. This property of the convergent system can be explained in two ways. Either this system is connected with a certain type of receptor, "a pin-prick light tap receptor", or the cells of one of the relays of the convergent afferent pathway need a rapid onset to be driven. In this case, the convergent afferent pathway is invaded by a message only when a rapid deformation of a variety of receptors gives rise to a burst of spikes because of the temporospatial convergence it puts in action.

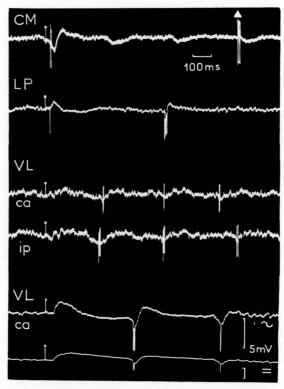

Fig. 17. Typical double response (CM, LP) or rhythmic responses (VL) recorded after a short electrical stimulation was applied to a peripheral area. In the lower tracing, DC recording was used. It shows that the inter-burst interval is accompanied by a hyperpolarization of the membrane

First inclined to accept the existence of a specific pin-prick-light-tap receptor, the ideas of the authors that have dealt with this problem changed when it was shown (see Mallart, 1967) that, to produce a response in CM-Pf, spatial or temporal convergence was necessary. The just supraliminal stimulation of two cutaneous nerve branches that give rise to responses in VP only and not in CM-Pf when individually stimulated, produces responses in CM-Pf when these branches are stimulated together. Thus, it is not the type of receptor put in action, but the convergence of messages, that seems to be the important factor in order to drive units in non-specific pathways. The cells of these convergent nuclei are not modality specific.

These facts, indisputable under chloralose anaesthesia, have however to be reconsidered in non-anaesthetized conditions. If, as we have verified, light taps are here again the easiest way to drive convergent cells, it is certain that some other types of stimuli (light stroking of hair (Fig. 16B), movements putting in action articulations or muscles) can be effective in the region of medial thalamus. As we have said, a systematic exploration performed with microelectrodes in chronic animals has still to be done.

Temporal Information Carried by the Messages and Special Rhythmic Organization of the Responses. At least in the anaesthetized animals, the duration of the stimulation is never represented at the convergent thalamic level because, whether the duration of the deformation is long or short, only a burst of spikes is provoked at the onset of the stimulus (Fig. 16A). However, in the chloralose anaesthetized or drowsy animal, a particular typical response appears in convergent type II zones. In CM-Pf, a second response appears after a delay of 200 to 1000 msec depending on the unit (ALBE-FESSARD and KRUGER, 1962) (Fig. 17).

In other regions (in VL in particular), rhythmic bursts of activity are provoked by one short stimulation. The occurence of this second response or of the rhythmic burst is unrelated to the duration of the stimulus. Similar rhythmic bursts can appear also spontaneously in the same regions.

The interburst interval is shorter in non-anaesthetized preparations. In CM-Pf as well as in VL, intracellular recordings have shown that these bursts are separated by a hyperpolarization of long duration (ALBE-FESSARD and KRUGER, 1962; MASSION et al., 1965b; NAKAMURA and SCHLAG, 1968). This rhythmic activity disappears in the awake alert animal to reappear during sleep (LAMARRE et al., 1971); it is only in abnormal cases, like Parkinson's disease in man or experimental tremor in animals (LAMARRE and CORDEAU, 1964, 1967), that such rhythms can appear during alertness.

Different interpretations have been given for the existence of these bursts during sleep (see MASSION, 1968; ANDERSEN and ANDERSSON, 1968; ALBE-FESSARD, 1971; ANDERSSON and MANSON, 1971). As we shall see later, the pathways that convey non-specific messages are under descending inhibitory control from cortical and brain-stem origins. It is interesting to note that the interburst intervals have a duration of the same order as those of inhibitory phenomena from central origin observed in animals without anaesthesia (150 msec) or with anaesthesia (250–500 ms depending on the depth and on the type of anaesthesia). One can thus assume that the rhythmicity is due to a reverberation of ascending impulses acting in the cord and/or in other relays.

f) Types of Peripheral Nerve Fibres Involved. It was shown (MALLART, 1967) that group II as well as group III cutaneous nerves send impulses to CM-Pf. In the muscle nerves, group I does not seem to send impulses to these regions, the role of group II was not clearly shown, and group III certainly conveys messages to CM-Pf and to VL.

4. Characteristics of Thalamic Regions Presenting Type I Heterotopic Convergence

In the thalamic regions where we have described type I convergence (see Fig. 5), evoked potentials are produced and units are driven most frequently from bilateral peripheral fields, and, in some cases, from the entire body surface. The latency, slow wave duration and recovery time (Figs. 5 and 18) are far shorter than in the convergent type II zone. Effects of anaesthesia and of natural sleep are also different (see Fig. 12A).

The general properties of the responses are more similar to those of responses appearing in primary relays. The convergent characteristic is the major difference

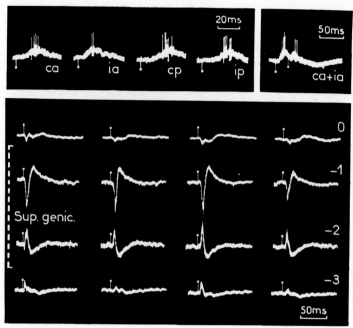

Fig. 18. Type I response recorded in the nucleus suprageniculatus of a macaca. Note the short duration of the slow wave convergent response, and the short recovery time when two shocks are applied on two different limbs (upper right corner tracing). Inferior group of tracings, each column corresponds respectively to ca, ia, cp, ip stimulations

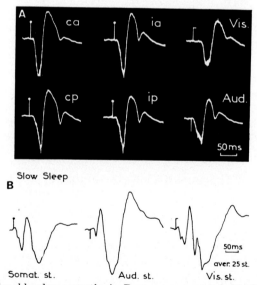

Fig. 19. A: Cat under chloralose anaesthesia. Responses are recorded in CM-Pf region not only with stimulation of four limbs, but also with visual and auditory stimuli. B: In a chronically implanted cat, averaged responses in CM-Pf to somatic, auditory and visual stimulations are recorded during slow sleep. (Modified from Guilbaud, 1968)

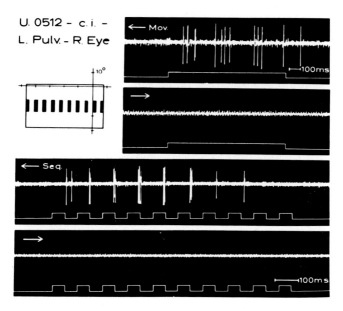

Fig. 20. Specific response of a pulvinar neuron to moving and sequential static visual stimuli. *Upper left:* Representation in the visual field of the area where the sequential stimulations (vertical rectangles) were placed. *Upper two tracings:* A moving stimulus is effective in one direction only. *Lower two tracings:* Sequential presentation of eight slits gives rise to response only if the direction of the sequence corresponds to the direction of the effective moving stimulus. (From VERAART et al., 1972)

between specific and type I convergent regions. Comparisons between properties of type I and type II structures at a thalamic level are rare in the literature. They are more numerous for telencephalic regions (see page 537).

5. Thalamic Regions Presenting Heterosensory Convergent Responses

1. In all type II convergent thalamic zones, responses can be recorded in cats under chloralose anaesthesia after stimulation of visual and auditory pathways. However the amplitudes of evoked potentials are not so large for visual and auditory stimuli as for somatic ones (Fig. 19).

For the VL, MASSION et al. (1965a) have shown analogous results with evoked potential techniques. The same authors, in a microphysiological study (1965b), found for 46 units, that 32 responded to somatic stimulation only, 7 to somatic, auditory and visual, 3 to somatic and auditory, and 4 to somatic and visual stimuli. Thus, if this group of convergent nuclei receives heterosensory afferents, it is certain that somatic stimulation is always better represented. An exception has however to be made for the n. GM magnocellularis which presents somatic, visual and auditory responses (WEPSIC, 1966), but in which the auditory inflow seems to be the most important. The characteristics of effective visual or auditory natural stimulation in type II regions have not yet been studied in detail.

2. Type I convergent zone receives also visual or auditory impulses or both. Nucleus suprageniculatus, nucleus posterior, part of lateralis posterior and part of Putamen adjacent to GL receive non-primary visual afferents, having however a certain organization (Meulders, 1970; Godfraind et al., 1969).

In recent work, Veraart et al. (1972) have found in these regions, among 730 neurones studied, one third responding to visual stimulation with a restricted contralateral receptive field (circular or oblong in form); those fields are generally made up of two regions, one responding with an "on" effect, the other with an "off", these regions being contiguous, but with some overlap (Fig. 20). It is thus certain that these visual projections are not totally non-specific; they have a specificity not as well developed as the primary one, but probably better developed than the convergent type II.

If work on the organization of non-specific auditory inflow is scarce at a thalamic level, we shall see that many studies on this subject exist for the cortex.

C. Afferent Pathways to Heterotopic and Heterosensory Thalamic Zones

1. Anatomical Knowledge on Somatic Inflow

a) Inflow from the Limbs and Trunk

(i) Specific Pathway without a Spinal Relay. It is well known that an important number of the myelinated axons which enter the spinal cord send a long branch without any relay in the spinal cord to the ascending dorsal column pathways. The terminals of 25% of the myelinated fibres entering the dorsal columns make contact with second order neurons in the dorsal column nuclei. From there they project through the medial lemniscus to the contralateral VP and the zona incerta (Boivie, 1971) and in suprageniculate (Bowsher, 1961). We shall refer to this pathway as the dorsal column pathway (DC) (Fig. 22 A).

This typical specific pathway, the internal organization of which is now well known (see Brown, Chapter 10), is not the only ascending one and others, relayed in spinal cord, have to be considered.

(ii) Pathways Relayed in the Spinal Cord. It is known from studies of Cajal (1909) that all the myelinated fibres entering the cord give ascending and descending branches, each of which present collaterals in five or six of the neighbouring segments. Thus long ascending branches enter the dorsal columns to terminate in dorsal column nuclei and their collaterals enter the spinal gray matter to make contact with cell bodies at different levels. Other fibres of the myelinated group will make contact only with spinal cells. The unmyelinated fibres are not represented in dorsal columns and make contacts only with cells of the two or three segments superior or inferior to their level of entry. The spinal terminals of afferent myelinated fibres are found in different layers of the cord (dorsal horn, but also ventral horn). The localization of terminals obtained by the Nauta technique is presented in Fig. 21 placed on a drawing presenting the different layers recognized in the spinal cord by Rexed (1952) using a cytoarchitectonic method.

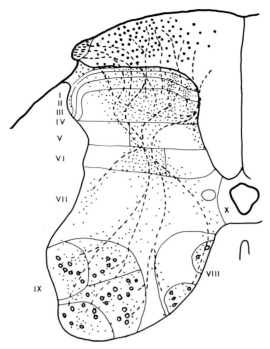

Fig. 21. Termination of fibres revealed in different layers of the cord (L6 segment) with the Nauta techniques after section of the ipsilateral dorsal root L6 (from SPRAGUE and HA, 1964). Terminal degeneration, small dots; fibres of passage, dash line; fibres in dorsal column, large dots

We shall not consider the crossed and uncrossed cerebellar pathways, but shall deal only with paths having a thalamic termination directly or through a bulbar relay.

1. Spinocervical Thalamic Tract (SCT) (see BROWN, Chapter 10). Physiological experiments, mainly based on antidromic activation techniques (ECCLES et al., 1960; FETZ, 1968) have shown that cells of lamina IV and, to a lesser degree, of lamine V, give rise to a tract situated in the dorsal horn just beneath the entrance of the dorsal roots. These fibres terminate in a slender column of nerve cells situated in the lateral funiculus in segments C_1 and C_2 (REXED and BRODAL, 1951; GRANT et al., 1968). The efferents leaving this nucleus cross in the upper cervical segments and ascend with those of the medial lemniscus (BUSCH, 1961).

This pathway, studied extensively in the cat (ANDERSSON, 1962; MORIN et al., 1963), is present but of less importance in monkeys (OSWALDO-CRUZ and KIDD, 1964). Its existence in man is an open question (HA and MORIN, 1964). The terminations of the spino-cervical thalamic pathway were traced by the degeneration technique to a restricted area of the nucleus ventralis posterior pars lateralis (BOIVIE, 1970).

2. Spinally Relayed Dorsal Column Pathway. Recent results from UDDENBERG (1968a and b) and PETIT and BURGESS (1968) have shown that postsynaptic fibres travel also in the dorsal columns. These fibres probably have their cells of origin in the dorsal horn (Cajal, 1909), although they have not been looked for in recent anatomical investigations. These fibres seem to end, like the DC fibres, in the dorsal column nuclei (Petit, 1971).

3. *Anterolateral Pathways.* In the anterolateral region of the cord, fibres from a contralateral and in less number from an ipsilateral origin ascend and terminate in different parts of the brain. Those fibres, which ascend directly to the thalamus, are called spino-thalamic fibres. The others are proprio-spinal and spino-reticular fibres. No spatial organization of these types of fibres seems to exist in the anterolateral bundle.

It is still a matter of discussion in which layers of the dorsal horn are found the cells of origin of these essentially crossed pathways. From Golgi studies it is said that cells send their axons from layers VI and VII to the contralateral side. Dilly et al. (1968), Trevino et al. (1971) have in the cat found, by antidromic activation, cells of origin of lemniscal fibres in layers V, VI and VII of the cervical and lumbar regions. From anatomical results the cells of origin of spino-reticular fibres may even be deeper in layer VII. Using the antidromic technique, we have ourselves found these cells in layers VII and VIII in the cat (Levante and Albe-Fessard, 1972) in layer V in the Monkey.

Spinothalamic Tracts: This tract is better developed in chimpanzee and man than in monkeys (Mehler, 1962). In cats, it seems to be composed of a relatively small number of fibres. This tract is divided into two components:

— the *neospinothalamic one,* ascending in the mesencephalic region just superior to the lemniscus has its termination throughout the VPl in clusters of fibres in rats (Mehler, 1966a; Lund and Webster, 1967) and in monkeys (Bowsher, 1961; Mehler, 1966a). This type of termination is however denied in cats by Boivie (1972), who has shown that the majority of the fibres terminate, not in the VPL itself, but in its posterior and anterior borders, i.e. in the region of posterior group and at the posterior limit of VL (Vim).

— the *paleo-spinothalamic* component has no terminations in or near VPL. It projects instead to the n. Parafascicularis, n. centralis lateralis, magnocellular region of GM, zona incerta, field of Forel H_1 and nucleus reticularis thalami. Thus the so-called paleo-spinothalamic component has its termination in the principal nuclei that present type II convergent responses. These terminations in the cat are essentially ipsilateral to the spinal pathway (Boivie, 1972). On the contrary, bilateral terminations were found in monkeys (Mehler et al., 1960; Bowsher, 1961) and in man (Bowsher, 1957; Mehler, 1962).

Spino-Reticular Inflow. Fibres ascending in the anterolateral quadrant terminate in the cat at two main levels, in the nucleus giganto-cellularis of the bulbar reticular formation and in the Pons (Rossi and Brodal, 1957; Anderson and Berry, 1959) and in smaller number at the mesencephalic reticular formation and the grisea centralis (Boivie, 1972). In rat and monkeys, Mehler et al. (1960), Mehler (1966a), in man, Bowsher (1957, 1962), Mehler (1962) have found a similar organization.

Cells in the same regions have long axons ascending beyond the mesencephalon. Following lesions of the reticular formation, different groups of authors, using the Golgi method (Scheibel and Scheibel, 1958; Valverde, 1961a) and

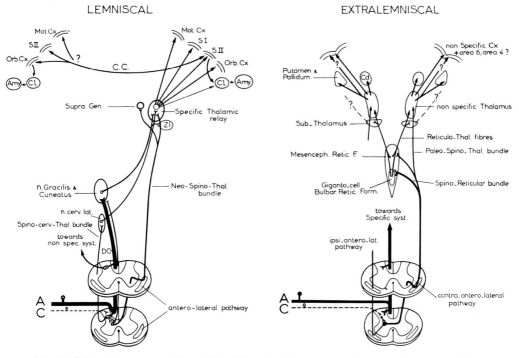

Fig. 22. Schematic representation of the different pathways conveying somatic messages from the trunk and limbs to the higher centres. They are divided into two categories, lemniscal and extralemniscal systems (see text)

the Nauta method (NAUTA and KUYPERS, 1958) have shown that fibres from the bulbar and pontine region end in the majority of the nuclei that present type II convergent responses (Parafascicularis, reticularis thalami, centralis lateralis, etc...). The same results were obtained by physiological methods (BOWSHER et al., 1968) which have shown that stimulation at the level of the bulbar reticular formation gives rise to large responses in CM-Pf.

b) Inflow from the Head. Impulses coming from the neck and posterior region of the head enter the cord between C8 and C1. The organization of the pathways conveying the impulses coming from this region is similar to the preceding ones.

The principal inflow from the face enters through the trigeminal nerve (see DARIAN-SMITH, Chapter 9). For this group of afferent fibres, an organization similar to the one found for the afferents from the body seems to exist.

Fibres conveying superficial and deep sensibility from the face, the cell bodies of which are in the semi-lunar or Gasserian ganglion, have two principal relays.

1. The *nucleus principalis or superior of the Vth nerve* which is the analogue of the dorsal column nuclei. From this nucleus a crossed pathway ascends in the medial lemniscus and goes to the ventralis posterior (a small uncrossed component exists however which does not have its equivalent in the DCN system).

2. The *spinal nucleus of the Vth nerve* receives collaterals of the large fibres that are going to the principal nucleus as well as other fibres and, in particular

non-myelinated ones. All these fibres constitute the spinal trigeminal tract that passes for some distance caudally in the medulla oblongata before entering the spinal nucleus. This nucleus is the homologue of the layers of gray matter where cells relaying ascending bundles are found in lumbar thoracic and low cervical cord.

— *Neospinothalamic inflow-* Fibres from all subdivisions of the spinal nucleus appear to ascend in close association with those of the medial lemniscus (Gordon et al., 1961; Darian-Smith and Yokota, 1964) and seem to terminate in the VPM only.

— *Paleo-spino-thalamic and spino-reticular fibres* come apparently only from nucleus caudalis. Crossed and uncrossed fibres coming from n. caudalis ascend in the reticular formation (Stewart and King, 1963) and give off terminals in the brain stem. Other fibres have thalamic terminals in all nuclei presenting type II convergence, and end also in zona incerta and the field of Forel H_1. In squirrel monkey, Shende, Stewart and King (1968) have shown that the principal terminations of pathways from nucleus caudalis are CM, Pf, and CL. Thus all of the major bundles carrying projections from the trunk and limbs are found as well for the face.

When we speak therefore of the grouping of these different bundles, in lemniscal and extralemniscal pathways, we will include both trigeminal and spinal systems.

2. Lemniscal and Extralemniscal Pathways

a) **Their Role in the Convergent Projections.** From the description we have just given, we may see that four spinal bundles send their afferents to the n. ventralis posterior through the lemniscus contralateral to the stimulated region: the DC direct bundle, the spinally relayed DC, the spinal-cervico-thalamic bundle, and the neo-spino-thalamic one. We will from now on speak of these 4 afferent systems as lemniscal inflow.

The other pathways, paleo-spino-thalamic and spino-reticulo-thalamic, constitute the extralemniscal one.

As we have just seen, anatomical findings have shown that this extralemniscal pathway projects to all those nuclei (except the VL) where we have described *convergent type II responses.* By physiological methods, Whitlock and Perl (1959), Perl and Whitlock (1961) have shown in cats and monkeys that units can be driven in convergent type II and type I nuclei in animals where only anterolateral pathways are left intact. That the spinal fibres conveying impulses to CM-Pf in the cat are located mainly in the anterolateral quadrant, essentially contralateral to the stimulated place with a small ipsilateral component, was demonstrated with the use of progressive sections of the spinal cord by Petit and Mallart (1964), Mallart (1968).

For the VL, Massion and Dormont (1966) have shown with the same technique that the major projection is also through the contralateral anterolateral pathway, but that messages also travel to this nucleus via the spino-cervico-thalamic bundle and through the crossed and uncrossed spino-cerebellar pathways. An important inflow to the VL region also comes through the cerebellum, the principal termination of brachium conjunctivum being this nucleus (see for the recent literature on the subject, ANGAUT, 1969; ANGAUT et al., 1968; CONDE and ANGAUT, 1970).

For the *type I convergent system* also, physiological studies have shown that the dorsal columns are not necessary for their appearance. In the cat, suprageniculate responses appear when the dorsal cord is severed (WHITLOCK and PERL, 1959). DENAVIT (1968) has shown that, in the subthalamus, the nucleus of the field of Forel receives its main inflow through the spino-cervico-thalamic pathway. In the region at the limit of VP and VL, LANDGREN et al. (1965) have described an inflow through the same pathway. All these findings are in good agreement with the anatomical results.

In the mesencephalic griseum centralis, LIEBESKIND and MAYER (1971) have described in rats evoked activities that present the characteristics of type I responses. Possibly, some of the type I convergent thalamic activities have a relay at this level.

In conclusion, the extralemniscal pathway seems to send, directly or through a relay in the bulbar or mesencephalic reticular formation, its afferents to the type II convergent thalamic regions. The neospinothalamic and the spino-cervico-thalamic tracts are the main pathway to convergent type I regions.

b) Number of Synapses in Lemniscal and Extralemniscal Pathways. For many years, it was believed that the non-specific convergent systems are fed through a multisynaptic pathway, in opposition to the specific system which has few synapses. The preferential effects of anaesthetics on the non-specific convergent system was attributed to this property. If we consider the anatomy of the two systems, we shall see that the difference in their number of synapses is less than was claimed. As classically known, the specific somatic pathways have a small number of relays before they reach the thalamus, either one relay (in the dorsal column nuclei or in the spinal cord), or two (in the spinal cord and superior cervical nucleus for the spino-cervico-thalamic bundle). If we consider as an example of non-specific pathways the one ending in the nucleus parafascicularis, we find that it has one or two synapses in the spinal gray matter and then, either the fibres pass directly to the nucleus parafascicularis, or they relay once again in the bulbar region. Thus, the number of synapses in this pathway is only slightly greater than in the specific pathway.

However, the types of synaptic connections are quite different in the two systems. In the specific relays, the conservation of a point-to-point organization all along the pathway means that a large number of axon terminals make powerful connections with a small number of postsynaptic neurons. This results in a high safety factor for synaptic transmission. These relays are, in the terms of MANNEN (1966) "closed nuclei". In contrast, in nonspecific relays, convergence is the rule and the terminals of a single axon are distributed to a very large number of neurons. The small safety factor thus reduces the probability of the message arriving by any one axon being transmitted to the next neuron; either convergence or some type of facilitation will be necessary to permit transmission at this type of synapse. The non-specific relays are "open nuclei" and it is this property, and not the supposed multiplicity of synapses, which makes them more susceptible to certain anaesthetics than are the specific structures. It is also in

33*

this way that the important variation of synaptic delay observed in the type II nuclei can be explained (see Fig. 6 and section 3a).

c) Connections Between Lemniscal and Extralemniscal Systems

Spinal Connections Through Collaterals of Dorsal Column Fibres. That lemniscal and extralemniscal pathways were anatomically connected was first hypothetized by Lindsley et al. (1949) and Starzl et al. (1951) on the basis of functional considerations. Collaterals from the lemniscal to the extralemniscal system were sought first at the level of the lemniscus itself, but the anatomical studies failed to reveal them there (Bowsher, 1958; Scheibel and Scheibel, 1958; Valverde, 1961a and b, etc...). Nevertheless, physiological results showed that these connections did in fact exist and that the error was only in regard to the level where they originally were hypothetized to be.

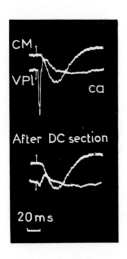

Fig. 23. Cat under chloralose anaesthesia. Responses simultaneously recorded in CM and VPl; stimulation of contralateral anterior limb before (upper) and after (lower) section of dorsal columns

It was first demonstrated that responses recorded under chloralose in type II thalamic nuclei are not affected when DC pathways are sectioned (Fig. 23). However, they still exist if the dorsal columns are dissected, two electrodes are placed on the bundle separated from the cord and a stimulation is applied to the dorsal columns isolated from the cord over a few segments. Thus afferents going through the DC to an extralemniscal path can produce responses in non-specific thalamus (Kruger and Albe-Fessard, 1960). Mallart and Petit (1963) and Mallart (1968) have shown that this result can be explained by the existence of collaterals from DC fibres which synapse in the dorsal horn a few segments after their entrance. Section of the ventral quadrant totally prevents a response in type II thalamic nuclei only if the section is made at least six segments higher than the level of the dorsal root entry when all the collaterals have left the dorsal columns (Fig. 24A). An alternative explanation for these results could be that some short fibres ascend in the DC before entering the dorsal horn. However the original hypothesis was proved to be correct by the fact that stimulation of the dorsal columns sectioned just below the level of the dorsal column nuclei evoked a response in centrum medianum due to collaterals activated by antidromic impulses travelling in dorsal column fibres. The long latency of the CM response obtained in this way, longer than the one obtained by stimulation of the same DC

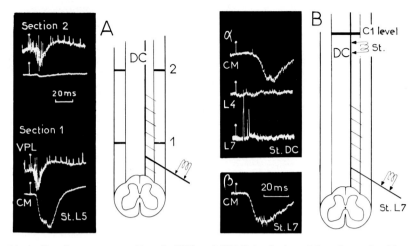

Fig. 24. A: Simultaneous recordings in VPl and CM. Stimulation of dorsal root L5. Note that response in CM is still present after section 1 and disappears after section 2. A fibre and its collateral are presented showing that, at level of section 2, collaterals are no longer there. B: a) Responses are recorded in CM when a localized stimulation of dorsal column at C_1 level gives rise to antidromic activation of L7 root and not in L4. b) Same L7 root stimulation gives rise to a similar response, but with a shorter latency (see text). (From MALLART, 1968)

fibre at its entrance in the cord, is the evidence for the relatively long conduction distance of antidromic impulses in DC fibres (Fig. 24 B).

Connections through Primary Areas. We shall see in the next paragraph that descending connections exist from the primary cortex to the cells of the cord that are probably at the origin of the extralemniscal pathways. Connections also exist between primary cortex and thalamic type II convergent nuclei, as well as between primary cortex and the reticular relays of these thalamic regions.

In some special conditions, when the excitability of primary cortical cells is especially high (injection of convulsant drugs, paradoxical sleep) it happens that lemniscal afferents are able to send impulses to nonspecific type II convergent nuclei through these cortico-spinal (BESSON and ABDELMOUMENE, 1970), cortico-reticular (ASCHER, 1964) or cortico-thalamic loops (GUILBAUD, 1968). These cortical loops are not always excitatory; in fact the majority of them are inhibitory. We shall deal in detail with these cortical reflex interactions in section D.

3. Organization of the Extralemniscal Pathway as a Function of the Type of Message

In man, an organization of the pathways conveying the messages giving rise to different sorts of sensation has been said to exist in the anterolateral quadrant on the basis of clinical findings. The fibres mediating sensations of pain and temperature appear to occupy the dorsolateral part of the anterolateral funiculus, those conveying sensations of touch and deep pressure are found in the ventro-medial part.

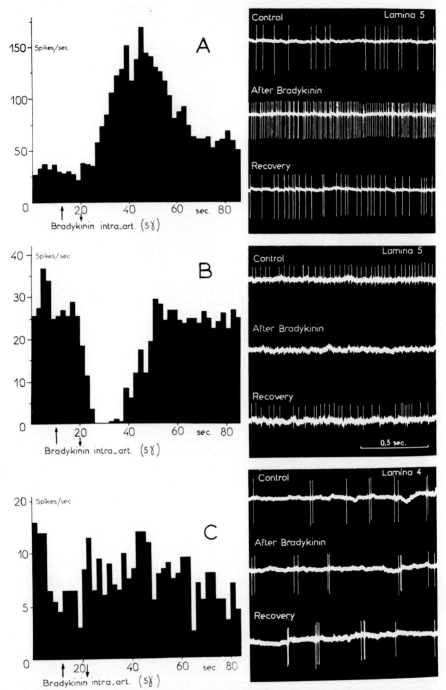

Fig. 25. Effects of intra-arterial injections of bradykinin on the activity of dorsal horn cells in non-anaesthetized cats (spinal transection at C_1). At left, diagrams showing the evolution of spike frequencies for three different cells. At right, examples taken for the same cells, before and after the injection. A and B: two cells of lamina V (previously recognized by their characteristic response to natural stimulation). Note that one is excited, the other inhibited by bradykinin. C: cell in lamina IV; no clear effect is observed. (Modified from BESSON et al., 1972)

These neurological findings have not yet been verified in animals. Lesions of the cord used to study the termination of degenerating fibres have always been a total section of the anterolateral bundle.

However, some knowledge can be deduced from experiments which studied the stimuli effective in driving units in the reticular formation. In the different parts of the bulbar and mesencephalic reticular formation where the spino-reticular pathway terminates, cells activated by light stimuli and by heavy ones were found to be intermingled (LAMARCHE and LANGLOIS, 1962; BECKER et al., 1969). In the gigantocellular nucleus of the awake cat, CASEY (1971a and b) found many cells uniquely responsive to noxious stimuli. Good localization also appears when afferents from the face are studied. For example, in the caudal part of the bulbar reticular formation of the cat, BURTON (1968) found units responding to heavy noxious stimuli only applied to the contralateral side of the face. Similar observations were made in the rat for the lateral bulbar reticular formation (NORD and KYLER, 1968; BENJAMIN, 1970).

Another technique seems to be promising for the identification of cells activated by painful stimuli, the intra-arterial injection of nociceptive drugs. This technique was first applied by LIM (1968) who utilised it to study the role of analgesic substances. He injected intra-arterially, small doses of bradykinin that gave in man a transitory pain and in animals vocalization, severe agitation and drastic changes in respiratory and cardiovascular functions.

In cats in which recordings of units of the spinal cord were performed, this type of injection was used (SATOH et al., 1971; BESSON et al., 1971, 1972). In the cord, cells in layer IV were rarely activated by bradykinin injections while cells in layer V were (BESSON et al., 1972, and Fig. 25). In the thalamus, LIM et al. (1969) have used the same method. In our group, the giganto-cellularis bulbar relay, CM-Pf, and VP were explored in the same way. Cells are activated in reticular nuclei and CM-Pf, but less frequently in VP. The central exploration is at its beginning, but it will certainly give an idea of the spinal and thalamic regions involved in the conduction or integration of noxious stimuli.

4. Control Exerted on the Extralemniscal Messages at Different Levels

a) Level of Spinal Relays

(i) Physiological Properties of the Cells in Different Spinal Cord Layers. Physiological results have shown that the messages which activate the antero-lateral pathway are probably delayed in the spinal cord itself by one or two synapses. Thus the neurons of origin of the anterolateral pathway fibres (whose place in layer VI, VII or VIII is still, as we have said, a subject of discussion) may receive some of their inflow from cells placed more dorsally in the cord.

CHRISTENSEN and PERL (1970) have recorded units in layer I, and showed that these cells are activated only by strong peripheral stimuli. Recordings in layers II and III are rare, and the majority of the authors have studied cells in layers IV, V, VI and VII. The cells of layers IV and V are the easiest to recognize by the characteristics of their natural excitatory field (WALL, 1960, 1967). In layer IV, cells are driven by light tactile stimulation with a small receptive field (very often

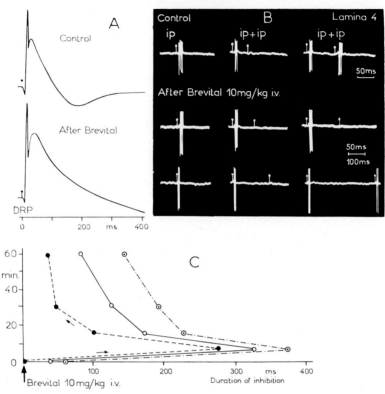

Fig. 26. Effect of barbiturate anaesthesia on duration of DRPs (A) and recovery period (B and C). A: Injection of Brevital produces an increase of the DRP negative phase duration. B: Measured by the double shock technique, the recovery period is short before injection (upper tracings). It becomes long after it (lower tracings). C: Three curves have been traces of the recovery period measured for three different cells with the method used in B. Note that, after injection of Brevital, the recovery phase attains nearly 400 msec, just like the duration of DRP negative phase

a few hairs) and no lateral inhibition. In layer V, the centre of the field may be of the light tactile type, but has always a peripheral region which is excited by a more intense stimulation (pinch, strong pressure). In decerebrate animals with an intact reticulo-spinal system, a surrounding field of inhibition exists (WALL, 1967; BROWN, 1970). Cells of this layer receive also visceral afferents (POMERANZ et al., 1968; SELZER and SPENCER, 1969a and b). In layer VI, cells are activated by the same stimulation as in V and also by muscular or articular afferents. Thus cells of layer VI seem to have an integrative role. The characteristics of natural stimulation that put in action layers VII and VIII have not yet been studied in detail.

(ii) General Knowledge on Spinal Controls. The "segmental" and central controls exerted on all these spinal cells have been extensively studied in recent years.

The "segmental" control initially studied by GASSER and GRAHAM (1933), BARRON and MATTHEWS (1936, 1938), LLOYD and MACINTYRE (1949) seems to be indubitably of presynaptic origin (Wall, 1958, 1964; Eccles et al., 1962; Eccles, 1964); the sign of its existence being the slow phase observed on the dorsal root after the afferent volley. These slow phases in the non-anaesthetized animal are diphasic negative-positive, and in the anaesthetized one are purely negative.

That the negative phase is accompanied by an inhibition of cellular activities was demonstrated by many authors. Similar conclusions can be deduced from experiments at unitary levels in spinal cats. Injection of barbiturates prolonged the recovery period measured with a double-shock technique, in the same way that it prolonged the negative phase of the DRP (Fig. 26) (Besson et al., 1970).

However discussion continues regarding the localization of the interneurons that are at the origin of the depolarization of terminals responsible for the negative DRP. For Wall (1962), Mendell and Wall (1964), Wall (1964), Melzack and Wall (1965), these interneurons are located in the substantia gelatinosa (layers II and III of Rexed). For others, they are in the inferior layers of the dorsal horn and the intermediate zone of Cajal (Eccles et al., 1962; Eccles, 1964).

The origin of the positive phase of the DRP is another point of discussion. Mendell and Wall (1964) have shown that uniquely positive DRPs can be obtained when myelinated fibres are blocked and unmyelinated ones are still conducting. This observation induced Melzack and Wall (1965) to propose that the action of messages coming through C fibres is to facilitate the spinal transmission (gate control theory) that was inhibited after the arrival of a message through myelinated fibres.

That non-myelinated fibres convey facilitatory messages was made doubtful by the fact that certain authors (Zimmermann, 1968; Franz and Iggo, 1968; Vyklický et al., 1969) were unable to find a positive DRP, when C fibres were stimulated alone. This point is still debated. However recent experiments of Hillman and Wall (1969), made at the level of layer V cells, demonstrate a complex interaction of inhibitory and excitatory effects. Besson et al. (1972), using activation of nociceptive afferents by intra-arterial injection of bradykinin (see Fig. 25 page 518), have found an activation of cells in layer V, in 50 % of the cases, but also in 25 %, they have observed a pure inhibition or an inhibition followed by an excitation, thus showing the complex role of presumed nociceptive messages at the spinal level.

(iii) Supraspinal Control at Spinal Cord Level. Hagbarth and Kerr (1954) have demonstrated that transmission giving rise to activity in the spinothalamic tract could be inhibited by stimulation of cortical sensorimotor areas and the reticular formation. Hagbarth and Fex (1959) have shown later that units in the dorsal horn could be both inhibited and facilitated by the same stimulation. Andersen et al. (1962, 1964), Carpenter et al. (1962a, 1963) have demonstrated that these controls are, at least in part, of presynaptic nature; dorsal root potentials being provoked by cortical stimulation. These authors have described, in the cat, the cortical regions from where these DRPs can be provoked (SI, SII and motor cortex). Abdelmoumene et al. (1970) have shown that, in the cat, the orbital cortex has to be added to these areas. In the monkey, a topic organization of the descending pathway is observed which is even clearer than in the cat (Fig. 27).

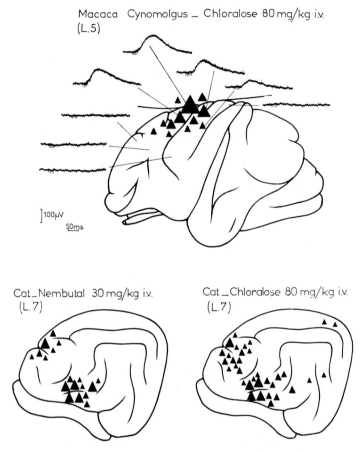

Fig. 27. Cortical areas the stimulation of which provokes DRPs at L5 level in macaque, at L7 in cats. (From ABDELMOUMENE et al., 1970)

In the cat, stimulation of precruciate cortex is less effective than that of postcruciate. Moreover, it seems that the stimulation of precruciate cortex is indirectly acting by stimulating the postcruciate cortex (ANDERSEN et al., 1964; MORRISON and POMPEIANO, 1965). The latency of these cortical DRPs are of the order of 20–30 msec, and their duration in the anaesthetized animal is of 150 to 300 msec. Here again, the DRPs, when recorded in cat under local analgesia, are diphasic negative-positive, and they become purely negative when anaesthetics are injected.

The pathway that mediates the impulses which provoke DRPs of cortical origin is principally the pyramidal tract. However, when the animal is anaesthetized with chloralose, DRPs can still be evoked by cortical stimulation after bilateral pyramidectomy. Thus other pathways, and in particular reticulospinal and rubrospinal ones, are involved in the central descending presynaptic control (CARPENTER et al., 1962b, 1966; HONGO and JANKOWSKA, 1967). There are reasons to

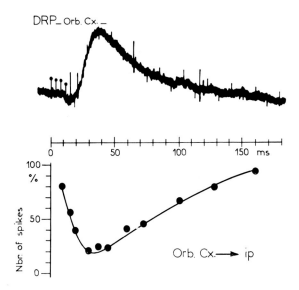

Fig. 28. Effects of orbital cortex stimulation at spinal level. *Upper trace:* DRP to orbital cortex stimulation. *Lower trace:* Reduction due to orbital cortex stimulation in number of spikes of the response of a layer IV cell to cutaneous electrical stimulation as a function of the interval between cortical and peripheral stimuli. Number of spikes expressed as a percentage of the control level (without cortical stimulation). Note the parallel time course of these processes. (Modified from MAILLARD et al., 1971)

think that the controls put in action by orbital cortex stimulation (MAILLARD et al., 1971) are mediated through the reticular formation.

DRPs can also be produced by the stimulation of regions of the body other than the one represented at the spinal level studied (heterosegmental controls, BERGMANS et al., 1964; MALLART, 1965). These facts were confirmed with unitary recordings in spinal cord (BESSON et RIVOT, 1972).

The effects of cortical stimulation were also studied at unitary level in the dorsal horn. Inhibitory and excitatory controls were demonstrated that seem to be well correlated with DRPs. Cells in layers IV, V and VI (WALL, 1967) and cells being at the origin of the spino-cervical tract (BROWN, 1970, 1971) are all under descending controls that are suppressed by section or cooling of the spinal cord.

In layer VI, the brain stem acts differently when the peripheral stimulus is tactile or muscular: inhibition is the rule for tactile inputs, facilitation for muscular ones (WALL, 1967). The inhibitory effects of cortical origin are maximal on the cells of layers IV and V. In layer IV, 66 % of the cells are inhibited by stimulation of the pyramidal tract (FETZ, 1968), and 40 % in layer V. By orbital stimulation, MAILLARD et al. (1971) have found 80 % and 60 % of the cells inhibited in layers IV and V respectively. The evolution and duration of the inhibitory phenomenon recorded at a unitary level after pyramidal stimulation (FETZ, 1968) or stimulation of orbital cortex (MAILLARD et al., 1971) (Fig. 28) are similar to the ones of the DRP provoked by the same stimulation. That these inhibitions are due to presynaptic action is thus probable. In layer VI, many cells are excited by central stimulations (Fetz, 1968).

(iv) Controls Exerted on Extralemniscal Messages at the Spinal Level. We will now examine what part the controls we have just described play on the transmission of anterolateral messages, thus finally on impulses going to convergent type II thalamic areas.

Several studies have shown that the cells which are at the origin of the spinocervical tract (SCT) are located in the more dorsal part of the dorsal horn (layer

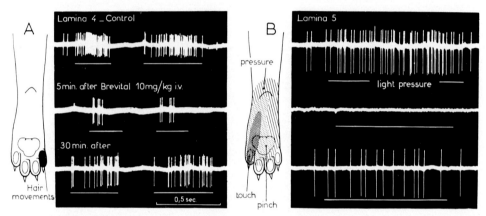

Fig. 29. Effects of an injection of Brevital on responses of two cells to natural stimulation.
A: cell in layer IV. B: cell in layer V

IV) (Brodal and Rexed, 1953; Morin, 1955; Oswaldo-Cruz and Kidd, 1964; Taub and Bishop, 1965; Fetz, 1968; Hongo et al., 1968). However, other electrophysiological findings have shown that the cells at the origin of the SCT respond differently from cells of layer IV, in particular to various somatic stimulations, and therefore are presumably located in another layer (Lundberg and Oscarsson, 1961; Burgess, 1965; Mendell, 1966; Wall, 1960, 1967; Fetz, 1968; Brown and Franz, 1969). In summary the problem of the functional role of the different dorsal horn cells remains complex and it is difficult to attribute a specific function in the conduction of ascending messages to cells of each of these layers.

We shall however consider schematically that the more dorsally located cells (of layer IV and some of layer V) are at the origin of the SCT, while the more ventrally located cells (V, VI) are the best candidates to be involved in the transmission of anterolateral messages.

This suggestion is made because cells at this level are activated by injection of nociceptive drugs, and also because Price and Wagman (1971) have shown that impulses travelling in the anterolateral pathways share characteristics with layer VI cells, and (Fields et al., 1970) with layer V cells. Cells in layer V are under inhibitory controls. Thus tactile and visceral afferents can be suppressed at the spinal level by descending impulses coming from primary cortices and also orbital cortex. This descending inhibition appears to be set in action by the specific afferent pathways.

If, as we are suggesting, layer V contains relay cells for the extralemniscal pathway, the inhibitory effect exerted through a lemniscal thalamo-cortico-pyramidal loop is an interesting finding. Effectively, the inhibitory action of specific afferents on nociceptive messages described long ago by the neurologists (HEAD, 1920; FOERSTER, 1936) has recently aroused a new interest (MELZACK and WALL, 1965; ALBE-FESSARD, 1967, 1968).

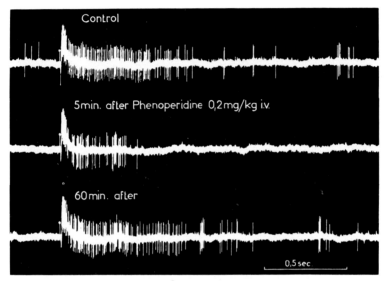

Fig. 30. Reduction by injection of phenoperidine of the response of a layer V cell to a strong electrical stimulation. (From MAILLARD et al., 1972)

(v) Effect of Anaesthetics and Analgesics on Messages Received at a Spinal Level by Extralemniscal Pathways. As we have said in section B3, the principal effect of anaesthetics on afferent messages has to be searched for at a spinal level. The results we have just described in this section give some information on this point.

1. During different types of anaesthesia (barbiturate, chloralose, halothane), a prolongation of the negative phase of the DRPs (corresponding to inhibition) appears (ECCLES et al., 1963) (see Fig. 26) and the positive phase (corresponding to a facilitation) disappears (MENDELL and WALL, 1964; BESSON et al., 1968b).

2. A general depressing effect is also exerted by anaesthesia on the activity of cells of layers IV and V (DE JONG and WAGMAN, 1968; DE JONG et al., 1969, 1970; BESSON et al., 1970; KITAHATA et al., 1971). This general depressing effect is demonstrated by reduction of spontaneous activity and of evoked responses. Drastic effects are observed on cells of layers IV and V (Fig. 29). Morphinomimetic agents present similar effects on layer V units (Fig. 30) activated by strong stimuli.

In conclusion, anaesthetic and analgesic drugs seem to have two effects in common at a spinal level: a reduction of the duration of the messages and a reduction in amplitude of its first phase. We have however to note that the reduction in amplitude of the first period of the message is more important under barbiturate anaesthesia than under chloralose (negative phases of DRPs are not increased in amplitude by chloralose injection). This fact may explain why under chloralose, because a first burst of spikes is always transmitted, short latencies responses still appear in convergent type II areas. The general effect of anaesthetics is due both to a hyperpolarization of the cellular membrane and to a modification of the duration of the controls exerted from segmental and supra-spinal regions.

b) Controls at the Level of the Spinal Trigeminal Nucleus. From what we have said in the anatomical part, the origin of the extralemniscal pathway for the face afferents takes place in the spinal trigeminal nuclei at the level of nucleus caudalis.

Hernández-Péon and Hagbarth (1955) found that it was possible to inhibit the central transmission of trigemnial impulses by stimulation of the sensorimotor areas or the reticular formation. Darian-Smith (1966), Dubner (1967) have shown in the cat that stimulation of the cortical face areas are the most effective for obtaining these modifications. That these effects are due in part, as in the cord, to presynaptic inhibition, was demonstrated by Darian-Smith and Yokota (1964) Darian-Smith (1966) and Stewart et al. (1967). Thus inhibitory and possibly facilitatory effects exist at this level which are reminiscent of what happens at the spinal level.

c) Controls Exerted on Convergent Type II Messages at the Level of Bulbar or Thalamic Relays

1. Controls Exerted at Thalamic Level Coming from Cortical Areas. Direct connections between the cortex and the medial and intralaminar thalamic zones (convergent type II) have been shown to exist by anatomical techniques in cats and monkeys (Mehler, 1966b; Rinvik, 1968, 1972; Scheibel and Scheibel, 1972; Petras, 1972). Albe-Fessard and Gillett (1961) using macroelectrode, then microelectrode recordings have shown that excitatory processes are produced at the same thalamic level by stimulation of the precruciate cortex. In a recent work (Albe-Fessard et al., 1972), it was suggested that among these excitatory processes, those having a latency of less than 2.5 msec correspond to direct descending pathways. Inhibitory processes with a similar latency which act on cells of the intralaminar nuclei may be due also to direct pathways.

In the VL, a direct connection exists coming from the same area (cruciate cortex) (Kusama et al., 1966; Nakamura and Schlag, 1968). This direct connection is inhibitory as many researches have shown (Cohen et al., 1962; Purpura et al., 1966; Massion and Dormont, 1966; Steriade and Briot, 1967; etc...). The region from whence the inhibitory pathway comes is about the same as the area on which projections from VL are terminating (Macchi, 1958).

2. Controls Probably Exerted Before the Thalamic Level. The somato-motor cortex and the primary areas have an important role to play in the control of convergent type II afferent pathways. This was demonstrated in acute animals by different groups of workers (ADEY et al., 1957; BORENSTEIN and BUSER, 1960; BAUMGARTEN et al., 1963; MEULDERS et al., 1963). Excitatory responses of long latencies (12 to 20 msec) were obtained at a unitary level in CM-Pf and intralaminar nuclei when SI, SII and orbital cortices were stimulated. These responses are certainly mediated through spinal or reticular relays.

That an inhibitory action from the primary cortical areas may act at the level of CM-Pf was demonstrated also in chronically implanted cats. As we have said (page 502), the evoked responses observed during sleep in this convergent type II area differ considerably from those observed in ventralis posterior in the same animals. The amplitudes of the responses recorded in both nuclei are affected in opposite directions during both rapid or slow wave sleep (FAVALE et al., 1963; ALBE-FESSARD et al., 1964; ALLISON, 1965; GUILBAUD, 1968, 1970) (see Fig. 12).

This fact and the recognition of the existence of different descending pathways from primary areas has led to the hypothesis (GUILBAUD, 1970) that the reduction in CM responses observed during the fast phase of sleep could be due to the increase of activity present during this time in the primary thalamic relays and cortical areas (also observed with microelectrodes during fast sleep, EVARTS, 1964; HODES, 1964; ALLISON, 1965). This hypothesis was confirmed when ablation of a well delineated area of precruciate cortex was shown to suppress the reduction of the CM responses observed during the fast phase of sleep (GUILBAUD and MENETREY, 1970). This demonstrated that an inhibitory pathway was acting from the precruciate cortex upon the somatic extralemniscal pathway. That these controls are set in action through a specific inflow was obvious since the same workers have found, after chronic sections of the lemniscal pathways, effects similar to those observed after precruciate cortex ablation.

This action is not due however to the direct pathway of which we have spoken just before. As we have said, in the CM-Pf, many cells are activated not only by somatic afferents, but also by visual and auditory ones. If the inhibitory effect exerted by the motor cortex acts at the CM-Pf level postsynaptically, it must act as well on the evoked activity provoked by the three types of afferents. It must be emphasized that, on the contrary, visual and auditory inputs are controlled respectively by their own primary areas of projection. First found in acute preparations (BUSER et al., 1963), this was demonstrated also in chronic animals (GUILBAUD et al., 1970).

Thus the cortical control acting during fast sleep on somatic afferents must be applied either presynaptically at the thalamic level or elsewhere on the ascending pathways (spinal cord or bulbar reticular formation).

In chronic animals again, it was shown that excitatory input arrives in VL from SI during fast sleep. That a facilitatory control is exerted on the medial thalamic inflow from the telencephalon can be deduced also from experiments of FEENEY et al. (1970) in non-anaesthetized animals, showing that rostral thalamic lesions produce a decrease in the evoked response of CM-Pf. However, as discussed by these authors, the role of a change in alertness due to the lesion can also possibly explain these modifications.

3. Inhibition of Caudate Origin Acting on the Extra-Lemniscal Pathway. In animals under chloralose anaesthesia, KRAUTHAMER and ALBE-FESSARD (1964, 1965) FELTZ et al. (1967), using macroelectrode and microelectrode derivations, have demonstrated that stimulation of the nucleus caudatus in its anterior lateral region can selectively suppress the convergent type II responses at thalamic and cortical levels (Fig. 31). The same observation was made in the bulbar reticular formation. Similar inhibition can be obtained in the cat from the n. entopeduncularis, which is the homologue in the cat of primate medial pallidum. Thus a pathway going through caudate and pallidum acts on the extralemniscal pathway.

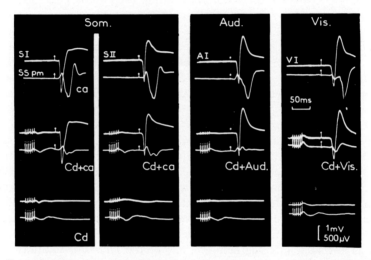

Fig. 31. Cat under chloralose anaesthesia. Recordings were taken simultaneously at cortical levels in SI, SII, auditory area I (AI) and visual area I (VI), and suprasylvian type II convergent area (SSpm). Stimulations were somatic, auditory and visual (first row). When this stimulation is preceded by a short train of stimuli applied to caudate nucleus, only the suprasylvian response disappears (second row). This caudate stimulation does not produce a response by itself (third row)

The exact site of action of this inhibitory pathway is not yet determined; spinal, reticular, thalamic levels are all possible candidates from latency calculations made by FELTZ et al. (1967). The existence of dorsal root potentials after stimulation of n. caudate was also demonstrated (BESSON et al., 1968a).

This inhibition acts equally upon visual, auditory and somatic afferents reaching the convergent structures of the medial thalamus. Similar effects have not been obtained for the extralemniscal messages which reach the VL nucleus. This nucleus is in this way different from the other type II convergent thalamic nuclei.

4. *Inhibition Produced by Stimulation of Hippocampus and Amygdala.* In chloralosed cats, hippocampal stimulation produces at medial thalamic level an inhibition with characteristics similar to those observed after caudate stimulation. However, the cell population on which both inhibitions are acting is not exactly the same. Some cells can be inhibited by both caudate and hippocampal stimulations; others by only one of them (MacKENZIE et al., 1971).

In awake monkeys, YOKOTA and MACLEAN (1968) have shown that hippocampal after-discharges inhibit cells of non-specific nuclei activated by fifth nerve stimulation, but not cells in specific nuclei. Stimulation of the amygdala was shown to have inhibitory effects on CM-Pf unitary responses (URABE and ITO, 1968). CAZARD and BUSER (1963), BUSER and VIALA (1963) have demonstrated hippocampal facilitatory controls on cortical and thalamic non-specific evoked responses.

5. Pathways for Visual and Auditory Non-Specific Thalamic Inflow

The non-specific pathways which bring to the thalamus visual and auditory impulses have not been so extensively studied as the somatic. MEULDERS (1970) has recently reviewed the literature on visual inflow. It is obvious that the reticular formation which receives both visual and auditory inflow plays a role in the transmission of these messages to the medial thalamus. However, it is not the only pathway involved because an inter-collicular section not only does not suppress, but increases the visual response in CM-Pf (MEULDERS, 1962).

The nucleus lateralis posterior receives a few direct retinal projections (ALTMAN, 1962; SUZUKI and KATO, 1969), but the majority of its inflow passes through the dorsal part of the n. geniculatus lateralis (GL) (BISHOP and CLARE, 1955; ALTMAN, 1962; VAN STRAATEN, 1962) or comes from the superior colliculus (ALTMAN and CARPENTER, 1961). The posterior nucleus is also connected with the same regions (KINSTON et al., 1969). The nucleus reticularis thalami receives impulses from the ventral GL (ALTMAN, 1962) and its dorsal portion (SCHEIBEL and SCHEIBEL, 1966). The pars magnocellularis of GM and the nucleus suprageniculatus receive their visual inflow from the superior colliculus (ALTMAN and CARPENTER, 1961; NIIMI et al., 1970) and also from the dorsal part of GL (ALTMAN, 1962). The VL nucleus receives its visual input directly from the GL, and by a detour through the nucleus ruber (MASSION, 1968).

Only few studies have been made on the pathway of auditory inflow. By lesions in the inferior colliculus, connections have been demonstrated between this region and both the medial geniculate body and posterior group (JANE et al., 1968).

Primary visual and auditory cortical areas exert, on non-specific visual and auditory inflows, controls that seem to be organized in approximately the same way as the controls exerted by primary somatic areas on the extralemniscal system. For more details on this subject, see BUSER and BIGNALL (1967), MEULDERS (1970).

D. Telencephalic Convergent Areas

The duality of convergent systems we have described at the thalamic level exists also at the telencephalic level. Here however the system is made more complex by the existence of intra-cortical connections.

1. Telencephalic Areas Presenting Type II Convergence in the Cat

a) Cortical Areas Presenting Total Heterosensory Convergence

1. Localization of these Areas. In animals anaesthetized with chloralose, four cortical areas present activities similar to those described in convergent type II nuclei of medial thalamus (Fig. 32, a, b, c, d).

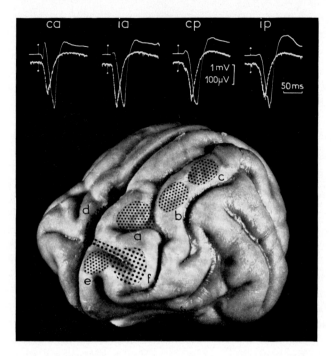

Fig. 32. Cortical areas of the cat where type II convergent responses can be recorded are designated a to e. Motor cortex area is designated f. *Above:* Recordings taken in a cat under chloralose anaesthesia from suprasylvian zone (c) and bulbar reticular formation (shorter latencies) showing the similarities of these responses

The first of these convergent areas was found by Amassian (1954) in the anterior part of the marginal gyrus; heterosensory impulses evoked slow wave activity at this level and units are driven by heterosensory messages. Studies of interaction between these messages were pursued at a unitary level in the same area by Rutledge (1963) and Dubner (1966). In anteromedial suprasylvian gyrus, two foci of heterosensory convergent type II activities can be observed, one anteriorly and one in the medial part (Bruner and Sindberg, 1962; Thompson et al., 1963a; Rutledge ,1963; Bruner, 1965). Another focus occurs on the interhemispheric cortex where photic evoked responses were described (Ingvar and Hunter, 1955; Harman and Berry, 1956; Hughes, 1959; Bruner, 1960) as well as auditory and somatic responses (Bruner, 1960; Thompson et al., 1963a).

In all these 4 regions, convergence between heterotopic somatic afferents was observed (Albe-Fessard and Rougeul, 1955, 1958; Thompson et al., 1963a; etc...). The latency of evoked activities (5 to 6 msec longer than in corresponding primary areas), the long duration of the positive evoked phase, the susceptibility to barbiturate anaesthesia, the type of effective natural somatic stimuli and the duration of recovery phases are all similar to that observed under chloralose anaesthesia in thalamic convergent type II zones and in particular in CM-Pf (Albe-Fessard and Rougeul, 1955, 1958; Thompson et al., 1963b) or in reti-

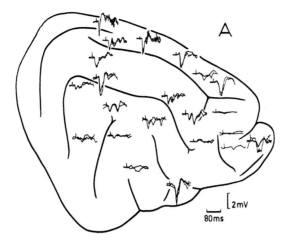

Thalamic ablation except GL

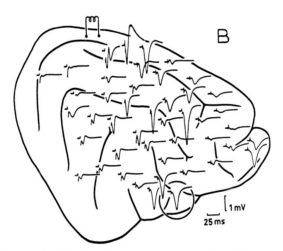

Fig. 33. A: Animal under local analgesia; responses to a flash of light from an animal where the thalamus was totally ablated with the exception of GL. Note that responses can be observed under these conditions in convergent type II areas. B: Animal under chloralose; total ablation of thalamus was made. Responses are recorded after stimulation of visual primary areas in different convergent zones. (From IMBERT, 1967)

cular relays to this thalamic region (see Fig. 32). Convergence was also found at these levels in awake animals (BUSER and BORENSTEIN, 1959).

2. Cortical Primary Areas and Convergent Type II Responses. It was originally thought that the impulses arriving in these convergent zones relayed in the primary cortical areas. The fact that convergent heterotopic responses can appear when primary somatic cortical areas are ablated (ALBE-FESSARD and ROUGEUL, 1958) demonstrated that this was not so. Similar observations were made for visual and

34*

auditory inflows (see Buser et al., 1959; Bignall et al., 1966). However, a series of experiments performed for the visual inflow has shown that evoked activities can appear in these regions when the thalamus was ablated except for the GL region (Fig. 33 A). Even when the entire thalamus was ablated, a stimulus applied to the primary visual area evoked a response in these cortical convergent zones (Fig. 33 B). From indirect and direct evidence (Poliakova, 1972) it seems that what was shown for visual inflow must also exist for auditory and somatic inflow.

Thus, in normal animals, the convergent type II cortical areas receive impulses through the typical extralemniscal pathways, but also from the primary thalamic relay and somatic primary areas through cortico-cortical connections. They receive input also (as described in section II) from primary specific areas through cortico-thalamic, cortico-reticulo-thalamic and cortico-spino-thalamic pathways. These regions thus seem to integrate complex messages from various sources. In animals deeply anaesthetized with chloralose, the recovery times are very similar for all inputs as they are in thalamic type II areas. When chloralose anaesthesia is lighter or when the animals are under local analgesia (certainly when all the afferent pathways which we have just described are functioning), the interactions between different inflows vary depending on the inflow itself and in which cortical area these interactions are studied. Differences in patterns of responses as well as interaction times were found at a unitary level (Dubner and Rutledge, 1964, 1965; Dubner, 1966; Rutledge and Duncan, 1966). Dubner and Rutledge (1964) have shown that with deepening of anaesthetic level, convergence shifted from unequal to equal input for polysensory neurons of type II convergent areas.

Recently, Dow and Dubner (1969) have studied the responsiveness of cells of the medial suprasylvian area to natural visual stimuli under light chloralose anaesthesia. Receptive field mapping has made it possible to recognize cells responding to stationary spots with enhanced responses when stimulus size is increased. Other cells respond to sudden movements and have on-off responses to stationary spots. Such cells also respond to click. Finally a last group of cells, totally independant of primary cortex integrity, responds to oriented edges. Thus cells in convergent areas demonstrate a certain specificity when natural stimuli are employed. Moreover such specificity does not depend only on cortico-cortical projections.

b) Special Cortical Convergent Type II Projection in Premotor and Somato-Motor Areas

1. *Premotor Projection.* In the most medial part of the precruciate cortex (e in Fig. 32), heterotopic responses were described (Albe-Fessard and Rougeul, 1958). Heterosensory afferents were also found at this level (Gastaut and Hunter, 1950; Hunter and Ingvar, 1955; Feng et al., 1956; Buser and Ascher, 1960; Thompson and Sindberg, 1960; Thompson et al., 1963a). The only characteristic that seems to differentiate this area from other convergent ones is the shorter latency observed for their evoked somatic responses.

2. *Special Case of Motor Cortex.* The motor area in the cat involves the two banks of the cruciate sulcus (cf. Fig. 32), the homologue of the Rolandic fissure

being a small dimple just posterior to the cruciate sulcus. At this level, heterotopic convergence can be observed. Some neurons present pure type II convergence. For others, in the same area, somatic inflow is conducted through both primary and extralemniscal pathways (ALBE-FESSARD and FESSARD, 1963).

In motor cortex, some studies have dealt with heterotopic somatic afferents (BROOKS et al., 1961a and b; ALBE-FESSARD and FESSARD, 1963; BROOKS, 1965; ALBE-FESSARD, 1967; TOWE et al., 1968) while others have examined hetero-sensory inflow (BUSER and IMBERT, 1961; KORNHUBER and DAFONSECA, 1964; BOISACQ-SCHEPENS et al., 1968, 1969; BOISACQ-SCHEPENS, 1971).

The cells in these regions present a complex heterosensory organization. In cats under chloralose anaesthesia, most units respond to photic and auditory stimuli. The proportion is however smaller in the work by BOISACQ-SCHEPENS et al. (1968) than in the work by IMBERT and BUSER (1961). This discrepancy can be explained in two ways. In the statistics of IMBERT and BUSER, cells of premotor area are possibly included. Differences in stimulating techniques also exist (see BOISACQ-SCHEPENS, 1971). In motor cortex, the heterosensory neurons are in general the heterotopic ones. This heterosensory convergent inflow to motor cortex seems to be reduced and even to disappear in animals under local analgesia. Here again, variations in the state of alertness during recordings can explain at least in part the discrepancies observed between the findings of different research groups.

At this cortical level, the arrival of vestibular inflow has also been demonstrated (KORNHUBER and DAFONSECA, 1964; BOISACQ-SCHEPENS, 1971).

In conclusion, while the somatomotor cortex presents type II convergence, this convergence is however different from that in other areas. The particular organization of the heterosensory inflow observed at this level is due probably to the VL origin of these messages (see next section).

c) Thalamic Pathways to Convergent Type II Areas in Cat. As we have said in the preceding section, the integrity of primary cortices is not necessary for the appearance of this type of projection in convergent areas. For heterotopic afferents in motor cortex of the cat, it has not been possible to demonstrate directly their lack of dependence on the sensory area by destruction of this latter region since sensory and motor areas are overlapped. However, this sort of demonstration was possible in monkeys (SINGER and BIGNALL, 1969, personal communication) where the two regions are more separated. It is thus probable that all the convergent cortical inflow we have described in cats is mediated through non-specific reticular or thalamic zones.

After sections of the dorsal column and spino-cervical bundle cortical heterotopic convergence still appears. This fact has proved here again that the principal afferent pathway to these regions is in the anterolateral quadrant. The next step was to decide if a direct reticulo-cortical pathway was responsible for the convergent responses or if this pathway relayed at a thalamic level.

A reticulo-cortical projection which does not relay in thalamic convergent regions seems to exist. Its intervention in the conduction of non-specific type II afferents cannot until now either be proved or disproved (see references and discussion on this point in BUSER and BIGNALL, 1967). On the other hand, the involvement of a thalamic relay was suggested by the fact that stimulation

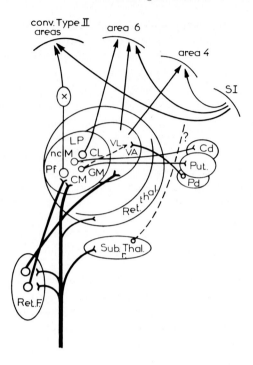

Fig. 34. Schematic representation of possible pathways in the cat between type II convergent thalamic nucleus and cortex

applied in CM-Pf in the area of maximal responses to peripheral stimulation evoked short latency responses in all cortical areas where typical convergent type II responses are observed (see Albe-Fessard and Rougeul, 1957; Albe-Fessard and Fessard, 1963).

For the somato-motor cortex, results were different; and when the stimulating technique was used, the region that was found to mediate the non-specific heterotopic inflow was in the VL (Jankowska and Albe-Fessard, 1961; Albe-Fessard, 1961). These facts are in good agreement with anatomical knowledge (by retrograde degeneration, Macchi, 1958; or by anterograde degeneration, Strick, 1970) and recent physiological work (Rispal-Padel and Massion, 1970).

The responses evoked by medial thalamic stimulation in the anterior marginal and suprasylvian area had relatively long latencies (3 to 4 msec). Shorter latency responses were only observed in the premotor area (2 msec). The fact that the blockage of CM-Pf by reversible cooling suppresses cortical convergent responses was the subject of discussion because definitive lesions of the same areas by coagulation (Bignall, 1967; Buser and Bignall, 1967) proved to have only a transitory effect. These transitory effects are easy to understand, now that we know that specific afferents can arrive at the same convergent areas through a cortico-cortical loop. The fact that we were obliged to use relatively low temperature (of the order of –5°C) in order to block CM-Pf has two possible explanations

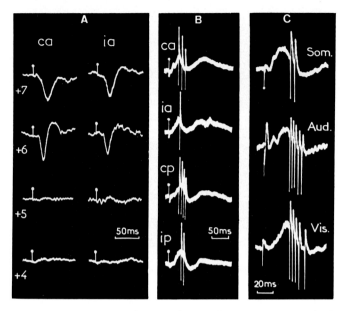

Fig. 35. Convergent type II responses from caudate nucleus. A: in a cat under local analgesia after cortical ablation of somato-motor cortex, responses to stimulation of anterior limbs recorded in the head of caudate nucleus. B and C: Cat under chloralose. B: A cell responds to stimulation of the 4 limbs. C: Another cell responds to heterosensory stimuli

1) the temperature has to be low because all of CM-Pf must be blocked; 2) the temperature has to be low, because it is fibres of passage that were blocked at the CM-Pf level (CONDE et al., 1968; BENITA and CONDE, 1971).

Relations between CM-Pf and cortical areas are in general denied by the anatomists (see references in ROSE and WOOLSEY, 1949; ALBE-FESSARD and ROUGEUL, 1957; BOWSHER, 1966; MEHLER, 1966b). The only direct projection known from CM is to Putamen. For this reason, it has often been said that, if a CM-Pf cortical pathway exists, it has to be through a relay (see Fig. 34). Relays in VA nucleus (DROOGLEEVER-FORTUYN and STEFENS, 1951) or in reticular thalamic nucleus were suggested.

That a direct connection between CM-Pf and anterior marginal and suprasylvian areas does not exist was also demonstrated by physiological techniques. The latency of the potential recorded in these cortical areas after CM-Pf stimulation makes this direct connection doubtful. No antidromic activation of units in CM-Pf after stimulation of anterior marginal and suprasylvian areas was found (BOWSHER and ALEXINSKY, quoted in BENITA and CONDE, 1971; ALBE-FESSARD et al., 1971). Thus a relay has to be sought between CM-Pf and marginal and suprasylvian cortex. We have called it x on the schema of Fig. 34.

Results are different when connections from the medial thalamic zone to premotor and motor cortex are considered. Premotor cortex, as we have said, responds with a short latency to CM-Pf stimulation. On the other hand, stimulations applied to precruciate cortex give rise to antidromic responses in CM-Pf.

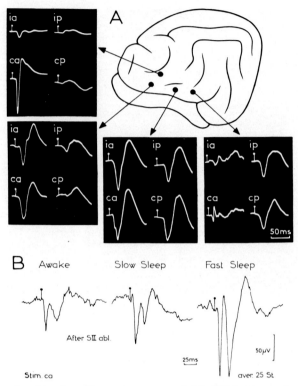

Fig. 36. A: Cat under chloralose. Responses are recorded in SII (upper tracings) and in orbital cortex (3 lower ones). B: Chronically implanted cat after SII ablation. Averaged responses from orbital cortex. Note its increase during fast sleep. (From Korn, 1967)

The latencies of these antidromic responses are compatible with a myelinated pathway from this medial thalamic region to precruciate cortex (Albe-Fessard et al., 1971). These facts are supported by recent anatomical data (Totibadze and Moniava, 1969); they do not exclude, as we have said before, that the same cortical areas receive an important non-specific inflow through VL nucleus (Benita and Conde, 1971; and page 534). That the relay between medial thalamus and other convergent type II areas is in the pericruciate region cannot be accepted, because these responses still exist when large ablations of pericruciate cortex are performed.

d) **Type II Convergence in the Corpus Striatum.** Responses similar to the heterosensory cortical ones appear in the head of nucleus caudatus, in the putamen and in the pallidum (Segundo and Machne, 1956). Responses in nucleus caudatus were more extensively studied (Albe-Fessard et al., 1960a, 1960b). Again these responses which exist in chloralosed animals can be recorded also in drowsy, acute, decorticated or chronically implanted cats (Fig. 35).

The projections do not depend on the integrity of the cortex although the n. caudatus receives afferents from the cortex (see Rocha-Miranda, 1961). Some of the afferent impulses to the n. caudatus certainly relay in the nucleus centralis medialis of the thalamus as confirmed by electrophysiological (ALBE-FESSARD et al., 1960 a) and anatomical studies (POWELL and COWAN, 1956).

2. Telencephalic Areas Presenting Type I Convergence in the Cat

Regions where convergence exists, but where responses have properties similar in duration, latency and recovery cycle, to the responses observed in primary areas exist in two adjacent cortical zones, SII and orbital gyrus (Fig. 36).

a) **The Second Somatic Area (SII)** is known from the early work of ADRIAN (1940, 1941) and of WOOLSEY (1943, 1944, 1947). The locus of the thalamic relay to SII cortex was for some time a subject of discussion. Recently, agreement has been reached that local stimulation of VP gives rise to responses in SII cortex as well as in SI, and that all the different parts of VP project to SII (GUILLERY et al., 1966). We came to the same conclusion using the cooling technique in VP nucleus (WENDT and ALBE-FESSARD, 1961).

Bilateral responses can be observed in SII, but this bilaterality involves only a portion of the cells. We have seen ourselves that at least a part of the ipsilateral inflow arrives through corpus callosum. ANDERSSON (1962) on the other hand has shown that the spino-cervico-thalamic bundle is involved in the SII projection. Thus a bilateral inflow to SII may derive from the type I convergent area described at the limit between anterior and posterior VL, or from the suprageniculate.

Short latency, click-evoked responses have been described in the anterior part of suprasylvian gyrus by BREMER (1952), MICKLE and ADES (1953), BREMER et al. (1954), LOMBROSO and MERLIS (1957), THOMPSON et al. (1963 a). This area overlaps with somatic area II (BERMAN, 1961 a and b). Thus a convergent zone exists in SII where pure contralateral dorsal column afferents are mixed with type I bilateral somatic inflow and auditory messages.

b) **Orbito-Insular Projection.** The posterior part of the orbital gyrus in the cat (which corresponds to the anterior extension of anterior sylvian gyrus limited above by the orbital sulcus) presents responses to three sensory modalities. Responses in this area have been reported to photic stimulation (DESMEDT and MECHELSE, 1959), to auditory stimulation (WOOLSEY, 1944, 1961; DESMEDT and MECHELSE, 1959) and to somatic stimulation (KORN et al., 1966). The somatic responses are almost totally bilateral, the amplitude of the responses for two symmetrical loci of stimulation being extremely similar. This fact differentiates orbital cortex from the adjacent SII zone (see Fig. 36). In the same region, an important interoceptive inflow is known to exist. BAILEY and BREMER (1938), DELL and OLSON (1951) and MASSION et al. (1966) have demonstrated the arrival of both rapid and slow vagal afferents at this level. BYSTRYCKA and KORN (1969) have also shown a splanchnic projection to the same area. With evoked potential and microelectrode techniques a focus of total heterotopic convergence was shown. It is surrounded anteriorly and posteriorly by more organized convergent somatic areas (Fig. 36 A).

Among the natural somatic messages that evoked unitary responses, the interoceptive were the most effective. The pathways of the contralateral somatic inflow (determined by stimulations and lesions) pass through the specific thalamic relay (KORN and RICHARD, 1968). The responses in orbital gyrus to stimulation

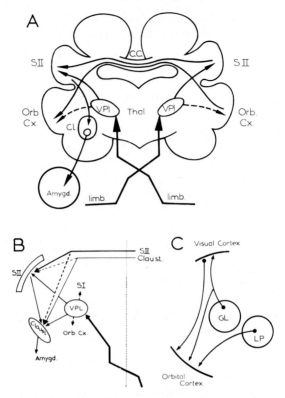

Fig. 37. Group of schemas demonstrating. A: Somatic pathways to SII and orbital cortex. B: Somatic pathways to claustrum (from Spector, 1967). C: Visual pathways to orbital cortex (from Imbert, 1967)

of the ipsilateral side of the body is due to a callosal transmission of messages coming from the opposite orbital area (Fig. 37 A). In the cord, the afferent messages follow the neo-spino-thalamic pathway. Ablation of SII does not modify somatic orbital responses.

The same orbital area receives direct projections from the lateral geniculate body (Bignall et al., 1966), the lateral posterior thalamus (Landau and Imbert, 1965) and the primary visual cortex (Imbert, 1967) (Fig. 37 C). For the auditory input, anatomical studies indicate projections from medial geniculate body (Rose and Woolsey, 1958; Diamond et al., 1958). The different types of sensory afferents do not seem to converge on a common cortical pool of neurons; they are distributed in a mosaic fashion (Batini and Imbert, 1965; Batini et al., 1965).

Thus the responses recorded in this area have the typical characteristics of what we have described at the thalamic level as type I convergence and in particular they have a low susceptibility to anaesthesia, are not suppressed by alertness or fast sleep (Fig. 36 B), etc.... However, the majority of the convergence observed there does not seem to take place at a thalamic level, but at a cortical one. Moreover there exists no true heterosensory convergence at the unitary level.

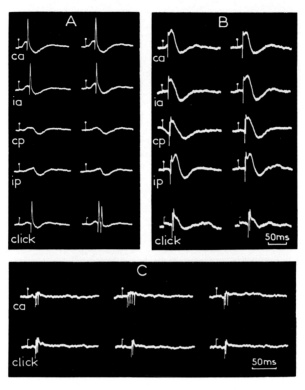

Fig. 38. Demonstration of somatic and auditory convergence at cellular level in claustrum. A and B: Cats anaesthetized with chloralose. C: Cat under local analgesia. (From SPECTOR, 1967). Two (A and B) or three (C) examples of the same response are given

c) **Claustrum Convergent Zone.** SEGUNDO and MACHNE (1956) found that convergence of a variety of sensory inputs appeared in claustral neurons. URBANO et al. (1966) observed that claustral units may be activated by stimulation of restricted somatic fields.

An evoked potential study (SPECTOR et al., 1970) has shown that, although multisensory heterotopic convergence is seen throughout the claustrum, it is nonetheless a regionally differentiated structure where a part of the somatic inflow is essentially of lemniscal origin. The pathways mediating the contralateral somatic inflow are multiple. A direct pathway was recognized from the VP and an indirect one from the VP through the SII area. The ipsilateral inflow arrives through the contralateral SII cortex, and is then conducted through the corpus callosum to the ipsilateral SII and then to claustrum (Fig. 37 A and B). For the auditory inflow, pathways through medial geniculate and auditory cortex were demonstrated. The visual inflow to claustrum is minimal. Thus the claustrum is a type I convergent structure where impulses of a specific type are received. But, here again, the convergence (that in this case, appears also at a cellular level, see Fig. 38) takes place in the structure itself or in SII, but not in the thalamus.

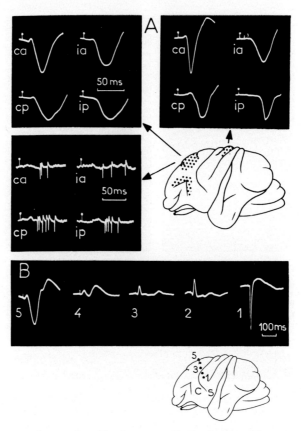

Fig. 39. Macaque monkey under chloralose anaesthesia. A: Type II convergent areas. Responses in areas 6 and 5 are presented. B: Response to contralateral stimulation of the hand recorded at 1 (primary projection) and at 5 (area 6, type II). Note absence of clear responses in between

Thus SII, orbital cortex and claustrum present heterosensory convergence (SII and claustrum being devoted to somato-auditory and orbital cortex to somato viscero-visual convergence). However they are not totally similar to the focus of type I convergence we have described in thalamus. They do not receive their main inflow from these thalamic zones. Even if convergent type I thalamic zones take some part in supplying these convergent cortical areas, they are not alone. Type I convergence is more characteristic of cortical areas than of thalamus.

d) A Special Convergent Area, the Nucleus Medialis of Amygdala. In this nucleus as well as in the nearby cortex, Wendt using macroelectrode recordings, observed large responses when the two anterior limbs were stimulated. This projection is mediated from the VP through the SII cortex. A pathway from SII through the claustrum was demonstrated. The ipsilateral projection observed in amygdala is mediated through the corpus callosum (Wendt and Albe-Fessard, 1961). Auditory and visual inflows also exist at this level. Units (Segundo and Machne,

1956; WENDT and ALBE-FESSARD, 1961) are driven by electrical peripheral stimuli. Responses in this region have some properties (short duration potentials, lemniscal pathways) in common with convergent cortical type I areas. However their high fatiguability and their susceptibility to anaesthetics make this area a special zone; the type of natural stimuli able to drive these cells has not yet been found.

e) **Suprasylvian Responses to Photic Stimulation Only.** A visual area of projection exists at the lateral border of the suprasylvian gyrus, just proximal to the auditory cortex. The evoked potentials recorded at this level persist after acute ablation of visual cortex (MARSHALL et al., 1943; DOTY, 1958; BIGNALL et al., 1966). This region is exclusively visual (THOMPSON et al., 1963b; BRUNER, 1965). It receives its visual inputs from GL and thalamus just medial to GL (Pulvinar and LP) (BRUNER, 1965), as well as from visual cortex (CLARE and BISHOP, 1954; HUBEL and WIESEL, 1965; BRUNER, 1965).

Anatomical pathways were described originating in pulvinar and LP and terminating at this level (WALLER and BARRIS, 1937; NIIMI et al., 1970; GRAYBIEL, 1970; HEATH and JONES, 1971). This area is just a special visual area receiving convergent visual messages from three main entrances of pure visual origin. No heterosensory convergence was found at this level.

We will not include in this review a description of convergent units in primary somatic, visual and auditory areas.

3. Cortical Areas Presenting Convergent Properties in the Monkey

Convergent heterotopic areas have been described in macaque monkeys, anaesthetized with chloralose, in parietal area 5 and premotor area 6 and near the sulcus arcuatus (Fig. 39) (ALBE-FESSARD et al., 1959).

Other types of convergence were found at the level of precentral cortex (WOOLSEY et al., 1947; RUCH et al., 1952; GARDNER and MORIN, 1953; MALIS et al., 1953; ADEY et al., 1954; KRUGER, 1956). This convergence is more organized than type II convergence. Often bilateral areas for hands or legs are separated. At a unitary level the convergence of afferents was shown to be frequently organized on the mode of reciprocal innervation; moreover the cells in these regions were driven essentially by peripheral movements and traction on muscle (ALBE-FESSARD and LIEBESKIND, 1966; O'BRIEN et al., 1971). A detailed examination of the characteristics of macaca motor cortex will not be made here.

We believe that only area 6, area 5 and the region of the arcuate sulcus are the homologue of the heterotopic zones of cortical type II convergence we have described in the cat (Fig. 39). This is suggested by the fact that the response characteristics (latency, waveform, fatigability) are similar. However, in the few experiments we have made, we were unable to find at these levels clear heterosensory convergence. BIGNALL and IMBERT (1969) on the other hand have found in macaca auditory responses at the level of the arcuate area of somatic heterotopic projections, but visual evoked responses were detected only in one of four animals studied and they were restricted to a small portion of this region. Thus species differences exist and if type II heterotopic convergence appears in macaque

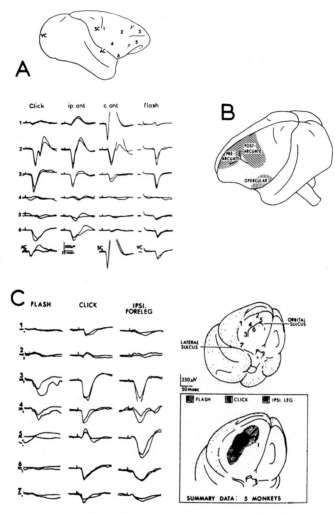

Fig. 40. Squirrel monkey under chloralose anaesthesia. A: Heterotopic and heterosensorial responses recorded in a frontal area. B: Regions where convergent responses are recorded in the superior surface of the hemisphere. C: Convergent heterosensory region at level of inferior frontal surface. (From Bignall and Imbert, 1969)

monkeys it lacks the total heterosensory convergent property it has in cat. Moreover the extension and the number of convergent zones are smaller.

In squirrel monkey, Bignall and Imbert (1969) have found different results. In these animals, where exploration of the entire frontal pole was made, four heterosensory zones were found (see Fig. 40):

— Two polysensory areas were described. One exists in the superior frontal surface extending onto the medial surfaces, possibly the homologue of the macaca area 6. Another was placed more anteriorly. Responses recorded at these two levels have many characteristics in common with type II convergent zones of the carnivores.

— Two other responsive areas were found: a fronto-opercular area, that perhaps extends deep in the insula and can be the homologue of the region called orbital cortex in the cat. This area presents also heterosensory convergence. Another area was found in the orbital cortex of the monkey (which shares only its name with orbital cortex of the cat). This region is probably also part of the convergent type II system.

The same authors have shown in squirrel monkey that primary sensory areas are not essential for elicitation of responses in frontal lobe, but they have shown also that cortico-cortical connections exist between primary and convergent areas. Thus, in this lower primate, regions having properties of cat convergent type II and type I cortical areas seem to exist.

E. On the Possible Functional Role of Convergent Systems

1. Influence of Anaesthetics

Convergent responses are not due, as it was often claimed, to an artefactual effect of chloralose anaesthesia. We hope that this fact is made obvious by the results presented in this article. Many of the figures illustrate convergent responses recorded in animals without anaesthesia and having only received spinal sections, cortical ablations or local analgesia. Other work, performed on chronically implanted animals, has given similar results. We want however to emphasize here that responses can be recorded in convergent type II zones only when the chronic animals are drowsy or in the slow wave stage of sleep, a fact that can explain the lack of results obtained when responses were looked for without regard to the state of alertness. Abnormal respiratory conditions can explain also certain of the discrepancies in the literature.

The results obtained under chloralose do not represent however a complete description of the properties of these complex areas which have convergent properties. They must not be discarded because certainly no new pathways can be created by an anaesthetic. Drugs can only exacerbate the role of these pathways (like chloralose) or suppress their invasion (like barbiturate). But, even if chloralose leaves intact the first burst of spikes which travels in the extralemniscal pathway, it provokes a general hyperpolarization of the membrane and silences many cells. It also prolongs strikingly all the inhibitory processes and thus distorts the unitary responses.

Hence, maps of pathways and studies of nuclear organization made under these anaesthetic conditions have to be considered essentially as a schema. On this schema, results of more sophisticated studies, using acute non-anaesthetized or chronic animals, have to be made to provide a better understanding of the role played by the convergent type II systems.

2. Role of Convergent Structures in Conditioning

That convergent structures play a role in sensory-sensory conditioning seems obvious. Indisputably, convergence between messages must occur somewhere in order for one type of nervous signal to replace another. This general opinion has frequently led to the hypothesis that such conditioning may be mediated by convergent type II areas in the reticular formation, thalamus or cortex. However, conditioning stimuli frequently possess specific properties (stimulus quality, or spatial and temporal characteristics) which are poorly or not at all represented in these convergent regions. If future studies in unanaesthetized animals fail to reveal a better specificity for convergent type II cells than is encountered under chloralose, other areas with greater properties of specificity must be found which permit nonetheless stimulus association and hence conditioning. The type I convergent system, and in particular its telencephalic component, seems on these grounds to be a promising candidate. As we have seen, specific messages can converge in these regions without much loss of qualitative, spatial and temporal information. Frequently pairs of modalities are represented (somatic-auditory, somatic-visual, etc...). A number of experiments have shown by the lesion technique the importance of the SII and orbital cortex as well as the claustrum in certain kinds of learning (see Albe-Fessard, 1971b). If the convergent type II system plays any role in conditioning of a sensory nature, it can only be when intensity is the relevant stimulus dimension, since this is the only stimulus characteristic clearly encoded by this system.

3. Role of Convergent Systems in Transmission of Sensory Messages

From clinical findings, it is well known that pathways in anterolateral columns are involved in mediating messages allowing pain and temperature perception. We will not examine here the problem of temperature which is treated elsewhere in this book, and examine only the problem of transmission of noxious messages. That the messages subserving pain (protopathic) are somewhere in the nervous system under the control of specific afferent systems (epicritic) is an old notion in neurology (see references in Albe-Fessard, 1967, 1968). From what we have said in section II, powerful controls coming from the specific systems are exerted in the spinal cord on messages transmitted by cells in layers IV and V, which send their impulses through the spino-cervico-thalamic bundle and the anterolateral pathways. All of these pathways therefore are candidates for mediating messages important for the appreciation of pain. The spino-cervico-thalamic tract seems at first examination not to be involved because of its ipsilateral dorsal position in the spinal cord and the knowledge that controlateral antero-lateral sections are the more effective in relieving patients from certain pain syndromes. However, since pain syndromes were studied in man whereas the position of the spino-cervico-thalamic tract was considered in cats we cannot discard without further examination the role in mediating noxious impulses of this pathway or its unknown homologue in Man.

The main termination of SCT and neo-spino-thalamic systems is as we have seen in the ventralis posterior and its supero-anterior border. This region, when considered alone, is in our opinion not involved in pain appreciation, because even very strong stimulation in this area (performed in patients with Parkinson's disease) never produced pain (Albe-Fessard et al., 1970b). On the contrary, stimulation in an area just inferior to ventralis posterior at the limit of thalamus and subthalamus, evokes pain sensation in patients having abnormal spontaneous pain (HASSLER, 1968; ALBE-FESSARD et al., 1970c) and even in patients without pain syndrome (HALLIDAY, 1971). If we consider that convergent type I responses of SCT and neo-spino-thalamic origin exist in cats and monkeys at this sub-VP level, we have reasons to believe that some convergent type I regions can be involved in pain appreciation. Cat orbital cortex seems to receive noxious stimuli also through the same sorts of pathways.

When noxious drugs are injected (technique proposed by LIM, 1968), unit responses often appear in convergent type II regions; thus the paleo-spino-thalamic and spino-reticulo-thalamic pathways are certainly also involved in the conduction of noxious stimuli. However, as we have said in the preceding section, these convergent type II regions cannot have a unique role in normal appreciation of pain, because this appreciation needs a certain specificity and local sign of which convergent type II responses are deprived.

The fact that CM-Pf was the first thalamic region to be clearly shown to receive anterolateral impulses has often led these nuclei to be considered as a pain appreciation centre. Admitting that the CM-Pf may have a role to play in this appreciation (see later), nevertheless we cannot consider it is the unique role in which this region is involved. Because, when stimuli are applied to a nerve in a cat through chronically implanted electrodes, large responses can be observed in CM for stimulus intensities that have no overt noxious effect. The animals seem to be unaffected by the stimulation and may even fall asleep under these conditions.

For all these reasons, if the convergent type II areas are involved in pain appreciation, it is not their only role and they are certainly not alone in serving such a function. Another system must be involved at the same time, one capable of analysing information concerning stimulus location and quality. This system must be the lemniscal one in the broad sense in which we have defined this term in section II (which differs from the classical one, see ROSE and MOUNTCASTLE, 1960).

If our explanation is correct, the sorts of stimuli, whose localization and temporal characteristics are appreciated in a lemniscal projection region, will result in a painful sensation only if some convergent nuclei receiving input through the antero-lateral bundle are also involved. That a complementary role in the awakening of pain sensation is played by dorsal column and antero-lateral pathways was also hypothetized on the basis of experimental cord sections performed in monkeys by VIERCK et al. (1970).

According to our hypothesis, pain will occur in two different situations.

1. *In Normal Man:* (1) if the stimulation is sufficiently strong to result in a converging inflow sufficiently powerful to outweigh the inhibitory controls exerted at the first spinal synapses of convergent pathways (WALL and TAUB, 1962) or (2) if facilitation through impulses conducted by slow myelinated or unmyelinated fibres appears at this level (MELZACK and WALL, 1965; HILLMAN and WALL, 1969).

2. *In Patients with Intractable Pain,* if some inhibition normally acting on these first spinal synapses is released, we know (see section II) that, at the level of first synapses in the cord, but also at bulbar, thalamic and cortical levels of the con-

vergent type II system, inhibitory actions occur coming from primary areas and driven by a lemniscal inflow. Thus we may suppose that this inhibition is released when a destructive lesion due to a disease process appears anywhere in this loop (peripheral nerve, dorsal roots, dorsal columns, ventralis posterior, cortex) or in the descending cortico-spinal or cortico-reticulo-spinal pathways.

A lesion produced at any point in the ascending portion of the loop will cause both a loss in discriminative sensibility and the appearance of poorly localized pain. The typical examples of these phenomena are the painful syndromes produced by: peripheral deafferentation, dorsal column interruption, lesions of bulbar or mesencephalic lemniscal pathways, or lesions involving ventralis posterior (the Dejerine-Roussy thalamic syndrome). If the origin of the appearance of abnormal pain has to be sought in a lack of inhibition acting on the synapses of the pathways to convergent areas, the same sort of consideration has driven people to seek the relief of painful syndromes by stimulating descending inhibitory pathways. Ervin et al. (1966) reported some success in relieving pain in man by stimulating the inhibitory system of caudate origin. In cases of pain due to deafferentation, Wall and Sweet (1967) had success in re-establishing segmental inhibitory phenomena, using light stimulation of the dorsal roots which gave rise to tactile sensation referred to the deafferented area (see also Shealy et al., 1971).

Recent studies reporting a marked augmentation in pain threshold by central stimulation in animals can certainly be explained in the same way (Reynolds, 1969; Mayer et al., 1971; Schmidek et al., 1971).

Finally, we must point out that facilitatory actions coming from cortex are exerted on different relays of pathways to convergent structures. The liberation of these facilitatory effects by suppression of inhibitory ones can explain the fact that central stimulation which in normal patients does not elicit pain, becomes extraordinary painful in patients suffering from spontaneous pain.

We wish to thank Dr. J. C. Liebeskind for his constructive advice and kind assistance in the organization of the English text, Mrs. C. De Besses for her invaluable help in preparing the bibliography and the text, Miss A. Trinson and Mr. J. L. Pierre, for their careful attention to the preparation of the illustrations.

References

Abdelmoumene, M., Besson, J. M., Aleonard, P.: Cortical area exerting presynaptic inhibitory action on the spinal cord in cat and monkey. Brain Res. **20**, 327–329 (1970).

Adey, W. R., Porter, R., Carter, I. D.: Temporal dispersion in cortical afferent volleys as a factor in perception; an evoked potential study of deep somatic sensibility in the monkey. Brain **77**, 344–352 (1954).

Adey, W. R., Segundo, J. P., Livingston, R. B.: Corticifugal influences on intrinsic brain stem conduction in cat and monkey. J. Neurophysiol. **20**, 1–16 (1957).

Adrian, E. D.: Double representation of the feet in the sensory cortex of the cat. J. Physiol. (Lond.) **98**, 16P (1940).

Adrian, E. D.: Afferent discharges to the cerebral cortex from peripheral sense organs. J. Physiol. (Lond.) **100**, 159–191 (1941).

Albe-Fessard, D.: Nouvelles données sur l'origine des composantes des potentiels évoqués somesthésiques. In: Actualités Neurophysiologiques, A. M. Monnier (ed.), vol. **3**, 23–59. Paris: Masson 1961.

Albe-Fessard, D.: Organisation of somatic central projections. In: Contribution to Sensory Physiology, W. D. Neff (ed.), **2**, 101–167. New York Academic Press 1965.

ALBE-FESSARD, D.: Central nervous mechanisms involved in pain and analgesia. In: Pharmacology of Pain, R.K.S. LIM (ed.), 131–168. Oxford-New York: Pergamon Press 1968.

ALBE-FESSARD, D.: Electrophysiologie cérébrale et électroencéphalographie. Encyclopédie Médico-Chirurgicale, 17031, 1 10, 1–12 (1971 a).

ALBE-FESSARD, D.: Multisensory projection areas and association phenomena. J. Activ. Nerv. Sup., Acad. Sci. U.R.S.S. **21**, 509–513 (1971 b).

ALBE-FESSARD, D., ARFEL, G., DEROME, P., DONDEY, M.: Electrophysiology of the human thalamus with special reference to trigeminal pain. In: Trigeminal Neuralgia, R. HASSLER and A.E. WALKER (eds.), 139–148. Stuttgart: Georg Thieme 1970 b.

ALBE-FESSARD, D., BESSON, J.M., ABDELMOUMENE, M.: Action of anesthetics on somatic evoked activities. In: International Anesthesiology Clinics: Anesthesia and Neurophysiology. H. H. YAMAMURA (ed.), vol. VIII, 129–166 (1970 a).

ALBE-FESSARD, D., BESSON, J.M., GUILBAUD, G., LEVANTE, A.: Cortical control of somatic inflow to medial thalamus. In Symposium on Corticothalamic Projections and Sensorimotor Activities. in press (1972).

ALBE-FESSARD, D., BOWSHER, D.: Responses of monkey thalamus to somatic stimuli under chloralose anaesthesia. Electroenceph. clin. Neurophysiol. **19**, 1–15 (1965).

ALBE-FESSARD, D., DONDEY, M., NICOLAIDIS, S., LE BEAU, J.: Remarks concerning the effect of diencephalic lesions on pain and sensitivity with special reference to lemniscally mediated control of noxious afferences. Confin. Neurol. **32**, 174–184 (1970 c).

ALBE-FESSARD, D., FESSARD, A.: Thalamic integrations and their consequences at the telencephalic level. Progr. Brain Res. **1**, 115–148 (1963).

ALBE-FESSARD, D., GILLETT, E.: Convergence d'afférences d'origine corticale et périphérique vers le CM du chat anesthésié ou éveillé. Electroenceph. clin. Neurophysiol. **13**, 257–269 (1961).

ALBE-FESSARD, D., KRUGER, L.: Duality of unit discharges from cat centrum medianum in response to natural and electrical stimuli. J. Neurophysiol. **25**, 1–20 (1962).

ALBE-FESSARD, D., LEVANTE, A., ROKYTA, R.: Cortical projections of cat medial thalamic cells. Int. J. Neurosci. **1**, 327–338 (1971).

ALBE-FESSARD, D., LIEBESKIND, J.C.: Origine des messages somato-sensitifs activant les cellules du cortex moteur chez le Singe. Exp. Brain Res. **1**, 127–146 (1966).

ALBE-FESSARD, D., MALLART, A., ALEONARD, P.: Réduction au cours du comportement attentif, de l'amplitude des réponses évoquées dans le centre médian du thalamus chez le chat éveillé libre, porteur d'électrodes à demeure. C.R. Acad. Sci. (Paris) **252**, 187–189 (1961).

ALBE-FESSARD, D., MASSION, J., HALL, R., ROSENBLITH, W.: Modifications au cours de la veille et du sommeil des valeurs moyennes des réponses nerveuses corticales induites par des stimulations somatiques chez le chat libre. C.R. Acad. Sci. (Paris) **258**, 353–356 (1964).

ALBE-FESSARD, D., OSWALDO-CRUZ, E., ROCHA-MIRANDA, C.E.: Activités évoquées dans le noyau caudé du chat en réponse à des types divers d'afférences. I. Etude macrophysiologique. Electroenceph. clin. Neurophysiol. **12**, 405–420 (1960a).

ALBE-FESSARD, D., OSWALDO-CRUZ, E., ROCHA-MIRANDA, C.: Activités évoquées dans le noyau caudé du chat en réponse à des types divers d'afférences. II. Etude microphysiologique. Electroenceph. clin. Neurophysiol. **12**, 649–661 (1960b).

ALBE-FESSARD, D., ROCHA-MIRANDA, C., OSWALDO-CRUZ, E.: Activités d'origine somesthésiques évoquées au niveau du cortex non-specifique et du centre médian du thalamus chez le singe anesthésié au chloralose. Electroenceph. clin. Neurophysiol. **11**, 777–787 (1959).

ALBE-FESSARD, D., ROUGEUL, A.: Activités bilatérales tardives évoquées sur le cortex du chat sous chloralose, par stimulation d'une voie somesthésique. J. Physiol. (Paris) **47**, 69–72 (1955).

ALBE-FESSARD, D., ROUGEUL, A.: Activités d'origine somesthésique évoquées sur le cortex non spécifique du chat anesthésié au chloralose: Rôle du centre médian du thalamus. Electroenceph. clin. Neurophysiol. **10**, 131–152 (1958).

ALLISON, T.: Cortical and subcortical evoked responses to central stimuli during wakefulness and sleep. Electroenceph. clin. Neurophysiol. **18**, 131–139 (1965).

ALTMAN, J.: Some fiber projections to the superior colliculus in the cat. J. comp. Neurol. **119**, 77–88 (1962).

Altman, J., Carpenter, M.B.: Fiber projections of the superior colliculus in the cat. J. comp. Neurol. **116**, 157–178 (1961).

Amassian, V.E.: Studies on organization of a somesthetic association area, including a single unit analysis. J. Neurophysiol. **17**, 39–58 (1954).

Andersen, P., Andersson, S.A.: Physiological basis of the alpha rhythm. A. Towe (ed.), 235 p. New York: Appleton-Century-Crofts 1968.

Andersen, P., Eccles, J.C., Sears, T.A.: Presynaptic inhibitory action of cerebral cortex on spinal cord. Nature (Lond.) **194**, 740–743 (1962).

Andersen, P., Eccles, J.C., Sears, T.A.: Cortically evoked depolarization of primary afferent fibres in the spinal cord. J. Neurophysiol. **27**, 63–77 (1964).

Anderson, F.D., Berry, C.M.: Degeneration studies of long ascending fiber systems in the cat brain stem. J. comp. Neurol. **111**, 195–229 (1959).

Andersson, S.A.: Projection of different spinal pathways to the second somatic sensory area in cat. Acta physiol. scand. **56**, Suppl. 194, 74 (1962).

Andersson, S.A., Manson, J.R.: Rhythmic activity in the thalamus of the unanaesthetized decorticate cat. Electroenceph. clin. Neurophysiol. **31**, 21–34 (1971).

Angaut, P.: Etude anatomique expérimentale des efférences cérébelleuses ascendantes. Analyse électroanatomique des projections cérébelleuses sur le noyau ventral latéral du thalamus. Thèse Sci. (Paris) 186 p. (1969).

Angaut, P., Guilbaud, G., Reymond, M.C.: An electrophysiological study of the cerebellar projections to the nucleus ventralis lateralis of thalamus in the cat. I. Nuclei Fastigii and Interpositus. J. comp. Neurol. **124**, 9–20 (1968).

Ascher, P.: Rôle de la voie lemniscale dans l'élaboration des réponses motrices extrapyramidales à des stimulations somesthésiques. J. Physiol. (Paris) **56**, 278 (1964).

Bailey, P., Bremer, F.: A sensory cortical representation of the vagus nerve. J. Neurophysiol. **1**, 405–412 (1938).

Barron, D.M., Matthews, B.M.C.: Electrotonus in ventral roots of the spinal cord. J. Physiol. (Lond.) **87**, 26–27 (1936).

Barron, D.M., Matthews, B.M.C.: The interpretation of potentials changes in the spinal cord. J. Physiol. (Lond.) **92**, 276–321 (1938).

Batini, C., Castellanos, G., Buser, P.: Activations directe et réflexe des projections corticales cérébelleuses issues du cortex moteur et du cortex orbitaire. Arch. ital. Biol. **104**, 50–72 (1965).

Batini, C., Imbert, M.: Efferences corticifuges "non pyramidales" au niveau du pédoncule cérébral. Arch. ital. Biol. **103**, 421–447 (1965).

Baumgarten, R.V., Mollica, A., Moruzzi, G.: Influence of the motor cortex on the spike discharges of bulbo-reticular neurons. Electroenceph. clin. Neurophysiol. Suppl. 3, 58–68 (1963).

Becker, D.P., Gluck, H., Nulsen, F.E., Jane, J.A.: An inquiry into the neurophysiological basis for pain. J. Neurosurg. **30**, 1–13 (1969).

Benjamin, R.M.: Single neurons in the rat medulla responsive to nociceptive stimulation. Brain Res. **24**, 525–529 (1970).

Benita, M., Conde, H.: Etude des efférences du noyau centre médian du thalamus du chat vers le cortex et les structures strio-pallidales. Exp. Brain Res. **12**, 204–222 (1971).

Bergmans, J., Colle, J., Lafere, Y.: Etude électrophysiologique des relations entre les membres antérieurs et postérieurs chez la grenouille. J. Physiol. (Paris) **56**, 290–291 (1964).

Berman, A.L.: Overlap of somatic and auditory cortical response fields in anterior ectosylvian gyrus of cat. J. Neurophysiol. **24**, 595–607 (1961a).

Berman, A.L.: Interactions of cortical responses to somatic and auditory stimuli in anterior ectosylvian gyrus of cat. J. Neurophysiol. **24**, 608–620 (1961b).

Besson, J.M., Abdelmoumene, M.: Modifications of dorsal root potentials during cortical seizures. Electroenceph. clin. Neurophysiol. **29**, 166–172 (1970).

Besson, J.M., Abdelmoumene, M., Aleonard, P., Conseiller, C.: Effects des anesthésiques sur les différentes composantes des potentiels de racine dorsale. J. Physiol. (Paris) **60**, 217 (1968b).

Besson, J.M., Abdelmoumene, M., Rivot, J.P., Conseiller, C., Aleonard, P.: Potentiels radiculaires dorsaux provoqués par la stimulation du noyau caudé. J. Physiol. (Paris) **60**, 350 (1968a).

Besson, J.M., Conseiller, C., Hamann, K.-F., Maillard, M.C., Aleonard, P.: Mcdifications de l'activité unitaire des neuroncs de la corne dorsale de la moelle sous l'effet de l'injection intra-artérielle de bradykinine au niveau du membre postérieur chez le chat. J. Physiol. (Paris) **63**, 171A–172A (1971).

Besson, J.M., Conseiller, C., Hamann, K.-F., Maillard, M.C.: Modifications of dorsal horn cell activities in the spinal cord, after intra-arterial injection of Bradykinin. J. Physiol. (Lond.) **221**, 189–205 (1972).

Besson, J.M., Rivot, J.P.: Heterosegmental, heterosensory and cortical inhibitory effects on dorsal horn interneurons in the cat's spinal cord. Electroenceph. clin. Neurophysiol. in press (1972).

Besson, J.M., Rivot, J.P., Abdelmoumene, M., Aleonard, P.: Etude de l'action des anesthésiques sur l'activité des cellules de la corne dorsale de la moelle. J. Physiol. (Paris) **62**, 350–351 (1970).

Bignall, K.E.: Effects of subcortical ablations on polysensory cortical responses and interactions in the cat. Exp. Neurol. **18**, 56–67 (1967).

Bignall, K.E., Imbert, M.: Polysensory and cortico-cortical projections to frontal lobe of squirrel and rhesus monkey. Electroenceph. clin. Neurophysiol. **26**, 206–215 (1969).

Bignall, K.E., Imbert, P., Buser, P.: Optic projections to non-visual cortex of the cat. J. Neurophysiol. **29**, 396–409 (1966).

Bishop, G.H., Clare, M.H.: Organization and distribution of fibers in the optic tract of the cat. J. comp. Neurol. **103**, 269–304 (1955).

Boisacq-Schepens, N.: Etude microphysiologique de l'organisation fonctionnelle du cortex sensori-moteur. Effects prolongés de stimulations sensorielles. Relation entre afférences sensorielles et efférence pyramidale. Thèse d'Agrégation (Bruxelles) 279 p., Vander Pub., (1971).

Boisacq-Schepens, N., Crommelinck, M., Hanus, M.: Relation au niveau des neurones du cortex précrucié du chat entre l'organisation des afférences sensorielles et le type de projection efférente testé au moyen de la stimulation électrique antidromique du faisceau pyramidal. J. Physiol. (Paris) **60**, 406–407 (1968).

Boisacq-Schepens, N., Crommelinck, M., Hanus, M.: Influence de la stimulation visuelle sur les réponses sensorielles somatiques des neurones du cortex moteur chez le chat identifiés par test antidromique. Arch. intern. Physiol. Biochem. **77**, 328–329 (1969).

Boivie, J.: The termination of the cervicothalamic tract in cat. An experimental study with silver impregnation method. Brain Res. **19**, 330–360 (1970).

Boivie, J.: The termination in the thalamus and the zona incerta of fibres from the dorsal column nuclei (DCN) in the cat. An experimental study with silver impregnation method. Brain Res. **28**, 459–490 (1971).

Boivie, J.: The termination of the spinothalamic tract in the Cat. An experimental study with silver impregnation methods. Exp. Brain Res. in press (1972).

Borenstein, P., Buser, P.: Observations sur les projections du cortex dans la formation réticulée mésencéphalique chez le Chat. C.R. Soc. Biol. (Paris) **154**, 38–40 (1960).

Bowsher, D.: Termination of the central pain pathway in man: the conscious appreciation of pain. Brain **80**, 606–622 (1957).

Bowsher, D.: Projection of the gracile and cuneate nuclei in Macaca Mulatta. An experimental degeneration study. J. comp. Neurol. **110**, 135–155 (1958).

Bowsher, D.: The termination of secondary somatosensory neurons within the thalamus of Macaca Mulatta: an experimental degeneration study. J. comp. Neurol. **117**, 213–228 (1961).

Bowsher, D.: The topographical projection of fibres from the antero-lateral quadrant of the spinal cord to the subdiencephalic brain stem in Man. Mschr. Psychiat. Neurol. **143**, 75–99 (1962).

Bowsher, D.: Some afferent and efferent connections of the Parafascicular — Centre Median complex. In: The Thalamus, D.P. Purpura and M.D. Yahr (eds.), pp. 99–108. New York-London: Columbia Univ. Press 1966.

Bowsher, D., Angaut, P., Conde, H.: Projections des noyaux cérébelleux sur le noyau ventro-latéral du thalamus: confrontation des résultats acquis par la technique anatomique et par la technique électrophysiologique. J. Physiol. (Paris) **57**, 570 (1965).

Bowsher, D., Mallart, A., Petit, D., Albe-Fessard, D.: A bulbar relay to the centre median. J. Neurophysiol. **31**, 288–300 (1968).

Bremer, F.: Les aires auditives de l'écorce cérébrale. 22 p. (Cours Intern. d'Audiologie Clinique) 1952.

Bremer, F., Bonnet, V., Terzuolo, C.: Etude électrophysiologique des aires auditives corticales du chat. Arch. intern. Physiol. **3**, 390–428.

Brodal, A.: Neurological anatomy in relation to clinical medicine. Second Edition, 807 p., Oxford: University Press 1969.

Brodal, A., Rexed, B.: Spinal afferents to the lateral cervical nucleus in the cat. An experimental study. J. comp. Neurol. **98**, 179–213 (1953).

Brooks, V. B.: Some factors governing sensory convergence in the cat's motor cortex. In: Studies in Physiology, D. R. Curtis and A. K. McIntyre (eds.), pp. 13–17. Berlin-Heidelberg-New York: Springer 1965.

Brooks, V. B., Rudomin, P., Slayman, C. L.: Sensory activation of neurons in the cat's cerebral cortex. J. Neurophysiol. **24**, 286–301 (1961a).

Brooks, V. B., Rudomin, P., Slayman, C. L.: Peripheral receptive fields of neurons in the cat's cerebral cortex. J. Neurophysiol. **24**, 302–325 (1961b).

Brown, A. G.: Effects of descending impulses on transmission through the spinocervical tract. J. Physiol. (Lond.) **219**, 103–125 (1971).

Brown, A. G., Franz, D. N.: Responses of spinocervical tract neurones to natural stimulation of identified cutaneous receptors. Exp. Brain Res. **7**, 231–249 (1969).

Brown, P. B.: Descending control of the spinocervical tract in decerebrate cats. Brain Res. **17**, 152–155 (1970).

Bruner, J.: Réponses visuelles et acoustiques au niveau de la face médiane antérieure du cortex chez le chat sous chloralose. J. Physiol. (Paris) **52**, 36 (1960).

Bruner, J.: Afférences visuelles non-primaires vers le cortex cérébral chez le Chat. J. Physiol. (Paris) **56**, 1–120 (Suppl. 12) (1965).

Bruner, J., Sindberg, R.: Différentiation de deux catégories de projections visuelles non-primaires sur le cortex associatif suprasylvien du Chat. Influences de la formation réticulée et du cortex visuel. J. Physiol. (Paris) **54**, 303 (1962).

Burgess, P. R.: A study of the transmission of sensory information in the cat spinal cord. New York: Ph. D. Thesis, Rockefeller Institute 1965.

Burke, R. E., Rudomin, P., Vyklicky, L., Zajac III, F. E.: Primary afferent depolarization and flexion reflexes produced by radiant heat stimulation of the skin. J. Physiol. (Lond.) **213**, 185–215.

Burton, H.: Somatic sensory properties of caudal bulbar reticular neurons in the cat (Felix Domestica). Brain Res. **11**, 357–372 (1968).

Busch, H. F. M.: An anatomical analysis of the white matter in the brain stem of the cat. Thesis, 116 p. Assen: Van Gorcum 1961.

Buser, P., Ascher, P.: Mise en jeu réflexe du système pyramidal chez le chat. Arch. ital. Biol. **98**, 123–164 (1960).

Buser, P., Bignall, K. E.: Non primary sensory projections on the cat neocortex. Int. Rev. Biol. **10**, 111–165 (1967).

Buser, P., Borenstein, P.: Réponses somesthésiques, visuelles et auditives recueillies au niveau du cortex "associatif" suprasylvien chez le chat curarisé non anesthésié. Electroenceph. clin. Neurophysiol. **11**, 299–304 (1959).

Buser, P., Borenstein, P., Bruner, J.: Etude des systèmes "associatifs" visuels et auditifs chez le chat anesthésié au chloralose. Electrocenceph. clin. Neurophysiol. **11**, 305–325 (1959).

Buser, P., Bruner, J., Sindberg, R. M.: Influences of the visual cortex upon posteromedial thalamus in the cat. J. Neurophysiol. **26**, 677–691 (1963).

Buser, P., Imbert, M.: Sensory projections to motor cortex in cats: a microelectrode study. In: Sensory Communication, W. A. Rosenblith (ed.), p. 607–626. Cambridge Mass.: M.I.T. Press 1961.

BUSER, P., VIALA, G.: Facilitation de réponses sous-corticales non spécifiques après tétanisation de l'hippocampe chez le Lapin. J. Physiol. (Paris) 55, 118 (1963).

BYSTRZYCKA, E., KORN, H.: Origine et topographie des projections du nerf splanchnique sur le cortex anterior chez le Chat. C.R. Acad. Sci. (Paris) 268, 566–568 (1969).

CAJAL, RAMÓN Y S.: Histologie du système nerveux de l'homme et des vertébrés. Maloine Ed. (Paris), Vol. I, 986 p. (1909).

CARPENTER, D., ENGBERG, I., LUNDBERG, A.: Presynaptic inhibition in the lumbar cord evoked from the brain stem. Experientia (Basel) 18, 450–451 (1962b).

CARPENTER, D., ENGBERG, I., LUNDBERG, A.: Primary afferent depolarization evoked from the brain and the cerebellum. Arch. ital. Biol. 104, 73–85 (1966).

CARPENTER, D., LUNDBERG, A., NORRSELL, U.: Effects from the pyramidal tract on primary afferents and on spinal reflex actions to primary afferents. Experientia (Basel) 18, 337–338 (1962a).

CARPENTER, D., LUNDBERG, A., NORRSELL, U.: Primary afferent depolarization evoked from the sensorimotor cortex. Acta physiol. scand. 59, 126–142 (1963).

CASEY, K.L.: Somatosensory responses of bulbo-reticular units in awake cat: relation to escape-producing stimuli. Science 173, 77–80 (1971a).

CASEY, K.L.: Responses of bulbo-reticular units to somatic stimuli eliciting escape behaviour in the cat. Int. J. Neurosci. 2, 15–28 (1971b).

CAZARD, P., BUSER, P.: Modifications des réponses sensorielles corticales par stimulation de l'hippocampe dorsal chez le lapin. Electroenceph. clin. Neurophysiol. 15, 413–425 (1963)

CHRISTENSEN, B.N., PERL, E.R.: Spinal neurons specifically excited by noxious or thermal stimuli: Marginal zone of the dorsal horn. J. Neurophysiol. 33, 293–307 (1970).

CLARE, M.H., BISHOP, G.H.: Responses from association area secondarily activated from optic cortex. J. Neurophysiol. 17, 271–277 (1954).

COHEN, B., HOUSEPIAN, E.M., PURPURA, D.: Intrathalamic regulation of activity in a cerebello-cortical projection system. Exp. Neurol. 6, 492–506 (1962).

CONDE, H., ANGAUT, P.: An electrophysiological study of the cerebellar projections to the nucleus ventralis lateralis of thalamus on the cat. II. Nucleus lateralis. Brain Res. 20 107–119 (1970).

CONDE, H., SCHMIED, A., BENITA, M.: Quelques données électrophysiologiques sur les efférences du centre médian du thalamus. J. Physiol. (Paris) 60, 420 (1968).

DARIAN-SMITH, I.: Neural mechanisms of facial sensation. Int. Rev. Neurobiol. 9, 301–395 (1966).

DARIAN-SMITH, I., PHILLIPS, G., RYAN, R.D.: Functional organization of the trigeminal main sensory and rostral spinal nuclei of the cat. J. Physiol. (Lond.) 168, 129–146 (1963).

DARIAN-SMITH, I., YOKOTA, T.: Cortically evoked depolarization of trigeminal cutaneous afferent fibers in the cat. J. Neurophysiol. 27, 78–91 (1964).

DE JONG, R.H., ROBLES, R., HEAVNER, J.E.: Suppression of impulse transmission in the cat's dorsal horn by inhalation of anesthetics. Anesthesiology 32, 440–445 (1970).

DE JONG, R.H., ROBLES, R., MORIKAWA, K.: Actions of halothane and nitrous oxide on dorsal horn neurons ("the spinal gate"). Anesthesiology 31, 205–212 (1969).

DE JONG, R.H., WAGMAN, I.H.: Block of afferent impulses in the dorsal horn of monkey. A possible mechanism of anesthesia. Exp. Neurol. 20, 352–358 (1968).

DELL, P., OLSON, R.: Projections secondaires mésencéphaliques, diencéphaliques et amygdaliennes des afférences viscérales vagales. C.R. Soc. Biol. (Paris) 145, 1088–1091 (1951).

DENAVIT, M.: Zone subthalamique intervenant dans le comportement de veille et de sommeil. Etude des afférences sensorielles qui l'activent. Thèse Sci., Paris, 171 p. (1968).

DENAVIT, M., KOSINSKI, E.: Somatic afferents to the cat subthalamus. Arch. ital. Biol. 106, 391–411 (1968).

DESMEDT, J.E., MECHELSE, K.: Mise en évidence d'une quatrième aire de projection acoustique dans l'écorce cérébrale du chat. J. Physiol. (Paris) 51, 448–449 (1959).

DIAMOND, I.T., CHOW, K.L., NEFF, W.D.: Degeneration of caudal medial geniculate body following cortical lesion ventral to auditory area II in the cat. J. comp. Neurol. 109, 349–362 (1958).

Dilly, P. N., Wall, P. D., Webster, K. E.: Cells of origin of the spinothalamic tract in the Cat and Rat. Exp. Neurol. **21**, 550–562 (1968).

Dormont, J. F., Massion, J.: Etude des relations entre les aires sensori-motrices et le noyau ventro-latéral du thalamus chez le Chat. J. Physiol. (Paris) **57**, 603–604 (1965).

Doty, R. W.: Potentials evoked in cat cerebral cortex by diffuse and by punctiform photic stimuli. J. Neurophysiol. **21**, 437–464 (1958).

Dow, B. M., Dubner, R.: Visual receptive fields and responses to movement in an association area of cat cerebral cortex. J. Neurophysiol. **32**, 773–784 (1969).

Drooglever-Fortuyn, J., Stefens, R.: On the anatomical relation of the intralaminar and midline cells. Electroenceph. clin. Neurophysiol. **3**, 393–400 (1951).

Dubner, R.: Single cell analysis of sensory interaction in anterior lateral and suprasylvian gyri of the cat cerebral cortex. Exp. Neurol. **12**, 255–273 (1966).

Dubner, R.: Interaction of peripheral and central input in the main sensory trigeminal nucleus of the Cat. Exp. Neurol. **17**, 186–202 (1967).

Dubner, R., Rutledge, L. T.: Recording and analysis of converging input upon neurons in cat association cortex. J. Neurophysiol. **27**, 620–634 (1964).

Dubner, R., Rutledge, L. T.: Intracellular recording of the convergence of input upon neurons in cat association cortex. Exp. Neurol. **12**, 349–369 (1965).

Eccles, J. C.: The Physiology of Synapses. 316 p. Berlin-Göttingen-Heidelberg-New York: Springer 1964.

Eccles, J. C., Eccles, R. M., Lundberg, A.: Types of neurone in and around the intermediate nucleus of the lumbosacral cord. J. Physiol. (Lond.) **154**, 89–114 (1960).

Eccles, J. C., Kostyuk, P. G., Schmidt, R. F.: Central pathways responsible for depolarization of primary afferent fibres. J. Physiol. (Lond.) **161**, 237–257 (1962).

Eccles, J. C., Schmidt, R. F., Willis, W. D.: Pharmacological studies on presynaptic inhibition. J. Physiol. (Lond.) **168**, 500–530 (1963).

Ervin, F. R., Brown, C. E., Mark, V. H.: Striatal influence on facial pain. 2nd Int. Symp. Steroeencephalotomy (Vienne, 1965). Confin. Neurol. (Basel) **27**, 75–86 (1966).

Evarts, E.: Temporal patterns of discharge of pyramidal tract neurons during sleep and waking in the monkey. J. Neurophysiol. **27**, 152–171 (1964).

Favale, E., Loeb, C., Manfredi, M.: Somatic responses evoked by central stimulation during natural sleep and during arousal. Arch. intern. Physiol. Biochem. **71**, 229–235 (1963).

Feeney, D. M., Schlag, J. D., Villablanca, J., Waszack, M.: Depression of centrum medianum complex response by rostral thalamis lesions. Exp. Neurol. **26**, 401–410 (1970).

Feldman, S., Porter, R. W.: Long latency responses evoked in the anterior brain stem under pentobarbital anesthesia. Electroenceph. clin. Neurophysiol. **12**, 111–118 (1960).

Feltz, P., Krauthamer, G., Albe-Fessard, D.: Neurons of the medial diencephalon. I. Somatosensory responses and caudate inhibition. J. Neurophysiol. **30**, 55–80 (1967).

Feng, T. P., Liu, Y. M., Shen, E.: Pathways mediating irradiation of auditory and visual impulses to the sensorimotor cortex. 20th Intern. Congr. Physiol. Sci., Brussels, Comm. p. 997 (1956).

Fetz, E. E.: Pyramidal tract effects on interneurons in the cat lumbar dorsal horn. J. Neurophysiol. **31**, 69–80 (1968).

Fields, H. L., Partridge, L. D., Jr., Winter, D. L.: Somatic and visceral receptive field properties of fibers in ventral quadrant white matter of the cat spinal cord. J. Neurophysiol. **33**, 827–837 (1970).

Foerster, O.: (Bumbke et Foerster, Handbuch der Neurologie) **5**, 1–403 (1936).

Franz, D. N., Iggo, A.: Dorsal root potentials and ventral root reflexes evoked by nonmyelinated fibres. Science **162**, 1140–1142 (1968).

French, J. D., Verzeano, M., Magoun, H. W.: An extralemniscal sensory system of the brain. Arch. Neurol. Psychiat. (Chic.) **69**, 505–518 (1953a).

French, J. D., Verzeano, M., Magoun, H. W.: A neural basis of the anesthetic state. Arch. Neurol. Psychiat. (Chic.) **69**, 519–529 (1953b).

Gardner, E. D., Morin, F.: Spinal pathways for projection of cutaneous and muscular afferents to the sensory and motor cortex of the monkey (Macaca Mulatta). Amer. J. Physiol. **174**, 149–154 (1953).

GASSER, M.S., GRAHAM, H.T.: Potentials produced in the spinal cord by stimulation of the dorsal roots. Amer. J. Physiol. **103**, 303–320 (1933).

GASTAUT, H., HUNTER, J.: An experimental study of the mechanism of photic activation in idiopathic epilepsy. Electroenceph. clin. Neurophysiol. **2**, 263–287 (1950).

GAZE, R.M., GORDON, G.: Representation of cutaneous sense in the thalamus of cat and monkey. Quart. J. exp. Physiol. **9**, 279–304 (1954).

GODFRAIND, J.M., MEULDERS, M., VERAART, C.: Visual receptive fields of neurons in Pulvinar, nucleus lateralis-posterior and nucleus suprageniculatus thalami of the Cat. Brain Res. **15**, 552–555 (1969).

GORDON, G., LANDGREN, S., SEED, W.A.: The functional characteristics of single cells in the caudal part of the spinal nucleus of the trigeminal nerve of the cat. J. Physiol. (Lond.) **158**, 544–559 (1961).

GRANT, G., BOIVIE, J., BRODAL, A.: The question of a cerebellar projection from the lateral cervical nucleus re-examined. Brain Res. **9**, 95–102 (1968).

GRAYBIEL, A.M.: Some thalamocortical projections of the pulvinar-posterior system of the thalamus in the cat. Brain Res. **22**, 131–136 (1970).

GUILBAUD, G.: Evolution au cours du sommeil naturel des réponses somatiques évoquées en différents niveaux corticaux et sous-corticaux chez le Chat. Thèse Sci., Paris, 93 p. (1968).

GUILBAUD, G.: Essai de classification des structures centrales au moyen des variations d'amplitude de leurs réponses évoquées somatiques au cours des cycles veille-sommeil. Electroenceph. clin. Neurophysiol. **28**, 340–350 (1970).

GUILBAUD, G., KREUTZER, M., MENETREY, D., GUANO, G.: Effets de l'ablation des aires corticales primaires sur les variations au cours du sommeil, des réponses évoquées au niveau du système extralemniscal par différentes modalités. J. Physiol. (Paris) **62**, 385–386 (1970).

GUILBAUD, G., MENETREY, D.: Rôle joué par les voies et aires de projection lemniscales dans le contrôle des afférences extralemniscales au cours du sommeil naturel chez le chat. Electroenceph. clin. Neurophysiol. **29**, 295–302 (1970).

GUILLERY, R.W., ADRIAN, H.O., WOOLSEY, C.N., ROSE, J.E.: Thalamic integration of sensory and motor activities. In: "The Thalamus", M.D. YAHR and D. PURPURA (eds.), pp. 197–207. New York-London: Columbia University Press 1966.

HA, H., MORIN, F.: Comparative anatomical observations of the cervical nucleus, N. cervicalis lateralis, of some primates. Anat. Rec. **148**, 374–375 (1964).

HAGBARTH, K.E., FEX, J.: Centrifugal influences on single units activity in spinal sensory paths. J. Neurophysiol. **22**, 321–338 (1959).

HAGBARTH, K.E., KERR, D.I.B.: Central influences on spinal afferent conduction. J. Neurophysiol. **17**, 295–307 (1954).

HALLIDAY, A.M.: Personal Communication (1971).

HARMAN, P.J., BERRY, C.M.: Neuroanatomical distribution of action potentials evoked by photic stimulation in cat fore- and midbrain. J. comp. Neurol. **105**, 395–416 (1956).

HASSLER, R.: Anatomy of the thalamus. In: "Introduction to stereotaxis with an atlas of the human brain. G. SCHALTENBRANDT and P. BAILEY. Stuttgart: Georg Thieme, p. 230–290, 1959.

HASSLER, R.: Interrelationship of cortical and subcortical pain systems. In: Pharmacology of Pain, R.K.S. LIM (ed.), pp. 219–229 Oxford-New York: Pergamon Press 1968.

HEAD, H.: Studies in Neurology. Londres, vol. I (1920).

HEATH, C.J., JONES, E.G.: An experimental study of ascending connection from the posterior group of thalamic nuclei in the cat. J. comp. Neurol. **141**, 397–426 (1971).

HERNÀNDEZ-PÈON, R., HAGBARTH, K.E.: Interaction between afferent and cortically induced reticular responses. J. Neurophysiol. **18**, 44–45 (1965).

HILLMAN, P., WALL, P.D.: Inhibition and excitation factors influencing the receptive fields of lamina 5 spinal cord cells. Exp. Brain Res. **9**, 284–306 (1969).

HODES, R.: Lower cortical threshold in rapid eye movements periods than during sleep. Fed. Proc. **23**, 208 (1964).

HONGO, T., JANKOWSKA, E.: Effects from the sensorimotor cortex on the spinal cord in cats with transected pyramids. Exp. Brain Res. **3**, 117–134 (1967).

Hongo, T., Jankowska, E., Lundberg, A.: Post-synaptic excitation and inhibition from primary afferents in neurones of the spinocervical tract. J. Physiol. (Lond.) 199, 569–592 (1968).

Hubel, D. H., Wiesel, T. N.: Receptive fields and functional architecture in two non-striate visual areas (18 and 19) in the cat. J. Neurophysiol. 28, 229–289 (1965).

Hughes, J. R.: Studies on the supra-callosal mesial cortex of unanesthetized conscious mammals. I. Cat. B. Electrical activity. Electroenceph. clin. Neurophysiol. 11, 459–469 (1959).

Hunter, J., Ingvar, D. H.: Pathways mediating metrasol induced irradiation of visual impulses. Electroenceph. clin. Neurophysiol. 7, 39–60 (1955).

Imbert, M.: Recherches sur l'organisation de l'aire motrice et du gyrus orbitaire du cortex cérébral chez le chat. Thèse Sci. 183 p., Paris (1967).

Ingvar, D. H., Hunter, J.: Influence of visual cortex on light impulses in the brainstem of the unanesthetized cat. Acta physiol. scand. 33, 194–218 (1955).

Jane, J. A., Yashon, D., Diamond, I. T.: An anatomic basis for multimodal thalamic units. Exp. Neurol. 22, 464–471 (1968).

Jankowska, E., Albe-Fessard, D.: Sur l'origine et l'interprétation de la seconde phase du potentiel évoqué primaire de l'aire somatique. J. Physiol. (Paris) 53, 374 (1961).

Jasper, H. H.: Unspecific thalamocortical relations. In: Handbook of Physiology, Neurophysiology, J. Field (ed.), p. 1307–1321. Baltimore: Williams and Wilkins 1960.

Jasper, H. H., Ajmone-Marsan, C.: A stereotaxic atlas of the diencephalon of the cat. Totonto: Univ. Toronto Press 1954.

Kinston, W. J., Vadas, M. A., Bishop, P. O.: Multiple projection of the visual field to the medial portion of the dorsal lateral geniculate nucleus and the adjacent nuclei of the thalamus of the cat. J. comp. Neurol. 136, 295–316 (1969).

Kitahata, L. M., Taub, A., Sato, L.: Lamina-specific suppression of dorsal horn unit activity by nitrous oxide and by hyperventilation. J. Pharmacol. exp. Ther. 176, 101–108 (1971).

Korn, H.: Organisation des projections somatiques et végétatives sur le cortex orbitaire et contrôle cortical des réflexes viscéro-moteurs chez le Chat. Thèse Sci., Paris, pp. 175 (1967).

Korn, H., Richard, P.: Participation des faisceaux spino-cervico-thalamique et néo-spino-thalamique à la transmission des messages somatiques vers le cortex orbitaire du Chat. Electroenceph. clin. Neurophysiol. 24, 514–531 (1968).

Korn, H., Wendt, R., Albe-Fessard, D.: Somatic projection to the orbital cortex of the Cat. Electroenceph. clin. Neurophysiol. 21, 209–226 (1966).

Kornhuber, H. H., Dafonseca, J. S.: Optovestibular integration in the cat's cortex: a study of sensory convergence on cortical neurons. In: The Oculo-Motor System, M. B. Bender (ed.), pp. 239–279 (1964).

Krauthamer, G., Albe-Fessard, D.: Electrophysiologic studies of the basal ganglia and striopallidal inhibition of non-specific afferent activity. Neuropsychologia 2, 73–83 (1964).

Krauthamer, G., Albe-Fessard, D.: Inhibition of non-specific sensory activities following strio-pallidal and capsular stimulation. J. Neurophysiol. 28, 100–124 (1965).

Kruger, L.: Characteristics of the somatic afferent projection to the precentral cortex in the monkey. Amer. J. Physiol. 186, 475–482 (1956).

Kruger, L., Albe-Fessard, D.: Distribution of responses to somatic afferent stimuli in the diencephalon of the cat under chloralose anesthesia. Exp. Neurol. 2, 442–467 (1960).

Kusama, T., Otani, K., Kawana, E.: Projections of the motor somatic, sensory and visual cortices in cats. In: Progress in Brain Research, T. Tokizane and J. P. Schadé (eds.), Vol. 21, Part A, pp. 292–322. Amsterdam: Elsevier Publishing Co 1966.

Lamarche, G., Langlois, J. M.: Les neurones de la formation réticulaire pontobulbaire et la stimulation trigéminale. Canad. J. Biochem. 40, 261–271 (1962).

Lamarre, Y., Cordeau, J. P.: Activités des neurones contraux chez le singe porteur d'un tremblement postural expérimental. J. Physiol. (Paris) 56, 589–591 (1964).

Lamarre, Y., Cordeau, J. P.: Etude du mécanisme physiopathologique responsable, chez le singe, d'un tremblement expérimental de type Parkinsonien. Actualités Neurophysiologiques, 7ème Série. Paris: Masson 1967.

Lamarre, Y., Filion, M., Cordeau, J. P.: Neuronal discharges of the ventrolateral nucleus of the thalamus during sleep and wakefulness in the cat. I. Spontaneous activity. Exp. Brain Res. 12, 480–498 (1971).

LANDAU, A., IMBERT, M.: Organisation des projections visuelles au niveau du cortex orbitaire chez le chat. J. Physiol. (Paris) **57**, 642 (1965).

LANDGREN, S., NORDWALL, A., WENGSTRÖM, C.: The location of the thalamic relay in the spino-cervico-lemniscal path. Acta physiol. scand. **65**, 164–175 (1965).

LEVANTE, A., ALBE-FESSARD, D.: Localisation dans les couches VII et VIII de Rexed des cellules d'origine d'un faisceau spino-réticulaire croisé. C.R. Acad. Sci. (Paris) **274**, 3007–3010 (1972).

LIEBESKIND, J.C., MAYER, D.J.: Somatosensory evoked responses in the mesencephalic central gray matter of the rat. Brain Res. **27**, 133–151 (1971).

LIM, R.K.S.: Neuropharmacology of pain and analgesia. In: Pharmacology of pain and analgesia, R.K.S. LIM, D. ARMSTRONG and E.G. PARDO (eds.), pp. 169–217. London: Pergamon Press 1968.

LIM, R.K.S., KRAUTHAMER, G., GUZMAN, F., FULP, R.R.: Central nervous system activity associated with the pain evoked by Bradykinin and its alteration by morphin and aspirin. Proc. nat. Acad. Sci. (Wash.) **63**, 705–712 (1969).

LINDSLEY, D.B., BOWDEN, J., MAGOUN, H.W.: Effect upon EEG of acute injury to the brain stem activating system. Electroenceph. clin. Neurophysiol. **1**, 475–486 (1949).

LLOYD, D.P.C., MACINTYRE, A.K.: On the origin of dorsal root potentials. J. gen. Physiol. **32**, 409–433 (1949).

LOMBROSO, C.T., MERLIS, J.K.: Suprasylvian auditory responses in the Cat. Electroenceph. clin. Neurophysiol. **9**, 301–308 (1957),

LUND, R.D., WEBSTER, K.E.: Thalamic efferents from the spinal cord and trigeminal nuclei. J. comp. Neurol. **130**, 313–238 (1967).

LUNDBERG, A., OSCARSSON, O.: Three ascending spinal pathways in the dorsal part of the lateral funiculus. Acta physiol. scand. **51**, 1–16 (1961).

MACCHI, G.: Organizazione morfologica delle connessioni thalamo-corticali (Analisi anatomo-comparative dei contributi sperimentali). Atti della Societa Italiana di Anatomia. 18° Convegno Sociale. Dott. Luigi Mairi, Firenze, pp. 25–124 (1958).

MAGOUN, H.W., MACKINLEY, W.A.: The termination of ascending trigeminal and spinal tracts in the thalamus of the cat. Amer. J. Physiol. **137**, 409–416 (1942).

MAILLARD, M.C., BENOIST, J.M., CONSEILLER, C., HAMANN, K.F., BESSON, J.M.: Effects de la phénopéridine sur l'activité des interneurones de la corne dorsale de la moelle chez le chat spinal. C.R. Acad. Sci. (Paris) **274**, 726–728 (1972).

MAILLARD, M.C., BESSON, J.M., CONSEILLER, C., ALEONARD, P.: Effets provoqués par la stimulation du cortex orbitaire sur les cellules des couches IV et V de la corne dorsale de la moelle chez le Chat. C.R. Acad. Sci. (Paris) **272**, 729–732 (1971).

MALIS, L.I., PRIBRAM, K.H., KRUGER, L.: Action potentials in "motor" cortex evoked by peripheral nerve stimulation. J. Neurophysiol. **16**, 161–167 (1953).

MALLART, A.: Heterosegmental and heterosensory presynaptic inhibition. Nature (Lond.) **206**, 119–120 (1965).

MALLART, A.: Projection des afférences somatiques vers les structures cérébrales spécifiques et non spécifiques. Thèse Sci., 125 p. (1967).

MALLART, A.: Thalamic projections of muscle nerve afferents in the cat. J. Physiol. (Lond.) **194**, 337–353 (1968).

MALLART, A., PETIT, D.: Afférences non spécifiques conduites par les collatérales spinales des voies longues des cordons postérieurs. J. Physiol. (Paris) **55**, 291–292 (1963).

MANNEN, H.: Contribution to the morphological study of dendritic arborization in the brain stem. Progr. Brain Res. **21A**, 131–162 (1966).

MARSHALL, W.H., TALBOT, S.A., ADES, H.W.: Cortical response of the anesthetized cat to gross photic and electrical afferent stimulation. J. Neurophysiol. **6**, 1–15 (1943).

MASSION, J.: Etude d'une structure motrice thalamique, le noyau ventro-latéral et sa régulation par les afférences sensorielles. Thèse, Sci., Paris (34 p.) (1968).

MASSION, J., ANGAUT, P., ALBE-FESSARD, D.: Activités évoquées chez le chat dans la région du nucleus ventralis lateralis par diverses stimulations sensorielles. I. Etude macrophysiologique. E.E.G. J. **19**, 433–451 (1965a).

Massion, J., Angaut, P., Albe-Fessard, D.: Activités évoquées chez le chat dans la région du nucleus ventralis lateralis par diverses stimulations sensorielles. II. Etude microphysiologique. Electroenceph. clin. Neurophysiol. **19**, 452–469 (1965b).

Massion, J., Dormont, J.F.: Localisation spinale et bulbaire des voies afférentes de la somesthésie vers le noyau ventral lateral du thalamus. Electroenceph. clin. Neurophysiol. **21**, 437–451 (1966).

Massion, J., Korn, H., Albe-Fessard, D.: Contribution à l'analyse des afférences vagales projetant sur le cortex antérieur du chat. Acta neuroveg. (Wien) **28**, 135–147 (1966).

Mayer, D.J., Wolfle, T.L., Akil, H., Carder, B., Liebeskind, J.C.: Analgesia from electrical stimulation in the brainstem of the rat. Science **174**, 1351–1354 (1971).

McKenzie, J.S., Gilbert, D.M., Rogers, D.K.: Hippocampal and neostriatal inhibition of extralemniscal thalamic unitary responses in the cat. Brain Res. **23**, 382–385 (1971).

Mehler, W.R.: The anatomy of the so-called "pain tract" in Man: An analysis of the course and distribution of the ascending fibers of the fasciculus antero-lateralis. In: Basic Research in Paraplegia, J.D. French and R.W. Porter (eds.), pp. 26–55. Springfield, Ill.: Charles C. Thomas 1962.

Mehler, W.R.: Some observations on secondary ascending afferent systems in the central nervous system. In: Pain, R.S. Knighton and P.R. Dunke (eds.), pp. 11–32. Little, Brown and Company, Boston, 1966a.

Mehler, W.R.: Further notes on the centre median, nucleus of Luys. In: The Thalamus. D.P. Purpura and M.D. Yahr (eds.), pp. 109–127. New York: Columbia Univ. Press 1966b.

Mehler, W.R., Feferman, M.E., Nauta, W.J.H.: Ascending axon degeneration following anterolateral cordotomy. An experimental study in the monkey. Brain **83**, 718–750 (1960).

Melzack, R., Wall, P.D.: Pain mechanisms: a new theory. Science **150**, 971–979 (1965).

Mendell, L.M.: Physiological properties of unmyelinated fiber projection to the spinal cord. Exp. Neurol. **16**, 316–332 (1966).

Mendell, L.M., Wall, P.D.: Presynaptic hyperpolarization: a role for fine afferent fibers. J. Physiol. (Lond.) **172**, 272–294 (1964).

Meulders, M.: Etude comparative de la physiologie des voies sensorielles primaires et des voies associatives. Thèse, Arscia, Maloine, Bruxelles, Paris, 192 p. (1962).

Meulders, M.: Integration centrale des afférences visuelles. J. Physiol. (Paris) **62**, Suppl. 1, 61–109 (1970).

Meulders, M., Massion, J., Colle, J., Albe-Fessard, D.: Effects d'ablations télencéphaliques sur l'amplitude des potentiels évoqués dans le CM par stimulation somatique. Electroenceph. clin. Neurophysiol. **15**, 29–38 (1963).

Mickle, W.A., Ades, H.W.: Spread of evoked cortical potentials. J. Neurophysiol. **16**, 608–633 (1953).

Morin, F.: A new spinal pathway for cutaneous impulses. Amer. J. Physiol. **183**, 245–252 (1955).

Morin, F., Kitai, S.T., Portnoy, H., Demirjian, C.: Afferent projections to the lateral cervical nucleus: a microelectrodes study. Amer. J. Physiol. **204**, 667–672 (1963).

Morrison, A.R., Pompeiano, O.: Pyramidal discharge from somatosensory cortex and cortical control of primary afferents during sleep. Arch. ital. Biol. **103**, 538–568 (1965).

Mountcastle, V.B., Henneman, E.: Pattern of tactile representation: in thalamus of cat. J. Neurophysiol. **12**, 85–100 (1949).

Mountcastle, V.B., Henneman, E.: The representation of tactile sensibility in the thalamus of the monkey. J. comp. Neurol. **97**, 409–440 (1952).

Nakamura, Y., Schlag, J.O.: Cortically induced rhythmic activities in the thalamic ventrolateral nucleus of the cat. Exp. Neurol. **22**, no 2, 209–221 (1968).

Nauta, W.J.H., Kuypers, H.G.J.M.: Some ascending pathways in the brainstem reticular formation. In: Reticular Formation of the Brain, H.H. Jasper and L.L. Proctor (eds.), Henry Ford Hospital Symposium, pp. 3–30. Boston: Little, Brown and Co. 1958.

Niimi, K., Miki, M., Kawamura, J.: Ascending projections of the superior colliculus in the Cat. Okajimas Folia anat. jap. **47**, 269–287 (1970).

Nord, S.G., Kyler, H.J.: Somatosensory mechanisms in brainstem reticular nuclei. Paper read at Meetings of the Eastern Psychological Association, Washington (1968).

O'Brien, J.H., Pimpaneau, A., Albe-Fessard, D.: Evoked cortical responses to vagal, laryngeal and facial afferents in monkeys under chloralose anaesthesia. Electroenceph. clin. Neurophysiol. **31**, 7–20 (1971).

Olszewski, S.: The thalamus of macaca mulatta, an atlas for use with the stereotaxic instrument, 93 p. Basel: Karger 1952.

Oswaldo-Cruz, E., Kidd, C.: Functional properties of neurons in the lateral cervical nucleus of the Cat. J. Neurophysiol. **27**, 1–14 (1964).

Percheron, G.: Etude anatomique du thalamus de l'Homme adulte et de sa vascularisation artérielle. Thèse Médicine, Paris, 350 p. (1966).

Perl, E.R., Whitlock, D.G.: Somatic stimuli exciting spino-thalamic projections to thalamic neurons in cat and monkey .Exp. Neurol. **3**, 256–296 (1961).

Petit, D.: Données nouvelles sur l'organisation des messages d'origine cutanée à la périphérie et dans les systèmes des colonnes dorsales. Thèse Sci., Paris, 191 p. (1971).

Petit, D., Burgess, P.R.: Dorsal column projection of receptors in cat hairy skin supplied by myelinated fibers. J. Neurophysiol. **31**, 849–855 (1968).

Petit, D., Mallart, A.: Voies spinales afférentes vers le noyau centre-médian du thalamus chez le Chat. J. Physiol. (Paris) **56**, 423–424 (1964).

Petras, J.M.: Corticostriate and corticothalamic connections in the gibbon and chimpanzee. In: Symposium on Corticothalamic and Sensorimotor activities, in press (1972).

Poggio, G.F., Mountcastle, V.B.: A study of the functional contributions of the lemniscal and spinothalamic systems to somatic sensibility. Bull. Johns Hopk. Hosp. **106**, 266–316 (1960).

Poggio, G.F., Mountcastle, V.B.: The functional properties of ventrobasal thalamic neurons studied in unanesthetized monkeys. J. Neurophysiol. **26**, 773–806 (1963).

Poliakova, A.G.: Origin of the early component of the evoked response in the association cortex of the cat. Electroenceph. clin. Neurophysiol. **32**, 129–138 (1972).

Pomeranz, B., Wall, P.D., Weber, W.V.: Cord cells responding to fine myelinated afferents from viscera muscle and skin. J. Physiol. (Lond.) **199**, 511–532 (1968).

Powell, T.P.S., Cowan, W.M.A.: A study of thalamo-striate relations in the monkey. Brain **79**, 364–390 (1956).

Powell, T.P.S., Mountcastle, V.B.: The cytoarchitecture of the post-central gyrus of the monkey macaca mulatta. Bull. Johns Hopk. Hosp. **106**, 108–131 (1959).

Price, D.D., Wagman, I.H.: Characteristics of two ascending pathways which originate in spinal dorsal horn of macaca mulatta. Brain **26**, 406–410 (1971).

Purpura, D.P., Frigyesi, T.L., McMurtry, J.G., Scarff, T.: Synaptic mechanisms in thalamic regulation of cerebello-cortical projection activity. In: The Thalamus, D.P. Purpura and M.D. Yahr (eds.), pp. 153–172. New York: Columbia University Press 1966.

Rexed, B.: The cytoarchitectonic organization of the spinal cord in the Cat. J. comp. Neurol. **96**, 415–496 (1952).

Rexed, B., Brodal, P.: The nucleus cervicalis lateralis. A spino-cerebellar relay nucleus. J. Neurophysiol. **14**, 399–407 (1951).

Reynolds, D.V.: Surgery in the rat during electrical analgesia induced by focal brain stimulation. Science **164**, 444–445 (1969).

Rinvik, E.: The corticothalamic projection from the precruciate and coronal gyri in the cat. An experimental study with silver-impregnation methods. Brain Res. **10**, 79–119 (1968).

Rinvik, E.: Organization of thalamic connections from motor and somatosensory cortical areas in the cat. 4th Symposium of the Parkinson's Disease Res. Center: "Corticothalamic projections and sensorimotor activities", Raven Press (1972) (in press).

Rispal-Padel, L., Massion, J.: Relations between the ventrolateral nucleus and the motor cortex in the Cat. Exp. Brain Res. **10**, 331–339 (1970).

Rocha-Miranda, C.E.: Electrofisiologia do nucleo caudato. Thesis Med. Sci., Univ. of Brasil — Institute of Biophysics, Rio de Janeiro (1961).

Roitback, A.I., Eristavi, N.: EEG and behavior reactions upon stimulation of nonspecific thalamic nuclei in unanesthetized cats. Acta Biol. exp. (Warszawa) **26**, 463–482 (1966).

Rose, J.E., Mountcastle, V.B.: The thalamic tactile region in rabbit and cat. J. comp. Neurol. **97**, 441–490 (1952).

Rose, J.E., Mountcastle, V.B.: Touch and Kinesthesis. In: Handbook of Physiology. Neurophysiology **1**, 387–430 (1960).

Rose, J. E., Woolsey, C. N.: Organization of the mammalian thalamus and its relationships to the cerebral cortex. Electroenceph. clin. Neurophysiol. **1**, 391–404 (1949).

Rose, J. E., Woolsey, C. N.: Cortical connections and functional organization of the thalamic auditory system of the cat. In: Biological and Biochemical Bases of Behavior, H. F. Harlow and C. N. Woolsey (eds.), pp. 127-150. Madison, Wisc.: Univ. Wisconsin Press 1958.

Rossi, G. F., Brodal, A.: Terminal distribution of spino-reticular fibres in the Cat. A.M.A. Arch. Neurol. Psychol. **78**, 439–453 (1957).

Ruch, T. C., Patton, H. D., Amassian, V. E.: Topographical and functional determinants of cortical localization patterns. Res. Publ. Ass. nerv. ment. Dis. **30**, 403–429 (1952).

Rutledge, L. T.: Interactions of peripherally and centrally originating input to association cortex. Electroenceph. clin. Neurophysiol. **15**, 958–968 (1963).

Rutledge, L. T., Duncan, J. A.: Extracellular recording of converging input on cortical neurones using a flexible microelectrode. Nature (Lond.) **210**, 737–739 (1966).

Satoh, M., Nakamura, N., Takagi, H.: Effect of morphine on bradykinin-induced unitary discharges in the spinal cord of the rabbit. Europ. J. Pharmacol. **16**, 245–247 (1971).

Segundo, J. P., Machne, X.: Unitary responses to afferent volleys in lenticular nucleus and claustrum. J. Neurophysiol. **21**, 325–339 (1956).

Scheibel, M. E., Scheibel, A. B.: Structural substrates for integrative patterns in the brainstem reticular core. In: Reticular Formation of the Brain, H. H. Jasper et al. (eds.), pp. 31–55. Boston: Little, Brown and Co. 1958.

Scheibel, M. E., Scheibel, A. B.: Cortical modulation of certain thalamic cell ensembles. In 4th Symposium of the Parkinson's Disease Research Center: "Corticothalamic projections and sensorimotor activities", Raven Press (in press) (1972).

Scheibel, M., Scheibel. A., Mollica, A., Moruzzi, G.: Convergence and interaction of afferent impulses on single units of reticular formation. J. Neurophysiol., **18**, 309–332 (1955).

Schmidek, H. H., Fohanno, D., Frank, R. E., Sweet, W. H.: Pain threshold alterations by brain stimulation in the monkey. J. Neurosurg. **35**, 715–722 (1971).

Selzer, M., Spencer, W. A.: Convergence of visceral and cutaneous afferent pathways in the lumbar spinal cord. Brain Res. **14**, 331–348 (1969 a).

Selzer, M., Spencer, W. A.: Interactions between visceral and cutaneous afferents pathways in the spinal cord: reciprocal primary afferent fibre depolarization. Brain Res. **14**, 349–366 (1969 b).

Shealy, C. N., Mortimer, J. T., Hagfors, N. R.: Dorsal column electroanalgesia. J. Neurosurg. **32**, 560–564 (1970).

Shende, M. C., Stewart, D. H., Jr., King, R. B.: Projections from the trigeminal nucleus caudalis in the squirrel monkey. Exp. Neurol. **20**, 655–670 (1968).

Singer, P., Bignall, K. E.: Multiple somatic projections to frontal lobe of the squirrel monkey. Personal Communication (1969).

Spector, I.: Organisation des projections somatiques et sensorielles au niveau du claustrum chez le Chat. Thèse Sci., Paris, 186 p. (1967).

Spector, I., Hassmannova, Y., Albe-Fessard, D.: A macrophysiological study of functional organization of the claustrum. Exp. Neurol. **29**, 31–51 (1970).

Sprague, J. M., Ha, H.: The terminal fields of dorsal root fibers in the lumbosacral fibers of the cat, and the dendritic organization of the motor nuclei. In: Organization of the spinal cord, J. C. Eccles and J. P. Schadé (ed.), Elsevier Publ. Co., pp. 120–152 (1964).

Starzl, T. E., Taylor, C. W., Magoun, H. W.: Collateral afferent excitation of reticular formation of brainstem. J. Neurophysiol. **14**, 479–496 (1951).

Steriade, M., Briot, R.: Convergences inhibitrices d'influx cérébelleux et corticaux au niveau du noyau rouge et du noyau thalamique ventral latéral. J. Physiol. (Paris) **59**, 298–299 (1967).

Stewart, D. H., Jr., Scibetta, C. J., King, R. B.: Presynaptic inhibition in the trigeminal relay nuclei. J. Neurophysiol. **30**, 135–153 (1967).

Stewart, W. A., King, R. B.: Fiber projections from the nucleus caudalis of the spinal trigeminal nucleus. J. comp. Neurol. **121**, 271–286 (1963).

Straaten, J. J. van: Relation between the secondary optic fibre system and the centrencephalic system. Arch. intern. Physiol. **70**, 483–495 (1962).

STRATFORD, J.: Cortico-thalamic connection from gyrus proreus and first and second somatic sensory areas of the cat. J. comp. Neurol. **100**, 1–14 (1954).

STRICK, P.L.: Cortical projections of the feline thalamic nucleus ventralis lateralis. Brain Res. **20**, 130–134 (1970).

SUZUKI, H., KATO, H.: Neurons with visual properties in the posterior group of the thalamic nuclei. Exp. Neurol. **23**, 353–365 (1969).

TAUB, A., BISHOP, P.O.: The spinocervical tract: dorsal column linkage, conduction velocity, primary afferent spectrum. Exp. Neurol. **13**, 1–21 (1965).

THOMPSON, R.F., JOHNSON, R.H., HOOPES, J.J.: Organization of auditory, somatic sensory and visual projection to association fields of cerebral cortex in the cat. J. Neurophysiol. **26**, 343–364 (1963a).

THOMPSON, R.F., SINDBERG, R.M.: Auditory response fields in association and motor cortex of cat. J. Neurophysiol. **23**, 87–105 (1960).

THOMPSON, R.F., SMITH, H., BLISS, R.: Auditory, somatic sensory and visual response interactions and interrelations in association and primary cortical fields of the cat. J. Neurophysiol. **26**, 365–378 (1963b).

TOTIBADZE, N.K., MONIAVA, E.S.: On the direct cortical connections of the nucleus centrum medianum thalami. J. comp. Neurol. **137**, 347–360 (1969).

TOWE, A.L., WHITEHORN, D., NYQUIST, J.K.: Differential activity among wide-field neurons of the cat post-cruciate cerebral cortex. Exp. Neurol. **20**, 497–521 (1968).

TREVINO, D.L., WILLIS, W.D., MAUNZ, R.A.: Location of cells of origin of the spinothalamic tract in the Cat. Proc. of the Int. Union of Physiol. Sci., **IX**, 569 (1971).

UDDENBERG, N.: Differential localization in dorsal funiculus of fibres originating from different receptors. Exp. Brain Res. **4**, 367–376 (1968a).

UDDENBERG, N.: Functional organization of long, second order afferents in the dorsal funiculus. Exp. Brain Res. **4**, 377–382 (1968b).

URABE, M., ITO, H.: Inhibitory effects of the limbic system on the nucleus centrum medianum of the thalamus. Physiol. Behav. **3**, 695–702 (1968).

URBANO, A., RAPISARDA, C., INFANTELLINA, F.: Etude microphysiologique des afférences somatiques au claustrum chez le Chat. Arch. Sci. biol. (Bologna) **50**, 41–54 (1966).

VALVERDE, F.: Reticular formation of the pons and medulla oblongata. A Golgi study. J. comp. Neurol. **116**, 71–100 (1961a).

VALVERDE, F.: A new type of cell in the lateral reticular formation of the brain stem. J. comp. Neurol. **117**, 189–195 (1961b).

VERAART, C., MEULDERS, M., GODFRAIN, J.M.: Visual properties of neurones in Pulvinar, nucleus lateralis posterior and nucleus suprageniculatus thalami in the cat (II. Quantitative investigation). Brain Res. (in press) (1972).

VIERCK, C.J., HAMILTON, D.M., THORNBY, J.: Pain reactivity of monkeys after lesions to the dorsal columns of the spinal cord. Exp. Brain Res. **13**, 140–158 (1971).

VYKLICKÝ, L., RUDOMIN, P., ZAJAC, F.E., BURKE, R.E.: Primary afferent depolarization evoked by a painful stimulus. Science **165**, 184–186 (1969).

WALKER, A.E.: The Primate Thalamus. Illinois: University of Chicago Press 1938.

WALL, P.D.: Excitability changes of primary afferents in relation with slow cord potentials. J. Physiol. (Lond.) **142**, 1–22 (1958).

WALL, P.D.: Cord cells responding to touch, damage and temperature of the skin. J. Neurophysiol. **23**, 197–210 (1960).

WALL, P.D.: The origin of a spinal cord slow potential. J. Physiol. (Lond.) 508–526 (1962).

WALL, P.D.: Presynaptic control of impulses at the first central synapse in the cutaneous pathway. In: Progress in Brain Research, J.C. ECCLES and J.P. SCHADÉ (eds.), Vol. **12**, Physiology of Spinal Neurons, pp. 92–118. Amsterdam: Elsevier 1964.

WALL, P.D.: The lamina organization of dorsal horn and effects of descending impulses. J. Physiol. (Lond.) **188**, 403–423 (1967).

WALL, P.D., SWEET, W.H.: Temporary abolition of Pain in Man. Science **155**, 108–109 (1967).

WALL, P.D., TAUB, A.: Four aspects of trigeminal nucleus and a Paradox. J. Neurophysiol. **25**, 110–126 (1962).

WALLER, J.M., BARRIS, R.W.: Relationships of thalamic nuclei to the cerebral cortex in the cat. J. comp. Neurol. **67**, 317–341 (1937).

Wendt, R., Albe-Fessard, D.: Sensory responses of the amygdala with special reference to somatic afferent pathways. Coll. Intern. CNRS, Montpellier, 24–25 Août 1961, pp. 172–200. Eds du CNRS.

Wepsic, J. G.: Multimodal sensory activation of cells in the magnocellularis medial geniculate nucleus. Exp. Neurol. **15**, 299–318 (1966).

Whitlock, D. G., Perl, E. R.: Afferent projections through ventrolateral funiculi to thalamus of cat. J. Neurophysiol. **22**, 133–148 (1959).

Woolsey, C. N.: "Second" somatic receiving areas in the cerebral cortex of cat, dog and monkey. Fed. Proc. **2**, 55 (1943).

Woolsey, C. N.: Additional observations on a "second" somatic area in the cerebral cortex of the monkey. Fed. Proc. **3**, 53 (1944).

Woolsey, C. N.: The somatic function of the central nervous system. Ann. Rev. Physiol. **9**, 525–552 (1947).

Woolsey, C. N.: Organization of cortical auditory system. In: Sensory Communication, Rosenblith, W. A. (ed.), pp. 235–257. Cambridge, Mass.: Technology Press 1961.

Woolsey, C. N., Chang, H. T., Bard, P.: Distribution of cortical potentials evoked by electrical stimulation of dorsal roots in Macaca Mulatta. Fed. Proc. **6**, 230 (1947).

Yokota, T., MacLean, P. T.: Fornix and fifth-nerve interaction on thalamic units in awake, sitting monkeys. J. Neurophysiol. **31**, 358–370 (1968).

Zimmermann, M.: Dorsal root potentials after C-fibre stimulation. Science **160**, 896–898 (1968).

Chapter 14

Electrical Recording from the Thalamus in Human Subjects

By

J. A. V. Bates, London (Great Britain)

With 7 Figures

Contents

A. Introduction

This chapter will discuss some of the findings made by microelectrode recordings from the third-order sensory neurones in the thalamus in man; in particular the spontaneous activity of neurones, the characteristics of effective stimuli and, as a separate aspect, the response in neurones. Finally, the difficulty in defining the location and arrangement of thalamic areas will be considered.

It is not technically difficult to make micro-electrode recordings from the thalamus of the awake human, and since the risk of complications is not increased and the results are helpful in guiding a stereotactic operation, the procedure is ethically justified. However, one cannot perform experiments on the brain in the operating theatre, and the value of the data is limited by the lack of histological verification of the site of recording. We should, nevertheless, consider any evidence of the behaviour of single neurones in an animal with whom we can talk and whose

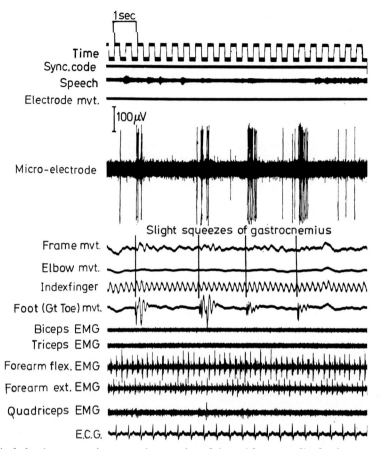

Fig. 1. A thalamic neurone in a conscious patient firing with an amplitude about ×5 background level, provoked by slight squeezes of the gastrocnemius indicated on the recording by the movement this imparted to an accelerometer on the contralateral great toe

feelings we can share. Observations on the normally conscious human should go beyond the demonstration that man is just another primate. This task inevitably involves discussing the variable rather than fixed behaviour of single neurones, and the difficulty of meeting strict criteria of scientific rigour must be accepted.

Thalamic recording in man was started from the need to reduce errors in stereotactic surgery. These arose from the variability in position between certain thalamic structures visible on a ventriculogram and those found empirically to be suitable targets for stereotactic surgery. It was realised that there were only two ways to reduce localisation errors; the first was to use proportionate rather than absolute measure in plotting targets from X-ray tracings, and the second to add the security of functional localisation by the techniques of stimulation and recording. In 1961 the first recordings of human thalamic neurones firing in response to sensory stimulation were reported by ALBE-FESSARD et al. (1962) and GUIOT et al. (1962). They used a stainless steel bipolar semi-microelectrode, and their success stimulated other groups to use finer etched tungsten monopolar microelectrodes of the kind described by HUBEL (1957). This electrode gives better resolution of the activity of single cells but opinion remains divided about which type gives the most useful information to the surgeon. In 1964 there were reports by JASPER and BERTRAND (1964) and GAZE et al. (1964), and these have been followed by others (BERTRAND, 1963; ALBE-FESSARD et al., 1966; CARRERAS et al., 1967; BATES, 1969; and HANKINSON et al., 1971).

The remarks that follow are based on an analysis of 147 selected recording tracks through 10–15 mm of the thalamus. They were obtained in 130 patients: 118 had Parkinson's disease; 10 had other disorders of a hyperkinetic nature; 2 had epilepsy. No sedation or general anaesthetic was used. The patients were lying on their backs with good access to the face and limbs. They were encouraged to talk and co-operate in testing. A modified Leksell stereotactic frame was applied and the thalamus was approached from a frontal burr-hole. In a typical case the electrode was advanced slowly at about one micron a second, and the recording took about 45 minutes. In an average electrode track 50–100 individual neurones could be identified because of their spontaneous discharge which appeared as spikes with an amplitude twice or more the background level. From the start a loudspeaker was used for monitoring neuronal activity which was continuously recorded on a U–V galvanometer and other channels using accelerometers and electromyography were added. A typical recording has the form shown in Fig. 1. The general procedure of examination was for the electrode advance to be halted whenever an active neurone was heard in isolation from the background. The patient was then examined to see if sensory stimulation could affect its firing. Two observers were always present and continuous dictation was recorded. First the limbs were examined by asking for a maximum voluntary effort against resistance, and if this failed, they were examined by palpation and passive movements. The patient was then asked to clench the teeth or swallow or put out the tongue and the face was touched. If the spontaneous discharge pattern seemed to be affected by any of these gross procedures, the examination was pursued until an end-point was reached at which no further progress in isolating the necessary stimulus condition could be made. Inevitably, some parts of the body were not adequately examined, notably the neck and axial musculature and the viscera. Somatosensory neurones were identified in 70 % of the recording tracks.

The practice of using physiological stimulation and of not examining the patient unless a neurone was actively discharging, gives a false impression that all sensory neurones are normally in a state of spontaneous activity. This procedure was adopted because sensory examination without an active neurone near the electrode seemed in practice to be unrewarding. Stimulation of the median nerve as an aid in finding sensory neurones of the upper limb was used by HANKINSON et al. (1971), and with this technique they found proportionately more neurones activated from small areas of the skin and fingers than there were in the present data. Thus, confining oneself to physiological stimulation only when the recording shows an active neurone, may result in some sensory neurones, particularly those related to skin sensation, being missed. Unfortunately, any practical method of procedure produces some bias in the sample of the whole population.

36*

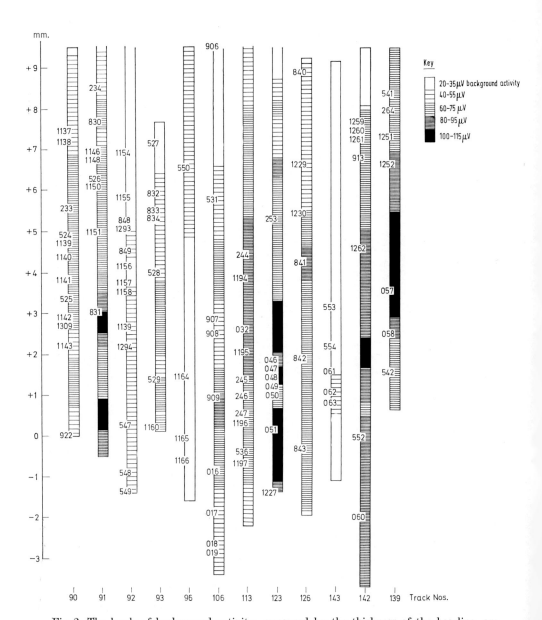

Fig. 2. The levels of background activity, measured by the thickness of the baseline, are indicated in twelve recording tracks to the same target at 'O', from Parkinsonian patients. The positions of provokable neurones are marked on the tracks; numbers 000–099 were neurones provoked by stimulating the face, 200–299 the upper arm and shoulder, 500–599 the wrist and hand, 800–899 the leg and 900–999 were responsive to whole body movements. Tremor phasic units firing at rates of 4–6 per sec are shown as 1000–1999

B. Spontaneous Activity

As the microelectrode was advanced from above downwards through the lateral mass of the thalamus, the overall impression of neuronal activity varied considerably from patient to patient. There was variation both in the density of actively discharging cells and in the discharge pattern of those that are within 50 μ of the tip. The more distant activity caused a thickening of the base-line and this varied both between individuals and between one part of the thalamus and another in the same individual. Measurements of this variation are illustrated in Fig. 2 which shows the range in twelve selected recordings from different individuals through the same part of the thalamus. Variation between individuals might be due to small differences in the taper and tip of the microelectrodes, but the experience in a few cases of making a second parallel track 3 mm away with the same electrode, and in other cases with a different electrode, and also of making a second recording in the same patient some months later, has suggested that the variation between patients is more related to differences in the thalamus rather than in the electrode. There is no reason to suspect considerable differences in the number of neurones in the thalamus from one patient to the next, and thus one infers that the majority of thalamic neurones in most cases are quiescent — presumably through active inhibition. Patients with hyperkinetic syndromes other than Parkinsonism tended to have the higher amplitude backgrounds, but we know nothing of the level of neuronal activity in the normal human thalamus and thus cannot evaluate this observation. Since all the patients were awake and in a normal state of sensory responsiveness, one must conclude that considerable differences in the number of spontaneously active neurones are not related to differences in the ordinary awareness of touch and movement. Sudden changes in background level were never encountered at one recording position. This is significant since sudden changes in arousal can greatly affect the E.E.G. and global changes might have been expected in a population of neurones intimately related to sensory function.

When an actively discharging neurone was within 50 μ of the electrode tip, the commonest type of activity was an irregular discharge at rates of 1–5 per sec. Rates above 20 per sec were rare. Some active neurones showing grouping of discharges into a burst-interval-burst or phasic pattern were found in all parts of most tracks. The rate of the bursts was usually in the range of 1–10 per sec, but within the burst the frequency could be as high as 200 per sec. Spontaneous burst activity in the range 4–6 per sec was common in Parkinsonian patients, as ALBE-FESSARD et al. (1962) first reported, but in one case a neurone firing in 5 per sec bursts was found in an epileptic patient without signs of Parkinsonism. Thus phasic activity at the frequency of the tremor is not necessarily pathological in type, though it may well be in amount in the Parkinsonian thalamus. Burst activity could come and go without any apparent alteration in the patient's state. At least half of the neurones in a state of active discharge within the sensory relay area were unaffected by sensory stimulation. The same observation has been reported by JASPER and BERTRAND (1966). In some instances two active neurones were being recorded at the same electrode position and one of them was affected by sensory stimulation and the other was unaffected.

In conclusion it can be said that observations on man have not so far contributed to an understanding of the functional role, if any, of the considerable amount of neuronal discharge that is characteristic of the awake brain. Further understanding will need techniques that enable a single neurone to be monitored for hours rather than minutes, for there seem to be no significant correlations with behavioural state in the "short-term".

C. Provoking Stimuli

In the present series a total of 244 thalamic neurones was found to be influenced by sensory stimulation; 85 (36%) by light touch, 20 (8%) by pressure, and the remaining 139 (56%) required some sort of movement. It is difficult to

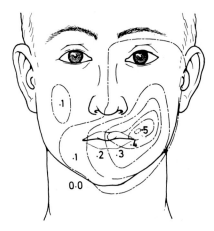

Fig. 3. Diagram based on recordings from 50 thalamic neurones provoked by stroking the face, to show the probability of a neurone being excited by stimulating an area of skin

form any idea of the bias in this sample and hence of the real proportionate differences in the whole population of sensory neurones in the normal human thalamus.

1. Light Touch

The firing rate of a single thalamic sensory neurone can be increased by the lightest of touches such as stroking an appropriate area of the skin with a camel hair brush – a procedure which gives rise to a conscious sensation of a minimal touch at the base of the nail, but a strong and unpleasant tickle on the lip. The smallest receptive field of a single unit was an area of about 1 mm² found both on the lip and at the base of the finger-nail. The largest field was an area of about 4×8 cm on the outer aspect of the upper arm. Although no precise measurements were possible, the receptive field to brush stimulation was typically rather sharp edged and a similar increase in firing occurred with moving contact anywhere within the field. There was never an impression of gradation of response with a zone of maximal affect in the centre. In parts of the thalamus related to the face, neurones responsive to stimulation of areas less than 2 mm² could be adjacent to others responsive to stimulation of a much larger field (up to 15 cm²) which contained the smaller field. In other words, there was no evidence of the collecting together of neurones provoked by small fields into one part, and of neurones with larger fields into another. The upper or lower lip commonly marked the edge of the field of a neurone, but 5 neurones with small fields were found which extended across the muco-cutaneous junction. The areas of the skin of the face from which 50 neurones in 21 patients could be excited were plotted and transferred onto a common diagram (Fig. 3), so that the innervation density of the face could be plotted as a contour map. It is interesting to note that the most dense area on the chart corresponds to the most sensitive area subjectively and that 50 % or more of the neurones in this small sample could be stimulated by contact within it.

2. Pressure

Neurones were found which were unaffected by the lightest contact but which could be excited by blunt pressure on the skin sufficient to cause a dimple of 1–2 mm. They were readily detected by tapping the skin. Others were provoked by a firm squeeze of the calf or the forearm. These neurones were unaffected by joint movement and probably were influenced by receptors in the deep fascia or periostium of the long bones. Surround inhibition is difficult to apply with physiological stimuli, but it was looked for in suitable cases and only one doubtful example was found. HANKINSON et al. (1971) reported finding it in one neurone in 107 which was sensitive to light pressure. If surround inhibition was a common feature of sensory mechanisms at the thalamic level, it could scarcely have been missed so consistently.

3. Joint Movement

Of the 244 sensory neurones, 139 (56 %) seemed necessarily to require some passive or active movement to affect their discharge rate. When this movement was confined to one joint, more than one of the movements possible at the joint was usually effective. In this case the effective receptor can be located at least to the immediate neighbourhood of the joint. When, however, the neurone was affected by a single movement only (e.g. flexion of the elbow and not extension), the anatomical location of the receptor remains uncertain, especially when the movement involves a two-joint system as in supination and pronation. In the present data 29 (12 %) were of the first type, that is to say the receptor had a definite location because the stimulating movement was complex. In such a case for example, any movement of the shoulder would make the neurone fire. Twenty of this group of 29 units could have been fired from one receptor site in, for example, a joint capsule, but for 9 of the neurones a single receptor was less easy to

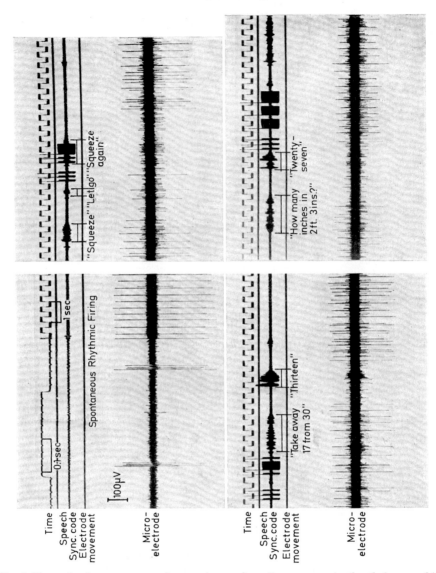

Fig. 4. Examples from one case of a spontaneously active neurone in the thalamus which stopped firing when the patient's attention was affected by a command or a question

locate, because although these neurones were showing a consistent response to the same peripheral disturbance, this was not a precise movement. It is possible to imagine in such cases that the stimulus might be of a higher order than a single discrete movement, such as a pattern of movement, but in only one case was a neurone found which suggested this explanation. The 'movement' in this case was voluntary 'piano-playing' involving alternate sequential flexions and extensions of the four fingers. Flexion and extension of each finger individually did not make this neurone fire. If neurones with this property exist the range of combinations of movement is so vast that it is very possible they would remain undetected.

The remaining 110 neurones comprised 63 (26 %) in which there was movement in a single direction about one axis, and these were mostly of the shoulder, elbow, wrist or ankle. A smaller group of 25 (10 %) had bidirectional movement about a single axis (e.g. flexion and extension of the elbow). In the case of 26 (11 %) the necessary movement was in one direction, but involved two adjacent joints. The remaining group of 8 (3 %) neurones required a movement of the whole limb. A typical dictation record of such a neurone reads: "There was a fine brush-like sound on flexion of the hip. It is most sensitive to abduction of the hip and it can also be made to fire by extension or flexion of the knee and also by squeezing the gastrocnemius". Within each group were neurones whose discharge was unaffected unless the movement was rapid. Other neurones were found in which the position at which the movement was started seemed critical. It was not possible in the circumstances of the operating theatre to make precise measurements of the necessary stimulating conditions of these more special units, but their existence in man is certain. When the 139 neurones affected by joint movement are considered as a group, no two neurones are alike when the stimulus conditions are fully specified.

4. "Psychic" Stimuli — Attention and Intention

When a neurone was consistently affected by touch or movement the subject's attention could readily be directed either to the stimulus or to the sound of his own responding unit in the loud speaker, or to neither, by asking a reply to some simple question requiring the minimum of mental effort (e.g. "spell your name backwards"). In no case did alterations of the mental state by such procedures affect the response to stimulation. This confirms a finding first reported by JASPER and BERTRAND (1964). A few neurones within the sensory relay area were found to respond by ceasing to fire when the subject's attention was directed to some simple task such as mental arithmetic. Neurones of this type were found in 4 patients and a set of observations on one case is illustrated in Fig. 4. No neurone was found in which 'attention' had the effect of increasing the rate of spontaneous irregular activity. Neurones apparently responsive to intention have been described by BERTRAND (1971) and his records are certainly suggestive of units with these properties. But in view of the known facts of sub-liminal changes in tension and preparatory set in the musculature and the great sensitivity of some thalamic neurones to slight movement, it would be difficult to establish 'intention' as a stimulus unless the unit was proved to be sufficiently far removed from other sensory neurones in the same recording.

D. Responses to Stimuli

1. Sensory Neurones with Consistent Responses

The responses of thalamic neurones to sensory stimulation suggest that they may vary in the degree of influence which a peripheral receptor can exert over their activity along a scale from complete domination to the scarcely detectable. It is well established that receptors vary from those with static or non-adapting properties to all degrees of dynamic or rapidly adapting response. If a neurone is one of those dominated by a receptor it will of course show the adaptive properties of the receptor. It is just those neurones behaving consistently like a peripheral receptor which are the easiest to locate and study, and as a consequence our picture of the sensory role of the thalamus may be greatly biased by the sample of neurones studied and reported on. Peripheral dependent neurones may, however, be a minority population among all third-order neurones.

Of the 244 sensory neurones in the present data 205 (88%) had a consistent response. The response was typically a significant acceleration of the rate of spontaneous firing up to a maximum of 100–150 per sec, often followed by a brief inhibitory interval; the latency being within the range 16–20 msec. Since no quantitative control of physiological stimuli in the operating theatre was attempted, only an approximate idea can be obtained of the relationship between the magnitude of the stimulus and the response in the thalamic neurone. In the case of neurones responsive to light touch, the increased rate of firing seemed to be a function of the speed of the moving light contact, and in the case of the pressure sensitive neurones the change in firing rate seemed to be a function of the amount and rate of deformation produced by pressure. In the group of thalamic neurones affected by movement, some were found which only responded to fast and not to slow movement over the range. Inhibition of spontaneous firing was only seen on one occasion when one neurone repeatedly ceased to discharge on squeezing the forearm, but was unaffected by touch or manipulation of the wrist or elbow. It is possible that a receptor was mechanically stressed in the resting position and the effect of the squeeze happened to relieve this stress. Presumably an explanation on these lines can always be applied to apparent inhibition from peripheral stimulation in the neighbourhood of a mechano-receptor, in which case it is surprising that the observation was not more common.

2. Neurones with Variable Responses

In the case of the remaining 39 (12%) neurones, the evidence of variable behaviour to a constant stimulus was sufficient to suggest that they might be a different group with less determinate properties. The variability was of two types best illustrated by the dictation record: "This neurone seemed responsive to any movement of the shoulder but most responsive to flexion, i.e. to lifting the elbow a fraction of an inch off the couch. The neurone was also responsive to depression and to lateral and medial rotation of the shoulder. After the examination had proceeded for some minutes the neurone slowly ceased to respond to any of these manoeuvres. It gave no signs of being penetrated. Its initial response was very sensitive." In this case the spontaneous activity of the neurone slowly declined and with it the responsiveness to stimuli which a few moments before had been very effective. In other cases the spontaneous activity continued while the neurone changed its responsiveness; e.g. "The neurone was spontaneously active and provoked by stroking the palmar surface of the left hand but after three or four bursts of firing to this stimulus, continued stroking of the palm did not affect the spontaneous activity." In this particular patient the above unusual behaviour was typical of four other sensory neurones, namely, that after a neurone had been found the effect of continuing to stimulate it was to make the reaction slowly vanish. Why this was so, of course, could not be determined, but it is typical of an impression, which it is impossible to quantify, that many of the records showed an individuality in the response characteristics of the neurones as well as in the level of background activity as already noted.

E. Sensory Transformation

One of the central unsolved problems of the sensory thalamus is what transformations occur there in the signal initiated in the receptor. When the receptor is below the skin there will always be a difficulty in specifying the stimulus with sufficient precision, and the problem will only be answered when simultaneous recording from a primary fibre and a third-order neurone on which it converges is technically possible.

A second question is whether one must visualise that neurones can show convergence by being responsive to disturbance at more than a single peripheral receptor site. In the 139 neurones affected by movement, all except two could have been affected from only one peripheral receptor site. In one of these exceptions, the neurone would fire either with external rotation of the shoulder, or with extension of the elbow, or with extension of the wrist. These are three movements which are fairly easy to perform in isolation, and the fact that a neurone would fire with any of them but not with the flexor or rotatory counterparts suggests that this neurone may have been demonstrating convergence from more than one site. The other neurone which possibly demonstrated convergence was that already mentioned as being responsive to 'piano-playing'. There were six other neurones in which the behaviour might have been evidence of convergence; for example, a neurone was found which was independently responsive either to extension of the wrist, or to flexion of the elbow, or to squeezing the hand (making a fist). The receptor site could be the fascia of the forearm. But on gripping, the wrist extensors and the elbow flexors commonly act synergically as fixators, so while this neurone could have been influenced from a single receptor in the forearm, it could also be seen as responsive to a common pattern involving three movements. In every case when the movement was complex, the neurone could have been responsive to a pattern or part of a pattern of movement, and there were no neurones found which were responsive to several separate movements independently, which, when combined, would result in an impossible or unnatural movement of the limb. For example, internal rotation of the shoulder and extension of the elbow might have been independently present, but this particular combination leads to an unnatural movement and it was not found. The conclusion at present must be that there is no way of deciding conclusively whether a complex stimulus is in fact exciting one receptor, or whether some neurones are being driven by particular patterns of movement. The absence of incongruous combinations of movement may slightly favour the latter hypothesis.

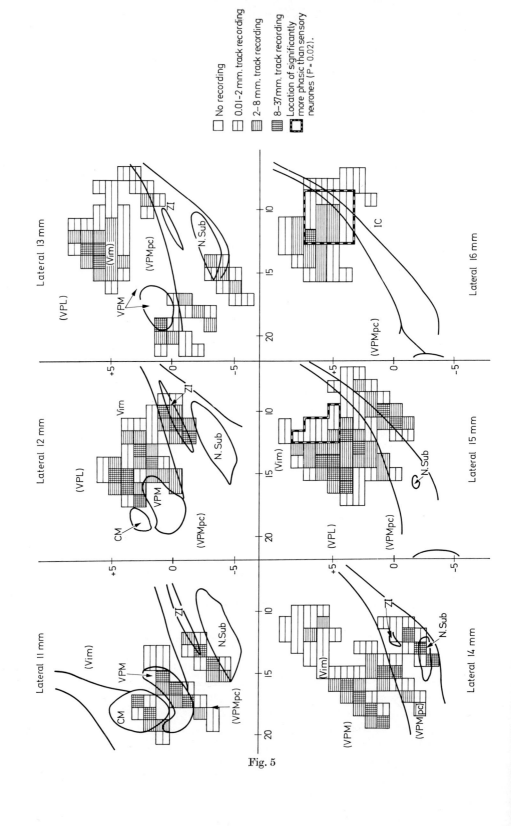

Fig. 5

Cases have been cited where the stimulus was applied constantly but the response faded. Neurones of this type were found more frequently as experience was gained, rather than less frequently. It is possible that, in the earlier recordings, neurones of this property were missed as the recording electrode was moved on immediately a definite result was obtained.

In arriving at an overall picture, one has to take into account the fact already mentioned that no sampling is random, and that any given set of testing methods will favour the discovery of neurones with certain properties, and act against the discovery of other types of neurones. These factors undoubtedly account for part of the population of spontaneously active neurones whose behaviour could not be affected. It seems possible to visualise the sensory thalamus as comprising a population made up of neurones with considerable variation in their properties. At one end of the spectrum the influence of the receptor is so prepotent that they always and instantly signal to a peripheral event. At the other end there is a population in whom the effect of any peripheral stimulus is so weak as to be in practice undetectable. These would be most of those spontaneously active neurones apparently unresponsive to any type of stimulation and which were possibly twice as numerous as neurones of the first type. In the intermediate range would be a third group in which the peripheral drive is moderate but fluctuating. These may be much more numerous than the data suggests as the method did not involve lingering in the presence of neurones which were spontaneously active but unresponsive to natural stimuli. It may be then that the type of neuronal behaviour on which a picture of a lemniscal relay in the thalamus is being built up is at one end of a distribution of properties and that attention is focussed on it because the only techniques available happen to favour its selection.

F. Location of Responsive Neurones

For the practical problems of stereotactic surgery, the position of the microelectrode throughout its travel must be known in a three-dimensional system based on absolute measurements along three defined rectangular co-ordinates. The details of how this is achieved in various systems need not concern us. But with a set of reference co-ordinates attached to each point on a track, there is data for computer processing. Ideally, one should be able to state for each point of the space so defined, a probability of being in a recognised anatomical area. This is at present impossible. It will require detailed histological study of sufficient brains sectioned in standard planes, and in the lateral and ventral-lateral mass of the human thalamus the present methods do not allow us to make correlations be-

Fig. 5. The extent of the sampling by all the electrode tracks of the sagittal planes from 11 mm to 16 mm from the midline is shown by the hatched areas. At 15 mm and 16 mm lateral is a zone where counts of phasic neurones are significantly in excess of sensory, as shown by a broken line (P = 0 · 02)

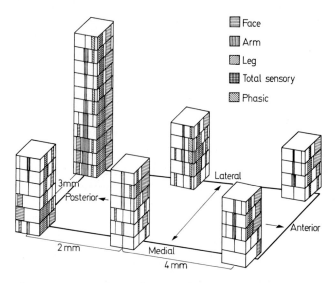

Fig. 6. The columns represent the tracks towards six target points. The horizontal blocks denote volumes which have been equally sampled. Within each block the relative number of different types of neurone is shown and comparisons between blocks can be made; see text p. 576

tween neuronal properties and appearance. Attempts to guess and 'jump the gun' should be resisted.

Three different types of locational analysis have been attempted. The first is to find if there are significant differences in the relative incidence of any two types of neurone in a defined three dimensional space. Significance tests can be done on counts. But counts do not include the relative frequency with which neurones of various types are found, because the amount of sampling in different areas is unequal. To overcome this difficulty a second type of analysis can be done in which the thalamus is parcelled off into a number of volumes of equal sampling, measured and computed so that each volume contains an equal number of 'track millimetres'. When this has been done one can give significance to counts of the

Fig. 7a. A diagrammatic representation of the 17 recording tracks (out of 145) in which sensory neurones related to different parts of the upper limb were encountered. The tracks have been vertically adjusted so that the mean position of the neurones related to the upper arm and shoulder (○) lie on the same horizontal line. The vertical scale is in millimetres measured along the electrode track. It is seen that neurones for the wrist and hand (⊖) are distributed so that 8 are above the horizontal line and 24 below. This difference is unlikely to have occurred by chance (P = 0.003). — Fig. 7b. 15 recording tracks aligned with respect to the mean position of neurones relating to the face. It shows the relatively close packing of these neurones and a tendency to be below other sensory neurones encountered on the same track. — Fig. 7c. 10 tracks with mixed phasic and sensory neurones to illustrate a tendency towards grouping of neurones of similar type. This is significant in the starred (*) tracks

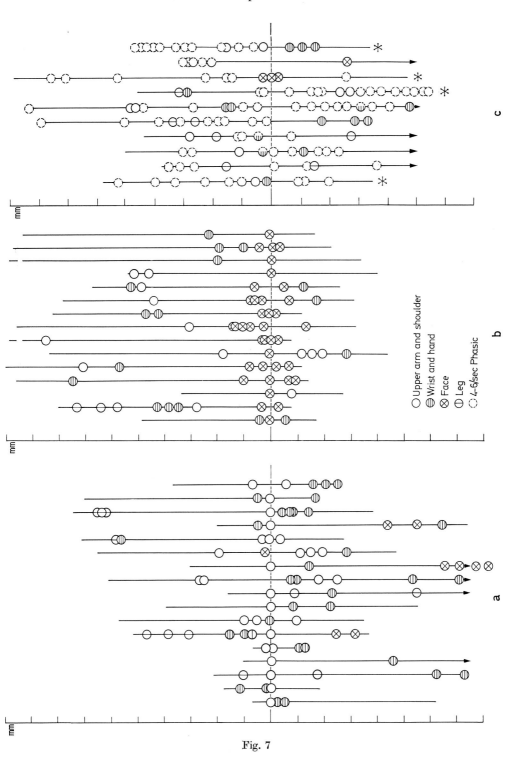

Fig. 7

same type of neurone and find the location of zones of maximum density for a particular type of neurone within the zones studied. The third type of analysis looks for consistent patterns in the relative location of neurones of different type along a succession of recording tracks. This type of analysis ignores the x, y, z information and can take a point of similar function, for example, the centre of points responsive to superficial stimulation of the face, and regardless of its parti-cular location one can express the relation of other points to it. The results of these three different types of analysis will now be briefly described.

1. The Location Zones of Maximum Density

By means of a computer program it is possible to plot the regions in which the electrode has been in each successive plane of laterality from 11–16 mm from the midline. These areas can be superimposed on outlined figures from the Atlas of Andrew and Watkins (1969). These outlines approximately embrace the 70 % of 27 specimens in their series. It is seen in Fig. 5 that the sampling was selective and secondly, that at lateral 15 and 16 there was a region where the computer's count of phasic neurones was significantly in excess of sensory. In other areas there was no significant difference in incidence of the neurones of these two types.

2. Relative Location by Normalised Density

The recordings towards one of six target points have been represented by columns erected on an imaginary horizontal plane (Fig. 6). The computer computes volumes or 'quanta' of equal recording. A quantum is expressed in a unit of 30 track millimetres. Each quantum is represented by a separate block, so that in each quantum we have counts of the total number of neurones of different types. The location of each quantum in x, y, and z is known, but not shown. It is seen on this analysis that the most anterior and lateral quanta have an excess of phasic over sensory neurones. With regard to parts of the body, it shows that the incidence of 'face' neurones is maximal postero-laterally, but that going 2 mm anteriorly and 3 mm laterally there is an excess of 'leg' neurones. This arrangement of the data shows that there are regions postero-medially where nothing but 'face', neurones were recorded, but lateral to this there are regions where 'face', 'arm' and 'leg' neurones were recorded. It also shows in the postero-lateral column that 'arm' and 'leg' neurones tended to be superior to 'face' neurones.

3. Location by Relative Position Along Recording Tracks

To investigate the relative location of neurones connected to different parts of the body, for example, the hand and arm in contrast to the elbow and shoulder, one can select a number of tracks which have both types of neurones and centre them along a zero line, and this is done in Fig. 7. We find there is a significant increase of 'wrist' and 'hand' representation below the upper arm. These kinds of plots, however, stress the great variability, and the fact that some tracks show the reverse of this. We can do the same thing with the face and locate tracks which include 'face' and 'hand' neurones and show that 'face' neurones tend to be rather closely distributed and that they tend to be significantly below the other sensory neurones. As regard the general arrangement of phasic and sensory neurones, one can see from selected plots to include neurones of both types, there is a tendency for neurones to occur in blocks. Simple statistics, show that the clumping is significant. Location of neurones confirms the general picture of a homunculus with a face medial and leg lateral and with the trunk superior and the distal parts inferior.

The general picture from location analysis that emerges at this stage is of sensory neurones grouped probably in many small interlaced plates, each plate containing neurones with one or more than one of the many possible attributes which these neurones can show. The primary attributes seem to be those of body-location (superficial versus deep, in its many varieties), somite (face to sacrum), axial versus distal, fixed versus free in relation to dependence on the periphery, and others yet to be discovered. The organisation of these permutations in three dimensions in the space of about one cubic centimetre is at present an unsolved mystery.

References

ALBE-FESSARD, D., ARFEL, G., GUIOT, G., HARDY, J., VOURC'H, G., HERTZOG, E., ALEONARD, P., DEROME, P.: Dérivations d'activités spontanées et évoquées dans les structures cérébrales profondes de l'homme. Rev. neurol. **106**, 89–105 (1962).

ALBE-FESSARD, D., ARFEL, G., GUIOT, G., DEROME, P., HERTZOG, E., VOURC'G, G., BROWN, H., ALEONARD, P., DE LA HERRAN, J., TRIGO, J.C.: Electrophysiological studies of some deep cerebral structures in man. J. Neurol. Sci. **3**, 37–51 (1966).

ALBE-FESSARD, D., GUIOT, G., LAMARRE, Y., ARFEL, G.: Activation of Thalamocortical Projections Related to Tremorogenic Processes. In: The Thalamus. Ed. by D.P. PURPURA and M.D. YAHR. pp. 237–253. New York: Colombia Univ. Press 1969.

ANDREW, J., WATKINS, E.S.: A Stereotaxic Atlas of the Human Thalamus and Adjacent Structures. Baltimore: The Williams & Wilkins Co. 1969.

BATES, J.A.V.: The Significance of Tremor Phasic Units in the Human Thalamus. 3rd Symp. Park. Dis. Edinburgh: Livingstone, pp. 118–123, 1969.

BERTRAND, C.: Discussion. J. Neurosurg. **20**, 882–883.

BERTRAND, G.: Studies of Unit Activity in the Human Thalamus during Stereotaxic Surgery. Proc. XXV Internat. Union of Physiol. Sci., VIII, 195–196 (1971).

CARRERAS, M., MANCIA, D., PAGNI, C.A.: Unit Discharges Recorded from the Human Thalamus with Microelectrodes. 3rd. Int. Symp. Stereoencephalotomy, Madrid 1967. Confin. neurol. (Basel) **29**, 87–89 (1967).

GAZE, R.M., GILLINGHAM, F.J., KALYANARAMAN, S., PORTER, R.W., DONALDSON, A.A., DONALDSON, I.M.L.: Microelectrode Recordings from the Human Thalamus. Brain **87**, 691–706 (1964).

GUIOT, G., HARDY, J., ALBE-FESSARD, D.: Délimitation précise des structures sous-corticales et identification de noyaux thalamiques chez l'homme par l'électrophysiologie stéréotaxique. Neurochirurgia (Stuttg.) **5**, 1–18 (1962).

HANKINSON, J., McCOMAS, A.J., WILSON, P.: Properties of somatosensory cells in the human thalamus. J. Physiol. (Lond.) **216**, 23P–24P (1971).

HUBEL, D.H.: Tungsten Microelectrode for Recording from Single Units. Science **125**, 549–550 (1957).

JASPER, H., BERTRAND, G.: Exploration of the Human Thalamus with Microelectrodes. Physiologist 7, 167 (1964a).

JASPER, H., BERTRAND, G.: Stereotaxic Microelectrode Studies of Single Thalamic Cells and Fibres in Patients with Dyskinesia. Trans. Amer. neurol. Ass. 79–82 (1964b).

JASPER, H., BERTRAND, G.: Thalamic Units Involved in Somatic Sensation and Voluntary and Involuntary Movements in Man. In: The Thalamus. Ed. by D.P. PURPURA and M.D. YAHR. 365–390. New York: Colombia Univ. Press 1966.

Chapter 15

Anatomical Organization of the Somatosensory Cortex

By

E. G. Jones, Dunedin (New Zealand) and T. P. S. Powell, Oxford (Great Britain)

With 8 Figures

Contents

Introduction

This chapter is primarily a review of experimental anatomical work carried out in the last five years with both light and electron microscopy. Throughout this account an attempt has been made to link these observations with known physiological properties and where a physiological correlation is wanting, to suggest possible directions for further study.

A. Somatic Sensory Representation in the Cerebral Cortex

In the somatic sensory cortex of all mammals except the monotremes (LENDE, 1964), the surface of the body is represented twice (Fig. 1A) (WOOLSEY, 1952,

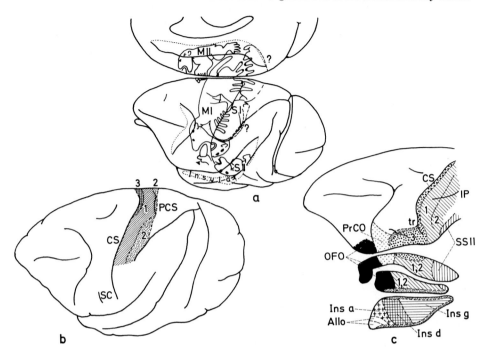

Fig. 1. a. The position and overall organization of the first (SI) and second (SII) somatic sensory areas of the cerebral cortex of the rhesus monkey as determined by the method of evoked potentials, and of the motor (MI) and supplementary motor (MII) areas as determined by electrical stimulation (Woolsey, 1958. Reproduced with permission of the publishers.) b. and c. The position and extent of the three architectonic subdivisions (areas 3, 1 and 2) of the postcentral gyrus and of the insulo-opercular region, after Powell and Mountcastle (1959a) (b), and Roberts and Akert (1963) (c). tr., the transitional field, area 3a, which for the greater part of its extent is buried in the depths of the central sulcus. (Reproduced with permission of the publishers)

1958). In the first area (SI), with the exception of regions related to areas in and around the mouth, in which neurons can be excited from bilateral and ipsilateral receptive fields, only the contralateral half of the body surface is represented (Woolsey, 1942, 1952, 1958). Within the overall map of SI as plotted in the "homuncular" form of Woolsey and his associates there is a precise mapping of individual dermatomes so that each dermatome is represented in serial order in such a way that its topographic relationships to neighbouring dermatomal areas are identical to those seen on the body surface (Werner and Whitsel, 1968). Individual dermatomal areas, however, overlap to a considerable extent (Celesia, 1963; Werner and Whitsel, 1968).

The boundaries of SI as determined by the method of evoked potentials fit remarkably well with certain anatomical boundaries described by workers who have studied the cytoarchitectonics of the region (Brodmann, 1909; Economo and Koskinas, 1925; Powell and Mountcastle, 1959a; Roberts and Akert, 1963; Hassler and Muhs-Clement, 1964) (Fig. 1B, C). SI encompasses three architectural fields, areas 3, 1 and 2, arranged in that order from before back. The caudal boundary of SI corresponds to the junction of area 2 with area 5 or area 7 of BRODMANN (1909; POWELL and MOUNTCASTLE, 1959a) and, anteriorly, it merges with the transitional field, area 3a, which separates area 3 proper ("area 3b") from the motor cortex, area 4. (It should be noted that area 3b is what most authors have referred to in the monkey simply as area 3.) The significance of these fields lies in the fact that within them neurons are aggregated according to their modality properties (POWELL and MOUNTCASTLE, 1959b). Thus in area 3b, the majority of single units are activated by light tactile stimuli, while in areas 1 and 2 most are driven by "deep" stimuli — i.e. by pressure or by movement of a joint (POWELL and MOUNTCASTLE, 1959b). In the cat and baboon, the transitional field (3a) is a receiving area for Group I muscle afferents (OSCARSSON and ROSÉN, 1966; JONES and POWELL, 1968b, 1969c; LANDGREN and SILFVENIUS, 1969; PHILLIPS et al., 1971). Throughout SI, an occasional unit is encountered which is excited by nociceptive stimuli and from wide peripheral receptive fields (POWELL and MOUNT-CASTLE, 1959b).

One as yet unresolved problem in regard to the representation of the body surface in SI is that, although with the method of surface recording of evoked potentials the dorsum of the back is represented caudally (in area 2) and the apices of the limbs rostrally (in area 3b) (WOOLSEY et al., 1942), yet with the method of single unit recording, each portion of the body surface appears to be represented as an antero-posterior strip spanning areas 3b, 1 and 2 (POWELL and MOUNTCASTLE, 1959b). Thus, light tactile units recorded in area 3b relate to the dorsum of the back as well as to the digits, and deep units relating to the feet and hands are found in area 2 along with those related to the back (POWELL and MOUNTCASTLE, 1959b). To some extent this problem has recently been clarified by PAUL et al. (1971). These workers have found that the hand is totally represented in area 3b and that this area does not merely represent an extension of the digits. A complete representation of the hand has also been found in area 1. Area 2 has not been explored completely because of its sensitivity to barbiturates but the limited data available from the rostral part of this area suggests that there is another representation here. As this systematic study has so far been limited to the hand area it is not justifiable to generalize these findings to the remainder of the body, and it is quite possible that the re-representation may be limited to certain parts of the body such as the distal parts of the limbs and face as the result of phylogenetic specialization. This finding of a multiple representation of the hand is not necessarily incompatible with the new and important concept of the representation of the limbs in SI proposed by WERNER and WHITSEL (1968), as there could either be a complete representation in the form proposed by these authors in *each* of the architectonic areas or within one common overall map in the postcentral gyrus there could be multiple representation of certain identical areas of the body surface (such as the hand).

A second somatic sensory area (SII) has been recognized in most mammals on the grounds of both evoked potentials (WOOLSEY, 1952, 1958; BLOMQUIST and LORENZINI, 1965) and cytoarchitecture (ROBERTS and AKERT, 1963; HASSLER and MUHS-CLEMENT, 1964). It lies below and behind SI such that the face areas of the two abut upon one another. There is a growing tendency in current papers to refer to SI as the "primary" and SII as the "secondary" somatic sensory area. In our opinion, this terminology should be avoided because it gives to the two areas a functional connotation which was never intended by Adrian (1940, 1941) who named them "first" and "second" only in a chronological sense. As each receives fibres from the main somatic sensory relay nucleus of the thalamus, the ventrobasal complex (Guillery et al., 1966; Morrison et al., 1968; Manson, 1969; Jones and Powell, 1969b, 1970a), for the present they are probably best regarded as but subdivisions of a single "primary" sensory area. The representation of the body surface in SII is a bilateral one (Woolsey, 1952, 1958) and is far less precise than in SI; the dermatomal regions, although still in serial order (Whitsel et al., 1969) are arranged with a far greater degree of overlap (Celesia, 1963; Whitsel et al., 1969). The properties of single neurons in SII are remarkably similar to those of neurons in SI in being excited by light tactile stimuli and occasionally by deep pressure applied to small, localized peripheral receptive fields (Carreras and Andersson, 1963; Whitsel et al., 1969). Each neuron of this type is usually fired by ipsi- and contralateral stimuli applied to approximately symmetrical peripheral fields and the cells have certain features suggestive of both lemniscal and antero-lateral inputs (Whitsel et al., 1969). No neurons responsive to joint movement have been recorded in SII of the monkey (Whitsel et al., 1969) and in the cat joint afferents project only to a small region in the vicinity of the representation of the apical portions of the limbs (Landgren et al., 1967a, b). At the posterior margin of SII proper, in both the cat and monkey, there is a small region intercalated between, and perhaps overlapping SII and the auditory cortex (Woolsey, 1961; Berman, 1961a, b; Carreras and Andersson, 1963; Whitsel et al., 1969; Heath, 1970; Heath and Jones, 1971). Here, convergence upon single neurons of somatic, auditory and even visual stimuli occurs, and neurons with wide, often discontinuous and asymmetrical peripheral receptive fields and responding to nociceptive stimuli, are common (Carreras and Andersson, 1963; Whitsel et al., 1969). Within, or overlapping, the head representation of SII of the cat and dog is another small area (the "third auditory area") in which auditory responses may be evoked (Woolsey, 1961).

A third somatic sensory area or "SIII" has been described in the cat by Darian-Smith and his colleagues (Darian-Smith, 1964; Darian-Smith et al., 1966). This occupies the rostral end of the middle suprasylvian gyrus immediately caudal to the part of SI related to the head and must lie within the architectonic field, area 5 (Hassler and Muhs-Clement, 1964; Jones and Powell, 1968b). In it there is a topographic mapping of the surface of the head and forelimbs almost as detailed as in SI itself and Darian-Smith has suggested that, like SI and SII, it receives fibres from the ventrobasal complex (Darian-Smith, 1964). Similarly, in man and in the squirrel monkey a "supplementary sensory area" has been described in which evoked sensations or evoked responses are referred to the limbs (Penfield and Jasper, 1954; Blomquist and Lorenzini, 1965). This also lies immediately behind SI and can be equated with area 5 (Jones and Powell, 1969c). In the sections which follow, evidence will be presented to show that these areas do not receive fibres from the thalamic somatic sensory relay nucleus, but that other pathways may account for the somatic sensory evoked responses and topographic mapping in each of them.

B. Pattern of Thalamic Projections to the Somatic Sensory Cortex

As the somatic sensory cortex consists of two main subdivisions (SI and SII) each containing a detailed representation of all or half of the surface of the body (WOOLSEY, 1952, 1958), a reasonable postulate in the 1950's was that each received a separate thalamic input (KNIGHTON, 1950). SI had been known for some time to be related to the ventrobasal complex from studies of cellular degeneration following cortical lesions, and in 1958 ROSE and WOOLSEY showed in the cat, that provided SII was destroyed in conjunction with the auditory cortex, then a different part of the thalamus underwent retrograde degeneration. This other region had earlier been called by ROSE (1942) the posterior group of thalamic nuclei and is a region of heterogeneous cell types and with ill-defined boundaries, essentially intercalated between the main somatic, auditory and visual relay nuclei at the caudal end of the thalamus. It is best known in the cat but there seems to be every reason for believing that a similarly organized posterior group is also a feature of the Primate brain (MEHLER, 1966; JONES and POWELL, 1970a).

Following the work of ROSE and WOOLSEY, it became obvious that the posterior group received afferents from the spinal cord (WHITLOCK and PERL, 1959; MEHLER et al., 1960; PERL and WHITLOCK, 1961) and subsequent anatomical work has demonstrated that there is a bilateral projection from the spinal cord and a crossed one from the dorsal column nuclei (MEHLER, 1966). The properties of posterior group neurons are such that they may, *a priori*, be considered as being involved in the more protopathic aspects of somatic sensation (POGGIO and MOUNTCASTLE, 1960). Thus, in contrast to ventrobasal neurons which are exclusively modality- and place-specific (POGGIO and MOUNTCASTLE, 1960, 1963), posterior group neurons are excited from wide, often bilateral, peripheral receptive fields, are sensitive to nociceptive stimuli and frequently show convergence of somatic, auditory and vibratory inputs (POGGIO and MOUNTCASTLE, 1960). Finally, there is some evidence for a topographic representation of the body surface in a region caudal to the ventrobasal complex (EMMERS, 1965; DAVIDSON, 1965). On the basis of this evidence, a reasonable prediction (POGGIO and MOUNTCASTLE, 1960) was that the ventrobasal complex received fibres primarily from the medial lemniscus, was concerned with the more discriminative aspects of somatic sensation and projected to SI, while the posterior group received mainly from the spinal cord, was concerned with protopathic sensibility and sent fibres mainly to SII and the auditory cortex. Such a suggestion is still not entirely ruled out, although it is obvious that the cortical and subcortical relations of the posterior group are rather more complex than those implied by this dual scheme.

1. Cat. In this review of the thalamo-cortical projections in the somatic sensory pathway, the cat and monkey will be described separately as certain irreconcilable differences make it difficult to generalize from the one animal to the other and suggest that a certain element of species variation may exist. It is becoming apparent that the concept of a dual thalamo-cortical system involving the ventrobasal complex and SI on the one hand and the posterior group and SII on the other is now unlikely. GUILLERY et al. (1966) have shown that following focal stimulation of the ventrobasal complex, evoked responses can be obtained in topographically related parts of both SI and SII. This demonstration that the ventrobasal complex does indeed project to both areas confirms an earlier report of Macchi, Angeleri and Guazzi (1959) who claimed that small lesions of SII, like those of SI, cause focal cellular degeneration in the ventrobasal complex. Their results, however, are open to criticism that the lesions employed could have interrupted fibres passing to SI. Recent anatomical studies have made use of the more sensitive Nauta technique. The fibre degeneration ensuing from a stereotaxic lesion of the ventrobasal complex of the cat is found in both SI and SII and there is a topographic distribution of such fibres corresponding to the dermatomal affinities of the damaged part of the ventrobasal complex (Jones and Powell, 1969b) (Fig. 2A). The degeneration in SII is finer and of about half the intensity

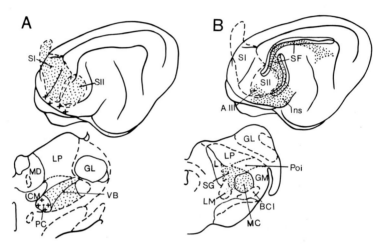

Fig. 2. A. The total cortical projection of the ventrobasal complex of the thalamus in the cat (stipple) and of the parvocellular component of the ventroposterior nucleus (crosses). B. The total cortical projection of the part of the posterior group consisting of the magnocellular division (MC) of the medial geniculate nucleus and the adjacent suprageniculate nucleus (SG). The cortical area involved comprises mainly the insular and suprasylvian fringe auditory areas (Woolsey, 1961) but overlaps into those parts of SII in which there is overlap and/or convergence of auditory and somatic sensory inputs (area AIII of Tunturi and possibly area SIIB of Carreras and Andersson)

of that in SI and the topographic distribution appears to be less precise in SII (Morrison et al., 1968; Jones and Powell, 1969b) in keeping with the greater degree of dermatomal overlap therein (Celesia, 1963; Whitsel et al., 1969). Within SI, areas 3b, 1 and 2 receive heavy and apparently equal projections composed of rather coarse fibres (Jones and Powell, 1969b). Even in those brains with small lesions of the ventrobasal complex some additional coarse but sparse degeneration always spreads forwards into the transitional field, area 3a, in a region continuous with that in SI proper (Jones and Powell, 1969b). There is no projection from the ventrobasal complex to the motor cortex (Jones and Powell, 1969b) so that somatic sensory evoked responses in area 4 must be mediated by other pathways (Malis et al., 1953). Similarly, fibre degeneration only occurs in area 5 when the rostral part of the lateroposterior nucleus is invaded by a lesion (JONES and POWELL, 1969 b), so that the basis for somatic evoked responses in this area cannot be direct thalamo-cortical pathways emanating from the ventro-basal complex.

Although the anatomical studies clearly show that the ventrobasal complex projects to both SI and SII, they obviously cannot in themselves indicate whether the same or a separate population of neurons in the ventrobasal complex send their axons to these two cortical areas. This problem has been resolved, however, by the work of MANSON (1969), who, in antidromically activating single ventro-basal neurons from the cortex, showed that about half of his sample projected to SI alone and of the remainder the vast majority sent branches to both SI and SII. Only a very small proportion sent axons solely to SII. The anatomical observation that the axonal degeneration in SII is approximately half that seen in SI following lesions of the ventrobasal complex (MORRISON et al., 1968; JONES and POWELL, 1969 b) could be in keeping with the observations of MANSON that only about half the neurons of the complex send axons to SII. This provides support for the con-cept of ROSE and WOOLSEY (1949, 1958) that some cortical areas receive "essen-tial" and others "sustaining" projections from a given thalamic nucleus. A com-mon interpretation of the latter type of projection is that it is a collateral one (ROSE and WOOLSEY, 1949, 1958).

The demonstration that the ventrobasal complex projects to both SI and SII still does not resolve the question of the cortical projections of the posterior group of thalamic nuclei. GUILLERY et al. (1966) observed responses in topographically related parts of SI and SII in two examples in which neurons in the magnocellular division of the medial geniculate nucleus were stimulated. MEHLER (1966) in referring to a single experiment, felt that the posterior group probably projected to SII and not to SI. However, ROWE and SESSLE (1968), in recording antidromic responses in the "posterior group", found a proportion of cells which seemed to project to quite wide areas of the cortex, including SI, SII, the auditory cortex and the anterior end of the suprasylvian gyrus.

The most recent evidence (HEATH, 1970; HEATH and JONES, 1971) (Fig. 2 B), obtained with the technique of axonal degeneration, is that destruction of that part of the posterior group consisting of the suprageniculate nucleus and the adjoining magnocellular division of the medial geniculate nucleus, causes degene-ration in a continuous band of cortex. This includes the insular and suprasylvian fringe auditory fields (WOOLSEY, 1961), the vestibular projection area (MICKLE and ADES, 1952), and partially overlaps the head and hindlimb representations of SII. That is, it incorporates the two regions in which overlap and/or convergence of somatic sensory and auditory impulses occurs (WOOLSEY, 1961; BERMAN, 1961 a, 1961 b; CARRERAS and ANDERSSON, 1963) and in one of which neurons possess properties similar to those of the posterior group. No degeneration has been found in SI nor in SII proper even after very large lesions of the posterior group. There is, therefore, in the somatic sensory system, a central core consisting of SI and the greater part of SII, which, in receiving fibres only from the ventrobasal complex, is relatively "modality-pure". But SII is surrounded and partially overlapped by a fringe area receiving fibres from the posterior group and exhibiting overlap and convergence of sensory modalities.

2. Monkey. The earlier work of Walker (1938), and Le Gros Clark and Boggon (1935), together with more recent studies (Le Gros Clark and Powell, 1953; Roberts and Akert, 1963) using the method of retrograde cellular degeneration has firmly established that the post-central gyrus, including all three of its cytoarchitectural subdivisions, is related to the ventrobasal complex. There have been no cellular studies which include SII within the cortical target of the ventrobasal complex. More recent work with the Nauta method following stereotaxic lesions in the thalamus of the monkey (Jones and Powell, 1970a) has shown that as in the cat, the ventrobasal complex sends fibres in a topographically orga-

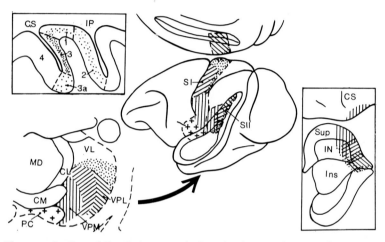

Fig. 3. The organization of the thalamo-cortical projections to the somatic sensory areas in the rhesus monkey. Trunk representation stippled; forelimb and hindlimb representations obliquely hatched; head and face representation vertically hatched; projection of the parvocellular component of the ventroposterior nucleus crosses. *Upper inset:* The relative distribution of terminal degeneration in SI following a lesion of the ventrobasal complex. Area 3b receives a heavy projection but that to areas 3a, 1 and 2 is relatively slight. *Lower inset:* A more accurate representation of the organization of the projection from the ventrobasal complex to SII shown on a reconstruction of the lateral sulcus. Note the extensive overlap. Sup., superior face; In., internal face; CS, central sulcus

nized fashion to both SI and SII (Fig. 3). As in the cat, the projection to SII is finer, sparser and the organization less precise.

The projection to SI is remarkably different from that of the ventrobasal complex to SI in the cat. Whereas in the cat, subareas 3b, 1 and 2 receive equally dense projections (Jones and Powell, 1969b), in the monkey only area 3b receives a heavy projection and this is made up of singularly coarse fibres some of which overlap into area 3a (Jones and Powell, 1970a) (Fig. 3). By contrast, areas 1 and 2 receive a very much smaller number of fibres all of which are of fine calibre and distribute only sparse terminal ramifications through the two areas. The intensity of degeneration in areas 1 and 2 does not increase when parts of the thalamus other than the ventrobasal complex are destroyed (Jones and Powell, 1970a) so that apparently they do not receive fibres from any other thalamic nuclei. The trajectory of the fine fibres passing to areas 1 and 2 is such as to suggest that they are branches of the coarser fibres entering area 3b, although actual branching has not been observed (JONES and POWELL, 1970a). If this suggestive observation should prove to be correct, it would lend direct support to certain conclusions of LE GROS CLARK and POWELL (1953) and of ROBERTS and AKERT (1963); using the method of retrograde cell degeneration, these authors deduced that the neurons of the ventrobasal complex send their axons primarily to area 3b and that areas 1 and 2 receive predominantly collaterals of these. If this is accepted, then to a cursory examination, a problem of considerable magnitude arises, for the response properties of a single neuron in the ventrobasal complex are identical to those of a neuron in area 3b or of one in areas 1 and 2 but it never seems to have characteristics proper to both (ROSE and MOUNTCASTLE, 1954; MOUNTCASTLE, 1957; MOUNTCASTLE and POWELL, 1959; POWELL and MOUNTCASTLE, 1959b; POGGIO and MOUNTCASTLE, 1960, 1963). That is, a ventrobasal neuron excited by joint movement and, therefore, presumably sending its axon to area 2, is not excited by light tactile stimuli. However, the problem may be more apparent than real for POWELL and MOUNTCASTLE (1959) emphasize that it is only the majority of neurons in area 3b which are excited by light tactile stimuli. A small proportion are still preferentially fired by deep stimuli. Conversely in areas 1 and 2, although most neurons respond only to deep stimuli, some are still specific for light tactile stimuli (POWELL and MOUNTCASTLE, 1959b). Thus most of the ventrobasal neurons may send their axons to areas 3b, 1 or 2 and not to two or all three of these, but a small as yet unidentified population could send branches to all three areas (and possibly to SII as well).

3. The Question of Area 3a. In both the cat and monkey, the transitional area, 3a (POWELL and MOUNTCASTLE, 1959a; ROBERTS and AKERT, 1963), receives a sparse but constant projection from the ventrobasal complex (JONES and POWELL, 1969b, 1970a). In the monkey, when more rostral portions of the ventroposterior nucleus are invaded by a lesion, the axonal degeneration in area 3a becomes intense (JONES and POWELL, 1970a), suggesting that the subnucleus ventralis posterolateralis, pars oralis (VPLo), which POGGIO and MOUNTCASTLE (1963) place outside the confines of the ventrobasal complex, is the main thalamic relay for area 3a. A number of pieces of admittedly circumstantial evidence militate in favour of area 3a receiving primarily from VPLo. First, it is a cortical receiving area for group I muscle afferents in the cat and baboon (OSCARSSON and ROSÉN, 1966; LANDGREN et al., 1967a; LANDGREN and SILFVENIUS, 1969; PHILLIPS et al., 1971) and of unspecified deep stimuli in the rhesus monkey (POWELL and MOUNTCASTLE, 1959b). In the cat, Group I muscle afferents relay in the rostral part of the ventrobasal complex (ANDERSSON et al., 1966) while in the monkey, VPLo is activated from deep tissues (POGGIO and MOUNTCASTLE, 1963; ALBE-FESSARD, 1967) and receives cerebellar as well as lemniscal afferents (TARLOV, 1969). Secondly, in the human thalamus a separate subnucleus, intercalated between the ventrobasal and ventrolateral complexes and possibly the homologue of VPLo, contains single neurons which are preferentially excited by muscle stretch and joint movement (JASPER and BERTRAND, 1966; GOTO et al., 1968). There thus appear to be some grounds for considering that it is the homologue of this nucleus which is projecting to area 3a in the cat and monkey. Furthermore, because the cortical connections of area 3a, both associational and callosal, are those of SI rather than those of the motor cortex (Jones and Powell, 1968b, 1968c, 1969c, 1969d), instead of being a vague transitional field, area 3a appears to be a further subarea of SI devoted to low threshold muscle afferents and with a separate thalamic dependency. In this context it is noteworthy that the cortical region which in the cat appears to be primarily concerned with controlling transmission in the dorsal spinocerebellar tract seems to fall within area 3a (Hongo et al., 1967). Area 3a may also be concerned with other corticofugal activities, for of a small sample of neurons which were antidromically activated from the dorsal column nuclei in the cat, the majority lay in this area, rather than in SI proper (Gordon and Miller, 1969).

4. Cortical Projections of Other Parts of the Ventroposterior Nucleus

The most medial, parvocellular part of the ventroposterior nucleus serves as the thalamic relay for taste afferents (Oakley and Benjamin, 1966; Benjamin et al., 1967; Benjamin and Burton, 1968) and, in not being excited by tactile or kinesthetic stimuli, forms a part of the ventromedial complex of Rose and Mountcastle (1952) which may be concerned with visceral impulses (Rose and Mountcastle, 1952) and with the vagus nerve in particular (Dell, 1952). It should be noted, however, that splanchnic nerve afferents relay in the ventrobasal complex itself (McLeod, 1958) and project to the trunk region of SI (Amassian, 1951). The cortical projection of the parvocellular part of the ventroposterior nucleus includes in the monkey (Jones and Powell, 1970a) those parts of areas 3, 1 and 2 which lie outside the confines of SI as determined by evoked potentials (Woolsey et al., 1942) — below and in front of the central sulcus and in the frontal operculum (Roberts and Akert, 1963). This region contains two projection areas for taste nerve afferents (Benjamin et al., 1967; Benjamin and Burton, 1968) and visceral sensations can be evoked from it in man (Penfield and Rasmussen, 1950). In the cat, the situation appears to be similar with a second taste area lying below SII, in the lateral bank of the presylvian sulcus and close to the claustrum (Benjamin and Burton, 1968; Jones and Powell, 1969b; Burton and Earls, 1970).

A further subnucleus of the ventroposterior nucleus, the nucleus ventralis posterior inferior (VPI) is obvious in the monkey (Olszewski, 1952) and is recognised by some workers in the cat (Rinvik, 1968a) and other animals. It is activated by somatic stimuli (Mountcastle and Henneman, 1952) but little is known of its connections except that the fore and hindlimb areas of SI send fibres to it (Jones and Powell, 1970a). Its efferent connections are unknown although Roberts and Akert (1963) predict on the basis of its topographic relationship to other thalamic nuclei that it should project to the insula.

C. Cortico-Thalamic Pathways

Electrical stimulation of the somatic sensory cortex has been reported to have a facilitatory or an inhibitory effect upon transmission in the ventrobasal complex (Shimazu et al., 1965; Andersen et al., 1967). Stimulation of SI will depolarize thalamo-cortical relay cells in the ventrobasal complex and facilitate the passage of a lemniscal volley (Andersen et al., 1967). It also causes excitation of small groups of neurons which in turn results in inhibition of surrounding neurons (Shimazu et al., 1965). These effects are not surprising in view of the well-known part played by descending fibres in controlling transmission at the spinal and dorsal column relay sites (Walberg, 1957; Kuypers, 1960; Towe and Jabbur, 1961; Andersen et al., 1964; Gordon and Jukes, 1964; Levitt et al., 1964;

DARIAN-SMITH and YOKOTA, 1966; NYBERG-HANSEN, 1966). In the last few years, the existence of cortico-thalamic fibres passing to the ventrobasal complex has been confirmed by experiments with the Nauta technique (KAWANA and KUSAMA, 1964; MEHLER, 1966; DE VITO, 1967; RINVIK, 1968b, 1968c; JONES and POWELL, 1968a, 1970a) and by the electron microscopic demonstration of degenerating axon terminals after cortical lesions (JONES and POWELL, 1968a, 1969a).

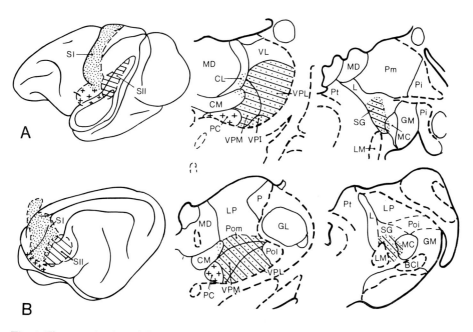

Fig. 4. The organization of the cortico-thalamic connections of SI and SII in the monkey (A) and cat (B). Both project to the ventrobasal complex and to a part of the medial division of the posterior group of thalamic nuclei (Pom). In the monkey this comprises mainly the ventral part of the suprageniculate nucleus (SG). SI has additional projections to the central lateral and centre median nuclei (probably from area 3a) and to the nucleus ventralis posterior, pars inferius (VPI). Projections from the taste and presumptive visceral regions at the lower end of the precentral gyrus and in the frontal operculum pass only to the parvocellular part of the ventroposterior nucleus

It has now been shown that both SI and SII of the cat and monkey project to the ipsilateral ventrobasal complex and to a restricted part of the ipsilateral medial division of the posterior group of thalamic nuclei (KAWANA and KUSAMA, 1964; MEHLER, 1966; DE VITO, 1967; RINVIK, 1968b, 1968c; JONES and POWELL, 1968a, 1970a) (Fig. 4). Although the projection of SII to the ventrobasal complex is less dense than that emanating from SI (JONES and POWELL, 1968a, 1970a), fibres from both SI and SII are distributed throughout the whole ventrobasal complex in a topographically organized fashion (RINVIK, 1968b, 1968c; JONES and POWELL, 1968a, 1970a) conforming to the evoked potential maps of ROSE and

Mountcastle (1952) and of Mountcastle and Henneman (1949, 1952), so that only those parts of the cortex receiving fibres from a given part of the ventrobasal complex send fibres back to that part (Jones and Powell, 1968a). The organization of the cortico-thalamic fibres passing to the ventrobasal complex is, therefore, very firmly governed by topographic relationships. There is little experimental evidence to support the view put forward by Tömböl (1967) on the basis of observations in Golgi-impregnated material, that cortico-thalamic fibres are distributed widely throughout a single nucleus and even to several nuclei. It is impossible with present anatomical methods to determine whether a given cortical neuron projects back to that cell in the thalamus from which it receives fibres, but the observation that all architectonic subdivisions of SI send fibres to the ventrobasal complex (Jones and Powell, 1968a) suggests that such an arrangement is by no means impossible. Centrifugal fibres, therefore, would respect both topographic and modality properties of single cells (or groups of cells) in the thalamic relay nuclei. Although it has been claimed by workers who have studied normal, Golgi-impregnated material that cortico-thalamic fibres are very thick (Cajal, 1911; Scheibel and Scheibel, 1966), electron microscopy shows that they are the smallest myelinated fibres in the nucleus, with a total diameter of 1–2 μ (Jones and Powell, 1969a). These fibres distribute very large numbers of axon terminals to the ventrobasal complex (the proportion from SII is less than from SI). The terminals of the cortico-thalamic fibres appear to exert their effect upon the dendrites of thalamo-cortical relay cells just beyond the synapse made by the incoming lemniscal fibres (Jones and Powell, 1969a).

Two authors have claimed that the ventrobasal complex receives a bilateral input from certain areas of the cerebral cortex. Chandler (cited by Bowsher (1966)) states that SII of the cat sends fibres to the ventrobasal complex of both sides, while Carreras et al. (1969) consider that "SIII" of Darian-Smith (1964, 1966) projects to both ventrobasal complexes as well as to the lateroposterior nucleus. A bilateral projection from SII has not been confirmed in four other studies (De Vito, 1967; Rinvik, 1968b, 1968c; Jones and Powell, 1968a, 1970a). In the case of projections from "SIII", the lesions mentioned by Carreras et al. (1969) must have invaded both SI and area 5. When SI is affected separately, the thalamic projection is strictly ipsilateral and passes only to the ventrobasal complex and to a part of the posterior group (Rinvik, 1968b, 1968c; Jones and Powell, 1968a, 1970a). When area 5 is affected separately (Jones and Powell, 1968a, 1970a), only the ipsilateral lateroposterior nucleus and another part of the posterior group contain degeneration.

As well as sending fibres to the ipsilateral ventrobasal complex, in both the cat and monkey SI and SII each project to the restricted part of the posterior group which receives ascending spinal and dorsal column fibres (Mehler, 1966). There is a little evidence for a topographic organization within the corticofugal projection (Rinvik, 1968b) and this would perhaps be in keeping with the second representation of the surface of the body demonstrated with evoked potentials in the caudal part of the thalamus of the rat (Davidson, 1965; Emmers, 1965). The projections of different cortical areas upon the posterior group appear to be rather precise, with only a little overlap between the projections of somatic, auditory and parietal cortex (Jones and Powell, 1968a, 1970a, 1971; Diamond et al., 1969), except when the region of overlap between auditory and somatic responses in the upper part of the anterior ectosylvian gyrus (BERMAN, 1961a, 1961b; CARRERAS and ANDERSSON, 1963) is considered, for its projection to the posterior group appears to overlap that of SII proper and that of the auditory cortex (RINVIK, 1968b; JONES and POWELL, 1968a; DIAMOND et al., 1969).

RINVIK in the cat (1968c) and PETRAS (1965) in the monkey have shown that a certain proportion of fibres from SI reach the caudal parts of the intralaminar and centre median nuclei. In the monkey the impression is gained that degeneration appears at the caudal ends of these nuclei if a lesion of SI encroaches upon area 3a (JONES and POWELL, 1970a). RINVIK (1968c) also notes in the cat that the motor cortex, as well as SI and SII, may send fibres to the ventrobasal complex in addition to its main relay nucleus, the ventrolateral complex. This could not be confirmed in the experiments of JONES and POWELL (1968a) in which all lesions of the "motor cortex" were confined to area 4. The inconsistency between these independent studies which in most other respects agree remarkably closely is probably in many ways an interpretative one, reflecting the belief of some workers that the junction between sensory and motor cortex in the cat is represented by the postcruciate dimple. Area 3a, however, extends for some distance in front of the postcruciate dimple (HASSLER and MUHS-CLEMENT, 1964); thus the interpretation of any experiments with lesions in the posterior sigmoid and coronal gyri will depend to a considerable extent upon whether area 3a is considered as a part of SI, as a transitional zone, or neglected altogether. In view of what has been said earlier, area 3a could project to a separate rostral part of the ventroposterior nucleus. Moreover, its close association with low threshold muscle afferents (OSCARSSON and ROSÉN, 1966; LANDGREN and SILFVENIUS, 1969; JONES and POWELL, 1968b, 1969c; PHILLIPS et al., 1971) could explain a connection with the caudal parts of the intralaminar nuclei which receive cerebellar as well as spinal afferents (MEHLER, 1966).

D. Organization of the Somatic Sensory Cortex

The basic unit of functional organization in SI and in SII appears to be a column of cells perpendicular to the surface and extending through all layers of the cortex (MOUNTCASTLE, 1957; POWELL and MOUNTCASTLE, 1959b; WERNER and WHITSEL, 1968). A single column contains cells with identical modality properties and similar topographic relationships. Hence, in area 3b of SI most columns are modality- and place-specific in relation to light tactile stimuli, while those in areas 1 and 2 are similarly related to deep stimuli, including joint movement (POWELL and MOUNTCASTLE, 1959b). All the cells in a column seem to be excited simultaneously as the first response to an incoming afferent impulse (MOUNTCASTLE, 1957; POWELL and MOUNTCASTLE, 1959b). In SII, there are similar columns responding to light tactile stimuli (CARRERAS and ANDERSSON, 1963; WHITSEL et al., 1969). Modality- and place-specific columns also appear to be the functional units of the visual cortex (HUBEL and WIESEL, 1962, 1965, 1969).

Recent anatomical studies on the connections of the somatic sensory cortex seem to fall naturally into three separate, though related spheres of interest. Two come under the heading of *ipsilateral association connections:* the first of these is more concerned with the detailed intrinsic organization of the somaesthetic areas and the connections involved may be termed *"intrinsic"*; the second is more concerned with the outward progression of impulses from the somatic sensory cortex and the connections involved may be considered as *"extrinsic"*. The third line of research has been devoted to the *interhemispheric connections* of the somatic sensory areas on the two sides of the brain. These subdivisions of the topic will be considered separately.

1. "Intrinsic" Association Connections. By electrically stimulating the somatic sensory cortex of the cat and recording the ensuing evoked potentials with surface electrodes, Sencer (1950) and Nakahama (1961) were able to demonstrate connections joining SI and SII to one another and to the motor cortex. Detailed studies of these connections have now been made in the cat and monkey (Jones and Powell, 1968b, 1969c) and as the findings in the two animals are identical (Fig. 5), the results may be considered together:

(i) A precisely organized set of reciprocal connections joins SI and SII to one another. Thus a lesion confined to one of the main topographic subdivisions of SI (leg, arm, trunk, head) causes axonal degeneration only in the part of SII related to the same part of the periphery and *vice versa*. Experiments in the monkey in which the architectonic (and functional) subdivisions of SI, areas 3b, 1 and 2, can be selectively damaged with greater facility, show that each of these areas projects to SII. SII, in turn, sends fibres to all three, and also to area 3a. It has not been possible to damage area 3a independent of the other fields in the monkey because of its position in the depths of the central sulcus, but there is reasonable evidence from the study on the cat that it projects back to SII.

(ii) Within SI, intrinsic association fibres join all parts of each of the main topographic subdivisions, but there are no connections with adjacent subdivisions. Hence, a lesion in the leg area causes degeneration throughout the leg area but not in the arm, trunk or head areas. Thus different parts of the peripheral representation seem to be kept separate in this part of the somatic sensory cortex. This demonstration of restriction within the boundaries of gross topographic regions offers confirmatory evidence for Woolsey's postulate (1952, 1958) that the two parts of the trigeminal nerve representation which appear to have been separated by expansion of the hand area in the primate (Woolsey et al., 1942) are, in fact, tenuously connected (Fig. 1A): following a lesion in the face area of the monkey (Jones and Powell, 1969c), intracortical degeneration spreads throughout the face area and up the caudal margin of the hand area to reach the region related to the occiput. There is some evidence from the smallest lesions in the monkey that the topographic segregation may be even more restricted. For example, a very small lesion confined to the representation of the forepaw digits causes a narrow band of axonal degeneration spanning the postcentral gyrus but not completely filling the forepaw representation (Jones and Powell, 1969c).

In view of the marked tendency for neurons to be aggregated in different architectonic fields of SI according to their modality properties (Powell and Mountcastle, 1959b), the connections of areas 3b, 1 and 2 are of interest. A small lesion of any one of these areas in the monkey (Jones and Powell, 1969c) causes axonal degeneration in a band stretching from area 3a in the fundus of the central sulcus across each of the others and back into area 5 of the superior parietal lobule. Often, there is an appearance of a focus of increased density in each of the individual fields. This indicates that all the fields of SI are reciprocally connected and has led to the suggestion (JONES and POWELL, 1969c) that one of the prime purposes of these intrinsic association fibres is to bring together columns of cells with different modality properties but lying within the same part of the topographic representation. Area 3a should probably also be included in this context for it receives fibres from each of the others and, at least in the cat (JONES and POWELL, 1968b), sends fibres to them.

(iii) The intrinsic connections of SII appear to be less precisely organized than those within SI (JONES and POWELL, 1968b, 1969c) in that a lesion anywhere in SII tends to cause Nauta-stained degeneration throughout the whole area, including the caudally situated overlap zone of BERMAN (1961a, 1961b) of CARRERAS and ANDERSSON (1963) and of WHITSEL et al. (1969). This is probably in keeping with the greater degree of dermatomal overlap in SII (CELESIA, 1963; WHITSEL et al., 1969). It should be noted, however, that the evidence upon which this rests is based upon experiments in which the lesions were relatively large (JONES and POWELL, 1968b, 1969c), so that it is possible that the use of smaller lesions might bring out some degree of organization akin to that in SI.

Intrinsic association fibres linking the parts of a topographic subdivision of SI or the whole of SII have an almost exclusively intracortical course, travelling for the most part in the bands of Baillarger. Fibres passing between SI and SII and between these areas and other parts of the cortex are invariably subcortical, running in the white matter, with their depth beneath the cortex generally dependent upon the distance which they have to travel (JONES and POWELL, 1968b, 1969c). The intracortical course of fibres within a functional division of the cortex and the subcortical course of fibres linking different subdivisions appears to hold as a general rule for the rest of the cortex (DIAMOND et al., 1968). A further small group of fine myelinated axons lies in the molecular layer immediately deep to the pia mater (DIAMOND et al., 1968; JONES and POWELL, 1968b, 1969c, 1970e). Following a lesion anywhere in the cortex these fibres degenerate up to a constant distance of about 5–7 mm on all sides of the lesion (JONES and POWELL, 1968b). Unlike most of the other intracortical fibres which remain within their functional subdivision, these fine fibres will cross architectonic boundaries and may, therefore, belong to some less specific intracortical association system. Because of their position and length, these axons could mediate the initial surface negative response which appears when the cortex is stimulated by surface electrodes (ADRIAN, 1936). This is caused by depolarisation of processes lying just beneath the surface, is rapidly attenuated and disappears at distances between 5–10 mm from the point of stimulation (BURNS, 1951).

2. "Extrinsic" Association Connections. *The total efferent cortical connections of SI* pass to area 5 of the parietal (monkey) or suprasylvian (cat) cortex, to the motor cortex (area 4) and to the supplementary motor cortex (JONES and POWELL, 1968b, 1969c) (Fig. 5). The other efferent projection, to SII, has been considered as an intrinsic connection. The projections from SI to area 5 and to the motor cortex are heavy, that to area 5 in particular being composed of singularly coarse fibres, but the projection to the supplementary motor area is sparse. As in the case of connections joining SI and SII, there is a detailed topographic organization of all these extrinsic projections from SI in that a lesion of one of its main subdivisions (leg, arm, trunk and head) causes degeneration only in the topographically related subdivision of the motor and supplementary motor areas. The projection to the motor cortex is especially precise and this is probably indicative of the high degree of interaction between somatic sensory and motor functions. However, these connections cannot account for the presence of somatic sensory evoked responses in the motor cortex for these responses survive ablation of the postcentral gyrus (Malis et al., 1953). There is a little overlap in the projections from

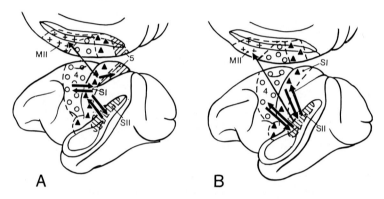

A   B

Fig. 5. A schematic diagram summarizing the ipsilateral cortical connections of SI (A) and SII (B). Reciprocal connections join SI and SII to one another and to the motor cortex (area 4). Each has an additional projection to the supplementary motor area (MII) but SI stands alone in sending fibres to area 5 of the parietal cortex

different subdivisions of SI to the supplementary motor area (Jones and Powell, 1969c), in keeping with the less detailed mapping of the periphery in this region (Woolsey, 1952, 1958). The projections of different parts of the peripheral representation to area 5 also show a certain amount of overlap, but a topographic segregation may still be discerned with the head region of SI sending fibres to the most lateral and the leg subdivision to the most medial part of area 5 (Jones and Powell, 1968b, 1969c). Hence, the topographic representation imposed upon area 5 by these projections is essentially continuous with that in SI itself. In the cat (Jones and Powell, 1968b), head and forelimb are "represented" in the part of area 5 contained in the suprasylvian gyrus, the trunk in the part in the depths of the ansate and lateral sulci, and the hindlimb in the part contained in the lateral gyrus. The suprasylvian part of area 5 conforms almost exactly with the "SIII" of Darian-Smith et al. (1964, 1966) and it seems significant that in this "SIII" responses are obtained only to stimulation of the head and forelimb, with those evoked from the head lying lateral to those evoked from the forelimb (Darian-Smith et al., 1966). Failure to obtain responses following stimulation of a hindlimb nerve may be added reason for equating "SIII" with area 5, for the part of area 5 related to the hindlimb lies in the lateral gyrus. This is not to say that the results of DARIAN-SMITH et al. are based entirely upon connections passing from SI, for in their experiments, cooling of SI did not abolish the evoked responses (DARIAN-SMITH et al., 1966). Because area 5 does not receive a thalamo-cortical input from the ventrobasal complex (JONES and POWELL, 1969b, 1970a), the most obvious pathway for such impulses would be *via* the superior colliculus and its projection to the lateroposterior nucleus (ALTMAN and CARPENTER, 1961), the latter then projecting to area 5 (JONES and POWELL, 1969b). In the monkey, area 5 occupies the greater part of the superior parietal lobule and the adjacent medial surface of the brain (BRODMANN, 1909). The hindlimb subdivision of SI sends fibres mainly to the part of area 5 on the medial surface, the trunk to the region behind the postcentral sulcus, the forelimb region to the exposed part on the lateral surface, and the head region to the part buried in the medial bank of the intraparietal sulcus (JONES and POWELL, 1969c). Because of its position and these connections, area 5 has been equated (JONES and POWELL, 1969c) with the "supplementary sensory area" first described in man (PENFIELD and JASPER, 1954) and subsequently in the squirrel monkey (BLOMQUIST and LORENZINI, 1965). If this is so, it is not surprising that sensations have never been referred to the head by stimulation of this region in man and evoked responses were not recorded in it following stimulation of the face in the monkey. In both man and the monkey, the relevant part of area 5 would be largely buried in the intraparietal sulcus (BRODMANN, 1909); in any case, because the "representation" in area 5 is essentially continuous with that in SI (JONES and POWELL, 1969c), responses in its "head region" could easily have been interpreted as being in SI itself.

All three architectonic subdivisions of SI, areas 3b, 1 and 2, and as far as can be ascertained, area 3a, have the same efferent connections (JONES and POWELL, 1969c). Lesions confined to areas 3b, 1 or 2 in the monkey show that as well as all sending fibres to SII, they project individually to the motor and supplementary motor areas and to area 5. Each field distributes fibres throughout the full rostro-caudal extent of the topographically related segment of areas 4 and 5. This would appear to indicate that individual neurons in areas 4 and 5 receive cortical afferents from somatic sensory neurons related to skin and deep tissues, suggesting that association fibres serve to bring together at these levels, as well as within SI, neuronal columns with different functional characteristics but related to the same part of the periphery.

The total efferent cortical connections of SII are with SI and with the motor and supplementary motor areas (JONES and POWELL, 1968b, 1969c) (Fig. 5). The connections with SI have been considered as intrinsic connections. The projections to the motor and supplementary motor areas are found in the cat and monkey and, allowing for the overlap present in the representation of the body form in SII, are just as precisely organized as those of SI. The most obvious difference between the ipsilateral connections of SI and SII is that SII does not project to area 5 nor to any other "association area". The entire cortical outflow from SII is to the motor and supplementary motor areas (JONES and POWELL, 1968b, 1969c).

The supplementary motor area and area 5 of the cat fall within the boundaries of three of the so-called "polysensory areas" of this animal — the precruciate and the anterior lateral and anterior middle suprasylvian polysensory areas (THOMPSON et al., 1963; DUBNER, 1966;

Bignall et al., 1966; Bignall, 1967; Rutledge and Shellenberger, 1968). In these areas, particularly under chloralose anaesthesia, there is convergence of somatic sensory, auditory and visual impulses upon single neurons. It is probable that both ascending and cortico-cortical pathways are important in the functioning of these cortical areas: for example, although the primary visual cortex is not essential for maintaining visual evoked responses in at least one of them, in its absence, the responses are modified (Bignall, 1967; Rutledge and Shellenberger, 1968). There is as yet no anatomical evidence for direct cortico-cortical convergence from the three primary sensory areas upon the polysensory areas. While the primary somatic, auditory and visual cortices send fibres to immediately adjoining regions at the rostral ends of the lateral and middle suprasylvian gyri, these projections do not overlap (Diamond et al., 1968; Garey et al., 1968; Jones and Powell, 1968b). Similarly, in the frontal lobe, all three areas project to parts of area 6 which lie within the precruciate polysensory area, but the projections do not obviously converge (Diamond et al., 1968; Garey et al., 1968; Jones and Powell, 1968b). The remaining polysensory area at the caudal end of the middle suprasylvian gyrus overlaps projection areas of the visual and auditory cortex (Diamond et al., 1968; Garey et al., 1968; Jones and Powell, 1968b) but no direct nor indirect cortical pathways from the somatic sensory cortex reach this region (Jones and Powell, 1968b).

The total afferent cortical connections of the somatic sensory areas. Only the motor cortex (area 4) projects back into SI and SII (Jones and Powell, 1968b, 1969c; Pandya and Kuypers, 1969) (Fig. 5). Thus, while the connections of the two somatic sensory areas with one another and with area 4 are reciprocal, those with area 5 and the supplementary motor area are not. This absence of fibres returning to the somatic sensory cortex from its cortical projection areas clearly distinguishes the cortical from subcortical levels of this sensory pathway, as thalamic, brain stem and spinal relay sites all receive such "centrifugal" fibres. The same is true in the visual and auditory pathways, and therefore this difference may provide an important clue to the differences in function between cortical and subcortical components of a sensory pathway. As in the case of the projections from SI and SII to it, the returning projection from the motor cortex is precisely organized according to the topographic representation of the periphery. The number of fibres passing from the motor cortex to SII is considerably less than that directed to SI. There are no direct connections between the primary somatic, visual and auditory cortices (Jones and Powell, 1968b, 1969c). Indeed, it has been shown that the efferent intracortical pathways leaving these areas pass through at least three independent architectonic fields before they start to converge within the cortex (Jones, 1969; Jones and Powell, 1970f).

3. Interhemispheric Connections. Following the work of Sperry (1961) and Myers (1962a) who showed the importance of the forebrain commissures in the interhemispheric transfer of learning based upon sensory cues, there has been a growing interest in the anatomical organization of such pathways. In the 1930's, Mettler (1935a, b) on the basis of his work with the Marchi technique, enunciated a dictum that "any given cortical point is in direct callosal relation with such points in the heterolateral cortex as are related to it homolaterally by short association fibers." This he called a principle of heterolateral association. The first indication that this was perhaps an over-simplification came from the work of Curtis (1940) who showed with the evoked potential technique that certain parts of the sensory-motor and visual areas of the cat received few or no callosal connections. More recently, in a Nauta study, Myers (1962b), showed that the greater part of the area striata did not receive commissural fibres and this has since been confirmed and extended (EBNER and MYERS, 1965; CHOUDHURY et al., 1965; BERLUCCHI et al., 1967; HUBEL and WIESEL, 1967; WILSON, 1968; GAREY et al., 1968; HUGHES and WILSON, 1969). In the somatic sensory cortex of both the cat and monkey (Fig. 6) it has been shown that the parts of SI and SII related to the more distal aspects of the fore- and hindlimbs do not receive fibres from the opposite cortex (EBNER and MYERS, 1962, 1965; PANDYA and VIGNOLO, 1968; JONES and POWELL, 1968c, 1969d). There are, however, heavy commissural projections to the head, trunk, tail and proximal limb regions. These anatomical observations receive

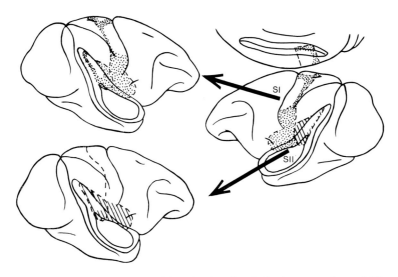

Fig. 6. A schematic diagram summarizing the interhemispheric connections of SI and SII. SI projects commissurally to both SI and SII of the opposite side. SII projects mainly to its counterpart only but sends additional fibres to the regions at the foot of the pre-central gyrus in which parts of the body are bilaterally represented. In both cases, however, regions related to the more distal aspects of the limbs neither send nor receive callosal fibres

support from the evoked potential study of TEITELBAUM et al. (1968). Experiments using small lesions confined to different parts of SI and SII (JONES and POWELL, 1968c, 1969d) have established the following pattern of connections: (i) the somatic sensory areas project callosally only to the somatic areas of the opposite cortex; there are no connections with the motor or parietal cortex. (ii) SI projects to both SI and SII of the opposite side; SII projects almost exclusively to its counterpart only, but its face region has an additional small projection to the portion of the opposite SI in which neurons can be excited by bilateral and ipsilateral stimuli applied to regions in and about the mouth. Thus, regions containing a contralateral representation (most of SI) receive a single callosal input (from SI); regions containing a bilateral representation (SII and the peri-oral part of SI) receive a double callosal input (from SI and SII). (iii) Within this pattern, only head, trunk, tail and proximal limb regions are connected, for the distal limb regions *neither send nor receive* commissural fibres (Fig. 6). This means that although SII receives a double callosal input, the commissural connections cannot account for the bilateral representation. The fact that certain important parts of the representation are not callosally connected, offers anatomical confirmation for the original observation of Woolsey and Wang (1945) that the bilateral representation is dependent upon other mechanisms. The available evidence also tends to exclude the thalamo-cortical and cortico-thalamic pathways, for the somatic sensory cortical areas are only directly related to the thalamus of the same side (Mehler, 1966; De Vito, 1967; Rinvik, 1968b, 1968c; Jones and Powell, 1968a, 1969b, 1970a). Therefore, the bilaterality of the representation in SII is probably engendered at the thalamic level or even lower. For example, a separate population of neurons in the ventrobasal complex or posterior group could be receiving afferent fibres from both sides of the body and projecting solely to SII. (iv) The connections between the representations of parts of the body lying in and adjacent to the midline are strictly organised (Jones and Powell, 1968c, 1969d). Thus, a tiny pinprick lesion in the middle of the head region of SI causes degeneration in an equally tiny portion of the opposite SI which is virtually a mirror image of the lesion, and in a further very small part of SII in which the same part of the periphery is represented. The callosal connection, therefore, assumes the nature of a point to point one. (v) Areas 3b, 1 and 2, each send fibres only to their counterparts in the opposite SI, but all three send fibres to the opposite SII (Jones and Powell, 1969d). A small amount of evidence from the cat suggests that area 3a projects to its homotopical field and to SII.

The intracortical course of commissural fibres in these functional subareas of SI is perpendicular and is so straight, with apparently so little branching (Jones and Powell, 1970e), that impulses carried in a single fibre can only influence a very restricted part of the cortex — though it has terminals in all layers (Jones and Powell, 1970e). The conclusion to be reached is that single commissural fibres passing to the architectonic subdivisions of SI must respect both the modality and topographic properties of single functional columns therein. In SII, the general topographic boundaries are respected, with some overlap, but within them the commissural fibres run an oblique course (Jones and Powell, 1969d) — though they still end in all layers (Jones and Powell, 1970e). This doubtless reflects the considerable overlap in the projection of individual dermatomes to SII (Celesia, 1963; Whitsel et al., 1969) and the modality convergence which must be occurring in SII as the result of all architectonic (and functional) subdivisions of SI projecting to it (Jones and Powell, 1968b, 1969c). All of these factors would suggest that in the unanaesthetised animal in which cortico-cortical activity is not depressed, the functional column in SII might be broader and less specific than that in SI.

It is obvious that all the influences crossing the midline at this cortical level are related solely to the axial and para-axial parts of the body, but it is difficult to decide whether it is the presence or absence of callosal connections which has the most important functional implications. In the visual system, where only the representations of the midline portions of the two visual fields are connected (Choudhury et al., 1965; Berlucchi et al., 1967; Hubel and Wiesel, 1967; Wilson, 1968; Garey et al., 1968; Hughes and Wilson, 1969), it is probably best interpreted as a mechanism for ensuring fusion of overlapping parts of the two images in the process of binocular vision. Whether the callosal connections of the somatic sensory cortex ensure that the nervous system's "view" of the axial parts of the body is a single, three dimensional one, cannot be answered.

The functional implications for the somatic sensory system of the lack of interhemispheric integration at this cortical level are far from obvious. It has been tentatively suggested that this lack could maintain the relative "purity" of centrifugal impulses emanating from the limb regions (JONES and POWELL, 1968c). Because centrifugal fibres appear to play a key role in controlling transmission at all levels in the sensory pathways (WALBERG, 1957; KUYPERS, 1960; TOWE and JABBUR, 1961; ANDERSEN et al., 1964; GORDON and JUKES, 1964; LEVITT et al., 1964; DARIAN-SMITH and YOKOTA, 1966; NYBERG-HANSEN, 1966) except the primary sensory cortex, this could be a factor in making the peripheral receptive fields of neurons related to the distal aspects of the limbs smaller than those related to other parts of the body (MOUNTCASTLE, 1957; POWELL and MOUNT-CASTLE, 1959b; POGGIO and MOUNTCASTLE, 1963; GORDON and JUKES, 1964). Such an arrangement would probably contribute to making the distal limb regions more sensitive in somaesthetic discrimination (POWELL and MOUNTCASTLE, 1959b). Could the corticofugal fibres carry back to the lower order neurons a reflection of central inhibitory processes which tend to be blurred by transcallosal influences? If as has been suggested (MOUNTCASTLE and POWELL, 1959), inhibition in the somatic sensory pathway serves to heighten stimulus contrast, such an interpretation would be by no means unlikely. The regions at which sensory information emanating from the apical limb segments is finally brought together across the midline are at present unknown but deserve further study, particularly in view of current interest in the interhemispheric transfer of learning. One possibility is that areas 5 and 6 of the parietal and premotor cortices are involved for there seem to be no gaps in their commissural connections (unpublished observations).

TEITELBAUM et al. (1968) find that unilateral destruction of SII in cats leads to a failure of transfer of acquired tactile discriminations from the damaged to the normal hemisphere, or *vice versa*. That is, a unilateral lesion of SII seems to have the same effect as section of the corpus callosum. Destruction of SI, by contrast, though leading to failure of transfer from the damaged to the undamaged hemisphere, does not interfere with transfer in the opposite direction. They, therefore, postulate that SII "plays a special role in this transfer as the recipient of tactile information flowing over the callosal pathways". It is difficult, however, to see this as being a direct transcallosal effect, for it was observed in experiments involving tactile discriminations in which the animal used its forepaws. Yet, the forepaw regions of SII are not commissurally connected (EBNER and MYERS, 1962, 1965; PANDYA and VIGNOLO, 1968; JONES and POWELL, 1968c, 1969d). It is obvious that the callosal is not the sole pathway for interhemispheric transfer of learned habits based on sensory cues, for GLICKSTEIN and SPERRY (1960) found that provided the somatic sensory cortex was damaged on one side after sectioning the corpus callosum, transfer would occur from the damaged to the undamaged hemisphere.

E. Differences between SI and SII

Obvious differences are seen in the anatomical connections of SI and SII. Ipsilaterally, each of these areas are firmly linked to one another and to the motor cortex but SI stands alone in sending a heavy, organized projection to the parietal field, area 5. This would imply that of the two, only SI is concerned with channelling somatic sensory information directly into "association" cortex. The main cortical outflow from SII is back to SI and to the motor areas. Because all architectonic fields of SI on *both* sides of the brain project to SII, the latter must be a region of convergence of impulses from skin, deep tissues and joints and also from muscles (i.e. from area 3a). In addition to receiving fibres from the opposite SII and from SI of both sides, SII shows a considerable overlap in the projection of ascending afferents (Carreras and Andersson, 1963; Whitsel et al., 1969). Presumably after integration within SII, this information from the body as a whole is made available *via* association fibres to both SI and the motor areas. There would, thus, be within the sensori-motor cortex a region for the integration of sensory information of all types and from both sides of the body at a relatively early stage of cortical function, although the only information from the distal aspects of the ipsilateral limbs would come *via* the (unknown) pathway responsible for the bilateral representation in SII. This can perhaps be envisaged as a collateral mechanism to the pathways involved in the onward progression of somatic sensory impulses from the first receiving area (SI) through the parietal, frontal and temporal association fields (Jones, 1969). Viewed in this light, SII might in a sense take the place of the association cortex in primitive mammals; this would not necessarily make it a more recent phylogenetic development than SI, for its thalamo-cortical connections seem to conform more to the primitive and generalized pattern of the opossum (Diamond and Uttley, 1963) and hedgehog (Diamond, 1967; Diamond and Hall, 1969; Hall and Diamond, 1968). Its activities in passing integrated somatic sensory information on to the motor areas might be more in the nature of a reflex rather than being involved in the "higher" qualities of perception and memory.

Whether SII is or is not a more recent development than SI is of course an open question but if the appearances of essential as opposed to sustaining thalamo-cortical projections is a newer phylogenetic development (Diamond, 1967; Diamond and Hall, 1969), SI would appear to be the more recent. Conceivably, SI has grown out of SII, or the two have developed from a common precursor during phylogeny. Indeed, all the primary sensory areas must have originally developed from the primitive dorsal pallium of the reptile (Smith, 1910; Goldby and Gamble, 1957), and the overlap of auditory, somatic, visual and motor areas in the alligator (Kruger and Berkowitz, 1960) and in primitive mammals such as the echidna (Lende, 1964) and opossum (Lende, 1963) is probably a reflection of this. Perhaps even more striking in the opossum (Lende, 1963) is the fact that SII falls completely within the anterior part of the auditory field, and the posterior part of the auditory field is overlapped by the visual areas. It is tempting to speculate that this is the part of the cortex most closely related to the common sensory cortex of the reptile and, if so, SII, the suprasylvian auditory fringe (Woolsey, 1961) and the lateral suprasylvian visual area (Vastola, 1961; Thompson et al., 1963; Hubel and Wiesel, 1969) all of which abut upon and perhaps overlap one another in the cat, could be the higher mammalian counterparts.

SII in having a less discrete topographic organization than SI, both in the projection of ascending afferents (Celesia, 1963; Whitsel et al., 1969) and in its cortical connections (JONES and POWELL, 1968b, 1969c), could be expected on *a priori* grounds to be less involved in the finer aspects of somaesthetic discrimination, whereas SI with its highly ordered topographic representation of the body form (CELESIA, 1963; WERNER and WHITSEL, 1968), discretely organized connections (JONES and Powell, 1968b, 1968c, 1969c, 1969d) and modality segregation (POWELL and MOUNTCASTLE, 1959b) could be expected to be more intimately concerned with such activities. There is a certain amount of evidence that this is so (ZUBECK, 1952; ORBACH and CHOW, 1959; SPERRY, 1959), although following lesions of SI, tactile discriminations can still be acquired provided that sufficient time is allowed to elapse after the operation (DIAMOND et al., 1964; TEITELBAUM et al., 1968). Because of the convergence on SII of impulses derived from all the different functional subdivisions of SI (JONES and POWELL, 1968b, 1969c), lesions of SII might be expected to result in more complex sensory defects, although if SII is no more than a relatively low-order reflex centre, such deficits might not be obvious. However, it is virtually impossible to analyse the functions of SI and SII in somaesthesis on the basis of selective ablations: *because of the strong reciprocal connections between them, interference with either must make the other abnormal on both sides of the brain.*

F. Analogy with the Visual Cortex

The organization of the connections of the somatic sensory areas has much in common with that of the visual areas of the cortex and suggests that to a considerable extent these may be based on a common plan. The closest analogy can be drawn in the cat: in three of the architectonic fields of the visual cortex (areas 17, 18 and 19), as in areas 3, 1 and 2, single columns of cells tend to be modality specific and are selectively activated by peripheral stimuli of different orders of complexity (HUBEL and WIESEL, 1962, 1965). These three fields are interconnected by association fibres, with one another and with a fourth — the lateral suprasylvian area (HUBEL and WIESEL, 1965; WILSON, 1968; GAREY et al., 1968; HEATH and JONES, 1970). Commissurally, areas 17, 18 and 19 project to their counterparts and to the lateral suprasylvian area, whereas the latter projects only to the opposite lateral suprasylvian area (HEATH and JONES, 1970). The similarity between areas 3, 1 and 2 and SII on the one hand, and areas 17, 18 and 19 and the lateral suprasylvian area on the other is striking. As the four visual areas each seem to contain separate representations of the retina (HUBEL and WIESEL, 1962, 1965, 1969) and as it now appears likely that areas 3, 1 and 2, as well as SII, may contain separate representations of at least some parts of the body, the analogy becomes even more striking.

The thalamic relationships of the somatic sensory and visual areas are less readily homologized but evidence is accruing to suggest that there are certain species differences in the pattern of thalamic projections to the cerebral cortex. In primitive mammals such as the opossum (DIAMOND and UTTLEY, 1963) and in those generalized mammals such as the hedgehog which lie closest to the basic mammalian stock (DIAMOND, 1967; HALL and DIAMOND, 1968; DIAMOND and HALL, 1969), it would appear that most thalamo-cortical projections are of the sustaining (collateral) type. The more specific or essential projections only seem to emerge on ascending the mammalian scale and may have appeared independently in different groups (DIAMOND and HALL, 1969). Certain irreconcilable differences between the thalamo-cortical projections in the visual and somatic systems of the cat and monkey seem to bear this out. In the cat, areas 3, 1 and 2 on the one hand (JONES and POWELL, 1968a) and areas 17, 18 and 19 on the other (GAREY and POWELL, 1967; WILSON and CRAGG, 1967), receive equally heavy and "essential" projections from the main thalamic relay nucleus, while SII and the lateral suprasylvian area receive less dense projections apparently of the "sustaining" type. In the monkey somatic sensory system, only area 3b appears to receive essential projections, areas 1 and 2, like SII, receiving a sustaining one (LE GROS CLARK and POWELL, 1953; ROBERTS and AKERT, 1963). This suggests that the somatic thalamo-cortical pathway has become more refined in respect of area 3. In the visual system of the monkey, although areas 17, 18, 19 and the homologue of the lateral suprasylvian area are present (CRAGG, 1969; ZEKI, 1969), the refinement may have proceeded a step further; here, only area 17 receives a direct thalamo-cortical input from the lateral geniculate body (WILSON and CRAGG, 1967; HUBEL and WIESEL, 1969) and this is of the essential type (POLYAK, 1957). Therefore, there may be no collateral thalamo-cortical projections in the monkey visual system. Areas 18 and 19 and the "lateral suprasylvian area" of the monkey undoubtedly receive a thalamo-cortical input, but this must be from parts of the thalamus which are not in direct receipt of retinal afferents; such afferents are distributed only to the lateral geniculate nucleus. To what extent these speculations are correct can only be determined by further detailed anatomical and physiological studies, but they have been put forward in the hope that they may stimulate investigations aimed to elucidate the interrelationships of the known subdivisions within each of the main sensory areas and also the possible homologies between those of different sensory systems.

G. The Intrinsic Organization of SI

The three architectonic subdivisions of SI, areas 3b, 1 and 2 have been known for many years from cyto- and myeloarchitectonic studies (BRODMANN, 1909; ECONOMO and KOSKINAS, 1925; POWELL and MOUNTCASTLE, 1959a; ROBERTS and AKERT, 1963; HASSLER and MUHS-CLEMENT, 1964). Area 3b is basically a granular field: i.e. there are greatly increased numbers of granule or stellate neurons in all six layers, leading to a blurring of lines of demarcation between adjacent laminae. Increased granularity in this and in the other primary sensory fields (visual, auditory) is generally held to betoken an increased number of thalamo-cortical afferents (ROSE, 1949). Areas 1 and 2, on the other hand, exhibit pyramidalization: i.e. on passing backwards from area 3 through areas 1 and 2, the number of granule neurons progressively diminishes and they are replaced by pyramidal neurons which progressively increase in size and in number. On passing out of area 2 into area 5, the classical six layered isocortex of the parietal lobe commences. Here, the granule or stellate cell layers (II and IV) and the pyramidal cell layers (III, V and VI) alternate in ordered fashion. It may be noted that although it is customary to refer to layer II as the outer granular layer, in fact the predominant cell in this layer is a small pyramid (CAJAL, 1911; SHOLL, 1956; JONES and POWELL, 1970c). Rostral to area 3b, between it and the motor cortex (area 4), the cortex of area 3a is transitional in structure. The marked fusion of layers II, III and IV which is characteristic of 3b is lost, and more pyramidal cells appear, some of which in layers III and V are quite large.

Numerous studies have been made of the cerebral cortex with the Golgi method which impregnates whole nerve cells and their processes. While a multiplicity of cell types has been described, a general consensus seems to have been reached that most fall into one of two classes — pyramidal or stellate (SHOLL, 1956; GLOBUS and SCHEIBEL, 1967). Pyramidal neurons in all layers have a stout apical dendrite which invariably ascends to ramify as a brush-like spray of finer branches in the molecular layer. Some side branches may be given off in intervening layers. From the basal part of the cell, short basal dendrites emerge but tend to remain within the layer containing the soma. Their lateral spread is rarely wider than that of the apical spray, so that a pyramidal neuron can in effect be considered as a cylinder of constant diameter (GLOBUS and SCHEIBEL, 1967). All dendrites have short spine-like appendages which are especially concentrated in the middle parts of the apical and basal dendritic trees (SHOLL, 1956; GLOBUS and SCHEIBEL, 1967; VALVERDE, 1968; VALVERDE and ESTEBAN, 1968). Pyramidal cells always send their axons outside the cortex but these may give off intracortical collaterals *en passant* (CAJAL, 1911; LORENTE DE NÓ, 1949; SHOLL, 1956; GLOBUS and SCHEIBEL, 1967). The latter may extend horizontally for long distances through a cortical layer (CAJAL, 1911; SHOLL, 1956). Stellate (or granule) neurons have many short dendrites which ramify in all directions but rarely extend much beyond the layer in which the soma lies (GLOBUS and SCHEIBEL, 1967; SHOLL, 1956). They have few or no dendritic spines. The axons of stellate neurons ramify mostly in the vicinity of the soma, although some may extend horizontally for several mms through a lamina and others may ascend vertically through several layers (CAJAL, 1911; LORENTE DE NÓ, 1949; SHOLL, 1956; GLOBUS and SCHEIBEL, 1967). Other cell types which have been described at intervals, form less than 2.5% of the total population and many of these may be distorted or incompletely impregnated stellate neurons (SHOLL, 1967).

With the application of the electron microscope to the study of the cortex, it has become possible to recognize more subtle differences between the pyramidal and stellate neurons and more importantly, some indication of their synaptic relations can now be given. First in the visual cortex (COLONNIER, 1968) and later in the somatic cortex itself (JONES and POWELL, 1969f, 1970b, c, d), it has been shown that the majority of synaptic contacts upon pyramidal cells are with dendritic spines (Fig. 8); only a few axon terminals make contact directly with the dendritic shafts or with the soma. By contrast, the dendrites and the somata of the stellate cells are simply covered in synaptic contacts. In aldehyde-fixed material, most terminals in the visual and somatic cortex fall quite cleanly into one of two categories: some contain synaptic vesicles which are spherical in shape while others have vesicles which are generally smaller and are ovoid, "flattened" or pleomorphic in shape (COLONNIER, 1968; JONES and POWELL, 1969f, 1970b) (Fig. 8). The significance of this finding lies in relation to the fact that in certain sites, notably the cerebellum (UCHIZONO, 1965, 1968; LARRAMENDI and VICTOR, 1967; LARRAMENDI et al., 1967; LEMKEY-JOHNSTON and LARRAMENDI, 1968) and olfactory bulb (PRICE, 1968), it is possible to equate terminals containing flattened vesicles with known inhibitory synapses and those containing spherical vesicles with excitatory synapses (see also BODIAN (1966) and WALBERG (1968)). In the cortex the terminals containing the two different types of synaptic vesicle can be related to one or other of the two types of synaptic complex originally described in the cortex by GRAY (1959). Terminals with spherical vesicles usually make contact with the postsynaptic element by means of contact zones which are *asymmetrical* in having a far greater accumulation of electron dense material attached to the postsynaptic membrane (type I of Gray) (COLONNIER, 1968; JONES and POWELL, 1970b). Terminals containing flattened vesicles on the other hand usually make synaptic contact by means of contact zones which are *symmetrical*, with smaller but equal amounts of electron dense material attached to both pre- and post-synaptic membranes (type II of Gray) (Colonnier, 1968; Jones and Powell, 1970b). The distribution of the two types of synapse in the somatic sensory cortex may be summarized as follows (Jones and Powell, 1969f, 1970b, c, d): every dendritic spine of the pyramidal cells receives at least one terminal containing spherical vesicles and ending in an asymmetrical contact. Few of this type of terminal end directly upon the shafts of the pyramidal cells but when they do, there is invariably a "spine apparatus" in the underlying dendritic cytoplasm. The organelle first described by Gray (1959) is present to some extent in all but the smallest dendritic spines (Jones and Powell, 1969f) so that its presence may be functionally associated with the asymmetrical synapses upon the pyramidal cells. A few dendritic spines (10–20%) may receive a second terminal which can be either of the type containing spherical vesicles and ending asymmetrically or of the type containing flattened vesicles and ending symmetrically (Jones and Powell, 1970b). The latter type of synapse forms the bulk of the small number of terminals making synaptic contacts directly upon the dendritic shafts of the pyramidal cells and is the only type to be found on the pyramidal cell soma (Jones and Powell, 1970b). Stellate cells, by contrast, receive synaptic contacts of both types all over their somata and dendrites. While these observations do not establish conclusively that one or other of these two types of synapse is excitatory and the other inhibitory, the evidence in other systems for flattened vesicles being associated with inhibitory synapses is so suggestive that it cannot be ignored. Moreover, it seems significant that in the cortex, terminals at these sites where they might be expected to have an inhibitory effect, notably on the axon hillocks and initial segments of axons leaving the pyramidal cells, regularly contain flattened vesicles and end in symmetrical contacts (Westrum, 1966; Jones and Powell, 1969e).

1. Laminar Pattern of Afferents in SI. Studies of the cerebral cortex with the light microscope in both normal and experimental material have suggested that

Fig. 7. A schematic representation giving the laminar pattern, mode of termination and a likely interpretation of the sites of termination upon the postsynaptic neurons, of thalamic, commissural and cortico-cortical fibres in SI. Commissural and cortico-cortical afferents and approximately 75% of the thalamic afferents terminate on dendritic spines, and, therefore, probably mainly on pyramidal cells (left). The remaining 25% of thalamic afferents end on stellate cells (right). All thalamic and the majority of commissural and cortico-cortical afferents terminate in a bilaminar pattern (hatching): in layer IV with overlap into layers III and V, and in the deep part of layer I. These two regions should contain the middle portions of the apical dendritic trees of pyramidal neurons of all layers (broken lines) suggesting that this is the main receiving surface of the pyramidal cell for extrinsic afferents. The axons of stellate neurons (right) are orientated both vertically and horizontally in the cortex and may provide for inhibition acting in these two directions within vertical columns based upon pyramidal cells of all layers. On the extreme right are shown the horizontally disposed bands of intracortical association fibres. T: tangential plexus of layer I; K: stria of Kaes; B′, B″: inner and outer bands of Baillarger; D: deep plexus of layer VI. (Reproduced, with permission, from the Philosophical Transactions of the Royal Society, **257**, 45–62, 1970)

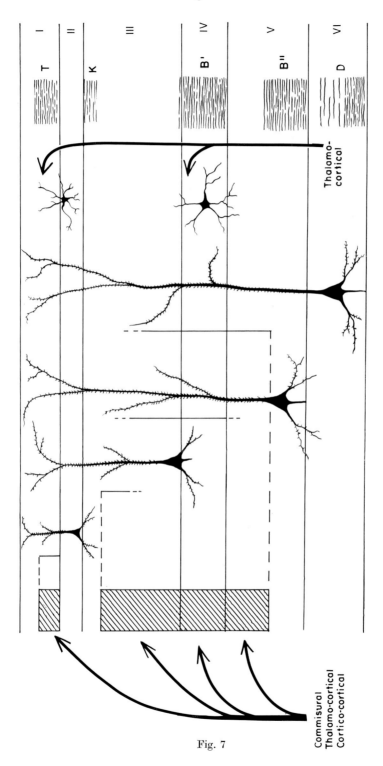

Fig. 7

the three sets of afferent fibres entering a particular cortical area — thalamic, associational and callosal — terminate in different patterns and in different cortical laminae. In particular, the study of Hubel and Wiesel (1969) should be noted for they have shown that following a small lesion in the lateral geniculate body, the Nauta-stained degeneration in the visual cortex is arranged as a mosaic of columns which they equate with the functional columns of physiological studies. Whether a similar organization could be demonstrated in the somatic cortex by appropriately placed lesions in the ventrobasal complex remains to be seen. However, only the electron microscope can conclusively demonstrate actual axon terminals and, when combined with a technique for experimental degeneration, which permits, as it were, a "labelling" of axon terminals derived from selected fibre systems, the exact sites and mode of termination within the different cortical layers can be determined. In electron microscopic studies of SI of the cat 2–6 days after selective interruption of thalamic, associational (from SII) and commissural fibres, certain differences in their laminar pattern of termination became obvious (Jones and Powell, 1970e) (Fig. 7). Thalamo-cortical afferents from the ventrobasal complex show a very clear-cut bilaminar distribution: the majority end in layer IV with overlap into adjacent parts of layers III and V but a small, though consistent number, terminate in the deep part of layer I. Commissural and association fibres have a less clear-cut pattern of termination: both distribute terminals to all layers but in both cases there are concentrations of terminals in the same two regions containing the thalamic terminals, i.e. in layer IV and adjacent parts of layers III and V, and in the deep part of layer I (Fig. 7). Unlike thalamic and association fibres whose preterminal ramifications branch quite extensively, the preterminal axon segments of commissural fibres are very short and as the commissural axon is vertically orientated within the cortex, it may therefore exert its effect on a single functional column only (Jones and Powell, 1970e).

2. Mode of Termination of Afferents in SI. An earlier view of the circuitry of the cortex, largely based upon a speculation of Ramón y Cajal (1911) was that thalamic afferents end upon stellate cells which send their axons in turn to terminate on pyramidal cells whose axons are the main efferent elements of the cortex, giving rise to projection, association and commissural fibres — even as the branches of a single axon (Lorente de Nó, 1949). On this basis, Colonnier (1966) has speculated that the morphological basis for the columnar functional unit of the cortex is a stellate type cell of layer IV which receives the thalamic terminals and sends a diffuse axonal spray upwards and downwards in a narrow column to synapse on pyramidal cells at all levels. This interpretation neglects the fact, however, that the columnar hypothesis is based upon an analysis of the first cortical response to a peripheral stimulus (Mountcastle, 1957; Powell and Mountcastle, 1959b) and "the latencies of cells along the vertical axis of the cortex [are] not significantly different for the neuronal elements of different layers" (Powell and Mountcastle, 1959b). Recently, it has been shown that the pyramidal cell has a more direct association with the thalamic afferents and an alternative hypothesis is now possible. Experimental Golgi studies of the visual cortex, in which certain proportions of the dendritic spines of pyramidal cells fail to impregnate following eye removal or sensory deprivation suggest that some at least of the thalamic afferents end directly on these cells (GLOBUS and SCHEIBEL, 1967; VALVERDE, 1968; VALVERDE and ESTEBAN, 1968), although changes affect the dendrites of stellate cells as well (COLEMAN and RIESEN, 1968). Electron microscopy (JONES and POWELL, 1970e; GAREY, 1970; GAREY and POWELL, 1971) shows that a high proportion (75%) of the thalamic terminals in the somatic sensory and visual areas of the cortex end on dendritic spines and, therefore, probably mainly on pyramidal cells but possibly on stellate cells as well (Fig. 7). The remaining 25% end mostly on the shafts of stellate cell dendrites (JONES and POWELL, 1970e; GAREY, 1970; GAREY and POWELL, 1971). All the commissural and association fibre terminals are on pyramidal cells — most on the spines but a few directly on the shafts as well (JONES and POWELL, 1970e). As far as can be ascertained, all the parent dendrites whose spines receive these terminals of the extrinsic afferents are of small to medium diameter, suggesting that these dendrites are somewhere in the middle of the dendritic tree of the pyramidal neurons, because dendrites taper in passing away from the soma or, if branches, from the parent trunk. Because few or no terminals of the three afferent systems end in layer VI which contains mainly basal dendrites, it seems probable that all those thalamic, associational and commissural fibres ending on the pyramidal cells, do so on the spines attached in the middle portion of the apical dendritic tree (JONES and POWELL, 1970e). Moreover, the bilaminar pattern exhibited so strikingly by the thalamic terminals but also to some extent by commissural and associational terminals as well, suggests that the three sets of afferents contact pyramidal cells of all layers, for the middle portions of the apical dendritic trees of pyramidal cells from layers II to VI would fall within the two bands of terminals common to all three systems (Fig. 7). It must be stressed that this *interpretation* of the level of termination upon the pyramidal cells is provisional only. Terminations upon pyramidal cells in all layers would, however, befit the columnar hypothesis more adequately than a system involving an initial relay from stellate to pyramidal cell. Although 25% of the thalamic terminals are on stellate cells, the essential bilaminar pattern of intracortical terminations also fits their distribution pattern, for these cells are concentrated in layers II and IV (CAJAL, 1911; SHOLL, 1956) and much of their dendritic ramifications falls within the two bands showing heaviest concentrations of the terminals of all three sets of extrinsic afferents. The fact that thalamo-cortical afferents terminate on stellate as well as pyramidal cells (JONES and POWELL, 1970e; GAREY, 1970; GAREY and POWELL, 1971) may be relevant to certain observations of HUBEL and WIESEL on functional columns in the visual cortex. HUBEL and WIESEL (1962, 1968) found that particularly in the visual cortex of the monkey, and to a lesser extent in that of the cat, "simple" cells (interpreted as receiving direct connections from neurons of the lateral geniculate nucleus) were concentrated in the parts of functional columns traversing layer IV. On the other hand, "complex" and "hypercomplex" cells (interpreted as receiving from many simple and complex cells respectively) were more common in layers II, III, V and VI. This would imply that afferents from the lateral geniculate nucleus end on simple cells which in turn send their axons on to complex and hypercomplex cells. Because stellate cells are especially concentrated in layer IV and almost certainly send their axons to terminate on pyramidal cells (CAJAL, 1911; LORENTE DE NÓ, 1949), they could be the simple cells and the pyramidal cells (receiving also from the thalamic relay cells) could be the complex and hypercomplex types.

What the other afferents to the pyramidal and stellate cells are has not been determined but only a small proportion of their axo-spinous and axo-dendritic synapses ever degenerate following interruption of all thalamic, association and callosal extrinsic afferents (JONES and POWELL, 1970e). This suggests that the majority of axon terminals on the cells of a functional area of the cortex have their origin within that area only.

The terminals of thalamic, commissural and association fibres all end in synaptic contacts which are of the asymmetrical type (JONES and POWELL, 1970e) and such terminals contain vesicles which are spherical. Therefore, if terminals of this type are taken to be excitatory, then all extrinsic influences upon the somatic sensory cortex should be excitatory in nature and some other mechanism must be available to give rise to the inhibition which can be demonstrated in the cortex following stimulation of the periphery (MOUNTCASTLE and POWELL, 1959) or the opposite hemisphere (CHANG, 1953; BREMER, 1958; ASANUMA and OKUDA, 1962). Inhibition in the somatic and visual areas of the cortex would, therefore, be mediated by axons arising and terminating within the sensory cortex itself. In view of this, it is important to note that in the regions showing maximal concentrations of extrinsic afferent terminals, there are many horizontally disposed unmyelinated axons which have multiple *en passant* terminals containing flattened vesicles and ending in symmetrical synaptic contacts on the dendritic shafts of pyramidal and stellate neurons (JONES and POWELL, 1970c, d). Other unmyelinated axons are orientated vertically, especially in layer III (JONES and POWELL, 1970d) and also give off multiple *en passant* terminals of this type to the dendrites of the pyramidal cells. These unmyelinated axons arise within the cortex (JONES and POWELL, 1970e) and may, therefore, be axons of stellate cells (Fig. 7). If their synapses are taken to be inhibitory, they could form the basis for an intracortical inhibitory mechanism acting both at right angles to, and within the functional columns. Stellate cells conform to the Golgi type II classification and there is increasing evidence, notably from work in the cerebellar cortex (ECCLES et al., 1967) that such cells do have inhibitory properties.

Possibly one of the important features of neuronal activity in the sensory areas of the cortex is the heightening of contrast, either between the "neural correlates" of two points applied close together to the skin in the somatic sensory system or between light and dark bars in the visual. MOUNTCASTLE and POWELL (1959) have discussed the role of surround inhibition in relation to two-point discrimination at all levels in the somatic sensory system and conclude that it is a function of "collateral mechanisms" at synaptic stations rather than of first order afferent fibres. It is also apparent that inhibitory mechanisms play a part in defining the nature of a visual stimulus in the lateral geniculate body and particularly in the visual cortex (HUBEL and WIESEL, 1961, 1962, 1965, 1968). If the short axon stellate cells are inhibitory by nature, this "heightening of contrast" could account for their concentration in the primary sensory areas. The area striata (area 17) is the granular area *par excellence* of the cortex (BRODMANN, 1909; CAJAL, 1911; OTSUKA and HASSLER, 1962) and the difference between the types of stimuli required to elicit responses therein as compared with the lateral geniculate body is remarkable.

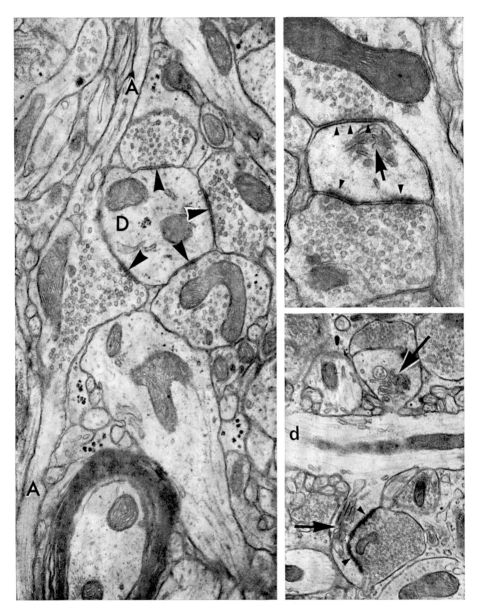

Fig. 8. Left: a small dendrite of a stellate cell (D) surrounded by axon terminals which end in a symmetrical manner (arrow heads). One is an *en passant* terminal of a small unmyelinated axon (A). × 30,000. (Reproduced, with permission, from the Philosophical Transactions of the Royal Society, **257**, 1–11, 1970.) Above right: dendritic spine in layer III of somatic sensory cortex contacted by two distinct types of axon terminals: one with symmetrical membrane thickenings and pleomorphic vesicles (above) and the other (below) with asymmetrical membrane thickenings and spherical vesicles × 84,000. Below right: dendrite of medium size (d) with a short pedunculated spine (above) and a sessile one (below) × 16,000. (arrow heads: membrane thickenings, arrow: spine apparatus). (Both figures on the right are reproduced, with permission, from the Journal of Cell Science, **5**, 509–529, 1969)

Single cells in the lateral geniculate respond to circular spots of light applied to peripheral fields of constant size and position (Hubel and Wiesel, 1961). Cells in the visual cortex on the other hand, "show a marked increase in the number of stimulus parameters that must be specified in order to influence their firing" (Hubel and Wiesel, 1962); in area 17 most are excited only by slits, edges or bars of light or dark whose shape, position and, particularly, orientation are critical. The conversion of the effective stimulus from a spot at the lateral geniculate nucleus to a specifically orientated slit at the cortical level must entail considerable changes in the patterns of afferent nervous activity within the visual cortex. If the stellate cells are inhibitory interneurons, it seems more than probable that they would play a large part in such a dramatic change. Beyond the sensory areas, granulation of the cortex progressively diminishes (Brodmann, 1909; Economo and Koskinas, 1925; Bonin and Bailey, 1947). Even within the visual cortex itself, there is a change in passing from area 17 to areas 18 and 19, for the latter are far less granular than area 17 (Otsuka and Hassler, 1962). It may be significant, therefore, that complex and hypercomplex cells are concentrated in areas 18 and 19 and that these cells are far less specific than "simple" cells, especially in regard to stimulus placement (Hubel and Wiesel, 1962, 1965, 1968). The similarities between the structure and the organization of the connections of the individual subdivisions of the somatic and visual areas of the cortex have already been discussed and it is tempting to suggest that the type of stimulus required to evoke responses of single cells in areas 1 and 2 of the somatic sensory cortex could also in a sense be considered as "complex" and "hypercomplex". Area 2 is chiefly concerned with receiving afferents from joints and because joints are situated at junctional regions between two topographic subdivisions of the body, doubtless integration of the parts of the body image is already occurring at this level. This could conceivably be the equivalent of the loss of specificity in regard to stimulus placement shown by the complex cells of area 18. Conversely, in area 3b where neurons are largely concerned with cutaneous afferents, heightening of contrast by inhibitory mechanisms, between trains of impulses evoked by stimuli applied to different spots on the skin could be highly important and a major factor in two-point discrimination (Mountcastle and Powell, 1959). This might then account for the large number of stellate cells in area 3b and for their marked diminution in area 2 (Powell and Mountcastle, 1959a; Hassler and Muhs-Clement, 1964). If these speculations are correct, it must be assumed that the granularity of the primary sensory areas is a reflection of the richness of local inhibitory circuits. Undoubtedly, inhibition plays an important role at all levels of cortical function, but it may be a more balanced one in the classical six-layered isocortex of the temporal, parietal and frontal lobes where stellate and pyramidal neurons alternate in a nicely ordered fashion.

Much of the foregoing discussion has been concerned with those anatomical features of the somatic sensory cortex which may be important in the processing of afferent impulses arriving at the primary cortex. The anatomical organization lends itself less to a correlation with the efferent activities of the primary sensory cortex. One feature, however, deserves comment. In view of the organization of the connections of the somatic sensory cortex which has already been discussed, the question may be asked whether the different connections — association and commissural cortical fibres and subcortical projection pathways — arise from different pyramidal cells or are all branches of the same cell. There is little or no evidence to favour either of these alternatives at present, but it should be possible by microelectrode recording and antidromic activation from more than one site to distinguish between these possibilities. A further point is whether the projection to different subcortical structures — striatum, thalamus, brain stem and spinal cord — are all branches of the same axon. There can be little doubt that the elucidation of this problem would have important consequences upon our understanding of the function of the efferent systems of the somatic sensory and other areas of the cortex.

Much further investigation using progressive refinements in technique will be required before the intrinsic organization of the cortex is finally understood. The fact that a huge number of normal synapses persist despite interruption of all extrinsic and a considerable number of the intrinsic afferents (JONES and POWELL, 1970e) is an indication of the magnitude of the task. One striking feature of the cortex is its relative simplicity, especially when compared with the thalamus. Apart from those endings on initial segments of other axons, most axon terminals are simply either axo-dendritic or axo-somatic. Obviously, special neuronal mechanisms are present: the dendritic spine cannot be simply a specialization for increasing the surface area available for synaptic contacts on pyramidal neurons and it may be part of an important mechanism for synaptic interaction between afferents from different sources and the neuron with which they make synaptic contact (SCHEIBEL and SCHEIBEL, 1968; JONES and POWELL, 1969f). (Is it to isolate, and make more effective, afferents from diverse sources at their site of termination upon the dendrite? DIAMOND and YASARGIL, 1969; DIAMOND et al., 1969). Moreover, some at least of the axo-dendritic and axo-somatic synapses may be inhibitory and others excitatory in nature. However, no axon terminals in the cortex enter into complex glomerular arrangements such as those seen in the thalamus and there are no axo-axonic synapses of the type thought to be concerned in presynaptic inhibition. It is perhaps apposite to conclude this review with one of the remarks of RAMÓN Y CAJAL upon the subject of neuronal organization in the cortex "... the functional superiority of the human brain is intimately linked up with the prodigious abundance and unaccustomed wealth of the so-called neurons with short axons" (RAMÓN Y CAJAL, 1937).

Abbreviations

Allo	allocortex
A III	third auditory area
BCI	brachium of inferior colliculus
CL	n. centralis lateralis
CM	n. centrum medianum
CS	central sulcus
GL	lateral geniculate nucleus
GM	medial geniculate nucleus, pars principalis
In	inner face of fronto-parietal operculum
Ins	insular cortex

Ins a   agranular insular cortex
Ins d   dysgranular insular cortex
Ins g   granular insular cortex
Ip   intraparietal sulcus
L   n. limitans
LM   medial lemniscus
LP   n. lateralis posterior
MC   magnocellular division of medial geniculate nucleus
MD   n. medialis dorsalis
MI, MII   motor and supplementary motor areas
OF ⎫
OFO ⎭   orbito-frontal cortex
P   pulvinar
PC   parvocellular division of n. ventralis posterior
PCS   postcentral sulcus
Pi   n. pulvinaris inferius
Poi, Pol, Pom intermediate, lateral and medial divisions of the posterior group
Pm   n. pulvinaris medialis
PrCo   precentral agranular cortex
Pt   pretectal area
SC   subcentral sulcus
SF   suprasylvian fringe
SG   n. suprageniculatus
Sup   superior face of fronto-parietal operculum
SI, SII   first and second somatic sensory areas
SSII   second somatic sensory area
Tr   transitional field, area 3a
VB   ventrobasal complex
VL   n. ventralis lateralis
VPI   n. ventralis posterior, pars inferius
VPL   n. ventralis posterior, pars lateralis
VPM   n. ventralis posterior, pars medialis

References

Adrian, E.D.: The spread of activity in the cerebral cortex. J. Physiol. (Lond.) 88, 127–161 (1936).
Adrian, E.D.: Double representation of the feet in the sensory cortex of the cat. J. Physiol. (Lond.) 98, 16P (1940).
Adrian, E.D.: Afferent discharges to the cerebral cortex from peripheral sense organs. J. Physiol. (Lond.) 100, 159–191 (1941).
Albe-Fessard, D.: Organization of somatic central projections. Contrib. sensory Physiol. 2, 101–177 (1967).
Altman, J., Carpenter, M.B.: Fiber projections of the superior colliculus in the cat. J. comp. Neurol. 116, 157–177 (1961).
Amassian, V.E.: Cortical representation of visceral afferents. J. Neurophysiol. 14, 433–444 (1951).
Andersen, P., Eccles, J.C., Sears, T.A.: Cortically evoked depolarization of primary afferent fibers in the spinal cord. J. Neurophysiol. 27, 63–77 (1964).

ANDERSEN, P., JUNGE, K., SVEEN, O.: Cortico-thalamic facilitation of somatosensory impulses. Nature (Lond.) **214**, 1011–1012 (1967).

ANDERSSON, S.A., LANDGREN, S., WOLSK, D.: The thalamic relay and cortical projection of Group I muscle afferents from the forelimb of the cat. J. Physiol. (Lond.) **183**, 576–591 (1966).

ASANUMA, H., OKUDA, O.: Effects of transcallosal volleys on pyramidal tract cell activity of cat. J. Neurophysiol. **25**, 198–208 (1962).

BENJAMIN, R.M., BURTON, H.: Projection of taste nerve afferents to anterior opercular-insular cortex in squirrel monkey (*Saimiri sciureus*). Brain Res. **7**, 221–231 (1968).

BENJAMIN, R.M., EMMERS, R., BLOMQUIST, A.J.: Projection of tongue nerve afferents to somatic sensory area I in squirrel monkey (*Saimiri sciureus*). Brain Res. **7**, 208–220 (1967).

BERLUCCHI, G., GAZZANIGA, M.S., RIZZOLATI, G.: Microelectrode analysis of transfer of visual information by the corpus callosum. Arch. ital. Biol. **105**, 583–598 (1967).

BERMAN, A.L.: Overlap of somatic and auditory cortical response fields in anterior ectosylvian gyrus of cat. J. Neurophysiol. **24**, 594–607 (1961 a).

BERMAN, A.L.: Interaction of cortical responses to somatic and auditory stimuli in anterior ectosylvian gyrus of cat. J. Neurophysiol. **24**, 608–620 (1961 b).

BIGNALL, K.E.: Comparison of optic afferents to primary visual and polysensory areas of cat neocortex. Exp. Neurol. **17**, 327–343 (1967).

BIGNALL, K.E., IMBERT, M., BUSER, P.: Optic projections to non-visual cortex of the cat. J. Neurophysiol. **29**, 396–409 (1966).

BLOMQUIST, A.J., LORENZINI, C.A.: Projection of dorsal roots and sensory nerves to cortical sensory motor regions of squirrel monkey. J. Neurophysiol. **28**, 1195–1205 (1965).

BODIAN, D.: Electron microscopy: two major synaptic types on spinal motoneurons. Science **151**, 1093–1094 (1966).

BONIN, G. VON, BAILEY, P.: The Neocortex of Macaca mulatta. Urbana. University of Illinois Press 1947.

BOWSHER, D.: Some afferent and efferent connections of the para-fascicular centre median complex. In: The Thalamus, pp. 99–108. Ed. by D.P. PURPURA and M.D. YAHR. New York: Columbia University Press 1966.

BREMER, F.: Physiology of the corpus callosum. Res. Publ. Ass. nerv. ment. Dis. **36**, 424–448 (1958).

BRODMANN, K.: Vergleichende Lokalisationslehre der Großhirnrinde in ihren Prinzipien dargestellt auf Grund des Zellenbaues. Leipzig: Barth 1909.

BURNS, B.D.: Some properties of isolated cerebral cortex in the unanaesthetized cat. J. Physiol. (Lond.) **112**, 156–175 (1951).

BURTON, H., EARLS, F.: Cortical representation of the ipsilateral chorda tympani nerve in the cat. Brain Res. **16**, 520–523 (1969).

CARRERAS, M., ANDERSSON, S.A.: Functional properties of neurons of the anterior ectosylvian gyrus of the cat. J. Neurophysiol. **26**, 100–126 (1963).

CARRERAS, M., CULZONI, V., EAGER, R.P., GUELI, O.: Cortico-cortical and cortico-thalamic connections of somatic sensory area III in the cat. Anat. Rec. **163**, 164 (1969).

CELESIA, G.G.: Segmental organization of cortical afferent areas in the cat. J. Neurophysiol. **26**, 193–206 (1963).

CHANG, H.T.: Cortical response to activity of callosal neurons. J. Neurophysiol. **16**, 117–131 (1953).

CHOUDHURY, B.P., WHITTERIDGE, D., WILSON, M.E.: The function of the callosal connections of the visual cortex. Quart. J. exp. Physiol. **50**, 214–219 (1965).

CLARK, W.E.J., LE GROS, BOGGON, R.H.: The thalamic connections of the parietal and frontal lobes of the brain in the monkey. Phil. Trans. B. **224**, 313–359 (1935).

CLARK, W.E.J., LE GROS, POWELL, T.P.S.: On the thalamo-cortical connections of the general sensory cortex of *Macaca*. Proc. roy. Soc. B. **141**, 467–487 (1953).

COLEMAN, P.D., RIESEN, A.H.: Environmental effects on cortical dendritic fields. I. Rearing in the dark. J. Anat. (Lond.) **102**, 363–374 (1968).

COLONNIER, M.: The structural design of the neocortex. In: Brain and Conscious Experience, pp. 1–23. Ed. by J.C. ECCLES. Berlin-Heidelberg-New York: Springer 1966.

COLONNIER, M.: Synaptic patterns on different cell types in the different laminae of the cat visual cortex. An electron microscope study. Brain Res. **9**, 268–287 (1968).

CRAGG, B. G.: The topography of the afferent projections in the circumstriate visual cortex of the monkey studied by the Nauta Method. Vision Res. **9**, 733–748 (1969).

CURTIS, H. J.: Intercortical connections of corpus callosum as indicated by evoked potentials. J. Neurophysiol. **3**, 407–413 (1940).

DARIAN-SMITH, I.: Cortical projections of thalamic neurons excited by mechanical stimulation of the face of the cat. J. Physiol. (Lond.) **171**, 339–360 (1964).

DARIAN-SMITH, I., ISBISTER, J., MOK, H., YOKOTA, T.: Somatic sensory cortical projection areas excited by tactile stimulation of the cat: a triple representation. J. Physiol. (Lond.) **182**, 671–689 (1966).

DARIAN-SMITH, I., YOKOTA, T.: Corticofugal effects on different neuron types within the cat's brain stem activated by tactile stimulation on the face. J. Neurophysiol. **29**, 185–206 (1966).

DAVIDSON, N.: The projection of afferent pathways on the thalamus of the rat. J. ccmp. Neurol. **124**, 377–390 (1965).

DE VITO, J.: Thalamic projection of the anterior ectcsylvian gyrus (somatic area II) in the cat. J. comp. Neurol. **131**, 67–78 (1967).

DELL, P.: Corrélations entre le système végétatif et le système de la vie de relation. Mésencéphale, diencéphale et cortex cérébral. J. Physiol. (Paris) **44**, 471–532 (1952).

DIAMOND, I. T.: The sensory neocortex. In: Contributions to Sensory Physiology, 2, pp. 51–100. Ed. by W. D. NEFF. New York: Academic Press 1967.

DIAMOND, I. T., HALL, W. C.: Evolution of neocortex. Science **164**, 251–262 (1969).

DIAMOND, I. T., JONES, E. G., POWELL, T. P. S.: The association connections of the auditory cortex of the cat. Brain Res. **11**, 560–579 (1968).

DIAMOND, I. T., JONES, E. G., POWELL, T. P. S.: The projection of the auditory cortex upon the diencephalon and brainstem in the cat. Brain Res. **15**, 305–340 (1969).

DIAMOND, I. T., RANDALL, W., SPRINGER, L.: Tactual localization in cats deprived of cortical areas SI and SII and the dorsal columns. Psychon. Sci. **1**, 261–262 (1964).

DIAMOND, I. T., UTTLEY, J. D.: Thalamic retrograde degeneration study of sensory cortex in opossum. J. comp. Neurol. **120**, 129–160 (1963).

DIAMOND, J. G., GRAY, E. G., YASARGIL, G. M.: The function of dendritic spines; An hypothesis. J. Physiol. (Lond.) **202**, 116 P (1969).

DIAMOND, J. G., YASARGIL, G. M.: Synaptic function in the fish spinal cord: dendritic integration. In: Prcgress in Brain Research, vol. 31, pp. 201–210. Mechanisms of Synaptic Transmission. Ed. by K. AKERT and P. G. WASER. Amsterdam: Elsevier 1969.

DUBNER, R.: Single cell analysis of sensory interaction in anterior lateral and suprasylvian gyri of the cat cerebral cortex. Exp. Neurol. **15**, 255–273 (1966).

EBNER, F. F., MYERS, R. E.: Commissural connections in the neocortex of monkey. Anat. Rec. **142**, 229 (1962).

EBNER, F. F., MYERS, R. E.: Distribution of corpus callosum and anterior commissure in cat and raccoon. J. ccmp. Neurol. **124**, 353–366 (1965).

ECCLES, J. C., ITO, M., SZENTÁGOTHAI, J.: The Cerebellum as a Neuronal Machine. Berlin-Heidelberg-New York: Springer 1967.

ECONOMO, C. VON, KOSKINAS, G. N.: Die Cytoarchitektonik der Hirnrinde der Erwachsenen Menschen. Berlin: Springer 1925.

EMMERS, R.: Organization of the first and the second somesthetic regions (SI and SII) in the rat thalamus. J. comp. Neurol. **124**, 215–228 (1965).

GAREY, L. J.: The termination of thalamo-cortical fibres in the visual cortex of the cat and monkey. J. Physiol. (Lond.) **210**, 15–17 P (1970).

GAREY, L. J., JONES, E. G., POWELL, T. P. S.: Interrelationships of striate and extrastriate cortex with the primary relay sites of the visual pathway. J. Neurol. Neurosurg. Psychiat. **31**, 135–157 (1968).

GAREY, L. J., POWELL, T. P. S.: The projection of the lateral geniculate nucleus upon the cortex in the cat. Proc. roy. Soc. B. **169**, 107–126 (1967).

GAREY, L. J., POWELL, T. P. S.: An experimental study of the termination of the lateral geniculo-cortical pathway in the cat and monkey. Proc. roy. Soc. B. **179**, 41–63 (1971).

GLICKSTEIN, M., SPERRY, R.W.: Intermanual somesthetic transfer in split-brain rhesus monkeys. J. comp. physiol. Psychol. **53**, 322–327 (1960).

GLOBUS, A., SCHEIBEL, A.B.: Pattern and field in cortical structure: the rabbit. J. comp. Neurol. **131**, 155–172 (1967).

GLOBUS, A., SCHEIBEL, A.B.: Synaptic loci on visual cortical neurons of the rabbit: the specific afferent radiation. Exp. Neurol. **18**, 116–131 (1967).

GOLDBY, F., GAMBLE, H.J.: The reptilian cerebral hemispheres. Biol. Rev. **32**, 383–420 (1957).

GORDON, G., JUKES, M.G.M.: Descending influences on the exteroceptive organizations of the cat's gracile nucleus. J. Physiol. (Lond.) **173**, 291–319 (1964).

GORDON, G., MILLER, R.: Identification of cortical cells projecting to the dorsal column nuclei of the cat. Quart. J. exp. Physiol. **54**, 85–98 (1969).

GOTO, A., KOSAKA, K., KUBOTA, K., NAKAMURA, R., NARABAYASHI, H.: Thalamic potentials from muscle afferents in the human. Arch. Neurol. (Chic.) **19**, 302–309 (1968).

GRAY, E.G.: Axo-somatic and axo-dendritic synapses in the cerebral cortex; an electron microscopic study. J. Anat. (Lond.) **93**, 420–433 (1959).

GUILLERY, R.W., ADRIAN, H.O., WOOLSEY, C.N., ROSE, J.E.: Activation of somatosensory areas I and II of cat's cerebral cortex by focal stimulation of the ventrobasal complex. In: The Thalamus, pp. 197–206. Ed. by D.P. PURPURA and M.D. YAHR. New York: Columbia University Press 1966.

HALL, W.C., DIAMOND, I.T.: Organization and function of the visual cortex in hedgehog. I. Cortical cytoarchitecture and thalamic retrograde degeneration. Brain Behav. Evol. **1**, 181–214 (1968).

HASSLER, R., MUHS-CLEMENT, K.: Architektonischer Aufbau des sensomotorischen und parietalen Cortex der Katze. J. Hirnforsch. **6**, 377–420 (1964).

HEATH, C.J.: Distribution of axonal degenerations following lesions of the posterior group of thalamic nuclei in the cat. Brain Res. **21**, 354–357 (1970).

HEATH, C.J., JONES, E.G.: Connections of area 19 and the lateral suprasylvian area of the visual cortex of the cat. Brain Res. **19**, 35–37 (1970).

HEATH, C.J., JONES, E.G.: An experimental study of ascending connections from the posterior group of thalamic nuclei in the cat. J. comp. Neurol. **141**, 397–426 (1971).

HONGO, T., OKADA, Y., SATO, M.: Corticofugal influences on transmission to the dorsal spinocerebellar tract from hindlimb primary afferents. Exp. Brain Res. **3**, 135–149 (1967).

HUBEL, D.H., WIESEL, T.N.: Integrative action in the cat's lateral geniculate body. J. Physiol. (Lond.) **155**, 385–398 (1961).

HUBEL, D.H., WIESEL, T.N.: Receptive fields, binocular interaction and functional architecture in the cat's visual cortex. J. Physiol. (Lond.) **160**, 106–154 (1962).

HUBEL, D.H., WIESEL, T.N.: Receptive fields and functional architecture in two non-striate visual areas (18 and 19) of the cat. J. Neurophysiol. **28**, 229–289 (1965).

HUBEL, D.H., WIESEL, T.N.: Cortical and callosal connections concerned with the vertical meridian of the visual fields in the cat. J. Neurophysiol. **30**, 1561–1573 (1967).

HUBEL, D.H., WIESEL, T.N.: Receptive fields and functional architecture of monkey striate cortex. J. Physiol. (Lond.) **195**, 215–243 (1968).

HUBEL, D.H., WIESEL, T.N.: Anatomical demonstration of columns in the monkey striate cortex. Nature (Lond.) **221**, 747–750 (1969).

HUBEL, D.H., WIESEL, T.N.: Visual area of the lateral suprasylvian gyrus (Clare-Bishop area) of the cat. J. Physiol. (Lond.) **202**, 251–260 (1969).

HUGHES, A., WILSON, M.E.: Callosal terminations along the boundary between visual areas I and II in the rabbit. Brain Res. **12**, 19–25 (1969).

JASPER, H.H., BERTRAND, G.: Thalamic units involved in somatic sensation and voluntary and involuntary movements in man. In: The Thalamus, pp. 365–390. Ed. by D.P. PURPURA and M.D. YAHR. New York: Columbia University Press 1966.

JONES, E.G.: Interrelationships of parieto-temporal and frontal cortex in the rhesus monkey. Brain Res. **13**, 412–415 (1969).

JONES, E.G., POWELL, T.P.S.: The projection of the somatic sensory cortex upon the thalamus in the cat. Brain Res. **10**, 369–391 (1968a).

JONES, E.G., POWELL, T.P.S.: The ipsilateral cortical connections of the somatic sensory areas in the cat. Brain Res. **9**, 71–94 (1968b).

Jones, E.G., Powell, T.P.S.: The commissural connections of the somatic sensory cortex in the cat. J. Anat. (Lond.) 103, 433–455 (1968c).

Jones, E.G., Powell, T.P.S.: An electron microscopic study of the mode of termination of cortico-thalamic fibres within the sensory relay nuclei of the thalamus. Proc. roy. Soc. B. 172, 173–185 (1969a).

Jones, E.G., Powell, T.P.S.: The cortical projection of the ventroposterior nucleus of the thalamus in the cat. Brain Res. 13, 298–318 (1969b).

Jones, E.G., Powell, T.P.S.: Connections of the somatic sensory cortex of the rhesus monkey. I. Ipsilateral cortical connections. Brain 92, 504–531 (1969c).

Jones, E.G., Powell, T.P.S.: Connections of the somatic sensory cortex of the rhesus monkey. II. Contralateral cortical connections. Brain 92, 717–730 (1969d).

Jones, E.G., Powell, T.P.S.: The synapses on the axon hillocks and initial segments of pyramidal cell axons in the cerebral cortex. J. Cell Sci. 5, 495–507 (1969e).

Jones, E.G., Powell, T.P.S.: Morphological variations in the dendritic spines of the neocortex. J. Cell Sci. 5, 509–529 (1969f).

Jones, E.G., Powell, T.P.S.: Connections of the somatic sensory cortex of the rhesus monkey. III. Thalamic connections. Brain 93, 37–56 (1970a).

Jones, E.G., Powell, T.P.S.: Electron microscopy of the somatic sensory cortex of the cat. I. Cell types and synaptic organization. Phil. Trans. B. 257, 1–11 (1970b).

Jones, E.G., Powell, T.P.S.: Electron microscopy of the somatic sensory cortex of the cat. II. The fine structure of layers I and II. Phil. Trans. B. 257, 13–21 (1970c).

Jones, E.G., Powell, T.P.S.: Electron microscopy of the somatic sensory cortex of the cat. III. The fine structure of layers III–VI. Phil. Trans. B. 257, 23–28 (1970d).

Jones, E.G., Powell, T.P.S.: An electron microscopic study of the laminar pattern and mode of termination of extrinsic afferent fibres in the somatic sensory cortex of the cat. Phil. Trans. B. 257, 45–62 (1970e).

Jones, E.G., Powell, T.P.S.: An anatomical study of converging sensory pathways within the cerebral cortex of the monkey. Brain 93, 793–820 (1970f).

Jones, E.G., Powell, T.P.S.: An analysis of the posterior group of thalamic nuclei on the basis of its afferent connections. J. comp. Neurol. 143, 185–216 (1971).

Kawana, E., Kusama, T.: Projection of the sensory motor cortex to the thalamus, the dorsal column nucleus, the trigeminal nucleus and the spinal cord in the cat. Folia psychiat. neurol. jap. 18, 337–380 (1964).

Knighton, R.S.: Thalamic relay nucleus for the second somatic sensory receiving area in the cerebral cortex of the cat. J. comp. Neurol. 92, 183–191 (1950).

Kruger, L., Berkowitz, E.C.: The main afferent connections of the reptilian telencephalon as determined by degeneration and electrophysiological methods. J. comp. Neurol. 115, 125–141 (1960).

Kuypers, H.G.J.M.: Central cortical projections to motor and somatosensory cell groups. An experimental study in the rhesus monkey. Brain 83, 161–184 (1960).

Landgren, S., Silfvenius, H.: Projection to the cerebral cortex in Group I muscle afferents from the cat's hind limb. J. Physiol. (Lond.) 200, 353–372 (1969).

Landgren, S., Silfvenius, H., Wolsk, D.: Somato-sensory paths to the second cortical projection area of the group I muscle afferents. J. Physiol. (Lond.) 191, 543–559 (1967a).

Landgren, S., Silfvenius, H., Wolsk, D.: Vestibular, cochlear and trigeminal projections to the cortex in the anterior suprasylvian sulcus of the cat. J. Physiol. (Lond.) 191, 561–573 (1967b).

Larramendi, L.M.H., Fickenscher, L., Lemkey-Johnston, N.: Synaptic vesicles of inhibitory and excitatory terminals in the cerebellum. Science 156, 967–969 (1967).

Larramendi, L.M.H., Victor, T.: Synapses of the Purkinje cell spines in the mouse. An electron microscopic study. Brain Res. 5, 15–30 (1967).

Lemkey-Johnston, N., Larramendi, L.M.H.: Types and distribution of synapses upon basket and stellate cells of the mouse cerebellum: an electron microscopic study. J. comp. Neurol. 134, 73–109 (1968).

Lende, R.A.: Sensory representation in the cerebral cortex of the opossum (Didelphys virginiana). J. comp. Neurol. 121, 395–404 (1963).

LENDE, R.A.: Representation in the cerebral cortex of a primitive mammal. Sensorimotor, visual and auditory fields in the echidna (*Tachyglossus aculeatus*). J. Neurophysiol. **27**, 37–48 (1964).

LEVITT, M., CARRERAS, M., LIU, C.-N., CHAMBERS, W.W.: Pyramidal and extrapyramidal modulation of somato-sensory activity in gracile and cuneate nuclei. Arch. ital. Biol. **102**, 197–229 (1964).

LORENTE DE NÓ, R.: Cerebral cortex: architectonics, intracortical connections. In: Physiology of the Nervous System, pp. 274–301. Ed. by J.F. FULTON. Oxford: Oxford University Press, third edition, 1949.

MACCHI, G., ANGELERI, F., GUAZZI, G.: Thalamo-cortical connections of the first and second somatic sensory areas in the cat. J. comp. Neurol. **111**, 387–405 (1959).

MALIS, L.I., PRIBRAM, K.H., KRUGER, L.: Action potentials in motor cortex evoked by peripheral nerve stimulation. J. Neurophysiol. **16**, 161–167 (1953).

MANSON, J.: The somatosensory cortical projection of single nerve cells in the thalamus of the cat. Brain Res. **12**, 489–492 (1969).

McLEOD, J.G.: The representation of the splanchnic afferent pathways in the thalamus of the cat. J. Physiol. (Lond.) **140**, 462–478 (1958).

MEHLER, W.R.: Some observations on secondary ascending afferent systems in the central nervous system. In: Pain, pp. 11–32. Ed. by R.S. KNIGHTON and P.R. DUMKE. Boston: Little, Brown 1966.

MEHLER, W.R., FEFERMAN, M.E., NAUTA, W.J.H.: Ascending axon degeneration following anterolateral cordotomy. An experimental study in the monkey. Brain **83**, 718–750 (1960).

METTLER, F.A.: Corticifugal fiber connections of the cortex of *Macaca mulatta*. The occipital region. J. comp. Neurol. **61**, 221–256 (1935a).

METTLER, F.A.: Corticifugal fiber connections of the cortex of *Macaca mulatta*. The parietal region. J. comp. Neurol. **62**, 263–291 (1935b).

MICKLE, W.A., ADES, H.W.: A composite sensory projection area in the cerebral cortex of the cat. Amer. J. Physiol. **170**, 682–689 (1952).

MORRISON, A.R., HAND, P.J., ELKINS, R.M.: Thalamocortical projections of nucleus ventralis posterolateralis (VPL) of the cat. Anat. Rec. **160**, 396 (1968).

MOUNTCASTLE, V.B.: Modality and topographic properties of single neurons of cat's somatic sensory cortex. J. Neurophysiol. **20**, 408–434 (1957).

MOUNTCASTLE, V.B., HENNEMAN, E.: Pattern of tactile representation in thalamus of cat. J. Neurophysiol. **12**, 85–100 (1949).

MOUNTCASTLE, V.B., HENNEMAN, E.: The representation of tactile sensibility in the thalamus of the monkey. J. comp. Neurol. **97**, 409–440 (1952).

MOUNTCASTLE, V.B., POWELL, T.P.S.: Neural mechanisms subserving cutaneous sensibility, with special reference to the role of afferent inhibition in sensory perception and discrimination. Bull. Johns Hopk. Hosp. **105**, 201–232 (1959).

MYERS, R.E.: Transmission of visual information within and between the hemispheres: a behavioral study. In: Interhemispheric Relations and Cerebral Dominance, pp. 51–73. Ed. by V.B. MOUNTCASTLE. Baltimore: Johns Hopkins University Press 1962a.

MYERS, R.E.: Commissural connections between occipital lobes of the monkey. J. comp. Neurol. **118**, 1–16 (1962b).

NAKAHAMA, A.H.: Functional organization of somatic areas of the cerebral cortex. Int. Rev. Neurobiol. **3**, 187–250 (1961).

NYBERG-HANSEN, R.: Functional organization of descending supraspinal fiber systems to the spinal cord. Anatomical observations and physiological correlations. Ergebn. Anat. Entwickl.-Gesch. **39**, 1–48 (1966).

OAKLEY, B., BENJAMIN, R.M.: Neural mechanisms of taste. Physiol. Rev. **46**, 173–211 (1966).

OLSZEWSKI, J.: The Thalamus of Macaca mulatta. New York: Karger 1952.

ORBACH, J., CHOW, K.L.: Differential effects of resections of somatic areas I and II in monkeys. J. Neurophysiol. **22**, 195–203 (1959).

OSCARSSON, O., ROSÉN, I.: Short-latency projections to the cat's cerebral cortex from skin and muscle afferents in the contralateral forelimb. J. Physiol. (Lond.) **182**, 164–184 (1966).

Otsuka, R., Hassler, R.: Über Aufbau und Gliederung der corticalen Sehsphäre bei der Katze. Arch. Psychiat. Nervenkr. **203**, 212–234 (1962).

Pandya, D., Kuypers, H. G. J. M.: Cortico-cortical connections in the rhesus monkey. Brain Res. **13**, 13–36 (1969).

Pandya, D., Vignolo, L. A.: Interhemispheric neocortical projections of somatosensory areas I and II in the rhesus monkey. Brain Res. **7**, 300–303 (1968).

Paul, R. L., Merzenich, M., Goodman, H.: Representation of slowly and rapidly adapting cutaneous mechanoreceptors of the hand in Brodmann's areas 3 and 1 of *Macaca mulatta*. Brain Res. **36**, 229–249 (1972).

Penfield, W., Jasper, H. H.: Epilepsy and the Functional Anatomy of the Human Brain. Boston: Little, Brown 1954.

Penfield, W., Rasmussen, T.: The Cerebral Cortex of Man. New York: Macmillan 1950.

Perl, E. R., Whitlock, D. G.: Somatic stimuli exciting spinothalamic projections to thalamic neurons in cat and monkey. Exp. Neurol. **3**, 256–296 (1961).

Petras, J. M.: Fiber degeneration in the basal ganglia and diencephalon following lesions in the precentral and postcentral cortex of the monkey (*Macaca mulatta*) with additional observations in the chimpanzee. In: Abstracts of the Eighth International Anatomical Congress, Wiesbaden, 1965.

Phillips, C. G., Powell, T. P. S., Wiesendanger, M.: Projection from low-threshold muscle afferents of hand and forearm to area 3a of baboon's cortex. J. Physiol. (Lond.) **217**, 419–446 (1971).

Poggio, G. F., Mountcastle, V. B.: A study of the functional contributions of the lemniscal and spinothalamic systems to somatic sensibility. Central nervous mechanisms in pain. Bull. Johns Hopk. Hosp. **106**, 266–316 (1960).

Poggio, G. F., Mountcastle, V. B.: The functional properties of ventrobasal thalamic neurons studied in unanaesthetized monkeys. J. Neurophysiol. **26**, 775–806 (1963).

Polyak, S.: The Vertebrate Visual System. Ed. by H. Klüver. Chicago: University of Chicago Press 1957.

Powell, T. P. S., Mountcastle, V. B.: The cytoarchitecture of the postcentral gyrus of the monkey *Macaca mulatta*. Bull. Johns Hopk. Hosp. **105**, 108–131 (1959a).

Powell, T. P. S., Mountcastle, V. B.: Some aspects of the functional organization of the cortex of the postcentral gyrus of the monkey: a correlation of findings obtained in a single unit analysis with cytoarchitecture. Bull. Johns Hopk. Hosp. **105**, 133–162 (1959b).

Price, J. L.: The synaptic vesicles of the reciprocal synapse of the olfactory bulb. Brain Res. **11**, 697–700 (1968).

Ramón y Cajal, S.: Histologie du Système Nerveux de l'Homme et des Vertébrés. Paris: Maloine 1909–1911, two vols.

Ramón y Cajal, S.: Recollections of my Life, translated by E. Horne Craigie. Cambridge, Mass.: M. I. T. Press 1937.

Rinvik, E.: A re-evaluation of the cytoarchitecture of the ventral nuclear complex of the cat's thalamus on the basis of corticothalamic connections. Brain Res. **8**, 237–254 (1968a).

Rinvik, E.: The corticothalamic projection from the second somatosensory cortical area in the cat. An experimental study with silver impregnation methods. Exp. Brain Res. **5**, 153–172 (1968b).

Rinvik, E.: The corticothalamic projection from the pericruciate and coronal gyri in the cat. An experimental study with silver impregnation methods. Brain Res. **10**, 79–119 (1968c).

Roberts, T. S., Akert, K.: Insular and opercular cortex and its thalamic projection in *Macaca mulatta*. Schweiz. Arch. Neurol. Neurochir. Psychiat. **92**, 1–43 (1963).

Rose, J. E.: The thalamus of the sheep: cellular and fibrous structure and comparison with pig, rabbit and cat. J. comp. Neurol. **77**, 469–523 (1942).

Rose, J. E.: The cellular structure of the auditory region of the cat. J. comp. Neurol. **91**, 409–440 (1949).

Rose, J. E., Mountcastle, V. B.: The thalamic tactile region in rabbit and cat. J. comp. Neurol. **97**, 441–489 (1952).

Rose, J. E., Mountcastle, V. B.: Activity of single neurons in the tactile thalamic region of the cat in response to a transient peripheral stimulus. Bull. Johns Hopk. Hosp. **94**, 238–282 (1954).

Rose, J.E., Woolsey, C.N.: The relations of thalamic connections, cellular structure and evocable electrical activity in the auditory region of the cat. J. comp. Neurol. **91**, 441–466 (1949).

Rose, J.E., Woolsey, C.N.: Cortical connections and functional organization of the thalamic auditory system of the cat. In: Biological and Biochemical Bases of Behaviour, pp. 127–150. Ed. by H.F. Harlow and C.N. Woolsey. Madison: University of Wisconsin Press 1958.

Rowe, M.J., Sessle, B.J.: Somatic afferent input to posterior thalamic neurones and their axon projection to the cerebral cortex in the cat. J. Physiol. (Lond.) **196**, 19–35 (1968).

Rutledge, L.T., Shellenberger, M.K.: The influence of visual cortex upon nonprimary area neurons. Arch. ital. Biol. **106**, 353–363 (1968).

Scheibel, M.E., Scheibel, A.B.: Patterns of organization in specific and nonspecific thalamic fields. In: The Thalamus, pp. 13–46. Ed. by D.P. Purpura and M.D. Yahr. New York: Columbia University Press 1966.

Scheibel, M.E., Scheibel, A.B.: On the nature of dendritic spines — report of a workshop. Commun. behav. Biol., Part A. **1**, 231–265 (1968).

Sencer, W.: Interconnections of somatic afferent areas I and II of the cerebral cortex of the cat. Amer. J. Physiol. **163**, 749 (1950).

Shimazu, H., Yanagisawa, N., Garoutte, B.: Cortico-pyramidal influences on thalamic somatosensory transmission in the cat. Jap. J. Physiol. **15**, 101–124 (1965).

Sholl, D.A.: The Organization of the Cerebral Cortex. London: Methuen 1956.

Smith, G.E.: The Arris and Gale lectures on some problems relating to the evolution of the brain. Lancet **1**, 1–6; 147–153; 221–227 (1910).

Sperry, R.W.: Preservation of high-order function in isolated somatic cortex in callosum-sectioned cat. J. Neurophysiol. **22**, 78–87 (1959).

Sperry, R.W.: Cerebral organization and behaviour. Science **133**, 1749–1757 (1961).

Tarlov, E.: The rostral projections of the primate vestibular nuclei: an experimental study in macaque, baboon and chimpanzee. J. comp. Neurol. **135**, 27–55 (1969).

Teitelbaum, H., Sharpless, S.K., Byck, R.: Role of somato-sensory cortex in interhemispheric transfer of tactile habits. J. comp. physiol. Psychol. **66**, 623–632 (1968).

Thompson, R.F., Johnson, R.H., Hoopes, J.J.: Organization of auditory, somatic sensory, and visual projection to association fields of cerebral cortex in the cat. J. Neurophysiol. **26**, 343–364 (1963).

Tömböl, T.: Short neurons and their synaptic relations in the specific thalamic nuclei. Brain Res. **3**, 307–326 (1967).

Towe, A.L., Jabbur, S.J.: Cortical inhibition of neurons in dorsal column nuclei of cat. J. Neurophysiol. **24**, 488–498 (1961).

Uchizono, K.: Characteristics of excitatory and inhibitory synapses in the central nervous system of the cat. Nature (Lond.) **207**, 642–643 (1965).

Uchizono, K.: Inhibitory and excitatory synapses in vertebrate and invertebrate animals. In: Structure and Function of Inhibitory Neuronal Mechanisms, pp. 33–60. Ed. by C. von Euler, S. Skoglund and U. Söderberg. Oxford: Pergamon Press 1968.

Valverde, F.: Structural changes in the area striata of the mouse after enucleation. Exp. Brain Res. **5**, 274–292 (1968).

Valverde, F., Esteban, M.E.: Peristriate cortex of mouse: location and the effects of enucleation on the number of dendritic spines. Brain Res. **9**, 145–148 (1968).

Vastola, E.F.: A direct pathway from lateral geniculate body to association cortex. J. Neurophysiol. **24**, 469–487 (1961).

Walberg, F.: Corticofugal fibres to the nuclei of the dorsal colums. An experimental study in the cat. Brain **80**, 273–287 (1957).

Walberg, F.: Morphological correlates of postsynaptic inhibitory processes. In: Structure and Function of Inhibitory Neuronal Mechanisms, pp. 7–14. Ed. by C. von Euler, S. Skoglund and U. Söderberg. Oxford: Pergamon Press 1968.

Walker, A.E.: The Primate Thalamus. Chicago: University of Chicago Press 1938.

Werner, G., Whitsel, B.L.: Topology of the body representation in somatosensory area I of primates. J. Neurophysiol. **31**, 856–869 (1968).

Westrum, L.E.: Synaptic contacts on axons in the cerebral cortex. Nature (Lond.) **210**, 1289–1290 (1966).

Whitlock, D.G., Perl, E.R.: Afferent projections through ventrolateral funiculi to thalamus of cat. J. Neurophysiol. 22, 133–148 (1959).

Whitsel, B.L., Petrucelli, L.M., Werner, G.: Symmetry and connectivity in the map of the body surface in somatosensory area II of primates. J. Neurophysiol. 32, 170–183 (1969).

Wilson, M.E.: Cortico-cortical connections of the cat visual areas. J. Anat. (Lond.) 102, 375–386 (1968).

Wilson, M.E., Cragg, B.G.: Projections from the lateral geniculate nucleus in the cat and monkey. J. Anat. (Lond.) 101, 677–692 (1967).

Woolsey, C.N.: Patterns of localization in sensory and motor areas of the cerebral cortex. In: The Biology of Mental Health and Disease, pp. 193–206. New York: Hoeber 1952.

Woolsey, C.N.: Organization of somatic sensory and motor areas of the cerebral cortex. In: The Biological and Biochemical Bases of Behaviour, pp. 63–81. Ed. by H.F. Harlow and C.N. Woolsey. Madison: University of Wisconsin Press 1958.

Woolsey, C.N.: Organization of cortical auditory systems: a review and a synthesis. In: Neural Mechanisms of the Auditory and Vestibular Systems, pp. 165–180. Ed. by G.L. Rasmussen and W.F. Windle. Springfield: Thomas 1961.

Woolsey, C.N., Marshall, W.H., Bard, P.: Representation of cutaneous tactile sensibility in the cerebral cortex of the monkey as indicated by evoked potentials. Bull. Johns Hopk. Hosp. 70, 399–441 (1942).

Woolsey, C.N., Wang, G.H.: Somatic sensory areas I and II of the cerebral cortex of the rabbit. Fed. Proc. 4, 79 (1945).

Zeki, S.M.: The secondary visual areas of the monkey. Brain Res. 13, 197–226 (1969).

Zubeck, J.P.: Studies in somesthesis: II. Role of somatic areas I and II in roughness discrimination in cat. J. Neurophysiol. 15, 401–408 (1952).

Chapter 16

Functional Organization of the Somatosensory Cortex

By

Gerhard Werner and Barry L. Whitsel, Pittsburgh (USA)

With 12 Figures

Contents

A. Introduction: The Concept of Functional Organization

The large segment of the attempts to gain an appreciation for the functional organization of the somatosensory cortex is based on the study of responses expressed as electrical activity, and engendered under specific, operationally defined stimulus conditions. The expectation that motivates these efforts is that it will be possible to analyze the pattern of flow and distribution of activity elicited by stimuli of known properties; to characterize the qualitative and quantitative relations between the stimuli used and the electrical responses obtained; and to fractionate the complex neural system into functionally and operationally distinct, though interacting, subunits. This latter objective is closely allied with the neuroanatomist's goal to describe and identify different morphological constituents and their geometric and possible synaptic relations to one another. Accordingly, the point of view that underlies the study of functional organization of neural systems is correlative in the sense of seeking to identify the role played by different structural components in the generation of the dynamic performance (i. e.: information flow) under controlled or natural perturbation by stimulus input.

This correlative approach has proven highly productive and informative, but there remains an element of doubt whether, by itself, it can go beyond establishing the possibility and sufficiency of structural-functional correlations. Conjectures regarding the "meaning" of these possible correlations require an additional frame of reference: namely, whether there are some aspects of somesthesis and the underlying structural architecture which become progressively emphasized in phylogeny, in parallel with evolving special functional capabilities; and to what extent the response characteristics of the somatosensory cortex in higher mammals, notably primates, reflect the coexistence and interaction between its early developed, and the phylogenetically more recent afferent components.

1. Background and Overview

The authors of the early neurophysiological studies of cortical somatosensory projection had valuable, though only approximate, guidelines at their disposal: POLIAK (1932) had already traced the cortical degeneration that follows interruption of thalamocortical fibers allegedly mediating deep and cutaneous sensibility, and thereby delineated a somesthetic projection area in the monkey, which extended "about equally, orally and caudally, from the sulcus centralis as well as over the internal face of the hemisphere where it reaches the sulcus cinguli". Additional details were known from tracing the retrograde degeneration in the thalamus following removal of one or another part of this cortical area (CLARK and BOGGON, 1935; WALKER, 1938). A possible role for this cortical area in somesthesis was suggested by the observations of CUSHING (1909), FOERSTER (1931) and PENFIELD and BOLDREY (1937) who elicited feelings of numbness and tingling, though rarely definite sensations comparable to those experienced in normal life, by stimulating the exposed cortex of human subjects in the course of operative procedures not involving the use of general anaesthetics. Moreover, DUSSER DE BARENNE (1924) had shown that local application of strychnine to certain parts of the cortex of cats and monkeys gives rise to signs of marked hyperesthesia to cutaneous tactile, thermal and nociceptive stimuli, and of deep structures to pressure: in the monkey, this cortical area included not only the entire parietal lobe with the cytoarchitectural areas 3, 1, 2, 5 and 7, but also the precentral areas 4 and 6, extending as far forward as the arcuate sulcus. BARD (1933) had discovered that the somesthetic cortex is an essential link in the mediation of a circumscript and highly specific function since ablation of the postcentral gyrus was followed by complete and permanent loss of placing reactions evoked by light contact (i. e. cutaneous tactile) stimulation; the loss of this reaction was entirely contralateral, and did not involve a deficiency of the motor mechanism.

The possibility for a more subtle and detailed analysis of the somesthetic functions of the postcentral gyrus arose with the discovery by GERARD et al. (1933, 1936) that gentle displacement of a few hairs on the body surface gives rise to a localized (evoked) electrical potential, clearly distinguishable from the ongoing "spontaneous" electrical activity. This suggested the fruitfulness of systematic and analytic explorations of the cortical neurophysiological mechanisms which might subserve somesthesis. The subsequent studies of evoked potentials in the somatosensory cortex have taken various directions, and underwent in the course of the intervening decades considerable methodologic and conceptual refinements. In chronological sequence, these studies first expounded greatly on the notion of an orderly, topographic organization of the afferent projection from the body to the postcentral gyrus which was already suggested, at least in rough form, by the earlier neuroanatomical work. The second mainstream of explorations was directed towards the characterization of the synaptic and neuronal events that underlie the evoked potentials, and the identification of the afferent pathways contributing to their generation. Finally, the introduction of microelectrodes in the early and mid 1950's in the laboratories of AMASSIAN (1953), JASPER (LI et al., 1956), and MOUNTCASTLE (1957) enabled not only a finer degree of experimental resolution of the questions raised by the evoked potential work, but led also to an experimental emphasis on qualitative and quantitative relations between stimuli and responses in individual neurons. This became the foundation for the more recent interest in stimulus coding and representation in the somatosensory cortex, with suggestive implications for the measurements of psychophysics and reference to body and surrounding space.

2. Evolutionary Aspects

The organization of the primate somesthetic system bears evidence that the early developed afferent components have been preserved, side by side with the phylogenetically more recent components. From the phylogenetic history, it might have been anticipated that the thalamus of mammals would contain at least two recipient stations: one, receiving the palaeosensory tract which was the only one reaching the thalamus in premammalian forms; the second receiving the mammalian neo-sensory tract for projection to neocortex. Peripheral sense organs of vertebrates had large fibre afferents developed before they had acquired a cortex to make use of them. The extension of these large fibre pathways through thalamus to cortex, and the acquisition everywhere in the cortex of an overlay of a large fibre component is in BISHOP's view (1959, 1961) an important clue to identify the new functions that have been added to the premammalian repertoire, and received emphasis in mammalian cortex. For, with the large fibres comes faster conduction and a higher synaptic safety factor : hence, specificity of response, where one or two neurons activate others across the synapse in a one-to-one sequence. The fibre size distribution within cortex itself reflects this increasing emphasis: for in cat and man, fibres up to 13 or 14 μ are present in the white matter below cortex, while in the turtle, most fibres are unmyelinated, and the remainder myelinated and small (BISHOP and SMITH, 1964).

Notwithstanding this emphasis on fast, lemniscal systems in mammalian encephalization (cf. NOBACK and SHRIVER, 1967, 1969), reticular pathways which constitute the basic matrix of the vertebrate nervous system (HERRICK, 1948) continue also to evolve and undergo their own adaptive radiations: having a long phylogenetic history does not necessarily preclude continuing evolution.

Thus, while lemniscal and reticular paths are organized in parallel along the longitudinal (rostrocaudal) extent of the central nervous system, there also developed mutual interactions at transverse, and between rostral and caudal, levels.

In discussions of the contrast between lemniscal and reticular afferent systems, the former appears with different connotations: NOBACK and SHRIVER (1969) emphasize as a common feature of all lemniscal pathways that they are composed of four orders of neurons. In the context of the somatic sensory system, the lemniscal component has received largely a functional characterization, based on the discreteness of receptive fields, modality specificity, and the ability of neurons to follow faithfully stimuli at high rate (MOUNTCASTLE, 1961; ROSE and MOUNTCASTLE, 1960).

Anatomical connections between lemniscal and extralemniscal paths were repeatedly proposed: they were first sought, but not found, at the level of the medial lemniscus itself (BOWSHER, 1958; SCHEIBEL and SCHEIBEL, 1958). Subsequent work in the laboratory of ALBE-FESSARD accumulated evidence for functional interrelations in the spinal cord (cf. ALBE-FESSARD, 1967). Moreover, descending pathways from primary cortex can control extralemniscal afferents: for example, ASCHER (1964) has shown an influence of somatic sensory area I on the nucleus gigantocellularies of the medulla obloganta; and LUNDBERG (1964) has shown descending inhibitory fibres which terminate at the level of the relay in the gray matter where the long fibres of the anterolateral columns have their origin.

In addition to the "myelinization" trend in evolution (cf. BISHOP, 1961), there appears also a characteristic trend in cytoarchitectonics in the form of increasing emphasis towards granularization of the cortex, culminating in the koniocortices of the primary sensory regions (SANIDES, 1969). In a comprehensive attempt to conceptualize the evolutionary trends of cortical differentiation, SANIDES (1968, 1970) proposed the hypothesis of concentrically developing growth rings of the neocortex: as a first stage of a laminated neocortex, the two strata (periarchicortex medially, and peripalaeocortex laterally) may have developed in reptiles. Next, the proisocortex consisting of the limbic cortex medially and insular cortex laterally, would appear as a second growth ring. There are regional differences within these five to six layered cortices, with the anterior cingulate gyrus being agranular, and the insula being dysgranular, notably where it borders the motor fields. The third growth ring, consisting of a paralimbic and a parinsular moiety, becomes the site of the supplementary motor and secondary sensory representations. Within these more primitive cortical regions, foci with denser thalamic input and intensive myelinization of subcortical fibres emerge as the highly specialized koniocortices of the primary sensory fields. In this light, the chemical senses, olfaction and gustation, remain less differentiated components of the parinsular and paralimbic growth ring of the telencephalon, along with the secondary and supplementary representations.

Though based on entirely different evidence, there appears a common denominator in this point of view, and that suggested by DIAMOND (1967): the primitive neocortex of hedgehog and opossum, although consisting completely of sensory and motor cortices, resembles more the part of the association cortex surrounding the sensory areas of higher mammals, than the sensory cortex of higher mammals. Thus, DIAMOND (1967) proposes that the specific sensory cortex of higher mammals was secondarily differentiated out of primitive cortex. In this process, the primary sensory cortices may acquire a more complex range of functions than merely signaling presence or absence of stimuli, and some intensity attribute. There is evidence for more intricate stimulus feature representation by neurons of the visual cortical areas, and for a role of auditory cortex in interpreting a sound image in terms of an attribute of locus in extra-corporeal space (cf. DIAMOND, 1967). The general implication may be that "sensory neocortex is not sensory at all" (DIAMOND, 1967), in the traditional sense. However, in the somatic sensory areas, the search for higher order stimulus transformations and more abstract stimulus coding has not yet been successful although the geometrical details of the cortical map (WERNER and WHITSEL, 1968; WERNER, 1970; WHITSEL et al., 1971 b) and the specificity of certain neurons for direction of motion in their receptive fields (WERNER and WHITSEL, 1970; WHITSEL et al., 1972) may be initial steps in this direction.

B. The Topography of Evoked Potentials in Somatosensory Area I

The technique for defining the afferent projection areas in the cortex by means of recording stimulus-evoked electrical activity from the cortical surface with electrodes covering a surface area in the order of 0.5 square millimeter, although of restricted capability for fine resolution, has given rise to most fundamental insights. The classical study by WOOLSEY et al. (1942) in the monkey has set the standards for execution of these experiments, and established the general principles governing the representation of tactile sensibility in the somatosensory cortex (Fig. 1). Under deep anaesthesia, with spontaneous electrical activity greatly reduced, point by point examination (within the limitations imposed by electrode size) of the cerebral cortex in terms of the peripheral cutaneous areas sending impulses to the cortical points examined revealed that the tactile system projects primarily to BRODMANN's areas 3, 1 and 2 of the contralateral hemisphere. Some evidence for ipsilateral representation of the head was obtained, but not for other

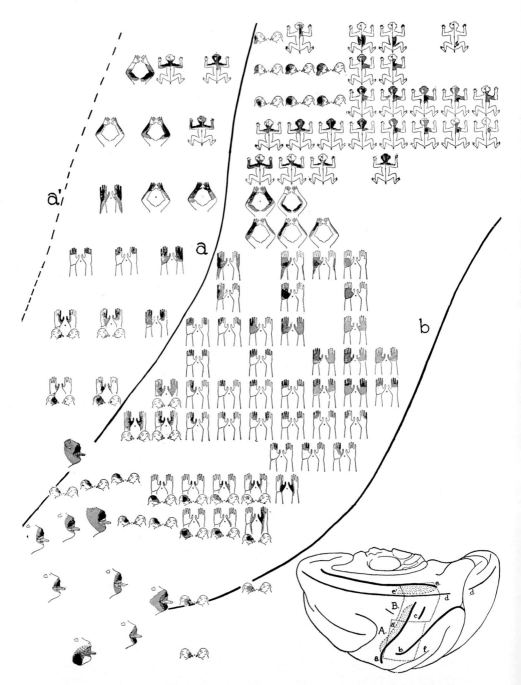

Fig. 1. The tactile sensory area of the monkey's cerebral cortex as indicated by cortical evoked potentials. 1A and 1B are figurine maps of approximately one-half of the total cortical area; their position with respect to the general topography of the cortex is indicated by the inset diagram in the lower right portion of 1A. The cutaneous receptive field which can evoke potentials at a cortical locus is indicated by the shaded region on the figurine which occupies

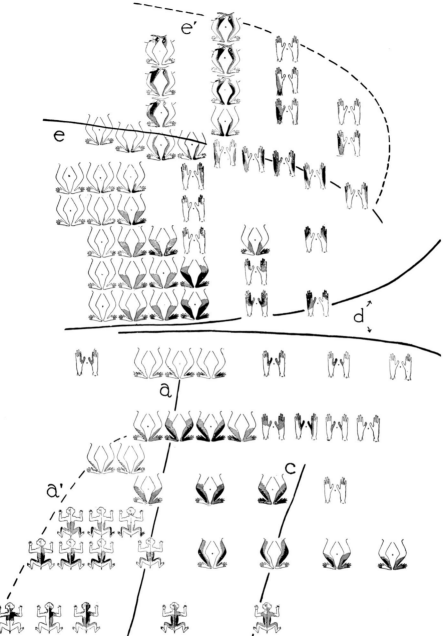

that cortical position. The right half of each figurine represents the dorsal surface, the left half the ventral surface of the body part illustrated. a: central fissure, a': bottom of central fissure, b: intraparietal sulcus, c: postcentral sulcus, d: rim of hemisphere separating dorsal and medial surfaces, e: sulcus callosus marginalis, e': bottom of sulcus callosus marginalis. The stippled areas are the posterior bank of the central fissure and the superior bank of sulcus callosus marginalis. The figurines are of such size that each would cover one square millimeter of cortex if the entire diagram were reduced to actual size. (From BARD, 1938). (Reproduced from MACLEOD's Physiology in Modern Medicine, 8th edit., C.V. Mosby Publ.)

parts of the body. Although there is some overlap, different body regions appear in the cortical representation in a characteristic sequence. The spinal segments from T-1 through the last caudal segment project to the (contralateral) postcentral gyrus in the same serial order in which they are arranged in the cord. At first, it was thought that the cervical segments, while retaining their serial order amongst themselves, would in the projection to the cortex reverse *en bloc*, thereby bringing cortical fields of the upper cervical segments into contiguity with the cortical fields of the upper thoracic segments, while the cortical field of C-8 would lie adjacent to the trigeminal field. Later investigations by WOOLSEY (1952) simplified this relation: it was found that the assumption of the reversal of the cervical segments was unnecessary, and that the body projection followed in its entirety the segmental order, with the trigeminal projection occupying the most lateral part of the body field in the postcentral gyrus, and *all* dermatomes projecting in their serial order, progressing from lateral to medial on the cortex.

The findings of these early mapping studies provided a very attractive explanation for the numerous clinical reports of cortical lesions giving rise to sensory disturbances of the axial type, that is: restricted to either the pre- or the postaxial portion of the limb, since the cortical fields of preaxial and postaxial limb dermatomes are separated by the relatively wide projection field of hand and foot, respectively.

The cortical projection areas of different dermatomes were found to vary widely in size: for example, a strip of cortex not more than 2.5 mm wide receives projections from all twelve thoracic segments, but the cortical fields of hand or foot dermatomes are, both, several millimeters wide. As might be expected, each cortical recording point is related to more than one dermatome so that, at least in evoked potential mapping, there is overlapping in the cortex similar to that in the skin. Nevertheless, the data suggested that the dermatomes are represented by overlapping bands of various width which parallel one another, and are arranged roughly at right angles to the central fissure.

The pioneering work of WOOLSEY et al. (1942) became a point of departure for several lines of investigations to elucidate the significance of the orderly, topographic projection pattern to the postcentral gyrus. One main thrust was based on the idea that the evoked potential technique would permit accurate and clear identification of homologous cortical regions in different species, thus circumventing uncertainties of cortical parcellation by cytoarchitectural criteria (WOOLSEY, 1958). By comparing different species, it would then be possible to inquire into a) relationships that might exist between localization patterns in homologous cortical fields; b) the elaboration of fissuration; and c) the role of the localization pattern for specific behavioral attributes or sensory capacities (WOOLSEY, 1960).

In the simple lissencephalic mammalian brains, of which the rat is an example, the representations of the different parts of the body in the cortical map are related to one another in much the same way as they are related on the body itself (WOOLSEY, 1952). For the purpose of these cortical representations, WOOLSEY and co-workers adopted the approach, introduced earlier by PENFIELD and BOLDREY (1937) for man, to represent the general arrangement of the cortical tactile localization pattern as an essentially continuous though metrically distorted image of the body. Concomitant with an increase of size of the cortical projection field for arm and face, the coronal sulcus appears in the cat and in the dog between these two cortical fields, at least as far as could be ascertained with the evoked potential method (WOOLSEY, 1958; PINTO HAMUY et al., 1956). However, recent degeneration studies employing circumscribed thalamic lesions indicate that, in the cat at least, S-I distal forelimb areas are not separated from facial areas by the coronal sulcus (HAND and MORRISON, 1969).

Concomitant with the remarkable development of a cortical forepaw field in the raccoon, there also appears a central sulcus in the cortical projection field (WELKER and SEIDENSTEIN, 1959). The extraordinary enlargement of the cortical sensory hand area is associated with extensive use of the forepaws in tactile exploration of the environment. Moreover, the sensory projection to the forepaw area is exquisitely discrete in the sense that there is minimal overlap of afferent input from different digits and the palm of the hand. Within this expanded cortical forepaw field of the raccoon, several subsidiary fissures appear which, despite variations in location, size and shape from animal to animal, regularly occur at boundaries between projections of different fingers or palm pads. The discreteness of projection and expansion of the cortical forepaw field enables one to recognize with the evoked potential method that some precise rules govern the mapping to the cortex: each digit appears in the cortical representation as if its cutaneous envelope was split down the middle of the dorsum, and spread out flat; the digits themselves are laid out in the cortex in the sequence in which they are on the hand, with the proximal portions of each digit adjacent to its palm pad.

The argument for the significance of this detailed projection pattern of the hand in the context of the raccoon's extensive tactile-exploratory behavior is strengthened by comparison with its close relative, the coatimundi: the different use of the forepaw in this species is associated with a much smaller cortical hand area, lacking the raccoon's detailed fissuration pattern (WELKER, 1959).

In some primates, the central fissure extends further medial on the cortex into the leg area, and establishes a complete separation between the pre- and the postcentral fields. Possibly, the caudal spur of the inferior precentral sulcus and the interparietal sulcus in M. mulatta can be considered remnants of the coronal sulcus since they separate the face and arm subdivision (WOOLSEY, 1960).

A well-documented case for a relation between local elaboration of cortical projection fields and specialization of function can also be made for the spider monkey (Ateles), when compared with Cebus and M. mulatta. In Ateles, the prehensile ability of the tail is developed to a degree which enables it to be used for the acquisition of a tactile roughness discrimination task (L.M. PUBOLS, 1966). This high degree of tactile acuity is accompanied by an expansion of the cortical tail field onto the dorsal aspect of the hemisphere, and a corresponding displacement of the leg and arm areas (CHANG et al., 1947). As a consequence, the face area is almost completely displaced from the postcentral position which it occupies in the macaque, whose prehensile tail function is minimal. The face area of Ateles is shifted, in part, into the Sylvian fissure, and to a larger extent, into a precentral position around the lower end of the central sulcus. Cebus occupies an intermediate position between Ateles and M. mulatta, both as regards prehensile tail capability, as well as with respect to the size of the cortical tail field and associated displacements of contiguous projection areas (HIRSCH and COXE, 1958).

Similar positive correlations between the differentiation of a particular peripheral receptive field in the species' life, and the relative size of this field's neocortical representation have also been established in other instances (Adrian, 1943; Woolsey and Fairman, 1946). Moreover, differences in the life style of different members of a species are also capable of introducing variations of the cortical fissuration pattern: domesticated animals usually have particular patterns of fissures which are unknown in their wild ancestors. Crossbreeding experiments between wild living and domesticated members of a species have shown that brain size, shape and patterns of fissures are determined by genetic factors which are independent of each other (Herre, 1967).

There are two general implications of these and related studies. In the first place, it appears that the tactile cortical projection areas need not be confined to cytoarchitecturally homogenous fields; for, in the case of *Cebus*, the cortical face field comes to lie within areas parietofrontalis and frontalis opercularis of von Bonin's (1938) cytoarchitectural map, whereas the tail, leg and arm representations occupy areas postcentralis granulosa and intermedia.

In the second place, there is cumulative evidence suggesting that new cortical sulci are formed at the boundaries of functional cortical subdivisions as if the dynamics of the sulcus formation were the expression of some form of "mushrooming" under the pressure from differential areal enlargements (Welker and Seidenstein, 1959). Pursuing this line of evidence, Welker and Campos (1963) argued convincingly that adjacent gyri within the somatosensory cortex receive separate bundles of afferents which project from distinct peripheral body regions; and that the growth of gyral crowns is, in some sense, a result of the space requirements to accommodate these different afferent fibre bundles in their cortical fields (Sanides, 1970). During early growth, when new cortical fissures begin to form, those zones of cortex lacking dense thalamo-cortical connections become the fundi of incipient sulci, while those with massive afferent connections expand. Thus, gyri would tend to become cortical fields with highly discrete tactile representations (and, accordingly, consist of neurons with small receptive fields and little receptive field overlap); and sulci would tend to represent body areas of low tactile discrimination capability. As a corollary, sulci would tend to separate the cortical fields of body areas which are in the periphery separated from one another by zones of low tactile discriminative capacity. In this sense, the cortical projection pattern is not only expressing body topography, but functional attributes as well, as Ruch et al. (1952) have argued.

C. Stimulus-Interactions in the Somatosensory Pathway: Overlap of Cortical Fields for Peripheral Cutaneous Regions

Although there was much emphasis in the classical mapping studies on the fact that stimuli in the form of small discrete displacements of hairs and skin were used to mimic the stimuli which occur in normal life, electrical stimulation of peripheral nerves or points on the skin was also employed as a source for some complementary data. To determine the effects of anaesthesia, Marshall et al. (1941) applied electrical shocks in pairs at controlled intervals to points on the skin, and recorded evoked responses from the appropriate cortical site. Under ether and nembutal anaesthesia, the latency of the primary cortical response to the first stimulus was some 17 msec, and very nearly identical with that measured in unanaesthetized preparations. The significant difference was in the time interval between consecutive electrical shocks required so that the second stimulus in a pair would also elicit a cortical response: this time was under ether anaesthesia about one third of that under nembutal anaesthesia where it lasted as long as 60 to 70 msec.

Under deep barbiturate anaesthesia, when spontaneous cortical activity is greatly reduced or abolished, the primary, predominantly surface positive (often nearly monophasic), sharply localized evoked potential is usually the only significant response elicited by weak cutaneous stimuli. In cats under chloralose anaesthesia, MARSHALL et al. (1941) observed, in addition, a secondary response of considerable variability in size, shape and latency, and irregular occurrence. In general, amplitudes and irregularities of this response are more prominent under light anaesthesia. Electrical stimulation of peripheral nerves sometimes gives rise to another form of secondary response which occurs also in deep anaesthesia and is probably related to the secondary response of FORBES and MORISON (1939). In summary, it appears that the primary cortical response itself is relatively little affected by the anaesthetic, but that events which follow it (including the recovery cycle) are markedly altered.

In the evoked potential mapping technique, each active cortical recording point is surrounded by a margin of submaximal response 0.5 to 4.0 mm wide. When the position of the tactile stimulus is moved a short distance, the cortical responses are found in a slightly different position, leaving a certain area of overlap. Thus, the question arose: do the stimuli of the two peripheral points activate the same neurons within the area of overlap? While this question received its definitive answers some 15 years later in the microelectrode studies of MOUNTCASTLE (1957) and MOUNTCASTLE and POWELL (1959b), it is still pertinent to discuss the conclusions of MARSHALL et al. (1941) and others, who used the primary evoked potential as response criterion.

The general principle of the method is to apply two discrete tactile stimuli at two adjacent peripheral points; one stimulus is timed to fall a certain interval after a preceding stimulus. In the study of MARSHALL et al. (1941) an interval of 25 msec was chosen in the anaesthetized preparation so that if any neurons were common to both reactions, the ones involved in the first reaction would be unresponsive when the second stimulus was delivered: thus, the second response would be reduced.

In the somatic sensory area I of the cat, reduction of the second response is a function of the distance between the peripheral points stimulated: the further they are apart, the smaller the interaction; but some reduction of the second response still occurs even when conditioning and test stimuli are applied to such widely separate areas as contralateral hindpaw and forepaw (MALCOLM and DA-RIAN-SMITH, 1958). Accordingly, certain neuronal elements within the central nervous system must be common to the pathway from these separate peripheral points. The evidence is that the reduction of the response to the second stimulus occurs at the thalamic relay station to the somatosensory cortex (KING et al., 1957; ANGEL, 1967). There are several neuronal mechanisms at this level to which this effect could be attributed. Of these, the presynaptic inhibition of fibres entering the ventrobasal thalamus (ANDERSEN et al., 1964) and the inhibitory feedback from the sensory cortex to the thalamus (ANGEL, 1963) are amongst the principal candidates.

D. The Multiplicity of Somatic Sensory Areas of the Cortex

ADRIAN (1941) discovered in the cat a "second" somatic area, lying next to the "classical" cortical body representation which came to be named "somatic sensory area II" (WOOLSEY, 1947). The second somatic area was in the cat identified at the rostral tip of the anterior ectosylvian gyrus. Subsequently, a second area was also identified in the rabbit (WOOLSEY and WANG, 1945), in the dog and in the monkey (WOOLSEY, 1943), in pig and sheep (WOOLSEY and FAIRMAN, 1946), man (PENFIELD and RASMUSSEN, 1950), marsupial (ADEY and KERR, 1954), porcupine (LENDE and WOOLSEY, 1956), raccoon (WELKER and SEIDENSTEIN, 1959) squirrel monkey (BENJAMIN and WELKER, 1957), and other species as well. As a result of these combined observations, a dual somesthetic projection to the cerebral cortex in the mammal became widely accepted.

The cortical localization patterns in S-I and S-II have certain similarities: in primates, for instance, the postaxial and preaxial arm and leg areas are separated by the representation of the respective digits; and the cortical areas devoted to the face and the occiput are separated by the projection from the forelimb. On the other hand, a marked difference appears to distinguish the map of the body in S-I from that in S-II: in the classical mapping experiments, the cortical recording site in S-II was not only activated by stimuli delivered to a particular contralateral body area as it is in S-I, but also to stimuli to a symmetrical, ipsilateral body region. The implication was either that individual neurons in S-II receive afferents from a contralateral peripheral field and its ipsilateral mirror image; or else, that the afferents from somatic contralateral and ipsilateral peripheral fields project to separate cortical neurons located in close proximity to one another. This question was decided in an exploration of S-II with microelectrodes in unanaesthetized preparations: the majority of neurons in S-II respond indeed with action potentials to gentle cutaneous stimulation of bilateral receptive fields (WHITSEL et al., 1969b).

Electrical stimulation of peripheral nerves in cats was shown to elicit evoked responses in S-I as well as in S-II, but the latter were more pronounced than the former (NAKAHAMA, 1958). Each of these areas was shown by this method to receive its separate afferent input; but, in addition, direct electrical stimulation of S-I can also evoke a response in ipsilateral S-II and vice versa (NAKAHAMA, 1960).

In the cat, but not in the primate (WHITSEL et al., 1969b), the second somatic area overlaps the cortical region responsive to click stimuli extensively in the anterior ectosylvian gyrus (BERMAN, 1961a): responses to click and somatic stimuli interact, at least in the transitional region between S-II and auditory area II (BUSER and HEINZE, 1954; PERL and CASBY, 1954; BERMAN, 1961b). Indeed, MICKLE and ADES (1952) suggested that this particular cortical zone may serve to correlate sensory information received through several different afferent channels. This suggestion was borne out for the cat by the microelectrode studies of CARRERAS and ANDERSSON (1963) who identified individual neurons in S-II with poly-sensory response characteristics. These poly-sensory neurons appeared diffusely distributed, though with some gradient of increasing density towards the posterior border of S-II. In the macaque, on the other hand, WHITSEL et al. (1969b) located the poly-sensory neurons exclusively posterior to the purely cutaneous S-II representation, in a cortical area whose rostral border coincides approximately with the cytoarchitectural transition between areas PF and PG of VON BONIN and BAILEY (1947). Possibly, this separation between purely cutaneous and polysensory neurons may be considered an instance of the general principle in cortical phylogeny that progressive cortical development consists of the increasing segregation of neurons into functionally and cytoarchitecturally differentiated zones (LENDE, 1963, 1969; GESCHWIND, 1965). In the second somatosensory area of primates this developmental trend would have resulted in two cortical zones containing neurons with distinctly different properties.

The demonstration of a sustaining projection from a portion of the posterior group nuclei of the thalamus to S-II in the cat is in accord with the observed stimulus interactions in this species: since this portion of the thalamus is intercalated between the ventrobasal complex and the medial geniculate nucleus it places the posterior group nuclei in a strategic position for tactile-auditory interactions (ROSE and WOOLSEY, 1958).

MARSHALL et al. (1941) made passing reference to a triple projection in the cat and in the monkey. Incidental observations of a third projection area appeared in subsequent years in the literature (MALCOLM and DARIAN-SMITH, 1958; OSCARSSON and ROSEN, 1963).

DARIAN-SMITH et al. (1966) finally established in the cat the existence of a somatic sensory projection area in the dorsal part of the anterior suprasylvian gyrus, representing face and forelimb independently of their projection to S-I and S-II. The neurons in this cortical projection field, which was designated S-III, have restricted cutaneous receptive fields, and are somatotopically arranged; the majority of the receptive fields are on the contralateral side of the body, but some have an ipsilateral extension. Most neurons are modality specific, responding only to tactile cutaneous stimulation; but some respond to auditory stimulation as well, much as do certain neurons in S-II of the cat.

JONES and POWELL (1968a) suggested that this third somatic sensory area of the cat is identical with cytoarchitectural area 5; and that this same cytoarchitectural area may also be equated with the "supplementary sensory area" described in man by PENFIELD and JASPER (1954), and in the squirrel monkey by BLOMQUIST and LORENZINI (1965). In both species, this region lies on the medial surface of the hemisphere immediately posterior to the leg area of S-I; it extends on to the dorsolateral surface, closely aligned with area 2, and largely buried in the intraparietal sulcus.

There remains one uncertainty in this argument of equating S-III with cytoarchitectural area 5: for, DARIAN-SMITH et al. (1966) secured electrophysiological evidence for a direct projection from the ventrobasal thalamic complex to S-III, whereas it has not as yet been possible to obtain anatomical evidence for the existence of pathways connecting the ventroposterior thalamic nuclei with area 5 (Jones and Powell, 1968a, 1969c, 1970c).

1. Latency Contour Maps of the Somatosensory Cortex

Since Woolsey, Marshall and Bard's (1942) classic work, the most widely used technique for mapping the cortical body representation has been based on determining the cortical foci of maximal peak-to-peak amplitudes of the primary evoked response to peripheral stimuli. An alternative way to study properties of the cortical body representation is to measure the latency of the cortical, surface positive response, and to join cortical points with equal latency by contour lines.

In the opossum, amplitude-based and latency-based cortical maps are aligned differently, most often to the extent of being mirror images of one another (Bode-mer and Towe, 1963). The latency contours define in the cat a small, discrete cortical area in the anterior part of the suprasylvian gyrus, distinct from both area I and II (Malcolm and Darian-Smith, 1958). Similarly, an area of short response latency was found to occupy, in the squirrel monkey, the region of cortex at, or slightly anterior to the central fissure. This region is immediately posterior to the precentral area which it overlaps (Zimmermann, 1968).

The separation of "minimal-latency" from "maximal-amplitude" foci suggest that the maps based on the one and the other of these two criteria reflect different aspects of the cortical projection: the one, the site of termination of the fastest pathway; the other, the site of maximal density of neural elements in the cortex, responsive to a particular stimulus mode and site. In the light of this, it appears possible that the short latency focus, at least in the squirrel monkey, reflects area 3a which receives the group Ia and Ib input from the periphery.

E. Relation Between Cortical Sensory and Motor Representations

It is now firmly established that the sensory cortical areas are not exclusively recipients of sensory projections, nor are the motor areas exclusively motor: hence, the concept has emerged that the Rolandic region is essentially a sensorimotor system, yet compounded of a number of distinguishable, individually complete, sensory-motor and motor-sensory representations, at least in placental mammals. There is a suggestion for an evolutionary trend in the relation between the sensory and the motor components: in the marsupial mammals (opossum and wallaby), one single area contains both the sensory and the motor representations of the various body parts, and this area is not divisible into predominantly sensory and predomi-nantly motor portions (Lende, 1963).

The somatic sensory areas I and II of placental mammals are matched by corresponding motor areas. In the basic plan of organization, these four Rolandic areas are laid down as mirror image patterns on opposite sides of a line which corresponds, in the macaque, to the bottom of the central sulcus (Fig. 2). But, the sensory areas contain motor elements and, on direct electric stimulation, can elicit movements. The principle that underlies the organization of motor pathways arising in S-I and S-II is simple: the peripheral site of origin of the afferent input to a sensory field and the destination of the motor outflow are nearly identical and related to the same body area (cf. WOOLSEY, 1958). The organization of sensory input to primarily motor cortex appears likewise orderly. In the cat's sigmoid cortex, there are two types of body representation, one grading over into the other: one to two millimeters posterior to a boundary running approximately parallel to the cruciate sulcus, somato-topically arranged receptive fields of individual neurons are discrete and of invariable size and modality. Detailed microelectrode studies established the existence of individual neuron pools whose afferent

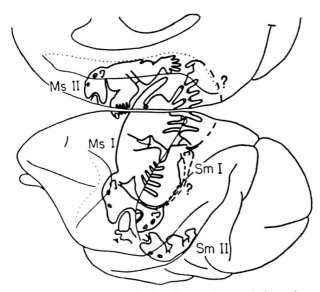

Fig. 2. Diagram of monkey cortex, showing locations and general plans of organization of the supplementary motor (MII), the precentral motor (MI), the postcentral tactile (SI) and the second sensory (SII) areas. The latter lies largely on the upper bank of the sylvian fissure adjacent to the insula and the auditory area on the lower bank (not illustrated). The anterolateral boundary of the first visual area (VI) is shown by the thin line, with an asterisk placed at the center of the macular projection area. (From WOOLSEY, 1958)

input and motor output are related to identical body areas. Accordingly, certain cell columns receive tactile sensory input from, and send motor output to the foot, and can thereby function as the operating unit of the cortical reflex which mediates the tactile placing reaction (WELT et al., 1967). Another circumstance which also enables a functional coordination between somatic sensory input and motor output at the cortical level is the somatotopic organization of the interconnections between sensory and motor cortex (JONES and POWELL, 1968a). The somatotopic specificity of these interconnections is of a considerable degree of refinement: small groups of neurons in S-I which receive afferent input from a particular peripheral locus send projections to a neuron group in motor cortex which receives sensory input from the same or a contiguous peripheral body region (BROOKS, 1969; THOMPSON et al., 1970).

Rostral to this region, neurons have large receptive fields which change size from time to time in the course of prolonged observation, and are polysensory (BROOKS et al., 1961a and b; BUSER and IMBERT, 1961). This cortical zone coincides with the gradual transition between sensory and motor cortex, as determined by the evoked potential methods (WOOLSEY, 1960), and by histological criteria (CAMPBELL, 1905). The multiple and disparate afferent inputs received by this transition zone may enable some integration of activity in diverse sensory channels prior to initiation of movement. However, human motor cortex appears to lack a comparable polysensory afferent projection, and even the specific sensory input of the type characteristic for S-I is less constant and reproducible than it is in the cat. This has led to the suggestion of a phylogenetic trend to separate sensory projections from direct access to motor cortex, with the latter becoming more exclusively a "final common path" determiner of movement (GOLDRING et al., 1970).

F. Evoked Potentials and Synaptic Organization in Somatosensory Cortex

The initially surface-positive evoked potential which forms the basis of the classical mapping studies with tactile or electrical stimulation of the skin is also recorded in S-I and S-II when the dorsal column nuclei, the ventrobasal thalamic nucleus, or cortical white matter are directly stimulated with electric pulses (PERL and WHITLOCK, 1955). Although the responses to synchronous corticipetal volleys do not permit insights into the function of neuron pools and pathways under the conditions of natural activation by temporally and spatially shifting peripheral stimulus patterns, they do permit a clearer display of the sequence of excitation and inhibition in different cortical laminae and neural structures.

In the surface positive response to stimulation of thalamic relays, PERL and WHITLOCK (1955) distinguished a brief, initially positive response (S) from two later waves (W1 and W2). Because of brief latency, high following rate to repetitive stimuli, and considerable resistance to anoxia and anaesthesia, the S-response was thought to be an expression of the incoming volley in thalamo-cortical afferents. The very early part of this response was attributed to the largest of the thalamo-cortical fibres, with diameters up to 4 micra or more, though their relative number is small (BISHOP and SMITH, 1964). The first axonal radiation spike may be followed by a series of smaller spikes, riding on the crest of the positive wave (LANDAU, 1967). The cortical field of the positive wave and the site of stimulation in the thalamus correspond to one another by both being activated from the same peripheral skin area. Under all but the deepest levels of anaesthesia, the surface positive wave is followed by a more variable negative wave, much as is seen with the primary response to peripheral stimuli.

The primary afferent surface response itself can be analyzed into at least two, sometimes three components: with gradual intensity increase of intradermally applied electrical stimuli, the evoked potential amplitude grows discontinuously as peripheral nerve fibre groups with different thresholds become engaged in the afferent volley (ROSNER et al., 1959).

Under all but the deepest levels of anaesthesia, the surface positive response to peripheral stimuli (and to stimulation of structures along the somesthetic pathway) is followed by a more variable negative wave. The analysis of this potential reversal with respect to the cortical depth at which it occurs, does not reveal differences which would correspond to the differential laminar distribution of the three sets of cortical afferents: the postsynaptic components of the responses to specific thalamo-cortical afferent volleys, to inter-areal afferent volleys and to callosal volleys all have virtually indistinguishable potential profiles in the cortical depth (PERL and WHITLOCK, 1955).

When explored in more detail by advancing a microelectrode tip progressively through consecutive cortical layers, a characteristic pattern is observed: at a depth between 200 to 500 μ beneath the pia-arachnoid surface, when spontaneously active and drivable single unit discharges appear in the record, the evoked potential wave becomes initially negative. This change occurs superficial to the main site of termination of specific thalamo-cortical afferents, and is accompanied by a shortening of the latency of the isopotential point between positive and negative wave (MOUNTCASTLE et al., 1957; AMASSIAN et al., 1955). This phenomenon can be interpreted to reflect the potential field distribution about an active dipole in a volume conductor, if one assumes that the nearly synchronous thalamo-cortical volley generates local postsynaptic responses in a column of cells extending from layer II downwards throughout the cellular thickness of the cortex (MOUNTCASTLE et al., 1957). Other observers, notably LI et al. (1956) noted complete potential reversal as deep as 800 to 1200 μ from the cortical surface and, therefore, attributed the surface positive wave to summed depolarization of the specific thalamo-cortical afferent terminals and Golgi type II cells, both prominent at that depth. However, there is some evidence that artefacts can shift the depth of potential reversal toward deeper cortical layers, notably when neurons in superficial layers become silent as result of deep anaesthesia or pressure damage to the cortical surface (MOUNTCASTLE, 1957; AMASSIAN, 1954).

Additional evidence for attributing the primary evoked response to summation of local postsynaptic activity in large numbers of cortical neurons near the recording electrode, including also neurons which sustain subthreshold membrane potential changes, comes from a computational model relating these potential changes to extracellular current flow and cortical fine structure (TOWE, 1966): the closeness of fit between the experimentally determined and the computed map of current flow supports the underlying assumption that the primary evoked response is, at least in large part, due to slow postsynaptic potential changes in active neurons.

AMASSIAN et al. (1955) emphasized that the earliest activity evoked in superficial neurons tends to occur several milliseconds after the activity onset in neurons below a depth of some 300 to 350 μ; accordingly, he suggested that neuronal dipoles are initially created close to the site of specific afferent terminations, and then transsynaptically generated at successively more superficial levels. In any case, if there is progressive recruitment of neurons towards the cortical surface and serial synaptic activation of more superficial portions of dendrites, it seems to involve but a minimal number of synapses, because of the lack of systematic variation of discharge latencies amongst neurons of individual cell columns (MOUNTCASTLE, 1957).

On the other hand, Towe et al. (1964) identified a subgroup of the neurons in the postcruciate area of cat's cortex with properties that appear to resemble those of the neurons sampled by Mountcastle (1957) in the post-dimple pericoronal area, at least on account of some somatotopic organization, and of similarities in stimulus evoked postsynaptic potentials (Whitehorn and Towe, 1968; Andersson, 1965). The density of this neuron population (the s-set of Towe et al.) increases towards the coronal cortex, in an area that might be considered a rostral and medial extension of area S-I, although there is some suggestion of differences in the modality composition. Operationally, these neurons are defined by responding to electrical stimulation of the contralateral forepaw, but not of any other body area. Under these conditions, the s-neurons are activated during the early part of a surface positive primary response to electrical stimulation of contralateral body areas, prior to activation of a more deeply located cell population (m-neurons) which responds also to ipsilateral stimulation. The distribution of spike density of s-neurons in response to electric stimuli in relation to depth in the cortex and time after stimulation suggests an apparent velocity of upward spread of neural activity, starting at 0.3 m/sec around 800 μ and decreasing to 0.05 m/sec at 200 μ from the cortical surface (Towe, 1968). Presumably, the s-neurons are the medium and small sized pyramids and stellate cells which are the prevailing cell types in the upper strata of the cat's cortex (Ramón-Moliner, 1961).

There is, then, some indication of the existence of a neuron population in which sequential activation along the surface-perpendicular cortical extension could occur, at least in the fringe zone of S-I, rostral to the dimple of the postcruciate gyrus (Kennedy and Towe, 1962), and under the condition of electrical stimulation of the periphery.

1. Slow Waves and Neuron Population Discharge

Data obtained in the past decade, recently summarized by Purpura (1967), have provided considerable information on the properties of dendrites, their role in the regulation of neuronal excitability, and their contribution to the generation of spontaneous and evoked electrical activities of the brain. The current view attributes a major role for determining the response pattern of a neuron to the net depolarizing activity of combinations of excitatory and inhibitory postsynaptic potentials at varying loci in dendritic elements; but contributions of axosomatic postsynaptic potentials in various proportions must also be taken into account, notably in the modulation of neuron responses by recruiting and augmenting activity (Purpura et al., 1964; Purpura and Shofer, 1964).

The relation between extracellular slow wave potentials and cell spike discharge patterns poses questions of considerable importance for the quantitative characterization of neural responses in studies of discriminative behavior. The principal question is: to what extent and in which manner do discharge patterns of individual neurons and evoked potential waves correspond to one another as potential "codes" of sensory behavior (Uttal, 1967)? Fox and O'Brien (1965) demonstrated under conditions of visual stimulation a very high correlation between the post-stimulus time histogram of neuron firing, and the slow wave potential record from the same cortical area; thus, the wave form of the evoked potential predicts the firing probability of individual cortical cells, at least statistically speaking. This correlation holds for both positive and negative potential deflections, as well as for its early and late components. Also during spontaneous neural activity (i. e.: in the absence of intentional stimulation), there is some "congruence" between extracellular slow voltage and neuronal firing probability, but the precise nature of the relation between potential level and firing probability may change from time to time during wakefulness (Fox and Norman, 1968). Such shifts in this relation do not occur during sleep or under anaesthesia.

Since in deep anaesthesia the summated postsynaptic potentials rarely reach the firing level of cortical neurons, it is possible to detect a high degree of correlation between the spindle waves recorded at the cortical surface, and the fluctuations of intracellularly recorded membrane potentials (cf. Creutzfeldt et al., 1966). Neurons in cat's somatosensory cortex under barbiturate anaesthesia can generate long lasting inhibitory postsynaptic potentials, either initially or subsequent to a transient depolarization, if the dorsal columns or the dorsal lateral funiculus are stimulated electrically (Andersson, 1965).

2. Ontogenesis of Cortical Synapses and Electrical Activity

Immature cortex is well suited to assist with the interpretation of the surface potentials in terms of synaptic activity, because synapses are present in relatively small number and in a distinct stratiform arrangement. As a general rule, cortical maturation begins deep in the cortical plate where the earliest cells form what may be considered the primordium of lamina V; subsequent maturation progresses successively through layers IV, III and II, while layer VI remains the last cortical lamina to mature (cf. Molliver and van der Loos, 1970). The earliest synapses in superficial neocortex of kittens are of the axodendritic type, primarily on dendrites of larger diameter; axosomatic synapses appear only in subsequent stages, after axodendritic synapses have become plentiful (Voeller et al., 1963). Superficial pyramidal cells develop their dendrites in a characteristic temporal sequence: at time of birth, apical dendrites prevail while large basilar dendrites are essentially missing (Noback and Purpura, 1961). Neurons in deeper cortical layers may follow a different pattern. In either case, dendrite maturation appears paralleled by synapse formation.

The different maturational gradients contribute at certain developmental stages to a characteristic localization of synapses in circumscribed cortical strata. In the neonatal dog, for instance, synapses are concentrated in three layers, separated from one another by well defined zones of low synaptic density: one, just beneath lamina I, presumably serving as the primordium of lamina II and upper lamina III; the other at the lower border of lamina V (Molliver and van der Loos, 1970). The development of the cortical lamination seems to depend upon the arrival of afferent fibers in the cortex, and follows a similar ontogenetic sequence (Marin-Padilla, 1970; Poliakov, 1967).

Stimulation of cutaneous sensory receptors evokes in midfoetal life a long latency, predominantly surface positive response (Molliver, 1967). In later foetal stages, a negative wave follows the initial surface positive deflection. This negative wave becomes increasingly more prominent as maturation progresses (Hunt and Goldring, 1951; Purpura, 1961; Myerson and Persson, 1969), until it entirely dominates the evoked response at the time of birth (Oeconomos and Scherrer, 1953; Scherrer and Oeconomos, 1955). The somatotopic organization of the evoked responses in S-I and S-II of newborn kittens is essentially identical with that of adult cats (Rubel, 1971).

The surface positive response in early foetal life appears to be attributable to the excitatory synaptic activity at the basal dendrites of deep pyramids which mature early in development. The transition to the predominantly surface negative evoked potential in later foetal life and at the time of birth occurs concomitantly with the emergence of the axodendritic synapses engaging the apical dendrites of superficial pyramids: hence the suggestion that excitatory postsynaptic potentials at these synapses are responsible for the negative component of the evoked potential (Molliver and van der Loos, 1970).

3. Modulation of Evoked Potentials by Non-specific Systems

Unless the animal is deeply anaesthetized both the size and the shape of the cortical evoked potential response to electric shock stimulation of peripheral nerve is highly variable, even when the parameters of the stimuli are kept constant and there are no obvious physiological changes in the general condition of the animal (cf. Bindman et al., 1964). Several factors appear to contribute to this variability.

For the present discussion it is pertinent to recall that Morison and Dempsey (1941) considered augmenting responses resulting from stimulation of the medial lemniscus-internal capsule relay, which are relatively localized in sensory motor cortex, to be distinctly different from recruiting responses evoked by midline thalamic stimulation. Indeed, augmenting waves have a profile of potential change in depth and time which reveals a short latency sink in layers III, IV and V of the cortex, while recruiting waves appear after a longer latent period, at first as a negativity in the most superficial cortical layers (Spencer and Brookhart, 1961a). But, while different synaptic organizations are involved initially, some interactions between these organizations is detectable in the later stages of the apical dendritic activation (cf. Purpura, 1959).

Based, in part, on observations by Brookhart and Zanchetti (1956), Purpura and Grundfest (1956) put forward additional evidence that augmenting and recruiting waves engage different synaptic organizations in the cortex: only the augmenting response initially involves elements in the cortical depth which axosomatically discharge cortico-spinal neurons. Spontaneous spindle waves, in turn, have potential-time profiles which contain components of both augmenting and recruiting waves (Spencer and Brookhart, 1961b).

The similarity between augmenting waves and primary evoked response is so striking as to suggest that both are the result of activity in a common class of thalamo-cortical afferents. Nevertheless, there is evidence from records of intracellular potentials in pyramidal cells of motor cortex that non-specific afferents have axodendritic synaptic contacts much further away from the soma than specific afferents (Nacimiento et al., 1964); moreover, axosomatic synaptic contacts are also involved (Purpura et al., 1964). This can give rise to the complex interactions between postsynaptic potentials elicited by specific and non-specific afferents which were studied in neurons of motor cortex (Lux et al., 1964): if the

EPSP's of specific origin fall on the rising phase of the EPSP's of non-specific origin, summation of depolarization and cell firing occurs; if, however, the inter-action occurs at the repolarization phase of the EPSP of non-specific origin, an EPSP amplitude becomes appreciably reduced, and an IPSP amplitude augment-ed. All in all, the interaction is non-additive; its magnitude and direction depend critically on the relative timing of arrival of the specific and the nonspecific volley. This is, at least in general terms, in line with JASPER's (1963) view that nonspecific activation may have a bimodal effect upon specific cortical responses: under appropriate circumstances increasing their effectiveness by a combination of inhibited spontaneous activity and facilitated specific response; and, with further increase in nonspecific activation, blurring specific responses by occlusion.

These considerations bear on the effect of sleep and arousal on cortical respon-siveness to somatic stimuli: cortical responsivity appears greatest during the light sleep phase; in deep sleep and in arousal as well, the amplitude of cortical responses to somatic stimuli is reduced (FAVALE et al., 1965). The interpretation of these relations is, however, obscured by the fact that the level of vigilance also signifi-cantly alters the transmission of somatic afferent volleys at subcortical relays. For instance, during bursts of REM sleep, transmission through the cuneate nucleus is depressed, both by pre- and postsynaptic inhibitory actions (CARLI et al., 1966). Moreover, polysynaptic activity initiated by cutaneous and high threshold muscle nerve volleys, and ascending in the ventral and lateral spinal funiculi is markedly depressed during desynchronized sleep, but not affected by synchronized sleep. On the other hand, monosynaptically transmitted activity in the ipsilateral ascending hindlimb pathway of the dorsal part of the lateral funiculus remains unaffected by changing sleep patterns (POMPEIANO et al., 1967).

Additional studies by CARLI et al. (1967) implicated the medial and descending components of the vestibular nuclei in the blockade of impulse transmission in dorsal column nuclei and polysynaptic reflex pathways during the REM phase of desynchronized sleep. Pathways originating from these nuclei ascend to sensory-motor cortex where activity is initiated which inhibits transmission of afferent impulses at the medullary and spinal level (POMPEIANO, 1970). Thus far, REM sleep is the only condition under which this mechanism has been found effective in modulating afferent activity in somatic sensory pathways. Whether this mecha-nism is also available for modulation of somatic sensory input by changing activity patterns in the vestibular organ remains an intriguing question, notably since WALBERG et al. (1958) established the projection of primary vestibular afferents to certain cell groups within the medial and descending vestibular nuclei.

Interhemispheric impulse traffic in the corpus callosum is, likewise, subject to variations with different phases of sleep and arousal: at the beginning of phases of desynchronized sleep, activity in callosal fibres is reduced, while phasic increases occur concomitant with high amplitude EEG spindles in synchronized sleep (BER-LUCCHI, 1965). Callosal fibres are largely silent under nembutal anaesthesia. Single stimulus volleys transmitted through the corpus callosum are not always effective in eliciting a primary discharge in neurons, but there is regularly a poststimulatory pause of several 100 msec duration in the spontaneous activity; however, repeti-tive stimuli at low repetition rate are more effective in driving the cortical neurons (CREUTZFELDT et al., 1956).

4. Barbiturates Spindles and Spinal Pathways

Peripheral stimuli may elicit over the entire cortex long lasting suppression of the spindle discharges, normally present in light barbiturate anaesthesia. This generalized effect of stimuli is absent after transection of the spinal cord, except for the dorsal funiculi: it is then merely possible to eliminate the spindles in the somatic sensory area; that is, that cortical area which is the projection area of the spinal pathways transmitting the neural activity from the periphery. Similarly, localized spindle suppression was obtained when afferent activity was confined to the spinal cervico-lemniscal path (Andersson, 1967). In contrast, generalized spindle suppression over the entire cortex required integrity of either the bilateral ventroflexion reflex tract in the ventral funiculus, or a pathway in the dorsal lateral funiculus consisting of thin, possibly unmyelinated fibres. Both pathways are activated by low and high threshold receptors in bilateral fields. The important point is that these experiments demonstrate the existence of somatic sensory pathways outside the specific projection system which can mediate long lasting generalized arousal not only from strong but also from gentle stimuli.

G. Patterns of Unit Responses to Electrical Stimulation

Although electrical stimulation fails to mimic the temporal and spatial conditions of natural stimulation, and can excite a spectrum of afferent fibres with functions and cortical projection patterns which depart from normal activity, it offers the possibility to measure precise response parameters, particularly if the responses of individual neurons are observed in isolation. Single electrical stimuli, applied either to a peripheral nerve trunk or to the skin, frequently generate repetitive responses (Mountcastle et al., 1957; Towe and Amassian, 1958; Mountcastle and Powell, 1959b). Typically, the response is a short train at high frequency, occasionally followed by a second group of discharges of the same neuron, after an interval which varies widely, from 40 to 150 msec. In contrast to the first train of discharges, the second group is best seen with rhythmic stimulation at about five per second; disappears at higher stimulus rates which are faithfully followed by the first response; and may appear at a stimulus intensity below threshold for the initial spike train. Therefore, it is possible that the late response train is attributable to activity which reaches the neuron via a different pathway, engaging a greater or more effective set of presynaptic terminals than those producing the early repetitive discharge (Amassian, 1953; Mountcastle et al., 1957).

The parameters of the early repetitive response depend in a characteristic fashion on the stimulus: both the latency and the number of responses elicited by each stimulus are sensitive to stimulus intensity, and to position of the stimulus in the receptive field (Mountcastle et al., 1957; Mountcastle and Powell, 1959b). Keeping the latter stimulus parameter constant, latency becomes shorter with increasing stimulus intensity. In the monkey, this reduction in latency occurs in two phases: near stimulus threshold latency varies greatly with stimulus intensity; once sufficiently above threshold intensity, there is only a minor additional reduction with further stimulus increment (Towe and Amassian, 1958). Occasionally, latency may again increase when stimulus intensity is raised to as

much as 10 times the threshold value, possibly due to involvement of high threshold inhibitory pathways (KENNEDY and TOWE, 1958). The latencies of the first
responses elicited in several cortical neurons by the same peripheral stimulus and
recorded simultaneously, are usually not correlated to any significant extent (cf.
AMASSIAN, 1961).

Presumably, the temporal distribution of activity in the presynaptic terminals
impinging on the neuron is a major factor determining discharge latency. Therefore, the degree of synchrony of activity in the stimulated nerve may be considered
of importance. TOWE and MORSE (1962) examined this proposition by stimulating
different strands of a peripheral nerve, while recording unit activity from its
cortical projection field. The result was in accord with the expectation: synchrony
in peripheral nerve activity is an important factor in shortening latency.

The capacity of the neurons of S-I to follow repetitive stimuli delivered to the
skin of their peripheral receptive fields depends on the anaesthetic state. At very
light levels of anaesthesia, these neurons follow the stimuli, beat for beat, up to
50–100 per second. At higher rates of stimulation and response commonly settles
after an initial period of higher response rate to an average discharge frequency in
which there is no longer any strict temporal relation between occurrence of individual shocks in the stimulus train, and the timing of neuronal discharges. Under
sodium pentobarbital anaesthesia, neurons follow slowly repeated stimuli faithfully, but cease to respond, and remain silent (or nearly so) throughout the duration of the stimulus train (MOUNTCASTLE and POWELL, 1959b) at high stimulus
frequencies.

Stimulation at certain sites within the receptive field evokes responses with a
shorter latency and with a higher probability of at least one discharge per stimulus, than does stimulation at other sites (MOUNTCASTLE et al., 1957; TOWE and
AMASSIAN, 1958). It appears that the position of the stimulus within the receptive
field is more sensitively reflected by the numer of repetitive discharges than by the
probability that at least one discharge will occur (MOUNTCASTLE and POWELL,
1959b).

These observations by themselves do not shed light on the specific role of the
somatosensory cortex in determining the response characteristics of its neurons:
for, the temporal pattern of the peripheral nerve activity elicited by the stimuli
has undergone some transformations prior to reaching the thalamocortical fibres.
Repetitive discharges in response to electrical stimuli applied to skin or nerve
trunks have indeed been observed at intermediate levels in the ascending somatic
system, such as the dorsal columns and the cuneate nucleus (AMASSIAN and DE
VITO, 1957), and the ventrobasal complex of the thalamus (ROSE and MOUNT-
CASTLE, 1960). Moreover, effects of anaesthesia on the recovery cycle of neurons in
the ventrobasal thalamus, and on their capacity to follow repetitive stimuli at
high frequency are virtually identical with those seen with cortical neurons (POG-
GIO and MOUNTCASTLE, 1963). It is, therefore, not precisely clear what contribution
the factors intrinsic to the cortex make to these response properties of cortical
neurons. Rather, they reflect to varying degrees the properties of the afferent
system as a whole. In one study, however, cortical neurons were activated monosynaptically by stimulation of the thalamic relay nucleus (LI et al., 1956): single
afferent volleys typically initiated repetitive unit responses; the shortest latency

responses were obtained in the immediate vicinity of the presynaptic terminals at a depth of 0.8 to 1.2 mm below the surface of the cortex. These experiments bear also on the question of transynaptic spread of excitation through the cortex, discussed earlier, since unit responses above and below the depth of minimal latency activity were consistently of much longer latency. There is doubt whether this finding is necessarily a valid argument for transynaptic spread of activity across the cortical depth; it would not be if the cortical neurons with long latency belonged to the cortical fringe zone of the thalamic site of stimulation (cf. Amassian, 1961).

In addition to those properties already discussed, cortical neurons exemplify one more functional characteristic which appears fundamental in all central components of the somatic sensory pathway: under suitable conditions, the electrical stimulation of nerve trunks (Amassian, 1953), or skin (Towe and Amassian, 1958; Mountcastle and Powell, 1959a, b) can cause inhibition of cortical neurons, manifested by reduction of probability of occurrence of at least one response, or by a reduction in the number of repetitive responses to a test stimulus. Inhibition occurs in some units when two different afferent sources are stimulated simultaneously; more commonly, however, the excitatory stimulus needs to trail the inhibitory stimulus by several milliseconds. This latter situation was encountered in approximately 10% of nearly 600 neurons studied in lightly anaesthetized macaques (Mountcastle and Powell, 1959a, b). If the stimuli are applied to the skin, it is invariably the case that the excitatory and the inhibitory fields are continuous. Most commonly, the inhibitory field surrounds, either partially or totally, the excitatory field. On the limbs, the inhibitory field may be axially opposed across the limb from that for excitation. This "afferent inhibition" possesses several of the properties of afferent excitation: temporal summation of the inhibitory effect produced by repetitive stimuli applied to a single site in the inhibitory field; spatial and temporal summation of the inhibitory effect of stimuli delivered to separate sites; and, for some neurons, adaptation to continuous stimulation of the inhibitory field. Morphological evidence appears to implicate an intracortical mechanism as contributory to this inhibition, for Jones and Powell (1970a) put forward evidence that inhibition within each cortical subdivision is mediated by axons of intrinsic origin.

H. Modality Representation in the Somatic Sensory Cortex, and Organization of Afferent Pathways

One of the current issues in somatic sensory cortical projections revolves around the question whether the modality distribution in the cortical projection areas reflects that of the peripheral innervation fields or should be viewed as a pattern, albeit one with continuous and graded transitions, of more or less discrete modality fields with separate projection pathways. More specifically, does the cortical representation primarily reflect the body form and its innervation pattern *per se*; or is the cortical map a composite of terminations of different afferent pathways, segregated from one another on the basis of modality and other properties of peripheral receptors, but aligned according to body geography?

1. Deep Modalities

MOUNTCASTLE et al. (1957) reported that gentle mechanical stimuli delivered to the receptors of periosteum, joint capsules and peritendinous connective tissue elicit responses in the somatic sensory receiving areas of deeply anaesthetized cats. The regions of cortex activated by these deep stimuli is roughly coextensive with the tactile projection area designated as S-I and S-II; in addition, it extends further dorsally, including the superior band of the most anterior extension of the suprasylvian sulcus which is also activated by electrical stimulation of the vestibular division of the eighth cranial nerve (WALZL and MOUNTCASTLE, 1949). In the phalanger, and in rabbit as well, the cortical areas activated by direct electrical stimulation of subcutaneous structures also extend beyond those receiving cutaneous, tactile input (ADEY and KERR, 1954).

In contrast to the representation of deep receptors in periost and connective tissue about tendons and joints, muscle stretch was not found to elicit cortical responses in the experiments of MOUNTCASTLE et al. (1952); electrical stimulation of the Group I afferents in fore- and hindlimb muscle nerves was also ineffective. Therefore, the conclusion at that time was that muscle receptors supplied by large-diameter afferents (muscle spindles and Golgi tendon organs) are not represented in the somatic sensory cortex.

Further studies by McINTYRE (1962a, 1962b) corroborated this view: stimuli applied to individual muscle nerves did not evoke cortical responses unless all the Group I fibres were activated. Further increases in stimulus strength led to progressively larger cortical positive waves, and the cortical responses became maximal only when the stimuli engaged Group III fibres of the muscle nerve. The conclusion was, therefore, that only the Group III and a few of the Group II afferents of muscle nerves project to the somatosensory cortices. Usually, the responses evoked in S-II were much larger than those in S-I. As regards the types of peripheral receptors involved in this projection to the cortex, McINTYRE (1962a, 1962b) concluded that muscle spindle receptors do not participate, at least as far as the hindlimbs are concerned; the few Group II fibres in muscle nerves which projected to the cortex were attributed to Pacinian corpuscles or joint receptors.

Weak mechanical pulses to individual Pacinian corpuscles situated near the cat's crural interosseous membrane are, indeed, capable of evoking surface positive cortical potentials in the contralateral S-II. The response to two pulses delivered to the same or different corpuscles at short stimulus intervals summate; as the interstimulus interval is changed there occasionally is a facilitation of the second response, and following each response there is always a period of several hundred milliseconds during which responses are depressed (McINTYRE et al., 1967). The Pacinian projection to S-II is most conspicuous in a region slightly caudal to the cutaneous projection field, between S-I, S-II and the auditory projections (SILFVENIUS, 1970).

Afferents of the Group II and III type in cutaneous nerves also have access to the contralateral somatic areas I and II, and to ipsilateral area II (MARK and STEINER, 1958). In addition to whatever direct ascending projection these fibres may have, they also converge together with large afferents onto spinal second-order neurons which respond to single primary afferent volleys of progressively greater size by firing repetitive trains of increasing length (McINTYRE, 1957). Thus, the smaller primary afferent fibres can exert effects at higher levels by way of tract units which are shared with fibres of larger diameter: the discharge pattern of second order neurons could in this manner signal the degree of involvement of different components of the peripheral nerve fibre spectrum. Moreover, if afferents from skin and muscle project to the same area of cortex, it is possible that volleys from the two sources may engage the same neural units, either at their cortical terminations or in some subcortical portion of the afferent pathway. Mountcastle et al. (1952) did, indeed, obtain some evidence that a Group II volley (largely engaging cutaneous fibres) leaves the ascending system refractory to a subsequent Group III volley for some 40 msec.

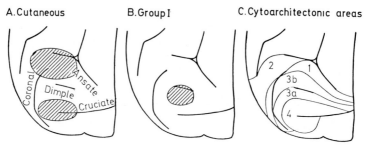

Fig. 3. The projection areas related to the contralateral forelimb of the cat. A, B, and C are dorsal views of the rostral pole of the right hemisphere. The ansate, coronal, and cruciate sulci as well as the postcruciate dimple are designated in A. Short latency surface-positive potentials are evoked in the hatched areas by volleys in cutaneous afferents (A) and by volleys in the Group I muscle afferents (B) of forelimb nerves. C illustrates the approximate extent of the cytoarchitectonic areas 3a, 3b, 1, 2 and 4 according to Hassler and Muhs-Clement (1964). (From Oscarsson, 1965)

2. Representation of Muscle Afferents

Oscarsson and Rosén (1963) confirmed earlier reports by Amassian and Berlin (1958a, b) that the Group I muscle afferents of the forelimb project to the cerebral cortex of the cat (Oscarsson and Rosén, 1966; Oscarsson et al., 1966). The potentials evoked by Group I muscle afferent volleys were located in the rostral part of the postcruciate gyrus, largely rostral to the postcruciate dimple, corresponding to area 3A of Hassler and Muhs-Clement (1964) (Fig. 3). The pathway mediating this response ascends through the dorsal funiculus of the spinal cord and relays in the cuneate nucleus. The Group I forelimb afferents with cortical projections supply slowly adapting muscle spindles in the periphery.

Latency measurements based on intra- and extracellularly recorded single neuron activity indicate that the majority of the forelimb Group I activated neurons are monosynaptically excited from thalamic fibres; accordingly, they represent the fourth-order neurons of the Group I forelimb projection system. The EPSPs evoked by stimulation of forelimb muscle nerves appear at very weak stimulus strengths and reach a maximum either before or concomitantly with the Group I component of the muscle afferent volley. The majority of the neurons in the Group I projection area receive only excitatory influences, but some receive exclusively inhibitory or mixed input. In the cat, the convergence of Group I input onto an individual neuron is usually extensive; i.e., from muscle groups working at different joints and from antagonistic muscle groups at the same joint. In addition, cutaneous afferents contribute synaptic actions of longer latency than the Group I inputs. Records obtained from single thalamocortical radiation fibres also display this complex convergence pattern, suggesting that the convergence had been effected at thalamic levels of the Group I projection system (OSCARSSON et al., 1966).

A projection of low threshold afferents from forelimb muscles and tendons was also established in the baboon: electric stimulation of the deep radial nerve at intensities below threshold of motor axons evoked a response in the forelimb region of area 3a, as did brief muscle pull and vibrations applied to the tendons of extensor digitorum communis (PHILLIPS et al., 1970).

At first, several studies failed to detect a cortical projection of the Group I hindlimb afferents. It was, therefore, considered that the cortical Group I representation from the forelimbs is of special functional significance, notably for the wide variety of fine movements which subserve the exploration of the environment. Moreover, the lack of a Group I hindlimb representation in the cortex was thought to limit this capability to the relatively crude performance levels which hindlimbs can achieve in such tasks. Recently, however, a cortical projection of the Group I hindlimb afferents has been described in the cat (LANDGREN and SILFVENIUS, 1969). These afferents as well as some from group II muscle and cutaneous receptors leave the dorsal columns at the level of L-3 to form synapses on neurons of the dorsal horn; their axons, in turn, project via the dorsolateral fasciculus to a group of neurons in the medulla (LANDGREN and SILFVENIUS, 1971), known as nucleus Z (BRODAL and POMPEIANO 1957). Finally, in the cortical projection, there appear two distinct and separate representations of hindlimb group I afferents in area 3a; one on the dorsal, the other on the medial surface of the hemisphere (LANDGREN and SILFVENIUS, 1969). Both hindlimb foci are medial to the projection area of groups I afferents from the forelimb (OSCARSSON et al., 1966).

These studies emphasize the separateness and discreteness of group I projections from fore- and hindlimb, which is most prominent at the spinal level where some of the hindlimb afferents join different spinal tracts according to modality and receptor adaptation properties (see section H-5). However, as regards the cortical projection, one can argue that the appearance of discreteness, based on experiments with electrical stimulation of peripheral nerves, obscures a much more striking property: namely, the continuity of transitions between neighboring projection fields which are aligned to one common and continuous body representation, notwithstanding the fact that their afferents travel in different pathways. This point of view will be more fully documented in section I.

3. Cytoarchitectural and Functional Specialization of Area 3a

In the primate, the junction of area 3 with the cortex of area 4 is marked by a short transition zone labeled 3a by the VOGTS (1919), and PA by VON BONIN and BAILEY (1947). For the most part this transitional area is situated at, and slightly behind the bottom of the central sulcus; laterally, area 3a forms most of its floor. At the medial end of the central sulcus, areas 3 and 3a jointly extend on to its anterior wall (POWELL and MOUNTCASTLE, 1959a). In the transition between areas 3 and 3a, there is progressive thinning of layer IV, and gradual reduction of granule cell density in layer III.

On the basis of its connections, area 3a can be considered an architectonic subdivision of somatic sensory area I: for it receives fibres from areas 3, 1 and 2 and, like these areas themselves, receives also afferents from area 4, from S-II and from the ventrobasal nuclei of the thalamus (JONES and POWELL, 1969 c). Accordingly, area 3a would function as a specific cortical projection area in S-I for Group I muscle afferents in much the same way as area 3 is the principal receiving area for cutaneous afferents, and areas 1 and 2 for afferents from joints and periosteum.

However, there is one important difference: impulses in Group I afferents cannot fulfill the role of discriminative stimuli for operant conditioning, even if the Group I activity elicits conspicuous cortical evoked potentials (SWETT and BOURASSA, 1967). In contrast, stimulation of Group II afferents which include fibres signaling joint position (BOYD and ROBERTS, 1953; GARDINER, 1948) is a discriminable cue. Moreover, there is evidence from human surgical cases that pulling tendons and stretching muscles is not perceived, as long as joint angles remain constant (GELFAN and CARTER, 1967); and PROVINS (1958) has shown that afferent activity from muscles cannot compensate for loss of joint position sense following conduction block in joint afferent nerves, at least at low angular velocities of joint movement. In contrast, there is now evidence for persistence of appreciable kinaesthesis after paralyzing joint afferents but preserving muscle afferents, provided joints are moved at velocities exceeding 5 or 10 degrees per sec (GOODWIN et al., 1972).

4. Sense Modality and Cortical Columns

The general trend in the modality distribution in the macaque's postcentral gyrus indicates a predominant cutaneous representation anteriorly, and a gradual increase of deep representation posteriorly. An additional, heavy representation of deep receptors in cytoarchitectural area 3a adjoins the rostral border of area 3, in the depth of the central sulcus (POWELL and MOUNTCASTLE, 1959b), to the cortex of the anterior bank of the macaque's central sulcus (ALBE-FESSARD, 1967).

The modality of temperature is commonly not thought to have a specific representation in S-I although there were occasions when observers recorded evoked activity in neurons of sensorimotor cortex in response to thermal stimulation of the tongue (COHEN et al., 1957; LANDGREN, 1957b) and of the skin (KREISMAN and ZIMMERMAN, 1971). In the monkey, ALBE-FESSARD and LIEBESKIND (1966) found the neural responses to thermal stimulation of the skin to be located in the pre-Rolandic cortex. Behavioral studies in primates do not lend support to the idea that cortex of the postcentral gyrus is significantly involved in temperature discrimination. However, the involvement of other cortical areas is suggested by the observation that corpus callosum section prevents transfer of a learned temperature discrimination from the trained hemisphere (which is contralateral to the trained hand) to the opposite side (CRAGG and DOWNER, 1967). Cortical and thalamic somatosensory lesions in the rat impair temperature sensitivity at most transiently and to a limited extent (FINGER and FROMMER, 1970).

Although the data obtained from gross potential mapping studies were suggestive, the question of whether or not deep and cutaneous receptors possess topographically separate representations within S-I and S-II was not answered definitively until the activity of individual cortical neurons was recorded in isolation and observed during mechanical stimulation of the periphery. In 1957, MOUNTCASTLE provided an extensive analysis of the modality and topographic attributes of the individual neurons comprising the posterior sigmoid, lateral sigmoid, and coronal gyri of anesthetized cats: within this region of cortex neurons are activated by only one mode of stimulation which may be either hair movement, pressure on the skin, or mechanical deformation of deep tissues. Furthermore, neurons of individual radial cell-columns are all activated from the same peripheral locus and by the same mode of stimulation. The three types of modality-pure cell-columns are intermingled in a mosaic-like fashion. The intermingling of columns is not random, however, for posteriorly (the cortex of the posterior sigmoid gyrus near the junction of the ansate and lateral sulci, for example) most cell columns represent hair movement or pressure; in contrast, further anterior (towards the postcruciate dimple) most of the columns contain neurons responding to stimuli classified as deep. The postcruciate dimple of the cat's cortex is believed to delineate the primary motor cortex from the primary somatic sensory cortex (MOUNTCASTLE, 1957; HASSLER and MUHS-CLEMENT, 1964).

The distribution of neurons belonging to various submodality classes within the postcentral gyrus of the macaque is similar and corresponds to the antero-posterior gradient in cortical cytoarchitecture (POWELL and MOUNTCASTLE, 1959a, b; MOUNTCASTLE and POWELL, 1959a). Receptors in joint capsules, peritendinous connective tissues, and muscle fascia were found to be represented, in the main, by the neurons positioned posteriorly (area 2); receptors from skin are represented anteriorly (chiefly in area 3); and the modality composition of the centrally located region (area 1) reflects a continuous gradient between the two bordering extremes. Neurons of the postcentral gyrus with receptive fields in the muscle tissue itself were not encountered (POWELL and MOUNTCASTLE, 1959b) nor were there any neurons that could be activated by muscle stretch (MOUNTCASTLE and POWELL, 1959a). This modality distribution in the postcentral gyrus is paralleled by characteristic differences in cortical cytoarchitecture (POWELL and MOUNTCASTLE, 1959a): area 3 is composed of koniocortex, as broadly defined by ROSE (1949), and receives a higher density of thalamic afferents than do areas 1 and 2 (WALKER, 1938; CLARK and POWELL, 1953); areas 1 and 2 are formed of cortex showing graded changes to the typical parietal cortex of areas 5 and 7, with area 2 being characterized by the increase in the number of large pyramidal cells in layers III and IV. The transition from area 1 to 2 is indicated by an increase in the thickness of all cortical layers, although the increase in layer III is most prominent. As in the cat, the neurons of a radial cell-column are related not only to the same submodality, but to nearly the same peripheral receptive field as well (POWELL and MOUNT-CASTLE, 1959b). This supports the idea of a vertical organization of the cortex and also indicates that the pattern of representation of the body form observed with surface recording extends throughout the depth of the cortex (Fig. 4).

The parcellation of cortex into cell columns according to functional criteria appears to be a general design principle of cortical organization (cf. CHOW and LEIMAN, 1970): current evidence favors the idea that it is significant for the orderly representation of particular stimulus features and attributes not only in the

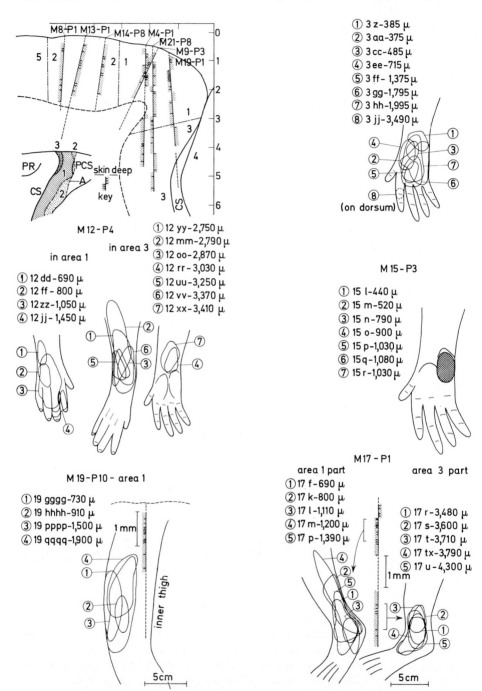

Fig. 4. The concept of the columnar organization of the postcentral gyrus in the monkey: a correlation of the findings obtained by single unit analysis with cytoarchitecture. At the top left portion of the figure is a reconstruction of seven microelectrode penetrations of the post-central gyrus of *Macaca mulatta*. The microelectrode tracks are displayed on a schematic

somaesthetic, but also in visual (HUBEL and WIESEL, 1962, 1963, 1969; BLAKE-MORE, 1970) and auditory cortex (HIND, 1960; OONISHI and KATSUKI, 1965; ABELES and GOLDSTEIN, 1970), and that it applies to motor cortex as well (SAKATA and MIYAMOTO, 1968). Cortical columns may be considered as functional modules, each of them centred around a pyramidal cell whose dendritic complex, characterized by a high density of spines, would encompass a cylinder of cortical tissue. Interspersed between these pyramidal cells are short axoned neurons whose dendrites do not have constant shape, size or directions: this class of cells could conceivably propagate activity between the modules to generate a depolarization sheet tangential to the cortical surface, whenever the pyramidal columns receive an afferent barrage of input over the specific thalamic afferents. The detailed panorama of the tangential activity sheet would then reflect the temporal and spatial pattern of excitation in a population of columnar modules (GLOBUS and SCHEIBEL, 1967a). The extent of interaction between modules is, however, restricted by the limited degree of connectivity of the cortex in the horizontal direction: even in layer I which was customarily considered a tangential connection system, fibre degeneration in isolated cortical slabs spreads generally only as far as 1.5 mm, and the total span of some large fibres may be estimated at 7 to 8 mm (SZENTÁGOTHAI, 1967). In Golgi stained material, specific thalamic afferents can be shown to terminate in a cylindrical plexus about 200 to 500 μ in diameter; the non-specific afferents spread their endings into 1 to 3 mm wide cylinders (SCHEIBEL and SCHEIBEL, 1971).

In an attempt to examine cortical tissue of macaque and man for a possible columnar organization, VON BONIN and MEHLER (1971) reconstructed three-dimensional displays from cresyl-violet and Golgi stained sections: groups, 2 to 6 cells in diameter, appeared to run vertically toward the cortical surface, separated from each other by radial fibre bundles and an intercolumnar neuropil. The columns appear some 80 μ apart, but do not always remain isolated: they may fuse or split apart.

drawing of a parasagittal section from the level marked A on the inset drawing of the dorsolateral surface of the cerebral cortex. Along each penetration, cross-hatching indicates the cortical location at which multiple neurons were observed to be activated by stimulation of the skin. Horizontal lines to the left indicate those locations at which a single neuron was isolated sufficiently long for its cutaneous receptive field to be mapped. Similar codes along the right of a track indicate the cortical location of neurons activated by stimulation of joint, periostial, and fascial receptors. The figurines of the various body parts outline the cutaneous receptive fields of single neurons which were isolated in penetrations of the macaque's postcentral gyrus. For each penetration the neurons which were studied are numbered and their depth below the cortical surface indicated. Superimposed drawings of receptive fields encountered in penetrations nearly normal to the cortical surface (M3–P6; area 1 part of M12–P4; M15–P3; M19–P1p; and area 1 part of M17–P1) show the essentially identical receptive fields of the neurons within a single column. The two penetrations displayed at the bottom of the figure (M19–P10 and M17–P1) are reconstructed in the manner described above. The sharp turnover in modality in the course of penetration M17–P1 indicates that this penetration crossed cell columns; for according to the concept of columnar organization the neurons comprising a cortical cell-column are modality pure. (Modified from POWELL and MOUNTCASTLE, 1959b)

As one particular aspect of the columnar organization in somatic sensory cortex, T.A. Woolsey and van der Loos (1970) analyzed in great detail the appearance of an especially prominent multicellular cytoarchitectonic unit in lamina IV of the face projection area in mouse cortex. In the reconstruction from Golgi and Nissl-Golgi stained tangential sections, neurons appear to be arranged in the form of "barrels", with a dense ring of cell bodies as the wall of the barrel, surrounding a central zone of lesser cell density; the barrels are separated from one another by a nearly acellular region, the septum. It appears that each barrel is the cortical correlate of one contralateral mystacial vibrissa. This high degree of cortical structural specialization in lamina IV which receives the afferents from thalamus, is possibly related to the considerable role which the mystacial vibrissae play in this species for the exploration of the environment

Notwithstanding these sources of suggestive evidence that cell columns are an integral part of cortical morphology, there are those who argue that patterning of neurons in functional vertical columns could result from a suitable interdigitation of horizontally and obliquely stratified structures (Ramón-Moliner, 1970). In any case, columns as defined by functional criteria do not necessarily need a counterpart in cortical morphology: for instance, the commissural fibres which ascend with constant diameter vertically through the cortex, are in a strategic position to influence activity within narrow vertical columns throughout the entire cortical depth (Jones and Powell, 1970a). However, at early stages of ontogeny, the cerebral cortex presages a columnar organization, be it morphological or functional: for, early in development, axons and apical dendritic shafts of pyramidal cells are oriented radially, and this stage precedes the emergence of lateral dendritic branches which occurs only during the postnatal period (Noback and Purpura, 1961; Schadé et al., 1962; Meller et al., 1968). Moreover, dendrites of Golgi type II neurons which play an important part in the tangential connectivity, develop much later than the dendrites of pyramidal cells (Morest, 1969).

5. Modality Segregation in Afferent Projections to S-I

During the past decade, the view prevailed that the modality classes of postcentral neurons replicate those of the myelinated first order fibres feeding the lemniscal system *via* the dorsal columns. (Rose and Mountcastle, 1960; Mountcastle, 1961; Bowsher, 1965; Mountcastle and Darian-Smith, 1968). The striking similarity of the modality representation in the ventro-posterior thalamic nucleus (VB) and in S-I is consistent with this view: i.e., 59% of the neurons in S-I (Powell and Mountcastle, 1959b) and 58% of the neurons in VP (Poggio and Mountcastle, 1963) receive input from receptors in the deep tissues of the periphery. Furthermore, approximately equal proportions (ca. 40%) of the deep neurons at the two levels are exclusively activated by joint movement (Powell and Mountcastle, 1959b; Poggio and Mountcastle, 1963). However, as previously discussed, single unit studies have demonstrated systematic variations in modality composition within the anteroposterior dimension of S-I, and in the dorso-ventral dimension of the ventroposterior nucleus of the thalamus as well. Poggio and Mountcastle (1963) suggested that this differential distribution of neurons representing different modalities can be interpreted as the central reflection of the regional differences in the modality composition of the peripheral innervation: the proximal body parts, which are dorsally represented in VB according to MOUNTCASTLE and HENNEMAN (1952) possess a proportionally greater innervation of deep structures than do the ventrally projecting distal parts, in which the richness of the skin innervation corresponds to their effectiveness as tactile organs. This thalamic pattern would fit with the differential projections of modalities to the postcentral gyrus (POWELL and MOUNTCASTLE, 1959b): there is suggestive evidence that the ventral and more posterior portion of the thalamic nuclear complex projects to area 3, and progressively more dorsal portions to areas 1 and 2 (WALKER, 1938). Accordingly, the gradient of increasing deep representation from rostral to caudal in the postcentral gyrus would correspond to a progression from ventral to dorsal in VB, and from distal to proximal along the limbs.

The elegance and simplicty of this conception rests on the postulate that preservation of body topography is the organizing principle of the medial lemsniscal system at all levels: all afferents entering the dorsal columns project rostrally according to this plan of organization, and the regional differences of modality composition merely reflect regional differences of receptor distribution in the body peripherey. The dermatomal segmentation of afferents from the body periphery, and the subsequent convergences between afferents from neighboring dermatomes, first recognized in the cortical mapping studies of WOOLSEY et al. (1942) and later partially obscured by the pictorial representations of the cortical projection pattern as replica of the body shape, tended to cloud the purity of this conception (cf. POWELL and MOUNTCASTLE, 1959b), though not to an extent that cast serious doubt on its general validity. However, more recent studies generated evidence which conflicts critically with some of the essential components of this conception.

Essentially, this evidence consists of gross discrepancies in modality and adaptation properties between neurons in S-I and afferents in the dorsal columns. Afferents supplying the hair follicles of down hairs (Type D) and touch corpuscles (Type I) are essentially absent at cervical levels of the dorsal columns of cat; as a consequence, there is a six fold increase in the proportion of afferents from the longest and thickest guard hairs (Type T) at the level of the cervical dorsal columns relative to the spectrum of cutaneous myelinated fibers as compared to peripheral nerve (BROWN, 1968). The afferents from Type D endings take in cat the alternate route of the spinocervical system; the rostral course of the slowly adapting Type I afferents in cat is still uncertain (BROWN and FRANZ, 1969). The second class of slowly adapting afferents, namely those originating from the intradermal endings (Type II) projects into the dorsal columns (PETIT and BURGESS, 1968), and is not represented in the spinocervical system (BROWN and FRANZ, 1969). In the primate, the exclusion of slowly adapting cutaneous afferents has been shown to occur in an, essentially, continuous progression from caudal to rostral: both Type I and Type II afferents from the hindlimb, at first, enter the dorsal columns at their respective segmental levels, ascend in the dorsal columns for a few segments, and then proceed to their rostral destinations outside the dorsal columns: hence, there are no slowly adapting cutaneous afferents from hindlimb at cervical levels of the dorsal columns, while there are still some from the forelimb (WHITSEL et al., 1969a).

In spite of these differences between carnivore and primate, there is a common principle involved: some property of peripheral receptors, unrelated to body topography, prescribes the spinal route taken by their afferents to reach their destination.

The ascending course of the afferents which innervate the joint capsules of the hindlimb also indicates that the dorsal column projection does not merely replicate the topographic variations in the peripheral innervation: Burgess and Clark (1969) demonstrated that only a small proportion of the fibres from the posterior and medial articular nerves of the cat and the posterior articular nerve of the squirrel monkey ascend to cervical levels within the dorsal columns. Those few joint afferents which ascend in the dorsal columns (8.6%) are of the rapidly adapting type, generally not considered to be directly concerned with position sense. Moreover, Whitsel et al. (1969a) provided data which also clearly indicate a segregation of afferents according to modality within the fasciculus gracilis of primates: the primary afferents innervating the joints, fascia and periostium of the hindlimb as well as those afferents supplying slowly adapting cutaneous afferent units enter the fasciculus at lumbosacral levels but leave prior to cervical levels of the spinal cord. It is possible that the ipsilateral spinovestibular pathway described in the cat by Pompeiano and Brodal (1957) may convey the deep modalities of the hindlimb which subserve somaesthesis (Whitsel et al., 1969a). The latter path lies in the dorsolateral funiculus in the cervical cord; a region in primates containing fibres which enable successful performance of discriminative hindlimb kinaesthetic tasks following total destruction of the cervical or thoracic dorsal columns (Gilman and Denny-Brown, 1966; Vierck, 1966).

These findings explain why transection of the dorsal columns at different levels of the spinal cord in macaques leads to contrasting deficits in the cortical representation of the hindlimb (Whitsel et al., 1971a; Dreyer et al., 1973). Specifically, a transection of the dorsal columns between segmental levels C_1 and T_3 leads to a marked diminution in the S-I representation of the rapidly adapting low threshold mechanoreceptors of the skin (this deficit is, in the main, confined to cytoarchitectural areas 1 and 3); yet the predominantly deep submodality representation of posterior area 1 and area 2 remains unaffected. In contrast, a lesion of the cervical spinal cord which includes both the dorsal columns and the dorsolateral funiculi (or a lesion interrupting the dorsal columns at upper lumbar levels) leads to a uniform and non-selective deficit in the cortical representation of low-threshold hindlimb mechanoreceptors within areas 3, 1, and 2. It was concluded that the deep submodality representation within area 3a apparently receives an appreciable input from crossed ventral spinal paths, for nearly complete hemisection of the ipsilateral cord failed to significantly alter the functional properties of the individual neurons located in area 3a. Moreover, although from 20—40% of the neurons located in anterior area 1 and area 3 in animals subjected to chronic cervical dorsal column transection could still be activated from the periphery, the great majority displayed functional properties distinct from those characteristic of S-I in unanaesthetized preparations (see Dreyer et al., 1973 for details). The spinal paths which conveyed such „non-lemniscal" input to the neurons of S-I were localized to the ventral cord; and there was no evidence for a significant contribution of anterolateral spinal paths to the „lemniscal" cutaneous representation in S-I. For a discussion of the effects of dorsal column lesions on S-I in the cat see LEVITT and LEVITT (1968a, b).

Concomitant with the segregation of modalities in the ascending course of fasciculus gracilis, there occurs also some rearrangement of the ascending fibres according to body topography: at the level of the dorsal root entry zone, fibres adjoin the fasciculus gracilis in dermatomal sequence, with further rostral segments coming to lie more lateral in the fascicle; in the rearrangement along the ascending course, the receptive fields of these fibres generate in the cross sectional plane, essentially, the outline of the cortical hindlimb map in S-I (WHITSEL et al., 1970). Different afferent pathways appear to project to slightly different cortical regions in S-I, although there is some interdigitation with continuous gradation and shifting overlap: in the cat, for instance, cutaneous afferents projecting via the dorsal funiculus terminate in the cytoarchitectural fields 3, 1 and 2, with the main focus centred on the caudal end of the coronal sulcus; on the other hand, the spinocervical cutaneous projection is restricted to the areas 1 and 2, its focus abutting the caudal edge of the dorsal funicular focus (OSCARSSON et al., 1966).

The pattern of afferent pathway terminations in the cortical receiving area replicates, essentially, that in the thalamus. Apart from the dorsal column projection to the central core of the ventroposterior thalamic nucleus with precise topographic organization (cf. POGGIO and MOUNTCASTLE, 1960, 1963) there is also a projection of the spinocervical tract, terminating in the ventro- and dorsolateral border zone of VP. The afferent input from this tract is complex, at least in the cat, for these neurons receive afferents from the hindlimbs and forelimbs (LANDGREN et al., 1965; ANDERSEN et al., 1966). Moreover, they can be antidromically activated from ipsilateral cortical foci corresponding closely to those cortical areas which receive the spinocervical projection pathway.

The neurons comprising the dorsomedial part of the shell around the central core of VP receive Group I afferents from muscles as well as skin afferents which ascend, in the cat, via the spino-cervical and the dorsal column paths. The thalamic Group I neurons for the forelimb project to two different cortical regions: one, in the region of the post-cruciate dimple; the other, in S-II; but, strangely, in that portion of S-II which CARRERAS and ANDERSSON (1963) identified as the hindlimb field. Collateral projections from thalamic neurons to S-I and S-II were described by MANSON (1969) and ROWE and SESSLE (1968). The significance of this dual cortical projection from thalamic neurons is uncertain; but the distinct differences in intracortical axonal degeneration patterns within S-I and S-II after small lesions in VB may provide morphological evidence that there are differences in the handling of incoming information (MORRISON et al., 1970).

The foregoing documented some of the principal evidence for a separation of afferents into different spinal pathways with separate rostral projections according to properties of peripheral receptors. As suggested in the introduction to this section, these findings conflict with the view that the modality and adaptation properties of neurons in S-I mirror those of afferents in the dorsal column pathway, and that the regional distribution of modality properties of S-I neurons merely reflect the distribution of different types of mechanoreceptors in the body periphery. However, the role of the body topography as an organizing principle of the projection to S-I remains valid, albeit in a modified form: shortly after entry into the dorsal columns the ascending collaterals of the fibres in each dorsal root are arranged to a fibre lamina with a dorsolateral to ventromedial orientation in the columns. Within each segmental lamina thus formed, the fibres are characteristically ordered: this is demonstrated by the fact that a recording microelectrode which advances perpendicular to the long axis of the lamina encounters a sequence of fibres whose receptive fields describe a continuous path on the body (the "dermatomal trajectory" of Werner and Whitsel (1967). Furthermore, each time the tip of the electrode crosses a boundary between consecutive segmental fibre laminae in the lumbar dorsal columns, there occurs an abrupt jump in the receptive field location which backtracks part of the peripheral path mapped in the preceding lamina, reflecting the overlap in the peripheral segmental innervation (Werner and Whitsel, 1967). As the dorsal column fibres ascend from lumbar to cervical levels, a significant change occurs, apart from the separation of submodalities described earlier in this section: the fibres of consecutive dermatomes rearrange to the extent that an electrode advancing through the cervical fasciculus gracilis encounters a sequence of fibres whose receptive fields form a smooth and continuous path on the body periphery (Whitsel et al., 1970). This process brings afferents from the same body regions into neighborhood and proximity relations which approach those of the neurons in S-I.

6. Sensory Functions of Somatic Afferent Pathways

Complete section of the dorsal columns at cervical levels impairs weight discrimination in primates only transiently, and there is evidence that an alternate pathway in the anterior columns contributes to the successful performance of this task (de Vito et al., 1964). After complete bilateral section of the posterior columns at the level of T6 to T7, macaques perform proprioceptive and vibratory discriminations in the hindlimb to preoperative criterion, though only after extensive retraining (Schwartzman and Bogdonoff, 1969). For certain tactile discrimination tasks, the integrity of the dorsal column pathways is also not essential: Tapper (1970) demonstrated in avoidance conditioning tests that transection of dorsal columns in cats leaves the discrimination of small indentations of single tactile pads in hairy skin unimpaired. Norrsell (1966) concluded that the spinocervical tract plays a primary, and the dorsal columns at best a secondary role in mediating conditioned reflexes to light tactile stimulation in the dog. However, the nature and intensity of the stimuli are of significance; for, neither of these pathways is essential when coarse stimuli are applied; on the other hand, roughness discrimination is acquired more rapidly, and attains a higher degree of resolution between small stimulus differences when the dorsal columns are intact (Kitai and Weinberg, 1968).

Semmes (1969) and Wall (1970) proposed recently an entirely different role for the dorsal columns: instead of signaling passively impressed peripheral stimuli to the cortical receiving areas, the dorsal columns would subserve the acquisition of sensory information which is generated by active and sequential exploration of stimulus objects. Their role in this process would be that of the afferent component in a neural subsystem that is concerned with search strategies leading to stimulus recognition (Schwartzman and Semmes, 1971). The implication is that the information transactions in which the dorsal column pathway and its cortical projection participate differ from those in projection areas of other somatic pathways concerned with the mere detection of stimuli, and of some quantitative gradation; there is, indeed, substantial evidence which attributes to S-II the principal role in passive, and to S-I the principal role in active tactile discrimination tasks (GLASSMEN, 1970).

These ideas about the operational mode of the dorsal column system appear to predispose it for playing a special role in the somatic sense of space (cf. REN-FREW and MELVILLE, 1960); and for the execution of serial acts of which accurate timing and sequencing of limb projections into extracorporeal space are important components (DUBROVSKY et al., 1971; MELZACK and BRIDGES, 1971). However, a particular aspect of somatic space, concerned with the bilateral symmetry of the body, requires normally the integrity of the neospinothalamic tract: for, lesions of the lateral lemniscal area in the brain stem through which the neospinothalamic tract courses (MEHLER et al., 1960; BOWSHER, 1961) causes a macaque to respond to bilateral simultenous tactile stimulation as if only one side of the body had been touched (extinction) (SCHWARTZ and EIDELBERG, 1968).

Recovery from this inability to recognize bilateral stimulation appears to require the dorsal column pathways for additional section of the latter restores extinction, possibly by creating a condition of perceptual rivalry such as obtained by SPRAGUE et al. (1963) in the cat with extensive lemniscal lesions, and described in man and macaque after extensive lesions of the parietal lobe (DENNY-BROWN and CHAMBER, 1958).

The common denominator that seems to emerge from these and similar studies underscores the difficulty of assigning a unique and specific sensory function to particular afferent pathways, as one may be inclined to do on the basis of their distinctive electrophysiological properties (cf. SCHWARTZMAN and SEMMES, 1971). On the one hand it becomes increasingly more appropriate to view the ascending spinal tracts as parallel systems with partial redundancy as regards the specific receptor types whose activity they transmit; on the other hand there is evidence that central pathways can assume a compensatory role after more extensive and prolonged training: for instance, the recovery of proprioceptive function in chimpanzee after medial lemniscal section in the medulla appears to be mediated by the dentato-rubro-thalamic tract (SJOQVIST and WEINSTEIN, 1942). This pathway was also thought to be involved in the gradual restoration of the ability to discriminate weights and textures after ablation of postcentral gyrus and parietal lobes (cf. RUCH et al., 1938). Both factors can contribute to restitution of behavioral capabilities (albeit after additional training) which, under normal circumstances, are carried out by one particular afferent tract: hence, the logic of denying to an afferent tract a certain function which can be regained after this tract's section, is not necessarily compelling; rather, it commonly turns out that permanent behavioral deficits presume lesions of several pathway whereby the mere quantitative imbalance of sensory input can, by itself, become a decisive factor (witness the condition of perceptual rivalry and neglect and the increased severity of unilateral as compared to bilateral lesions (MELZACK and BRIDGES, 1971; GILMAN and DENNY-BROWN, 1966). However, a more positive assertion suggests itself as well: if different afferent pathways can take each other's place in accomplishing a particular behavioral end, one can argue that their relationship in the cortical projection areas must be intimate, as would be the case if the respective cortical receiving areas were capable of operating as one functional unit (see section I).

7. Commissural Connection of S-I

A further differentiation in the afferent projections to S-I is introduced by the selective distribution of callosal fibres which appears related to patterns of evolution. In the macaque the terminal degeneration resulting from ablation of the opposite S-I occupies three main regions of S-I: a region on the medial wall of the hemisphere which included the lateral part of the upper bank of the cingulate sulcus and the immediately adjoining part of the marginal gyrus; a region on the medial portion of the dorsal surface of the hemisphere which stretches from the fundus of the central sulcus across the posterior bank of the postcentral sulcus; and a region which spans the entire postcentral gyrus below the level of the anterior end of the intraparietal sulcus and extends forwards around the lower end of the central sulcus. In addition, the three disjoint antero-posterior strips described above are connected via a tenuous but continuous band of degeneration running along the entire posterior margin of S-I from the cingulate sulcus to the end of the intraparietal sulcus (Ebner and Myers, 1962, 1965; Pandya and Vignolo, 1968; Jones and Powell, 1969c). Ebner (1969) suggested that commissure-free neocortex (namely: foot and head representations in S-I of cat and macaque) appear at a later stage of evolution than do the commissure-interconnected regions (the trunk, proximal hindlimb and proximal forelimb representations). The sequence of development appears to proceed from a state in which all regions within the primary projection field are commissure-interconnected (Ebner, 1967) to the form (represented by S-I of cat, raccoon, and primate) in which the body regions possessing a high degree of sensory acuity, and positioned remote from the body midline, are represented by cortical areas devoid of interhemispheric connections.

In cat (Jones and Powell, 1968c) and macaque (Jones and Powell, 1969a), S-I projects to both S-I and S-II of the opposite side; on the other hand, S-II projects merely to its opposite counterpart. Within those portions of S-I which possess callosal connections, the interhemisperic connections are discretely organized in that each cytoarchitectural field sends fibres only to the homotypical architectural field of the opposite side. In contrast, all cytoarchitectural areas of S-I project to the opposite S-II in an overlapping fashion.

The normally occurring transfer of a tactile discrimination habit from one hand to the other, which is mediated by the corpus callosum (Stamm and Sperry, 1957; Ebner and Myers, 1962a, b) requires that S-II of the recipient hemisphere, and both S-I and S-II of the transmitting hemisphere be intact (Teitelbaum et al., 1968). However, the transfer in these tasks involves skills executed by distal body regions which lack callosal connections in their somatosensory cortical areas; hence, one must assume that the interhemispheric transfer occurs between cortical regions outside the main sensory areas (cf. Jones and Powell, 1969a).

Electrophysiological and anatomical studies in the squirrel monkey determined the existence of interhemispheric connections from somatic sensory cortex to areas 4 and 6 which traverse the corpus callosum rostrally, presumably as slowly conducting fibers. In addition, there are interhemispheric connections to S-I and to the postcentral dimple of the parietal lobe (Boyd et al., 1971), in violation of the more conventional notion of homotopy of callosal connections (cf. BREMER, 1958).

Within neocortex of cat and macaque, commissural fibers have a laminar distribution in which layer IV and deep layer III are the principal sites of fibre termination (JONES and POWELL, 1969a, 1970a; KAROL and PANDYA, 1971).

8. Afferent Pathways and the Body Representation in S-I

The evidence presented in the preceding sections suggests in final analysis that different afferent fibre tracts, as well as different submodality components of one and the same fibre tract, terminate separately in the somatic area I, preferentially in relation to certain cytoarchitectural subdivisions of the cortex. The Group I afferents, conveyed by a dorsolateral funicular path, project to the rostral border of S-I which is cytoarchitectural area 3a; the cat's spinocervical projection and the quickly adapting cutaneous dorsal column projection favors areas 3 and 1; and the joint and periosteal component of a pathway which ascends outside the dorsal columns forms a second deep modality zone in area 2, at the caudal border of S-I.

The definitive establishment of these relations, and their generality, is complicated by what appear to be marked evolutionary changes in relatively recent phylogeny: this appears most clearly in the case of the commissural connections of S-I, with the commissure-free neocortex being a more recent phylogenetic acquisition. Furthermore, there is the replacement of the spinocervical tract by the direct access line elaborated in primate evolution in the form of the neospinothalamic system.

In spite of evidence for separate pathway termination, modality separation and, possibly, some functional specialization of pathways, there is one overriding principle which dominates the S-I body representation: that is, some coherence in terms of body topography. This leads to the question how the mapping process from body periphery to cortex can be conceptualized, and what the essential aspects of the topographic orderliness in the body representation are. This will be the subject of section I.

9. Projections from the Tongue Nerve

The most anterior part of the body projection to the postcentral gyrus receives bilateral input from each of the three tongue nerves: in the squirrel monkey, the chorda tympani receives afferents from the anterior lip and the sides of the tongue, and also from the posterior tongue near the circumvallate papillae; the lingual tonsillar branch of the IXth nerve, likewise, receives afferent input from two distinct areas of the oral cavity, from the posterior third of the tongue and from the tonsils, palate and fauces; finally, the lingual nerve supplies the anterior tongue and also the floor of the mouth and gums near the midline. Mechanical, thermal and (perhaps with the exception of the lingual nerve) gustatory stimuli elicit the activity in these nerves (BENJAMIN et al., 1968).

In the squirrel monkey and macaque, but not in the rat (BENJAMIN and PFAFFMAN, 1955), cat (PATTON and AMASSIAN, 1952) and dog (SANTIBANEZ et al., 1960), the chorda tympani projects contralaterally to two spatially separated cortical fields within the confines of the intraoral somatotopic projection pattern of the postcentral gyrus: a more rostrally located chorda tympani field overlaps the

IXth nerve projection, and a further posterior chorda tympani field falls within the lingual nerve projection. In contrast, the chorda tympani projects on the ipsilateral side to one continuous field which entirely overlaps with the projection areas of the other two lingual nerves (BENJAMIN et al., 1968). The high degree of tactile discriminatory capacity of the tongue (RINGEL and EWANOWSKI, 1965) which exceeds the two-point discrimination limen of the fingertips, is presumably related to the relatively large expansion of these cortical fields (see also: WOOLSEY and FAIRMAN, 1946).

Ablation of all cortical tongue nerve areas in the somatosensory cortex does not cause retrograde degeneration in the ventral medial thalamic complex which is thought to be the thalamic relay for gustatory activity in the squirrel monkey (BENJAMIN, 1963), but there is retrograde degeneration in the ventrobasal complex which contains neurons responsive to thermal and mechanical stimulation of the tongue (POULOS and BENJAMIN, 1968). This suggests that taste is not represented in the somatosensory projection field.

Retrograde degeneration in the ventromedial complex can, however, be obtained when the anterior opercular-insular cortex is ablated in addition to the cortical tongue nerve field in the somatosensory cortex (BENJAMIN and BURTON, 1968). Therefore, BENJAMIN and BURTON (1968) suggested that the cortical projection from the ventromedial thalamus is of the sustaining type, which is in line with the general notion that most of the thalamic input to insular and opercular cortex in the macaque is of this nature (LOCKE, 1967; ROBERTS and AKERT, 1963). Accordingly, axons from neurons in the ventromedial thalamus would bifurcate and send one branch, each, to opercular-insular and to somatosensory cortex. This leaves at present unresolved why and how the somatosensory and the opercular-insular projection fields could represent a different spectrum of sense modalities: if the neurons of the ventromedial thalamus signal gustatory stimuli, and their axon collaterals terminate in the postcentral somatosensory area, one would also expect some involvement of this latter area in the representation of taste. At least in the primate, there is no evidence for this, but it is clearly established that electric stimulation of taste nerves elicits responses in the opercular-insular region which is, at the same time, unresponsive to mechanical stimulation of the tongue. In the cat, however, neurons were identified in the chorda tympani field of the somatosensory cortex which did respond to gustatory stimuli (COHEN et al., 1957), in some instances with convergence of tactile, thermal and gustatory impulses onto the same neurons (LANDGREN, 1957a).

10. Modality and Afferent Pathways in the S-II Projection

Evoked potential mapping studies identified certain similarities between the S-I and S-II cortical localization patterns: for instance, the postaxial and preaxial arm and leg areas in both S-I and S-II are separated by the representation of the digits; and the cortical areas devoted to the face and the occiput are separated by the projection from the forelimb. On the other hand, a marked difference distinguishes the map of the body in S-I from that in S-II: in the classical mapping experiments, a cortical recording site in S-II was not only activated by stimuli delivered to a particular contralateral body area, as it is in S-I, but also by stimuli to a symmetrical, ipsilateral body region (BENJAMIN and WELKER, 1957; WOOLSEY,

1952). The implication was either that individual neurons in S-II receive afferents from a contralateral peripheral field and its ipsilateral mirror image; or else that the afferents from symmetrical contralateral and ipsilateral peripheral fields project to separate cortical neurons located in close proximity to one another. The experiments of CARRERAS and ANDERSSON (1963) did not support either of these contentions: an extensive analysis of individual neurons in the anterior ectosylvian gyrus of anaesthetized cats did not detect a sufficiently large population of neurons with ipsilateral receptive fields to account for the complete ipsilateral body representation seen in the classical mapping experiments.

To account for this discrepancy, CARRERAS and ANDERSSON (1963) suggested that activity in the ipsilateral projection to S-II may not result in action potentials of cortical neurons, but instead may only evoke non-propagated membrane potential changes which can be detected at the cortical surface. However, as the great majority of S-II neurons in unanaesthetized preparations possess bilateral receptive fields (WHITSEL et al., 1969b), a more likely explanation is that the ipsilateral projection to S-II is considerably more susceptible to blockade by anaesthetic agents than is the contralateral projection. According to this view, therefore, anaesthesia introduces a distortion in the balance between ipsi- and contralateral driving of neurons in S-II.

The neurons of S-II in cats or primates can be categorized into several groups, according to the properties of their receptive fields and the stimulus modality they represent. In unanaesthetized macaques (WHITSEL et al., 1969b) there is a clear delineation of the cortical area commonly designated as S-II into a portion extending several millimeters posterior to the Horsley-Clark coronal plane 0.0, and into a rostral portion (designated as S-II/r by WHITSEL et al., 1969b) extending to the level of the central sulcus. The posterior zone whose rostral border coincides approximately with the cytoarchitectural transition between areas PF and PG of VON BONIN and BAILEY (1949), consists of i) neurons with polysensory modality convergence, ii) neurons responding to nociceptive mechanical stimuli, and iii) neurons with wide cutaneous, often discontinuous, and asymmetrical receptive fields. This population of neurons closely resembles that described by POGGIO and MOUNTCASTLE (1960) in the posterior group of thalamic nuclei. Neurons with these properties were also identified by CARRERAS and ANDERSSON (1963) in S-II of the cat. However, there was no suggestion in their study that these neurons are arranged in a well-localized, restricted, and homogeneous neuronal pool in the cat as they are in the macaque; rather, there was only a gradient of increasing density of polysensory cell columns extending from the rostral limit of S-II to its posterior border.

In the cortical zone anterior to the coronal Horsley-Clarke plane 0.0 (S-II/r), neurons with two types of receptive fields are encountered: large bilateral receptive fields with connections across the body midline, smaller bilateral receptive fields with connections across the body midline, and disjoint bilateral receptive fields symmetrically positioned toward the apices of the extremities. As regards the adequate stimulus, however, there is considerable uniformity: 8 out of 10 neurons, on the average, respond to gentle tactile stimuli when precautions were taken to maintain the stimulus threshold at uniformly low levels. There is a complete absence of joint representation, but in 13% of the S-II/r neurons, WHITSEL et al. (1969b) were unable to decide whether they would exclusively respond to pressure on periosteum or deep fascia, or to cutaneous stimuli of higher intensity. The neurons of this category respond with rapid adaptation to maintained pressure.

In the cat electrophysiological recordings obtained from anaesthetized preparations with various spinal lesions indicate that the dorsal columns, the spinocervical pathway, and the ventral funiculi all convey fibres which ultimately reach S-II. Of these pathways, only the dorsal columns are implicated in afferent inhibition; and both the dorsal columns and the spinocervical tract project to S-II neurons with small receptive fields on the distal portions of the limbs. The ventral funiculi mediate S-II responses which appear with long latency, require strong mechanical stimulation of large receptive fields, and are easily suppressed by anaesthetics (Andersson, 1962). The characteristics of the S-II responses to inputs ascending in the ventral funiculi in the cat resemble those detected by Whitsel et al. (1969b) in the posterior portion of S-II in macaques.

The three different spinal pathways described above reach S-II through at least two thalamic projection systems: in the first place, via the thalamic ventrobasal complex to all of S-II; and in the second place via the posterior group of thalamic nuclei to the posterior part of S-II (Macchi et al., 1959; Guillery et al., 1966; Jones and Powell, 1969b; O'Donoghue et al., 1970; Hand and Morrison, 1970). The latter thalamic nucleus receives in the cat afferent input from the dorsal columns, from the contralateral (and to a lesser extent the ipsilateral) dorsolateral funiculus, and from the ventrolateral quadrant of the cord which includes the spinothalamic tract (Curry, 1971).

The projections from the ventrobasal thalamic complex to S-II are topographically organized (Guillery et al., 1966). The interhemispheric connections of S-II are, in certain respects, similar to those described for S-I: those regions of S-II representing the distal portions of the limbs do not receive nor do they send interhemispheric projections (cf. Jones and Powell, 1969a). In addition to giving rise to interhemispheric projections, S-II also projects to the ventrobasal complex and the posterior nuclear group of the thalamus (DeVito, 1967) as well as to a variety of other cortical areas (cf. Jones, 1969; Jones and Powell, 1969c). The corticofugal influences from somatic cortex to the posterior thalamic nucleus are powerful and are probably mediated by cortico-thalamic fibres (Curry, 1971) which have been demonstrated anatomically (Jones and Powell, 1968b).

There is experimental evidence that the cutaneous S-II field in the cat is surrounded in the depths of the suprasylvian fold by cortex which receives convergent projections from the Group I muscle afferents and joint afferents of the forelimbs, as well as the afferents of the vestibular and cochlear nerve and also from the chorda tympani (Landgren et al., 1967a, b). There is, thus, a suggestion that this cortical field may play a role in the orientation of the body and head towards various stimulus sources. Vestibular afferents project in the macaque to the posterior part of the postcentral gyrus at the base of the intraparietal sulcus between the first and second somatosensory field (Fredrickson et al., 1966). This vestibular projection field is cytoarchitecturally distinct from the neighboring areas 2, 5, 7 and 19. The neurons in this area receive convergent input from the vestibular organ and from one or several joints (Schwarz and Fredrickson, 1971).

Consequently, this specialized cortical area of the macaque may subserve the same function that was postulated for the depth of the suprasylvian fold in the cat.

11. Viscero-sensory Representation

It has been known for some time that the principal sensory fibres from the upper abdominal viscera course with the sympathetic motor nerves, primarily in the splanchnic trunks (see WHITE, 1942). Therefore, stimulation of the splanchnic nerves has been extensively employed to study the cortical representation of visceral sensibility, although there are also several cortical receiving areas for afferent vagal activity (AUBERT and LEGROS, 1970a, b).

The early cortical response typically elicited by single electric shock stimulation of the splanchnic nerve is a brief, initially surface positive wave, limited to a localized region of the contralateral sensory areas I and II (AMASSIAN, 1951a). The latency of the primary response in area I is, in the cat, 8 to 12 msec; that of the response in contralateral area II between 6.7 and 10.5 msec, and thereby intermediate between the latencies from electric stimulation of the ulnar (5 to 6 msec) and the sciatic (10 msec) nerves. Under light anaesthesia, there is also a cortical response evoked in ipsilateral area II, but its amplitude is lower, and its latency slightly longer (10 to 14 msec) than the contralateral area II response (see also: DOWNMAN, 1951). Neurons of cat sensori-motor cortex, responsive to sciatic nerve stimulation, can be conditioned to respond also to splanchnic nerve stimulation (ADAM et al., 1966).

The deeper the anaesthesia, the more clearly is the cortical field of the responses to splanchnic stimulation restricted to the trunk region in the cortical body representations. Under otherwise comparable conditions, the relative magnitudes of evoked potentials in areas I and II differ in a characteristic fashion from species to species: area I responses prevail by far over area II responses in the monkey; on the other hand, area I responses are virtually absent in the rabbit. The cat and the dog occupy an intermediate position (AMASSIAN, 1951a).

The afferent fibres of the splanchnic nerve fall into three classes, namely: $A\beta_1$, $A\beta_2$ and C fibers, corresponding to three elevations in the splanchnic nerve action potential (GERNANDT and ZOTTERMAN, 1946; AMASSIAN, 1951b; LANGHOF and RUBIA, 1969). Of these afferent fibre groups, the $A\beta$ class is responsible for generating the primary cortical responses (AMASSIAN, 1951b). However, this fibre class can itself be differentiated in three subclasses ($A\beta_1$, $A\beta_2$ and $A\beta_3$); each of them making a different contribution to the cortical evoked responses: the contralateral somatic sensory area II appears to receive principally the activity travelling over the fastest component of the A group (i.e. $A\beta_1$ fibres). The cortical response in the ipsilateral area II grows continuously as progressively higher threshold fibres of the $A\beta$ group are excited by the peripheral stimulus; thus, the entire range of $A\beta$ fibres appears to project to this area. Contralateral S-I appears not to be reached by activity in peripheral fibres of the lowest threshold end of the spectrum. Therefore, the fastest fibres of the splanchnic nerve do not seem to affect S-I, in contrast to their conspicuous contribution to the response in S-II (LANGHOF and RUBIA, 1969). This corresponds to DOWNMAN's finding (1951) that the contralateral area II response in cat is more constantly present, and occurs at lower stimulus intensity than the area I response. These and other forms of evidence

(e. g. the short latency of the contralateral S-II response and its relatively large resistance to the depressant effect of anaesthetics) led to the supposition that the large peripheral fibres in the splanchnic nerve posses a powerful synaptic linkage to contralateral S-II. There are, however, substantial species differences in the fiber composition of splanchnic nerve: in the monkey, the number of large myelinated fibers is extremely reduced as compared to cat (Gardner et al., 1955).

The identification of the end organs of the fast and secure visceral afferent projection is incomplete: Pacinian corpuscles certainly contribute, but there is reason to believe that the splanchnic afferent projection may be only partially derived from them (Sheehan, 1932). Bessou and Perl (1966) identified in cat mesenteric nerve small myelinated afferent fibres with 5 to 10 m/sec conduction velocity, which responded to gentle pressure and signaled rate of inflation or deflation of an intestinal balloon; their receptive fields consisted usually of several discrete sensitive points, each point situated in the vicinity of a mesenteric artery branch. This class of afferent fibres appears to function primarily as movement detectors. It is certain that impulses giving rise to painful sensations are also conducted in the splanchnic nerve, for direct stimulation in the human gives rise to pain (Leriche, 1937), and pain sense from the abdominal viscera is abolished by splanchnicectomy (Ray and Neill, 1947). In any case, the $A\gamma\delta$ fibres of splanchnic nerve which are activated by pinching and squeezing of the intestines in the cat (Gernandt and Zotterman, 1946) contribute to the cortical evoked response which, in contralateral S-I appears with a latency of some 30 msec (Langhof and Rubia, 1969; Amassian, 1951a). The fibres are also included in the splanchnic projection to the posterior ventral nucleus of the thalamus (McLeod, 1958).

The visceral afferents do not remain isolated on their pathway to the cortical projection area: activity in somatic afferents elicited, for instance, by a mechanical tap of the skin can markedly reduce the response to subsequent electrical stimulation of the splanchnic nerve. Certain combinations of afferent sources show strong evidence for inhibition in area II: for instance, activity in the dorsal cutaneous branch of the ulnar nerve and in the volar branch of the splanchnic nerve interact very strongly (Amassian, 1952). There is, indeed, some convergence of splanchnic and cutaneous afferent activity on individual neurons of both sensory cortical areas (Newman, 1962). At least some of this convergence occurs at subcortical levels, for McLeod (1958) observed it with neurons in the ventroposterior thalamic nucleus of the cat, and Selzer and Spencer (1969a) found it with neurons in the dorsal horn lamina V of Rexed. In addition to convergence which leads to occlusion, there exists also some reciprocal inhibition between the incoming cutaneous and visceral A fibres (Selzer and Spencer, 1969b). These experimental studies have suggestive implications for the phenomena of "referred pain" and "counter-irritation".

12. Cortical Association Connections of Somatic Sensory Areas

Areas 3, 1 and 2 are interconnected with one another, and also with area 3a, by intracortical association fibres. These connections, together with those passing between S-I and S-II form the *intrinsic* connections, in distinction from those joining S-I and S-II to cortical areas outside the somatic sensory region. This latter class of fibres is regarded as the *extrinsic* connections (Jones and Powell, 1969c).

A characteristic attribute of the intrinsic connections is that they join reciprocally the architectonic subdivisions of S-I within cortical zones which represent identical body areas. JONES and POWELL (1969 a) therefore suggest that the significance of these connections lies in enabling an interaction between cortical cell columns whose afferent input comes from identical body regions, but is segregated into the different cytoarchitectonic divisions according to modality.

Apart from reciprocal connections between the somatic sensory areas and the motor area across the central sulcus, extrinsic cortical connections consist of a local projection from S-I to area 5 and to the supplementary motor area. Area 5, in turn, projects to a second field in the parietal lobe, namely area 7; to the supplementary motor, and to an additional part of area 6 in the frontal lobe. Area 5 and 6 are then interconnected. This basic sequence is then repeated by a local projection from area 7 to the floor of the superior temporal sulcus, and the rostral projection to the upper part of area 46, with the latter returning fibres to area 7 (JONES and POWELL, 1970 b).

In general terms, a chain of projections originating from S-I reaches in successive steps distinct and circumscript areas in both the parieto-temporal and the frontal lobes. At each successive step, the frontal and the parietal-temporal fields are then reciprocally interconnected. The projection areas of somatic sensibility remain in this stepwise progression separated from the pathway of vision and audition (JONES and POWELL, 1970 b; KUYPERS et al., 1965; CRAGG, 1969; PANDYA and KUYPERS, 1969); but the topographic orderliness of the body representation in S-I is not retained beyond the area 5. The overlap in the representation of different body regions in the sequentially following parieto-temporal projection fields may signify the fusion of information from different body regions in preparation for the generation of a total body scheme, but convergence still remains within the somatic sense modality: an example is the neurons in area 5 which respond to rotation of different joints, or to combined cutaneous and joint input (DUFFY and BURCHFIEL, 1971). On the other hand, polysensory interactions of different sense modalities take place in motor cortex (BROOKS et al., 1961 a, b; BUSER and IMBERT, 1961) and in several areas of the frontal lobe (BIGNALL and IMBERT, 1969), some of which appear to be in the vicinity of the frontal projection fields with input from S-I (JONES and POWELL, 1970 b).

I. The Mapping of the Body Topography to Somatic Sensory Cortex

Several essential aspects of the cortical localization pattern in the postcentral gyrus have been firmly established by the numerous studies carried out during the three decades since its discovery by WOOLSEY et al. (1942): in the first place, there is abundant evidence that it is comprised of radial cell columns which extend through all six cortical layers which, in turn, receive afferents of identical submodality from nearly identical peripheral receptive fields (POWELL and MOUNTCASTLE, 1959 b). Secondly, there is evidence that the map of the body in the postcentral gyrus owes its essential topographic properties to the serial and overlapping projection of the dorsal roots (WOOLSEY et al., 1942; CELESIA, 1963). Thirdly, the various types of mechanoreceptive afferents project differentially to the cytoarchitectonic fields which comprise S-I (Powell and Mountcastle, 1959a, b); a process which is foreshadowed by the resorting of afferents according to modality and adaptation properties in the ascending pathways of the spinal cord (see Section H-8). As a result, the full mechanoreceptive modality spectrum within each dorsal root is represented in the postcentral gyrus as a band of cell columns with an anteroposterior orientation. Specifically, afferents from deep receptors of a segment project chiefly to cytoarchitectural areas 2 and 3a; afferents related to the skin chiefly to area 3; with area 1 representing a gradient between the two bordering extremes.

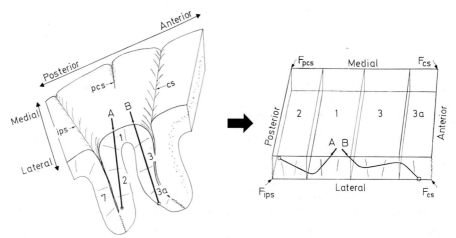

Fig. 5. Two schematic microelectrode penetrations as they would appear in the naturally enfolded cortex of S-I (on the left) and as they would appear if this cortical region were unfolded onto a plane (on the right). The radial lines crossing the cut lateral edge of the cortical mantle indicate the orientation of the cortical cell columns. Penetrations A and B were performed at the same mediolateral level and combine to form a continuous path from the posterior to the anterior extremes of S-I at that level, passing through the cell columns of cytoarchitectural areas 2, 1, 3 and 3a. F = fundus; ips = intraparietal sulcus; pcs = postcentral sulcus; cs = central sulcus. (From Whitsel et al., 1971b)

These findings which were documented in preceding sections sketch the outline of the organizational scheme of the body representation in S-I: i. e., the dorsal roots project in serial order, albeit with appreciable overlap, to the mediolateral dimension of the postcentral gyrus; and the full spectrum of mechanoreceptor afferents from each dorsal root are differentially distributed within cortical bands oriented perpendicular to the mediolateral dimension of the map.

With this general view as a starting point, Werner and Whitsel (1968) and Whitsel et al. (1971b) designed experiments to ascertain (a) whether this scheme of general organization of S-I could be validated in all details; (b) whether some general rules of mapping could be recognized which, if operative in morphogenesis, would generate a body representation of the form encountered in S-I; and, finally, (c) whether such mapping rules would also apply to other body representations in the cortex, notably in somatic sensory area II (Whitsel et al., 1969b).

The experiments by Werner and Whitsel (1968) and Whitsel et al. (1971b) were based on two principal considerations: firstly, the receptive field and modality of a neuron encountered at any depth of a cortical cell column is representative for the receptive field location and modality of all neurons of that same cell column. The second consideration relates to the enfolding of the four cortical cytoarchitectural fields comprising S-I. Fig. 5 schematically illustrates the natural folding of the cortex in that portion of S-I which was studied with microelectrode penetrations. Penetration A is directed down the anterior bank of the intraparietal sulcus and cuts across a continuous sequence of progressively more posterior cell columns belonging initially to area 1 and, subsequently, to area 2. Penetration B, on the other hand, at first traverses the cell columns of the most rostral portion of area 1 and, with further advance, cuts continuously across the cell columns of area 3 and 3a, in that order. The unfolded view of the postcentral gyrus shown on the right of Fig. 5 makes it apparent that upon appropriate reconstruction, a composite of two or more microelectrode penetrations at the same mediolateral level can reveal the detailed sequence of receptive fields represented by the arrangement of cell columns within the entirety of the anteroposterior dimension of S-I.

A composite of the results obtained in the macaque by WERNER and WHITSEL (1968) and WHITSEL et al. (1971b) in a total of 150 microelectrode penetrations in the course of which close to 1500 neurons were characterized with respect to receptive field location and modality, is depicted in Fig. 6.

A characteristic feature of the hindlimb projection, as well as of the entire body representation, is the projection of the dermatomes in their serial order, as indicated by the brackets to the left in the Fig. 6. The sacral dermatomes project medially to the cortex, with the preaxial fringes of these dermatomes occupying the rostral and the caudal borders of their representation; the lumbar dermatomes project further laterally on the cortex with their postaxial fringes occupying the rostral and caudal borders in the map. Within each dermatomal band in the cortical map there is a particular sequence of receptive fields as one traverses that band from medial to lateral: in the cortical region of the sacral dermatomes the receptive fields progress from proximal to distal on the leg; on the other hand, in the cortical dermatomal bands of the segments L-6 and L-5, the receptive fields progress from distal to proximal on the leg.

The position of the foot in the map between post- and preaxial dermatomal projection is in accord with its principal dermatomal affiliation to the dermatome L-7. The receptive fields of the neurons of this latter dermatomal band move from lateral to medial on the foot as one traverses its cortical map from medial to lateral. As a result of this, the totality of all receptive fields represented in any mediolateral traverse of the cortical map describes a continuous spiral path around the limb. This receptive field sequence is most clearly recognizable in the cutaneous portion of the cortical map (i. e. cytoarchitectural area 1 and 3), because of the more precise definition of receptive field location. However, the same sequence appears also rostrally and caudally in the map (i. e. in cytoarchitectural areas 2 and 3a), though less precisely defined because of the deep location of the receptive fields.

This way of looking at the relation between the body and its cortical image is the reverse of the experimental approach: instead of determining the projection from the body to the cortex, WERNER and WHITSEL (1968) based their interpretation on the relation between linear arrays of cortical neurons and the peripheral

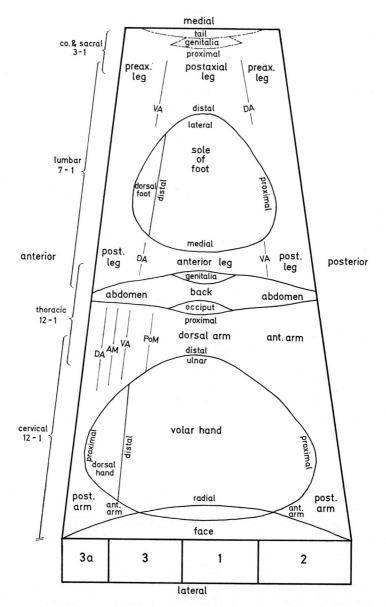

Fig. 6. Schematic unfolded view of the body representation in the postcentral gyrus of *Macaca mulatta*. The labels positioned external to the map (MEDIAL, LATERAL, ANTERIOR and POSTERIOR) indicate the orientation of the map on the cortex. The brackets to the left of the figure identify the serially overlapping anteroposterior regions to which the dorsal roots project. The labels contained within the map designate the body parts represented by the cell columns occupying that cortical location. The overlap of the face and radial hand areas in the central portion of the map (areas 1 and 3) is intended to reflect the disjoint character of the RF's observed at this location. PREAX. = preaxial; POST. = postaxial; ANT. = anterior; DA = dorsoaxial line; VA = ventroaxial line; AM = anterior midline; POM = posterior midline. The numerals (2, 1, 3 and 3a) along the cut lateral edge of the map indicate the cyto-architectural fields which comprise S-I. The lines which subdivide the foot and hand areas

patterns made up from the totality of the receptive fields of these same arrays of cells. The schematic displays of Fig. 7 are predictions of this relation, based on the experimentally determined landmarks of the cortical map. The mediolateral cortical traverse in Fig. 7 (left) corresponds to a hairpin-like peripheral path, crossing the sole of the foot from lateral to medial; another cortical traverse is seen to involve receptive fields from sole and dorsum of foot, in that sequence (Fig. 7 right). These and all other peripheral paths which correspond to mediolateral cortical traverses have in common that they progress on the leg from proximal to distal, traverse the foot from lateral to medial, and ascend the limb from distal to proximal.

A common characteristic of penetrations which traverse the hindlimb area in the rostro-caudal direction is that the sequence of consecutive receptive fields describe circular paths around the limb: for instance, in a region of the cortical map situated lateral to the foot representation, the cell columns of cytoarchitectural area 2 represent receptive fields at the postaxial leg; moving further anteriorly towards the central sulcus, the receptive fields cross the ventro-axial line, occupy the anterior leg and finally shift continuously to the hindlimb's posterodorsal surface; in this traverse, the modality distribution changes towards an increase in the representation of deep receptors as areas 3 and 3a are approached.

The largest contribution to the foot representation is made by the sole, with the lateral edge coming to lie in juxtaposition to the postaxial leg. In the posteroanterior extent of the map, each toe is traversed on the plantar surface in the direction from proximal to its tip as one advances in the map from posterior to anterior; finally, upon reaching cytoarchitectural area 3 and 3a, the dorsal surface of that same toe is reached.

The middle portion of the back region of the trunk projects mainly to area 1; rostrally as well as caudally in the map, the receptive fields shift progressively towards the abdomen.

The arm is represented immediately lateral to the trunk. The progression of receptive field locations along the electrode tracks define a topographic organization of the arm representation which is analogous to that of the hindlimb: the receptive fields shift along the long axis of the forelimb from proximal to distal when the electrode advanced from medial to lateral in the cortex. When the different cytoarchitectural areas are traversed the receptive fields progress around the circumference of the arm: the anterior area 1 accommodates the quickly adapting cutaneous submodalities from the posterior surface of the arm, and areas 3 and 3a accommodate the ventral, anterior, dorsal and, again, the posterior aspects of the arm in that order, with a gradually increasing preference for the deep submodalities.

Penetrations directed through a wide band of the posterior bank of the central sulcus lateral to the forelimb representation encounter neurons with receptive

---

overlie those cell columns which represent the very tips of the digits. If the map were refolded to the configuration of the postcentral gyrus, its anterior edge would lie at the fundus of the central sulcus (areas 3a and 3 comprise the anterior wall of the gyrus); and its posterior edge would occupy the fundus of the intraparietal sulcus laterally and the postcentral sulcus medially. (From WHITSEL et al., 1971b)

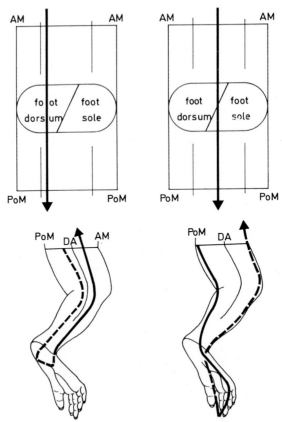

Fig. 7. Schematic display of two medio-lateral traverses through the hindlimb portion of the somatic sensory area I. The figures at the bottom show the paths on the body, consisting of the totality of receptive fields which one would encounter in microelectrode penetrations that cross the cortical map in the manner indicated in the figures at the top. The dotted portion of the path in the periphery traverses body regions which cannot be seen in the view presented.
AM = anterior midline; PoM = posterior midline; DA = dorso-axial line

fields on the hand: the ulnar hand is represented medially within the cortex of the gyral crown and the radial hand laterally. Penetrations which traverse the anterior portion of the gyral crown and the anterior wall of the postcentral gyrus without interruption reveal further details of the representation. As regards the digits, such penetrations present the following characteristics: superficially in anterior area 1 the neurons possess receptive fields located on the volar surface of a digit; and with electrode advance to and through area 3 the receptive fields shift continuously to the dorsum of that same digit. With even further advance through area 3 and into 3a receptive fields shift proximally on the dorsum of the same digit and may even extend to reach the distal forearm itself. In general, therefore, it is as if the hand were cut along its proximal, medial and lateral borders, unfolded with the finger-tips serving as a hinge, and laid out flat on the posterior bank of the central sulcus. In the process, the volar surface becomes superimposed upon areas 1 and superficial 3, and the dorsum upon the deep portion of area 3 as well as area 3a.

In the posterior continuation of hand and arm representations from area 1 into area 2, there appears anterior arm medially, and posterior arm laterally to the hand field. Accordingly, posterior area 1 and area 2 contain a "split" representation of the arm: i. e., the arm is represented by cell columns situated both medial and lateral to the hand representation. In this respect, the hand and arm representations of both the anterior and posterior walls of the postcentral gyrus are alike, except that (a) the posterior arm representation is more extensive and predominantly of the deep modality, and (b) the posterior hand representation consists primarily of neurons with receptive fields on the proximal volar surface of the hand. Within the cortical bands located medial and lateral to the hand representation, the receptive fields spiral around the circumference of the arm as one traverses the cortex from anterior to posterior in the course of crossing from area 1 to area 2.

The receptive fields of neurons in the posterior bank of the central sulcus at the junction of the radial hand and face representation present unusual features: these neurons of areas 3 and 3a possess large receptive fields in some instances extending continuously from the distoradial hand over the arm to the lateral aspect of head and face (WHITSEL et al., 1971b). In contrast, the cortex of the anterior gyral crown at this mediolateral level is characterized by a complete lack of neurons with receptive fields on the arm. Instead, neurons in the transition zone between hand and face in area 1 possess disjoint receptive fields: i. e., the receptive fields of the neurons in this region mapped a discrete locus on the radial hand as well as a locus on the lateral aspect of the head or face.

A schematic overview over these details of the body representation brings several general aspects into focus: one essential ingredient of the map is the fact that each dorsal root projects to an anteroposterior band of cell columns extending across all the cytoarchitectural areas comprising S-I (see brackets to the left of Fig. 6). Within each anteroposterior band, there is a characteristic sequence of receptive fields as one traverses that band from medial to lateral: e. g., within the foot and hand areas the receptive fields progress from lateral to medial: and within the trunk area they progress from caudal to rostral. The direction of receptive field progression within those bands representing the axial portions of the fore- and hindlimbs depends upon the cortical position of that band: i. e., if it lies medial to the hand or the foot representation the receptive field progression is from proximal to distal; but if it lies lateral the receptive fields shift from distal to proximal on the limb. As a result of this internal organization of the anteroposterior bands devoted to various body parts, the totality of all receptive fields represented by a continuous mediolateral array of cell columns describes a continuous trajectory on the body. Starting with the tip of the tail, it progresses from proximal to distal on the hindlimb, crosses the foot from lateral to medial, advances from distal to proximal on the hindlimb, ascends the trunk from caudal to rostral, proceeds from proximal to distal on the forelimb, crosses from the ulnar to the radial hand, and finally, ascends the forelimb to reach the face (Fig. 8).

A comparison of this organization of the cortical map with the arrangement of primary afferent fibres in the dorsal columns of the spinal cord led to the following concept of the mapping process: shortly after entry into the dorsal columns the ascending collaterals of the fibres in each dorsal root are arranged in a fibre lamina with a dorsomedial to ventrolateral orientation in the columns. Within

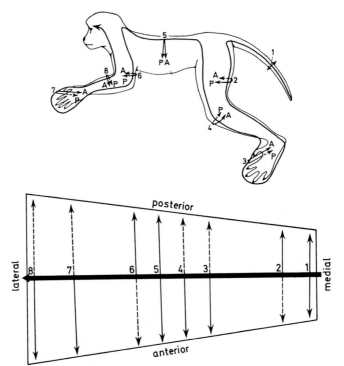

Fig. 8. The local neighborhood relations of the S-I MAP. The labels located external to the map indicate its orientation on the cortex. The heavy uninterrupted arrow which crosses the map corresponds to a continuous mediolateral array of cell columns which (a) extends across the entirety of S-I, and (b) maps the sequence of body regions encountered along the heavy arrow drawn upon the figurine displayed at the top. The narrow arrows drawn orthogonal to the heavy arrow in the lower portion of the figure correspond to linear arrays of neurons aligned in the anteroposterior dimension of S-I. The interrupted portions of these narrow arrows correspond to those parts of the body surface hidden from the view illustrated at the top; and indicate the cortical cell columns which represent those same regions. The labels at the extremes of the peripheral paths drawn orthogonal to the heavy arrow indicate the body regions encountered as one moves in the anteroposterior dimension of the S-I map. A = anterior in S-I; P = posterior in S-I. (From Whitsel et al., 1971b)

each segmental lamina thus formed, the fibres are characteristically ordered: this is demonstrated by the fact that a recording microelectrode which advances perpendicular to the long axis of the lamina encounters a sequence of fibres whose receptive fields describe a continuous path on the body (the "dermatomal trajectory" of Werner and Whitsel, 1967). Furthermore, each time the tip of the electrode crosses a boundary between consecutive segmental fibre laminae in the lumbar dorsal columns, there occurs an abrupt jump in the receptive field location which backtracks part of the peripheral path mapped in the preceding lamina, reflecting the overlap in the peripheral segmental innervation (Werner and Whitsel, 1967). As the dorsal column fibres ascend from lumbar to cervical levels, a significant change occurs, apart from the separation of submodalities: i. e., the fibres of consecutive dermatomes rearrange to the extent that an electrode advancing through the cervical fasciculus gracilis encounters a sequence of fibres whose receptive fields form a smooth and continuous path on the body periphery. The conclusion is, therefore, that the fragmentation of the body representation at the dorsal root entry zone is undone by resorting of fibres (WHITSEL et al., 1971 a). Generally speaking, the mapping principle appears to consist of the arrangement of primary afferents to "subassemblies" (the dermatomal trajectories), which then function as the elementary units of the mapping process (WERNER, 1972). The orderly recombination of these trajectories, evident already at the upper lumbar level of the spinal cord, insures that certain paths on the body periphery (namely, those formed by a succession of aligned dermatomal trajectories) map as a continuous receptive field sequence on the cortex. Moreover, in this conceptualization, the mapping of the body upon the cortex represents the family of these paths rather than the body topography as such; a circumstance which suggested a topological interpretation of the mapping process (WERNER, 1970).

While this interpretation accounts for the general features of the mapping process, there is one departure from the general rule which is possibly attributable to the behavioral specialization of the body region concerned: the region of the postcentral gyral crown in Ateles which maps the radial hand in apposition to the lateral aspect of the head has been cited as evidence for a discontinuity in the S-I cortical localization pattern (PUBOLS and PUBOLS, 1971) on the basis that this region lacks an intervening representation of the arm, at least as far as could be ascertained in records from neuron clusters. In the macaque, there is now evidence from microelectrode studies that continuity is preserved, albeit in an unusual manner: the receptive fields of neurons in the cell columns between the radial hand and the lateral head area encompass both body regions at the same time, either by neurons with very large receptive fields extending continuously from hand to face, or by neurons with disjoint receptive field components on hand and face.

A comparison between forelimb and hindlimb projection patterns provides a clue for the nature of the regional specialization of the hand-face area in S-I (WHITSEL et al., 1971 b). In the hindlimb area, the localization pattern is determined by a) the segmentation of primary afferents into dorsal roots; b) the highly structured overlap in the cortical projection of the consecutive dermatomes; and c) the relative density of the afferents from different body regions: hence, the "split" representation of the hindlimb in which the foot projection separates the leg representation into a medial and a lateral band in S-I. The same general principle of a "split" representation appears also in the forelimb area of the map, except that the afferents from hand and head apparently came to outnumber those from the arm by far, as a result of increasing behavioral specialization. As a consequence, there is competition for occupancy of available cortical cell columns, with an increasing tendency for face and hand afferents to occupy "arm" cell columns. In this process, a solution evolves which enables expansion of hand and face representation and, at the same time, insures continuity in the map: cell columns come to receive afferents from both hand and face at the same time.

On the basis of these considerations WHITSEL et al. (1971 b) suggested that "selective growth pressure" associated with functional differentiation in the periphery can introduce regional departures from one of the rules of mapping between body and cortex: for in these parts of the cortical map, the local neighborhood relations are no longer a continuous transformation of the fibre arrangement in the dorsal columns. Nevertheless, it appears that the mapping process tends to retain the connectivity of body regions along the path that traverses the entire longitudinal body extent, shown in Fig. 8.

1. Dermatomal Overlap in the Somatosensory Area I

Maps of electrical potentials evoked in the somatosensory area I by electrical stimulation of dorsal roots clearly prove that dermatomes project in an overlapping manner, and that this overlap extends over several neighboring segments (Celesia, 1963). In addition, the studies of Werner and Whitsel (1968) and of Whitsel et al. (1971 b) show that the receptive field sequence of neurons in this mediolateral direction of the cortex traces an essentially continuous path on the body. To make this possible, dermatomal overlap must be of a high degree of order: the suggestion is that the dermatomes overlap in the cortical projection as is indicated schematically in Fig. 9: the afferents from the dermatomal trajectories in each loop around the limb assemble according to the body region of origin, and thereby map each loop as a linear array of neurons, oriented from medial to lateral on the cortex. Thus, in the projection from the periphery to the cortex, the body is first segmented into a series of overlapping dermatomes whereby the afferents from each dermatome retain a specific order; namely, that of the dermatomal trajectories. In the projection of the cortex, the trajectories from consecutive dermatomes superimpose partially with the result that they map a continuous path on the body. It appears that the body and the cortical map can both be considered a composite of dermatomal trajectories; and that each dermatomal trajectory is treated in the projection as a unit, and maps as a whole. Accordingly, while the map itself is somatotopic in the sense that afferents from different dermatomes can converge to identical points in the map (cf. Pubols and Pubols, 1969), it is dermatomal by virtue of the mapping process which generates it.

2. Topology of the Somatosensory Projection to S-I

The geometrical properties of the two-dimensional cortical body map appear quite different from those of the three-dimensional body. This is for several reasons: first, cutaneous and deep receptors project onto one common plane; therefore, the projection from the skin does not appear in the cortical map as a continuous boundary enclosing the deep structures, as it does in the body of our perceptual experience. A second reason for this difference is that relations of proximity and distance between points on the body do not consistently remain preserved in the cortical map: for instance, receptive fields on the heel of the foot and on the dorsum of the ankle are closely adjacent or contiguous on the body, but they map to the far ends of the anterior and posterior edges, respectively, of the cortical projection of the dermatome L-7. Moreover, one and the same place on the body will, in general, have several representations in the cortical map: particularly when its afferents are part of trajectories of different dermatomes which project to the cortex sufficiently far apart. Such multiple representations were, indeed, observed by Woolsey et al. (1942) with evoked cortical potentials, and by Werner and Whitsel (1968) and Whitsel et al. (1971 b) with microelectrode penetrations.

These apparent discrepancies between geometrical properties of the body and its map preclude a simple correspondence between the two, at least in the frame-

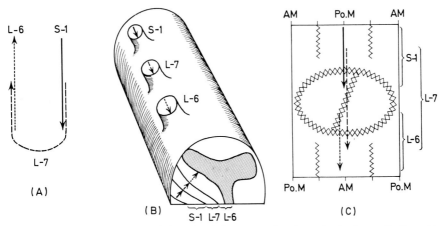

Fig. 9. A schematic illustration of the role of dermatomal trajectories in the medial lemniscal projection. (A) represents a hairpin-like path around the hindlimb. The path consists of receptive fields which project to three different spinal cord segments. Each dermatome is marked by a different shading of its contribution to the peripheral path. In (B) the afferents from the three dermatomes are shown to retain their sequential fibre order which is indicated by arrows in the cross-sections through the dorsal roots near their entry zone, and through the corresponding fibre laminae in the posterior funiculi. (C) shows, schematically, how the dermatomal trajectories combine in the cortical projection to a continuous and linear representation of the path of part (A) around the hindlimb; AM = anterior midline, PoM = posterior midline

work of ordinary spatial intuition which is based on the metric structure of space, i. e., on relations of proximity and distance of points. However, for the purpose of examining the mapping of one space to another, it is possible to conceive of spaces with different and more general properties than that of possessing a metric. It is then merely necessary that both the object space and the image space consist of sets of elements, and that the sets in the two spaces correspond to one another, one by one (WERNER, 1970).

The considerations of the previous section suggest that the dermatomal trajectories are the sets of elements that satisfy this requirement, for both the body and the cortical map can be shown to be a composite of dermatomal trajectories, with each trajectory mapping as a whole.

In the framework of topology, WERNER and WHITSEL (1968) proposed to interpret the body as an aggregate of receptive fields which combine to ordered sets in the form of the dermatomal trajectories. Similarly, the cortical map is considered as an aggregate of neurons, which also combine to ordered sets, each set receiving afferents from one dermatomal trajectory. When object and image space are conceptualized in this way, body and cortical map are topologically equivalent, for each set of elements in the periphery corresponds to one set of elements in the cortex, and vice versa. As a consequence, the neighborhood of two receptive fields in the periphery is always preserved in the projection when these receptive fields are adjacent members of one trajectory; but two adjacent peripheral receptive fields which do not belong to the same trajectory need not be neighbours in the cortical map.

43*

3. Mapping of Body Surface in S-II/r

In S-II/r each neuron maps a contralateral peripheral field as well as its ipsi-lateral mirror image: for the small receptive fields at the apices of the extremities the matching ipsi- and contralateral fields are disjoint, whereas the large symme-trical fields near the body axis are joined across the body midline.

In the mapping of the body surface upon the cortex, two geometric transforma-tions occur: the surface of the two body halves superimpose, with the craniocaudal axis of the body as the axis of symmetry; and the contiguity of body regions becomes disjoint in two places in the map, for the body surface appears in the cortical map laid out as in S-I (see Fig. 8). The longitudinal path along the body, shown in this figure, traces the body regions in the sequence in which they adjoin each other in S-II/r, which is also the same sequence as in S-I: starting with the face, descending the anterior chest to the dorsum of the forearm, looping around the hand, ascending to occiput, linking the latter via the trunk with a loop around the hindlimb, and terminating in the tail. The conclusion is that, with respect to this path along the body surface, cortical map and body space are of equal connectivity, i. e., adjacent body regions along the path are also adjacent in the cortical map.

The sequence of body regions along this path in the cortical map of S-II/r is that of the spinal cord segments to which the afferents from these body regions project. Accordingly, the connectivity and neighborhood relations in the cortical map are determined by the peripheral segmental innervation. As in the cortical map of S-I, dermatomal overlap in the cortical projection to S-II is extensive but somatotopically organized (Whitsel et al., 1969b).

4. Is There a Common Principle in Somatosensory Mapping?

The experimental results reviewed in the preceding sections ascribed a specific connotation to the general idea of "topographic orderliness" of cortical represen-tation: in the first place, this orderliness reflects in S-I the fact that the net shift of receptive fields along linear arrays of cortical cell columns traces a continuous path on the body; and, secondly, it is as if, for the purpose of mapping, the body periphery were decomposed into more or less narrow linear bands; and as if the afferents from these same bands assembled again in the cortical receiving areas to terminate on corresponding linear arrays of cell columns. It is now established that the projection to the second somatic area (Woolsey, 1943; Woolsey and Fairman, 1946) follows the same rules of mapping, except for the deletion of the "deep" submodality, and for introducing the bilateral symmetry of the cutaneous representation (Whitsel et al., 1969b).

In the projection to the first and second somatic sensory areas, certain neigh-borhood relations are rigorously preserved: they are reflected by the longitudinal path along the body, depicted in Fig. 8. Except for one area in the cortical map in S-I (namely the hand-face junction), this is also the order in which the ascending afferents within each segment arrange to form "dermatomal trajectories", and in which these trajectories combine to produce a continuous body representation (see Fig. 9). It is as if each afferent possessed some label signaling its position along the path in Fig. 8; and as if this label determined the place of that afferent along the mediolateral dimension of the cortical map. The place of projection of that afferent in the rostro-caudal dimension of the cortical map is then determined by modality, by the pathway the afferent courses, and by the cytoarchitectural area of termination. The important point is that the mapping process is topological in the sense of preserving the connectivity of the body along the longitudinal path depicted in Fig. 8, without regard to metric relations on the body itself. As a consequence, one and the same body area may appear in the map several times in disjoint locations, each time in a different context of adjacent body regions (WERNER et al., 1971).

Another implication of this mapping process is that the receptive fields at rostral and caudal borders of the cortical map approach the same regions on the body (albeit in S-I with some differences in the modality distribution). Thus, the cortical map is in some sense continuous: as a hypothetical observer capable of "reading" the receptive field labels of neurons moves within the cortical map at one medio-lateral coordinate towards one border, he "sees" the same body regions as he does on the opposite border. At least within certain regions, this imparts to the map the property of a non-orientable surface, in the topological sense. The suggestion has been made that the tactile-kinaesthetic representation in one common map which lacks boundaries (i.e., is non-orientable) is the mechanism by which the central nervous system combines contactual information about objects in space external to the body, and of geometric information from within the body into *one* common space, suited to reflect haptic stimulus information (WERNER, 1970).

J. Stimulus Coding in the Somatosensory Cortex

In the attempts to recognize in neural activity the features which represent the properties of stimuli, several experimental approaches in neurophysiology have been found informative: on the one hand, electrical responses in populations of neurons recorded as evoked potentials can be taken as indicative of location and magnitude of a neural response to a stimulus. On the other hand, the stimulus response of individual neurons can be observed with microelectrodes. In this case, it is possible to analyze the neural response in terms of a mean discharge rate and, in addition, in terms of variability and sequential ordering of the neuron discharges since these aspects of the neural activity might bear some relation to particular stimulus attributes. Evoked surface potentials and single neuron discharges need not necessarily reflect the same aspect of stimuli, or be an equivalent quantitative measure of stimulus magnitudes, for they are two different kinds of neural event which are not under all circumstances correlated with one another: namely, summated postsynaptic potentials on the one hand, and propagated spike discharges on the other.

This line of inquiry parallels essentially the traditional approach of the psychophysicist, except that the latter tried to correlate stimulus values with sensation magnitudes, while the neurophysiologist correlates stimulus values with differences in the neuronal responses: a distinct stimulus attribute with well defined physical properties is selected, and the magnitude of this stimulus attribute varied over a range of values. For instance, in the case of tactile stimuli restricted to a point of the skin, the displacement of the skin (measured in units of length), or the frequency of vibration may constitute suitable scales for the quantitative characterization of the stimulus. The next step is to measure the stimulus-evoked neural activity, and to seek a correspondence between the stimuli of different values on their measurement scale, and the neural responses they evoke.

This raises a source of considerable complexity. The questions are: What is an appropriate way to "measure" neural activity? And, what is a suitable rule to assign numerical values to neural activity, such that differences in "magnitude" of neural activity can be represented as relations of "greater" and "smaller" and, under more exacting conditions, as numerical differences on a continuous and monotonic scale?

In the absence of a suitable conceptual framework to guide in the selection of an appropriate scale for measuring neural activity, the procedure is purely experimental and pragmatic. It is necessary to vary the stimulus, to "measure" the neural activity in several ways, and to establish which scale of neural activity measurement makes the functional relation between stimulus and magnitude of the neural response correspond with the relation between the stimulus and a psychophysical measurement of sensation.

The ultimate goal is to find a particular way for characterizing neural responses in quantitative terms (i. e.: a scale to measure neural responses) such that the functional relation between stimulus and neural response is of the same form as the relation of stimulus to "sensation", measured in an independent psychophysical or behavioral experiment. It can then be said that this particular functional relation between stimulus and neural response qualifies as the "neural code" of the stimulus attribute under study (cf. WERNER, 1971).

1. Evoked Potential Studies of Somatic Stimulus-Intensity Functions

The evaluation of cortical evoked potentials in terms of quantitative relations to stimulus intensity was largely dependent on the development of suitable automatic averaging techniques (DAWSON, 1954), enabling a statistically valid measurement of the specific, stimulus evoked potential, separated from incidental potential fluctuations unrelated to the stimulus. SHAGASS and SCHWARTZ (1961, 1963) and UTTAL and COOK (1962) applied this method to record extra-cranial somatic evoked responses to percutaneous electrical stimulation of peripheral nerves. In the latter study, the cortical response to single stimuli was composed of three distinct potential deflections: two positive deflections of latency and amplitude varying widely from subject to subject; followed by a long, negative-positive wave. Although the subjects could grade the stimuli in psychophysical measurements over a large range of intensities, there was only a surprisingly narrow range over which the cortical potential deflection varied monotonically with increasing stimuli: at psychophysical threshold, amplitudes of the cortical responses were already over half of their maximum, and full amplitude was attained well below the stimuli which elicited maximal subjective sensation. Thus, the dynamic range of the cortical potential was much narrower than that of the sensation estimates.

Careful selection of the appropriate electrode location on the human scalp (GOFF et al., 1962) and randomization of stimulus intensities in each recording session (ALLISON, 1962) enabled a finer resolution of the average evoked responses into, essentially, five distinct components of which the fifth is often separated into two positive deflections, labeled 5a and 5b; is more widely distributed over the scalp; and also appears ipsilateral to the site of stimulation (ROSNER and GOFF, 1967). When the amplitude of the evoked potential components 4, 5A and 5B was plotted as function of the stimulus intensity on logarithmic scales, there was a discontinuity in the slope at about four times the threshold stimulus strengths. The data points fitted best a power function relationship: the low intensity part of the curve with an exponent between 0.8 and 1.5; at the high intensity part with an exponent of 0.1 to 0.2. The important point of this quantitative relation is that it matches relatively closely that between stimulus intensity and subjective magnitude estimation of the sensation elicited by the same stimuli. The earlier components in the evoked cortical response (i. e.: deflections 1 and 2 of ROSNER et al., 1963), possibly reflecting activity in thalamo-cortical afferents and early cortical postsynaptic activity in the specific somatic projection area, reach maximal amplitudes at low stimulus intensity, as did the responses evaluated by UTTAL and COOK (1962).

These considerations have important implications: they would suggest that the cortical site of the specific, topographically organized somatic pathway do not mediate the entire range of the subjective, psychophysical intensity function. Instead, this seems to be the role of the more widely distributed neural system which supports the late potential deflections with extensions to the ipsilateral cortex. There is also the possibility that the early potential waves with saturation of amplitude and low stimulus intensity are more concerned with representing the place of the peripheral stimulus, as distinct from its intensity which is more accurately reflected in the later potential waves (cf. ROSNER and GOFF, 1967).

Vibratory stimuli have also been employed in studies of the cortical evoked potential: typically, the first positive deflection appears some 70 msec after stimulus onset in synchrony with the stimulus, but its amplitude does not correlate with stimulus intensity. On the other hand, the magnitude of a subsequent negative deflection is a power function of stimulus intensity (KEIDEL, 1968).

To assess the relation between magnitude of evoked potentials and perceived stimulus intensity, FRANZEN and OFFENLOCH (1969) compared the former with the latter in human subjects under identical test conditions: perceived stimulus intensity was determined by the method of magnitude estimation (STEVENS, 1957); and the electrical responses were recorded from the scalp, and measured as the difference between the largest positive and negative deflections in each response. The psychophysical as well as the neuroelectric responses are both power functions of stimulus intensity (i. e.: skin indentation at the volar surface of digits) with nearly the same exponent (FRANZEN, 1970). Also, when vibratory stimuli of 300 cycles/sec frequency and varying amplitude were applied, there was close correspondence between the neurophysiologically and psychophysically determined power functions (FRANZEN, 1969). Simultaneous stimulation of two or more neighboring areas on the skin is reflected by an increase of apparent stimulus intensity and evoked electrical response; this increase amounts to a factor of $\sqrt{2}$ or $\sqrt{3}$, respectively, depending on the number of skin regions stimulated simultaneously. In formal, mathematical terms, it is as if the responses to the simultaneously applied stimuli were composed of a linear vector sum of the responses to each stimulus in isolation.

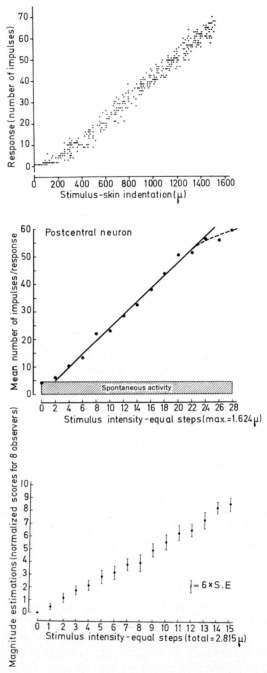

Fig. 10. Top: the linear stimulus-response relation for a slowly adapting myelinated mechanoreceptive fibre innervating the glabrous skin of the monkey's hand. Stimuli were step indentations of the skin of 600 msec duration; and delivered in random order as regards intensity at a
repetition rate of 12 per min. The stimulator tip was 2 mm in diameter, machined to a one-
third spherical surface. The number of impulses evoked by each indentation is plotted as a

Records of evoked potentials from the scalp fail to detect sharply localized cortical responses of low amplitude (GEISLER and GERSTEIN, 1961). Placement of the recording electrode subdurally, directly on the pia-arachnoid surface of the postcentral gyrus, enabled LIBET et al. (1967) to extend the range of cortical evoked potential studies to stimuli which were below threshold for sensation although still eliciting a cortical electrical response. Such electrical responses were deficient in late components. The suggestion, therefore, is: a) that evoked potentials in somato-sensory cortex of awake and attentive subjects can occur in the absence of subjective sensation; and b) that the appearance of late components of the evoked potential seems to be at least of equal, and possibly of greater importance for conscious processes than the primary response itself (LIBET, 1965a, b).

Correlations of this kind between electrical responses and subjective sensation magnitudes are of considerable significance for the understanding of neural events in sensation, although they do not penetrate into the finer subtleties of the information transactions in which the somatic sensory cortex may be involved. A program of research initiated by MOUNTCASTLE and coworkers (MOUNTCASTLE et al., 1963, 1966; WERNER and MOUNTCASTLE, 1965, 1968; MOUNTCASTLE, 1967) has shown that an approach of some heuristic and explanatory value is to compare measures of the human sensory performance when dealing with certain kinds of natural stimuli, with the neural events elicited by those same stimuli in the somatic afferent system of monkeys. These investigations documented examples of the neural representation of the intensity attribute of stimuli which did not require more than measuring the mean rate of discharges, or the average number of responses of individual neural elements to obtain a correspondence between neural and psychophysical stimulus-response relationships. Thus, depending on the test situation, mean discharge rate and average response numbers can be considered to be a neural code for stimulus intensity, at least at the levels of the mechanoreceptive afferent pathways at which these measurements were taken.

The slowly adapting mechanoreceptive afferents which probably originate in the expanded tip endings at the base of the intermediate dermal ridges in glabrous skin, are exquisitely sensitive to skin indentation. The relation between skin displacement by a stimulator probe and the mean discharge rate of the primary afferent fibres is linear over a wide stimulus range (MOUNTCASTLE et al., 1966): thus, the initial transfer from mechanical deformation of the skin to a neural code in the first order afferents is linear. Comparable experiments carried out with

---

function of the intensity of that stimulus. (From MOUNTCASTLE et al., 1966). Middle: the stimulus-response relation of a mechanoreceptive neuron in the postcentral gyrus of the unanaesthetized monkey. The receptive field of this neuron was located on the palmer skin of the contralateral hand. The experimental design was similar to that described above. The curved, dotted line at the top right of the figure indicates that for this, as for many postcentral neurons, the linear stimulus-response function tends to saturate when very strong stimuli are employed. (From MOUNTCASTLE and DARIAN-SMITH, 1968). Bottom: the results of a psychophysical experiment in human beings in which the subject is asked to rate stimuli numerically along an intensive continuum. The stimulator employed and the experimental design were identical to those of the experiments illustrated in the top and middle figures. The points represent means for eight healthy young adults after normalization of individual subjective scales. (From MOUNTCASTLE and DARIAN-SMITH, 1968)

neurons of the postcentral gyrus of unanaesthetized monkeys, also yielded a linear relation between skin indentation and neuronal mean discharge rate (MOUNTCASTLE and DARIAN-SMITH, 1968): hence, the conclusion that the impulse transmission across the intervening nuclear relays and the activation of cortical neurons in S-I imposes at most a linear, if any, transformation on the first-order input, as regards stimulus intensity. Even more significantly, psychophysical measurements in man, employing the same stimuli used in the experiments with monkeys, also establish a linear relation between stimulus intensity and sensation magnitude estimates. The implication is that the stimulus-response relation of the subjective experience for cutaneous sensory stimuli is set by the transfer properties of the peripheral receptors themselves (Fig. 10) (MOUNTCASTLE, 1967; MOUNT-CASTLE and DARIAN-SMITH, 1968).

A more complex relation between stimuli and cortical neural responses became apparent in the investigations of MOUNTCASTLE et al. (1969) on the cutaneous sense of flutter vibration. The conclusion of these studies was that the perception of regular oscillatory movements of the skin depends upon the appearance of periodic trains of nerve impulses in primary afferent nerve fibres, with the periodicity in the impulse train reflecting the stimulus frequency. Two classes of afferent fibres can be distinguished: those originating from the glabrous skin and most sensitive to frequencies of 5 to 40 cycles/second, and those originating from deep cutaneous tissue, and responding in a frequency range of 60 to 300 cycles/second (TALBOT et al., 1968).

In the projection to the somatosensory area I of the postcentral gyrus, the two classes of afferents remain essentially distinct, and activate different cortical neurons. One class of quickly adapting cortical neurons follows readily the sinusoidal mechanical stimulus of the skin over a frequency range of 5 to 80 cycles/seconds, with a periodic recurrence of impulses at intervals close to the cycle length of the vibratory stimulus. Thus, information on stimulus frequency remains preserved in the form of the temporal discharge pattern of these cortical neurons. This suggests that the capability of discriminating frequencies of vibratory stimuli in behavioral and psychophysical tests may be attributable to a central neural mechanism which can detect differences between the period lengths in impulse trains of this class of neurons.

The situation is different with another class of cortical neurons which receives its afferent input from the Pacinian corpuscles located in the deeper cutaneous layers. Vibratory stimuli of 80 to 400 cycles/seconds frequency, which entrain periodic discharges in the afferents originating from Pacinian corpuscles are reflected merely by an increase of discharge rates in these cortical neurons. But there is no relation between the magnitude of the increase in firing rate and the stimulus frequency, nor is there any periodicity in the discharges which would reflect the stimulus frequency. Yet, the human observer is capable of discriminating between different frequencies of vibratory stimuli, irrespective of whether the stimuli engage, according to their frequency, the quickly adapting system of afferents from the glabrous skin, or the Pacinian elements.

The general implication is that a certain stimulus attribute which, by virtue of the choice of the selected physical measure (e. g. frequency, as in the case under consideration) can be represented on a continuous and monotonic scale, need not

Unit : 69-6-B
Bin width : 50 msec

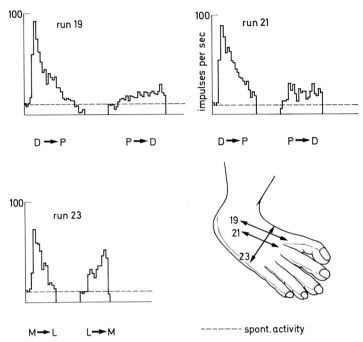

Fig. 11. The response of a neuron located in S-I (lamina V, cytoarchitectural area 1) of an unanaesthetized macaque to movement of a fine brush across the dorsum of the contralateral foot. The stimulus was delivered by a mechanical stimulator which permitted precise replication of the velocity and position of the moving brush. The bargraphs illustrate the neural response elicited when the brush traversed the receptive field at the three different orientations shown on the figurine in the lower right: the height of a vertical bar in these displays represents the number of discharges in a 50 msec bin during the stimulus motion, averaged over 25 consecutive and identical stimuli, and expressed as discharges per second. The stimuli moved at a constant velocity of 55 mm per sec. The spontaneous activity of the neuron was 11 impulses per sec and is indicated by the dotted line in each bargraph. The arrows below each bargraph designate the direction of stimulus movement: P → D = proximal-to-distal; M → L = medial-to-lateral; etc. (From WERNER et al., 1972)

be processed by the nervous system in an equally continuous and homogeneous fashion. Instead, different ranges of a particular attribute may be represented by the nervous system by means of entirely different kinds of codes. In the extreme, a mode of neural representation may be adopted which is entirely unlike the scales of sensory experiences, or the conventional measures of stimulus properties.

2. Stimulus Feature Detection by Neurons in Somatic Sensory Areas I and II

The central theme of a large segment of investigations in quantitative sensory neurophysiology is the proposition that mean rate and periodicity of neural discharges can represent stimulus intensity and frequency, respectively. As

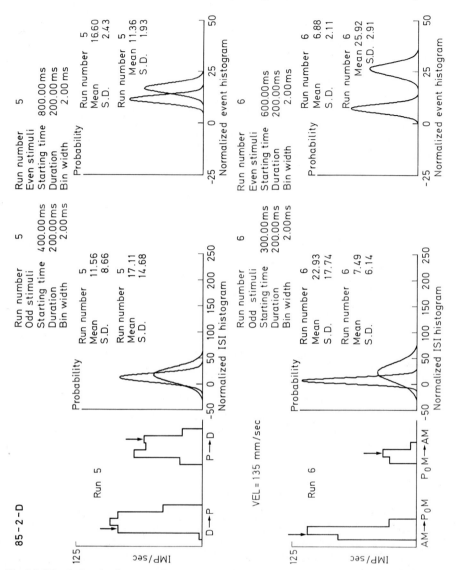

Fig. 12. Discrimination between the responses of a single S-I neuron (lamina III, cytoarchitectural area 1) to movement of a fine brush in opposite directions over the contralateral thigh. On the left are the bargraphs (bin width 200 msec) which depict the neural response elicited by the moving stimuli: D → P distal-to-proximal; AM → POM anterior midline-to-posterior midline of the thigh. The normalized ISI and event distributions to the right of the bargraphs are intended to compare the effectiveness of neural stimulus coding based on counting discharges over fixed short periods of time, with stimulus coding based on the assumption that the distribution of the intervals themselves are the physiological carrying code. For this purpose, the bins of the bargraphs which correspond to identical portions of the receptive field are selected (indicated by ↓). In RUN 5, the P → D movement is compared with the D → P movement: over the selected bin (specified by starting time and duration in the figure) the computer registers the interval and event distributions generated by the neuron in 25 replications of the stimulus. The probability distributions are computed from mean and standard deviation, assuming normality. The figure illustrates that, in RUN 5, neither an event nor an

demonstrated in the previous section, this general concept satisfies certain kinds of experimental data; however, it does not exhaust the scope of stimulus encoding by the central nervous system. There are now a number of instances known which attest to a different principle: namely, that neurons, notably in cortical sensory receiving areas, respond quite specifically to more complex "stimulus features". The relative selectivity with which neurons in the somatic sensory area I respond to cutaneous stimuli moving in a particular direction across the receptive field on the skin is an example of this type of coding (WERNER and WHITSEL, 1970; WHITSEL et al., 1972).

Some neurons in somatosensory area I which respond to punctate stimulation from cutaneous receptive fields, can be shown to be "triggered" to discharge at a high rate when a fine hair or brush is moved across the receptive field at constant velocity in certain directions, but not in others. There is some gradation of the density of discharges with variation of the direction of stimulus motion, but there exists for these neurons a clearly defined direction of stimulus movement which elicits a maximal discharge (Fig. 11). Thus, such neurons can be classified according to their "best" stimuli. A response less than maximal indicates only departure from the optimal stimulus, but not the direction of departure. The occurrence of the maximal discharge in a particular neuron can be thought of as the "code" of the particular stimulus context which this neuron represents.

In a smaller proportion of S-I neurons, this "trigger" feature is also sensitive to the velocity of stimulus motion. It is then possible to show that the peak discharge rate increases much faster with increasing stimulus velocity if the motion occurs in a certain direction, than it does with motion in other directions. Judged by the peak discharge rate attained, the receptive field "seen" by the neuron if stimuli move at high velocity tends more towards the shape of a narrow band or edge, in contrast to the receptive field shape of the same neuron registered at low stimulus velocity, or determined with punctate stimulation; the latter being mostly round or oval shaped (WERNER et al., 1972). The range of optimal stimulus velocities for sharpening the receptive field contour in this manner is in the order of 100 mm/sec which is also the velocity at which best texture discrimination of moving surfaces by palpation can be achieved in psychophysical tests (KATZ, 1925).

These observations with neurons in S-I bear also on another aspect of the neural coding of sensory information: namely, whether sensory information is transmitted by a frequency code, in the sense that neural discharges in a sensory channel are counted over fixed, short intervals of time; or else, whether the discharge intervals themselves are the physiological signal carrying code (cf. PER-

---

interval code would permit reliable discrimination of the direction of stimulus movement as indicated by the overlap of the distribution curves. On the other hand, the event distributions generated for the two directions of stimulus movement applied in the orthogonal axis of the same receptive field are clearly separated (lower right plot). Thus, we could select a "decision criterion" which would permit reliable differentiation of direction of stimulus movement on the basis of counts of neural discharges over a selected observation period. Over these same observation periods, however, an interval detecting device would confuse the direction of stimulus movement in a large number of cases as is indicated by the overlap of the ISI distribution curves (center plot in the lower row). (From WHITSEL et al., 1972)

kel and Bullock, 1968). Simple neural counting schemes have been found sufficient to account for signal detection (Fitzhugh, 1957) and information transmission (Werner and Mountcastle, 1965) in sensory systems. The cortical neurons of S-I with trigger properties sensitive to direction of stimulus motion provide an example for greater efficiency of a code based on counts of discharges over fixed periods of time, than one based on registering discharge intervals. To demonstrate this, Whitsel et al. (1972) compared the distributions of time intervals generated by the neuronal discharge when the stimulus moved across a selected portion of a field first in one and then in the opposite direction, with the distribution of events counted when moving over the same receptive field portion. The interspike interval histograms and the event histograms corresponding to the two directions of motion, displayed in Fig. 12 serve as an example, and were obtained from a neuron in S-I. The result is characteristic in that it shows the lack of overlap of the two event histograms; suggesting that a neural counting device could reliably differentiate the two directions of motions from one another. On the other hand, the interspike intervals, which correspond to the two directions of motion, overlap. Consequently, a spike interval registering device would in a high proportion of instances confuse the two directions of motion, irrespective of where along the interval continuum a decision criterion would be set. This implies that an event counting mechanism affords the possibility for a deterministic detection of motion direction, while an interval measuring mechanism would operate with stochastic indeterminacy.

Neurons in S-II signal not only the direction of stimulus motion, but also the side of the body to which the stimulus is applied. Individual neurons represent these stimulus features in concatenation, with each neuron reflecting several of these stimulus properties at once; for instance, a neuron may be directionally sensitive when the stimulus is applied on the contralateral side, but simultaneous ipsilateral stimulation may cause occlusion. Another neuron may be a directional for contralateral stimulation, and facilited for one direction of motion when simultaneously stimulated on the ipsilateral side. One can visualize that a population of such neurons, in conjunction, could "compute" complex logical functions over the stimulus categories of direction of stimulus motion and sidedness on the body (Werner and Whitsel, 1970; Werner et al., 1972).

3. Principles of Stimulus Transformations in Somatic Sensory Cortex

The representation of cutaneous stimulus properties in the somatosensory cortex emphasizes a piecemeal fragmentation and fractionation of a peripheral stimulus into distinct attributes and components, with different neuron groups quite specifically responding to one or another property of the stimulus, or to particular spatio-temporal contexts or concatenations of such properties. Thus, the overriding property of the stimulus representation in the somatic sensory cortical areas, as seen from the point of view of individual neurons, is that it displays little resemblance to the global stimulus properties; but that different sets of neurons reflect distinct aspects of the stimulus in isolation. In this respect, all sensory cortices seem to be in principle alike at least as studied thus far (Hubel and Wiesel, 1969; Evans, 1968; Werner et al., 1972).

EBNER, F. F., MYERS, R. E.: Commissural connections in the neocortex of monkey. Anat. Rec. **142**, 229 (1962a).

EBNER, F. F., MYERS, R. E.: Corpus callosum and the interhemispheric transmission of tactual learning. J. Neurophysiol. **25**, 380 (1962b).

EBNER, F. F., MYERS, R. E.: Distribution of corpus callosum and interior commissure in cat and raccoon. J. comp. Neurol. **124**, 353 (1965).

EVANS, E. F.: Upper and Lower Levels of the Auditory System: A Contrast of Structure and Function. In: Neural Networks, p. 24. Berlin-Heidelberg-New York: Springer 1968.

FAVALE, E., LOEB, C., MANFREDI, M., SACCO, G.: Somatic afferent transmission and cortical responsiveness during natural sleep and arousal in the cat. Electroenceph. clin. Neurophysiol. **18**, 354 (1965).

FINGER, S., FROMMER, G. P.: Effects of cortical and thalamic lesions on temperature discrimination and responsiveness to foot shock in the rat. Brain Res. **24**, 69 (1970).

FITZHUGH, R.: The statistical detection of threshold signals in the retina. J. gen. Physiol. **40**, 925 (1957).

FOERSTER, O.: The cerebral cortex in man. Lancet **221**, 309 (1931).

FORBES, A., MORISON, B. R.: Cortical response to sensory stimulation under deep barbiturate narcosis. J. Neurophysiol. **2**, 112 (1939).

FOX, S. S., O'BRIEN, J. H.: Duplication of evoked potential waveform by curve of probability of firing of a single cell. Science **147**, 888 (1965).

FOX, S. S., NORMAN, R. J.: Functional congruence — an index of neural homogeneity and a new measure of brain activity. Science **159**, 1257 (1968).

FRANZEN, O.: On spatial summation in the tactual sense. Scand. J. Psychol. **10**, 193 (1969).

FRANZEN, O.: Neural activity in the somatic primary receiving area of the human brain and its relation to perceptual estimates. IEEE Transactions, Vol. MMS-11, p. 115, 1970.

FRANZEN, O., OFFENLOCH, K.: Evoked response correlates of psychophysical magnitude estimates for tactile stimulation in man. Exp. Brain Res. **8**, 1 (1969).

FREDRICKSON, J. M., FIGGE, U., SCHEID, P., KORNHUBER, H. H.: Vestibular nerve projection to the cerebral cortex of Rhesus monkey. Exp. Brain Res. **2**, 318 (1966).

GARDINER, E.: Conductic rates and dorsal root inflow of sensory fibres from the knee joint of the cat. Amer. J. Physiol. **152**, 436 (1948).

GARDNER, E., THOMAS, L. M., MORIN, F.: Cortical projection of fast visceral afferents in the cat and monkey. Amer. J. Physiol. **183**, 438 (1955).

GEISLER, C. D., GERSTEIN, G. L.: The surface EEG in relation to its sources. E.E.G. clin. Neurophysiol. **13**, 927 (1961).

GELFAN, S., CARTER, S.: Muscle sense in man. Exp. Neurol. **18**, 469 (1967).

GERARD, R. W., MARSHALL, W. H., SAUL, L. J.: Cerebral action potentials. Proc. Soc. exp. Biol. (N.Y.) **30**, 1123 (1933).

GERARD, R. W., MARSHALL, W. H., SAUL, L. J.: Electrical activity of the cat's brain. Arch. Neurol. Psychiat. (Chic.) **36**, 675 (1936).

GERNANDT, B., ZOTTERMAN, Y.: Intestinal pain: an electrophysiological investigation on mesenteric nerves. Acta physiol. scand. **12**, 56 (1946).

GESCHWIND, N.: Disconnexion syndromes in animals and man. Brain **88**, 237 (1965).

GILMAN, S., DENNY-BROWN, D.: Disorders of movement and behavior following dorsal column lesions. Brain **89**, 397 (1966).

GLASSMAN, R.: Cutaneous discrimination and motor control following somatosensory cortical ablation. Physiol. Behav. **5**, 1009 (1970).

GLOBUS, A., SCHEIBEL, A. B.: Pattern and field in cortical structure: the rabbit. J. comp. Neurol. **131**, 155 (1967a).

GOFF, W. R., ROSNER, B. S., ALLISON, T.: Distribution of cerebral somatosensory evoked responses in normal man. Electroenceph. clin. Neurophysiol. **14**, 697 (1962).

GOLDRING, S., ARAS, E., WEBER, P. C.: Comparative Study of Sensory Input to Motor Cortex in Animals and Man. E.E.G. clin. Neurophysiol. **29**, 537 (1970).

GOODWIN, G. M., McCLOSKEY, D. I., MATTHEWS, P. B. C.: The persistence of appreciable kinesthesis after paralyzing joint afferents but preserving muscle afferents. Brain Res. **37**, 326 (1972).

GUILLERY, R.W., ADRIAN, H.O., WOOLSEY, C.N., ROSE, J.E.: Activation of Somatosensory Areas I and II of Cat's Cerebral Cortex by Focal Stimulation of the Ventrobasal Complex. In: The Thalamus, p. 197. New York: Columbia 1966.

HAND, P.J., MORRISON, A.R.: Thalamocortical projections in the cat. Ann. N.Y. Acad. Sci. **167**, 258 (1969).

HAND, P.J., MORRISON, A.R.: Thalamocortical projections from the ventrobasal complex to somatic sensory areas I and II. Exp. Neurol. **26**, 291 (1970).

HASSLER, R., MUHS-CLEMENT, K.: Architektonischer Aufbau des sensomotorischen und parietalen Cortex der Katze. J. Hirnforsch. **6**, 377 (1964).

HERRE, W.: Einige Bemerkungen zur Modifikabilitaet, Vererbung und Evolution von Merkmalen des Vorderhirns von Säugetieren. p. 162–174. In: Evolution of the forebrain, R. HASSLER and H. STEPHAN, edits. New York: Plenum Press 1966.

HERRICK, C.J.: The Brain of the Tiger Salamander. Chicago: Univ. of Chicago Press 1948.

HIRSCH, J.F., COXE, W.S.: Representation of cutaneous tactile sensibility in cerebral cortex of cebus. J. Neurophysiol. **21**, 481 (1958).

HIND, J.E.: Unit Activity in the Auditory Cortex. In: Neural Mechanisms of the Auditory and Vestibular Systems, p. 201. Springfield: Thomas 1960.

HUBEL, D.H., WIESEL, T.N.: Receptive fields, binocular interaction and functional architecture in the cat's visual cortex. J. Physiol. (Lond.) **160**, 106 (1962).

HUBEL, D.H., WIESEL, T.N.: Shape and arrangement of columns in the cat's striate cortex. J. Physiol. (Lond.) **165**, 559 (1963).

HUBEL, D.H., WIESEL, T.N.: Anatomical demonstration of columns in the monkey striate cortex. Nature (Lond.) **221**, 747 (1969).

HUNT, W.E., GOLDRING, S.: Maturation of evoked response of the visual cortex of postnatal rabbit. E.E.G. clin. Neurophysiol. **3**, 465 (1951).

JASPER, H.H.: Studies of non-specific afferents upon electrical responses in sensory system. Progr. Brain Res. **1**, 273 (1963).

JONES, E.G.: Interrelationships of parieto-temporal and frontal cortex in the rhesus monkey. Brain Res. **13**, 412 (1969).

JONES, E.G., POWELL, T.P.S.: The ipsilateral cortical connexions of the somatic sensory areas in cat. Brain Res. **9**, 71 (1968a).

JONES, E.G., POWELL, T.P.S.: The projection of the somatic sensory cortex upon the thalamus in the cat. Brain Res. **10**, 369 (1968b).

JONES, E.G., Powell, T.P.S.: The commissural connections of the somatic sensory cortex of cat. J. Anat. (Lond.) **103**, 433 (1968c).

JONES, E.G., POWELL, T.P.S.: Connexions of the somatic sensory cortex of the rhesus monkey. II. Contralateral cortical connexions. Brain **92**, 717 (1969a).

JONES, E.G., POWELL, T.P.S.: The cortical projection of the ventroposterior nucleus of the thalamus in the cat. Brain Res. **13**, 298 (1969b).

JONES, E.G., POWELL, T.P.S.: Connexions of the somatic sensory cortex of the rhesus monkey. I. Ipsilateral cortical connexions. Brain **92**, 477 (1969c).

JONES, E.G., POWELL, T.P.S.: An electron microscopic study of the laminar pattern and mode of termination of afferent fibre pathways in the somatic sensory cortex of the cat. Phil. Trans. B. **257**, 45 (1970a).

JONES, E.G., POWELL, T.P.S.: An anatomical study of converging sensory pathways with the cerebral cortex of monkey. Brain **93**, 793 (1970b).

JONES, E.G., POWELL, T.P.S.: Connexions of the somatic sensory cortex of Rhesus monkey. III. Thalamic Connexions. Brain **93**, 37 (1970c).

KAROL, E.A., Pandya, D.N.: The distribution of the corpus callosum in the Rhesus monkey. Brain **94**, 471 (1971).

KATZ, D.: Der Aufbau der Tastwelt. Leipzig: Barth 1925.

KEIDEL, W.D.: Electrophysiology of Vibratory Perception. In: Contributions to Sensory Physiology, Vol. 3, p. 1. New York Academic Press 1968.

KENNEDY, T.T., TOWE, A.L.: Response of somatosensory cortical units to variations in stimulus intensity. Fed. Proc. **17**, 85 (1958).

KENNEDY, T.T., TOWE, A.L.: Identification of a fast lemniscocortical system in the cat. J. Physiol. (Lond.) **160**, 535 (1962).

KING, E. E., NAQUET, R., MAGOUN, H. W.: Alterations in somatic afferent transmission through the thalamus by central mechanisms and barbiturates. J. Pharmacol. exp. Ther. **119**, 48 (1957).

KITAI, S. T., WEINBERG, J.: Tactile discrimination study of the dorsal column — medial lemniscal system and spino-cervico-thalamic tract in cat. Exp. Brain Res. **6**, 234 (1968).

KREISMAN, N. R., ZIMMERMAN, I. D.: Cortical unit responses to temperature stimulation of skin. Brain Res. **25**, 184 (1971).

KUYPERS, H. G. J. M., SZWARCBART, M. K., MISHKIN, M., RESVOLD, H. E.: Occipito temporal cortico-cortical connections in the Rhesus monkey. Exp. Neurol. **11**, 245 (1965).

LANDAU, W. M.: Evoked Potentials. In: The Neurosciences — A Study Program, p. 469. New York: Rockefeller University Press 1967.

LANDGREN, S.: Convergence of tactile, thermal and gustatory impulses on single cortical cells. Acta physiol. scand. **40**, 210 (1957a).

LANDGREN, S.: Cortical reception of cold impulses from the tongue of the cat. Acta physiol. scand. **40**, 202 (1957b).

LANDGREN, S., NORDWALL, A., WENGSTRÖM, C.: The location of the thalamic relay in the spino-cervico-lemniscal path. Acta physiol. scand. **65**, 164 (1965).

LANDGREN, S., SILFVENIUS, H.: Projection to cerebral cortex of Group I muscle afferents from the cat's hindlimb. J. Physiol. (Lond.) **200**, 353 (1969).

LANDGREN, S., SILFVENIUS, H.: Nucleus Z, the medullary relay in the projection path to the cerebral cortex of group I muscle afferents from the cat's hindlimb. J. Physiol. (Lond.) **218**, 551 (1971).

LANDGREN, S., SILFVENIUS, H., WOLSH, D.: Somatosensory paths to the second cortical projection area of the group I muscle afferents. J. Physiol. (Lond.) **191**, 543 (1967a).

LANDGREN, S., SILFVENIUS, H., WOLSH, D.: Vestibular, cochlear and trigeminal projections to the cortex in the anterior suprasylvian sulcus of the cat. J. Physiol. (Lond.) **191**, 561 (1967b).

LANGHOF, H., RUBIA, F. J.: Splanchnic afferents on the cerebral cortex of the cat. Pflügers Arch. **312**, 18 (1969).

LENDE, R.: Cerebral cortex: a sensorimotor amalgam in the marsupialia. Science **141**, 730 (1963).

LENDE, R. R.: A comparative approach to the neocortex: localization in monotremes, marsupials and insectivores. Ann. N.Y. Acad. Sci. **167**, 262 (1969).

LENDE, R. R., WOOLSEY, C. N.: Sensory and motor localization in cerebral cortex of porcupine (Erethizon Dorsatum). J. Neurophysiol. **19**, 544 (1956).

LERICHE, R.: Des douleures provoquées per l'excitation du bent central des grands splanchniques ou cours des splanchnicotomies. Presse méd. **45**, 971 (1937).

LEVITT, M., LEVITT, J.: Sensory hind-limb representation in SMI cortex of the cat. A unit analysis. Exp. Neurol. **22**, 259 (1968a).

LEVITT, M., LEVITT, J.: Sensory hind-limb representation in the SMI cortex of the cat after spinal tractotomies. Exp. Neurol. **22**, 276 (1968b).

LI, C. L., CULLEN, C., JASPER, H. H.: Laminar microelectrode studies of specific somatosensory cortical potentials. J. Neurophysiol. **19**, 111 (1956).

LIBET, B.: Brain stimulation and the threshold of conscious experience. In: Brain and conscious experience, edit. J. C. ECCLES, Springer 1965a.

LIBET, B.: Cortical activation in conscious and unconscious experience. Perspect. Biol. Med. **9**, 77 (1965b).

LIBET, B., ALBERTS, W. W., WRIGHT, E. W., FEINSTEIN, B.: Responses of human somatosensory cortex to stimuli below threshold for conscious sensation. Science **158**, 1597 (1967).

LOCKE, S.: Thalamic connections to insular and opercular cortex of monkey. J. comp. Neurol. **129**, 219 (1967).

LUNDBERG, A.: Supraspinal control of transmission in reflex paths to motoneurons and primary afferents. Progr. Brain Res. **12**, 197 (1964).

LUX, H. D., NACIMIENTO, A. C., CREUTZFELDT, O. D.: Gegenseitige Beeinflussung von postsynaptischen Potentialen corticaler Nervenzellen nach Reizen in unspezifischen und spezifischen Kernen des Thalamus. Pflügers Arch. ges. Physiol. **281**, 170 (1964).

MACCHI, G., ANGELERI, F., GUAZZI, G.: Thalamo-cortical connections of the first and second somatic sensory areas in the cat. J. comp. Neurol. **111**, 387 (1959).

Malcolm, J.L., Darian-Smith, I.: Convergence within the pathways to cat's somatic sensory cortex activated by mechanical stimulation of the skin. J. Physiol. (Lond.) **144**, 257 (1958).

Manson, J.: The somatosensory cortical projection of single nerve cells in the thalamus of the cat. Brain Res. **12**, 489 (1969).

Marin-Padilla, M.: Prenatal and early postnatal ontogenesis of the human motor cortex; a Golgi study. Brain Res. **23**, 167 (1970).

Mark, R.F., Steiner, J.: Cortical projection of impulses in myelinated cutaneous afferent nerve fibres of the cat. J. Physiol. (Lond.) **142**, 544 (1958).

Marshall, W.H., Woolsey, C.N., Bard, P.: Observations on cortical somatic sensory mechanisms of cat and monkey. J. Neurophysiol. **4**, 1 (1941).

McIntyre, A.K.: Symbolic mechanisms in biology. Aust. J. Sci. **19**, 171 (1957).

McIntyre, A.K.: Central Projection of Impulses from Muscle Receptors Activated by Muscle Stretch. In: Symposium on Muscle Receptors, p. 19. Hong Kong: Hong Kong University Press 1962a.

McIntyre, A.K.: Cortical projection of impulses in the interosseous nerve of the cat's hindlimb. J. Physiol. (Lond.) **183**, 46 (1962b).

McIntyre, A.K., Holman, M.E., Veale, J.L.: Cortical responses to impulses from single pacinian corpuscles in the cat's hindlimb. Exp. Brain Res. **4**, 243 (1967).

McLeod, J.G.: The representation of the splanchnic afferent pathways in the thalamus of the cat. J. Physiol. (Lond.) **140**, 462 (1958).

Mehler, W.R.: The mammalian "pain tract" in phylogeny. Anat. Rec. **127**, 332 (1957).

Mehler, W.R.: Some observations on secondary ascending afferent systems in the central nervous system. In: Pain, p. 11. Ed. by R.S. Knighton and P.R. Dumke. Boston: Little Brown Co. 1966.

Mehler, W.R., Feferman, M.E., Nauta, W.J.H.: Ascending axon degeneration following anterolateral cordotomy. An experimental study in the monkey. Brain **83**, 718 (1960).

Meller, K., Breipohl, W., Glees, P.: Synaptic organization of the molecular and outer granular layer in the motor cortex in the white mouse during postnatal development. Z. Zellforsch. **92**, 217 (1968).

Melzack, R., Bridges, J.A.: Dorsal column contribution to motor behavior. Exp. Neurol. **33**, 53 (1971).

Mickle, W.A., Ades, H.W.: A composite sensory projection area in the cerebral cortex of the cat. Amer. J. Physiol. **170**, 682 (1952).

Molliver, M.E.: An ontogenetic study of evoked, somesthetic cortical responses in sheep. Progr. Brain Res. **26**, 78 (1967). Ed. by C.G. Bernhard and J.P. Schadé.

Molliver, M.E., Van der Loos, H.: The ontogenesis of cortical curcuitry. The spatial distribution of synapses in somesthetic cortex of newborn dog. Ergebn. Anat. Entwickl.-Gesch. **42**, 7 (1970).

Morest, D.K.: The growth of dendrites in the mamalian brain. J. Anat. Entwickl.-Gesch. **128**, 290 (1969).

Morin, F.: A new spinal pathway for cutaneous impulses. Amer. J. Physiol. **183**, 245 (1955).

Morison, R.S., Dempsey, E.W.: A study of thalamo-cortical relations. Amer. J. Physiol. **135**, 281 (1941).

Morrison, A.R., Hand, P.J., O'Donoghue, J.: Contrasting projections from the posterior and ventrobasal thalamic nuclear complexes to the anterior ectosylvian gyrus of the cat. Brain Res. **21**, 115 (1970).

Mountcastle, V.B.: Modality and topographic properties of single neurons of cat's somatic sensory cortex. J. Neurophysiol. **20**, 408 (1957).

Mountcastle, V.B.: Some Functional Properties of the Somatic Afferent System. In: Sensory Communication, p. 403. New York: M.I.T. and Wiley 1961.

Mountcastle, V.B.: The Problem of Sensing and the Neural Coding of Sensory Events. In: The Neurosciences, p. 393. New York: Rockefeller 1967.

Mountcastle, V.B., Covian, M.R., Harrison, C.R.: The central representation of some forms of deep sensibility. Res. Publ. Ass. nerv. ment. Dis. **30**, 339 (1952).

Mountcastle, V.B., Davies, P.W., Berman, A.L.: Response properties of neurons of cat's somatic sensory cortex to peripheral stimuli. J. Neurophysiol. **20**, 374 (1957).

MOUNTCASTLE, V.B., DARIAN-SMITH, I.: Neural Mechanisms in Somesthesis. In: Medical Physiology, 12th edit. p. 1372. St. Louis: Mosby 1968.

MOUNTCASTLE, V.B., HENNEMAN, E.: The representation of tactile sensibility in the thalamus of the monkey. J. comp. Neurol. **97**, 409 (1952).

MOUNTCASTLE, V.B., POGGIO, G.F., WERNER, G.: The relation of thalamic cell response to peripheral stimuli varied over the intensive continuum. J. Neurophysiol. **26**, 807 (1963).

MOUNTCASTLE, V.B., POWELL, T.P.S.: Neural mechanisms subserving cutaneous sensibility, with special reference to the role of afferent inhibition in sensory perception and discrimination. Bull. Johns Hopk. Hosp. **105**, 201 (1959a).

MOUNTCASTLE, V.B., POWELL, T.P.S.: Neural mechanisms subserving cutaneous sensibility with special reference to the role of afferent inhibition on sensory perception and discrimination. Bull. Johns Hopk. Hosp. **105**, 201 (1959b).

MOUNTCASTLE, V.B., TALBOT, W.H., KORNHUBER, H.H.: The Neural Transformation of Mechanical Stimuli Delivered to the Monkey's Hand. In: Touch, Heat and Pain, p. 325. Boston: Little Brown 1966.

MOUNTCASTLE, V.B., TALBOT, W.H., SAKATA, H., HYVARINEN, J.: Cortical neuronal mechanisms in flutter-vibration studied in unanaesthetized monkeys. Neuronal periodicity and frequency discrimination. J. Neurophysiol. **32**, 452 (1969).

MYERSON, B.A., PERSSON, H.E.: Evoked unitary and gross electric activity in the cerebral cortex in early prenatal ontogeny. Nature (Lond.) **221**, 1248 (1969).

NACIMIENTO, A.C., LUX, H.D., CREUTZFELDT, O.D.: Postsynaptische Potentiale an Nervenzellen des motorischen Cortex nach elektrischer Reizung specifischer und unspecifischer Thalamuskerne. Pflügers Arch. ges. Physiol. **281**, 152 (1964).

NAKAHAMA, H.: Contralateral and ipsilateral cortical responses from somatic afferent nerves. J. Neurophysiol. **21**, 611 (1958).

NAKAHAMA, H.: Cerebral response in somatic area I of ipsilateral somatic II origin. J. Neurophysiol. **23**, 75 (1960).

NEWMAN, P.P.: Single unit activity in the viscero-sensory areas of the cerebral cortex. J. Physiol. (Lond.) **160**, 284 (1962).

NOBACK, C.R., PURPURA, D.P.: Postnatal ontogenesis of neurons in cat neocortex. J. comp. Neurol. **117**, 291 (1961).

NOBACK, C.R., SHRIVER, J.E.: Phylogenetic and ontogenetic Aspects of the Lemniscal Systems and the Pyramidal System. In: Evolution of the Forebrain, p. 316. New York: Plenum 1967.

NOBACK, C.R., SHRIVER, J.E.: Encephalization and the lemniscal systems during phylogeny. Ann. N.Y. Acad. Sci. **167**, art. **1**, 118 (1969).

NORRSELL, U.: The spinal afferent pathway of conditioned reflexes to cutaneous stimulation in the dog. Exp. Brain Res. **2**, 269 (1966).

O'DONOGHUE, J., MORRISON, A.R., HAND, P.J.: Contrasting cortical projections from the ventrobasal (VB) and posterior (PO) thalamic complexes of the cat. Anat. Rec. **166**, 356 (1970).

OECONOMOS, D., SCHERRER, J.: Étude des potentiels évoqués corticaux somésthesiques des le chat nouveau-né. C. R. Soc. Biol. (Paris) **147**, 1229 (1953).

OLSZEWSKI, J.: The Thalamus of *Macaca mulatta*. Basel: Karger 1952.

OONISHI, S., KATSUKI, Y.: Functional organization and integrative mechanism of the auditory cortex of cat. Jap. J. Physiol. **15**, 342 (1965).

OSCARSSON, O.: Proprioceptive and Exteroceptive Projections to the Pericruciate Cortex of the Cat. In: Studies in Physiology, p. 221. Berlin-Heidelberg-New York: Springer 1965.

OSCARSSON, O., ROSÉN, I.: Projection to cerebral cortex of large muscle-spindle afferents in forelimb nerves of the cat. J. Physiol. (Lond.) **169**, 924 (1963).

OSCARSSON, O., ROSÉN, I.: Short-latency projections to the cat's cerebral cortex from skin and muscle afferents in the contralateral forelimb. J. Physiol. (Lond.) **182**, 164 (1966).

OSCARSSON, O., ROSÉN, I., SULG, I.: Organization of neurones in the cat cerebral cortex that are influenced from Group I muscle afferents. J. Physiol. (Lond.) **183**, 189 (1966).

OSCARSSON, O., ROSÉN, I., UDDENBERG, N.: A comparative study of ascending spinal tracts activated from hindlimb afferents in monkey and dog. Arch. ital. Biol. **102**, 137 (1964).

Pandya, D.N., Vignolo, L.A.: Interhemispheric neocortical projections of somatosensory areas I and II in the rhesus monkey. Brain Res. **7**, 300 (1968).

Pandya, D.N., Kuypers, H.G.J.M.: Cortico-cortical connections in the rhesus monkey. Brain Res. **13**, 13 (1969).

Patton, H.D., Amassian, V.E.: Cortical projection zone of chorda tympani nerve in cat. J. Neurophysiol. **15**, 245 (1952).

Penfield, W.G., Boldrey, E.: Somatic motor and sensory representation in the cerebral cortex of man as studied by electrical stimulation. Brain **60**, 389 (1937).

Penfield, W., Rasmussen, T.: The Cerebral Cortex in Man. New York: McMillan 1950.

Penfield, W., Jasper, H.H.: Epilepsy and the functional anatomy of the human brain. Boston: Little, Brown and Co. 1954.

Perkel, D.H., Bullock, T.H.: Neural Coding. Neurosci. Res. Progr. **6**, 221 (1968).

Perl, E.R., Casby, J.U.: Localization of cerebral electrical activity: the acoustic cortex of cat. J. Neurophysiol. **17**, 429 (1954).

Perl, E.R., Whitlock, D.G.: Potentials evoked in cerebral somatosensory region. J. Neurophysiol. **18**, 486 (1955).

Perl, E.R., Whitlock, D.G.: Somatic stimuli exciting spinothalamic projections to thalamic neurons in cat and monkey. Exp. Neurol. **3**, 256 (1961).

Petit, D., Burgess, P.R.: Dorsal column projection of receptors in cat hairy skin supplied by myelinated fibres. J. Neurophysiol. **31**, 849 (1968).

Phillips, C.G., Powell, T.P.S., Wiesendanger, M.: Projection from low threshold muscle afferents of hand and forearm to area 3a of baboon's cortex. J. Physiol. (Lond.) **210**, 59P (1970).

Pinto Hamuy, T., Bromiley, R.B., Woolsey, C.N.: Somatic afferent areas I and II of dog's cerebral cortex. J. Neurophysiol. **19**, 485 (1956).

Poggio, G.F., Mountcastle, V.B.: A study of the functional contributions of the lemniscal and spinothalamic systems to somatic sensibility. Central nervous mechanisms in pain. Bull. Johns Hopk. Hosp. **106**, 266 (1960).

Poggio, G.F., Mountcastle, V.B.: The functional properties of ventrobasal thalamic neurons studied in unanaesthetized monkey. J. Neurophysiol. **26**, 775 (1963).

Poliak, S.: The Main Afferent Fibre Systems of the Cerebral Cortex in Primates. Berkeley: Univ. of Calif. Press 1932.

Poliakov, G.I.: Embryonal and postembryonal development of neurons in the human cerebral cortex. p. 249. In: Evolution of the forebrain. Ed. by R. Hassler and H. Stephan. New York: Plenum Press 1967.

Pompeiano, O.: Mechanism of sensorimotor integration during sleep. In: Prog. Physiol. Psychol. Vol. 3, p. 3. Ed. by E. Stellar and J.M. Sprague. New York: Academic Press 1970.

Pompeiano, O., Brodal, A.: Spino-vestibular fibres in the cat. An experimental study. J. comp. Neurol. **108**, 353 (1957).

Pompeiano, O., Carli, G., Kawamura, H.: Transmission of sensory information through ascending spinal hindlimb pathways during sleep and wakefulness. Arch. ital. Biol. **105**, 529 (1967).

Poulos, D.A., Benjamin, R.M.: Response of thalamic neurons to thermal stimulation of the tongue. J. Neurophysiol. **31**, 28 (1968).

Powell, T.P.S., Mountcastle, V.B.: The cytoarchitecture of the postcentral gyrus of the monkey Macaca mulatta. Bull. Johns Hopk. Hosp. **105**, 108 (1959a).

Powell, T.P.S., Mountcastle, V.B.: Some aspects of the functional organization of the cortex of the postcentral gyrus of the monkey: a correlation of findings obtained in a single unit analysis with cytoarchitecture. Bull. Johns Hopk. Hosp. **105**, 133 (1959b).

Pribram, K.H.: The Amnestic Syndromes: Disturbances in Coding? In: The Pathology of Memory, p. 127. New York and London: Academic Press 1969.

Provins, K.A.: The effect of peripheral nerve block on the appreciation and execution of finger movements. J. Physiol. (Lond.) **143**, 55 (1958).

Pubols, B.H., Pubols, L.M.: Forelimb, hindlimb, and tail dermatomes in the spider monkey (Ateles). Brain Behav. Evol. **2**, 132 (1969).

Pubols, B.H., Pubols, L.M.: Somatotopic organization of spider monkey somatic sensory cerebral cortex. J. comp. Neurol. **141**, 63 (1971).

Talbot, W.H., Darian-Smith, I., Kornhuber, H.H., Mountcastle, V.B.: The sense of flutter vibration: comparison of the human capacity with response patterns of mechano-receptive afferents from the monkey hand. J. Neurophysiol. **31**, 301 (1968).

Tapper, D.N.: Behavioral evaluation of the tactile pad receptor system in hairy skin of cat. Exp. Neurol. **26**, 447 (1970).

Teitelbaum, H., Sharpless, S.K., Byck, R.: Role of somatosensory cortex in interhemispheric transfer of tactile habits J. comp. physiol. Psychol. **66**, 623 (1968).

Thompson, W.D., Stoney, S.D., Asanuma, H.: Characteristics of projections from primary sensory cortex to motor sensory cortex in cats. Brain Res. **22**, 15 (1970).

Towe, A.L.: On the nature of the primary evoked response. Exp. Neurol. **15**, 113 (1966).

Towe, A.L.: Neuronal Population Behavior in the Somatosensory Systems. In: The Skin Senses, p. 552. Springfield: Thomas 1968.

Towe, A.L., Amassian, V.E.: Patterns of activity in single cortical units following stimulation of the digits in monkeys. J. Neurophysiol. **21**, 292 (1958).

Towe, A.L., Morse, R.W.: Dependence of the response characteristics of somatosensory neurons on the form of their afferent input. Exp. Neurol. **6**, 407 (1962).

Towe, A.L., Patton, H.D., Kennedy, T.T.: Response properties of neurons in the pericruciate cortex of the cat following electrical stimulation of the appendages. Exp. Neurol. **10**, 325 (1964).

Truex, R.C., Taylor, M.J., Smythe, M.Q., Gildenberg, P.L.: The lateral cervical nucleus of cat, dog and man. J. comp. Neurol. **139**, 93 (1970).

Uttal, W.R.: Evoked Brain Potentials — Signs or Codes. Perspect. Biol. Med. **10**, 627 (1967).

Uttal, W.R., Cook, L.: Systematics of the evoked somatosensory cortical potentials. IBM J. Res. Develop. **6**, 179 (1962).

Vierck, C.J.: Spinal pathways mediating limb position sense. Anat. Rec. **154**, 437 (1966).

Voeller, K., Pappas, G.D., Purpura, D.P.: Electron microscope study of development of cat superficial neocortex. Exp. Neurol. **7**, 107 (1963).

Vogt, C., Vogt, O.: Allgemeine Ergebnisse unserer Hirnforschung. J. Psychol. Neurol. (Lpz.) **25**, 279 (1919).

Walberg, F., Bowsher, D., Brodal, A.: The termination of primary vestibular fibres in the vestibular nuclei of the cat. J. comp. Neurol. **110**, 391 (1958).

Walker, A.E.: The primate thalamus. Chicago: Univ. of Chicago Press 1938.

Wall, P.D.: The sensory and motor role of impulse traveling in the dorsal column towards cerebral cortex. Brain **93**, 505 (1970).

Walzl, E.M., Mountcastle, V.B.: Projection of vestibular nerve to cerebral cortex of the cat. Amer. J. Physiol. **159**, 595 (1949).

Welker, W.I.: Comparative study of physiology and morphology of somatic cerebral cortex of procyonidae. Physiologist **2**, 121 (1959).

Welker, W.I., Campos, G.B.: Physiological significance of sulci in somatic sensory cerebral cortex in mammals of the family Procyonidae. J. comp. Neurol. **120**, 19 (1963).

Welker, W.I., Seidenstein, S.: Somatic sensory representation in the cerebral cortex of the raccoon (Procyon lotor). J. comp. Neurol. **111**, 469 (1959).

Welt, C., Aschoff, J.C., Kameda, K., Brooks, V.B.: Intracortical Organization of Cat's Motorsensory Neurons. In: Neurophysiological Basis of Normal and Abnormal Motor Activity, p. 255. Hewlett: Raven 1967.

Werner, G.: The Topology of the Body Representation in the Somatic Afferent Pathway. In: The Neurosciences, 2nd Study Program New York: Rockefeller University Press, edit. F. O. Schmitt et al. 1970.

Werner, G.: The Study of Sensation in Physiology: Psychophysical and Neurophysiologic Correlations. In: Medical Physiology 13th edit. Ed. by V.B. Mountcastle. St. Louis: Mosby 1971.

Werner, G.: Somatotopic Projections. Neurosciences Res. Progr. Bull. Vol. 10, No. 3. 1972.

Werner, G.: Neural Information Processing with feature extractors. In: The Neurosciences, Third Study Program. Ed. by F.O. Schmitt and F. Worden. Cambridge: MIT Press 1973.

Werner, G., Mountcastle, V.B.: Neural activity in mechanoreceptive cutaneous afferents: stimulus-response relations, Weber functions and information transfer. J. Neurophysiol. **28**, 359 (1965).

WERNER, G., MOUNTCASTLE, V.B.: Quantitative Relations Between Mechanical Stimuli to the Skin and Neural Responses Evoked by Them. In: The Skin Senses, p. 112. Springfield: Thomas 1968.

WERNER, G., WHITSEL, B.L.: The topology of dermatomal projection in the medial lemniscal system. J. Physiol. (Lond.) **192**, 123 (1967).

WERNER, G., WHITSEL, B.L.: Topology of the body representation in somatosensory area I of primates. J. Neurophysiol. **31**, 856 (1968).

WERNER, G., WHITSEL, B.L.: Stimulus Feature Detection by Neurons in Somatosensory Areas I and II of Primates. IEEE Trans. MMS-11, p. 36, 1970.

WERNER, G., WHITSEL, B.L., PETRUCELLI, L.M.: Data Structure and Algorithms in the Primate Somatosensory Cortex. In: Brain and Human Behavior. Ed. by A. KARCZMER and J.C. ECCLES. Berlin-Heidelberg-New York: Springer 1972.

WHITE, J.C.: Sensory innervation of the viscera. Res. Publ. Ass. nerv. ment. Dis. **23**, 373 (1942).

WHITEHORN, D., TOWE, A.L.: Postsynaptic potential patterns evoked upon cells in sensorimotor cortex of cat by stimulation at the periphery. Exp. Neurol. **22**, 222 (1968).

WHITLOCK, D.G., PERL, E.R.: Thalamic projections of spinothalamic pathways in monkey. Exp. Neurol. **3**, 240 (1961).

WHITSEL, B.L., DREYER, D.A., ROPPOLO, J.R.: Determinants of the Body Representation in the Postcentral Gyrus of Macaques. J. Neurophysiol. **34**, 1018 (1971b).

WHITSEL, B.L., PETRUCELLI, L.M., SAPIRO, G.: Modality representation in the lumbar and cervical fasciculus gracilis of squirrel monkeys. Brain Res. **15**, 67 (1969a).

WHITSEL, B.L., PETRUCELLI, L.M., WERNER, G.: Symmetry and connectivity in the map of the body surface in somatosensory area II of primates. J. Neurophysiol. **32**, 170 (1969b).

WHITSEL, B.L., PETRUCELLI, L.M., SAPIRO, G., HA, H.: Fibre sorting in the fasciculus gracilis of squirrel monkeys. Exp. Neurol. **29**, 227 (1970).

WHITSEL, B.L., PETRUCELLI, L.M., HA, H., DREYER, D.A.: The resorting of spinal afferents as antecedent to the body representation in the postcentral gyrus. Brain Behav. Evol. **5**, in press (1973).

WHITSEL, B.L., ROPPOLO, J.R., WERNER, G.: Cortical information processing of stimulus motion on primate skin. J. Neurophysiol. **35**: 691 (1972).

WOOLSEY, C.N.: "Second" somatic receiving areas in the cerebral cortex of cat, dog and monkey. Fed. Proc. **2**, 55 (1943).

WOOLSEY, C.N.: Patterns of sensory representation in the cerebral cortex. Fed. Proc. **6**, 437 (1947).

WOOLSEY, C.N.: Patterns of Localization in Sensory and Motor Areas of the Cerebral Cortex. In: The Biology of Mental Health and Disease, p. 193. New York: Hoeber 1952.

WOOLSEY, C.N.: Organization of Somatic Sensory and Motor Areas of the Cerebral Cortex. In: Biological and Biochemical Bases of Behavior, p. 63. Madison: Univ. of Wisconsin Press 1958.

WOOLSEY, C.N.: Some Observations on Brain Fissuration in Relation to Cortical Localization of Function. In: Structure and Function of the Cerebral Cortex, p. 64. Amsterdam: Elsevier 1960.

WOOLSEY, C.N.: Cortical localizations as defined by evoked potential and electrical stimulation studies. In: Cerebral localization and organization; G. SCHALTENBRAND and C.N. WOOLSEY, edits. University of Wisconsin Press 1964.

WOOLSEY, C.N., FAIRMAN, D.: Contralateral, ipsilateral and bilateral representation of cutaneous receptors in somatic areas I and II of the cerebral cortex of pig, sheep, and other mammals. Surgery **19**, 684 (1946).

WOOLSEY, C.N., MARSHALL, W.H., BARD, P.: Representation of cutaneous tactile sensibility in the cerebral cortex of the monkey as indicated by evoked potentials. Bull. Johns Hopk. Hosp. **70**, 399 (1942).

WOOLSEY, C.N., WANG, G.H.: Somatic sensory areas I and II of the cerebral cortex of the rabbit. Fed. Proc. **4**, 79 (1945).

WOOLSEY, T.A., VAN DER LOOS, H.: The structural organization of layer IV in the somatosensory region (S-I) of mouse cerebral cortex. Brain Res. **17**, 205 (1970).

ZIMMERMAN, I.D.: A triple representation of the body surface in the sensorimotor cortex of the squirrel monkey. Exp. Neurol. **20**, 415 (1968).

Chapter 17

Somatosensory Cortex: Descending Influences on Ascending Systems

By

Arnold L. Towe, Seattle (USA)

With 6 Figures

Contents

A. Introduction

In view of its limited interconnections with other than adjacent cerebral tissue, the somatic sensorimotor cortex may be regarded as an almost isolated unit of cerebral tissue — a unit interacting extensively with subcortical structures, but having little direct commerce with other regions of the cerebral mantle. A recent paper by Myers (1967) highlights the almost complete isolation of several cerebral regions, one from the other, and hints that the brain may be organized after the manner of the inflorescence of an umbelliferous plant. However, somatic sensorimotor cortex is a different sort of unit; it straddles two lobes, receives input from adjacent tissue in both lobes, and has a conspicuous one-way internal connection. Part of its output — the pyramidal tract — is the only one known in detail, and hence will occupy a prominent place in this chapter.

In the higher primates, which are almost the only mammals to have a clear mediolateral central fissure, the sensorimotor cortex includes both the precentral and the postcentral gyri. The pyramidal tract arises mainly from these two gyri, with only minor contributions from other cerebral regions. Primary evoked responses may be recorded in both gyri following cutaneous or deep stimulation, and discrete muscle contractions may be produced by direct stimulation of either gyrus (Woolsey, 1958). To be sure, there are variations within the region; both the latency and configuration of the primary evoked responses and the stimulus intensities necessary to produce observable muscle contractions differ between the two gyri. Nonetheless, the two gyri are united through their distinctive topographical organization and, as will become evident in this chapter, through their effects on subcortical structures.

Few mammals other than the higher primates present such a complete overlap of sensorimotor properties, with superimposed maps of the contralateral skin and of the muscles laid out along the rostral border of the parietal lobe, duplicated again as a mirror image along the caudal border of the frontal lobe, and with the pyramidal tract arising from the entire region. In particular, the felids present a less integrated picture, with the pyramidal tract arising primarily from the rostral half of the somatosensory cortex, as defined through the primary evoked response. On the other hand, the electrically excitable motor cortex of felids is almost coextensive with the somatosensory cortex (GAROL, 1942; WOOLSEY, 1958). The terms motorsensory (Ms) and sensorimotor (Sm) have been introduced to emphasize this overlap and at the same time to recognize the differences between the two regions. The terms are evidently appropriate for all placental mammals, but not for the marsupials or the monotremes, which present a single topographic map oriented in a way that is characteristic of the rostral border of the parietal lobe of placental mammals (LENDE, 1963a, 1963b, 1964). Thus it is important to keep in mind both the animal species and the cerebral sites under consideration. This chapter will be restricted mainly to the domestic cat and the rhesus monkey, because descending influences on ascending systems have received only scant attention in other animals.

It is important to recognize that the carnivores and the primates represent different structural adaptations to widely divergent life styles, the two lines having gone separate ways since early in the Cenozoic era. The structural patterns leading to the later carnivores and those leading to the primates can be recognized in fossils from Middle Paleocene beds; the tusk-like canines and distinctive carnassials of the archaic carnivores and the peculiar rodent-like incisors of the Paleocene primates are mute evidence of their different life styles (ROMER, 1966). Thus, any inclination to generalize from one mammalian family to the next must be tempered by the realization that the somatosensory system and the sensorimotor cortex might play somewhat different roles in the lives of the members of these two mammalian lines. Most importantly, the internal organization at each stage of the somatosensory system and the pattern of descending influences within the system might reflect these differences.

B. Descending Pathways

The sensorimotor cortex, like neopallium in general, sends fibers back to its own thalamic projection nuclei. In addition, it sends fibers to other thalamic nuclei, to parts of the basal ganglia, to midbrain, pontine and bulbar cell clusters and to the spinal cord (KAWANA, 1969; KAWANA and KUSAMA, 1964; KUYPERS, 1958a, 1958b, 1960; KUYPERS and BRINKMAN, 1970; KUYPERS and TUERK, 1964; NIIMI, KISHI, MIKI and FUJITA, 1963). However, the physiology of the corticofugal output from that portion of the sensorimotor cortex which is regarded as primarily sensory in character has been largely ignored, more attention having been given to sensation as output than to its corticofugal discharge. Only the pyramidal tract has been extensively studied, and its diffuse and far-flung terminations may account for most of the known terminations of fibers emanating from this part of the brain. Certainly, each new study shows the sphere of influence of the pyramidal tract to be broader than had previously been suspected (WIESEN-DANGER, 1969; TOWE, 1972). More than half of the corticofugal output from sensorimotor cortex goes by way of pyramidal tract fibers, and among these fibers, a large number terminate in cell clusters that make up the ascending somatosensory system.

1. Dorsal Column Nuclei

REDLICH (1897) and PROBST (1903) were among the first to realize that many fibers of cerebral origin terminate among cells in the ventral part of the cuneate and gracile nuclei. BROUWER (1932, 1933) was well aware of the implications of such an arrangement, though his specific interests centered on the dorsal thalamus. He stated that: "The corticofugal systems descending to the thalamus may not only regulate striatal movements, but must also have an influence on purely sensory functions." WALLENBERG, HEAD, BROUWER and many others were convinced that centrifugal effects exist in sensory systems; they spoke of both facilitatory and inhibitory processes and of "attention" in connection with these effects. Yet, serious interest in the study of centrifugal influences on ascending systems did not develop among physiologists until mid-century, when several provocative papers appeared (AUSTIN, 1952; BAUMGARTEN, MOLLICA and MORUZZI, 1954; HAGBARTH and KERR, 1954; HERNÁNDEZ-PEÓN, 1955; HERNÁNDEZ-PEÓN and HAGBARTH, 1955). These papers marked the beginning of a greater awareness that the brain may not behave simply as a passive recipient of sensory information. A flood of papers followed, especially concerning the effects of cerebral stimulation on the excitability of neurons in the dorsal column nuclei.

As expected from the relative efficacies of excitatory and inhibitory processes, the first and most conspicuous effect observed in the dorsal column nuclei was a reduction in the gross field potential evoked by cutaneous stimulation following iterative conditioning stimulation of the brain stem reticular formation and of the sensorimotor cortex itself (DAWSON, 1958; GUZMÁN-FLORES, BUENDÍA, ANDERSON and LINDSLEY, 1961; HERNÁNDEZ-PEÓN, SCHERRER and VELASCO, 1956; MAGNI, MELZACK, MORUZZI and SMITH, 1959; SCHERRER and HERNÁNDEZ-PEÓN, 1958). However, by 1959 (JABBUR and TOWE) it had been established that not only are some neurons of the dorsal column nuclei inhibited, but also that many are directly excited by stimulation of the sensorimotor cortex. Thus, DAWSON's (1958) earlier speculation about an occlusive interaction between cerebral and cutaneous inputs to explain the reduction in the gross field potential became more plausible.

Fig. 1 illustrates the response of a cuneate neuron to cutaneous and to cerebral stimulation, the particular neuron being a "double burster" to cutaneous stimulation (TOWE, 1968). Some neurons respond to a single cerebral shock, some require a brief train of stimuli (Fig. 1) and others fail to discharge, showing instead an early facilitation in a conditioning-testing (cerebral-cutaneous) situation. However, each of these neurons is said to receive excitation from the cerebral cortex. If at least some of the cerebral sites tested yield excitation or facilitation on a particular neuron, and none yields inhibition, then that neuron is said to be exclusively

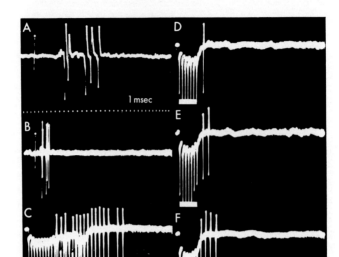

Fig. 1. Response of cat cuneate neuron to stimulation of ipsilateral forepaw (A & B) and contralateral postcruciate cortex (C–F). A: Supramaximal IFP shock. B: Same as in A, but at slower sweep speed. C: 20 shocks (312/sec) at 0.8 msec duration each, applied to contralateral postcruciate cortex. D–F: 7 shocks (312/sec) at 0.4 msec (D), 0.6 msec (E) and 0.8 msec (F) duration each

excited by the cerebral cortex. This terminology can be misleading, for a period of reduced excitability usually follows the response to cerebral stimulation; the expression refers to the *initial* effect of cerebral stimulation.

Fig. 2 illustrates the decrease of excitability for some cuneate neurons that follows cerebral stimulation. With strong cutaneous testing shocks, the inhibitory interaction is usually found to be weak; following an extended train of cerebral conditioning shocks, the response to a cutaneous test shock is usually slightly delayed and consists of fewer spikes (Fig. 2A). For some neurons, a brief train of cerebral shocks blocks responsiveness entirely (Fig. 2B), and for a few, a single cerebral shock is effective. Whatever the intensity of the interaction, if inhibition occurs, and no excitation or facilitation can be found from any cerebral testing site, the neuron is said to be exclusively inhibited from the cerebral cortex. However, if excitation or facilitation occurs from stimulation at some cerebral sites, and inhibition from others, then the neuron in question is said to receive a mixed influence. The initial inhibition gives way to a period of increased excitability. This subsequent facilitation manifests itself by an increased number of spikes and a shorter initial spike latency to the standard cutaneous testing stimulus. The time course of the initial inhibition is commensurate with a presynaptic inhibitory process, though its onset may occasionally be so abrupt that direct inhibition is implicated.

The following general features of sensorimotor cerebral influence on neurons of the dorsal column nuclei of the cat have been well established (JABBUR and

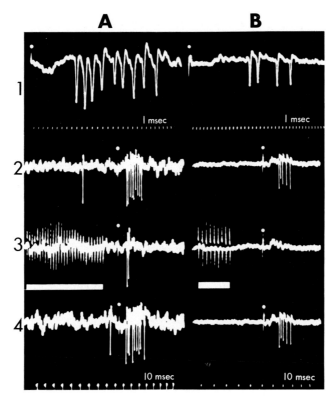

Fig. 2. Responses of two cat cuneate neurons to stimulation of ipsilateral forepaw, and their blocking by cerebral conditioning stimulation. 1: Weak IFP shock. 2: Same as in 1, but at slower sweep speed. 3: Reduction (A) and elimination (B) of response to weak IFP shock by 312/sec conditioning stimulation of postcruciate cortex. 4: Weak IFP shock, 1 sec after conditioning stimulation

Towe, 1961; Levitt, Carreras, Liu and Chambers, 1964; Towe and Jabbur, 1961): 1) Nearly all neurons of the dorsal column nuclei come under cerebral influence. 2) A neuron may be either excited (facilitated) or inhibited by cerebral stimulation, but rarely shows mixed influences. 3) A neuron may be influenced from both cerebral hemispheres, though the contralateral influence is more effective. 4) Stimulation medially on sensorimotor cortex primarily influences neurons in the gracile nucleus, whereas more lateral stimulation influences cuneate neurons. 5) Inhibition is usually produced by stimulation in the neighborhood of the cruciate sulcus (area 4), whereas excitation is apparently most readily produced by stimulation slightly more caudally (area 3a: see Gordon and Miller, 1969; and Levitt et al., 1964). 6) Transection of the medullary pyramid ipsilateral to the site of cerebral stimulation abolishes excitation in the contralateral dorsal column nuclei, though cerebral stimulation ipsilateral to the nuclei remains effective. 7) Transection of the medullary pyramid diminishes inhibition according to the level of the transection: the more rostral the transection, the greater the disruption of cerebrally induced inhibition. 8) Transection of the brain stem,

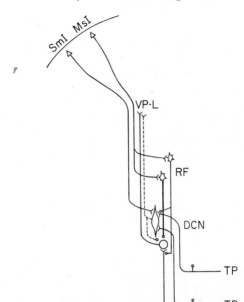

Fig. 3. Schematic arrangement of synaptic connections in the cat dorsal column nuclei (DCN), showing cortical excitatory influence (SmI) on the TP-sensitive neurons and cortical inhibitory influence (MsI) via bulbar reticular neurons (RF) directly onto HS-sensitive neurons and presynaptically onto both TP and HS afferent terminals

sparing the pyramidal tract, has no effect on excitation, but interferes with inhibition: the more rostral the transection, the lesser the disruption. These last two observations suggest that the inhibitory effect is relayed by neurons of the reticular formation. The schematic arrangement shown in Fig. 3 is probably descriptive for the domestic cat, for it incorporates most of the above features.

Some additional features of the cat dorsal column nuclei are suggested in Fig. 3 (Gordon and Jukes, 1964a, 1964b; Gordon and Miller, 1969; Gordon and Paine, 1960; Gordon and Seed, 1961; Perl, Whitlock and Gentry, 1962): 1) Nearly all neurons can be excited by some form of peripheral stimulation; most[1] are primarily sensitive either to hair-bending (HS) or to light touch or pressure (TP). 2) The TP neurons are isolated preferentially in the rostral part of the nuclei, but stretch caudally along the ventral aspect of the nuclei; they have large excitatory receptive fields and show facilitatory "surrounds" beyond the borders of their excitatory fields. 3) About half of the TP neurons project to the thalamus; some apparently have an inhibitory effect on HS cells, and all can be excited by cerebral stimulation. 4) The pyramidal tract fibers that excite TP neurons are not corticospinal collaterals, but rather are corticobulbar fibers of termination. 5) The HS neurons are usually isolated in the middle one-third of each nucleus; they have

---

1 Many neurons are excited by muscle, tendon and joint receptors; cerebral influences on such neurons in the dorsal column nuclei have received scant attention.

small excitatory receptive fields and show afferent inhibition beyond the borders of their excitatory fields. 6) Nearly all HS neurons project to the thalamus, and most can be inhibited by cerebral stimulation; the few HS neurons that lack afferent inhibition show a facilitatory "surround," and can be excited by cerebral stimulation. Fig. 3 shows inhibitory collaterals from the TP neurons as the only means by which the HS neurons can be inhibited from the periphery. However, some HS neurons can be inhibited by light deflection of hairs, as well as by frank tactual stimulation.

All of these "characteristic" features of neurons in the dorsal column nuclei are statistical abstractions, for exceptions can be found to each of them. It is the existence of the exceptions, as will be discussed shortly, that may provide the basis for continuing evolution among the mammals. It is also the existence of the exceptions that makes it difficult, if not impossible, to evaluate other possible networks to describe the organization of the dorsal column nuclei. In this connection, the arrangement proposed by ANDERSEN, ECCLES, SCHMIDT and YOKOTA (1964) comes to mind. They conceived the idea that the cerebral cortex acts to inhibit transmission through the dorsal column nuclei, and that the neurons excited by pyramidal tract fibers are interneurons that transduce the excitatory effect of the pyramidal system into an inhibitory effect on the neurons that project to the thalamus. Though they present observations that are consistent with this idea, the major features of the cat dorsal column nuclei as outlined above are not consistent with such an arrangement. However, by selection among the neurons that have been observed, it is possible to find a subset that meets the requirements. Thus, even though it is clear that the idea proposed by ANDERSEN et al. (1964) is not generally descriptive for the organization of the dorsal column nuclei of the domestic cat, it cannot be denied that such an arrangement might exist among some collection of neurons within the dorsal column nuclei. The net effect of direct and prolonged pyramidal tract stimulation seems to be an enhancement of transmission through the somatosensory system, for the cutaneous excitatory receptive fields of most somatosensory cerebral neurons are thereby increased in size (ADKINS, MORSE and TOWE, 1966).

Anatomical studies of the dorsal column nuclei of the cat provide an adequate substrate for the physiological findings. The bulk of the nuclei consists of small round cells with dense, bushy dendrites (cluster neurons); an abundance of triangular, multipolar and fusiform cells is disposed along the ventral aspect and rostral pole of the nuclei. Transection of the medial lemniscus yields acute retrograde changes in all cluster neurons and in all but a portion of the latter cell group, suggesting that some of the latter may not contribute to the medial lemniscus or that they may collateralize profusely within the nuclei (KUYPERS and TUERK, 1964). Pyramidal tract fibers enter the nuclei mainly from the ventral side to terminate extensively among the triangular, multipolar and fusiform cells (WALBERG, 1957; KUYPERS, 1958a; KUYPERS and TUERK, 1964), and the extended dendritic fields of these cells suggest that their excitatory receptive fields might be larger than those of the cluster neurons. As shown in Fig. 3, these cells probably are the large field TP neurons that are excited by the cerebral cortex and that apparently send inhibitory collaterals to the HS cells. On the other hand, the cluster neurons rarely receive pyramidal tract terminals; they receive dense terminal plexuses

45*

from small bundles of dorsal root fibers (CAJAL, 1952). These probably are the small-field HS neurons that are inhibited from the cerebral cortex via cells of the brain stem reticular formation (CESA-BIANCHI and SOTGIU, 1969)[2] and via some TP cells, and that are inhibited by skin stimulation primarily via the postulated inhibitory collaterals of some TP cells. As suggested in Fig. 3, both direct and presynaptic inhibition are implicated in the descending system. The putative inhibitory interneurons that operate to transduce the excitatory effect of reticular neurons on the dorsal column nuclei are not shown in Fig. 3. Direct inhibition following skin stimulation, again said to be mediated via local interneurons, is well documented (ANDERSEN, ECCLES, OSHIMA and SCHMIDT, 1964); only recently have data been brought forth suggesting that a presynaptic mechanism may also be at work (JABBUR and BANNA, 1970; ANDERSEN, ETHOLM and GORDON, 1970).

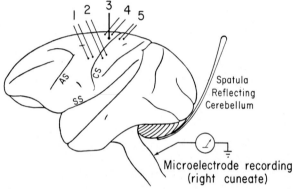

Fig. 4. Experimental arrangement for studying cerebral influence on cuneate neurons of the monkey. A neuron isolated in the right cuneate nucleus is tested for excitation, facilitation or inhibition from 1: precentral arm, 2: postcentral arm, 4: precentral leg, and 5: postcentral leg foci on the left cerebral hemisphere and for antidromic activation from 3: left thalamic nucleus VPL

In further agreement with the physiological findings, KUYPERS (1958a) reported that fibers originating medially from cerebral cortex concentrate in nucleus gracilis, whereas those originating laterally project mainly to nucleus cuneatus. Although the cerebral projections are primarily to the contralateral nuclei, some ipsilateral projections also exist.

Although the anatomical situation in the rhesus monkey is similar to that in the cat (FERRARO and BARRERA, 1935; KUYPERS, 1958b, 1960; KUYPERS, FLEMING and FARINHOLT, 1962), the physiological condition is quite different. In an as yet unpublished study of the cuneate nucleus of *M. mulatta*, TOWE, HARRIS, JABBUR, MORSE and BIEDENBACH recorded the responses of over 2000 neurons following stimulation of the ipsilateral forepaw and the contralateral sensorimotor cortex (Fig. 4). Complete testing for cerebral influences was accomplished on 1431 neu-

---

2 HERNÁNDEZ-PEÓN, SCHERRER and VALESCO (1956) suggest that these fibers may come from medial reticular cell clusters, whereas MAGNI, MELZACK, MORUZZI and SMITH (1959) implicate more lateral cell clusters.

rons, with the following results: 1) Only 416 of the neurons could be influenced by stimulation at the hand and foot foci of the precentral and postcentral gyri. 2) Excitation or facilitation occurred exclusively on 117 neurons, inhibition exclusively on 253 neurons, and mixed effects occurred on 46 neurons. 3) Excitation, facilitation, or inhibition did not necessarily occur from all four cerebral testing sites on each of the 416 neurons. 4) The probability of exciting or facilitating a cuneate neuron was about twice as great from the two hand foci as from the two foot foci. 5) The probability of inhibiting a cuneate neuron was about the same over the four cerebral testing sites, though somewhat larger at the postcentral hand focus. 6) Known cuneothalamic projection neurons were affected by cerebral stimulation in all the ways found on other neurons. 7) Neurons with small excitatory receptive fields were rarely affected by cerebral stimulation, and were most

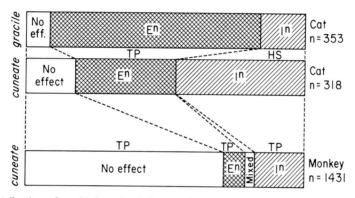

Fig. 5. Distribution of cerebral cortex influences in the dorsal column nuclei of the cat and cuneate nucleus of the monkey. E^n: excitation or facilitation; I^n: inhibition. Relative percentages represented by areas within each rectangle. HS = hair sensitive neuron, TP = touch/pressure neuron, n = number of neurons tested

often touch- or pressure-sensitive neurons. 8) Touch- or pressure-sensitive neurons were dominant in all categories of cerebral influence, hair-sensitivity being found in only 16% of the sample (and 33% of these also responded to tactual stimulation). 9) Some cuneothalamic projection neurons were excited monosynaptically by the most rapidly conducting fibers issuing from the cerebral cortex (HARRIS, JABBUR, MORSE and TOWE, 1965). It was presumed, but not shown, that these fibers were part of the pyramidal system, as in the cat. However, from the observations cited above it is obvious that any generalization from the cat to the monkey could be quite misleading.

Our current anatomical knowledge does not adequately explain the physiological findings in the rhesus monkey. The sparse projection from medial cerebral tissue into the contralateral cuneate nucleus, compared with the dense projection from more lateral cerebral tissue to the same nucleus, is not commensurate with the observed frequencies of cerebral excitation of cuneate neurons. A spatial bias in the sample was not involved, for the entire nucleus was sampled on a 0.5 mm grid of electrode tracks, referenced to the obex. Granting the anatomical findings, it seems necessary to make the unlikely propositions that "foot" cortex fibers have a more potent influence in the cuneate nucleus than do "hand" cortex fibers, or perhaps that the dendrites of cerebrally excited neurons transgress the nuclear boundaries. At least the location of cerebrally excited neurons within the nucleus agrees with that expected from anatomical work. However, there is not enough information in hand to suggest the circuitry of the monkey cuneate nucleus. The time course of cerebrally evoked inhibition suggests that both direct and presynaptic mechanisms (FELIX and WIESENDANGER, 1970) are at work, as in the cat; similarly, a presynaptic inhibitory effect seems to be evoked by cutaneous stimulation (FELIX and WIESENDANGER, 1970; BIEDENBACH, JABBUR and TOWE, 1971).

The distributions of cerebral influence on the dorsal column nuclei of the domestic cat and the rhesus monkey are shown in Fig. 5. The differences cannot be adequately explained by differences in sampling procedure; it seems necessary

Table 1. *Percentage of cells in the cuneate nucleus classed jointly by cutaneous sensitivity and by cerebral effect*

	A. Monkey		B. Cat	
cerebral/cutaneous	TP	HS	TP	HS
No effect	65	6	17–x	x
Excitation	7	1	33	4
Mixed E & I	3	1/3	∼0	∼0
Inhibition	14	4	0	46

to think of the process of differentiation into different cell types and the formation of different synaptic arrangements between the two species. The sensory information relevant to a monkey is probably different from that which is relevant to a cat. In optimizing the adaptation of an interbreeding population of animals to a particular life style (which itself may be slowly changing), there must be selection for the development of different "functional cell types" in particular proportions. These proportions may differ widely across mammalian orders, yielding different "circuitry" from the "same" embryonic collection of nerve cells. Thus, while the monkey makes good use of cuneate cells with mixed cerebral influences, the cat apparently has no need for them. However, the cerebral cortex of the cat can modify the excitability of 83% of its cuneate neurons, whereas the monkey gets along well by influencing only 29% of its cuneate neurons. Even within the cat, information from the hindpaw is evidently processed differently than that from the forepaw, for 76% of the gracile neurons have their excitability raised by the cerebral cortex, whereas that fraction drops to 37% among the cuneate neurons.[3]

Table 1 shows the distribution of neurons by the dual categories of cutaneous and cerebral influence. For the monkey, the neurons responding to touch (61%), pressure (12%) or both (11%) were lumped together in the TP category, and the

---

3 These statements presume a uniform sampling bias across cell types, an as yet unproven presumption. KUYPERS and TUERK (1964) offer a different explanation for the differences found between nuclei cuneatus and gracilis of the cat.

exclusively hair-sensitive neurons (11%) were put in the HS category. The neurons that responded to both touch and hair stimulation (5%) were not included in Table 1. For the cat, no data were available for parcelling the cutaneous inputs among the neurons that were not influenced by cerebral stimulation. Nonetheless, the data illustrate some significant points. Fully 71% of the cuneate neurons tested in the monkey could not be influenced by cerebral stimulation. If these neurons could have been influenced by stimulation deep in the central fissure, then they would constitute a special set. The patterns of cerebral influence that were found among cuneate neurons is consistent with this conclusion. The much greater prevalence of TP neurons in the monkey, compared to the cat, is commensurate with the larger proportion of glabrous skin and lower density of hairs in the monkey. Cerebral inhibition is relatively more prominent among HS neurons (HS:TP = 1:3.5) than are the other types of effect (HS:TP $\simeq$ 1:10), a situation somewhat reminiscent of the cat. On the other hand, apparently no TP neurons in the cat

Table 2. *Distribution of cerebral influences among cuneothalamic projection (CTN) and other neurons in the monkey, expressed as percentages*

	CTN	Other
No effect	51.5	72.7
Excitation	6.4	3.6
Mixed E & I	8.3	5.4
Inhibition	33.8	18.3

dorsal column nuclei come under an inhibitory influence from the cerebral cortex, quite unlike the situation in the monkey. This raises the question whether the foetal cat suppresses an existing mechanism for developing neurons that allow or attract such connections, or whether the cat does not possess such a mechanism. In the latter case, one avenue of future evolution is closed — no future "cat" could process cutaneous information like a monkey. The existence in the cat of a small but non-zero number of neurons having mixed cerebral influences promises that a selective process could work to increase that population of cells, should greater numbers of such cells ever be of advantage to future "cats." In existing animals, variations in these small populations at many levels of the central nervous system might account for many of the individual differences observed among members of the same species.

Table 2 casts the monkey cuneate nucleus in yet another perspective. Of the 1431 neurons thoroughly tested for cerebral influence in the unpublished study by Towe et al., 1145 were also adequately tested for antidromic activation from nucleus VPL of the thalamus. The 204 neurons thus activated were classified as cuneothalamic projection neurons (CTN). The remaining 941 neurons do not comprise a homogeneous group; they are classed as "other" for this discussion.[4] From Table 2 it is clear that all types of cerebral influence affect the CTN neurons.

---

4 Reticular neurons, identified on the basis of their response properties, were excluded from the study. The interested reader should consult the paper by DARIAN-SMITH and YOKOTA (1966a) for some idea of the shape of the classification problem.

Further, while half of the CTN neurons receive some form of cerebral influence, only one-fourth of the "other" neurons are affected. However, because of the highly restricted nature of the VPL stimulus, many cuneothalamic projection neurons were not antidromically activated, and hence appear in the "other" category. Careful study of Table 2 reveals that if about 56% of the "other" category contains true CTN neurons, then the true non-CTN neurons receive no cerebral influence at all. Wherever the answer lies, between these two limits, the condition in the cuneate nucleus of the monkey is strikingly different from that of the cat. On the other hand, this condition in the cuneate nucleus of the monkey bears some resemblance to that found in the trigeminal nuclei of the cat.

2. Trigeminal Nuclei

The general pattern of cerebral influence found in the dorsal column nuclei has also been found in the sensory nuclei of the fifth cranial nerve of the cat. Excitation and inhibition have been obtained by stimulation primarily of the coronal gyrus (SmI face area), but also by stimulation laterally on the sigmoid gyri and on the anterior ectosylvian gyrus (somatosensory area II)[5]. Even some mixed effects have been observed. However, the distribution of effects within the trigeminal nuclei is markedly different from that in the dorsal column nuclei. For example, in the study by DARIAN-SMITH and YOKOTA (1966a), 92% of the neurons classed as trigemino-thalamic projection neurons and 93% of those classed as interneurons showed afferent (or "surround") inhibition from the skin. From the cerebral cortex, 54% of the projection neurons and 42% of the interneurons were excited, while 63% of the projection neurons and 66% of the interneurons showed some form of inhibition. These data were taken from nuclei oralis and caudalis of the spinal trigeminal nucleus. DUBNER (1967) and WIESENDANGER and FELIX (1969) have reported a similar condition for the main sensory nucleus of the trigeminal nerve. All have found that the cerebrally excited neurons, though widely distributed, are concentrated a little more ventromedially in the nucleus than the neurons that are exclusively inhibited from the cerebral cortex.

This arrangement has led to an attempted association of histological with functional cell type, as has also been attempted in the cuneate nucleus. Many corticofugal fibers from the lateral parts of the sigmoid gyri and from the coronal gyrus in the cat project to the triangular, multipolar and fusiform cells disposed all along the ventromedial aspect of the main sensory nucleus and the three spinal trigeminal nuclei (BRODAL, SZABO and TORVIK, 1956; KAWANA and KUSAMA, 1964; KUYPERS, 1958a; NIIMI et al., 1963). They terminate more densely in the contralateral than in the ipsilateral nuclei, and most sparsely in the nucleus interpositus of the spinal trigeminal complex — a nucleus that may contribute primarily to the cerebellum (CARPENTER and HANNA, 1961) rather than to the thalamus. A differential distribution of fibers within the spinal trigeminal complex has been reported (KAWANA and KUSAMA, 1964), but no physiological correlates have yet been recognized. The possible association between histological and functional cell types comes from a number of studies which seem to suggest an organization much

---

5 Though fibers from anterior ectosylvian gyrus also project into the dorsal column nuclei (KAWANA, 1969), the pattern of influence from that region has not been investigated.

like that found in the dorsal column nuclei of the cat (DARIAN-SMITH and YOKOTA, 1966a, 1966b; DUBNER, 1967; HAMMER, TARNECKI, VYKLICKÝ and WIESENDANGER, 1966; HERNÁNDEZ-PEÓN, O'FLAHERTY and MAZZUCHELLI-O'FLAHERTY, 1965; HEPP-REYMOND and WIESENDANGER, 1969; STEWART, SCIBETTA and KING, 1967; WIESENDANGER and FELIX, 1969; WIESENDANGER, HAMMER and TARNECKI, 1967). The primary features of this organization include: 1) excitation of the triangular, multipolar and fusiform cells by pyramidal tract fibers, 2) direct inhibition of the more dorsolaterally located small, round neurons by the pyramidal tract, probably via interneurons, and 3) presynaptic inhibition of the cutaneous input via some nonpyramidal pathway affecting nearly all neurons in the various trigeminal nuclei. However the relatively clean separation between excitation of TP neurons and inhibition of HS neurons that characterizes the dorsal column nuclei does not hold in the case of the trigeminal nuclei. Nor is the direct inhibitory effect exclusive to trigemino-thalamic projection neurons, as seems to be the case in the dorsal column nuclei. On the contrary, all types of cerebral influence can be found among all types of neurons in the trigeminal nuclei. A simple explanation of cerebral modulation, featuring signal enhancement through contrast effects, may rest comfortably with the dorsal column nuclei, but seems impossible to fit onto the trigeminal nuclei. No amount of "tinkering" could improve this situation, for even after removing the spinal trigeminal neurons that project into the cerebellum, the medial reticular formation, and other cell clusters, there remain the known trigemino-thalamic projection neurons, which receive all types of cerebral influence.

3. Non-lemniscal Sensory Systems

Other cell clusters having centrally directed axons have received scant investigation from the point of view of cerebral modulation. CLARE, LANDAU and BISHOP (1964) demonstrated the existence of pyramidal tract collaterals into nucleus VPL of the cat thalamus, and SHIMAZU, YANAGISAWA and GAROUTTE (1965) confirmed this finding. The latter authors, using extracellular recording methods, showed that many neurons in nucleus VPL can be excited by activation of pyramidal tract fibers, and they proposed that these neurons in turn inhibit other VPL neurons. They also found a prolonged period of decreased responsiveness to cutaneous stimulation following antidromic activation of VPL neurons, hinting that a presynaptic inhibitory process may also be at work.

The lateral cervical nucleus, which receives fibers from the dorsolaterally disposed spinocervical tract and which joins the medial lemniscus to project into nucleus VPL of the thalamus, has apparently received no attention from the point of view of cerebral modulation. The pattern of influence, if any, would be of considerable interest, because cells in that nucleus seem to require repetitive input to discharge briskly, and they show a novel sort of cutaneous inhibitory receptive field — one which does not "surround" the excitatory field, but rather is displaced to one side (TAUB, 1964). FEDINA, GORDON and LUNDBERG (1968) have found that both direct and presynaptic inhibition are at work in this nucleus.

Cerebral modulation of neuronal excitability occurs throughout the spinal cord, the effects being mediated not only by corticospinal fibers, but also via a system that relays in the brain stem. In 1954, HAGBARTH and KERR demonstrated that stimulation at a number of central sites reduces or abolishes the responses evoked in the ventral and lateral funiculi by dorsal root stimulation. Stimulation of the anterior and posterior sigmoid gyri and the anterior cingulate gyrus, the anterior ectosylvian gyrus, the anterior cerebellar vermis, and the midbrain and bulbar reticular formation was most effective, the contralateral effect being more intense than the ipsilateral. LINDBLOM and OTTOSSON (1956) showed that at least a part of the cerebrally induced effect depends upon the corticospinal tract. Later, HAGBARTH and FEX (1959) essentially repeated the early work, this time using single neuron recording methods; they found that direct excitation, as well as inhibition, is a feature of this central modulation. The modulating effects from cerebral cortex appear to be somatotopically organized in the cat, and are known to be so in the monkey (ABDELMOUMÈNE, BESSON and ALÉONARD, 1970).

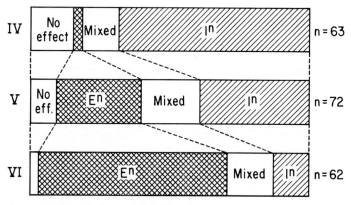

Fig. 6. Distribution of corticospinal tract influences in the dorsal horn of the cat spinal cord. IV, V, and VI are spinal laminae of Rexed. Relative percentages represented by areas within each rectangle. Abbreviations as in Fig. 5

    In 1968, FETZ published the most detailed study of this corticospinal modulatory effect, showing that the sign of the corticospinal influence on dorsal horn neurons in the cat changes from predominantly inhibitory in lamina IV of REXED (1952) to predominately excitatory in lamina VI. Some neurons showed mixed effects, and a few showed no detectable changes following stimulation of the pyramidal tract. The distributions of these pyramidal tract effects by laminae are shown in Fig. 6. Lamina IV neurons usually had small cutaneous excitatory receptive fields, and probably had an afferent or "surround" inhibition (TAUB, 1964), similar to that seen in the dorsal column nuclei. The lamina V cells showed larger cutaneous excitatory receptive fields that graded gradually to a weak inhibitory "surround" area. On the other hand, many lamina VI cells responded not only to cutaneous input, but also to movement of limb joints. Such cells had both their cutaneous and their joint inputs either enhanced or depressed by pyramidal tract stimulation; a differential effect was not observed. FETZ concludes that the excitatory effects reflect a direct corticospinal excitation of the cells, but thinks that the inhibitory effects could involve interneurons. It was possible, in these experiments, that stimulation of the pyramidal tract transynaptically excited bulbospinal neurons that mediated the inhibitory effects. Lamina IV cells provided the main contribution to the dorsolateral ascending tracts; these cells were usually inhibited by pyramidal tract stimulation.

C. Concluding Remarks

The list of known corticofugal effects on subcortical structures is long, only a few selected sites having been touched here. In each instance, we must admit to inadequate knowledge of the "functional" role(s) of the structure in the operation of the nervous system. The idea of "attention" implies central modulation of input, and hence is attractive in this connection. The idea of "feedback" in relation to a number of possible processes is also attractive. It implies closed loops, but there is evidence to support almost any loop that one might care to suggest. The notion that central modulation of input may have something to do with the integration and coordination of movements finds some experimental support. LUSCHEI and CLARK (personal communication) have found a decrease in cutaneous sensitivity beginning about 60 msec prior to the first electromyographic response in a simple reaction time paradigm. The change is specific to the hand that is used in the movement — even though much of the body musculature is involved in even such a simple "movement" as raising a hand from a key. Similarly, GHEZ and LENZI (1970) found a reduction in the medial lemniscus response to a standard radial nerve stimulus prior to and during movement by a cat in a simple reaction time paradigm. The decrease in the test response began about 150 msec prior to the onset of the measurement[6]. Whether this effect depends on the cerebral cortex has yet to be discovered; it may possibly account for much of the pyramidal tract cell activity that has been shown to precede movement, but which is much too feeble to be directly responsible for the movement itself (TOWE, 1973).

The idea of "set" is somewhat akin to the idea of "attention", though it stresses a readiness to act rather than a readiness to receive. From a phylogenetic point of view, the two ideas of "attention" and "set" are exceedingly attractive possibilities in explaining corticofugal modulation of subcortical structures. The capability of rapid identification of a signal and rapid mobilization of the appropriate response mechanism would confer a clear selective advantage to an animal over its fellows. Indeed, partial disruption of this descending system increases response time, especially when a decision must be made (BECK and CHAMBERS, 1970; LAURSEN and WIESENDANGER, 1967), and LAURSEN (1970) has shown for the monkey that this increase is specific to internal processing time in a disjunctive reaction time paradigm. The old view of the mammal as a passive receiver and responder has long since been supplanted by our current view of the mammal as an active experiencer. In interacting with its environment, the mammal seeks input and indeed "expects" specific inputs, especially as a consequence of specific output.

---

6 Limb contact with the apparatus, rather than the electromyographic response, evidently constituted the time reference, and may account for the apparently long reaction time.

References

Abdelmoumène, M., Besson, J.-M., Aléonard, P.: Cortical areas exerting presynaptic inhibitory action on the spinal cord in cat and monkey. Brain Res. **20**, 327–329 (1970).

Adkins, R.J., Morse, R.W., Towe, A.L.: Control of somatosensory input by cerebral cortex. Science **153**, 1020–1022 (1966).

Andersen, P., Eccles, J.C., Oshima, T., Schmidt, R.F., Mechanisms of synaptic transmission in the cuneate nucleus. J. Neurophysiol. **27**, 1096–1116 (1964).

Andersen, P., Eccles, J.C., Schmidt, R.F.: Yokota, T.: Identification of relay cells and interneurons in the cuneate nucleus. J. Neurophysiol. **27**, 1080–1095 (1964).

Andersen, P., Etholm, B., Gordon, G.: Presynaptic and post-synaptic inhibition elicited in the cat's dorsal column nuclei by mechanical stimulation of skin. J. Physiol. (Lond.) **210**, 433–455 (1970).

Austin, G.M.: Suprabulbar mechanisms of facilitation and inhibition of cord reflexes. Res. Publ. Ass. nerv. ment. Dis. **30**, 196–222 (1952).

Baumgarten, R. von, Mollica, A., Moruzzi, G.: Modulierung der Entladungfrequenz einzelner Zellen der Substantia reticularis durch cortico-fugale und cerebelläre Impulse. Pflügers Arch. ges. Physiol. **259**, 56–78 (1954).

Beck, C.H., Chambers, W.W.: Speed, accuracy, and strength of forelimb movement after unilateral pyramidotomy in rhesus monkeys. J. comp. physiol. Psychol. **70**, 1–22 (1970).

Biedenbach, M.A., Jabbur, S.J., Towe, A.L.: Afferent inhibition in the cuneate nucleus of the rhesus monkey. Brain Res. **27**, 179–183 (1971).

Brodal, A., Szabo, T., Torvik, A.: Corticofugal fibers to sensory trigeminal nuclei and nucleus of solitary tract. An experimental study in the cat. J. comp. Neurol. **106**, 527–555 (1956).

Brouwer, B.: Certain aspects of the anatomical basis of the phylogeny of encephalization. Proc. Ass. Res. nerv. ment. Dis. **13**, 3–25 (1932).

Brouwer, B.: Centrifugal influence on centripetal systems in the brain. Arch. Neurol. Psychiat. (Chic.) **30**, 456–460 (1933).

Cajal, S.R.: Histologie du Système Nerveux de l'Homme et des Vertébrés. Madrid: Instituto Ramón y Cajal 1952.

Carpenter, M.B., Hanna, G.R.: Fiber projections from the spinal trigeminal nucleus of the cat. J. comp. Neurol. **117**, 117–131 (1961).

Cesa-Bianchi, M.G., Sotgiu, M.L.: Control by brain stem reticular formation of sensory transmission in Burdach nucleus. Brain Res. **13**, 129–139 (1969).

Clare, M.H., Landau, W.M., Bishop, G.H.: Electrophysiological evidence of a collateral pathway from the pyramidal tract to the thalamus in the cat. Exp. Neurol. **9**, 262–267 (1964).

Darian-Smith, I., Yokota, T.: Cortically evoked depolarization of trigeminal cutaneous afferent fibers in the cat. J. Neurophysiol. **29**, 170–184 (1966a).

Darian-Smith, I., Yokota, T.: Cortifugal effects on different neuron types within the cat's brain stem activated by tactile stimulation on the face. J. Neurophysiol. **29**, 185–206 (1966b).

Dawson, G.D.: The central control of sensory inflow. Proc. roy. Soc. Med. **51**, 531–535 (1958).

Dubner, R.: Interaction of peripheral and central input in the main sensory trigeminal nucleus of the cat. Exp. Neurol. **17**, 186–202 (1967).

Fedina, L., Gordon, G., Lundberg, A.: The source and mechanisms of inhibition in the lateral cervical nucleus of the cat. Brain Res. **11**, 694–696 (1968).

Felix, D., Wiesendanger, M.: Cortically induced inhibition in the dorsal column nuclei of monkeys. Pflügers Arch. **320**, 285–288 (1970).

Ferraro, A., Barrera, S.E.: The nuclei of the posterior funiculi in Macacus rhesus. An anatomic and experimental investigation. Arch. Neurol. Psychiat. (Chic.) **33**, 262–275 (1935).

Fetz, E.E.: Pyramidal tract effects on interneurons in the cat lumbar dorsal horn. J. Neurophysiol. **31**, 69–80 (1968).

Garol, H.W.: The "motor" cortex of the cat. J. Neuropath. exp. Neurol. **1**, 139–145 (1942).

Ghez, C., Lenzi, G.L.: Modulation of afferent transmission in the lemniscal system during voluntary movement in cat. Brain Res. **24**, 542 (1970).

Gordon, G., Jukes, M.G.M.: Dual organization of the exteroceptive components of the cat's gracile nucleus. J. Physiol. (Lond.) **173**, 263–290 (1964a).

Gordon, G., Jukes, M.G.M.: Descending influences on the exteroceptive organization of the cat's gracile nucleus. J. Physiol. (Lond.) **173**, 291–319 (1964b).

Gordon, G., Miller, R.: Identification of cortical cells projecting to the dorsal column nuclei of the cat. Quart. J. exp. Physiol. **54**, 85–98 (1969).

Gordon, G., Paine, C.H.: Functional organization in nucleus gracilis of the cat. J. Physiol. (Lond.) **153**, 331–349 (1960).

Gordon, G., Seed, W.A.: An investigation of nucleus gracilis of the cat by antidromic stimulation. J. Physiol. (Lond.) **155**, 589–601 (1961).

Guzmán-Flores, C., Buendía, N., Anderson, C., Lindsley, D.B.: Cortical and reticular influences upon evoked responses in dorsal column nuclei. Exp. Neurol. **5**, 37–46 (1962).

Hagbarth, K.E., Fex, J.: Centrifugal influences on single unit activity in spinal sensory paths. J. Neurophysiol. **22**, 321–338 (1959).

Hagbarth, K.E., Kerr, D.I.B.: Central influences on spinal afferent conduction. J. Neurophysiol. **17**, 295–307 (1954).

Hammer, B., Tarnecki, R., Vyklický, L., Wiesendanger, M.: Corticofugal control of presynaptic inhibition in the spinal trigeminal complex of the cat. Brain Res. **2**, 216–218 (1966).

Harris, F., Jabbur, S.J., Morse, R.W., Towe, A.L.: The influence of the cerebral cortex on the cuneate nucleus of the monkey. Nature (Lond.) **208**, 1215–1216 (1965).

Hepp-Reymond, M.-C., Wiesendanger, M.: Pyramidal influence on the spinal trigeminal nucleus of the cat. Arch. ital. Biol. **107**, 54–66 (1969).

Hernández-Peón, R.: Central mechanisms controlling conduction along central sensory pathways. Acta neurol. lat.-amer. **1**, 256–264 (1955).

Hernández-Peón, R., Hagbarth, K.E.: Interaction between afferent and cortically induced reticular responses. J. Neurophysiol. **18**, 44–55 (1955).

Hernández-Peón, R., O'Flaherty, J.J., Mazzuchelli-O'Flaherty, A.L.: Modifications of tactile evoked potentials at the spinal trigeminal sensory nucleus during wakefulness and sleep. Exp. Neurol. **13**, 40–57 (1965).

Hernández-Peón, R., Scherrer, H., Velasco, M.: Central influences of afferent conduction in the somatic and visual pathways. Acta neurol. lat.-amer. **2**, 8–22 (1956).

Jabbur, S.J., Banna, N.R.: Presynaptic inhibition of cuneate transmission by widespread cutaneous inputs. Brain Res. **10**, 273–276 (1968).

Jabbur, S.J., Towe, A.L.: Blocking and excitation of cuneate neurons by sensori-motor cortical stimulation in the cat. Fed. Proc. **18**, 73 (1959).

Jabbur, S.J., Towe, A.L.: Cortical excitation of neurons in dorsal column nuclei of cat, including an analysis of pathways. J. Neurophysiol. **24**, 499–509 (1961).

Kawana, E.: Projections of the anterior ectosylvian gyrus to the thalamus, the dorsal column nuclei, the trigeminal nuclei and the spinal cord in cats. Brain Res. **14**, 117–136 (1969).

Kawana, E., Kusama, T.: Projection of the sensory motor cortex to the thalamus, the dorsal column nucleus, the trigeminal nucleus and the spinal cord in the cat. Folia psychiat. neurol. jap. **18**, 337–380 (1964).

Kuypers, H.G.J.M.: An anatomical analysis of cortico-bulbar connexions to the pons and lower brain stem in the cat. J. Anat. (Lond.) **92**, 198–218 (1958a).

Kuypers, H.G.J.M.: Some projections from the peri-central cortex to the pons and lower brain stem in monkey and chimpanzee. J. comp. Neurol. **110**, 221–255 (1958b).

Kuypers, H.G.J.M.: Central cortical projection to motor and somato-sensory cell groups. Brain **83**, 161–184 (1960).

Kuypers, H.G.J.M., Brinkman, J.: Precentral projections to different parts of the spinal intermediate zone in the rhesus monkey. Brain Res. **24**, 29–48 (1970).

Kuypers, H.G.J.M., Fleming, W.R., Farinholt, J.W.: Subcorticospinal projections in the rhesus monkey. J. comp. Neurol. **118**, 107–137 (1962).

Kuypers, H.G.J.M., Tuerk, J.D.: The distribution of the cortical fibres within the nuclei cuneatus and gracilis in the cat. J. Anat. (Lond.) **98**, 143–162 (1964).

Laursen, A.M.: Selective increase in choice latency after transection of a pyramidal tract in monkeys. Brain Res. **24**, 541–559 (1970).

Laursen, A.M., Wiesendanger, M.: The effect of pyramidal lesions on response latency in cats. Brain Res. **5**, 207–220 (1967).

Lende, R.A.: Sensory representation in the cerebral cortex of the opossum (*Didelphis virginiana*). J. comp. Neurol. **121**, 395–403 (1963a).

Lende, R.A.: Motor representation in the cerebral cortex of the opossum (*Didelphis virginiana*). J. comp. Neurol. **121**, 405–415 (1963b).

Lende, R.A.: Representation in the cerebral cortex of a primitive animal: Sensorimotor, visual, and auditory fields in the echidna (*Tachyglossus aculeata*). J. Neurophysiol. **27**, 37–48 (1964).

Levitt, M., Carreras, M., Liu, C.N., Chambers, W.W.: Pyramidal and extrapyramidal modulation of somatosensory activity in gracile and cuneate nuclei. Arch. ital. Biol. **102**, 197–229 (1964).

Lindblom, U.F., Ottosson, J.O.: Influence of pyramidal stimulation upon the relay of coarse cutaneous afferents in the dorsal horn. Acta physiol. scand. **38**, 309–318 (1956/1957).

Magni, F., Melzack, R., Moruzzi, G., Smith, C.J.: Direct pyramidal influences on the dorsal-column nuclei. Arch. ital. Biol. **97**, 357–377 (1959).

Myers, R.E.: Cerebral connectionism and brain function. In: Brain Mechanisms Underlying Speech and Language. New York: Grune & Stratton 1967.

Niimi, K., Kishi, S., Miki, M., Fujita, S.: An experimental study of the course and termination of the projection fibers from cortical areas 4 and 6 in the cat. Folia psychiat. neurol. jap. **17**, 167–216 (1963).

Perl, E.R., Whitlock, D.G., Gentry, J.R.: Cutaneous projection to second-order neurons of the dorsal column system. J. Neurophysiol. **25**, 337–358 (1962).

Probst, M.: Ueber die anatomischen und physiologischen Folgen der Halbseitendurchschneidung des Mittelhirns. Jb. Psychiat. Neurol. **24**, 219–325, 3 pl. (1903).

Redlich, E.: Über die anatomische Folgeerscheinungen ausgedehnter Exstirpationen der motorischen Rindencentern bei der Katze. Neurol. Centralbl. **16**, 818–883 (1897).

Rexed, B.: The cytoarchitectonic organization of the spinal cord in the cat. J. comp. Neurol. **96**, 415–496 (1952).

Romer, A.S.: Vertebrate Paleontology. Chicago: Univ. of Chicago Press 1966.

Scherrer, H., Hernández-Peón, R.: Hemmung postsynaptischer Potentiale im Nucleus Gracilis. Pflügers Arch. ges. Physiol. **267**, 434–445 (1958).

Shimazu, H., Yanagisawa, N., Garoutte, B.: Cortico-pyramidal influences on thalamic somatosensory transmission in the cat. Jap. J. Physiol. **15**, 101–124 (1965).

Stewart, D.H., Jr., Scibetta, D.J., King, R.B.: Presynaptic inhibition in the trigeminal relay nuclei. J. Neurophysiol. **30**, 135–153 (1967).

Taub, A.: Local, segmental and supraspinal interaction with a dorsolateral spinal cutaneous afferent system. Exp. Neurol. **10**, 357–374 (1964).

Towe, A.L.: Neuronal population behavior in the somatosensory systems. In: The Skin Senses. Springfield: CC Thomas 1968.

Towe, A.L.: Motor cortex and the pyramidal system. In: Efferent Organization and Motor Behavior. New York: Academic Press 1973 (in press).

Towe, A.L., Jabbur, S.J.: Cortical inhibition of neurons in dorsal column nuclei of cat. J. Neurophysiol. **24**, 488–498 (1961).

Walberg, F.: Corticofugal fibers to the nuclei of the dorsal columns. An experimental study in the cat. Brain **80**, 273–287 (1957).

Wiesendanger, M.: The pyramidal tract. Recent investigations on its morphology and function. Ergebn. Physiol. **61**, 72–136 (1969).

Wiesendanger, M., Felix, D.: Pyramidal excitation of lemniscal neurons and facilitation of sensory transmission in the spinal trigeminal nucleus of the cat. Exp. Neurol. **25**, 1–17 (1969).

Wiesendanger, M., Hammer, B., Tarnecki, R.: Corticofugal control of presynaptic inhibition in the spinal trigeminal nucleus of the cat. The effect of pyramidotomy and barbiturates. Schweiz. Arch. Neurol. Neurochir. Psychiat. **100**, 255–276 (1967).

Woolsey, C.N.: Organization of somatic sensory and motor areas of the cerebral cortex. In: Biological and Biochemical Bases of Behavior. Madison: Univ. of Wisconsin Press 1958.

Chapter 18

Somesthetic Effects of Damage to the Central Nervous System

By

Josephine Semmes, Bethesda (USA)

With 3 Figures

Contents

A. Introduction

Studying the alterations of behavior resulting from central nervous system lesions as a means of uncovering mechanisms of sensation has a long history. The method originated from the "experiments of Nature" provided by patients with local injury or disease. Neurologists made the basic behavioral observations which established the broad functional divisions of the somatic inflow, and it was they who formulated the fundamental ideas which remain influential among modern investigators using many different techniques. Around the turn of the century, this type of study evolved into true experiments directed toward discovering deficits produced by surgical lesions in trained animals.

Far from being merely a historical milestone, as it is currently viewed by many who favor other approaches, the general method of behavioral analysis following ablations or transections has considerable potential for further development and should help to answer not only the question of "Where ?" (localization) but also the more interesting question of "How ?" (neural coding). Full exploitation of the method in animal studies depends, on the one hand, upon relating behavioral results to anatomical and physiological properties of tracts and areas, and on the other, upon advancing behavioral techniques. Ideally, once it has been found that a selected lesion produces impairment on a test, the analytical task has only begun. It proceeds in two directions, toward identifying the critical feature of the lesion and toward defining as precisely as possible the function impaired. For example, if ablating a cortical area is followed by a behavioral deficit, the lesion-analysis might be pursued by destroying parts of the input to or the output from the area, by varying the size of the original lesion, by removing other areas of the same size but with different properties, or even by removing all other cortex leaving only the original area intact. The complementary deficit-analysis might proceed by employing a variety of tests in order to determine the category on which the subject fails *vs.* those on which he succeeds, by varying the original test to make it easier or more difficult on the stimulus side or on the response side, by altering motivation-reinforcement conditions, or by manipulating the subject's "set" through pretraining. The procedures enumerated are of course not exhaustive — what is tried depends on the ingenuity and insight of the experimenter.

A particularly effective combination of lesion- and deficit-analyses is aimed at establishing "double dissociation" of impairments, i.e., the simultaneous demonstration that lesions in locus A impair performance on test X but not on test Y, whereas lesions in locus B produce the converse results. Double dissociation (between groups of subjects) provides unequivocal evidence for functional distinctness of the loci ablated; single dissociation, i.e., a greater effect of one lesion than another on a single test, provides less convincing evidence for a qualitative difference. Where the double form can be demonstrated, the greater the similarity between sites of lesion, and between the tests used, the more revealing it is. It would be useful to apply this method more deliberately in attempts to differentiate functionally the various components of the somatic sensory apparatus.

Most of the studies to be described in this section are characterized not only by the use of a particular technique but also by the concentration on a particular aspect of somesthesis — discrimination of objects and object qualities by the hand, with the aim of approximating natural activities. Although other somesthetic capacities (e.g., pain and sexual feelings) are more closely tied to survival of the individual and the race, it is the discriminative activities of the hand, made possible by the bipedal stance, which are thought to be of prime importance in man's evolution. When the hands were freed to manipulate objects, manual sensation became comparable to vision as a means for exploring the environment, and these two modalities act together in many forms of eye-hand coordinations. It is worth noting that the preferential use of the hand, rather than the muzzle, for exploration cannot be traced to an advantage in sensitivity, since even in man, the tactile threshold is higher for the fingers than for the region around the mouth and nose (Weinstein, 1968). The dominance of vision over olfaction in the primate may have been a factor in the choice of the hand, thus leading to a visual-manual, rather than an olfactory-oral, acquaintance with objects (Semmes, 1967). Besides its suitability for cooperating with vision, the hand is a highly articulated and motile appendage capable of supplementing cutaneous information with a rich inflow from its joint receptors. The resulting tactual-kinesthetic complex appears to be especially effective in perception of the spatial qualities of objects — their shape, position, and orientation. The well-known superiority of an active exploration over a passive tactual impression of a pattern must reflect in part the contribution of kinesthesis.

It would be a mistake, however, to conceive of how we discriminate objects as dependent simply on an appreciation of joint position combined with a pattern of pressures. GIBSON (1962) has emphasized the implications of the fact that active touch, like active visual scanning, is not a purely receptive sense. When an unseen object is examined, the stimulation received depends not only on the features of the object itself, but also on what movements the subject makes. These movements are selective and purposive in the sense that they seem to be aimed at enhancing some features of the potential stimulation and reducing others. What the subject does is complex and never twice the same on different occasions: for example, he may use both hands or only one; he may trace the outline of the object with a single fingertip; or he may employ various combinations of rubbing, pressing, and grasping, perhaps using the palm and several fingertips at once.

An adequate neural theory of object perception in somesthesis (and probably in vision also) must therefore encompass phenomena such as the continuous interplay between sensation and movement, the integration of events occurring in both hemispheres simultaneously, the reconstruction of a spatial configuration from a temporal sequence of stimulations of the same point, and the equivalence of various movement-complexes in yielding samples of information sufficient to specify, rather than represent, the object. No simple notion of spatial isomorphism between a pattern of receptor stimulation and its projection in the somatotopically-organized sensory cortex appears adequate to account for the facts of behavior, just as similar notions have been judged to be inadequate to explain visual pattern perception (HEBB, 1949). Likewise, it appears doubtful that a satisfactory theory will emerge automatically from neurophysiological studies of single-cell activity, valuable though these studies are in their own right.

The assumption that the single cortical cell is the perceptual unit, and hence that only those cells which carry specific information about stimulus quality and position can contribute to discrimination, is not obligatory. In fact, this view implies that a large proportion of the afferent inflow, made up of cells which are relatively nonspecific for mode and place, constitutes "noise" which must be inhibited to permit accuracy of discrimination. ERICKSON (1968) has criticized this uneconomical conception of stimulus coding and presents the alternative hypothesis that perceptual information exists in the form of relative amounts of activity across many neurons, the "across-fiber pattern". Thus broadly-tuned cells — those that respond to a relatively great range of the stimulus dimension to be encoded, or even to more than one dimension — may be as capable in the aggregate of mediating fine discrimination as are narrowly-tuned cells. In vision, for example, a "vertical edge detector", so-called because its peak of responsiveness is to the vertical, participates in distinctive across-fiber patterns representing lines of many different orientations. In the somesthetic pathways, there are many such broadly-tuned neurons, and a recognition of their possible role in across-fiber patterns representing perceptual variables might drastically change current views, especially with regard to the extra-lemniscal inflow. As mentioned above, the lack of specificity of many extra-lemniscal elements has led to the view that their activity is unhelpful, or even detrimental, to discriminative processes and consequently that they must function only in mediating pain and other "affective" or "protopathic" modes of sensation. SEMMES (1969) has criticized this view, basing her arguments on the phylogenetic history of the lemniscal and extra-lemniscal systems, the anatomical interrelations between them, and clues to their function from behavioral studies. Reinterpretation of the contrasting physiological properties of these systems may be needed, and ERICKSON's suggestion (derived from theories of YOUNG and HELMHOLTZ for color vision and of PFAFFMANN for taste quality) provides a potentially valuable first step. It is perhaps encouraging that hypotheses similar to ERICKSON's have been found useful in constructing neural models for functions other than discrimination, namely, memory and reinforcement (PFAFF, 1969).

Such hypotheses are directly testable only by neurophysiologic methods. The question of whether or not methods of coding other than single-neuron specificity are needed to explain discrimination can be attacked by lesion studies, however. If the lemniscal system, which contains the narrowly-tuned cells, is solely responsible for the discriminative aspects of sensation, then one would expect these capacities to be permanently lost following interruption of this input, or following removal of its cortical projection with consequent degeneration of the thalamic target of the medial lemniscus. Conversely, one would expect discrimination to be normal after lesions of the cortical areas which receive the broadly-tuned afferents of the extra-lemniscal system. It will be apparent from the studies to be described that these expectations are not borne out. Furthermore, as indicated above, since discrimination appears to involve an active, directed search for certain kinds of information about objects, it would be surprising if it were found to depend only on the vertical afferent systems; the supposition that horizontal cortico-cortical connections also contribute to the discriminative process is substantiated.

B. Effects of Lesions in the Lemniscal System

The lemniscal pathway, defined in the strict classical sense, consists of the dorsal columns of the spinal cord, their medullary nuclei (gracile and cuneate) which give rise to the medial lemniscus, the posteroventral thalamic nucleus and its radiations, and finally, the postcentral gyrus of the cerebral cortex. It is generally taught that this system is essential for fine tactual sensitivity, acuity, and localization, for position sense, and for stereognosis. Since electrophysiological experiments showed that the neurons of this pathway are arranged somatotopically, that they are the most specific with respect to the type of stimulation, that they have the smallest peripheral receptive fields, and that they are the most subject to orderly inhibitory processes (at least at the cerebral level), the evidence seemed compelling that it was these characteristics that made discrimination possible. Yet there is increasing evidence from direct studies of sensation in man and of discriminative behavior in animals that destruction of this pathway does not lead to severe and persisting impairment of the capacities for which it is said to be the neural substrate.

1. The Spinal Level

RABINER and BROWDER (1948) and COOK and BROWDER (1965) have studied the sensory status of human cases with surgical interruption of the dorsal column

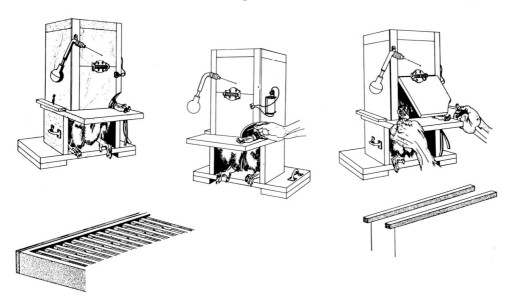

Fig. 1. Apparatus designed to permit passive stimulation of monkey's hand. Upper left, restraint box with subject seated inside. One hand protrudes through opening at right and is held by leather straps. Bulb at left is used to deliver a puff of air to subject's face as punishment for an error (pushing the hinged door open on a negative trial, i.e., one in which no tactile stimulus had been administered). Middle, experimenter about to stimulate subject's palm with one of a graded series of nylon filaments (shown in the case at lower left and individually at lower right). Small bulb mounted on right side of box is illuminated when hinged door is barely opened. Upper right, subject opening door on a positive trial and receiving a food reward. If the subject refrains from opening the door for 5 sec on a negative trial, he receives a food reward through the open top of the box. (From Schwartzman, R.J. and Semmes, J. The sensory cortex and tactile sensitivity. Exp. Neurol. **33**, 147–158, Fig. 1, 1971. Copyright 1971, Academic Press)

performed in the attempt to relieve pain from a cramped, abnormal posture of a phantom part. Although neurological examination showed that there was transient impairment of postural appreciation and of various forms of tactual discriminative sensation, permanent deficits were minimal or absent. One patient in the latter study is of particular interest since three fingers were intact on the same side as the section of the cuneate tract; the only persisting abnormality at 11 months after operation was a slight increase in the two-point threshold (from 4 mm to 6 mm).

It might be possible to dismiss these results as based on unverified lesions if the results in animals with verified dorsal column section were not highly confirmatory. Such a section in the monkey need not interfere permanently with weight discrimination (De Vito, 1954) nor with considerable recovery of proprioceptive placing (Christiansen, 1966). In monkeys trained to discriminate joint position, interruption of this path produced no elevation of threshold at the knee (Vierck, 1966) and only a slight elevation at the toe (Schwartzman and Bogdonoff, 1969). Vibration sense was also tested in the latter study, and no permanent deficit was noted. The results for the two-point threshold likewise indicated only slight or transient impairment (LEVITT and SCHWARTZMAN, 1966). Fig. 1 illustrates a technique devised by these investigators for testing the monkey's discrimination of a variety of passively-received tactual stimuli; the figure depicts a modification of the original apparatus now in use for testing the sensitivity of the hand to light touch (SCHWARTZMAN and SEMMES, 1971).

The conclusion is inescapable that the dorsal column-medial lemniscus pathway does not have the unique role that has been attributed to it, although evidence from the same studies suggests that it did participate in the formation and stability of the original gross discrimination habits which preceded the threshold determinations, as well as in the ultimate refinement of discrimination achieved. The maintenance or recovery of function demonstrated by the studies cited above, however, indicates that there must be other routes capable of sustaining a high level of discriminative sensation. In some of these studies, the dorsal column lesion was combined with interruption of the spinocervical or anterolateral tracts or both. The data show that marked and persistent deficits can be obtained when the spinocervical tract is included, but that total loss of function ensues only when the anterolateral paths are sectioned in addition (VIERCK, op. cit.; LEVITT and SCHWARTZMAN, op. cit.). An anterolateral lesion by itself does not impair limb position sense or two-point discrimination. Unfortunately, the effects on these abilities of sectioning the spinocervical tract by itself have not been determined.

This question is of particular interest since the results of studies on dogs and cats indicate that the spinocervical tract may be more important than the dorsal column. NORRSELL (1966) found that conditioned reflexes to light tactual stimuli (air puffs) on the hindleg in dogs were unaffected by unilateral or bilateral lesions of the dorsal column, but that unilateral destruction of the spinocervical tract did produce a deficit, although a transient one. That the dorsal column may serve the function in the absence of the spinocervical tract is suggested by the production of a severe, and in some cases, permanent impairment by a combination of the two lesions. The results of KITAI and WEINBERG (1968) provide an even clearer indication that the spinocervical tract plays the predominant role. Studying roughness discrimination of different degrees of difficulty in cats, these investigators showed that severance of this tract was followed by inability to learn even the easiest of the tasks, and that performance was as poor after this restricted lesion as after a tractotomy which included the dorsal column in addition; severance of only the dorsal column retarded the rate of learning, as compared with the rate in a sham-operated group, but did not affect the eventual level of performance. The authors note that the dorsal column-medial lemniscus pathway is phylogenetically newer than the lateral column system, of which the spinocervical tract is a part; the former is not well developed in animals below mammals, whereas the latter is prominent in lower species (based on KAPPERS, HUBER and CROSBY, 1936). It is possible that further development of the newer system has taken place in evolution, leading to dominance of the dorsal column in primates; the smallness of the deficit resulting from interruption of this path in man suggests, however, that even in the human species, another system must be capable of mediating a high degree of discrimination.

2. The Thalamo-Cortical Level

From its original anatomic meaning, the term "lemniscal" has been extended to designate a set of physiological properties characteristic of many individual neurons in the dorsal column-medial lemniscus system; the contrasting term "anterolateral" refers to the widely different properties of many neurons in the spinothalamic pathway (see POGGIO and MOUNTCASTLE, 1960). Thus any somatic afferent tract (or center) may be called lemniscal in this extended sense, if its neurons have at least some of the requisite properties. By this criterion, the spino-cervical tract and the neospinothalamic path in the anterolateral funiculus (as well as the cortical area S II) are classified by some authors as belonging to the lemniscal system (e.g., ALBE-FESSARD, 1967), although they may actually represent types of neuronal populations intermediate between the extremes along several, more or less independent, physiological dimensions. An additional reason for classing the tracts mentioned with the dorsal column is that, unlike the remaining somatic afferent channels, they all have as their thalamic target n. ventralis posterior. Their terminations within this nucleus are not identical, however, and BOWSHER (1965) suggests further that their cortical projections are partially separable, with S I being mainly activated by the dorsal column-medial lemniscus pathway and S II receiving its input mainly from the spinocervical and neospinothalamic components. If this suggestion is correct, then cortical ablations restricted to one or the other of these areas should have effects that correspond at least approximately to those obtained after selective transections of the spinal sensory tracts.

For lesions of S I as compared with dorsal column section, the results are consistent with the hypothesis. In man, surgical excisions invading the postcentral gyrus have been found to produce manual sensory deficits, especially in two-point discrimination and point localization (CORKIN et al., 1964), a finding which may be comparable to the residual elevation of the two-point threshold observed after interruption of the dorsal column. In experimental animals, it will be recalled that dorsal column section appeared to produce no permanent impairment, and likewise the deficits after S I ablation are generally described as transient. Since the work of RUCH and FULTON in the 1930's, it has been known that removal of the postcentral gyrus (which at that time was thought to be the only cortical projection area for somesthesis) has no permanent effects on weight or roughness discrimination; although sensitive measures of capacity (difference thresholds) were employed in their studies, the monkey and chimpanzee subjects showed only a temporary loss, regaining in a period of weeks their preoperative levels. The effects on other types of discrimination, not so far investigated after spinal tractotomies, have also been largely negative. COLE and GLEES (1954) made unilateral lesions of the postcentral hand area in monkeys trained to discriminate shapes (cone vs. pyramid); although all subjects initially showed a complete loss of the habit, more than half could be retrained to perform the task as well, or nearly as well, as they did preoperatively. An essentially similar result for temperature discrimination has recently been reported by CRAGG and DOWNER (1967). Monkeys were trained by approximation to discriminate with one hand between stimuli differing by about $1°C$ ($20°$ vs. $21°$). Removal of the postcentral gyrus, contralaterally or bilaterally, either failed to affect the threshold at all or elevated it by no more than $1°$, although extensions of the lesion posteriorly produced a somewhat greater loss.

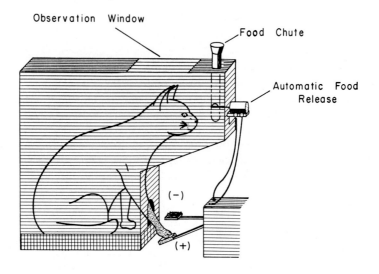

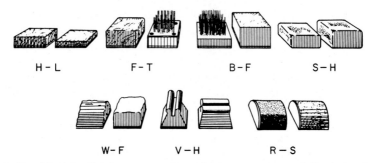

Fig. 2. Simplified sketch of apparatus for training cats on tactual discriminations. Pairs of interchangeable pedal mountings are shown at bottom. H–L, high *vs.* low pedal. F–T, flat wood *vs.* tines of plastic. B–F, bristles *vs.* flat wood. S–H, soft rubber *vs.* wood, both cloth covered. W–F, wedgeshaped block *vs.* flat block, both plastic covered. V–H, vertical *vs.* horizontal wooden ridges. R–S, rough ♯7 sandpaper *vs.* smooth wood, both half cylinders. (Adapted from Sperry, R.W. Cerebral organization and behavior. Science **133**, 1749–1757, Fig. 5, 1961. Copyright 1961, AAAS)

In other studies, ablations of S I have been made for the purpose of comparison with S II removals. On the basis of Bowsher's proposal that S II receives input originating mainly from the spinocervical tract, which at least in the dog and cat appears to be more important than the dorsal column, one would expect that lesions of S II might have greater effects than lesions of S I. Evidence bearing out this expectation has been obtained in some studies, but not in others. After bilateral removal of S I in dogs, Allen (1947) found loss but fairly rapid recovery of differential responses to brushing the skin of the back with the grain *vs.* against it, or with the grain at two different rates; bilateral removal of S II produced greater difficulty in relearning. ZUBEK's (1952) study in the cat also suggested that S II might be more important than S I for fine roughness discrimination. ORBACH and CHOW (1959) came to a different conclusion, however, from a study using monkeys tested on a variety of discriminations, including both easy and difficult roughness differences as well as size and form. In this study, bilateral S II lesions were found to have little if any effect, but bilateral lesions of S I produced deficits in retention and relearning. It is unclear whether or not the species difference can account for the apparent discrepancy in results, since more recent work in the cat tends to confirm the findings in the monkey, although the tasks used may not have been comparable to those which had revealed deficits after S II lesions in the earlier studies. Thus TEITELBAUM et al. (1968), employing a number of multiple-cue discriminations in cats, found no deficit in performance with the foreleg after contralateral or ipsilateral lesions of S II (see Fig. 2 for illustration of apparatus used), although the study did point to an important function of this area, to be discussed later. Contralateral removal of the foreleg area of S I was also found to be compatible with rapid acquisition of the same discrimination habits, if some weeks were allowed for recovery from the gross effects of this lesion, e.g., absent or deficient placing and hopping reactions.

The earlier positive results after lesions of S II might be ascribable to inadvertent interruption of fibers in their course to S I, a possibility recognized by many investigators but one which is difficult to evaluate without more detailed histological data than are presently available. Evidence bearing on this question might be obtained, however, by determining the effects of S II lesions in combination with removal of S I. If S II contributes to tactual discrimination, the combined lesion should produce greater decrement than removal of S I alone. Furthermore, on the assumption that such a combined lesion would completely destroy the lemniscal projection (even in the extended sense of the term "lemniscal"), its effects would indicate whether this projection is essential for discrimination; to permit an affirmative conclusion, it should be shown that discriminative capacities are abolished by destroying these areas in the contralateral hemisphere alone.

Although both ALLEN (op. cit.) and ZUBEK (op. cit.) found that animals with combined removal of S I and S II bilaterally were unable to reacquire the respective habits required (whereas preservation of either area made recovery possible), only ALLEN compared the effects of contralateral and bilateral lesions. The results showed that the lesions had to be bilateral in order to produce such a severe effect, thus indicating an extra-lemniscal contribution to discrimination, since the lemniscal projection is said to be restricted to the contralateral hemisphere. The findings of ORBACH and CHOW (op. cit.), based exclusively on bilateral lesions, raise other problems for the lemniscal theory of discrimination. These investigators found that combined removal of S I and S II was no more detrimental than removal of S I alone and that neither the single nor the combined lesion prevented relearning of any of the discriminations employed. Although the discrepant results of this and ALLEN's study on the contribution of S II remain unexplained, they agree in showing that there is considerable preservation of discriminative capacity after the lemniscal projection to the cortex has been destroyed.

Other studies dealing with the effects of bilateral combined lesions tend to reinforce this conclusion. Diamond et al. (1964) studied tactual localization in cats, the cues being repeated stimulation of the hindleg *vs.* alternating stimulation of the foreleg and hindleg. Combined removal of S I and S II caused loss of the habit, but relearning occurred as rapidly as had the original learning before operation; a subsequent transection of the dorsal columns (performed to interrupt fibers possibly transmitting to other cortical areas via the cerebellum) likewise failed to prevent relearning. Benjamin and Thompson (1959) showed that depriving infant cats of the lemniscal projection to S I and S II did not interfere with normal performance on any but the most difficult of a series of roughness discriminations, although their findings on most cats operated in adulthood agreed with those of Zubek (op. cit.), mentioned earlier.

One possibility of explaining the degree of discriminative ability remaining after removal of S I and S II opposite the tested limb is that a sufficient number of fibers of the lemniscal system to support discrimination terminate in other cortical areas. Support for this possibility is provided by the experiments of Norrsell (1967 a and b). Studying the same conditioned reflex — to light touch on the hindlimb — as the one he had previously employed to determine the most important spinal pathways (see above), he found that removal of the hindlimb portions of S I and S II produced only a transient deficit. Yet when dogs with this lesion were subjected to section of the spinocervical tract and the dorsal columns, a more marked and permanent impairment resulted, leading Norrsell to conclude that, "... the functional significance of the spinocervical tract and the dorsal columns for the tactile conditioned reflex may derive from sustaining transmission to central nervous loci other than S I and S II ..." (1967b, p. 86). With respect to the role of the sensory areas, Norrsell suggests two ways in which his findings can be viewed; either these areas are normally a part of the conditioned reflex circuit, but other tissue can substitute in their absence; or they are not normally a part of this circuit, but they exert a facilitating influence on it.

Insofar as complete removal of the recognized cortical sensory projection areas fails to reproduce the full effect of combined section of the two major spinal tracts classified as "lemniscal", as much of the evidence cited here suggests, one must agree with Norrsell that these tracts convey sensory information to other areas. To accept the conclusion that cortical areas lacking the properties of somatotopic organization and orderly inhibitory interaction can mediate discriminative sensation, however, is to give up some of the principles of the lemniscal theory of discrimination concerning stimulus coding. This is not to say that the organizational properties of S I and S II are without value in the processes underlying discrimination, but only to question whether the properties are as critical as proposed.

But in accounting for the surprisingly small effects of lesions of S I and S II so far demonstrated, another possibility deserves consideration. Not only may lemniscal fibers project to cortical areas other than S I and S II, but extra-lemniscal fiber-systems may be capable of mediating discrimination. Allen's finding that *bilateral* lesions of S I and S II are necessary to produce inability to relearn differential reactions to tactile stimuli seems to admit of no other explanation, if the current view is correct that the lemniscal projection is restricted to the contralateral hemisphere (but cf. GAZE and GORDON, 1954; COHEN, 1955). Likewise, since spinal lesions interrupting the anterolateral funiculus have been found in some instances to add to the deficit produced by section of the spinocervical tract and the dorsal columns (see above), it is not certain whether the exacerbation was due to involvement of the neospinothalamic component (which is considered "lemniscal") or of extra-lemniscal pathways. Lesions of the thalamic nucleus ventralis posterior, which receives the output from all three "lemniscal" tracts, would provide a conclusive test of the lemniscal theory of discrimination. If it were found that discriminative sensation is not abolished by destruction of this nucleus, it would have to be concluded that even the lemniscal properties relating to single units (place and mode specificity) are not essential to the residual ability, but that alternative methods of coding stimuli can be employed. Although no such studies have been reported as yet, evidence already exists indicating that section of the medial lemniscus (presumably including the neospinothalamic fibers and those emanating from the lateral cervical nucleus) does not abolish the ability of primates to discriminate weights (SJÖQVIST and WEINSTEIN, 1942). It would be useful to explore further the behavioral effects of lemniscus section using other somatic discriminations and other testing methods (e.g., passive rather than active tests).

With respect to the cortex, if regions other than S I and S II are part of the substrate of discriminative sensation, these regions must be identified and the nature of their contributions assessed before proceeding to the questions of the connections responsible and the code (or codes) by which information is received and transmitted further. It must be admitted that little definitive data are available even on the preliminary questions, although experiments have yielded potentially valuable facts and theories.

C. Effects of Cortical Lesions Outside the Lemniscal Projection Areas

1. The Motor Areas

The experiment of SJÖQVIST and WEINSTEIN (op. cit.) revealed that a combined section of the lemniscus and of the brachium conjunctivum produced a much greater impairment of weight discrimination than lemniscus section alone, suggesting that motor systems, by virtue of their afferent supply, play a role in sensory function. Analogous experiments at the cortical level (combined lesions of sensory and motor areas) have been attempted, but the results are difficult to evaluate because of the paralysis and ataxia that follow motor area lesions. RUCH and FULTON (1935) removed the anterior wall of the central fissure (the part of the motor area receiving the heaviest projection from the thalamus) after a previous ablation of the postcentral gyrus but were unable to detect any subsequent rise of weight discrimination thresholds. On the other hand, KRUGER and PORTER (1958) reported that only combined ablation of rolandic sensory and motor hand areas, generously defined, produced complete loss of discrimination between an erect and an inverted L-shape. Since the authors note, however, that the lesion caused the monkey subjects to have difficulty in finding and adequately palpating the stimulus objects, it is possible that the severity of the effect was attributable to the addition of a motor defect rather than to an increase in the sensory loss; or put differently, the effect may have resulted from loss of efferent fibers from, rather than afferent fibers to, the motor cortex. This question might be resolved by selective destruction of the output *vs.* the input of this area (an example of lesion-analysis) or by substituting a conditioned response to passive stimulation for the active discrimination test employed (an example of deficit-analysis).

There is still another possibility, however. The role of the motor cortex in sensory function might be viewed, not primarily in terms of its afferent or efferent connections with lower structures, but in terms of its participation in central processes. As pointed out earlier, the discrimination of objects and patterns suffers greatly when active exploration is not permitted. If the processes underlying "active touch" (Gibson, op. cit.) depend on central interaction between motor and sensory systems, then a lesion involving the motor cortex might have detrimental effects on discrimination by precluding, or reducing, such interaction. These effects could derive in part from loss of a "corollary discharge" (see Teuber, 1960), a postulated discharge from motor into sensory regions, occurring at the start of an active movement, which brings about changes in the central effects of the sensory input. This notion, which has proved useful in attempts to account for visual phenomena, such as the various "constancies", is at least equally likely to be relevant to somesthetic perception, considering the close relation between the somatic motor and sensory systems. Interaction in the opposite direction — from sensory into motor regions — might be assumed on the basis of the motor effects of lesions of postrolandic cortex. e. g., slight weakness, abnormalities of muscle tone, ataxia, impaired dexterity, and loss of certain postural reactions (see Cole and Glees, op. cit.). Semmes (1969, op. cit.) has suggested that the rolandic sensory and motor systems, with their similar somatotopic organizations and massive interconnections, evolved as one complex concerned with increasing the precision of sensory control over motor function and of motor control over sensory function. When this complex is damaged, other less efficient mechanisms of sensorimotor interaction presumably operate, either independently of or in conjunction with remaining rolandic tissue. Such auxiliary mechanisms may not be adequate for discrimination tasks like that used by Kruger and Porter, in which the differentiating cue must be obtained by active comparison of only certain corresponding parts of the stimulus objects.

Without further investigation, then, it cannot be assumed that the afferent projection to the motor cortex is responsible for recovery of function after removal of S I and S II, although the motor system may make an important contribution to active somesthetic discrimination by virtue of its connections with the sensory apparatus.

2. The Posterior Parietal Region

Among non-rolandic regions, the principal candidate for a critical role in somesthesis is the region just behind the postcentral gyrus, the so-called somesthetic association area. Damage to this region has long been known to produce defects, although, as is the case for the motor cortex, the nature of these defects and the related question of what connections make this region important are not fully understood. An old but still influential conception, deriving largely from neurological case studies, is that the posterior parietal cortex integrates the output from the postcentral gyrus and therefore mediates a higher level of function than that served by the primary projection area. In the ideal case, a pure posterior parietal lesion would therefore be expected to produce inability to perceive a pattern of somatic stimulation — such as an object, a shape, or an outline — despite preservation of sensitivity to touch, pain, warmth, and cold, as well as the ability to resolve and localize these stimuli; moreover, there should be no general disturbance of perception or mentation sufficient to account for the somesthetic impairment. It should be noted that this conception of the deficit after posterior parietal damage does not detract from the lemniscal theory of discrimination, since, stated more explicitly, the hypothesis implies that this region contains cells which "recognize" patterns of lemniscal activity.

Although it is doubtful that any clinical case which meets the above behavioral criteria has ever been observed, the presence of additional deficits at both lower and higher levels of complexity is generally ascribed to encroachments of the lesion on areas serving functions other than somesthetic integration. Turning to animal studies in which accurate placement of the lesion is achieved by surgery, the results are interpreted by some investigators as supporting the hypothesis, and by others, as denying it.

This line of research began with the study of BLUM et al. (1950) in which massive removals were made of posterior association cortex (including lateral temporal and preoccipital as well as parietal tissue) and impairments were found on both visual and somesthetic discrimination tasks. The visual impairment appeared to be more consistent and severe than the somesthetic and has proved to be the less difficult to analyze. CHOW (1951) and MISHKIN (1954) showed that the deficits on visual tasks could be attributed to removal of the inferior temporal region, and subsequent studies (PRIBRAM and BARRY, 1956; WILSON, 1957; BATES and ETTLINGER, 1960) demonstrated double dissociation of visual and somesthetic deficits following inferior temporal and posterior parietal lesions, respectively. Although this finding justifies the conclusion that these two parts of the posterior association cortex serve different functions, questions remain about the nature of each of these deficits, about whether or not they represent comparable losses in the two modalities, and about what connections enable these regions to contribute to discrimination learning.

WILSON (1965) suggests that the somesthetic deficits following posterior parietal ablation in monkeys are analogous to tactual agnosia in man, in the sense that the meaning of the stimulus objects (i. e., their significance for reward or non-reward) fails to develop at the normal rate. She supports this view by an analysis showing that these subjects exhibit weaker-than-normal responsiveness to all aspects of a tactual learning situation — the stimulus objects themselves, the position in which they are presented, and the reward contingencies — and thus are retarded in attaining the optimal strategy; in contrast, such animals are normally responsive to analogous aspects of a visual learning situation. This analysis, though ingenious and valuable, fails to answer the question of *why* animals with this lesion are relatively unreactive under the conditions of tactual testing employed, i.e., in the dark. Wilson rejects the notion that the lack of reactivity is attributable to a simple sensory loss, since these animals do not show a clear abnormality in spontaneous tactual preferences and aversions (Wilson and Wilson, 1964) or more than a slight deficit in roughness discrimination (Wilson et al., 1960).

Other investigators, more impressed with the disturbances seen outside of formal testing situations as a result of posterior parietal removal, disagree with Wilson's interpretation. These disturbances are loosely referred to as "sensory ataxias" and include a variety of phenomena such as awkwardness and poverty of movement, gross inaccuracy in reaching for desired objects, and often striking spatial disorientation (e.g., difficulty in finding the home cage when the monkey is released in an adjoining enclosure). It has been suggested that the key to the impairment in somesthetic discrimination learning lies in this group of more basic disturbances, although particular investigators take somewhat different views of the relationship. Pasik et al. (1958) were unable to detect an impairment after posterior parietal lesions on form or roughness discrimination tasks, ". . . if symptoms of ataxia were not allowed to interfere with performance in the test situation" (p. 435). This negative result is reminiscent of the failure of Ettlinger and Wegener (1958) to demonstrate an impairment on form or length discrimination in monkeys whose earlier training on a non-tactual task may have helped them to compensate for their "ataxia". Perhaps to be similarly explained is the finding of Pribram and Barry (op. cit.) that only the first of two somesthetic discriminations retested postoperatively revealed an impairment, regardless of whether this task involved differentiating forms or weights; however, the same animals did show a clear deficit on a later discrimination of lengths, a task which may have required more exploration and which was presented for initial postoperative learning rather than retention.

On the basis of the poverty of movement resulting from posterior parietal ablation, Bates and Ettlinger (op. cit.) suggest that impairment in tactual discrimination learning reflects a "selective motor retardation", which is especially prominent when animals are not permitted to use vision, and that such retardation might prevent them from exploring the test objects sufficiently to discriminate them. Ettlinger and Kalsbeck (1962), studying posterior parietal ablations made successively in the two hemispheres, found additional support for this idea, in that their monkeys made errors predominantly on trials when the positive stimulus was on the side contralateral to the more recent lesion. These authors also propose that a central disturbance of position sense results from this lesion, a disturbance which accounts for the inaccuracy of reaching even when vision is permitted; the evidence for this proposal was that, after a unilateral ablation, only the contralateral hand is inaccurate, and its inaccuracy is equally great regardless of whether the target is presented in one visual half-field or the other. Impaired position sense is not assumed to play any part in the somesthetic discrimination deficit, however, since ratings of inaccuracy of reaching and learning scores on discrimination tasks are not highly correlated. Nevertheless, an attempt by Moffett et al. (1967) to dissociate these two kinds of deficit by partial lesions of the posterior parietal region was unsuccessful: the abilities tapped by the discrimination and the reaching tasks seemed not only to share the same focus (which the authors believe to be the anterior parts of the inferior and superior parietal lobule) but also a similar gradient across the entire region.

Still a different view of deficits in somesthetic discrimination is held by SEMMES (1965) on the basis of studies in human subjects with brain injuries. She presents evidence that two factors enter into impaired discrimination of shapes by palpation: one factor is sensory deficit of the hand tested, and the other is a disorder in dealing with spatial relationships, which affects performance of both hands alike. Although the sensory factor was found to affect a variety of somesthetic discriminations, the spatial factor was specific to those involving shape (2-dimensional patterns and 3-dimensional forms), not affecting discriminations of roughness, texture, or size. SEMMES et al. (1955) had found earlier that the spatial disorder was supramodal, rather than restricted to behavior guided by vision (as orientational difficulties are classically assumed to be) or by touch (as might be assumed from its relation to tactual shape discrimination). It was proposed that such a disorder might operate in the miniature space encompassed by the hand just as it does in locomotor space. The two determinants of impaired shape discrimination were both associated with parietal lobe injury, although they seemed to be independent and additive: either was sufficient by itself to produce a significant deficit in appreciating differences between shapes, but when both were present, the deficit was greater than with either alone.

The wide diversity of opinion concerning the nature of the deficit in somesthetic discrimination after posterior parietal lesion is reflected in equally great differences in neural mechanisms suggested to account for it. WILSON's view that the deficit is akin to tactual agnosia is in harmony with the classical idea that this region integrates the outflow from the postcentral gyrus. But against this conception is, first, the paucity of fibers passing from the postcentral gyrus posteriorly (COLE and GLEES, op. cit.); in particular, these authors deny that any such fibers terminate in the inferior parietal area, yet lesions restricted to this locus produce at least as severe a deficit in discrimination as superior parietal removals (MOFFETT et al., op. cit.). And second, the deficits observed do not conform to those expected on the assumption that the posterior region is simply an integrative area for somesthesis alone. Impairment may be found in relatively simple somesthetic discriminations, as well as in those which would seem to require integration of cues (BLUM, 1951). Furthermore, the lesion appears to produce disabilities both in elementary sensation and in non-sensory functions to which the discrimination impairments can be linked.

Among the non-sensory disabilities, motor retardation and spatial disorientation have been implicated. The former is attributed to loss of the outflow from the posterior parietal region into the corticospinal tract (BATES and ETTLINGER, op. cit.), whereas the latter is thought to be based on the heterosensory inflow to this region (SEMMES, 1965). The relation of the motor and the spatial impairments to performance on somesthetic tasks indicates that the posterior parietal contribution does not rest simply on its cortico-cortical connections with the lemniscal system.

Evidence has been cited for a loss in proprioceptive sensibility, produced maximally by lesions of the same subareas as those which produce the maximal discrimination deficits. Although such loss after damage to area 5 (BRODMANN) could be explained by its projection from the thalamic nucleus of the lemniscal system (Krieg, 1963), the finding of a similar loss after damage confined to area 7, which receives no projection from this nucleus (and none from the postcentral gyrus), implicates an extra-lemniscal pathway. The early work of Ruch and Fulton likewise pointed to the importance of the extra-lemniscal input. Finding that posterior parietal removal was at least as damaging to weight and roughness discrimination thresholds as was ablation of the postcentral gyrus, and that combined lesion of the two areas resulted in more severe and permanent deficit, they concluded that, "The experiments are difficult to interpret by the traditional concept of a postcentral gyrus which receives all sensory impulses and transmits them to the posterior parietal association area ... Both subregions appear capable of independent function, which implies that the posterior parietal lobule receives an independent projection" (Fulton, 1943, pp. 362–363). The independent projection was thought to be that arising from n. lateralis posterior, one of the group of nuclei whose cells have markedly different properties from those of cells in the lemniscal nucleus (Poggio and Mountcastle, op. cit.). These data and their implications emphasize the need to consider other methods of stimulus coding than those characteristic of the lemniscal system in accounting for discriminative sensation.

3. The Ipsilateral Sensorimotor Region

Although it has long been known that there are somatic afferents from the limbs, as well as the face, terminating in the ipsilateral hemisphere (in S II, the motor areas, the association cortex, and even some in S I), it has been assumed that this projection plays no part in sensory discrimination. This assumption rested on three lines of evidence: human cases studied by neurological examination, in which one side of the body is customarily used as a control for the other; single-unit analyses in animals, showing that cells with ipsilateral or bilateral receptive fields exhibit little specificity for mode or place; and a few behavioral studies, in which negative results were obtained with ablations ipsilateral to the part tested (e.g., Allen, op. cit.; Ettlinger and Kalsbeck, op. cit.; Kruger and Porter, op. cit.). In Allen's study, however, it was found that contralateral lesions were followed by recovery, whereas bilateral lesions produced an apparently complete and permanent deficit, as previously mentioned. Norrsell (1966a), studying bilateral successive lesions, also found evidence for an ipsilateral contribution, manifested chiefly in the more pronounced and lasting effects on a given limb of a contralateral lesion added to an ipsilateral than of a contralateral lesion alone.

Detrimental effects of lesions which seemed to be restricted to the ipsilateral hemisphere were noted by Semmes et al. (1960) in a study of brain-injured human cases which employed an appropriate normal control group. Ipsilateral deficits were found mainly on a passive test of point localization, a result which was later confirmed by Corkin et al. (op. cit.) on subjects with surgical excisions, although effects on other discrimination tasks have also been shown (Weinstein et al., 1958; Vaughan and Costa, 1962; Semmes, 1965).

Since the presumed unilaterality of the lesion in the human subjects was not verified histologically, Semmes and Mishkin (1965) undertook a study in monkeys. Performance on the battery of somesthetic discrimination tasks shown in Fig. 3

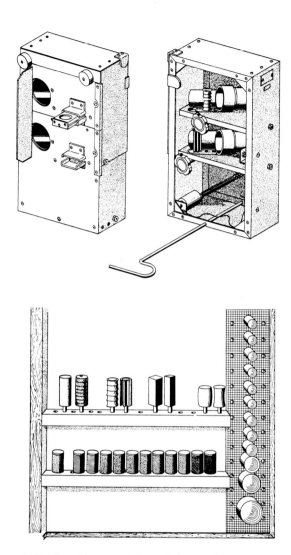

Fig. 3. Apparatus and stimulus objects used for training monkeys on tactual discriminations. Top left, monkey's view of discrimination box. Subject reaches between bars of his cage to insert his left arm into one or the other of the tubes; the bend in the tubes (45° plumber's elbows), together with the barrier at extreme left, precludes vision of the stimulus objects. Food-drawers are on right, with upper one protruded and containing a peanut. Top right, experimenter's view of box. A pair of stimulus objects is shown in place, with the upper one advanced as though the subject had made the correct instrumental pulling response. Small light bulb at inside right is illuminated when either the positive or negative object is pulled forward far enough to barely expose the edge of the food-well. Handle inserted through lower frame of box is used to move the box forward and backward on tracks. Lower sketch shows some of the stimulus objects used. On upper shelf are, from left to right, Hard-Soft, Horizontal-Vertical, Square-Diamond, and Convex-Concave. At extreme right are a series of cylinders, differing in diameter, used in determining size thresholds. On lower shelf are a series of cylinders, identical in size but covered with different grades of sandpaper, used in determining roughness thresholds

was compared in three groups — unoperated animals, animals with removal of the entire sensorimotor cortex (S I, S II, M I, M II, and the posterior parietal region) of the hemisphere ipsilateral to the hand tested, and animals with removal of the remainder of the same hemisphere (the prefrontal, temporal, occipital, and cingulate regions, together with a nearly complete section of the corpus callosum). Although the sensorimotor lesion group learned the initial easy tasks with normal facility, they were significantly impaired in learning more difficult form discriminations and showed a marked elevation of roughness thresholds. In contrast, there was no decrement on any task in the nonsensorimotor lesion group, despite the greater mass of tissue destroyed. The results show that unilateral lesions affect the hand on the same side in some of its discriminative functions. Among the possible explanations of the effect that were considered, loss of the ipsilateral projection seemed the most probable. On the basis of the lack of effect of the sensorimotor lesion on size discrimination thresholds (presumably a test of position sense of the fingers), the authors suggest that the ipsilateral projection contributes less to kinesthesis than to touch-pressure sensibility.

4. The Nonsensorimotor Cortex

The technique of combining section of the forebrain commissures with a massive unilateral ablation sparing only an island of cortex has been useful in attacking the question of whether or not regions outside the recognized sensory projection zones are necessary for discrimination learning and memory. For vision, the answer is assuredly in the affirmative, as shown by the detrimental effects of isolating the striate cortex using this technique (Sperry et al., 1960), as well as by effects demonstrated in other studies to follow bilateral extrastriate lesions. For somesthesis, however, Sperry (1959) came to the opposite conclusion on the basis of failure to detect deficits in cats with isolation of the sensorimotor region contralateral to the tested paw. The inapplicability of this conclusion to monkeys, evident in the deficits after bilateral posterior parietal or ipsilateral sensorimotor lesions already mentioned, may be the consequence of the widely different organization of the carnivore and primate brains (Diamond and Hall, 1969). That the substrate of somesthetic discriminative behavior in the monkey extends even beyond these additional areas was shown in a study by Semmes et al. (1968), modelled after Sperry's, but with modifications of the lesion such that the posterior parietal region was included in the spared island and the prefrontal region excluded. This study revealed a severe deficit on the first two of a battery of somesthetic tasks, which was interpreted as difficulty in acquiring the basic strategies of learning by palpation, possibly stemming from a condition akin to unilateral "neglect". In an extension of the study, Semmes et al. (1969) found that the deficit was attributable equally to the prefrontal and the temporal parts of the nonsensorimotor removal. The results agree with previous reports of deficit on somesthetic discrimination tasks after bilateral prefrontal removals (Ettlinger and Wegener, op. cit.; Orbach and Fischer, 1959; Iversen, 1964) and may also be related to the impairment of tactual reversal learning found after destruction of the hippocampus (Teitelbaum, 1964; Webster and Voneida, 1964); in addition, since the effects are obtainable by unilateral ablation plus commissurotomy as well as by bilateral ablation, they appear to be based on interruption of connections within the telencephalon probably between the sensorimotor cortex governing the tested hand and the critical prefrontal and temporal loci.

The use of the split-brain preparation has also led to evidence possibly implicating the nonsensorimotor cortex in recall of a somesthetic discrimination habit. Research using this preparation to investigate memory has focussed on habit transfer from a trained to an untrained hand, a phenomenon which has been taken to indicate that unimanual learning sets up a memory trace not only in the "trained hemisphere" but also in the "untrained". This research can be divided into two categories: one in which the commissurotomy is performed prior to training of the first hand, and the other in which the first hand is trained prior to operation, thus allowing the trace to be formed normally in the intact brain.

Experiments of the first category have shown repeatedly that the corpus callosum is important in setting up the trace in the untrained hemisphere (STAMM and SPERRY, 1957; GLICKSTEIN and SPERRY, 1960; EBNER and MYERS, 1962; MEIKLE et al., 1962; LEE-TENG and SPERRY, 1966). MYERS and EBNER (1962) found that the posterior body of the callosum was critically involved. Since the two S I hand areas are not directly connected across the callosum (EBNER and MYERS, op. cit.; PANDYA and VIGNOLO, 1968), it was clear that the callosal path concerned in intermanual transfer must arise and terminate elsewhere. For the cat, TEITELBAUM et al. (op. cit.) found that a unilateral lesion of S II in either hemisphere mimics the effect of callosal section, preventing transfer in both directions, whereas a lesion of the forepaw area of S I blocks transfer from the damaged to the normal hemisphere but not vice versa. The results suggested that the transcallosal paths the authors had demonstrated by electrophysiological methods (from S I and S II of one hemisphere to the opposite S II) are necessary for transfer; nevertheless, since lesions of these areas had little or no effect on learning or retention with the first paw, neither S I nor S II can be considered the site of the memory trace in the trained hemisphere.

For the monkey, ETTLINGER (1962) presented evidence that either bilateral or unilateral posterior parietal removal impairs intermanual transfer. However, when ETTLINGER and MORTON (1966) attempted to confirm this effect and compare it with that following callosal section, they found that neither the lesion nor the section interfered with transfer. Since in two of their animals the interthalamic commissure (GLEES and WALL, 1948) had been sectioned along with the callosum, they favor the view that the ipsilateral sensory projection is capable under some conditions of setting up the memory trace in the untrained hemisphere. It should be noted further that even in the studies which revealed the importance of the callosal connections (see above) there was partial transfer in some of the subjects, suggesting an alternative route. If the ipsilateral projection is responsible for the residual capacity, it would imply an extra-lemniscal contribution to formation and maintenance of the memory trace.

Experiments of the second category (in which commissurotomy is performed after the original unimanual training) are based on the assumption that for some habits the memory trace is formed entirely or predominantly in the hemisphere contralateral to the experienced hand, even though the interhemispheric commissures are intact. Thus when the inexperienced hand is tested, the hemisphere governing it has to "reach across" the callosum in order to have access to the trace. For vision, Myers (1957) showed that commissurotomy after training of the first eye in chiasma-sectioned cats impaired interocular transfer of a difficult pattern discrimination. Myers and Sperry (1958) then attempted to localize the memory trace by ablating parts of the trained hemisphere instead of sectioning the commissures; they concluded that the visual trace is localized in the visual receptive cortex on the basis of comparisons between lesions restricted to this area *vs.* more extensive removals including it. For somesthesis, Semmes and Mishkin (1965) performed a somewhat similar experiment in monkeys, with the difference that sensorimotor lesions of the trained hemisphere (including the entire parietal lobe and the motor areas) were compared with non-overlapping removals of the remainder of this hemisphere. Equal deficits in recall (i. e., transfer) of a difficult form discrimination were obtained from the two lesions, and each appeared to reproduce the full effect of commissurotomy. Since the sensorimotor ablation was found later to affect original learning of the same discrimination with the ipsilateral hand (the one tested for transfer), the apparent deficit in recall may actually have been of a different nature. The nonsensorimotor lesion, however, does not affect learning or performance with the hand on the same side, and hence the deficit cannot be explained away in the same manner. Damage to limbic structures, notably those deep in the temporal lobe, are known to affect learning and retention without regard to modality, at least in man; although memories established prior to damage (as was the case for the habits in the study just described) are thought to be undisturbed, such a dissociation of effects is difficult to establish with certainty. In any case, the apparent discrepancy between vision and somesthesis in effects of lesions outside the receptive areas remains unresolved, and it is fair to conclude that no general principle governing localization of memory for a discrimination habit has emerged.

5. Concluding Comment

It is clear that much remains to be done before the neural basis of somesthetic discrimination can be understood. On the basis of existing evidence, however, it can be said that the identification of discriminative sensation solely with the lemniscal system (whether in the strict or the extended sense of the term) is too narrow a view. Although the physiological properties of this system, as contrasted with those of extra-lemniscal pathways, have been thought to be the *sine qua non* of discrimination, the lemniscal method of stimulus coding is obviously neither the only possible one nor the only one actually employed by the nervous system in serving various kinds of discrimination in other sensory modalities. However plausible the lemniscal theory of discrimination may appear when only the electrophysiological evidence is taken into account, behavioral studies of the effects of central nervous damage provide direct evidence against it. Experiments on spinal tractotomies have shown that little permanent impairment of discriminative capacities results from interruption of the dorsal columns, which possess the lemniscal properties to the highest degree, and have further indicated that a phylogenetically older pathway, the spinocervical tract, may be more important in conveying discriminative information, at least in the cat and dog. The results of cortical excisions likewise show that the areas to which tracts with lemniscal properties are known to project — namely, S I and S II — are not essential for discrimination. Excisions of these areas may result in loss of habits acquired preoperatively, and they may retard reacquisition even of gross discriminations; nevertheless, the available evidence indicates that, with time and retraining, a high level of discrimination can be achieved.

The lemniscal theory of discrimination is weakened not only by the absence of severe and permanent deficits in discrimination after lesions of S I and S II but also by the presence of deficits after lesions sparing these areas. Posterior parietal ablations are followed by marked impairment of position sense (shown by inaccuracy of reaching for targets) and by elevation of thresholds for discriminating differences in weight, roughness, and temperature, although compensation for deficits after this lesion also takes place. Evidence from combined removal of postcentral and posterior parietal regions suggests that the latter is an extralemniscal projection area and that some of the effects of the removal stem from loss of this projection. An even clearer indication of an extralemniscal contribution to discrimination is found in the impairments of touch-pressure sensibility (noted chiefly in point localization and in roughness thresholds) following lesions of the sensorimotor region ipsilateral to the tested hand, impairments which are not dependent on interruption of callosal connections. Thus the intactness of the lemniscal system is not sufficient to guarantee that the sensory processes underlying discrimination are normal.

If the lemniscal theory does not fully encompass such sensory processes, still less does it offer a satisfactory account of the larger topic of how objects are perceived and discriminated. Characteristically, perceiving an object by touch is not a mere "recognition" of a pattern by master cells onto which lemniscal units converge, but rather a reconstruction, influenced by already existing perceptual schemata, from partial impressions gained through active exploration. Brain lesions which disrupt such schemata (e.g., those which produce the supramodal form of spatial disorientation) or those which interfere with exploratory activity therefore impair somesthetic perception of objects. The contribution of non-sensory, as well as sensory, factors to such perception may account for the results of lesion studies which have revealed the participation of widespread regions of the brain.

References

ALBE-FESSARD, D.: Organization of somatic central projection. In: Contributions to sensory physiology. Vol. 2. New York: Academic Press 1967.

ALLEN, W.F.: Effect of partial and complete destruction of the tactile cerebral cortex on correct conditioned differential foreleg responses from cutaneous stimulation. Amer. J. Physiol. 151, 325–337 (1947).

BATES, J.A.V., ETTLINGER, G.: Posterior biparietal ablations in the monkey. A.M.A. Arch. Neurol. 3, 177–192 (1960).

BENJAMIN, R.M., THOMPSON, R.F.: Differential effects of cortical lesions in infant and adult cats on roughness discrimination. Exp. Neurol. 1, 305–321 (1959).

BLUM, J.S.: Cortical organization in somesthesis: effects of lesions in posterior associative cortex on somatosensory function in Macaca mulatta. Comp. Psychol. Monog. 20, 219–249 (1951).

Blum, J.S., Chow, K.L., Pribram, K.H.: A behavioral analysis of the organization of the parieto-temporo-preoccipital cortex. J. comp. Neurol. 93, 53–100 (1950).

Bowsher, D.: The anatomophysiological basis of somatosensory discrimination. Int. Rev. Neurobiol. 8, 35–75 (1965).

Chow, K.L.: Effects of partial extirpations of the posterior association cortex on visually mediated behavior in monkeys. Comp. Psychol. Monog. 20, 187–217 (1951).

Christiansen, J.: Neurological observations of macaques with spinal cord lesions. Anat. Rec. 154, 330 (1966).

Cohen, S.M.: Ascending pathways activating thalamus of cat. J. Neurophysiol. 18, 33–43 (1955).

Cole, J., Glees, P.: Effects of small lesions in sensory cortex in trained monkeys. J. Neurophysiol. 17, 1–13 (1954).

Cook, A.W., Browder, E.J.: Function of posterior columns in man. Arch. Neurol. 12, 72–79 (1965).

Corkin, S., Milner, B., Rasmussen, T.: Effects of different cortical excisions on sensory thresholds in man. Trans. Amer. neurol. Ass. 112–116 (1964).

Cragg, B.G., Downer, J. de C.: Behavioral evidence for cortical involvement in manual temperature discrimination in the monkey. Exp. Neurol. 19, 433–442 (1967).

DeVito, J.: Study of sensory pathways in monkeys, Ph. D. thesis, University of Washington 1954.

Diamond, I.T., Hall, W.C.: Evolution of neocortex. Science 164, 251–262 (1969).

Diamond, I.T., Randall, W., Springer, L.: Tactual localization in cats deprived of cortical areas SI and SII and the dorsal columns. Psychon. Sci. 1, 261–262 (1964).

Ebner, F.F., Myers, R.E.: Corpus callosum and the interhemispheric transmission of tactual learning. J. Neurophysiol. 25, 380–391 (1962).

Erickson, R.P.: Stimulus coding in topographic and nontopographic afferent modalities: on the significance of the activity of individual sensory neurons. Psychol. Rev. 75, 447–465 (1968).

Ettlinger, G.: Interhemispheric integration in the somatic sensory system. In: Interhemispheric relations and cerebral dominance. Baltimore: Johns Hopkins Press 1962.

Ettlinger, G., Kalsbeck, J.E.: Changes in tactile discrimination and in visual reaching after successive and simultaneous bilateral posterior parietal ablations in the monkey. J. Neurol. Neurosurg. Psychiat. 25, 256–268 (1962).

Ettlinger, G., Wegener, J.: Somaesthetic alternation discrimination and orientation after frontal and parietal lesions in monkeys. Quart. J. exp. Psychol. 10, 177–186 (1958).

Fulton, J.F.: Physiology of the nervous system, Second Edition. New York: Oxford University Press 1943.

Gaze, R.M., Gordon, G.: The representation of cutaneous sense in the thalamus of the cat and monkey. Quart. J. exp. Physiol. 39, 279–304 (1954).

Gibson, J.J.: Observations on active touch. Psychol. Rev. 69, 477–491 (1962).

Glees, P., Wall, P.D.: Commissural fibers of the macaque thalamus — an experimental study. J. comp. Neurol. 88, 129–137 (1948).

Glickstein, M., Sperry, R.W.: Intermanual somesthetic transfer in "split-brain" rhesus monkeys. J. comp. physiol. Psychol. 53, 322–327 (1960).

Hebb, D.O.: The organization of behavior: a neuropsychological theory. New York: John Wiley and Sons 1949.

Iversen, S.D.: Tactile learning and memory in baboons after temporal and frontal lesions. Exp. Neurol. 18, 228–238 (1967).

Lee-Teng, E., Sperry, R.W.: Intermanual stereognostic size discrimination in split-brain monkeys. J. comp. physiol. Psychol. 62, 84–89 (1966).

Levitt, M., Schwartzman, R.J.: Spinal sensory tracts and two-point tactile sensitivity. Anat. Rec. 154, 377 (1966).

Kitai, S.T., Weinberg, J.: Tactile discrimination study of the dorsal column-medial lemniscus system and spino-cervico-thalamic tract in cat. Exp. Brain Res. 6, 234–246 (1968).

Krieg, W.J.S.: Connections of the cerebral cortex. Evanston, Ill.: Brain Books 1963.

Kruger, L., Porter, P.: A behavioral study of the functions of the rolandic cortex in the monkey. J. comp. Neurol. 109, 439–469 (1958).

MEIKLE, T. H., JR., SECHZER, J. A., STELLAR, E.: Interhemispheric transfer of tactile conditioned responses in corpus callosum-sectioned cats. J. Neurophysiol. **25**, 530–543 (1962).

MISHKIN, M.: Visual discrimination performance following partial ablations of the temporal lobe: II. Ventral surface vs. hippocampus. J. comp. physiol. Psychol. **47**, 187–193 (1954).

MOFFETT, A., ETTLINGER, G., MORTON, H. B., PIERCY, M. F.: Tactile discrimination performance in the monkey: the effect of ablation of various subdivisions of posterior parietal cortex. Cortex **3**, 59–96 (1967).

MYERS, R. E.: Corpus callosum and interhemispheric communcation: enduring memory effects. Fed. Proc. **16**, 92 (1957).

MYERS, R. E., EBNER, F. F.: Localization of tactual gnostic functions in corpus callosum. Neurology **12**, 303 (1962).

MYERS, R. E., SPERRY, R. W.: Interhemispheric communication through the corpus callosum. Arch. Neurol. Psychiat. (Chic.) **80**, 298–303 (1958).

NORRSELL, U.: The spinal afferent pathways of conditioned reflexes to cutaneous stimuli in the dog. Exp. Brain Res. **2**, 269–282 (1966).

NORRSELL, U.: A conditioned reflex study of sensory defects caused by cortical somatosensory ablations. Physiol. Behav. **2**, 73–81 (1967a).

NORRSELL, U.: Afferent pathways of a tactile conditioned reflex after cortical somatosensory ablations. Physiol. Behav. **2**, 83–86 (1967b).

ORBACH, J., CHOW, K. L.: Differential effects of resections of somatic areas I and II in monkeys. J. Neurophysiol. **22**, 195–203 (1959).

ORBACH, J., FISCHER, G. J.: Bilateral resections of frontal granular cortex. A.M.A. Arch. Neurol. **1**, 78–86 (1959).

PANDYA, D. N., VIGNOLO, L. A.: Interhemispheric neocortical projections of somatosensory areas I and II in the rhesus monkey. Brain Res. **7**, 300–303 (1968).

PASIK, P., PASIK, T., BATTERSBY, W. S., BENDER, M. B.: Visual and tactual discriminations by macaques with serial temporal and parietal lesions. J. comp. physiol. Psychol. **51**, 427–436 (1958).

PFAFF, D.: Parsimonious biological models of memory and reinforcement. Psychol. Rev. **76**, 70–81 (1969).

PRIBRAM, H. B., BARRY, J.: Further behavioral analysis of parieto-temporo-preoccipital cortex. J. Neurophysiol. **19**, 99–106 (1956).

RABINER, A. M., BROWDER, E. J.: Concerning conduction of touch and deep sensibilities through spinal cord. Trans. Amer. neurol. Ass. **73**, 137 (1948).

RUCH, T. C., FULTON, J. F.: Cortical localization of somatic sensibility; the effect of precentral, postcentral and posterior parietal lesions upon the performance of monkeys trained to discriminate weights. Res. Publ. Ass. nerv. ment. Dis. **15**, 289–330 (1935).

SCHWARTZMAN, R. J., BOGDONOFF, M. D.: Proprioception and vibration sensibility discrimination in the absence of the posterior columns. Arch. Neurol. **20**, 349–353 (1969).

SEMMES, J.: A non-tactual factor in astereognosis. Neuropsychologia **3**, 295–315 (1965).

SEMMES, J.: Manual stereognosis after brain injury. In: Oral sensation and perception. Springfield: C. C. Thomas 1967.

SEMMES, J.: Protopathic and epicritic sensation: a reappraisal. In: Contributions to clinical neuropsychology. Chicago: Aldine 1969.

SEMMES, J., MISHKIN, M.: Somatosensory loss in monkeys after ipsilateral cortical ablation. J. Neurophysiol. **28**, 473–486 (1965).

SEMMES, J., MISHKIN, M.: A search for the cortical substrate of tactual memories. In: Functions of the corpus callosum. London: J. and A. Churchill 1965.

SEMMES, J., MISHKIN, M., COLE, M.: Effects of isolating sensorimotor cortex in monkeys. Cortex **4**, 301–327 (1968).

SEMMES, J., MISHKIN, M., DEUEL, R. K.: Somesthetic discrimination learning after partial nonsensorimotor lesions in monkeys. Cortex **5**, 331–350 (1969).

SEMMES, J., WEINSTEIN, S., GHENT, L., TEUBER, H. L.: Somatosensory changes after penetrating brain wounds in man. Cambridge, Mass.: Harvard University Press 1960.

SEMMES, J., WEINSTEIN, S., GHENT, L., TEUBER, H. L.: Spatial orientation in man after cerebral injury: I. Analyses by locus of lesion. J. Psychol. **39**, 227–244 (1955).

SJÖQVIST, O., WEINSTEIN, E. A.: The effect of section of the medial lemniscus on proprioceptive functions in chimpanzees and monkeys. J. Neurophysiol. **5**, 69–74 (1942).

SPERRY, R. W.: Preservation of high-order function in isolated somatic cortex in callosum-sectioned cat. J. Neurophysiol. **22**, 78–87 (1959).

SPERRY, R. W., MYERS, R. E., SCHRIER, A. M.: Perceptual capacity of the isolated visual cortex in the cat. Quart. J. exp. Psychol. **12**, 65–71 (1960).

STAMM, J. S., SPERRY, R. W.: Function of corpus callosum in contralateral transfer of somesthetic discriminations in cats. J. comp. physiol. Psychol. **50**, 138–143 (1957).

TEITELBAUM, H.: A comparison of effects of orbitofrontal and hippocampal lesions upon discrimination learning and reversal in the cat. Exp. Neurol. **9**, 452–462 (1964).

TEITELBAUM, H., SHARPLESS, S. K., BYCK, R.: Role of somatosensory cortex in interhemispheric transfer of tactile habits. J. comp. physiol. Psychol. **66**, 623–632 (1968).

TEUBER, H. L.: Perception. In: Handbook of Physiol. Neurophysiol. Vol. III. Washington, D. C.: Amer. Physiol. Soc. 1960.

VAUGHAN, H. G., JR., COSTA, L. D.: Performance of patients with lateralized cerebral lesions. J. nerv. ment. Dis. **134**, 237–243 (1962).

VIERCK, C. J.: Spinal pathways mediating limb position sense. Anat. Rec. **154**, 437 (1966).

WEBSTER, D. B., VONEIDA, T. J.: Learning deficits following hippocampal lesions in split-brain cats. Exp. Neurol. **10**, 170–182 (1964).

WEINSTEIN, S.: Intensive and extensive aspects of tactile sensitivity as a function of body part, sex, and laterality. In: The Skin Senses. Springfield: C. C. Thomas 1968.

WEINSTEIN, S., SEMMES, J., GHENT, L., TEUBER, H. L.: Roughness discrimination after penetrating brain injury in man: Analysis according to locus of lesion. J. comp. physiol. Psychol. **51**, 269–275 (1958).

WILSON, M.: Effects of circumscribed cortical lesions upon somesthetic and visual discrimination in the monkey. J. comp. physiol. Psychol. **50**, 630–635 (1957).

WILSON, M.: Tactual discrimination learning in monkeys. Neuropsychologia **3**, 353–361 (1965).

WILSON, M., STAMM, J. S., PRIBRAM, K. H.: Deficits in roughness discrimination after posterior parietal lesions in monkeys. J. comp. physiol. Psychol. **53**, 535–539 (1960).

WILSON, M., WILSON, W. A.: Visual and tactual preferences in normal and brain-operated monkeys. Anim. Behav. **12**, 227–230 (1964).

ZUBEK, J. P.: Studies in somesthesis. II. Role of somatic sensory areas I and II in roughness discrimination in cat. J. Neurophysiol. **15**, 401–408 (1952).

Chapter 19

Electrical Stimulation of Cortex in Human Subjects, and Conscious Sensory Aspects

By

Benjamin Libet, San Francisco (USA)

With 7 Figures

Contents

A. Introduction

Most problems in neurophysiology can be attacked more fruitfully in animals other than man, for the obvious reasons of controllability of conditions and of our moral restraints on the experimental procedures which are tolerable for human studies. But if one wants to investigate cerebral mechanisms underlying subjective experience (of sensation, in the present context), it should also be obvious that recourse must be had to human subjects for primary validation of the subjective phenomenon under study. Direct approaches to the brain of waking subjects are of course limited by compatibility with therapeutic procedures and by the patient's condition and informed consent. Electrical stimulation of (and, more recently, recording from) the cerebral cortex and deeper structures has provided one approach which, when suitably utilized, makes possible informative studies with no irreversible effects on the subject. The problems susceptible to investigation can be much broader than the initial classical one of the topographical relations of cortical sites to the body sites of the subjectively referred sensations, and some of these problems will be considered in this article.

B. "Excitable" Somatosensory Cortex

1. Topography

Since the initial experiments by Fritsch and Hitzig (1870) on electrical stimulation of the cerebral cortex of dogs, it has been recognized that only certain cortical areas would give rise to motor responses, when stimulated with subconvulsive strengths of current. Later, Cushing (1909) demonstrated that sensory experiences without movement also could be elicited in conscious patients upon stimulation of postcentral gyrus[1]. The areas of "excitable" cortex in man, that is those areas where electrical stimulation gives rise to motor or conscious sensory responses, were subsequently enlarged (Fig. 1) especially by the extensive investigations of Foerster (1936a, b, c) and of Penfield and his collaborators (Penfield and Boldrey, 1937; Penfield and Rasmussen, 1950; Penfield and Jasper, 1954; Penfield, 1958). The extent of such areas may vary with the condition of the subject, particularly as to whether his pathological disorder is one (like epilepsy) which affects cortical excitability; and it may vary with the stimulus parametric values employed, i. e., in relation to the range between threshold values (for motor, sensory or evoked electrical responses) and the values for producing seizure activity (either overt motor or sensory, or local electrical convulsive-type wave patterns).

Using stimulus trains at strengths below electrical seizure-wave production, the Penfield group (see Fig. 1) could consistently elicit motor responses in epileptic subjects only when applying such stimuli to the Rolandic region (mainly in precentral areas) and to supplementary motor area (superior mesial surface of cortex anterior to the precentral gyrus; see Penfield and Welch, 1951; Ber-

---

[1] A historical summary of the initial studies of motor and sensory responses to cortical stimulation in animals and man is given by Penfield and Boldrey (1937), Penfield and Rasmussen (1950), and Penfield and Jasper (1954). Therefore, reference will be made here to the earlier works only incidentally, to help clarify points under discussion.

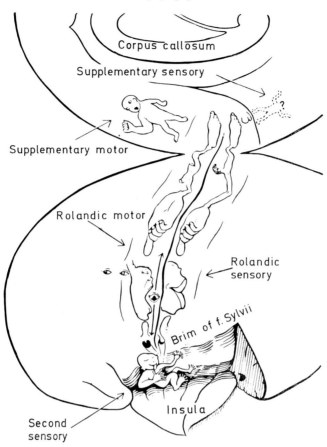

Fig. 1. Somatic figurines drawn on the left hemisphere. (1) *Rolandic Figurines*. The size and position of the figurine parts correspond roughly with the extent of Rolandic cortex devoted to the sensation or movement, respectively, of those parts. (Tongue, pharynx and intra-ab-dominal areas are indicated below the face region). (2) *The Second Sensory Figurine*. This indicates only that the face is above arms and arms above legs and that the representation is, to a larger extent, contralateral and, to a lesser extent, ipsilateral. The tips of fingers and toes are made to seem important. (3) *Supplementary Figurines*. These are represented on the medial aspect of the hemisphere, flipped upwards in the diagram. The *motor* figure is assuming the posture most often produced by stimulation, but no fixed topographical localization of the parts of the body or of vocalization, autonomic sensation, and inhibition were established by PENFIELD and JASPER. (See also TALAIRACH and BANCAUD, 1966). In regard to the *sensory* figure, PENFIELD and JASPER's observations were not yet sufficient to justify conclusion as to form or exact position. The positions of the parts of these figurines must not be considered topographically accurate in any precise way. The figurines are rough indicators of what has been generally observed. (From PENFIELD and JASPER, 1954, by permission of Little, Brown & Co.)

TRAND, 1956; TALAIRACH and BANCAUD, 1966). Occasionally stimulation of the second sensory area (lateral and posterior to postcentral gyrus) produced some trembling movements, and stimulation of an area of the mesial surface of the temporal lobe produced at times a stiffening of the limbs (PENFIELD, 1958, p. 15).

Results obtained from stimulation studies of the frontal and parietal areas of non-epileptic subjects, with peak currents limited to about 3 times the threshold level required at precentral gyrus (Libet et al., 1964; Alberts et al., 1967) were in more or less agreement with those from Penfield's group, except that only a tremor-like movement could be obtained by stimulating postcentral gyrus (see below). With apparently stronger stimuli Foerster (1936a, c) had additionally produced rather generalized movements in epileptic patients by stimulation of rather large "extrapyramidal" areas, expecially in the superior frontal and parietal regions. In unanesthetized monkeys and cats, stimulation within wide areas of cortex is reportedly capable of eliciting movements, although often with threshold intensities greater than those required at the primary motor area (see Brown, 1916; Doty, 1969). This is in contrast to the relatively small extent of the excitable areas for motor responses in human cortex, when using moderate stimulation.

The extent of the "excitable" areas for eliciting conscious somatosensory responses in man is even more limited than for motor responses; it is essentially restricted to Rolandic cortex (Foerster, 1936b, c; Penfield and Boldrey, 1937), perhaps to the postcentral gyrus portion of this, i.e. somatosensory area I (SS-I) in non-epileptics (Libet et al., 1964; Alberts et al., 1967), and to somatosensory area II located inferiorly to SS-I, i.e. more laterally (Penfield and Rasmussen, 1950; Penfield and Jasper, 1954; see further below). Foerster (1936b) reported that strong stimulation of area 5, in the superior parietal region posterior to the upper part of postcentral gyrus, could also elicit sensations over the whole body, initially contralaterally; this area overlapped with that producing whole body extrapyramidal type movements. However, Penfield and Boldrey (1937, p. 411) reported only an uncertain production of an epigastric aura for this area.

A relatively large proportion of human cerebral cortex is thus "inexcitable" or "silent". No subjective experiences or obvious behavioral changes of any sort have been elicited in these "inexcitable" areas, with some notable exceptions. The latter include the striking instances of various psychical responses (memories, hallucinations, etc.) aroused by stimulation of temporal lobe cortex in certain epileptic patients (Penfield and Rasmussen, 1950; Penfield and Jasper, 1954); and the negative or aphasic-like effects in certain association areas, such as the arrest of speech produced by stimulation at several regions (in Broca's area; in an inferior parietal area near the sensory area; and in an area in posterior temporal cortex — Penfield and Rasmussen, 1950). Much of the "silent" cortex is apparently also "dispensable", in the sense that excision or pathological destruction of individual portions of it does not produce defects in sensation or motor control, as occurs in the case of the Rolandic region (Penfield and Rasmussen, 1950). Of course, neither the "inexcitability" nor the "dispensability" as defined above, prove that "silent" cortex could not respond to suitable stimulation or does not have significant and important functions related to sensory input or motor output. Indeed it had been proposed by J. Hughlings Jackson (see Foerster, 1936c) and others that the whole cortex may be thought to contain nervous arrangements that mediate sensory impressions and movements, whether in a specific or more generalized manner.

Responses of "silent" cortex to stimulation, other than direct motor acts or reports of subjective experience, can in fact be detected. For example, local electrophysiological changes termed direct cortical responses (DCR) are elicited by relatively weak stimuli at all cortical areas in animals (PURPURA, 1959; OCHS, 1962), and they are recordable on human cortex as well (PURPURA et al., 1957 b; GOLDRING et al., 1958, 1961; LIBET et al., 1967). Additionally, electrical stimuli applied to virtually any cortical area can be utilized successfully to establish conditioned behavioral responses in cats and monkeys (e.g., DOTY, 1969).

2. Adequacy and Limitations of Electrical Stimulation; Interference with Normal Functions

The "inexcitability" of extensive areas of the cerebral cortex is probably not due to an actual and special nonresponsiveness of these neurons to electrical stimulation. It is perhaps more appropriate to view such cortical "inexcitability" as a reflection of (a) the inadequacy of the stimuli employed and/or (b) the inadequacy of the kinds of observations employed to detect changes in behavioral or unconscious psychical processes.

Electrical stimuli, as ordinarily applied on the cortical surfaces, can only influence the mass of underlying neurons in a manner that is relatively non-selective and gross, compared to the organized spatial-temporal patterns of activities that presumably go on during normal functioning. There is, for example, evidence that different groups of cells in different cortical layers are selectively acted upon in certain sequences, by the arriving ascending impulses from natural peripheral sensory stimulation (TOWE et al., 1968; WHITEHORN and TOWE, 1968). The significant kinds of electrical changes may be difficult or impossible to produce with ordinary stimuli; for example, local postsynaptic potentials in dendrites etc. can be generated only indirectly by activating appropriate synaptic inputs rather than by direct electrical fields. The density of the particular units, that must be suitably affected in order to produce the response, may be too low in any given area of "silent" cortex for sufficient activation by the usual type of electrode. (An electrical converse of this latter possibility has been demonstrated in attempting to record ongoing activity instead of to elicit a response by a stimulus: A small electrode on the cortical surface could not record the dominant EEG rhythms that could be recorded with a scalp electrode, unless a number of the small suitably-placed cortical electrodes were connected together in parallel — DELUCCHI et al., 1962). In addition, the electrical stimulus may excite both excitatory and (when stronger) inhibitory presynaptic fibers to local or distant neurons (e.g., LI and CHOU, 1962; KRNJEVIĆ et al., 1966; PHILLIS and YORK, 1967; PRINCE and WILDER, 1967; OCHS and CLARK, 1968 b), and may do so in a manner that is not conducive to developing a functional response.

Aside from these hypothetical possibilities for inadequacy, there is actual evidence that electrical stimuli can in fact interfere with or repress the normal function of a cortical area (PENFIELD, 1958). Stimulation of postcentral gyrus often produces a feeling of numbness in the referred bodily site (although this subjective response does not, by itself, necessarily indicate that an actual hypesthesia to peripheral stimulation has been produced). Stimulation of auditory cortex, i.e., on temporal lobe close to the sylvian fissure, has at times produced feelings of being deaf (Penfield and Rasmussen, 1950, Chapter VIII). Penfield (1958) states that stimulation of the calcarine cortex not only produces conscious sensory visions of lights, etc., but also makes the patient blind in that part of the visual field during stimulation. In this circumstance, then, the cortical stimulus elicits a positive sensory experience even when it is simultaneously interfering with sensation elicited by the peripheral sensory stimulus. An example of interference with normal motor functions is seen in the arrest of speech, without any direct motor responses to account for this arrest, when stimulating Broca's areas, etc. (Penfield and Rasmussen, 1950, Chapter V). It has been suggested (Penfield and Rasmussen, 1950) that this interference phenomenon may be related to the complete loss of normal sensibility to peripheral stimuli which occurs when there is seizure activity in the respective sensory cortex (i.e., somatic, visual, or auditory).

A more quantitative study of this interaction between cortical stimulation and responsiveness to peripheral input has now been carried out for the somatosensory system in non-epileptic subjects (Libet et al., 1972a; see further below, under "retroactive masking"). The conditioning stimulus to postcentral gyrus consisted of a train of pulses; the test stimulus was a single pulse applied to the skin, within the referral area of sensation elicited by the cortical stimulus. When a threshold test stimulus to skin was delivered during the conditioning cortical stimulus, the conscious sensory experience otherwise elicited by the skin stimulus was absent. This suppression of the sensory response to threshold skin stimuli could occur even with strengths of cortical stimulus only slightly above the liminal intensity for cortical production of a conscious sensory response (see below, "parametric values"). The effect on skin threshold occurred not only when the cortical stimulus elicited a feeling of numbness but also when it elicited positive or even natural-like sensory experiences (e.g., "rolling"; "wave-like").

The mechanism of depression of peripheral sensibility by cortical stimuli remains an open question. Cortical efferent systems that are inhibitory to the subcortical sensory relay stations have been found in animals (Hagbarth and Kerr, 1954; see also Wiesendanger, 1969) and probably function in man as well (Hagbarth and Höjeberg, 1957; Jouvet et al., 1960). Production of local intracortical inhibitory actions by cortical stimuli has already been discussed above. Interference could also result from production of local cortical discharges which may disorganize neuronal activity or response patterns (e.g., Penfield, 1958; Phillips, 1966). Such disorganizing effects would no doubt explain the loss of normal cortical functions during strong cortical stimulation or seizure activity. But their significance is less obvious when considering the interference with peripheral sensibility by cortical stimuli which are at only the liminal current strengths required for eliciting conscious sensory responses (see above; Libet et al., 1972a). The interference is probably not due to a Leaõ-type spreading depression; the latter requires much stronger stimulation as well as other differences in experimental conditions. Recordings of the direct cortical responses, to trains of pulses near the liminal intensity for conscious sensory responses, have shown no changes in ongoing rhythms and no steady potentials shifts that characterize spreading depression (LIBET et al., 1972a). The possibility of producing spreading depression must be kept in mind, however, when rather long periods of apparent inhibition (some minutes) are produced by stimulation, especially of exposed cortex (see MARSHALL, 1959).

In view of the theoretically possible deficiencies of electrical stimulation at the surface of somatosensory cortex, as well as the actually observed depression of peripheral sensibility, it is perhaps surprising that any subjective sensory experiences can be elicited at all by such stimuli. The fact that responses are elicited may be a reflection of the relatively simple input-response relationship in a primary sensory area compared to that in "silent" cortex. For example, the stimulus might intracortically excite some of the neural elements normally involved in mediating the responses to the afferent projections in a sensory system (see further below). However, even for sensory cortex, the inability to elicit in any controllable manner each different quality of conscious somatic sensation (see below) could be a function of inadequately sophisticated spatial and temporal patterns of applied stimuli. Where more complex responses have been elicited, e.g. psychical responses to stimulation of temporal cortex in epileptics, it has been suggested that the stimulus may simply be triggering-off an established pattern in an abnormally irritable cortex (PENFIELD and RASMUSSEN, 1950). Probably this is true, in a sense, for responses elicited by stimuli at all points in the sensory system; that is, the stimuli may activate existing patterns of neuronal function by adequately exciting a suitable input at the site of stimulation. For example, direct surface stimulation of somatosensory cortex undoubtedly excites neural elements at a step beyond the ascending specific afferent projection fiber; even so, the requirements for adequate stimulation of either postcentral gyrus or of the specific afferent projection in n. VPL (thalamus) were found to be generally similar (LIBET et al., 1964, 1967; see below).

It has been argued that surface stimulation of "excitable" cortex never evokes natural functioning of the cortical neuronal apparatus, since the motor or sensory responses that are elicited have unnatural characteristics (e.g. PENFIELD, 1958; PHILLIPS, 1966). While this may be true in a strict sense, it may nevertheless be possible to approximate the evocation of natural functions to a greater degree than has been thought feasible. For example, most types of specific somatosensory qualities (rather than merely parasthesias) can in fact be elicited by stimulation of postcentral gyrus (see below).

3. Topographical Representation of Somatosensory Responses in SS-I Area

Upon stimulating postcentral gyrus of conscious human subjects, CUSHING (1909) obtained reports of parasthesia sensations (tingling, etc.) referred to the contralateral side, with no visible movements. FOERSTER (1936b) extended these observations to show that the representation, for body sites to which the sensations were referred, was similar to that for the motor responses from the precentral gyrus; i.e., leg area was near the longitudinal fissure on top, and head area below towards the Sylvian fissure. PENFIELD and his colleagues have made extensive and closely observed investigations of the responses to electrical stimuli that were near threshold or at least sufficiently moderate in intensities so as not to produce local seizure activity. (Fig. 1 shows their summary of the topographical representation for stimuli at different points on postcentral gyrus, in the form of a homunculus drawing; a more detailed homuncular drawing is given by Penfield and Rasmussen, 1950, p. 44). There is not any strict correspondence between this cortical sensory sequence and the sensory representation by spinal segment. Responses to stimulating postcentral gyrus are strictly contralateral, except for the face area where about 10 % of the responses were either bilateral or ipsilateral (e.g. Penfield and Rasmussen, 1950). It should be added that stimulation of the "bank" of the postcentral gyrus, down in the central sulcus, elicited responses with sites comparable to those obtained from the free surface; this could be accomplished in some patients after removal of the precentral gyrus. There were also no systematic differences in the referral sites of responses, or in the threshold intensities required, with stimulation of different points along the antero-posterior axis on the exposed face of the postcentral gyrus (Penfield and Rasmussen, 1950; Libet et al., 1964).

4. Variation in Responses to Stimuli at a Given Cortical Point

The precise referral sites of the sensation elicited by stimulating a given point on the postcentral gyrus may vary, partly as a function of previous stimuli at this or at other points in the vicinity. (1) In successive tests with the same stimulus to the same cortical point, the somatic sites to which the sensation is subjectively referred can at times shift or change in size. This occurs even though the threshold intensity requirement for any response can remain remarkably stable (Libet et al., 1964). Such changes perhaps reflect fluctuating degrees of spatial and temporal facilitation of the cortex in the vicinity of the electrode (see below for further quantitative aspects of such facilitations). (2) An initially subthreshold stimulus at a given cortical point can often elicit a response after it is repeated a number of times at sufficiently short intervals ("primary" facilitation; see TRR section below). (3) A type of "secondary" facilitation by a responsive cortical point (A) on another initially unresponsive point (B) has also been observed (Penfield and Boldrey, 1937; Penfield and Welch, 1949). When stimulation of a point (B) along the antero-posterior axis of the post-central gyrus gives no response with reasonable stimulus strengths (i.e. relative to the threshold values for points that do give responses), it may be induced to give responses if stimulated shortly after repeated stimulation of an adjacent point (A) which does give a response initially (see Penfield and Boldrey, 1937, p. 402). In addition, when stimulation of a point (B) does elicit a sensory response, the somatic site to which the sensation is referred can be changed by prior stimulation of another point (A). For example, if stimulation of point B elicited a sensation in the thumb, while that of point A was referred to the lower lip, then stimulation of B following a series of stimuli at A could now elicit a sensation in the lower lip instead of the thumb (Penfield and Welch, 1949). Such a shift in the referral site, produced by conditioning stimuli at another point, was termed "deviation of sensory response". Since the sensory response in the original referral site for point B is absent during such a "deviation" Penfield and Welch (1949) suggested that the process includes a form of "sensory inhibition". (Such a cerebral inhibitory mechanism could be related to "surround inhibition" that was initially found with peripheral stimuli, e.g. Towe and Amassian, 1958; Mountcastle and Powell, 1959b, and later demonstrated in cortical areas adjacent to a cortical stimulus by Li and Chou, 1962; Krnjević et al., 1966; Phillis and York, 1967; Prince and Wilder, 1967; Ochs and Clark, 1968b). On the other hand, the change in referral site of the sensory response when stimulating point B after conditioning point A is presumably accomplished by a lasting state of facilitation at point A; i.e., weak presynaptic input to point A that can be initiated by stimulating at point B now becomes sufficient to generate the usual response at point A. Similar instabilities of threshold and site had been observed for motor responses to stimuli at points in precentral gyrus in man, by Penfield and Boldrey (1937) and Penfield and Welch (1949), and previously in the anthropoid brain by Leyton and Sherrington (1917). (4) Referral site may also be affected by the polarity and diameter of a surface unipolar electrode (Libet et al., 1964). Shifting from cathodal to anodal polarity pulses can shift the site of referral. An increase in diameter of unipolar electrode, for example from 0.25 to 2 mm, tends to enlarge the referral site; but it was surprising to find how little actual change in referral site did occur, even with electrode diameter raised to as much as 10 mm, if stimulus strengths were carefully kept to the threshold or liminal level for each electrode (Libet et al., 1964, and unpubl.; see further below).

It should be obvious from all this that the detailed representation of responses to stimuli is not a rigidly fixed condition but depends on past history of activity, area of electrode, polarity, etc. The site and total area of referral can fluctuate even with threshold level stimuli, and even when sufficiently long inter-stimulus time intervals are employed so that there is no evidence of any incidence of seizure-like activities. However, the quality of the sensation reported, in contrast to the referral site, tends to remain relatively constant for threshold stimuli applied to a given area of postcentral gyrus (see further below).

5. Uniqueness of Responses to Postcentral vs. Precentral Stimulation

Motor responses to stimulation of postcentral gyrus can be obtained (Foerster, 1936a; Penfield and Boldrey, 1937) but they differ in stimulus requirements (Foerster, 1936b, c) and in character (Libet et al., 1964) from those elicited at area 4 on precentral gyrus. Application of a single 0.5 msec constant current pulse of sufficient intensity to postcentral gyrus produces a twitch, but this is a very weak and restricted response compared with the twitch obtainable with a pulse at precentral gyrus. When trains of pulses (e.g. 60 pps) are applied to precentral gyrus, the response is a pyramidal-type, smoothly developing contraction with no intermittency, even when stimulus intensity is near threshold. With postcentral gyrus, trains of stimulus pulses generally elicit no motor responses when the intensity is near threshold level for conscious sensation or near the threshold level for precentral motor responses (Libet et al., 1964). The latter difference, between pre- and postcentral thresholds, had been noted earlier, in apes (Leyton and Sherrington, 1917) and in man (Foerster, 1936a). Stimulating postcentral gyrus in man with a train of pulses at much higher intensities could elicit only a series of slowly repeating weak twitches, occurring in the same body region as the referred sensations produced by the lower intensity (Libet et al., 1964). (Not infrequently postcentral stimuli could initiate a somewhat irregular tremor, or exaggerate an ongoing one in Parkinsonians, often with stimulus intensities not far above threshold for sensation and in some cases at or below this threshold.) By contrast, Penfield and Rasmussen (1950, p. 211) stated that stimulation of postcentral gyrus (in epileptic subjects) produced movement that was similar in character to the response from stimulation of precentral gyrus. However, in describing an instance of a motor response to postcentral stimulation, Penfield and Boldrey (1937, p. 426) called it "up and down vibratory movements" associated with a tingling. Foerster (1936a, c) described only isolated focal twitches produced by galvanic (single pulse) stimulation of postcentral gyrus, when precentral pyramidal outflow was intact. He also noted that the motor part of seizures that originated in postcentral gyrus often began with a tremor, unlike precentral seizures.

On the possibility of eliciting *sensory* responses by stimulating *pre*central gyrus reports differ, perhaps in relation to whether epileptic subjects were tested. In non-epileptic patients, Libet et al. (1964) could not elicit any non-motion sensations that were unrelated to production of movement itself; no tingling etc. accompanied any motor response or appeared without the latter. The sensory responses to precentral stimulation that were reported by Penfield and Boldrey (1937) could not be explained as due to spread of stimulus or of neural excitation to the postcentral gyrus, for they could still be elicited after excision of the latter (Penfield and Rasmussen, 1950, p. 59). It should be noted further that somatosensory responses can be obtained with relatively strong stimulation of widely scattered points on the cortex of epileptics (Penfield and Rasmussen, 1950, p. 132) but not in nonepileptics (Libet et al., 1964; Alberts et al., 1967).

The pre- and postcentral areas adjoining the central fissure appeared to share functions sufficiently to be referred to as the "sensorimotor strip" by Penfield et al. (Penfield and Rasmussen, 1950; Penfield and Jasper, 1954) and by Foerster (1936b), although it was recognized that the primary (more indispensable) motor area was precentral and the primary somatosensory area was postcentral. However, on the basis of findings in non-epileptic subjects, and with close attention to threshold stimulus values (Libet et al., 1964), the functional distinction between these two areas in the adult human cortex appears to be even sharper than previously seemed to be the case. This is further supported by the results of excision, that of area 4 producing relatively little or no loss in sensibility (Foerster, 1936b; Penfield and Rasmussen, 1950) and that of areas 3-1-2 producing no motor losses except for some ataxia, an effect that may be assignable to the sensory loss, and some light spasticity (Foerster, 1936b). On the other hand, certain kinds of motor responses can be elicited by strong stimulation of postcentral gyrus even in non-epileptics (Libet et al., 1964), and generalized extra-pyramidal-type movements under certain conditions (Foerster, 1936a, c). It has, of course, been known for some time that the postcentral gyrus contributes fibers to the pyramidal tract, although it now appears that these may be at least in part a descending inhibitory outflow to sensory input stations (see Wiesendanger, 1969); and that the gyrus has cortico-cortical U-fiber connections to precentral gyrus (e.g. Penfield and Jasper, 1954, p. 57). Also, group I afferents from muscle spindles project to the vicinity of somatosensory cortex, even though they appear

to elicit no conscious sensory responses (see next section, below). There are therefore reasons for thinking that postcentral gyrus may have some functional roles in
the organizing of motor patterns, as already envisioned by FOERSTER (1936a, c),
and by PENFIELD (e.g. 1958), and even earlier by J. HUGHLINGS JACKSON (see
FOERSTER, 1936c).

6. Relation of Sensory Responses to Representation of Evoked Potentials

Mapping of topographical representation of somatic sensory projections to the
cortex can be carried out using, as the response indicators, the recordings of the
early-latency or "primary" evoked potentials. This was initially carried out in
animals including primates (see WOOLSEY, 1952), and then in man (WOOLSEY and
ERICKSON, 1950; JASPER et al., 1960; KELLY et al., 1965). The topographical
representation of the body parts on the postcentral gyrus produced by this method
is in generally good accord with that obtained by the mappings of the body parts
to which subjective sensory responses are referred, when the latter are elicited by
stimulation of points on the postcentral gyrus (e.g. JASPER et al., 1960). The
existence of another somatosensory area ("SS-II") was indicated by ADRIAN's
(1941) observations of evoked potentials in a region below area SS-I in the cat,
and it was then extensively mapped with this technique by WOOLSEY and collaborators (WOOLSEY, 1952). In SS-II the representation for head is oriented anter-
omedially and for legs posterolaterally, and evoked potentials are obtainable
ipsilaterally and contralaterally. Stimulation of the apparently homologous cortical area in man (see Fig. 1) has elicited subjective sensory responses with a roughly
appropriate representation, though only on the contralateral side of body (PEN-
FIELD and RASMUSSEN, 1950; PENFIELD and JASPER, 1954). However excision
of the regions lying in the presumed area SS-II did not produce any obvious loss
of subjective sensibility (PENFIELD and RASMUSSEN, 1950), in contrast to the
losses incurred when SS-I (postcentral gyrus) is removed in man.

While cortical evoked potentials to peripheral stimuli have been appropriately
recordable wherever it has been possible to elicit conscious sensory responses by
cortical stimuli, the converse is not true.That is, conscious sensory responses cannot be elicited at all the cortical areas that do respond with recordable evoked
potentials. Evoked potentials, particularly later components with latencies greater
than that of the specific primary response (about 20 msec $\pm$), can be recorded
over regions outside areas SS-I and SS-II. This is true for both scalp and subdural
electrodes (see DONCHIN and LINDSLEY, 1969; McKAY, 1969) and for intracortical
electrodes (WALTER, 1964); the scalp site at the vertex yields prominent evoked
potentials with somatic (and other) peripheral sensory stimuli and is commonly
employed especially in psychophysical studies (e. g. KATZMAN, 1964; COBB and
MOROCUTTI, 1968; MACKAY, 1969; DONCHIN and LINDSLEY, 1969). Direct cortical
stimulation of sites external to SS-I and SS-II has not elicited conscious sensory
responses, as already noted above; this includes the cortical area in the vicinity of
the vertex (e.g. PENFIELD and RASMUSSEN, 1950; LIBET et al., 1972b).

It has been argued that the evoked potentials elicited by somatic stimuli
and recorded over non-sensory cortex actually originate only in the primary somatosensory areas (MACKAY, 1969, pp. 201–203; STOHR and GOLDRING, 1969; VAUG-

han, 1969). This question cannot be considered fully here. However, there now appears to be good evidence for at least some other cortical sources for somatosensory evoked potentials. Large evoked potentials are recordable at supplementary motor cortex in man and have been found to show a subcortical reversal of polarity, in accord with Stohr and Goldring's criterion (Libet et al., 1972b). Indeed, the origination of evoked potentials by this area makes it a prime candidate for the actual source of at least some of the recorded evoked potentials at the vertex. Yet, no conscious sensory responses can be elicited by stimulation of supplementary motor cortex (Penfield and Jasper, 1954; Talairach and Bancaud, 1966; Libet et al., 1972b). Penfield and Rasmussen, 1950, pp. 62–3, elicited some vague sensations there but these were similar to those experienced by the patients at the time of an epileptic attack. Evoked potentials can also originate in wide "polysensory" areas of the frontal lobe, in at least some primates (squirrel and rhesus monkeys), as has been shown by Bignall and Imbert (1967); these responses also show reversal of polarity subcortically and they remain even when the primary sensory areas have been ablated. These frontally originating evoked potentials may be related to those recorded in man by Walter (1964). There are further indicators of multiple generators of evoked potentials from the distributions of the recorded fields, especially for different components of the evoked potentials (Vaughan, 1969; Broughton, 1969; Libet et al., 1972b).

Finally, it must be noted that although some group I muscle afferent fiber inputs from the periphery have been found to elicit evoked responses in primary somatosensory or closely related cortex (Amassian and Berlin, 1958; Oscarsson and Rosén, 1963, 1966; Albe-Fessard, 1967; Swett and Bourassa, 1967), these inputs do not elicit any subjective experience of motion, position, muscle length or other in man (Brindley and Merton, 1960; Gelfan and Carter, 1967). The group I afferent inputs, in contrast to other somatic inputs, could not produce behavioral (Giaquinto et al., 1963) or conditional learned responses in the cat (Swett and Bourassa, 1967). The group I projection of muscle spindle afferent impulses to the cortex may therefore serve in the integration and organization of movements mediated by the cortex, without giving rise to any subjective sensory experience (e.g. Oscarsson, 1965; Albe-Fessard, 1967). The actual subjective experience of position and movement would depend on other inputs, especially those originating in and about the joints (Skoglund, 1956; Provins, 1958; Mountcastle and Powell, 1959a). Oscarsson (1965) has suggested that the projection of *cutaneous* afferents to the primary *motor* area may also serve for motor rather than conscious sensory functions; this would fit with the inability to elicit conscious sensory responses by stimulation of precentral gyrus in nonepileptic human subjects (Libet et al., 1964; Libet, 1966). (See above.)

It should be realized, then, that it is possible for somatic sensory inputs to elicit, in the cerebral cortex, evoked potentials that represent processes whose functional roles are not necessarily involved in production of conscious sensory experience. Mountcastle (p. 228 in MacKay, 1969) notes that the elucidation of these other functions provides a challenging task at present. Clearly, caution must be used when interpreting psychophysical correlations, between evoked potentials and the production of conscious sensory responses, in terms of cerebral mechanisms underlying subjective sensory experiences. The demonstrated experimental potentiality for error in such interpretations illustrates the point made below ("criteria for conscious sensory response") about the necessity for distinguishing experimentally among the different classes of detection indicators of sensory inputs.

C. Significant Stimulus Parameters for Threshold Conscious Sensation

Clarification of the significant stimulus parameters and their values for producing conscious sensory responses is important for achieving adequate control and reproducibility of stimulation of sensory cortex for experimental and clinical purposes, and to avoid possible production of seizures or damage. There is the more interesting possibility, however, that an analysis of the "adequate" stimulus might be helpful in problems related to the dynamics rather than topography of cortical function (see Libet et al., 1964; Libet, 1965, 1966). For example, what can the differences between stimuli that are adequate and those that are inadequate, tell us about the requirements of sensory cortex for neural inputs that can elicit a conscious sensory experience? Can we elicit the different specific qualities of somatic sensation with uniquely different kinds of adequate stimuli? Although direct cortical stimulation has limitations, as already noted, it bypasses the unknown modifications imposed on the original peripheral sensory input by various subcortical mechanisms. It thus provides a possible route for analysing the more immediate requirements of cortical activation in the production of sensory experiences.

1. Criteria for Threshold Level of Conscious Sensory Response

This issue provides an exercise in the philosophy of scientific method, since it raises the problem of the validity of the evidence in relation to question under investigation. When the objective is to investigate conscious sensory responses to cortical (or other) stimuli, it should be clear that the indication to the experimental observer that the response has occurred must be based on the introspective experience of the subject (see Eccles, 1966; Libet, 1966). There are many possible response indicators that might show that a stimulus had affected the subject, i.e. that it had been "detected" in some way. Responses could range from internal and autonomic ones (such as cortical evoked potentials, changes in heart rate, galvanic skin responses etc.) to alterations in external behavior, either as overt actions or as covert modifications of the behavior that was expected without the cortical stimulus. But a clear distinction should be made between responses that indicate one of these kinds of detection of the stimulus, as utilized in detection theory studies (Green and Swets, 1966), and those that indicate the specific kind of detection represented in the subject's awareness of a sensory experience. There is considerable evidence that behavioral responses can occur in normal subjects without awareness (Eriksen, 1956; Adams, 1957; Goldiamond, 1958; Raab, 1963; Bevan, 1964; Shevrin and Fritzler, 1968); there are also the automatisms and responses without awareness in certain types of epilepsies (e.g. Penfield and Jasper, 1954). Thus, many indicators of detection may or may not be accompanied by subjective experience of the sensory stimulus. (See also section above on "Relation of sensory responses to representation of evoked potentials.") The cerebral processes that mediate subjective experience may have some unique differences from those that mediate responses without such awareness, i.e. from those responses in which the subject is "unconscious" of the stimulus itself. It is precisely such possible differences that are of great interest (for further discussion of this issue see Raab, 1963; Libet, 1965, 1966; Krech, 1969). Some of the physiological significance of the suggested distinction will become apparent in the discussion below (see also above, on evoked potentials). The failure to make the distinction can lead to a fundamental error in the validity of conclusions drawn from stimulus detection studies.

The distinction between these two classes of detection (conscious vs. other) has been made by psychophysicists on the basis of differences in "criterion" levels, allegedly adopted by the subjects for making a response at some point in what is regarded by those investigators as a stimulus response continuum (e.g. Swets, 1961; Eijkman and Vendrik, 1963; Sutton, 1969). The threshold level for a report of conscious experience is considered by them to be an arbitrary one, with each subject setting his own "criterion" for the level at which he will report subjective experience (e.g. Sutton, 1969; it should be noted, however, that there is no evidence for any such conscious deliberate action by the subject). On this view it would be argued that demonstrations of actual signal detection of some kind (e.g. by forced-choice responses or by the appearance of an evoked potential response, etc.) indicate that the subject really did have a conscious subjective experience even when the subject reports flatly and consistently that he had none. Such an argument would appear to constitute an unwarranted distortion of the primary evidence in order to make it fit a preconceived theoretical framework (Libet, 1965, 1966).

In determining threshold levels on the basis of reports of subjective experience, a subject may be asked to report (a) whether he did feel or experience the sensation in question (no matter how weakly), or (b) whether he is uncertain about having felt it, or (c) whether he definitely did not feel it (Libet et al., 1964). Speediness of report, for example by pressing a switch as soon as possible, is to be avoided as a potentially complicating factor; it is possible that speedy reports, at least at the instant they are made, could indicate detection without actual subjective awareness (see further below). Both the upper limit (a) and lower limit (c) can be approached by descending from a superthreshold value, or by ascending from a subthreshold value. The threshold level has often been specified as the level at which the subject makes the response in 50% of the tests, i.e. within the range of uncertainty.

In actual practice the threshold levels for conscious sensory responses can be very stable (5–10%) over periods of an hour or more (Libet et al., 1964). There has usually been no important difference between the limiting values obtained by either ascending or descending approaches, except when using cortical stimuli with a low pulse frequency, < 15 per sec (Libet et al., 1964). Re-establishing the threshold by presentation of stimuli with values more randomly distributed among the tests, and with false tests (no stimuli) thrown in at times, has usually not affected the values achieved with the method of approaching limits. The range of intensity for uncertainty of response, i.e. the difference between the upper limit (a, 100% positive) and the lower limit (c, virtually 100% negative), has turned out to be relatively small, i.e. about 10% of the stimulus intensity for the upper limit; and there remains a considerable range below the lower limit (c) in which the subject reports that he definitely feels nothing. This contrasts with the results obtained when a forced-choice answer is requested without any necessary regard to conscious sensory awareness (e.g. SWETS, 1961; EIJKMAN and VENDRIK, 1963; see also KIETZMAN and SUTTON, 1968).

The nature of the warning signal before a stimulus appears to have no major influence in a generally attentive and cooperative subject. However, it appears to be necessary that the subject focus his attention on the precise somatic site of the sensation and becomes familiarized in a few initial trials with the very weak sensory experiences generated by near-threshold stimuli. When the sensory experience is a very short-lasting one, e.g. with a single pulse to the skin, the degree of attention during the precise time period, in which the stimulus occurs, apparently becomes more significant. This could be seen when, instead of presenting the stimulus at some variable moment during a period of several seconds following the usual alerting auditory signal, the latter is followed at a fixed interval by a brief light. The light signal indicates the time period during which the stimulus is actually delivered (LIBET et al., 1972a). With this combination of indicator signals, the threshold values for brief skin stimuli could be reduced by some 10% (or more in some instances).

Somewhat surprisingly, a shift in the general state of "arousal" from that of EEG "alpha-blocked" (eyes open, alerting signals, etc.) to that with "alpha rhythm present" (eyes closed and no immediate alerting signal) had no significant effect on threshold values for stimulation of cortex or skin with pulse trains (LIBET et al., 1964); in the case of "alpha present" the subject was queried just after the stimulus was delivered so that any alerting could only be "retroactive". This kind of result provides another experimental difference between a conscious sensory response and other kinds of detection indicators. For example, reaction times have been found to change with such a shift in EEG "arousal" state (LANSING et al., 1959).

2. Definitions of Threshold Terminology

Different types of psychological and electrophysiological responses to stimuli in the sensory system (conscious sensory experience, forced choice detection, DCR's, evoked potentials, etc.) may have different stimulus threshold requirements. To avoid confusion and repeated qualifiers, the threshold levels for eliciting a conscious sensory experience will be referred to as *threshold-c*. Threshold-c level can refer to the middle of the usually small range of uncertainty, between the lower (0 response) and upper (100% responses) levels. However, it is useful for certain purposes to specify the threshold-c level as the lower or upper limit itself.

The term threshold as applied to the stimulus can and will be used in the broad sense of the just adequate levels of all significant parameters of a stimulus. For threshold-c, the significant parameters of electrical stimuli (rectangular wave pulses) applied to somatosensory cortex include not merely intensity, i.e. peak current (I), but also polarity (with unipolar surface electrode), pulse duration (PD), pulse frequency (PF, i.e. pulse repetition rate) for a stimulus made up of a train of pulses, train duration (TD), train repetition rate (TRR, the reciprocal of the interval between successive delivery of stimulus trains), and the contact area of the electrode (especially for surface unipolar electrodes). Since the threshold value for each parameter depends on the values selected for the other parameters in the set, it is desirable to adopt the usage of LILLY et al. (1952) which was applied to their study of threshold movements produced by stimulation of cortex. A

Table 1. *Summary of parametric regions for threshold stimuli*

	Region A	Region B	Region C
I	Liminal	2 or more times that in A	Intermediate range, between A and B
TD	> 0.5–1 sec	< 0.1–0.3 sec; or single pulse	0.5 to 5 sec, at 8 pulses/sec 0.1 to 0.5 sec at PF $\geq$ 15 pulses/sec
PF	$\geq$ 15 pulses/sec (can get with 8 pulse/sec if TD > 5–10 sec)	Any	Probably any, but best seen in low range (< 15 pulses/sec)
Facilitation evident with TTR = 1 per 30 sec	Usually none	Usually considerable	Usually present
Response at threshold	Purely somatosensory (no motor)	Observable muscular contraction	No observable contraction; sensation often has aspect of motion (at 15 pulses/sec often has slow pulsatile quality)

I = peak current; TD = train duration; PF = pulse repetition frequency; TTR = train repetition rate. (From LIBET et al., 1964, by permission of J. Neurophysiology).

"parametric point" is the group of simultaneously assigned single values, one for each parameter of a set. A "parametric line" is a set of parameters all of whose values are fixed except for one, e.g. peak current. (The threshold value of a given parameter is ordinarily determined with respect to a given parametric line.) A "parametric region" is determined by the simultaneous choices of an upper and lower limit (i.e., a range) for the values of each parameter of a set; as a consequence of such choices there is a "region" in which parametric points fall within the limits chosen for the various parameters.

3. Parametric Regions for Threshold Stimuli

It has been found useful to characterize threshold-c stimuli to somatosensory cortex into three parametric regions, according to some features of both the stimuli (especially their train duration) and the nature of the responses, as shown in Table 1 (LIBET et al., 1964). Parametric *region A* includes all threshold stimuli with the relatively longer TD's ($>$ 0.5 sec), higher pulse frequencies ($>$ 15 per sec) and lowest possible peak currents (i.e., liminal I; see below). Since the responses are all purely sensory, region A encompasses the kinds of stimuli which should generally be employed for somatosensory investigations. For stimuli in *region B*, the peripheral afferent input, generated by the observable muscular contraction that is produced at threshold, is probably responsible for any conscious sensory responses. This distinction of parametric regions clarifies an observation reported by FOERSTER (1936a, b, c,) that when brief galvanic (dc) stimuli of sufficient intensity were applied to postcentral gyrus in man they could only elicit localized motor responses; and that faradic stimuli (i.e. repetitive pulses) were required to elicit sensation. The conscious sensory responses elicited in *region C* often had an aspect of motion ("quiver", "pull", "drawing in") even when this quality was not elicited in *region A* in the same subject; with PF's of 8 per sec or lower, pulsatile sensations (having a subjective frequency of about 1 per sec irrespective of the actual PF) were commonly reported. However, no muscular contractions could ordinarily be detected by the external observer. The possibility that the sensations in region C may, at least in part, be due to undetected small but deep muscular responses has not been resolved. (The findings with short TD's of stimuli in the thalamus, see below, are relevant to this issue.) It should be clear, then, that particular attention must be paid to the TD, PF, and I combinations of the electrical stimuli employed, if one wants to relate mechanisms in somatosensory cortex to production of conscious sensory experience.

4. Train Duration (TD) and Intensity (I)

Holding other parametric values constant, the peak current values (I) for a threshold-c response can be determined for stimuli of different TD's. A plot of these parametric points (Fig. 2) shows that once the TD reaches a certain value, the threshold I requirement does not change with further increase in TD. This feature appears analogous to the rheobasic current level given by the curve for intensity vs. *pulse*-duration obtained for the threshold excitation of nerve or muscle fibers. The minimum intensity level in the I-TD curves for cortical stimuli has been termed "liminal I"; and the minimum TD that is required when using pulses with liminal I peak currents, has been termed the "utilization-TD" (LIBET et al., 1964; the significance of the utilization-TD is taken up below). With TD's less than utilization-TD, not only is threshold-I greater but the response is often different (already described above, under "parametric regions"). The unique nature of the I-TD relationship for threshold-c stimuli at somatosensory cortex may be compared to that for motor cortex and for two subcortical sites in the somatosensory pathway, namely the ventroposterolateral nucleus (n. VPL) in thalamus and the skin.

a) Motor Cortex. An I-TD curve has now been carefully determined for motor cortex in one unanesthetized human subject using cathodal 0.5 msec pulses at a PF of 60 pps (LIBET et al., 1972a). In contrast to sensory cortex, the peak current required at precentral gyrus for a threshold motor response was already liminal with very short TD's of about 0.05 sec (actually 4 pulses); i.e. longer TD's (up to 2 sec) required the same liminal I. Threshold I for a single pulse was greater than liminal I. Thus the "utilization-TD" was very short, resembling that for the skin (see below). On the other hand, for motor cortex in the anesthetized cat Lilly et al. (1952) found that the threshold I (for PF's of 20–100 pps) progressively decreased with increasing TD's over the range of 0.1 to 20 sec that was studied. In spite of the difference in utilization-TD's required for motor responses from precentral gyrus as compared to sensory responses from postcentral gyrus, which we found

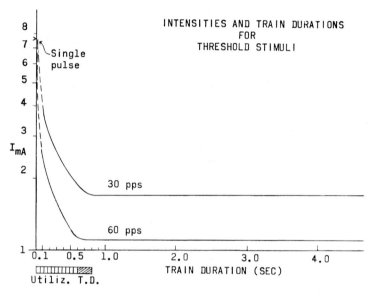

Fig. 2. Intensity-train duration combinations for stimuli (to postcentral gyrus) just adequate to elicit a threshold conscious experience of somatic sensation. Curves are presented for two different pulse repetition frequencies, employing rectangular pulses of 0.5 msec duration. "Utilization train duration" is discussed in the text. (From Libet, 1966)

in human subjects, the liminal I (min. threshold-I with trains) was not much different for these two test situations in the same subject, using similar electrodes and stimulus parameters (Libet et al., 1964; see also Penfield and Boldrey, 1937). However, with brief galvanic current (i.e. single dc pulse) Foerster (1936a,c) observed that the threshold for eliciting a motor twitch response from postcentral gyrus was two or three times as great as that for precentral gyrus.

b) **Thalamus, n. VPL.** The I-TD relationship for threshold-c stimuli in n. VPL does show a leveling off of liminal I with TD's longer than about 0.5–1 sec. The utilization-TD is thus similar to that for somatosensory cortex. Stimuli with shorter TD's and higher threshold I's have often produced some motor response in addition to sensory ones, if unipolar or even bipolar electrodes with appreciable separation (e.g. 3 mm) were used (Guiot et al., 1962; Johansson, 1969). However, with a coaxial type electrode motor responses did not appear, indicating that with the other electrodes there was spread of stimulating current to internal capsule (LIBET et al., 1967; see also GUIOT et al., 1962). With the coaxial electrode, a single pulse stimulus did not elicit either a muscular twitch or any conscious sensory response, with peak currents even up to 20 or more times the liminal I level (LIBET et al., 1967, 1972a). [This finding is different from that for postcentral gyrus, where there are evidently some motor efferent elements that can respond to a single pulse; it supports the suggestion that any sensory response to a single pulse at postcentral gyrus is due purely to peripheral sensory impulses set up by the motor response, rather than to an activation of the somatosensory mechanism in the cortex.] On the other hand, stimulation of n.VPL with TD's as short as 0.05 sec (i.e. 3 pulses, at 60 pps) and sufficiently supraliminal I could produce conscious sensory responses, though also without any movement. The subjective

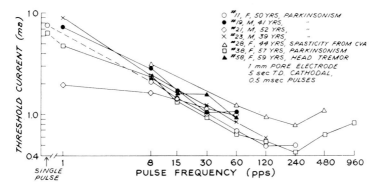

Fig. 3. Liminal I values (i.e., threshold peak currents required to elicit a sensation using 5-sec train durations in these tests) at different pulse frequencies (0.5 msec PD, 1 mm cathodal electrode). Each curve represents a set of determinations made at one session for each of the seven subjects in the graph. (From LIBET et al., 1964, by permission of J. Neurophysiology)

quality of the responses to these stimuli with short TD's (equivalent to parametric region C for cortex) was similar to that reported by the same subjects for stimuli with utilization-TD's or longer TD's and liminal I (equivalent to parametric region A); the sensory responses were all parasthesia-like in nature, i.e. tingling, numbness, or electricity (LIBET et al., 1972b). The findings with n.VPL showed that stimuli with TD's less than the utilization-TD could elicit pure sensory responses in the absence of any motor response (compare above, "parametric regions" for cortical stimuli).

c) **Skin.** The threshold-c peak currents for different TD's with electrical stimuli applied to the skin also level off to a minimum or liminal-I value, but this occurs at a relatively short utilization-TD of about 0.1 sec or less. That is, threshold-c I is the same for all TD's of about 0.1 second and longer (LIBET et al., 1964, 1967). Threshold-c I for a single pulse is generally only 110–130% that of liminal I. Thus while repetition of pulses does somewhat increase the effectiveness here, it is relatively unimportant when compared to the case of somatosensory cortex or n.VPL.

5. Pulse Frequency (PF) and Liminal I

Holding other parametric values constant (and using TD's longer than utilization-TD), the relationship between liminal I and PF for eliciting threshold-c responses is shown in Fig. 3 (Libet et al., 1964). The relationship may reflect a temporal facilitation, such as has been seen with suitable intervals between two pulses (Rosenthal et al., 1967). Such a facilitation may be significant in at least the early portion of the stimulus train of pulses (see below, "direct cortical responses").

6. Pulse Duration (PD) and Liminal I

When PD for the individual pulses in the stimulus trains was changed from 0.1 msec to 0.5 msec liminal I decreased about 25–50% (Libet et al., 1964). Increases in PD between 0.5 and 5.0 msec produced relatively little further decrease in liminal I. The longer PD's above 1 msec and especially at 5 msec or more, introduce the possibility of repetitive discharge of some neuronal elements with each pulse (e.g. Phillips, 1969). This, in effect becomes equivalent to stimulating with a train of short pulses of unknown train duration. Therefore PD's for controlled stimuli with the lowest liminal I requirements should be in the vicinity of 0.5 msec. (See below for PD vs. total coulombs passed and possible damage.)

7. Polarity of Pulses and Liminal I

With unipolar electrodes on the exposed surface postcentral gyrus, surface cathodal polarity required uniformly lower liminal I values than did surface anodal polarity for threshold-c stimuli (Libet et al., 1964). The mean ratio of cathodal/anodal values was about 0.7 (range 0.6–0.9), for 0.5 msec pulses and PF's of 8–60 pps. For threshold I's with single pulses (which produce a motor response) the mean ratio was about 0.9. On precentral gyrus, the mean ratio was also about 0.9 for threshold motor responses, whether stimulating with trains or single pulses. Cathodal pulses thus seem to be distinctly more effective than anodal ones for producing conscious sensory responses but not for motor responses. The near parity of cathode vs. anode for observable motor responses fits with the findings for precentral gyrus in monkey (Mihailović and Delgado, 1956; but see Lilly et al., 1952) and in baboon (Hern et al., 1962; Phillips, 1969). With more sensitive endpoints than an observable twitch (e.g. EPSP's in spinal motoneurones), or with certain positionings of the electrode, Hern et al. (1962) found the anode distinctly more effective.

8. Unipolar vs. Bipolar Electrode, and Liminal I

For threshold-c stimulus trains to somatosensory cortex, the liminal I requirement for a unipolar electrode (0.5 mm diameter) was roughly similar to that for bipolar electrodes (Libet et al., 1964). This relationship was obtained with a 1.5 mm separation between the bipolar contracts and with the cathodal member of the pair employed as the surface cathode in the unipolar tests. For eliciting movements by stimulating the motor cortex of baboon, Phillips and Porter

(1962) found that a similar bipolar arrangement required stronger currents than a unipolar one of either polarity.

9. Area of Unipolar Electrode and Liminal I: Spatial Facilitation

An increase in diameter of the electrode contact from 1 mm increased the liminal I requirement (for a conscious sensory response) about twofold for a 2 mm electrode, and about fourfold for a 10 mm electrode (LIBET et al., 1964). However, the current density at the electrode, i.e. liminal I per mm² of contact area, was markedly lower with the larger electrodes; it was reduced to about 50% of the value for a 1 mm electrode when the latter was replaced by a 2 mm electrode, and down to about 4 % when replaced by a 10 mm electrode. Because of lateral spread, the current density calculated for the contact area of a surface electrode would reflect the actual current density through the cortical tissue less accurately for a smaller than for a larger electrode. Nevertheless, it is safe to assume that the maximal current density through some area of cortex is considerably greater under a 1 mm than under a 10 mm electrode.

Although the liminal current density was lower with the larger electrode, the size of the body area to which the subjective sensation was referred did not decrease; if anything, there was a small increase of the referral area in some cases. The ability of the large electrode to produce a similar sensory response but with much lower current density would appear to represent a form of spatial facilitation. Under the large electrode there may be an initial activation of certain lower threshold neuronal elements, which are present in a lower density over the wider area of cortex. Excitation of these elements may induce the sufficient activation of certain neuronal elements that can lead eventually to a conscious sensory response.

10. Neural Elements Initially Excited

In an analysis of the latency and other characteristics of pyramidal cell responses to surface stimulation of motor cortex, PHILLIPS and his colleagues (HERN et al., 1962; PHILLIPS, 1969) concluded that a unipolar anode excited the axons of pyramidal cells directly, but that a unipolar cathode acted on them indirectly by exciting elements that lie more superficial and are presynaptic to the pyramidal cells. This appeared to hold at least for stimulus strengths that are near threshold levels. In producing conscious sensory responses by threshold stimulation of somatosensory cortex, the distinctly lower threshold currents required of surface cathodal as opposed to anodal pulse trains thus indicate that these responses involve the initial excitation of presynaptic fibers. Since the threshold intensities for sensory responses are similar when determined with bipolar or with unipolar cathodal stimuli (see above), the relevant presynaptic fibers initially excited probably lie very close to the cortical surface, i.e. in layer I. This conclusion would follow from the supposition that the fields of stimulus current would be very similar immediately below the cathodes of both a surface bipolar or unipolar electrode arrangement, but that the fields would be dissimilar elsewhere in the cortex (cf. GLEASON, 1970, for fields of applied currents). While the possibility of direct excitation of pyramidal cell axons cannot be excluded even with bipolar surface electrodes (e.g. Patton and Amassian, 1954; Rosenthal et al., 1967; Phillips, 1969), it would seem to be an improbable occurrence under the conditions of liminal stimulation required at sensory cortex (see Phillis and Ochs, 1971).

These parametric stimulus relationships, for cathode-anode polarity and for uni- vs. bipolarity would not distinguish between alternative anatomical orientations of the relevant presynaptic fibers in layer I, i.e. as to whether the orientation is tangential (horizontal) or vertical (radial or perpendicular to the surface). Fibers in layer I are predominantly tangential and each can spread for a distance of several mm in this direction (Colonnier, 1966), but they could be excited as they turned vertically to enter or leave layer I. Fibers below layer I are oriented predominantly in the vertical direction. However, there is little doubt that under the large, 10 mm electrode the relevant presynaptic fibers would be excited along a vertically oriented course, since the bulk of the lower density current at threshold-c must be taking a purely vertical path in the upper cortical layers directly below this electrode.

Axons in layer I are apparently derived from ascending intracortical axons originating mainly from cells in the deeper layers, V and VI (Colonnier, 1966). There may also be a contribution from axons of stellate cells particularly the fusiform type in layers II, III, and IV. Other vertically oriented fibers in primary sensory cortices would include the specific thalamo-cortical afferents, which appear to terminate on stellate cells and on the middle regions of apical dendrite shafts, most heavily in layer IV; nonspecific afferents from reticular core of brain stem and thalamus, ending diffusely on the entire apical shaft; and transcortical and transcallosal fibers terminating in all layers below I, but heavily in the lower layers (see Chow and Leiman, 1970). It would appear unlikely that surface stimuli at threshold-c intensities are exciting the specific afferents, because of the latter's depth and because of the form of the direct cortical response evoked by such stimuli (see below). The most likely elements initially excited by trains with liminal I strength would appear to be the axons of intracortical origin which enter into layer I. (See also Burns, 1958, and Ochs and Clark, 1968a, b, in relation to production of direct cortical responses by surface stimuli.) Excitation of other vertically oriented elements that rise through the upper layers to levels below layer I cannot, of course, be excluded, especially under the large 10 mm electrode. The location and nature of the *post*synaptic elements, that are innervated by the presynaptic fibers presumed to be excited initially, is considered below under "direct cortical responses".

11. Train Repetition Rate (TRR) and Liminal I: Temporal Facilitation

A 30 sec interval between successive stimulus trains is generally sufficient to prevent any progressive reduction in liminal I, with stimuli in parametric region A (Libet et al., 1964); the minimum interval for constancy of liminal I has not been established. However, with stimuli in parametric regions B and C repeated at a TRR of 2 per min there is often a progressive reduction in threshold-c I to a new level; also, repetition of stimuli with initially subthreshold-c I values at this TRR can achieve a threshold-c response without a change in I. Such changes are not observed when the TRR is slowed to 0.25–1 per min.

There are several points of interest in this post-stimulus facilitatory effect. (1) A sufficiently long stimulus interval, depending on the parametric region, must obviously be allowed if constancy of threshold is desired. (2) The use of peak currents greater than liminal I appeared to be more important for this effect than the total amount of activation. With stimulus currents initially at liminal I there was no evidence of any progressive change in threshold I at a TRR of 2 per min, whether the stimulus TD's were 0.5 sec or 5.0 sec. (3) A post-stimulus facilitatory effect with a duration of minutes must have a basis different from the type of facilitation that is a function of the pulse repetition rate during the stimulus train (see above under PF and liminal I). Whatever the synaptic mechanisms are for the former long-lasting type, they are probably related to the "primary" facilitation observed in motor and sensory cortex (BROWN, 1915; LEYTON and SHERRINGTON, 1917; LILLY, 1952; PENFIELD and WELCH, 1949). At motor cortex, repetition of such stimuli at shorter intervals can, of course, lead into a seizure pattern in unanesthetized individuals. (The possibility of a post-stimulus "surround inhibition" should also be borne in mind; see above under "Variation in responses etc.".)

12. Neuronal Injury and Parameters of Stimulation

It is generally agreed that irreversible injury due to passage of electrical current is chiefly a function of the number of unidirectional coulombs passed by the stimuli (McINTYRE et al., 1959). (This is apart from the possibility of injury from release of products at the metal-solution interface of the electrode, or from the generation of sufficient heat, as in the case of passage of currents in the radiofrequency range.) No injury has been found in brain when the total unidirectional charge passed is less than about 2.5 millicoulombs, with the ordinary macroscopic electrode exposure (McINTYRE et al., 1959). As pointed out by LILLY (1961), injury can be avoided by using a "balanced" diphasic pulse form with phases of opposite polarity separated by about 100 μsec, so that charges passed in both directions are equal. An interval as long as 50 msec between the alternate phases of bidirectional stimuli has been found to be effective for this purpose (ROWLAND et al., 1960). This permits one to adapt the usually available rectangular stimulus pulses by alternating the polarity of successive pulses in a train (ALBERTS, 1958). An alternating polarity of pulses could involve alternating shifts in the site of intracortical excitation with the successive pulses. This may not be a serious problem for many purposes; with surface stimulation of somatosensory cortex the values of stimulus parameters for threshold-c sensory responses (in parametric region A) have been found to fall into the same general range of values that are obtained when using unidirectional pulses.

The coulomb content of threshold-c stimuli was found to vary within the range of values for each parameter (LIBET et al., 1964). Coulombic content for threshold-c stimuli is lower (even though liminal I is greater) with lower pulse frequencies and with shorter pulse durations. Thus, the total amount of coulombs of unidirectional current could be minimized by proper selection of ranges used. In addition, coulombs passed may be minimized by using TD's that are no longer than utilization-TD (of 0.5–1 sec) whenever possible, since longer TD's merely give a longer-lasting sensory response with no decrease in liminal I (i.e. in the peak current required; see TD, above).

D. Potentials Evoked in Somatosensory Cortex by Threshold-c Stimuli

The electrophysiological responses of somatosensory cortex may provide some further indications of the kinds of neuronal activity that are involved in mediating conscious sensory experience. The potentials elicited there by stimuli that are adequate for producing a conscious sensory response may be compared to those elicited by inadequate or subthreshold-c stimuli.

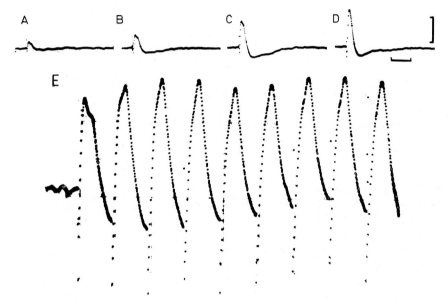

Fig. 4. Direct cortical responses (DCR) evoked in somatosensory cortex by adjacent direct stimuli (0.3-msec pulses). Subject is a parkinsonian patient, unanesthetized. Each tracing in A–D is the average of 18 responses at 0.5 per second; horizontal bar in D indicates 100 msec. A, stimulus current 0.3 ma; B, 0.8 ma (equal to liminal I, see E); C, 1.7 ma; D, 5.0 ma (4 ma gave a similar response). Subject reported not feeling any of these "single pulse" stimuli, in A to D. Vertical bar, 200 μvolt. (From LIBET et al., 1967, by permission of Science). E, averaged response to 10 separate trains, 0.5 sec TD, PF of 20 pps and I of 0.8 ma peak currents; i.e. stimulus with utilization-TD at liminal I, each eliciting a conscious sensory response in the same subject as in A–D. Lines indicate time intervals of 55 msec. (From LIBET et al., 1972a)

1. Direct Cortical Responses; Postsynaptic Neuronal Elements Mediating Conscious Sensory Response

As found in animal studies (e.g. PURPURA, 1959; OCHS, 1962), the DCR recorded unipolarly on the surface of human cerebral cortex, adjacent to a bipolar stimulus, shows an initial surface negative component (N), followed by a smaller, longer-lasting positive (P) component and, with stronger stimuli, a slow negative wave (PURPURA et al., 1957b; GOLDRING et al., 1958, 1961). During a train of repetitive pulses, a slow negative shift builds up and the faster N response to each pulse tends to decrease concomitantly (GOLDRING et al., 1958, 1961). The N and P potentials are largely generated as a result of postsynaptic responses to the excitation of presynaptic fibers by the stimulus (ECCLES, 1951; PURPURA, 1959; OCHS and CLARK, 1968 a). There is general agreement that the N wave represents a response of apical dendrites, with some additional evidence that this may include production of a decrementally propagating dendritic action potential or local response (OCHS and CLARK, 1968 b; PHILLIS and OCHS, 1971). The P component apparently reflects a depolarizing response of pyramidal soma-dendritic regions in somewhat deeper cortical layers (IWAMA and JASPER, 1957; BINDMAN et al., 1962; SUZUKI and OCHS, 1964; LANDAU, 1967) and perhaps IPSP responses in the apical shafts as well (PURPURA, 1959; LI and CHOU, 1962; CREUTZFELDT et al., 1966; OCHS and CLARK, 1968 b).

The threshold-I levels needed for eliciting DCR-N and P responses were found to be below the liminal I values that were required to elicit conscious sensory responses by cortical stimulus trains of 20 or 30 pps in parametric region A, as in Fig. 4 (LIBET et al., 1967). On the other hand, liminal I for sensory responses was found to be below the strength required for producing maximal N and P waves, and it was below the threshold I for producing any slow negativity in single DCR responses. When stimulating with a 20–30 pps train of liminal I pulses, which become adequate for conscious sensation after a utilization-train duration of about 0.5 sec (as in Fig. 4), there were no striking changes in the DCR responses during or at the end of such a train (LIBET, 1965; LIBET et al., 1972 a). In addition, no after-waves could be detected after such stimulus trains. Nor was there any correlation between threshold-c stimulus adequacy and the appearance of a negative steady potential shift during such trains. There is, therefore, no evidence in the surface recorded DCR's of any unique neuronal response that appears to be correlated with the attainment of adequacy, by the cortical stimulus, for eliciting subjective sensory experience (see further discussion of this below, in section on utilization-TD).

One approach to discovering which components of a compound neuronal response may at least be necessary, for the production of the conscious sensory response, lies in applying selective blocking agents to the tissue. Gamma-aminobutyric acid (GABA) appears to mimic or in fact be an inhibitory synaptic transmitter in the cerebral cortex (KRNJEVIĆ and SCHWARTZ, 1967; CURTIS et al., 1970); it hyperpolarizes and increases ionic conductance of postsynaptic membranes and should, therefore, depress the excitability of postsynaptic structures as well as the amplitudes of postsynaptic potentials. The application of GABA to the cortical surface can produce a suppression of the DCR-N wave, or a reversal of its polarity to surface positivity (PURPURA et al., 1957 a; IWAMA and JASPER, 1957; OCHS, 1962); surface negative components of evoked potentials responding to peripheral sensory stimuli, and of other evoked or spontaneous potentials also are depressed or inverted to positivity. The best explanation of these effects of GABA is that, when applied to the cortical surface, it penetrates only into the uppermost layers and depresses postsynaptic responses there. The unaffected postsynaptic responses of the deeper layers still contribute to the surface recordings and thus account for the change in surface polarity (IWAMA and JASPER, 1957; BINDMAN et al., 1962;

Ochs and Clark, 1968a). GABA does not interfere with excitation of superficial fibers and transmission of their presynaptic impulses to adjacent areas, where they can still elicit normal DCR responses (Iwama and Jasper, 1957; Ochs and Clark, 1968a).

GABA has now been applied to somatosensory cortex of human subjects, in a manner sufficient to abolish the DCR-N wave or invert the polarity of this response (Libet et al., 1972b). Under such conditions, no significant changes were produced in the ability of surface cortical stimuli to elicit conscious sensory responses; i.e. there was no effect on the liminal I or the utilization-TD required for threshold-c trains, or on the quality of the conscious sensory responses to such cortical stimuli. Nor were any changes observed by the subjects in their peripheral somatic sensibility (e.g. there were no reports of "numbness"), and preliminary tests in a few cases for thresholds with von Frey hairs and for 2-point discrimination showed no obvious changes.

These findings indicate that postsynaptic responses of apical dendrites and other neuronal elements in the superficial cortical layers of sensory cortex (including the neuropil of the molecular layer) are not necessary for the production of a subjective sensory experience. Instead, it would seem that postsynaptic responses of neurons or parts thereof that lie below the upper few layers are probably more directly involved in mediating the conscious sensory response. Such neuronal elements could presumably be acted upon by presynaptic fibers that are initially excited by the surface stimuli (see above), e.g. by fibers in the molecular layer that dip down vertically to end on deeper neuronal elements (Ochs and Clark, 1968a, b) or by radially ascending fibers. The findings with GABA might be taken to support Penfield's contention (e.g. Penfield, 1958) that, to elicit a sensory response, the cortical stimulus directly excites corticofugal fibers, and that the primary sensory cortex should be regarded as a simple relay station. However, the other available evidence, from stimulus parameter requirements and from analyses of responses in cortex of lower animals, points to a presynaptic site for the initial excitatory action of the cortical stimulus (see above). Additional evidence is accumulating which suggests (e.g. Towe et al., 1968; Whitehorn and Towe, 1968) that the primary sensory cortex has a more elaborate function than that of a simple distributory relay station. On the other hand, any such functions of sensory cortex are quite compatible with a requirement for eventual efferent discharge, from sensory cortex to other cerebral areas, as part of the processes mediating conscious sensory experience.

2. Evoked Potentials, with Stimulation of Skin or n. VPL

When single pulse stimuli are applied to the skin (or to a peripheral nerve), evoked potentials can be detected with electrodes on the scalp with the aid of averaging techniques (e.g. Katzman, 1964; Cobb and Morocutti, 1968; Donchin and Lindsley, 1969). With suitable placement of electrodes, even the short latency (20 $\pm$ msec) relatively localized, surface-positive component can be detected (e.g. Giblin, 1964; DeBecker et al., 1965). The thresholds for scalp-recorded evoked potentials have been reported to coincide reasonably well with those for eliciting a conscious sensory response (Shagass and Schwartz, 1961);

evoked potentials could also be detected in the "uncertainty" range of stimulus intensities, in which some but not all the stimuli are felt by the subject (DEBECKER et al., 1965), and even at about the "absolute threshold for psychophysical detection" (ROSNER and GOFF, 1967). But it was also reported that scalp-evoked potentials could be reduced to the vanishing level by inhalation of cyclopropane without markedly depressing the psychophysical detection of the stimulus by the subjects (CLARK et al., 1969).

However, recordings of evoked potentials on the scalp are considerably attenuated as compared to those recordable on the cortex directly (e.g. HEATH and GALBRAITH, 1966; LIBET et al., 1967; BROUGHTON, 1969); this is especially the case for the early, more localized components (see also GEISLER and GERSTEIN,

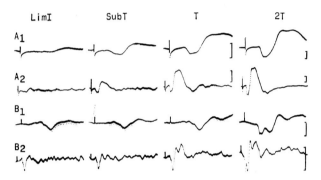

Fig. 5. Averaged evoked potentials of somatosensory cortex in relation to threshold stimuli at skin. Each tracing is the average of 500 responses at 1.8 per second. Total trace length is 125 msec in A_1 and B_1 and 500 msec in A_2 and B_2; beginning of stimulus artifact has been made visible near start of each tracing. A and B, separate subjects, both parkinsonian patients. Vertical column T: threshold stimuli, subjects reporting not feeling some of the 500 stimuli. Column 2T: stimuli at twice threshold current; all stimuli felt distinctly. Column SubT: subthreshold stimuli, none felt by subject; current about 15 percent below T in subject A, 25% below T in B. Column LimI: subthreshold stimuli at "liminal intensity" (see text), about 25% below T in subject A, about 35 to 40% below T in B. Polarity, positive downward in all figures. Vertical bars in A, under T, indicate 50 μvolt in A_1 and A_2 respectively, but gains are different in 2T as shown; for B_1 and B_2, 20-μvolt bars. (Calibration obtained by summating 500 sweeps of calibrating signal.) (From LIBET et al., 1967, by permission of Science)

1961; CELESIA et al., 1968; STOHR and GOLDRING, 1969; VAUGHAN, 1969). Scalp recordings may also be contaminated with potentials originating extracranially (BICKFORD et al., 1964; CELESIA et al., 1968; VAUGHAN, 1969). When recordings are made subdurally the position of the electrode on the skin can be matched with the referred location of the conscious sensory response obtainable by directly stimulating the cortical electrode; this can improve the cortical recording of highly localized responses to skin stimulation (see also JASPER et al., 1960). Subdural recording can also obviate the problem of extracranial potentials.

With subdural recordings at a point on postcentral gyrus and with the locus for the skin stimulus matched to the referral from this cortical point, it was found that an averaged evoked potential could be detected with stimulus strengths that were distinctly below the lower limit for threshold-c level (see Fig. 5). That is, evoked potentials could be detected with skin stimuli which were well below the range of uncertainty and which never elicited any conscious sensory responses (Libet et al., 1967). The evoked potentials produced by such single subthreshold-c pulses to skin consist mainly of an initial or primary surface positive component; the later components only appear at about the threshold-c level (though the first negative component that follows the primary positive one has at times also been evident with subthreshold-c strengths). This finding indicates (a) that the neuronal activity represented by the primary component of the evoked potential is not sufficient for initiating the cerebral events involved in the appearance of the conscious sensory response (see further below, under n.VPL); and it suggests (b) that the later components represent activity that may be necessary for such a response, as has also been suggested more indirectly from other types of findings (Davis, 1964; Haider et al., 1964; Wagman and Battersby, 1964; Donchin and Cohen, 1967).

The skin threshold strength for detection of some cortical evoked potentials did coincide roughly with the liminal I value for conscious sensory response, as seen in Fig. 5 (Libet et al., 1967); liminal I is obtained when the stimulus is a brief train of pulses at 60 pps instead of a single pulse. This indicated that a single pulse (i.e. repeated at 1 pps or less), which has a somewhat higher threshold-c I than liminal I for the train, has to excite more than one cutaneous sensory nerve fiber in order to elicit a conscious sensory response, even in subjects who are closely attentive to the stimulus (Libet et al., 1967). Such a conclusion is in accord with the quantitative peripheral nerve studies of Buchthal and Rosenfalck (1966). With recordings from an exposed cutaneous nerve bundle in trained human subjects, Hensel and Boman (1960) concluded that one nerve impulse in one sensory fiber might be sufficient to produce a conscious sensation, although they admit the possibility that additionally excited fibers may not have been included in the recorded bundle.

In n.VPL, a single pulse of relatively high current is ineffective for eliciting a conscious sensory experience (see above section on "train duration"). Nevertheless, such a pulse can produce a large evoked potential in the appropriate area of human somatosensory cortex (Libet et al., 1967), as was to be expected from studies on animals (Dempsey and Morison, 1943; Andersen and Andersson, 1968). The primary surface-positive component of these evoked potentials is presumably elicited in the same cortical elements and by the same specific projection fibers to the cortex as is the primary component elicited by a skin stimulus. The primary evoked potential elicited by single pulse-stimuli to n.VPL can attain an amplitude that is greater than the one elicited by a skin stimulus that is well above threshold-c level for skin, as seen in Fig. 6 (Libet et al., 1967). The absence of a conscious sensory response to a single pulse in n.VPL, therefore, establishes even more firmly the conclusion that the primary component is not sufficient to initiate subjective experience (see above, "evoked potentials with the skin stimuli").

It follows from these considerations, that the presence or amplitude of an evoked potential, particularly of the primary component, cannot be assumed to be an indicator of the occurrence or intensity of subjective sensory experience without other validation under the conditions of study (see also, section above on "relation of sensory responses to representation of evoked potentials").

E. Significance of Utilization-TD

The utilization-TD, i.e. the minimum train duration required for cortical stimuli at liminal I strength (parametric region A) to elicit a conscious sensory response, appears to be a physiologically significant phenomenon and quantity. Values for utilization-TD have fallen mostly in the range of 0.4–1.0 sec (clustering at 0.5–0.6 sec) for all subjects. The value is relatively constant for a given subject. Changes in other stimulus parameters have little or no effect on utilization-TD, even when they markedly affect the liminal I requirements. The value for utiliza-

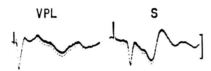

Fig. 6. Evoked potentials of somatosensory cortex in response to thalamic (VPL) and skin stimuli in the same subject (patient with heredofamilial tremor). Each tracing is the average of 250 responses at 1.8 per second; total trace length, 125 msec. VPL: stimuli in ventral poster-olateral nucleus of thalamus; subject reported not feeling any of these stimuli, though current was 6 times liminal I for VPL electrode (liminal I being minimum current to elicit sensation with 60 pulses per second trains of stimuli). S: stimuli at skin; current at twice threshold, all stimuli felt. Vertical bar, 50 μvolt. Note the shorter latency of the primary (positive) evoked response to VPL stimulus. (From LIBET et al., 1967, by permission of Science)

tion-TD is relatively independent of PF's (except for the range below 10 pps, where it seems to be distinctly longer, — see LIBET et al., 1964). Values for utiliza-tion-TD were found to be in the usual range whether the stimulus pulses were cathodal or anodal in surface polarity (unidirectional pulses), alternating in pola-rity, had pulse durations varying from 0.1–0.5 msec, or were applied via bipolar instead of unipolar electrodes, or by larger (up to 10 mm) electrodes instead of smaller ones (down to 0.25 mm).

The relatively large utilization-TD (about 0.5 sec) for eliciting conscious sen-sory responses with stimuli at sensory cortex, as compared to skin (0.1 sec), is not a peculiarity due to "abnormal" routes of input that may be excited by the surface cortical electrode; similarly long values were found with stimulation of the ascend-ing projection system, both in n.VPL and in the subcortical white matter below somatosensory cortex (LIBET et al., 1964, 1967). Incidentally, the finding that the same subject shows a large difference, between the utilization-TD's for skin and cortical stimuli, rules out a possible contention that the longer utilization-TD is due to an arbitrary criterion level, for some minimal duration of the sensation, before the subjects are willing to report the experience of a conscious sensory response.

49*

The longer utilization-TD for stimuli in the cerebral portions of the somatosensory system is not a peculiar requirement for all types of stimulus-response processes at these levels. For, the motor cortex required only a very brief utilization-TD for liminal stimuli in the unanesthetized human subject, and it showed no definable utilization-TD in the anesthetized cat (see above). In addition, the effect of prolonging the stimulus TD beyond 0.5–1 sec is strikingly different for sensory and motor areas in man. For somatosensory cortex, stimuli with TD's longer than the utilization-TD, but at the same liminal I strength, simply elicit longer-lasting conscious sensory experiences without any change in subjective intensity. For motor cortex, stimuli kept at a liminal-I value elicit motor responses that progressively increase in intensity and in extent of responding body musculature as the TD is lengthened. Indeed, motor responses to longer trains of even relatively weak stimuli tend to progress into seizures, even in non-epileptic patients.

A utilization-TD of about 0.5 sec for eliciting a conscious sensory experience would indicate a requirement of a surprisingly long period of "activation" of somatosensory cortex, at least for near-liminal inputs. It has been postulated that such a period of activation, of the cortical areas that may be involved, is a fundamental physiological requirement for the mediation of conscious sensory and other subjective experiences (Libet et al., 1964; Libet, 1965, 1966). If one accepts the relatively long period of activation as a requirement for conscious experience of at least near-threshold sensory stimuli, then a number of interesting psychological and philosophical inferences arise (Libet, 1965, 1966). One of these is that the conscious sensory response at threshold has a kind of all-or-nothing aspect to it; "activation" below the minimum, either in duration or intensity, would not give rise to any conscious experience, as defined here, although they are generating demonstrable neural responses in the cortex.

Evidence for such a minimum time requirement for the experience also of peripheral sensory inputs is presented below ("Retroactive masking"). Peripheral stimuli to skin require only a very short utilization-TD (0.1 sec) and a single pulse stimulus can easily be made adequate for a sensory response, but this does not exclude the postulated cortical requirement. Peripheral sensory nerve impulses may, by various routes, initiate cortical activations that outlast the initial short-latency cortical response (e.g. Wagman and Battersby, 1964; see also Katzman, 1964; Bergamini and Bergamasco, 1967; Cobb and Morocutti, 1968; Donchin and Lindsley, 1969; MacKay, 1969). Even a single pulse stimulus to skin, at or just above threshold-c intensity, has been shown to elicit at the cortex a sequence of evoked potential components that may have a total duration of several 100 msec or more (Libet et al., 1967, and 1972b; see also Giblin, 1964, DeBecker et al., 1965, and others, for scalp recordings on this point).

At least two alternative possibilities exist to describe the nature of the physiological "coding" of the conscious sensory experience, when a relatively long utilization time of about 0.5 sec is required: (a) Some special neuronal event is triggered at the end of the adequate period; or (b), the occurrence of a series of certain similar neuronal events for a given period itself constitutes the code. With stimulus sites at sensory cortex or n.VPL, where the actual utilizations-TD's are long, one can have more direct control of the period of activation. As already indicated, no distinctive differences can be seen between the DCR's elicited by trains of liminal I pulses that are shorter, equal to, or somewhat longer than utilization TD. Nor have any unique new potentials or after-waves been detected following completion of a utilization-TD, at least in surface recordings from somatosensory or other cortical areas (LIBET, 1966; LIBET et al., 1967, and 1972a). This absence of distinctive changes in the recorded electrical responses during and after the utilization-TD is in accord with the absence of any progressive build-up in subjective intensity of the sensory experience when cortical stimulus trains longer than the utilization-TD are delivered. (The relationships between stimulus train, DCR's and "appearance" of conscious sensory response are diagrammed in Fig. 7).

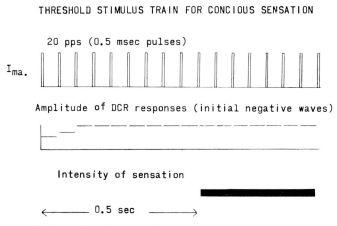

THRESHOLD STIMULUS TRAIN FOR CONCIOUS SENSATION

20 pps (0.5 msec pulses)

$I_{ma.}$

Amplitude of DCR responses (initial negative waves)

Intensity of sensation

←——— 0.5 sec ———→

Fig. 7. Diagram of relationships between the train of 0.5 msec pulses at liminal intensity applied to postcentral gyrus, and the amplitudes of the direct cortical responses (DCR) recorded nearby. (A train of actual DCR's elicited by an adequate stimulus train is seen in Fig. 4 E). The third line indicates that no conscious sensory experience is elicited until approximately the initial 0.5 sec of events has elapsed, and that the just detectable sensation appearing after that period remains at the same subjective intensity while the stimulus train continues. (From LIBET, 1966)

Similarly, the evoked potentials which are elicited at sensory cortex by a utilization-TD stimulus to n.VPL show no unique components at the end or after the train (LIBET et al., 1972a, b). Such evidence appears to favor alternative (b) for the "coding mechanisms", but this can only be regarded as indicative rather than conclusive. Obviously, DCR's and evoked potentials are incomplete representations of the neuronal events that may be occurring in the somatosensory cortex or elsewhere in the brain at such times.

1. Retroactive or Backward Masking, by a Second Stimulus, of the Conscious Sensory Response to a Preceding Stimulus

It has been demonstrated that a second but stronger peripheral stimulus (S_2) can in various ways mask or completely blank out the awareness of a *preceding* relatively weak and shorter-lasting peripheral stimulus (S_1) (see review by RAAB,

1963). With visual stimuli the backward masking effect can be obtained with the conditioning stimulus S_2 following the test stimulus S_1 by about 100 to 200 msec or more, in the so-called Crawford effect (Crawford, 1947; see also Wagman and Battersby, 1964). Backward masking effects with auditory stimuli have generally been shown for intervals of about 50–100 msec, but some effects have been reported for intervals as long as 1000 msec (see Raab, 1963; Békésy, 1971). Cutaneous backward masking has been less frequently studied but has been demonstrated for intervals of about 50 to 100 msec (see Raab, 1963; Melzack and Wall, 1963). The question of the nature and location of the neural elements and processes involved in retroactive masking is complicated by the fact that there are both peripheral and central contributions possible (see Crawford, 1947; Raab, 1963). This complication could be avoided if backward masking could be demonstrated when the conditioning or second stimulus S_2 is applied directly to a cortical site, in a known temporal relationship to the initial arrival at the cortex of the afferent projection of impulses initiated by S_1.

2. Retroactive Masking by a Cortical Stimulus

Positive results with such a retroactive masking paradigm have now been achieved (Libet et al., 1972a). The conditioning or delayed stimulus S_2 was applied directly to somatosensory cortex (postcentral gyrus) in human subjects. It consisted of a brief train (usually of 0.5 sec TD) of pulses (60 pps), with peak currents at about 1.3–1.5 times the liminal I that was required by this cortical stimulus for eliciting a conscious sensory response. The test or first stimulus S_1 was a single pulse at threshold-c intensity; it was applied to the skin inside the body area to which was referred the sensory response elicited by the cortical stimulus. The sensations generated by S_1 and S_2 separately could usually be distinguished readily, by their different qualities and extent of somatic area. The S_1–S_2 interval in this procedure refers to the time between S_1 (single pulse) and the *beginning* of the S_2 train of pulses.

The conscious sensory response obtained with S_1 alone completely vanished when S_1 and S_2 overlapped in time (see above, "Adequacy of electrical stimulation . . ."). Response to S_1 continued to be masked, however, when the S_1–S_2 interval was increased up to 125–200 msec for most subjects, and up to 500 msec in one subject; i.e. at these intervals only a single sensory response was reported which was identical with that elicited by S_2 alone. When the interval was greater, or when the strength of S_1 was raised sufficiently, the subjects experienced both of the sensations in the same temporal order as the responsible stimuli. When S_2 was a single pulse stimulus to the cortex it appeared to be ineffective for masking; the minimum S_2 train duration that is needed in order to achieve retroactive masking, and therefore the total effective interval for masking, is yet to be determined. The latency to the beginning of the primary evoked potential produced at somatosensory cortex by S_1 (when applied to the hand) is about 20 msec, and this should be subtracted from the total effective interval. Fortunately, the latent periods of the early evoked potential components do not vary significantly with the strength of peripheral somatic stimuli (Giblin, 1964; Libet et al., 1967), and are not increased even for skin stimuli at threshold-c levels or below (Libet et al., 1967; In prep. b); this is unlike the increase in latencies of the visual evoked response with decreasing intensities of light flash (e.g. VAUGHAN et al., 1966).

Retroactive masking of the peripheral (S_1) sensation by a later stimulus (S_2) directly to somatosensory cortex, with S_1–S_2 intervals of up to 200 msec or more, could only be due to interference with some late components of the brain responses to S_1 that are necessary for the mediation of a conscious sensory response. The mechanism of such interference is an open question. It seems probable that the maximum potential S_1–S_2 interval for effective backward masking is greater than that achieved, as it is unlikely that all of the potentially effective cortex was stimulated by the S_2 stimulus that was applied. In any case, the extent of retroactive masking that could be demonstrated provides powerful support for the hypothesis that a relatively long period of suitable cerebral activations is a necessary feature of the processes mediating conscious sensory experiences (LIBET et al., 1964; LIBET, 1965, 1966).

F. Qualities of Sensory Responses to Cortical Stimuli

The discussion thus far has considered the relationship between stimulation of somatosensory cortex and the production of some conscious sensory experience, but without any special consideration of the way in which specific subjective qualities of sensory experiences may be related to such stimulation. The latter consideration relates to the question of what the specific spatial-temporal configurations of neuronal activity are that provide the coding for the subjective experiences of different sensory qualities in general. For the differences among the more general modalities (i.e. somatic, visual, auditory, olfactory, gustatory), a modified version of Johannes Müller's Doctrine of Specific Nerve Energies would still appear to satisfy the findings obtained by electrical stimulation of the cortex. MÜLLER (1843) had observed that the general quality of a sensation depended on the specific nerve that was excited rather than on the nature of the stimulus, e.g. a visual experience resulted whether the eye was stimulated by light or mechanically. He concluded that: "Sensation consists in the sensorium receiving through the medium of the nerves, and as the result of the action of an external cause, a knowledge of certain qualities or conditions, not of external bodies, but of the nerves of sense themselves; and these qualities of the nerves of sense are in all different, the nerve of each sense having its own peculiar quality or energy" (Book VI, p. 712). He added with some perspicacity that "it is not known whether the essential cause of the peculiar 'energy' of each nerve or sense is seated in the nerve itself, or in the parts of the brain and spinal cord with which it is connected" (p. 714). The unique relationship between the subjective experience of a given modality and an afferent pathway appears to hold, at least crudely, for the primary sensory receiving areas of the cerebral cortex. Direct electrical stimulation of each such cortical area not only elicits subjective sensory experiences but does so only within the one general sensory modality associated with the specific afferent projection to that area (e.g. PENFIELD and RASMUSSEN, 1950). Convergence of different sensory inputs has been found in wide areas of cortex outside the primary sensory areas (e.g. BUSER and BIGNALL, 1967; BIGNALL and IMBERT, 1969), but the relation of such polysensory projections to subjective modalities is yet to be determined. (See also section above, on "Relation of sensory responses to representation of evoked potentials.") The questions about (a) whether a given peripheral afferent fiber or a given ascending fiber in the CNS can be involved in the mediation of more than one quality of sensory experience, and (b) the nature and extent of the interaction of effects among different inputs and ascending pathways in relation to modalities, have been considered elsewhere in this volume.

It is theoretically possible that suitably sophisticated stimulation of the "silent" cortical areas would elicit subjective experiences that could include sensory ones in some form, as already indicated above (section on "Limitations of electrical stimulation"). However, the present results of cortical stimulation and excision (or pathological damage) would support a re-stated version of Müller's Doctrine — namely, that the quality of a sensation depends on the activation of specific cerebral areas by the sensory nerve fibers mediating that quality. Such a view would not exclude the possibility that temporal and/or spatial patterns of the inputs to such cerebral areas play a significant role in determining quality. Nor would it rule out the possibility that cerebral areas other than the primary sensory areas of cortex play a role, whether activated through a primary area or otherwise. But such a view does continue the Müllerian idea that the site(s) of the cerebral neurones activated is (are) of critical significance in mediating quality; in this view, any spatio-temporal patterns of inputs that might be specifically involved in mediating a given sensory quality would be effective only if imposed on certain specified groups of cerebral neurones, not on any nonspecified groups anywhere in the cortex or subcortex.

The question to be considered more fully in the present context is that of the production, by stimulation of somatosensory cortex, of subjective experiences of the subqualities within the modality of somatic sensation (i.e. touch, pressure, motion, heat, cold, pain, etc.). Earlier investigators have emphasized the generally non-specific qualities of the responses, i.e. that the experiences were usually of parasthesia-like character (tingling, electric shock, etc.), although other more natural-like qualities were elicited by them at times (e.g. Foerster, 1936b; Penfield and Rasmussen, 1950). Penfield and Boldrey (1937) summarized the qualities described by their subjects in a total of 426 responses. (Since their compilation evidently included many stimulus responses at various cortical sites in a given individual, the total number of individual subjects was presumably much smaller than 426). Of the 426 responses, 335 responses were called tingling or electricity or numbness (131 being numbness). Of the remaining 91 responses that did not have a purely parasthesia-like quality, 49 were described as a "sense of movement" when no change in position was observed; 13 were called "coldness", most of these in the face region (though Penfield and Boldrey suggested that it seemed possible that tingling may have been called or taken for coldness); 2 were called heat; 10 were described as a "sense of blood rushing"; 6 were termed thickness or swelling, all in connection with the tongue. For 11 responses the word "pain" was used, but the "pain" was never severe and never caused the patient to object; they concluded that pain has "little if any true cortical representation". (A subjective "desire-to-move", without resultant movement was reported a number of times with stimuli on the precentral cortex.) Seizures involving the

Table 2.[a] *Incidence of responses among subjects, to stimulation of postcentral gyrus*[b]

Type of response	(X) Stimulus parametric region A[c]		(Y) Subdural testing[d]	(Z) Exploring electrode[e]
A. "Parasthesia-like" (totals)	41		47	40
B. "Natural-like" (totals)	64		51	18
a) something "moving inside"		17	15	5
b) feeling of movement of part		15	17	3
c) deep pressures		12	8	7
d) surface mechano-type		6	6	2
e) vibration		4	2	–
f) warmth		8	3	1
g) coldness		2	–	–
Actual number of subjects, in the stimulus and response categories Totals (164)	60		64	50
I. Subjects reporting parasthesias *only*		12	24	33
II. Subjects reporting "natural-like" qualities *only*[f]		14	21	10
III. Subjects reporting parasthesias plus any non-parasthesias[g]	34		19	7
III'. Subjects reporting parasthesias plus only *one* non-parasthesia[h]		(17)[8]	(15)[8]	

[a] Data from LIBET et al. (1972b).

[b] Each type of response is counted only once for a given subject, even if it was elicited repeatedly by multiple tests in that subject. However, if a given subject experienced more than one type of response he was listed in each appropriate category. The actual numbers of subjects in each general category are given below. Referral sites for almost all responses were in the upper extremity, mostly in the regions of the hand and fingers.

[c] Stimulus values were all at threshold-c in parametric region A, i.e. at liminal I carefully determined for trains with PF's > 15 pps and train durations > 0.5 sec. All tests in a given subject were usually applied at the same cortical site with the electrode stationary.

[d] Stimuli were applied via a subdural Delgado-type electrode, usually as part of procedure of localizing area SS-I for evoked potential studies (LIBET et al., 1967); stimulus values were in parametric region A except that intensity may have been greater than liminal I by some unknown but usually not large fraction.

[e] Stimuli applied via a stigmatic hand-held electrode to points on postcentral gyrus; trains of 60 pps with variable durations and with intensities generally fixed at reasonable values that were usually in the range of being superthreshold, though not strongly so.

[f] In these subjects, with sensory responses that did not include any parasthesias, the qualities reported were almost all of the types in B-a and/or B-c.

[g] In subjects listed as reporting both parasthesias and natural-type (non-parasthesia) qualities for their responses the two different types of qualities often were elicited independently, by separate stimulus tests with a given subject, as well as jointly by the same test (i.e. as one response with several qualities distinguishable in it).

[h] This group is, of course, a subgroup of group III and is already included in the total given for group III.

Rolandic area, pre- and postcentral gyri, give rise to sensory experiences that are not far different in their distribution of qualities from those obtained by subconvulsive cortical stimulation in epileptics (Penfield and Jasper, 1954; Penfield and Kristiansen, 1951). Most of the experiences reported with seizure activity were parasthesia-like, i.e. tingling, numbness, pins and needles. However a small minority of the seizure experiences were not of this type (Penfield and Kristiansen, 1951), and included "throbbing", "sensation of movement", and temperature sensations (although the 4 subjects reporting the latter all had lesions in the temporo-parietal region).

The relative incidence and variety of natural-like qualities have since been found to be considerably greater by Libet et al. (1972b; see also Libet, 1959). In their studies, parametric values of the stimuli to somatosensory cortex were carefully controlled for proximity to liminal levels, and the subjects were not

Table 3. *Kinds of descriptions included in each category of qualities*[a]

A. *Parasthesia-like:* tingling; electric shock; pins and needles; prickling; numbness.

B. *"Natural-like" sensory responses*
    a) Something "moving inside": wave moving along inside through the affected part; or wavy-like feeling inside; or wavy "like a snake back's" motion; rolling or flowing motion inside; moving back and forth inside; circular motion inside; crawling under the skin, or more deeply.
    b) Feeling of movement of the part (but with no actual motion observable to outsider): quiver; trembling; shaking; flutter; twitching; jumping; rotating; jerking; pushing; pulling; straightening; floating, or sensation of hand raising up, or lifting.
    c) Deep pressures: throb; pulsing; swelling; squeeze; tightening.
    d) Surface mechano-type: touch; tapping; hairs moving; rolling (a ball etc.) over surface; water running over surface; talcum powder sprinkling on; light brushing of skin; holding a ball of cotton; rubbing something between thumb and index finger.
    e) Vibration: vibration, buzzing (distinct from tingling, etc.).
    f) Warmth, or warming.
    g) Coldness.

[a] Data from Libet et al. (1972b).

epileptics. Table 2 presents a summary of the reports of qualities in these studies. It may be seen that, for the 124 subjects with stimulation in parametric region A, at or not far above the liminal levels, the incidence of natural-like qualities was in fact greater than that of parasthesia-like ones. For most of the subjects both categories of responses were elicited, even though the stimulus site was usually stationary. In a minority of cases only parasthesia-like responses were reported, but an approximately equal minority reported only natural-like responses. For subjects in the last column (Z) of Table 2, the manner of stimulating postcentral gyrus more or less resembled that usually employed by other investigators; in this column, the relative incidence of parasthesia-like and natural-like qualities also more closely resembled that given for all responses by Penfield and Boldrey (1937).

The large variety of the sensory descriptions, on which the sub-categories of natural-like stimuli under B of Table 2 are based, is indicated in Table 3. Pen-

FIELD and RASMUSSEN (1950) had concluded that "the tactile and proprioceptive sensation is detailed only in regard to the location of the part of the body represented (p. 158)", and they stated that "the patient never suggested that something rough or smooth or warm or cold had actually touched the part (p. 217)". By contrast, descriptions of detailed sensory qualities, in addition to their precise locations, were obtained among the responses summarized in Table 2, columns X and Y. For example, descriptions included statements such as "like talcum powder being sprinkled" on the index finger; or "like rolling a deodorant jar lightly over the surface" of the base of the last three fingers; or "crinkling touch, like picking up a paper thing" with the whole hand (see further examples in Table 3). The experiences of "warmth" and "coldness", although relatively infrequently obtained, appeared to the subjects to be qualitatively similar to their natural sensations. (It should be noted that FOERSTER, 1936b, reported obtaining descriptions of vibration, waves, tickle, burning and cold, though he did not specify their rate of incidence among the total number, which were "mostly tingling, etc.".) However, in agreement with other investigators (PENFIELD group; FOERSTER, 1936b), no definite sensations of pain were ever elicited by stimulating postcentral gyrus. (Stimulation of n.VPL in thalamus similarly never elicits pain in "normal" subjects, i.e. who are not suffering from intractable pain — ALBE-FESSARD and BOWSHER, 1968; LIBET et al., 1972a). A large fraction of the natural-like sensory responses involved some sort of motion quality (B–a and B–b in Table 2), although only about one half of these involved any kind of feeling of actual movement of a part (B–b), such as might be related to the "sense of movement" that predominated among the non-parasthesia-like responses reported by the PENFIELD group (e.g. PENFIELD, 1958).

It should be made clear that the so-called "natural-like" sensory responses were usually peculiar and different from all of the normal sensory experiences of the subject, even though they resembled the specific normal qualities and were clearly in a different category from what are defined here as parasthesia-like qualities (LIBET et al., 1972b). The "natural-like" qualities were often difficult for the subjects to describe except by indicating similarities to or analogies with naturally occurring ones, and the subjects often insisted that these descriptions were really inadequate. This situation provides a fascinating illustration of the breakdown in the ability of one person to communicate the content of his primary subjective experience to another person, when both individuals have not experienced similar situations in common. In spite of these difficulties, many subjects used similar verbal expressions to describe their sensory responses; for example, an experience of "a wave moving inside", from one site to another in the arm or hand, was one of the more commonly reported ones.

It appears, then, that most of the various qualities that are at least related to natural somatosensory experiences (except for pain) can be elicited by liminal stimulation of somatosensory cortex. The large fraction of responses to cortical stimuli that are parasthesia-like, and clearly un-natural in quality, may be a result of inadequately sophisticated stimulation (see below) rather than due to an actual lack of representation of the various specific qualities in postcentral gyrus. This conclusion about representation of qualities would suggest that the function of the primary somatosensory cortex is not limited to that proposed by PENFIELD and colleagues (e.g. PENFIELD and JASPER, 1954, pp. 68–69), i.e. to the discriminative aspects of sensation (localization and sense of position and movement) that are involved in perceiving the form of objects. It is true that the long-term defect that remains following ablation of postcentral gyrus is primarily an astereognosis of the affected part of the body, involving loss of two-point discrimination and of sense of position and movement (e.g. PENFIELD and RASMUSSEN, 1950, p. 184). But FOERSTER (1936b) emphasized the fact that there are losses of all somatic sensory qualities, including those of warm, cold and even pain, for some variable time after ablation. He regarded this as understandable in terms of some kind of representation of all somatosensory qualities in the postcentral gyrus, although he noted that nothing was then known about how the various qualities were arranged in the gyrus (FOERSTER, 1936b, p. 431). Representation of specific somatosensory qualities in the SS-I area has also been demonstrated by recording of evoked potentials in response to some individual natural sensory stimuli at the periphery (e.g. MOUNTCASTLE, 1967), including cortical evoked responses to radiant thermal stimulation of the skin (MARTIN and MANNING, 1969). However, as already noted above, the appearance of evoked potentials is not necessarily matched by an ability to elicit conscious sensory experience.

1. Cortical Mechanisms Mediating Specific Qualities

If there is a representation of the various specific somatic sensory qualities in postcentral gyrus, what is the nature of this representation and why has it not been possible by electrical stimulation of the gyrus to elicit specific natural-like qualities more regularly and predictably ? Two alternative hypotheses have been proposed in relation to cortical mechanisms for specific somatosensory qualities: (a) Each of several "basic" qualities is represented in a separate type of vertical (radial) column of cells in the cortex. Such a functional columnar arrangement was demonstrated by POWELL and MOUNTCASTLE (1959), for at least the different types of mechanoreceptors in the skin, by single unit electrical recordings of cortical responses to peripheral stimuli. Columnar organization is also discernable histologically, with an apparent columnar width (horizontally) of the order of 100 microns (e.g. COLONNIER, 1966; BONIN and MEHLER, 1970), but with impreciseness of borders as seen in the extension of horizontally oriented elements through more than one column. This hypothesis would extend Müller's Doctrine to a uniqueness of different microscopic sites, within the somatosensory cortex, for the different qualities of somatic sensation. The hypothesis also has a further basis in the present evidence for specificity of first order afferent fibers in relation to the different natural stimuli (IGGO, 1965; BURGESS et al., 1968; BESSOU and PERL, 1969). (b) In the second hypothesis, the production of each specific quality of somatic sensation depends on an appropriate patterning of incoming impulses for each quality, rather than on activation of a specific site. The patterning could involve specific configurations of temporal and/or spatial distributions. Such a viewpoint has been advocated by WEDDELL (1961) and others for the coding of the afferent discharges in first order afferent fibers, each of which was hypothesized to respond nonspecifically to different physical stimuli at the periphery; the present evidence, however, favors the concept of specificity, rather than non-specificity, of function for individual first order afferent fibers (IGGO, 1965; PERL, 1968). With either hypothesis (a) or (b), one is referring to those activities occurring only at the level of somatosensory cortex, which enable this area to participate suitably in the overall cerebral processes that mediate the subjective experience of a given quality.

If specific somatosensory qualities are represented separately in different vertical columns of cortex, i.e. on hypothesis (a) above, it ought to be possible to elicit some specific quality (not a parasthesia) in all tests by adequately localizing the stimulus. When the exposure of a unipolar electrode on the pia-arachnoid surface was reduced from 1 mm to 0.25 mm in diameter, there was in fact no significant difference in the incidence of parasthesia-like qualities of the responses to stimuli in parametric region A (LIBET et al., 1972 b). However, even the smaller surface electrode probably excites neural elements in many vertical columns, even in areas outside the area of electrode contact (see LANDGREN et al., 1962, and STONEY et al., 1968, for examples of such spread in motor cortex). Adequate localization of stimulating current to one vertical column would undoubtedly require the use of intracortical microelectrodes, as has been achieved for motor cortex (ASANUMA and SAKATA, 1967; STONEY et al., 1968). Stimulation with microelectrodes has been employed in n.VPL of the thalamus in waking human subjects, by MARG and DIERSSEN (1966). They obtained mostly reports of parasthesia-like qualities for superficial cutaneous responses although rare reports of some more natural-like ones also occurred (e.g. tickle, light touch, warmth); they also obtained some deep pressure responses. Macroelectrode stimulation of n.VPL, with trains carefully adjusted to liminal I levels, also elicited chiefly parasthesia-like sensations, though there were also rare reports of warmth or position change (ALBERTS et al., 1966; LIBET et al., 1972 b). It may be that the much closer packing of neurones of different types, in the thalamic nucleus as opposed to cortical area SS-I, does not permit a sufficiently selective stimulation even with microelectrodes. On the other hand, it is possible that the specific projection nucleus in thalamus transmits information only of a localizing, epicritic nature (as suggested by MARG and DIERSSEN, 1966), but that somatosensory cortex receives a greater variety of inputs that encompasses information about the various qualities of somatic sensation.

Although reducing the number of excited vertical columns in the cortex is technically difficult, one should be able easily to increase the number of responding columns by raising the intensity of the stimulus. If one makes the assumption that stimulation of a larger group of presumably mixed types of columns would be more likely to elicit a parasthesia-like experience, then the latter should appear more readily when intensity of stimulation is raised to supraliminal levels. This assumption would be in accord with the common experience of tingling or electric shock, etc. when a mixed peripheral nerve is stimulated, especially with a train of pulses, (e.g. COLLINS et al., 1960); it contrasts with responses to stimulation of the skin, where presumably more selectively uniform fibers are excited by near-threshold stimuli and give rise to more natural-like sensations (e.g. SIGEL, 1953). When stimulating somatosensory cortex it was indeed found that raising the intensity of a stimulus train to 1.5–2 times liminal I did change the quality of the sensory response to a parasthesia-like one, when the response at liminal I strength had a specific or natural-like quality (Libet et al., 1972b). A less direct demonstration of this may also be deduced from Table 2; for the group in column (Z), in which the stimulus intensities were often likely to be distinctly supraliminal, the incidence of parasthesia-like qualities predominates (cf. columns X and Y). The effects of raised stimulus intensities therefore do provide some indirect support for the columnar specificity hypothesis (a), above.

If the different somatosensory qualities depend upon specific temporal patternings of neuronal activation in somatosensory cortex and perhaps elsewhere (hypothesis b, above), rather than on the sites of activation, there are at least two kinds of direct cortical tests that might be applied. (1) It ought to be possible to alter the quality elicited by a peripheral sensory stimulus by simultaneously introducing inputs via cortical electrical stimulation which would change any naturally specific input patterns. This test is difficult to apply, since cortical stimuli tend to mask or inhibit the conscious sensory response to a peripheral stimulus (see above). (2) It should also be possible to elicit different specific qualities of responses to cortical electrical stimuli by changing the various parametric values of the stimulus in some appropriate manner. Test number (2) has been applied in a limited way by Libet et al. (1972b), by investigating the influences of changes in various parametric values of the cortical stimuli on the quality of the conscious sensory responses. With stimuli in parametric region A, at their respective liminal I values, differences in pulse frequency over a large range (15 to 120 pps), train duration, polarity, etc. did not result in changes in quality. When different qualities of responses were reported by a given subject in different tests with a stationary electrode, there was no apparent correlation of the different quality reports with any changes in stimulus parameters, except for two limited alterations with two parametric changes. One of these is the conversion of a specific quality to one of a parasthesia by raising intensity above liminal I, as already discussed above. Another effective change in parametric values was found to be the lowering of pulse frequency to the range below approximately 10 pps (part of parametric region C). Stimuli with PF's of 8, 6, or 1 pps, using 5 sec TD's and peak currents near the liminal I for such PF's, elicited sensory responses which often had a subjective quality of pulsation; no actual movement in the part was apparent (Libet et al., 1964). This was often described as an internal arterial-like beat, with a frequency of about 1 per sec regardless of the stimulus PF. It remains to be determined whether this sensation was simply elicited indirectly by actual deep small muscle contractions which could not be detected by the observer, rather than by direct activation of the sensory cortex. The pulsation frequency of about 1 per sec does in fact resemble that of the series of observable muscular twitches which are elicited by a train of higher PF's (e.g. 60 pps) when the peak current is raised to that of the threshold-I for a single pulse (see section on stimulus parameters above).

It would appear, then, that the particular subjective quality of a conscious sensory experience is relatively independent of the nature of the stimulus to somatosensory cortex, at least within the limits of the variations in parametric values tested thus far (Libet et al., 1959; and 1972b). If this is correct it would favor hypothesis (a) above, as opposed to (b). However, it would be desirable to extend the presently limited studies to include further kinds of stimulus patterning, for example by temporal groupings of pulses into bursts or modulations of intervals between pulses or bursts within a given stimulus train. This will become more feasible as clues to possible significant patternings of afferent inputs become available (e.g. IGGO, 1964; BULLOCK, 1968). It is important to note, however, that even if specific patterns of sensory nerve discharge were found to be characteristically correlated with different types of natural peripheral stimuli, it would not necessarily follow that such patterns were meaningful for CNS function (e.g. BULLOCK, 1968). This caution would apply particularly to the production of the different subjective qualities of sensory experience; significance for subjective experience would have to be established by appropriate studies in conscious human subjects. Particularly instructive on this point is the ability of an actual cooling of the skin to elicit subjective sensory experiences of pressure. This phenomenon is known as "Weber's deception" and is discussed by HENSEL and ZOTTERMAN (1951) and HENSEL and BOMAN (1960), as it relates to their findings that mechanoreceptor fibers can often also respond to thermal stimuli though with a lower degree of sensitivity (see also IGGO, 1965). They conclude (HENSEL and BOMAN, 1960) that certain mechanoreceptor fibers arouse a subjective sensory response of touch or pressure whether these fibers are excited either by pressure or by cooling! Their observation incidentally also provides an elegant demonstration of Müller's Doctrine at the level of a single sensory fiber.

2. Perseveration of Quality

A surprising requirement for the production of a pulsatile quality, in the response to a stimulus at low pulse frequency, was found to be an interval of at least 4–5 min after any preceding test with a higher PF (60 pps) stimulus (LIBET et al., 1964; this feature has already been referred to above, in the section on TRR and temporal facilitation). If a shorter period of time was allowed, the same quality (e.g. tingling) that was elicited by a 60 pps train at its liminal I was also elicited by a succeeding 8 pps train at its liminal I. (The absence of changes in the subjective quality of sensory responses with changes in stimulus values within parametric region A, as described above, was not due to a similar perseveration; it was found to hold even in those instances when intervals of 4 min or more between tests did occur.) This perseveration or persistence of the given subjective quality occurs without any concomitant changes in the respective threshold-c requirements of the different stimuli; temporal facilitation as evidenced by a change in liminal I following a stimulus in parametric region A persists for less than 0.5 min, and for about 2–3 min after a stimulus in parametric region C (see TRR section). (However, it seems likely that the persistence of a given quality applies only for the change to a pulsatile quality, when shifting to a low pulse frequency, and not to changes among other qualities in the range of stimulus pulse frequencies of 15–120 pps, — LIBET et al., 1972b). An analogous perseveration of subjective experiences was described by PENFIELD (1958, p. 37; see also in Discussion after the paper by LIBET, 1966), for "psychic" responses to stimulation of the temporal lobe cortex. These responses could include experiences of elaborate memory "flash backs" as well as a variety of types of illusions. PENFIELD reported that, after a given subjective experience was produced by stimulation at a given site, the same experience was often produced again from the same point or even from other points unless there was a considerable lapse of time. The mechanism providing for cortical changes lasting many minutes could have a possible general significance. In any case, the perseveration of changes over long inter-stimulus intervals is a variable that must be considered when studying responses to cortical stimulation.

Acknowledgements

The author is indebted to his colleagues in the Mount Zion Neurological Institute, W. Watson Alberts, Bertram Feinstein, Mary Lewis and Elwood W. Wright, Jr., for permission to include much of our as yet unpublished work and also expresses his gratitude to them and to an additional colleague, Curtis Gleason, for helpful discussion of issues presented in this article. This work was supported in part by U.S.P.H.S. Research Grant NS0601 from the National Institute for Neural Diseases and Stroke and by National Science Foundation Grant GB-30552X1.

References

Adams, J.K.: Laboratory studies of behavior without awareness. Psychol. Bull. **54**, 383–405 (1957).

Adrian, E.D.: Afferent discharges to the cerebral cortex from peripheral sense organs. J. Physiol. (Lond.) **100**, 159–191 (1941).

Albe-Fessard, D.: Organization of somatic central projections. In: Contributions to sensory physiology, **2**, 101—167. Ed. by W.D. Neff. New York: Academic Press 1967.

Albe-Fessard, D., Bowsher, D.: Central pathways for painful messages. Proc. Int. Congr. Physiol. Sci. XXIV, Washington, D.C. **6**, 241–242 (1968).

Alberts, W.W.: A stimulus pulse polarity reversal unit. Electroenceph. clin. Neurophysiol. **10**, 172–173 (1958).

Alberts, W.W., Feinstein, B., Libet, B.: Electrical stimulation of "silent" cortex in conscious man. (abs) Electroenceph. clin. Neurophysiol. **22**, 293 (1967).

Alberts, W.W., Feinstein, B., Levin, G., Wright, E.W., Jr.: Electrical stimulation of therapeutic targets in waking dyskinetic patients. Electroenceph. clin. Neurophysiol. **20**, 559–566 (1966).

Amassian, V.E., Berlin, L.: Early cortical projection of Group I afferents in forelimb muscle nerves of cat. J. Physiol. (Lond.) **143**, 61P (1958).

Andersen, P., Andersson, S.A.: Physiological basis of the alpha rhythm. New York: Appleton-Century-Crofts 1968.

Asanuma, H., Sakata, H.: Functional organization of a cortical efferent examined with focal depth stimulation in cats. J. Neurophysiol. **30**, 35–54 (1967).

Békésy, G. von: Auditory backward inhibition in concert halls. Science **171**, 529–536 (1971).

Bergamini, L., Bergamasco, B.: Cortical evoked potentials in man. Springfield: Charles C. Thomas 1967.

Bertrand, G.: Spinal efferent pathways from the supplementary motor area. Brain **79**, 461–473 (1956).

Bessou, P., Perl, E.R.: Response of cutaneous sensory units with unmyelinated fibers to noxious stimuli. J. Neurophysiol. **32**, 1025–1043 (1969).

Bevan, W.: Subliminal stimulation: a pervasive problem for psychology. Psychol. Bull. **61**, 81–99 (1964).

Bickford, R.G., Jacobson, J.L., Cody, D.T.R.: Nature of average evoked potentials to sound and other stimuli in man. In: Sensory evoked response in man. Ed. by R. Katzman. Ann. N.Y. Acad. Sci. **112**, 205–223 (1964).

Bignall, K.E., Imbert, M.: Polysensory and cortico-cortical projections to frontal lobe of squirrel and rhesus monkeys. Electroenceph. clin. Neurophysiol. **26**, 206–215 (1969).

Bindman, L.J., Lippold, O.C.J., Redfearn, J.W.T.: The non-selective blocking action of γ-aminobutyric acid on the sensory cerebral cortex of the rat. J. Physiol. (Lond.) **162**, 105–120 (1962).

BONIN, G. von, MEHLER, W. R.: In: The structural and functional organization of the neocortex. Ed. by K. L. CHOW and A. L. LEIMAN. Neurosci. Res. Prog. Bull. **8**, 174–175 (1970).

BRINDLEY, G. S., MERTON, P. A.: The absence of position sense in the human eye. J. Physiol. (Lond.) **153**, 127–130 (1960).

BROUGHTON, R. J.: In: Averaged evoked potentials. Methods, results, and evaluation. Ed. by E. DONCHIN and D. B. LINDSLEY. Washington, D.C.: NASA SP-191 (1969) pp. 79–84.

BROWN, T. G.: Studies in the physiology of the nervous system. XXII: On the phenomena of facilitation. I. Its occurrence in reactions induced by stimulation of the "motor" cortex of the cerebrum in monkeys. Quart. J. exp. Physiol. **9**, 81–99 (1915).

BROWN, T. G.: Studies in the physiology of the nervous system. XXVII: On the phenomena of facilitation. 6. The motor activation of parts of the cerebral cortex other than those included in the so-called "motor" areas in monkeys; with a note on the theory of cortical localization of function. Quart. J. exp. Physiol. **10**, 103–143 (1916).

BUCHTHAL, F., ROSENFALCK, A.: Evoked action potentials and conduction velocity in human sensory nerves. Brain Res. **3**, 1–402 (1966–1967).

BULLOCK, T. H.: Representation of information in neurons and sites for molecular participation. Proc. nat. Acad. Sci. (Wash.) **60**, 1058–1068 (1968).

BURGESS, P. R., PETIT, D., WARREN, R. W.: Receptor types in cat hairy skin supplied by myelinated fibers. J. Neurophysiol. **31**, 833–848 (1968).

BURNS, B. D.: The mammalian cerebral cortex. London: Arnold 1958.

BUSER, P., BIGNALL, K. E.: Nonprimary sensory projections on cat neocortex. Int. Rev. Neurobiol. **10**, 111–165 (1967).

CELESIA, G. C., BROUGHTON, R. J., RASMUSSEN, T., BRANCH, C.: Auditory evoked responses from the exposed human cortex. Electroenceph. clin. Neurophysiol. **24**, 458–466 (1968).

CHOW, K. L., LEIMAN, A. L., eds.: The structural and functional organization of the neocortex. Neurosci. Res. Prog. Bull. **8**, 153–220 (1970).

CLARK, D. L., BUTLER, R. A., ROSNER, B. S.: Dissociation of sensation and evoked responses by a general anesthetic in man. J. comp. physiol. Psychol. **68**, 315–319 (1969).

COBB, W., MOROCUTTI, C., eds.: The evoked potentials. Electroenceph. clin. Neurophysiol. Suppl. No. 26. Amsterdam: Elsevier 1968.

COLLINS, W. F., NULSEN, F. E., RANDT, C. T.: Relation of peripheral nerve fiber size and sensation in man. Arch. Neurol. (Chic.) **3**, 381–385 (1960).

COLONNIER, M. L.: The structural design of the neocortex. In: Brain and conscious experience, pp. 1–23. Ed. by J. C. ECCLES. Berlin-Heidelberg-New York: Springer 1966.

CRAWFORD, B. H.: Visual adaptation in relation to brief conditioning stimuli. Proc. roy. Soc. B. **134**, 283–302 (1947).

CREUTZFELDT, O. D., WATANABE, S., LUX, H. D.: Relations between EEG phenomena and potentials of single cortical cells. I. Evoked responses after thalamic and epicortical stimulation. Electroenceph. clin. Neurophysiol. **20**, 1–18 (1966).

CURTIS, D. R., DUGGAN, A. W., FELIX, D., JOHNSTON, G. A. R.: GABA, bicuculline and central inhibition. Nature (Lond.) **226**, 1222–1224 (1970).

CUSHING, H.: A note upon the faradic stimulation of the postcentral gyrus in conscious patients. Brain **32**, 44–54 (1909).

DAVIS, H.: Enhancement of evoked cortical potentials in humans related to a task requiring a decision. Science **145**, 182–183 (1964).

DEBECKER, J., DESMEDT, J. E., MANIL, J.: Sur la relation entre le seuil de perception tactile et les potentiels évoqués de l'écorce cérébrale somato-sensible chez l'homme. C.R. Acad. Sci. (Paris) **260**, 687–689 (1965).

DELUCCHI, M. R., GAROUTTE, B., AIRD, R. B.: The scalp as an electroencephalographic averager. Electroenceph. clin. Neurophysiol. **14**, 191–196 (1962).

DEMPSEY, E. W., MORISON, R. S.: The electrical activity of a thalamocortical relay system. Amer. J. Physiol. **138**, 283–296 (1943).

DONCHIN, E., COHEN, L.: Averaged evoked potentials and intramodality selective attention. Electroenceph. clin. Neurophysiol. **22**, 537–546 (1967).

DONCHIN, E., LINDSLEY, D. B.: Averaged evoked potentials. Methods, results, and evaluation. Washington, D.C.: NASA, SP-191 (1969).

Doty, R.W.: Electrical stimulation of the brain in behavioral context. Ann. Rev. Physiol. **20**, 289–320 (1969).

Eccles, J.C.: Interpretation of action potentials evoked in the cerebral cortex. Electroenceph. clin. Neurophysiol. **3**, 449–464 (1951).

Eccles, J.C.: Conscious experience and memory. In: Brain and conscious experience, pp. 314–344. Ed. by J.C. Eccles. Berlin-Heidelberg-New York: Springer 1966.

Eijkman, E., Vendrik, A.J.H.: Detection theory applied to the absolute sensitivity of sensory systems. Biophys. J. **3**, 65–78 (1963).

Eriksen, C.W.: Discrimination and learning without awareness. Psychol. Rev. **67**, 279–300 (1956).

Foerster, O.: Motorische Felder und Bahnen. In: Handbuch der Neurologie, vol. 6, pp. 1–357. Ed. by O. Bumke und O. Foerster. Berlin: Springer 1936a.

Foerster, O.: Sensible corticale Felder. In: Handbuch der Neurologie, vol. 6, pp. 358–448. Ed. by O. Bumke and O. Foerster. Berlin: Springer 1936b.

Foerster, O.: The motor cortex in man in the light of Hughling Jackson's doctrines. Brain **59** (2), 135–159 (1936c).

Fritsch, R., Hitzig, E.: Über die elektrische Erregbarkeit des Großhirns. Arch. f. Anat., Physiol. u. wissensch. Med. **37**, 300–332 (1870).

Geisler, C.D., Gerstein, G.L.: The surface EEG in relation to its sources. Electroenceph. clin. Neurophysiol. **13**, 927–934 (1961).

Gelfan, S., Carter, S.: Muscle sense in man. Exp. Neurol. **18**, 469–473 (1967).

Giaquinto, S., Pompeiano, O., Swett, J.E.: EEG and behavioral affects of fore- and hindlimb muscular afferent volleys in unrestrained cats. Arch. ital. Biol. **101**, 133–148 (1963).

Giblin, D.: Somatosensory evoked potentials in healthy subjects and in patients with lesions of the nervous system. In: Sensory evoked response in man. Ed. by R. Katzman. Ann. N.Y. Acad. Sci. **112**, 93–142 (1964).

Gleason, C.: The use of applied DC fields in the analysis of interictal epileptiform discharges. In: The nervous system and electric currents, pp. 93–98. Ed. by N.L. Wulfson and A. Sances, Jr. New York: Plenum Press 1970.

Goldiamond, I.: Indicators of perception: I. Subliminal perception, subception, unconscious perception. An analysis in terms of psychophysical indicator methodology. Psychol. Bull. **55**, 373–411 (1958).

Goldring, S., O'Leary, J.L., King, R.B.: Singly and repetitively evoked potentials in human cerebral cortex with D.C. changes. Electroenceph. clin. Neurophysiol. **10**, 233–240 (1958).

Goldring, S., Jerva, M.J., Holmes, T.G., O'Leary, J.L., Shields, J.R.: Direct response of human cerebral cortex. Arch. Neurol. (Chic.) **4**, 590–598 (1961).

Green, D.M., Swets, J.A.: Signal detection theory and psychophysics. New York: Wiley 1966.

Guiot, G., Albe-Fessard, D., Arfel, G., Hertzog, E., Vourc'h, G., Hard, Y., Derome, P., Aleonard, P.: Interpretation of the effects of thalamus stimulation in man by isolated shocks. C.R. Acad. Sci. (Paris) **254**, 3581–3583 (1962).

Hagbarth, K.-E., Höjeberg, S.: Evidence for subcortical regulation of the afferent discharge to the somatic sensory cortex in man. Nature (Lond.) **179**, 526–527 (1957).

Hagbarth, K.-E., Kerr, D.I.B.: Central influences on spinal afferent conduction. J. Neurophysiol. **17**, 295–307 (1954).

Haider, M., Spong, P., Lindsley, D.B.: Attention, vigilance, and cortical evoked-potentials in humans. Science **145**, 180–182 (1964).

Heath, R.G., Galbraith, G.C.: Sensory evoked responses recorded simultaneously from human cortex and scalp. Nature (Lond.) **212**, 1535–1537 (1966).

Hensel, H., Boman, K.K.A.: Afferent impulses in cutaneous sensory nerves in human subjects. J. Neurophysiol. **23**, 564–578 (1960).

Hensel, H., Zotterman, Y.: The response of mechanoreceptors to thermal stimulation. J. Physiol. (Lond.) **115**, 16–24 (1951).

Hern, J.E.C., Landgren, S., Phillips, C.G., Porter, R.: Selective excitation of corticofugal neurons by surface-anodal stimulation of the baboon's motor cortex. J. Physiol. (Lond.) **161**, 73–90 (1962).

IGGO, A.: Temperature discrimination in the skin. Nature (Lond.) **204**, 481–483 (1964).

IGGO, A.: The peripheral mechanisms of cutaneous sensation. In: Studies in Physiology, pp. 92–100. Ed. by D.R. CURTIS and A.K. MCINTYRE. Berlin-Heidelberg-New York: Springer 1965.

IWAMA, K., JASPER, H.: The action of gamma aminobutyric acid upon cortical electrical activity in the cat. J. Physiol. (Lond.) **138**, 365–380 (1957).

JASPER, H., LENDE, R., RASMUSSEN, T.: Evoked potentials from the exposed somatosensory cortex in man. J. nerv. ment. Dis. **130**, 526–537 (1960).

JOHANSSON, G.C.: Electrical stimulation of a human ventrolateral-subventrolateral thalamic target area, I–IV. Acta physiol. scand. **75**, 433–475 (1969).

JOUVET, M., LAPRAS, C., TUNISI, G., WERTHEIMER, P.: Mise en evidence chez l'homme au cours d'enregistrements stereotaxiques thalamiques d'un contrôle central des afférences somesthésiques. Acta neurochir. (Wien) **8**, 287–292 (1960).

KATZMAN, R., ed.: Sensory evoked responses in man. Ann. N.Y. Acad. Sci. **112**, 1–546 (1964).

KELLY, D.L., GOLDRING, S., O'LEARY, J.L.: Averaged evoked somatosensory responses from exposed cortex of man. Arch. Neurol. (Chic.) **13**, 1—9 (1965).

KIETZMAN, M.L., SUTTON, S.: The interpretation of two-pulse measures of temporal resolution in vision. Vision Res. **8**, 287–302 (1968).

KRECH, D.: Does behavior really need a brain? In: WM. JAMES: Unfinished business. Ed. by R.B. MCLEOD. Washington: Amer. Psychol. Assoc. 1969.

KRNJEVIĆ, K., RANDIĆ, M., STRAUGHAN, D.W.: An inhibitory process in the cerebral cortex. J. Physiol. (Lond.) **184**, 16–48 (1966).

KRNJEVIĆ, K., SCHWARTZ, S.: The action of gamma-aminobutyric acid on cortical neurones. Exp. Brain Res. **3**, 320–326 (1967).

LANDAU, W.M.: Evoked potentials. In: The neurosciences, pp. 409–482. Ed. by G.C. QUARTON, T. MELNECHUK and F.O. SCHMITT. New York: Rockefeller Univ. Press 1967.

LANDGREN, S., PHILLIPS, C.G., PORTER, R.: Cortical fields of origin of the monosynaptic pyramidal pathways to some alpha motoneurones of the baboon's hand and forearm. J. Physiol. (Lond.) **161**, 112–125 (1962).

LANSING, R.W., SCHWARTZ, E., LINDSLEY, D.B.: Reaction time and EEG activation under alerted and non-alerted conditions. J. exp. Psychol. **58**, 1–6 (1959).

LEYTON, A.S.F., SHERRINGTON, C.S.: Observations on the excitable cortex of the chimpanzee, orang-utan, and gorilla. Quart. J. exp. Physiol. **11**, 135–222 (1917).

LI, C.-L., CHOU, S.N.: Cortical intracellular synaptic potentials and direct cortical stimulation. J. cell. comp. Physiol. **60**, 1–16 (1962).

LIBET, B.: Cortical activation in conscious and unconscious experience. Perspect. Biol. Med. **9**, 77–86 (1965).

LIBET, B.: Brain stimulation and the threshold of conscious experience. In: Brain and conscious experience, pp. 165–181. Ed. by J.C. ECCLES. Berlin-Heidelberg-New York: Springer 1966.

LIBET, B., ALBERTS, W.W., WRIGHT, E.W., JR., DELATTRE, L., LEVIN, G., FEINSTEIN, B.: Production of threshold levels of conscious sensation by electrical stimulation of human somatosensory cortex. J. Neurophysiol. **27**, 546–578 (1964).

LIBET, B., ALBERTS, W.W., WRIGHT, E.W., JR., LEVIN, G., FEINSTEIN, B.: Sensory perception by direct stimulation of human cerebral cortex: stimulus parameters. Fed. Proc. **18**, 92 (1959).

LIBET, B., ALBERTS, W.W., WRIGHT, E.W., JR., FEINSTEIN, B.: Responses of human somatosensory cortex to stimuli below threshold for conscious sensation. Science **158**, 1597–1600 (1967).

LIBET, B., ALBERTS, W.W., WRIGHT, E.W., JR., FEINSTEIN, B.: Cortical and thalamic activation in conscious sensory experience. In: Neurophysiology Studied in Man, pp. 157–168. Ed. by G.G. SOMJEN. Amsterdam: Excerpta Medica 1972a.

LIBET, B., ALBERTS, W.W., WRIGHT, E.W., JR., LEWIS, M., FEINSTEIN, B.: Some cortical mechanisms mediating conscious sensory responses and the somatosensory qualities in man. In: Somatosensory System. Ed. by H.H. KORNHUBER. Stuttgart: Georg Thieme (In press, 1972b).

Lilly, J.C.: Injury and excitation by electric currents. A. The balanced pulse-pair waveform. In: Electrical stimulation of the brain, pp. 60–64. Ed. by D.E. Sheer. Austin: Univ. of Texas Press 1961.

Lilly, J.C., Austin, G.M., Chambers, W.W.: Threshold movements produced by excitation of cerebral cortex and efferent fibers with some parametric regions of rectangular current pulses (cats and monkeys). J. Neurophysiol. 15, 319–341 (1952).

MacIntyre, W.J., Bidder, T.G., Rowland, V.: The production of brain lesions with electric currents. Proc. Nat. Biophys. Conf. 1st, 1957 (pub. 1959) pp. 723–732.

MacKay, D.M.: Evoked brain potentials as indicators of sensory information processing. Neurosci. Res. Prog. Bull. 7, 184–276 (1969).

Marg, E., Dierssen, G.: Somatosensory reports from electrical stimulation of the brain during therapeutic surgery. Nature (Lond.) 212, 188–189 (1966).

Marshall, W.: Spreading cortical depression of Leaõ. Physiol. Rev. 39, 239–279 (1959).

Martin, H.F., III, Manning, J.W.: Peripheral nerve and cortical responses to radiant thermal stimulation of skin fields. Fed. Proc. 28, 458 (1969).

Melzack, R., Wall, P.D.: Masking and metacontrast phenomena in the skin sensory system. Exp. Neurol. 8, 35–46 (1963).

Mihailović, L., Delgado, J.M.R.: Electrical stimulation of monkey brain with various frequencies and pulse durations. J. Neurophysiol. 19, 21–36 (1956).

Mountcastle, V.B.: The problem of sensing and the neural coding of sensory events. In: The neurosciences, pp. 393–408. Ed. by G.C. Quarton, T. Melnechuk and F.O. Schmitt. New York: Rockefeller Press 1967.

Mountcastle, V.B., Powell, T.P.S.: Central nerve mechanisms subserving position-sense and kinesthesis. Bull. Johns Hopk. Hosp. 105, 173–200 (1959a).

Mountcastle, V.B., Powell, T.P.S.: Neural mechanisms subserving cutaneous sensibility, with special reference to the role of afferent inhibition in sensory perception and discrimination. Bull. Johns Hopk. Hosp. 105, 201–232 (1959b).

Müller, J.: Elements of physiology., transl. by W. Baly, Lea, and Blanchard. Book VI, Of the senses (1843).

Ochs, S.: Analysis of cellular mechanisms of direct cortical responses. Fed. Proc. 21, 642–647 (1962).

Ochs, S., Clark, F.J.: Tetrodotoxin analysis of direct cortical responses. Electroenceph. clin. Neurophysiol. 24, 101–107 (1968a).

Ochs, S., Clark, F.J.: Interaction of direct cortical responses — a possible dendritic site of inhibition. Electroenceph. clin. Neurophysiol. 24, 108–115 (1968b).

Oscarsson, O.: Proprioceptive and exteroceptive projections to the pericruciate cortex of the cat. In: Studies in physiology, pp. 221–226. Ed. by D.R. Curtis and A.K. McIntyre. Berlin-Heidelberg-New York: Springer 1965.

Oscarsson, O., Rosén, I.: Projection to cerebral cortex of large muscle-spindle afferents in the forelimb nerves of the cat. J. Physiol. (Lond.) 169, 924–945 (1963).

Oscarsson, O., Rosén, I.: Short latency projections to the cat's cerebral cortex from skin and muscle afferents in the contralateral forelimb. J. Physiol. (Lond.) 182, 164–184 (1966).

Patton, H.D., Amassian, V.E.: Single- and multiple-unit analysis of cortical stage of pyramidal tract activation. J. Neurophysiol. 17, 345–363 (1954).

Penfield, W.: The excitable cortex in conscious man. Liverpool: Liverpool Univ. Press 1958.

Penfield, W., Boldrey, E.: Somatic motor and sensory representation in the cerebral cortex of man as studied by electrical stimulation. Brain 60, 389–443 (1937).

Penfield, W., Jasper, H.: Epilepsy and the functional anatomy of the human brain. Boston: Little, Brown & Co. 1954.

Penfield, W., Kristiansen, K.: Epileptic seizure patterns. Springfield: Thomas 1951.

Penfield, W., Rasmussen, T.: The cerebral cortex of man. New York: Macmillan 1950.

Penfield, W., Welch, K.: Instability of response to stimulation of the sensorimotor cortex of man. J. Physiol. (Lond.) 109, 358–365 (1949).

Penfield, W., Welch, K.: The supplementary motor area of the cerebral cortex. Arch. Neurol. Psychiat. (Chic.) 66, 289–317 (1951).

Perl, E.R.: Relation of cutaneous receptors to pain. Int. Union Physiol. Sci., 24th, Washington, D.C. 6, 235–236 (1968).

Phillips, C.G.: Changing concepts of the precentral motor area. In: Brain and conscious experience, pp. 389–421. Ed. by J.C. Eccles. Berlin-Heidelberg-New York: Springer 1966.

Phillips, C.G.: Motor apparatus of the baboon's hand. Proc. roy. Soc. B. **173**, 141–174 (1969).

Phillips, C.G., Porter, R.: Unifocal and bifocal stimulation of the motor cortex. J. Physiol. (Lond.) **162**, 532–538 (1962).

Phillis, J.W., Ochs, S.: Occlusive behavior of the negative wave direct cortical response (DCR) and single cells in the cortex. J. Neurophysiol. **34**, 374–388 (1971).

Phillis, J.W., York, D.H.: Cholinergic inhibition in the cerebral cortex. Brain Res. **5**, 517–520 (1967).

Powell, T.P.S., Mountcastle, V.B.: Some aspects of the functional organization of the cortex of the postcentral gyrus of the monkey: a correlation of findings obtained in a single unit analysis with cytoarchitecture. Bull. Johns Hopk. Hosp. **105**, 133–162 (1959).

Prince, D.A., Wilder, B.J.: Control mechanisms in cortical epileptogenic foci; "surround" inhibition. Arch. Neurol. (Chic.) **16**, 194–202 (1967).

Provins, K.A.: The effect of peripheral nerve block on the appreciation and execution of finger movements. J. Physiol. (Lond.) **143**, 55–67 (1958).

Purpura, D.P.: Nature of electrocortical potentials and synaptic organizations in cerebral and cerebellar cortex. Int. Rev. Neurobiol. **1**, 47–163 (1959).

Purpura, D.P., Girado, M., Grundfest, H.: Selective blockade of excitatory synapses in the cat brain by γ-aminobutyric acid. Science **125**, 1200–1202 (1957a).

Purpura, D.P., Pool, J.L., Ransohoff, J., Frumin, M.J., Housepian, E.M.: Observations on evoked dendritic potentials of human cortex. Electroenceph. clin. Neurophysiol. **9**, 453–459 (1957b).

Raab, D.: Backward masking. Psychol. Bull. **60**, 118–129 (1963).

Rosenthal, J., Waller, H.J., Amassian, V.E.: An analysis of the activation of motor cortical neurons by surface stimulation. J. Neurophysiol. **30**, 844–858 (1967).

Rosner, B.S., Goff, W.R.: Electrical responses of the nervous system and subjective scales of intensity. In: Contributions to sensory physiology, 2, pp. 169–221. Ed. by W.D. Neff. New York: Academic Press 1967.

Rowland, V., MacIntyre, W.J., Bidder, T.G.: The production of brain lesions with electric currents. II. Bidirectional currents. J. Neurosurg. **17**, 55–69 (1960).

Shagass, C., Schwartz, M.: Evoked cortical potentials and sensation in man. J. Neuropsychiat. **2**, 262–270 (1961).

Shevrin, H., Fritzler, D.E.: Visual evoked response correlates of unconscious mental processes. Science **161**, 295–298 (1968).

Sigel, N.: Prick threshold stimulation with square wave current: a new measure of skin sensibility. Yale J. Biol. Med. **26**, 145–154 (1953).

Skoglund, S.: Anatomical and physiological studies of knee joint innervation in the cat. Acta physiol. scand. **36**, Suppl. 124, 1—101 (1956).

Stohr, P.E., Goldring, S.: Origin of somatosensory evoked scalp responses in man. J. Neurosurg. **31**, 117–127 (1969).

Stoney, S.D., Jr., Thompson, W.D., Asanuma, H.: Excitation of pyramidal tract cells by intracortical microstimulation: effective extent of stimulating current. J. Neurophysiol. **31**, 659–669 (1968).

Sugaya, E., Goldring, S., O'Leary, J.L.: Intracellular potentials associated with direct cortical response and seizure discharge in cat. Electroenceph. clin. Neurophysiol. **17**, 661–669 (1964).

Sutton, S.: The specification of psychological variables in an average evoked potential experiment. In: Averaged evoked potentials. Methods, results, and evaluation, pp. 237–297. Ed. by E. Donchin and D.B. Lindsley. Washington, D.C.: NASA, SP-191 1969.

Suzuki, H., Ochs, S.: Laminar stimulation for direct cortical responses from intact and chronically isolated cortex. Electroenceph. clin. Neurophysiol. **17**, 405–413 (1964).

Swets, J.A.: Is there a sensory threshold? Science **134**, 168–177 (1961).

Swett, J.E., Bourassa, C.M.: Comparison of sensory discrimination thresholds with muscle and cutaneous nerve volleys in the cat. J. Neurophysiol. **30**, 530–545 (1967).

Talairach, J., Bancaud, J.: The supplementary motor area in man. Int. J. Neurol. (Monte-video) **5**, 330–347 (1966).

Towe, A. L., Amassian, V. E.: Patterns of activity in single cortical units following stimulation of the digits in monkeys. J. Neurophysiol. **21**, 292–311 (1958).

Towe, A. L., Whitehorn, D., Nyquist, J. K.: Differential activity among wide-field neurons of the cat postcruciate cerebral cortex. Exp. Neurol. **20**, 497–521 (1968).

Vaughan, H. G., Jr.: The relationship of brain activity to scalp recordings of event-related potentials. In: Averaged evoked potentials. Methods, results, and evaluation, pp. 45–94. Ed. by E. Donchin and D. B. Lindsley. Washington, D.C.: NASA, SP-191 1969.

Vaughan, H. G., Jr., Costa, L. D., Gilden, L.: The functional relation of visual evoked response and reaction time to stimulus intensity. Vision Res. **6**, 645–656 (1966).

Wagman, I., Battersby, W. S.: Neural limitations of visual excitability. V. Cerebral after-activity evoked by photic stimulation. Vision Res. **4**, 193–208 (1964).

Walter, W. G.: The convergence and interaction of visual, auditory, and tactile responses in human nonspecific cortex. Ann. N.Y. Acad. Sci. **112**, 320–361 (1964).

Weddell, G.: Receptors for somatic sensation. In: Brain and Behavior, vol. I, pp. 13–48. Ed. by M. A. B. Brazier. Washington, D.C.: Amer. Inst. Biol. Sci. 1961.

Whitehorn, D., Towe, A. L.: Postsynaptic potential patterns evoked upon cells in sensori-motor cortex of cat by stimulation at the periphery. Exp. Neurol. **22**, 222–242 (1968).

Wiesendanger, M.: The pyramidal tract. Recent investigations on its morphology and function. Ergebn. Physiol. **61**, 72–136 (1969).

Woolsey, C. N.: Patterns of localization in sensory and motor areas of the cerebral cortex. In: The biology of mental health and disease, Chap. 14. New York: Hoeber 1952.

Woolsey, C. N., Erickson, T. C.: Study of the postcentral gyrus of man by the evoked potential technique. Trans. Amer. neurol. Ass. **75**, 50–52 (1950).

Author Index

Page numbers in *italics* refer to the bibliography

Bowman, J. P., see Engel, R. T. 284, *307*

Bowsher, D. 331, *333*, 385, 390 —392, 400, 423, 427, 431, 432, 438, *466*, 510, 512, 516, 535, *549*, 590, *613*, 624, 652, 657, *689*, 725, 726, *740*

Bowsher, D., Albe-Fessard, D. 428, 438, *466*, 494

Bowsher, D., Albe-Fessard, D., Mallart, A. 400, *466*

Bowsher, D., Alexinsky, T. 535

Bowsher, D., Angaut, P., Conde, H. *550*

Bowsher, D., Mallart, A., Petit, D., Albe-Fessard, D. 400, 423, 427—429, 431—434, 438, *466*, 513, *550*

Bowsher, D., Petit, D. 400, 423, 427—429, 431—433, *466*

Bowsher, D., Westman, J. 383, 385, 391, *466*

Bowsher, D., Westman, J., Grant, G. 391, *466*

Bowsher, D., see Albe-Fessard, D. 400, 423, 430, 432, 437, 438, 462, *463*, 496, *547*, 779, *784*

Bowsher, D., see Clarke, W. B. 289, 299, *305*

Bowsher, D., see Walberg, F. 641, *699*

Bowsher, D., see Westman, J. 383, 391, *488*

Boyd, E. H., Pandya, D. N., Bignall, K. E. 658, *689*

Boyd, E. S., Meritt, D. A., Gardner, L. C. 164, 186, 187, *195*

Boyd, I. A. 44, *73*, 114, 116, *134*

Boyd, I. A., Roberts, T. D. M. 113, 115, 116, 119, *134*

Boyd, J. A., Roberts, T. D. M. 648, *689*

Bradley, K., Eccles, J. C. 443, *466*

Bradley, P. B., Dhawan, B. N., Wolstencroft, J. H. 420, *466*, *467*

Bradley, P. B., Mollica, A. 420, *467*

Bradley, P. B., Wolstencroft, J. H. 420, *467*

Brännström, M. 280, *305*

Branch, C., see Celesia, G. C. 769, *785*

Brazier, M. A. 153, *195*

Brearley, E. A., Kenshalo, D. R. 105, *106*

Brearley, E. A., see Kenshalo, D. R. 89, 105, 106, *109*

Breipohl, W., see Meller, K. 652, *694*

Bremer, F. 537, *550*, 608, *613*, 659, *689*

Bremer, F., Bonnet, V. 398, 401, *467*

Bremer, F., Bonnet, V., Terzuolo, C. 490, 537, *550*

Bremer, F., see Bailey, P. 537, 548

Bridges, J. A., see Melzack, R. 657, *694*

Brindley, G. S., Merton, P. A. 406, *467*, 754, *785*

Brinkman, J., see Kuypers, H. G. J. M. 702, *717*

Briot, R., see Steriade, M. 526, 558

Britton, S. W., see Cannon, W. B. 409, *468*

Brocklehurst, R. J., see Bazett, H. C. 88, *106*

Brodal, A. 283, *305*, 340, 356, 361, *373*, 382—386, 388, 390—393, 426, *467*, 492, *550*

Brodal, A., Pompeiano, O. 130, *134*, 408, *467*, 647, *689*

Brodal, A., Pompeiano, O., Walberg, F. 455, *467*

Brodal, A., Rexed, B. 321, *333*, 524, *550*

Brodal, A., Rossi, G. F. 299, *305*, 385, 392, 426, 427, *467*

Brodal, A., Saugstad, L. F. 283, *305*

Brodal, A., Szabo, T., Torvik, A. 285, *305*, 712, *716*

Brodal, A., Taber, E., Walberg, F. 452, *467*

Brodal, A., Walberg, F., Blackstad, T. 362, 364, *374*

Brodal, A., see Brodal, P. 355, 356, *374*

Brodal, A., see Grant, G. 511, *553*

Brodal, A., see Jansen, J. 340, 341, 355, 361, 362, *376*

Brodal, A., see Nyberg-Hansen, R. 237, *250*, 388, *482*

Brodal, A., see Pompeiano, O. 388, 455, *483*, 654, *696*

Brodal, A., see Rossi, G. F. 388—391, 393, *485*, 512, 558

Brodal, A., see Sousa-Pinto, A. 361, 362, 367, *380*

Brodal, A., see Torvik, A. 239, *252*, 385—388, 390, 392, 426, 427, 451, *487*

Brodal, A., see Walberg, F. 641, *699*

Brodal, P., Marsala, J., Brodal, A. 355, 356, *374*

Brodal, P., see Rexed, B. 511, *557*

Brodmann, K. 580, 581, 595, 602, 608, 610, *613*, 625, 733

Broere, G., see Voogd, J. 344, *380*

Broggi, G., see Baldissera, F. 172, 188, 189, *194*, *195*

Bromiley, R. B., see Pinto Hamuy, T. 629, *696*

Brookhart, J., Livingston, W. K., Haugen, F. P. 280, *305*

Brookhart, J. M., Zanchetti, A. 640, *689*

Brookhart, J. M., see Cook, W. A. 169, *197*

Brookhart, J. M., see Fadiga, E. 160, *199*

Brookhart, J. M., see Spencer, W. A. 400, *486*, 640, *698*

Brooks, C. McC., see Andersen, P. 191, *194*, 632, *688*

Brooks, C. McC., see Kleyntjens, F. 451, 456, *475*

Brooks, C. McC., see Koizumi, K. 451, *475*

Brooks, V. B. 533, *550*, 635, *689*

Brooks, V. B., Rudomin, P., Slayman, C. L. 533, *550*, 636, 665, *689*

Brooks, V. B., see Welt, C. 635, *699*

Brouchon, M., see Paillard, J. 130, 131, *136*

Broughton, R. J. 754, 769, *785*

Broughton, R. J., see Celesia, G. C. 769, *785*

Brouwer, B. 703, *716*

Browder, E. J., Gallagher, J. P. 320, *333*

Browder, E. J., see Cook, A. W. 320, *334*, 722, *740*

Browder, E. J., see Rabiner, A. M. 722, *741*

Brown, A. G. 52, *73*, 142, 146, 153, 190, 191, 318—320, 324, 325, 327, *333*, *334*, 510, 511, 523, *550*, 653, *689*

Subject Index

Numbers in *italics* refer to pages containing illustrations

54*